A Textbook of Epilepsy

A Textbook of Epilepsy

EDITED BY

John Laidlaw FRCP(Edin)
Formerly Consultant Physician to the Epilepsy Centre, Quarrier's Homes, Bridge of Weir, Scotland;
Formerly Physician-in-charge of the Chalfont Centre for Epilepsy,
Chalfont St Peter, Buckinghamshire, and Honorary Consultant to the National Hospitals,
London, UK

Alan Richens PhD FRCP
Professor of Pharmacology and Therapeutics, University of Wales College of Medicine,
Heath Park, Cardiff, UK

Jolyon Oxley MA MRCP
Medical Director, National Society for Epilepsy, Chalfont Centre for Epilepsy, Chalfont St Peter,
Buckinghamshire, UK

FOREWORD BY
Denis Williams CBE MD DSc FRCP

THIRD EDITION

CHURCHILL LIVINGSTONE
EDINBURGH LONDON MELBOURNE AND NEW YORK 1988

CHURCHILL LIVINGSTONE
Medical Division of Longman Group UK Limited

Distributed in the United States of America by Churchill
Livingstone Inc., 1560 Broadway, New York, N.Y. 10036,
and by associated companies, branches and representatives
throughout the world.

First edition 1976
Second edition 1982
Third edition 1988

ISBN 0-443-03667-5

British Library Cataloguing in Publication Data
A Textbook of epilepsy. – 3rd ed.
  1. Epilepsy
  I. Laidlaw, John   II. Richens, Alan
  III. Oxley, Jolyon
  616.8'53 RC372

Library of Congress Cataloging in Publication Data
A Textbook of epilepsy.
  Includes bibliographies and index.
  1. Epilepsy. I. Laidlaw, John.   II. Richens, Alan.
III. Oxley, Jolyon. [DNLM: 1. Epilepsy. WL 385 T355]
RC372.T48 1988   616.8'53   87-18379

Printed in Great Britain at The Bath Press, Avon

Foreword

The epilepsies have been classified and reclassified upon the basis of each of their attributes – seizure pattern, temporal occurrence, etiology and accompaniments. There are quite clearly as many classifications as there are needs to classify. Although this volume deals with all aspects of epilepsy, its authors have managed to conceal the classifications in the logical framework of their chapters; and yet this division of the subject is inevitable, for the epilepsies involve so much of the whole person and his whole life. This is part of their fascination to the neurologist.

The polymorphous nature of the subject is seen also in the evolution of our knowledge of it. First, there was the description of the observed and sensed events of the ictus itself, which slowly changed epilepsy into the epilepsies, and which so blurred its boundaries that physiogenesis and psychogenesis became indistinguishable. Later there was the identification of the ictal events with cerebral morphology, and consequently with recognised disease forms. This was encouraged by the sequential gain in knowledge of cerebral function. Encouragement of specific research into the nature of epilepsy seemed to be unnecessary, for the disease itself was the research tool for the early neurophysiologists.

Then with the advent of controlled anaesthesia the advance in knowledge was in the hands of physiologically orientated neurosurgeons, working mainly in North America, but following the English tradition of identification of the site of the epileptogenic lesion. This work was much helped by the development of the electroencephalogram shortly before World War II, and afterwards by electrophysiological ways of recording from the surface of the exposed human brain, and later within its depth. At this time, provision was not made for research into epilepsy as such, because the ictus, since it was a research tool, was a model of the behaviour of that part of the cortex – albeit a caricature of the function involved. Still, it was a tiny window into the brain which gave a view of its function. This, of course, was distorted by circumstance, for which the observer had to allow, both at the time of his observations and later in the holistic deductions he drew from them.

Neurosurgery taught us much about the focal fit, something about the general epilepsies, and furthered knowledge of cerebral function. The unfortunate genitor of the attacks may have had rather less attention though, as has the patient who is regarded by his physician as 'an interesting case'. Simultaneously, by good fortune, the drug treatment of epilepsy was advanced by the use of the hydantoins for major, and the diones for minor, epilepsy. But a third of a century had to pass before the pharmacology of these drugs began to be understood and a wider variety of anti-epileptic drugs became available. This delay on both sides of the Atlantic was caused mainly by the war: not merely the five years of war but the length of time it took afterwards for a new generation to emerge from training to ask themselves: *why*? This trend is *pari passu* with the enormous increase in knowledge in neurochemistry. In this subject, epilepsy is no longer the tool as it was for the neurophysiologist, but it is the object towards which the advances of neurochemistry itself are directed.

The fit itself continues to fascinate physiologists as well as clinicians, not so much for its pattern but for the circumstances of its occurrence, why it starts at all (for it must always have a final precipitant, the reflex epilepsies being exceptional stereotyped examples), and why it stops spontaneously, which is more important to the therapist.

There is so much to intrigue everyone in the very occurrence of epilepsy that scientific enquiry generates itself. But there has been a major change in attitude to the epilepsies in our own time, a change fostered by those who live with people with epilepsy, in the home, in society at large, in clinics and hospitals, and in special centres. This change is reflected in booklets for the layman, in special societies, in congresses, in the social services, and in scientific publications such as this. It consists of putting the person with epilepsy before his handicap. The change is worldwide and pervades the whole of the society which is involved in the problem of epilepsy. This may be partly because now we are in general more liberal; we are certainly more egalitarian; we may have, as a whole society, more regard for the handicapped; and clearly we have greater material resources and knowledge. We also have a limitless capacity for communication through the community so that education in the home is commonplace. More than all these, those who work in the field of epilepsy have come to learn that regard for the personal problems of the patient and knowledge of the psychological consequences of the affliction (caused both by disordered brain and disquiet mind) are of primary importance in treatment. After our scientific enquiry into the physical causes of the epilepsy, we use medical methods of treatment, and perhaps later on may use surgical procedures, but throughout we attend to the needs of the whole person, the person with epilepsy.

I was honoured to be asked in 1976 to write the foreword to the first edition of this textbook, which has become a best seller in this particularly wide field of medicine – a field which demands the labour and the love of people from several disparate scientific disciplines. That is not

surprising, for after all, the brain, to which the disability epilepsy is unique, pervades every aspect of living. Communally, it dominates society too, or should.

I wrote in the Second Edition, of 1982, 'The authors have faced up to the task of casting their net more widely to include our recently won knowledge, as you will see from the many new authors. The titles of sections shows that they have also used a finer mesh to enable them to include such diverse topics as traumatic and photosensitive epilepsy, telemetry, adverse therapeutic effects, and cerebellar stimulation. The first edition came to be used as a standard work of reference, as well as of education. Now the informed can take the second edition from its shelf with some confidence when searching for the up-to-date or the more esoteric topics. The introduction of so much which is new mirrors the change that there can be in modern medicine, even in six short years – a change in the depth of understanding as well as in the breadth of knowledge.'

In the transient quinquennium since then our basic knowledge of how the brain works in health and in disease has extended so quickly that communication itself has been diminished, and specialists within their disciplines must talk down to those without, to enable understanding, the ultimate beneficiary here being the therapist and so the patient. So a third edition has become imperative to distil the language of Babel.

The editors have been recognised by us all to be eminently suited for the task of selection and presentation which they have undertaken, and they and the contributors deserve our thanks.

I can have no more to say than that I am honoured that they should once more have remembered me, for even half a century seems ages to the medical scientist. When Hughlings Jackson and his contemporaries were laying our first foundations I was still quite young.

1988   Denis Williams

Preface

The most notable change in this further expanded third edition has been the addition of a third, and younger, editor. We hope that he will continue to supervise further editions well into the 21st century.

Again there has been a major revision. Although many of our earlier authors have updated their contributions, new authors have been introduced: Dr Wallace for children and Dr Binnie for EEG. Dr Rimmer has joined Professor Richens for the important chapter on clinical pharmacology and therapeutics. There are several new chapters: genetics (Anderson and Hauser) and medical services (Shorvon). The chapter about developing countries has been expanded to include a section from Dr Bittencourt on South America, and an overview by Professor Meinardi, who has a particular interest in them. Another new chapter on special problems includes sections on mental handicap (Corbett), problems for women (Cleland and Espir) and a different section on dental problems (Addy). A major new chapter on social aspects (Craig and Oxley) deals with employment, previously by Dr Rodin, and more systematically with the subjects considered by the Laidlaws in the earlier editions. As a coda the Laidlaws try to look at epilepsy as seen, not by the experts, but through the eyes of the person with epilepsy.

There is an introductory chapter on the vexed question of classification, in which the divergent views of Drs Parsonage and Porter are expressed, together with, we hope, a diplomatic editorial comment.

From the first edition our aim has been that experts should write so as to inform those in other disciplines interested in epilepsy. We hope that again we have succeeded. However, in this edition there are some chapters which should be of value also to professionals in the same discipline: for example, those on EEG and social aspects of epilepsy.

Reviewing this edition in relation to the first, written over a decade ago, it is exciting to record the increase in the knowledge and the understanding of epilepsy. Let us hope that this augurs well for the person with epilepsy. In particular we might note the increasing broadening of approach from the purely medico-scientific to the socio-medical.

As always we would like to thank all those people, un-named in the credits, without whom this book would never have been produced.

1988

J. L.
A. R.
J. O.

Contributors

Martin Addy MSc PhD FDSRCS
Reader and Honorary Consultant, Department of
Periodontology, Dental School, University of
Wales College of Medicine, Cardiff, UK

V. Elving Anderson PhD
Professor of Genetics, Dight Laboratories and
Comprehensive Epilepsy Program, University of
Minnesota, Minneapolis, Minnesota, USA

Tim A. Betts FRCPsych
Senior Lecturer in Psychiatry, University of
Birmingham; Visiting Senior Research Fellow in
Epilepsy, University of Aston in Birmingham;
Consultant Psychiatrist, Central Birmingham
Health District, UK

Colin D. Binnie MD MA BChir
Consultant Clinical Neurophysiologist, The
Bethlem Royal Hospital and The Maudsley
Hospital, London

Paulo Rogério M. Bittencourt MD PhD
Head of Clinical Neurology Unit, Hospital
Nossa Senhora das Graças, Curitiba, Paraná,
Brazil

Benjamin Chandra MD PhD
Professor and Head of Department of
Neurology, University of Airlangga, Surabaya,
Indonesia

Peter G. Cleland MRCP
Consultant Neurologist, Sunderland District
General Hospital and Newcastle General
Hospital; Clinical Lecturer in Neurology to the
University of Newcastle upon Tyne, Sunderland,
UK

John A. Corbett MRCP FRCPsych DCH
Professor, Department of Mental Handicap,
Birmingham University, Lea Castle Hospital,
Nr. Kidderminster, UK

Andrew Gordon Craig PhD PGCE DipHlthEd
MIHE
Advisor in Health Education, National Society
for Epilepsy, UK

Carl B. Dodrill PhD
Professor of Neurological Surgery, University of
Washington School of Medicine, Seattle,
Washington, USA

Michael Espir FRCP
Honorary Consultant Neurologist, Charing Cross
Hospital, London, UK

W. Allen Hauser MD
Professor of Neurology and Public Health
(Epidemiology), Sergievsky Center, Faculty of
Medicine, Columbia University, New York

Brian Kendall FRCP FRCR
Consultant Neurologist, Lysholm Radiological
Department, the National Hospitals, London,
UK

John Laidlaw FRCP(Edin)
Formerly Consultant Physician to the Epilepsy
Centre, Quarrier's Homes, Bridge of Weir,
Scotland; Formerly Physician in charge of the
Chalfont Centre for Epilepsy, Chalfont St Peter,
Buckinghamshire, and Honorary Consultant to
the National Hospitals, London, UK

Mary V. Laidlaw SRN
Formerly Rehabilitation Adviser to the Epilepsy
Centre, Quarriers Homes, Bridge of Weir,
Scotland, and to the Chalfont Centre for
Epilepsy, Chalfont St Peter, Buckinghamshire

C. David Marsden DSc FRCP FRS
University Department of Neurology, the
National Hospitals for Nervous Diseases,
London, UK

Gordon Mathieson MSc FRCP(C)
Professor and Chairman Discipline of Pathology,
Memorial University of Newfoundland, St
John's, Newfoundland, Canada

Harry Meinardi MD PhD
Professor of Epileptology, Catholic University of
Nijmegen; Director of Epileptology, Instituut
voor Epilepsiebestrijding, Heemstede, The
Netherlands

Brian S. Meldrum PhD
Reader in Experimental Neurology, Institute of
Psychiatry, University of London, The Bethlem
Royal Hospital and The Maudsley Hospital,
London, UK

Jolyon Oxley MA MRCP
Medical Director, National Society for Epilepsy,
Chalfont Centre for Epilepsy, Chalfont St Peter,
Buckinghamshire, UK

Maurice Parsonage BSc FRCP DCH
Formerly Consultant Physician, Neurological
Department, Leeds General Infirmary; Formerly
Director, Neuropsychiatric Unit and Special
Centre for Epilepsy, Bootham Park Hospital,
York, UK

Charles E. Polkey MD FRCS
Consultant Neurosurgeon, The Neurosurgical
Unit, The Maudsley Hospital, London, UK

Roger J. Porter MD
Chief, Medical Neurology Branch, Intramural
Research Program, National Institute of
Neurological and Communicative Disorders and
Stroke, NIH, Bethesda, Maryland, USA

Edward H. Reynolds MD FRCP FRCPsych
Consultant Neurologist, Maudsley and King's
College Hospitals, London; Honorary Senior
Lecturer, University Department of Neurology,
Institute of Psychiatry and King's College
Hospital Medical School, London, UK

Alan Richens PhD FRCP
Professor of Pharmacology and Therapeutics,
University of Wales College of Medicine,
Cardiff, UK

E. M. Rimmer MD MRCP
Research Fellow, Department of Pharmacology
and Therapeutics, University of Wales College of
Medicine, Cardiff, UK

Simon Shorvon MA MD MRCP
Senior Lecturer in Neurology and Honorary
Consultant Neurologist, Institute of Neurology
and the National Hospitals for Nervous
Diseases, London, and the Chalfont Centre for
Epilepsy, Chalfont St Peter, Buckinghamshire,
UK

Michael Trimble FRCP FRCPsych
Consultant Physician in Psychological Medicine,
and Raymond Way Senior Lecturer in
Behavioural Neurology, the National Hospitals
for Nervous Diseases, London, UK

Sheila J. Wallace FRCP(Edin)
Consultant Paediatric Neurologist, University
Hospital of Wales, Cardiff, UK

Janusz J. Zielinski MD DM DSc
Director of Clinical Studies, Epilepsy Center of
Michigan, Detroit; Associate Clinical Professor
in Neurology, Wayne State University School of
Medicine, Detroit, USA

Contents

1

Classification of the epileptic seizures

The patterns of clinical presentation of epileptic seizures are many and complex. Although a number of clearly defined seizure patterns are recognized, e.g. the classical petit mal absence or tonic-clonic (grand mal) seizure, many epileptic phenomena defy rigid classification. The classification originally developed by Henri Gastaut (1969) and adopted by the International League Against Epilepsy (ILAE) went far in rationalizing the terminology and providing a common language in books and scientific papers. Weaknesses in the scheme, however, have been the subject of continuous debate by the ILAE's Commission on Classification and Terminology and, in 1981, a revised classification of epileptic seizures was proposed (Commission 1981). In our view, this newer version has produced further problems. For example, it has redefined the terms 'simple' and 'complex' which had by general usage acquired very specific meanings in the original classification. Furthermore, it recommends distinguishing simple partial seizures from complex partial seizures by whether consciousness is altered or not. As all gradations of altered consciousness occur in relation to epileptic seizures we do not see how a clear separation can be made on this subjective criterion. One consequence would be that many of our patients will have both simple and complex partial seizures according to whether the focal discharge spreads far enough in a given attack to produce perceptible alteration of consciousness. This will lead to much confusion and future generations of readers looking back at the published literature of the 1980s will have little idea of which way these terms have been used by individual authors unless it has been clearly stated.

The two classifications are discussed in detail in the contributions that follow. We must leave the reader to make up his own mind on which he prefers, but for the sake of clear communication we felt that we ought to state our own editorial policy. The original classification of Gastaut (1969), shown in Table 1.1, has been used in all the chapters except Chapter 5, in which Professor Marsden and Dr Reynolds present their own simplified version. They avoid the terms 'simple' and 'complex', which in the light of current confusion is perhaps the best policy, and is suggested also as one option by Dr Parsonage in the following section.

John Laidlaw
Alan Richens
Jolyon Oxley

REFERENCES

Commission on Classification and Terminology of the International League against Epilepsy 1981 Proposal for revised clinical and electroencephalographic classification of epileptic seizures. Epilepsia 22: 489–501

Gautaut H 1969 Clinical and electroencephalographical classification of epileptic seizures. Epilepsia 10 (suppl): S2–S13

Table 1.1 Clinical and electroencephalographical classification of epileptic seizures recommended by the *International League Against Epilepsy*, the *World Federation of Neurology*, the *World Federation of Neurosurgical Societies* and the *International Federation of Societies for Electroencephalography and Clinical Neurophysiology*

I. PARTIAL SEIZURES OR SEIZURES BEGINNING LOCALLY

Seizures in which the first clinical changes indicate activation of an anatomical and/or functional system of neurones limited to a part of a single hemisphere; in which the inconsistently present electrographic seizure patterns are restricted, at least at their onset, to one region of the scalp (the area corresponding to the cortical representation of the system involved); and in which the initial neuronal discharge usually originates in a narrowly limited or even quite diffuse cortical (the most accessible and vulnerable) part of such a system.

Clinical seizure type	Electroencephalographic seizure type	Electroencephalographic interictal expression*	Anatomical substrate	Etiology	Age
Elementary or complex symptomatology depending on the discharge of a system localized in one or, sometimes, both hemispheres	Rhythmic discharge of spikes and/or of more or less slow waves, more or less localized over one or, sometimes, both hemispheres	Intermittent local discharges, generally over one hemisphere only	Various cortical and/or subcortical regions corresponding with functional representation in one hemisphere	Usually related to a wide variety of local brain lesions (cause known, suspected or unknown). Constitutional factors may be important	Possible at all ages but more frequent with increasing age.
A. Partial seizures with elementary symptomatology (generally without impairment of consciousness)	local contralateral discharge starting over the corresponding area of cortical representation (not always recorded on the scalp)	local contralateral discharges	usually in the cortical region of one hemisphere corresponding to functional representation	as above	as above

1. With motor symptoms
  (i) focal motor (without march), including localized epileptic myoclonus
  (ii) jacksonian
  (iii) versive (generally contraversive)
  (iv) postural
  (v) somatic inhibitory(?)
  (vi) aphasic
  (vii) phonatory (vocalization and arrest of speech)
2. With special sensory or somatosensory

Clinical seizure type	EEG seizure	EEG interictal	Anatomical substratum

(i) somato-sensory
  (ii) visual
 (iii) auditory
 (iv) olfactory
  (v) gustatory
 (vi) vertiginous
3. With autonomic symptoms
4. Compound forms**
		as above	as above

B. Partial seizures with complex symptomatology* (generally with impairment of consciousness; may sometimes begin with elementary symptomatology)
 	
1. With impaired consciousness alone
2. With cognitive symptomatology
  (i) with dysmnesic disturbances (conscious amnesia, 'déjà vu', 'déjà vécu' . . .)
 (ii) with ideational disturbances (including 'forced thinking', dreamy state . . .)
3. With affective symptomatology
4. With 'psychosensory' symptomatology
  (i) illusions (*e.g.*) macropsia, metamorphopsia)
 (ii) hallucinations
5. With 'psychomotor' symptomatology (automatisms)
6. Compound forms
	unilateral or bilateral discharge, diffuse, or focal in temporal or fronto-temporal regions	unilateral or bilateral, generally asynchronous, focus; usually in the temporal region(s)	usually cortical and/or subcortical temporal or fronto-temporal regions (including rhinencephalic structures), unilateral or bilateral

* The incidence of interictal abnormalities varies; they may be absent.
** Compound implies a joining together of elementary or (and/or) complex symptoms.
*** Complex vs. elementary, implies an organized, high-level cerebral activity.

Table 1.1 (cont'd)

Clinical seizure type	Electroencephalographic seizure type	Electroencephalographic interictal expression*	Anatomical substrate	Etiology	Age
C. Partial seizures secondarily generalized (all forms of partial seizures, with elementary or complex symptomatology, can develop into generalized seizures, sometimes so rapidly that the focal features may be unobservable. These generalized seizures may be symmetrical or asymmetrical, tonic or clonic, but most often tonic-clonic in type)	above discharge becomes secondarily and rapidly generalized	⟶		refer to partial seizures in general	

II. GENERALIZED SEIZURES, BILATERAL SYMMETRICAL SEIZURES OR SEIZURES WITHOUT LOCAL ONSET

Seizures in which the clinical features do not include any sign of symptom referable to an anatomical and/or functional system localized in one hemisphere, and usually consist of initial impairment of consciousness, motor changes which are generalized or at least bilateral and more or less symmetrical and may be accompanied by an 'en masse' autonomic discharge; in which the electroencephalographic patterns from the start are bilateral, grossly synchronous and symmetrical over the two hemispheres; and in which the responsible neuronal discharge takes place, if not throughout the entire grey matter, then at least in the greater part of it and simultaneously on both sides.

Clinical seizure type	Electroencephalographic seizure type	Electroencephalographic interictal expression*	Anatomical substrate	Etiology	Age
Convulsive or non-convulsive symptomatology, without sign referable to a unilateral system localized in one hemisphere	Bilateral, essentially synchronous and symmetrical discharge from the start	Bilateral, essentially synchronous and usually symmetrical discharges	Unlocalized (? meso-diencephalon)	No cause found or: (i) diffuse or multiple bilateral lesions, and/or: (ii) toxic and/or metabolic disturbances, and/or: (iii) constitutional, often genetic factors (epileptic predisposition)	All ages
1. Absences (a) Simple absences, with impairment of consciousness only	1. with rhythmic 3 c/s spike and wave discharge ('petit mal' or typical absence)	spike and waves and/or polyspike and wave discharges	as above	as above (organic etiology is unusual)	especially in children

Clinical seizure	EEG (ictal)	EEG (interictal)	Pathological substratum	Etiological factors	Age
2. without 3 c/s spike and wave (variant of 'petit mal' or atypical absence)	(i) low-voltage fast activity or rhythmic discharge at 10 or more c/s, or (ii) more or less rhythmic discharge of sharp and slow waves, sometimes asymmetrical	more or less rhythmic discharges of sharp and slow waves, sometimes asymmetrical	as above	as above (organic etiology is usual; cerebral metabolic disturbances superimposed on previous brain lesion may be important)	especially in children
(b) Complex absences, with other phenomena associated with impairment of consciousness (i) with mild clonic components (myoclonic absences) (ii) with increase of postural tone (retropulsive absences) (iii) with diminution or abolition of postural tone (atonic absences) (iv) with automatisms (automatic absences) (v) with autonomic phenomena (e.g. enuretic absences) (vi) as mixed forms			as above	as above	as above
2. Bilateral massive epileptic myoclonus (myoclonic jerks)	polyspike and waves or, sometimes, spike and waves or sharp and slow waves	polyspike and waves, or spike and waves, sometimes sharp and slow waves	as above	as above	all ages
3. Infantile spasms	flattening of the hypsarhythmia during the spasm, or exceptionally more prominent spikes and slow waves	hypsarhythmia		as above (cerebral metabolic disturbances superimposed on previous brain lesion may be important)	infants only

Table 1.1 (cont'd)

Clinical seizure type	Electroencephalographic seizure type	Electroencephalographic interictal expression*	Anatomical substrate	Etiology	Age
4. *Clonic seizures*	Mixture of fast (10 c/s or more) and slow waves with occasional spike and wave patterns	spike and waves and/or polyspike and wave discharges	as above	as above	especially in children
5. *Tonic seizures*	low voltage fast activity or a fast rhythm (10 c/s or more) decreasing in frequency and increasing in amplitude	more or less rhythmic discharges of sharp and slow waves, sometimes asymmetrical	as above	as above (organic etiology is usual)	especially in children
6. *Tonic-clonic seizures* ('grand mal' seizures)	rhythm at 10 or more c/s, decreasing in frequency and increasing in amplitude during the tonic phase, interrupted by slow waves during the clonic phase	polyspike and waves and/or spike and waves or, sometimes, sharp and slow wave discharges	as above	as above	less frequent in young children than other forms of generalized seizures. All ages except infancy
7. *Atonic seizures* sometimes associated with myoclonic jerks (myoclonic-atonic seizures) (a) of very brief duration (epileptic drop attacks)	polyspike and waves (more waves than in the myoclonic polyspike and wave)	polyspike and wave			
(b) of longer duration (including atonic absences)	rhythmic spike and wave (3 to 1 c/s) or mixture of fast and slow waves with occasional spike and wave patterns	polyspike and waves and/or spike and waves or, sometimes, sharp and slow wave discharges	as above	as above (organic etiology is usual)	especially in children
8. *Akinetic seizures* (loss of movement without atonia)	rhythmic spike and wave (3 to 1 c/s) or mixture of fast and slow waves with occasional spike and wave pattern	polyspike and waves and/or spike and waves or, sometimes, sharp and slow wave discharges	as above	as above	especially in children

III. UNILATERAL OR PREDOMINANTLY UNILATERAL SEIZURES

Seizures in which the clinical and electrographic aspects are analogous to those of the preceding group (II), except that the clinical signs are restricted principally, if not exclusively, to one side of the body and the electrographic discharges are recorded over the contralateral hemisphere. Such seizures apparently depend upon a generalized or at least very diffuse neuronal discharge which predominates in, or is restricted to, a single hemisphere and its subcortical connections.

A. Characterised by clonic, tonic or tonic-clonic convulsions, with or without an impairment of consciousness, expressed only or predominantly in one side. Such seizures sometimes shift from one side to the other but usually do not become symmetrical

(i) partial discharge very rapidly spreading over only one hemisphere (corresponding with only contralateral seizures), or:	focal contralateral discharges	cortical and/or subcortical region in one hemisphere	wide variety of focal, unilateral lesions, generally in immature brain (constitutional factors may be important)	almost exclusively in very young children
(ii) discharges generalised from the start but considerably predominant over one hemisphere, susceptible to change from one side to the other at different moments (corresponding to alternating seizures)	bilateral and synchronous symmetrical or asymmetrical discharges of spike and waves and/or polyspike and waves	unlocalized (? mesodiencephalon)	no cause found, or: (i) diffuse or multiple bilateral lesions, and/or: (ii) toxic metabolic perturbations, and/or: (iii) constitutional, often genetic factors (epileptic predisposition), generally in immature brain	almost exclusively in very young children
(iii) partial discharge, susceptible to change, from time to time, in morphology and topography (from area to area and, sometimes, from one side to the other)	focal discharges, susceptible to change, from time to time, in morphology and topography	cortical and/or subcortical region in one or both hemispheres, or unlocalized	focal or diffuse lesions of diverse etiology or metabolic and/or toxic. Constitutional factors and cerebral immaturity are important	limited virtually to the new-born

IV. UNCLASSIFIED EPILEPTIC SEIZURES

Includes all seizures which cannot be classified because of inadequate or incomplete data.

PART TWO
M. Parsonage

CLASSIFICATION OF EPILEPTIC PHENOMENA

The construction of a generally acceptable classification of the clinical manifestations of epilepsy in all its forms remains a challenge, and no doubt will continue to do so as long as knowledge grows and new facts come to light. However, the growth of knowledge has probably encouraged the tendency in recent years to propose classifications of increasing complexity, especially in the case of the epilepsies (epileptic syndromes). Undoubtedly, the latter are harder to classify than epileptic seizures since there are more variables and a greater lack of knowledge to be taken into account. Nevertheless, if the desire for comprehensiveness is pursued at the expense of practicality the likely result will be unwieldiness and failure to gain sufficiently widespread acceptance, and the whole object of achieving a reasonable degree of uniformity of terminology will be jeopardized. Of course, there are limits to be imposed upon the needs of practical usage to ensure that proper recognition is given to important factual information, however discrepant it may appear to be. Even so, a reasonable degree of simplification is preferable to the construction of an all-embracing classification which by trying to take everything into account only succeeds in being too complicated for everyday use.

The task of devising an acceptable classification is much more than a mere academic pursuit. Not only should it be a stimulus to accuracy and clear thinking, it should also be a worthwhile one, both in the interests of communication and collation and in the incorporation of current knowledge and understanding. When undertaking this task it is important not to lose sight of the distinction between classifications of epileptic seizures and classifications of epileptic syndromes. Seizure classifications are primarily concerned with clinical manifestations of individual seizures and their distinctive features, and to a lesser extent with their known or presumed neurophysiological basis. Classifications of the epilepsies are concerned with additional criteria, especially aetiology and natural history, and are therefore of particular value to the clinician.

CLASSIFICATION OF EPILEPTIC SEIZURES

Since its publication in 1969, the scheme for the classification of epileptic seizures recommended by the International League Against Epilepsy (ILAE) (Gastaut 1969a) has proved useful and has been widely used. Thus, the division of seizures into the two main groups of *partial* and *generalized* has long been recognized as basic and the further subdivision of the former into 'simple' (elementary symptomatology) and complex (complex symptomatology) has long been widely accepted. It has also continued to be readily recognized that any partial seizure may become generalized (secondary generalization), being then converted most commonly into the familiar generalized tonic-clonic seizure. In these circumstances, the accompanying initial localized seizure discharge spreads rapidly to involve both the cerebral hemispheres and deep midline structures. Indeed, the spread usually occurs so rapidly that the initial localizing features are obscured and this may be a source of difficulty in identification. Furthermore, the resulting seizure may sometimes be asymmetrical or even unilateral, especially in children.

Partial seizures – general considerations

The classification of partial seizures is based on the longstanding traditional concept of their local, or relatively localized, origin in cerebral grey matter. This still seems to be a workable concept and, no doubt, will continue to be so, even though it is not a wholly accurate term; for example, its application in the case of seizures of temporal lobe origin is open to question in view of their frequently somewhat diffuse origin. The further subdivision of simple partial seizures into motor, sensory, autonomic and compound forms, has also survived as an acceptable arrangement embodying, as it does, all the common types of seizure.

The situation with regard to the classification of complex partial seizures is not so straightforward however. Basically, their status as seizures involving high level cerebral activity, as distinct from that which is implicated in simple partial seizures, is a distinction which is widely understood since it rests upon sound clinical and experimental evidence. In other words, neurophysiologically, these seizures involve neuronal systems which are of greater complexity and subserve more highly organized functions than the primary motor and sensory reception areas. They would naturally, therefore, be expected to give rise to more complex manifestations when their functions are activated or disrupted by seizure discharge. These so-called higher centres of neuronal function are clearly of later acquisition in the evolutionary history of man and help to endow him with the great flexibility and finesse which are so characteristically human. Anatomically, although the areas of cerebral cortex involved are not clearly defined, in essence they correspond to the so-called association neocortical areas of the frontal, temporal and parietal lobes and also the allocortex in the anteromedial portion of the temporal lobes.

Partial seizures associated with impaired consciousness

Certain problems arise with regard to the subdivision of complex partial seizures into those with impaired consciousness alone and those with cognitive, affective, psychosensory and psychomotor symptomatology (Table 1.2). Thus, some would doubt the existence of the first of these which have sometimes been referred to as 'temporal lobe absences'. Indeed, characteristically, they are frequently associated, not only with features of other types of complex partial seizure, but with confusion and automatisms; this would suggest, at least widely diffused rather than localized seizure discharge which most commonly involves the temporal lobes and connected deep structures with masking of any localized origin. In other words, seizures of this kind might reason-

Table 1.2 ILAE 1969 classification of partial seizures with complex symptomatology

1. With impaired consciousness alone
2. With cognitive symptomatology:
    i. with dysmnesic disturbances (conscious amnesia, déjà vu, déjà vécu)
    ii. with ideational disturbances (including forced thinking, dreamy state)
3. With affective symptomatology
4. With psychosensory symptomatology:
    i. illusions (macropsia, metamorphosia)
    ii. hallucinations
5. With psychomotor symptomatology (automatisms)
6. Compound forms

ably be regarded as verging on, if not actually, secondarily generalized partial seizures, and it has even been asserted that they may sometimes be primarily generalized (Penfield & Jasper 1954). Furthermore, it should be emphasized that *all* partial seizures, irrespective of their sites of origin, may become associated with impairment or loss of consciousness when the seizure discharge has become sufficiently widespread. It is, of course, well known that this is particularly likely to occur in seizures arising in the temporal lobes, with their widespread neuronal connections via the amygdaloid complexes. It would seem therefore that their frequent association with affective, cognitive and psychomotor components should facilitate more precise categorization (Gastaut & Broughton 1972).

It must nevertheless be pointed out that Gloor et al (1980) have reported instances of seizures of temporal lobe origin in which loss of consciousness (defined as unresponsiveness) was virtually the only clinical sign. Even so, in the majority of seizures studied by these observers the accompanying epileptic seizure discharges involved both temporal lobes widely, as well as limbic and neocortical structures. There was, however, at least one instance in which there appeared to be only minimal limbic movement and more recent observations have confirmed that unresponsiveness may occur when the seizure discharge is confined to one temporal lobe (Gloor 1986). This raises the problem as to whether unresponsiveness should be equated with loss or impairment of consciousness and this a matter which will be referred to again later.

Seizures with cognitive, affective and psychosensory symptomatology

In the ILAE 1969 classification *cognitive* complex partial seizures may be associated with either dysmnesic disturbances (conscious amnesia, déjà-vu experiences, etc) or with ideational disturbances (forced thinking, dreamy states). Those with *affective symptoms* are most commonly manifested as spontaneous feelings of fear and less commonly as feelings of pleasure, joy or elation and, on rare occasions, of rage. Lastly, *psychosensory* complex partial seizures are subdivided into those which give rise to illusional experiences (macropsia, etc) and those characterized by organized hallucinatory experiences which usually involve several sensory modalities. This subdivision of complex partial seizures has generally been regarded as reasonably satisfactory, if not without its critics, and some possible modifications will be discussed later.

Psychomotor seizures

The so-called *psychomotor* seizure (ictal automatism) has long been widely regarded as a distinct variety of complex partial seizure, as in the 1969 ILAE Classification. Gastaut & Broughton (1972) have maintained that motor activity accompanying them is the direct result of the state of confusion associated with these seizures, thus causing loss of higher control and the emergence of more primitive automatic behaviour. These authors point out, however, that the association of automatic behaviour and confusion may also be encountered in prolonged absences or as post-ictal phenomena, as may, for example, be seen after generalized tonic-clonic seizures. Furthermore, these authors remind us that the automatisms occurring in psychomotor seizures should be distinguished from the usually rhythmic motor activity to be seen, for example, arising from discharge in the lower Rolandic region. In the latter circumstance it should properly be regarded as a primary motor phenomenon as might be seen in a somatomotor seizure.

The automatisms seen in association with psychomotor seizures may consist of the continuation of activity which began at the time of onset of the seizure; or they may be characterized by

new activity which can take many forms. These have been variously described as alimentary (smacking of the lips, etc), mimetic (reflecting the individual's emotional state), gestural (hand-wringing, rearranging clothing, etc), ambulatory (walking in circles, cycling, etc) and vocal (mumbling, humming tunes, etc). Such seizure manifestations are, of course, most commonly associated with discharge arising in or adjacent to medial temporal lobe structures (amygdala, etc). Nevertheless, they may also occur in association with seizures arising in the anterior frontal and supplementary motor areas (Penfield & Jasper 1954) and should not be regarded as exclusively of temporal lobe origin.

In the past it has been clearly demonstrated that seizures of psychomotor pattern are accompanied by widespread seizure discharges involving both cortical and diencephalic structures (Jasper 1964, Penfield 1969). It might therefore seem questionable to classify them as partial seizures (Parsonage 1979) if the latter are to be defined as seizures in which the initial neuronal discharge arises in a narrow, limited, or even quite diffuse, cortical area (1969 ILAE Classification). Indeed, there is something to be said for regarding them as generalized seizures and, as mentioned earlier, it has been claimed that they can occasionally be primarily generalized (Penfield & Jasper 1954). On the other hand, Gloor (1986) takes the view that they should be regarded as partial seizures, even if the initial seizure discharge may spread rather widely.

Generalized seizures

In the 1969 classification generalized, bilateral symmetrical seizures are subdivided into non-convulsive (various types of absence) and convulsive varieties (seven in all). Absences are further subdivided into simple and complex varieties in accordance with whether or not there are such additional features as myoclonus, alterations in muscle tone, automatisms and autonomic phenomena. The convulsive group of seizures include the myoclonic, tonic-clonic and atonic varieties; it also includes two entities – infantile spasms and akinetic seizures – whose place in this group has often been questioned, but for different reasons. In the former case, most would now agree that the term 'infantile spasms' should more properly be regarded as an epileptic syndrome embodying more than one type of seizure in addition to other characteristic features. In the latter case, the so-called 'akinetic seizure' has often been regarded as a somewhat dubious entity, since its features (loss of movement without atonia in association with loss of impairment of consciousness) would appear to make it virtually indistinguishable from a variety of simple absence.

Revised classification of partial seizures

In 1981, the Commission on Classification and Terminology of the International League Against Epilepsy submitted new proposals for the classification of epileptic seizures which were subsequently officially adopted in 1982. However, both before and since, they have been subjected to certain criticisms which have not yet been fully met and which have prevented them from being generally accepted.

The most radical of the new proposals are embodied in a revised classification of partial seizures. It is now recommended that these be subdivided into 'simple' and 'complex' on the basis of whether consciousness is preserved or lost, irrespective of their other features. This has highlighted the continuing problem as to how consciousness should be defined, and also the question of whether it can be used effectively as a valid criterion in the classification of seizures. Furthermore, the new proposals introduce a new interpretation of the terms 'simple' and 'complex'. The classification of the former in the new scheme is given in Table 1.3.

Table 1.3 1982 ILAE classification of simple partial seizures

1. With motor signs: focal motor etc
2. With somatosensory or special sensory symptoms: somatosensory, visual etc
3. With autonomic symptoms
4. With psychic symptoms:
   a. dysphasic
   b. dysmnesic
   c. cognitive
   d. affective
   e. illusions
   f. structured hallucinations

Dealing first with the definition of consciousness, this is still a state which cannot yet be satisfactorily accounted for in neurophysiological terms, nor can it be defined in generally agreed clinical terms. For the purposes of the 1981 ILAE Classification, it is defined operationally as the degree of awareness and/or responsiveness in an individual. However, this has been criticized as being open to misinterpretation and being too restricted. For example, an individual who appears to be unresponsive may not necessarily be unaware of his surroundings, since he may have been merely aphasic or inattentive. Conversely, a person who appears responsive during a given period may afterwards make it clear that he was not really aware of his surroundings at the time. With regard to the criticism of restrictiveness, it can be argued that unconsciousness may more properly be regarded as a combination of unawareness, loss of (or reduced) responsiveness and subsequent amnesia for the events which occurred during the episode in question, automatisms being a common accompaniment.

It would therefore seem that differentiating partial seizures on the grounds of whether they are associated with preservation of consciousness ('simple' partial seizures) or with its loss ('complex' partial seizures), raises more problems than it solves. Furthermore, since loss of consciousness is at least a potential development in *all* partial seizures, it seems hardly logical to use it as a means of differentiating them, irrespective of how it may be defined.

With regard to the proposed new interpretation of the terms 'simple' and 'complex', if the latter term is to be used only when consciousness is affected at some stage, it would now be the case that seizures with psychic symptoms (including those characterized by illusional and highly organized hallucinatory states) are designated as simple in type. Such a change of definition has led to some confusion in view of the long-established understanding concerning higher and lower cerebral activity. Clearly, there are significant distinctions between the anatomical and physiological substrates of higher integrative cerebral activity as opposed to those related to lower level motor and sensory functions, distinctions which are long established in their own right. It is inevitable therefore that there should be objections to a re-defining of these two terms in this way.

In the interests of clarity it does now seem desirable that authors aspiring to publication should state whether they are using the 1969 or the 1981 ILAE Classification of partial seizures when submitting their presentations. The need for this is underlined by the fact that there still appear to be quite a number who are still adhering to the 1969 Classification, either on the grounds of non-acceptance or perhaps because of unawareness of the new proposals.

Further proposals for the classification of partial seizures

If there is to be any further attempt to achieve a consensus concerning seizure classification it might be worthwhile considering the possibility that a compromise between the 1969 and 1981 partial seizure classifications might pave the way towards overcoming the objections.

Since opposing opinions seem firmly entrenched, there might now be a case for abandoning the terms 'simple' and 'complex' altogether (Parsonage 1979; J. Stevens 1983 personal communication) and save further confusion. For example, a classi-fication such as the one listed in Table 1.4 might be acceptable, since it jettisons these terms while retaining psychomotor seizures (automatisms) and seizures with impairment of consciousness as the initial or only symptom in the partial seizure group. In this classification scheme allowance can be made for the fact that all partial seizures may occur both with or without impairment or loss of consciousness and also with or without secondary motor generalization. If no such compromise as this should prove acceptable then both the 1969 and 1981 classifications may well continue to be used, at least for the time being. However, such

Table 1.4 Alternative classification of partial seizures

1. With motor signs: focal motor, etc
2. With somatosensory or special sensory symptoms
3. With autonomic symptoms
4. With psychic symptoms: dysphasic, dysmnesic, cognitive, etc
5. Impairment of consciousness as the initial or only manifestation
6. Automatisms

an outcome might result in their inadequacies continuing to be the subject of debate which could be salutary in the long term.

In concluding this discussion on the classifi-cation of seizures, consideration must also be given to some minor questions of terminology which have arisen in recent years. These concern the classification of seizure types listed under the headings of aphasic, dysmnesic, illusional and hallucinatory and these will be considered briefly in turn. These terms are listed in Table 1.5 in accordance with the ways in which they may be used.

In the 1969 ILAE classification, seizures mani-fested by aphasic disturbances, irrespective of whether they are minimal or global, are classified as a variety of simple partial seizure with motor symptoms. In contrast, in the 1981 classification they are classified as a variety of psychic simple partial seizure with dysphasic manifestations. However, since the latter reflects disturbances of higher cerebral function, it is arguable whether they should be termed 'simple'.

Seizures characterized by *illusions of per-ception* (déjà-vu, jamais-vu, etc) are classified as cognitive complex partial seizures with dysmnesic disturbances in the 1969 classification, whereas in the 1981 classification they are listed as dysmnesic psychic simple partial seizures. Since seizures of this kind involve disturbances of both memory and perception they can be regarded as either dysmnesic or illusional. Thus, Gastaut & Broughton (1972) have suggested that they might be designated 'aperceptual' or 'agnosic' illusory experiences which, when in attenuated form with illusions of incoherence and depersonalization, become the basis of epileptic dreamy illusions (dreamy state of Jackson). The latter states are classified as cognitive seizures with ideational disturbances in the 1969 classification. On the other hand, in the 1981 classification they are categorized as psychic 'simple partial seizures' with either dysmnesic symptoms or cognitive disturbances, whereas feelings of depersonaliz-ation come under the latter heading. It would seem, however, that they might all be regarded as illusions of perception.

Seizures characterized by so-called 'forced thinking' (Penfield 1969), in which an obsessional idea or thought imposes itself in the individual's mind, are included with 'dreamy states' under the heading of 'cognitive complex partial seizures with ideational disturbances' in the 1969 classification. However, in the 1981 classification they would appear to be regarded as psychic simple partial seizures with dysmnesic symptoms. Perhaps they should be regarded as cognitive disturbances.

So-called *panoramic memory* seizures (flashbacks) are regarded by some observers as dysmnesic in nature, while others would regard them as hallucinatory. The latter view would appear to be the case in the 1969 Classification which is in keeping with the highly complex nature of the recalled experiences. In contrast, in the 1981 classification they are regarded as a form of 'forced thinking' and categorized as psychic simple partial seizures with dysmnesic symptoms. In fact, they can justifiably be regarded as either dysmnesic or hallucinatory varieties of partial seizure.

CLASSIFICATION OF THE EPILEPSIES (EPILEPTIC SYNDROMES)

For practical purposes, in any classification of the epilepsies, prime consideration needs to be given to aetiology. This embraces natural history and, to a lesser extent, prognosis, features which are of particular importance to the clinician. There are,

of course, other criteria which may be taken into account, such as age, the circumstances under which seizures habitually occur or the agents which precipitate them. However, the attempts to extend classifications in this way carry with them the risk of making them too complicated and therefore unwieldy. For such reasons the temptation to include an over-abundance of criteria is best avoided.

Over a very long period there have been many attempts to classify the epilepsies. From earliest times they have usually been based on the practical concept that some epilepsies could be attributed to recognizable gross cerebral lesions (symptomatic epilepsies), as opposed to those in which there was no identifiable cause (idiopathic epilepsies). Even though the latter group has tended to shrink as more causes have become recognized, this mode of classification has become enshrined by tradition and its usefulness remains undisputed.

By definition, the term 'idiopathic' refers to a primary morbid state neither consequent upon nor symptomatic of another disease. Nevertheless, it has sometimes been argued that all epilepsies are symptomatic, in the sense that they are manifestations of cerebral disorder; indeed, they may be rightly termed syndromes but this does not detract from the usefulness of distinguishing between those epilepsies in which the cause can be ident-

Table 1.5 Terminology in relation to aphasic, dysmnesic and cognitive partial seizures

Seizure type	1969 ILAE classification	1982 ILAE classification	Compromise classification
Aphasic	Simple partial seizure with motor manifestations	Psychic simple seizure with dysphasic symptoms	Partial seizure with dysphasic manifestations
Déjà vu, déjà entendu, jamais vu, etc	Cognitive complex partial seizures with dysmnesic disturbances	Dysmnesic psychic simple partial seizures	Psychic partial seizures with dysmnesic or illusional symptoms
Illusions of incoherence, unreality, depersonalization (dreamy state)	Cognitive complex partial seizures with ideational disturbances	Psychic simple partial seizures with dysmnesic, cognitive or illusional symptoms	Psychic partial seizures with illusional symptoms
Forced thinking	Cognitive complex partial seizure with ideational disturbances	Psychic simple partial seizure with dysmnesic symptoms	Psychic partial seizure with cognitive disturbances
Panoramic memory	Psychosensory complex partial seizure with hallucinatory features	Psychic simple partial seizure with dysmnesic symptoms	Cognitive partial seizure with dysmnesic or hallucinatory features

ified and those in which it can, for practical purposes, be regarded as a primary condition, given the present state of our knowledge.

The results of research into the genetics of the epilepsies have added impetus to the tendency to equate those epilepsies in which such factors appear to be aetiologically of prime importance with the so-called 'primary epilepsies'. However, there is need for continuing research in this field in order to elucidate the precise nature of the underlying basis. Furthermore, it has to be remembered that genetic factors may be operative in many so-called symptomatic epilepsies in which an underlying structural cause can be identified. The term 'primary' therefore becomes relative but this does not detract from the practical value of the view that in some epilepsies genetic factors appear to be of paramount importance.

In the meantime, it may be noted that in the past 30 or so years there have been two developments concerning the concepts of generalized epilepsies. The first is the realization that seizures which are generalized from the onset are seen not only in the primary generalized epilepsies: they may also reflect diffuse organic cortical disease which usually also gives rise to partial seizures. In the second place, increasing recognition has been given to the fact that the so-called 'focal epilepsies' may also be of primary (genetic) origin and not exclusively due to identifiable focal cortical lesions (Gastaut 1983). The benign partial epilepsies of childhood afford the best examples in this context.

In general terms, it may be stated that not all primary epilepsies are exclusively functional (non-lesional) or entirely benign in nature, indeed, cerebral lesions may contribute to their aetiology. Similarly, the generalized and partial epilepsies of lesional origin are not always exclusively so determined, nor are they invariably severe. In constructing classifications it therefore needs to be emphasized that the distinction between primary and secondary epilepsies must be regarded as a relative one; it is so often essentially a matter of preponderance of one set of aetiological factors or another.

Gastaut (1983) has proposed a scheme to complete his previously proposed international classification of the epilepsies (Gastaut 1969b). While preserving the basic distinction between generalized and partial epilepsies, it embodies the concept of primary and secondary epilepsies, be they generalized or partial. Thus, the primary generalized (functional, benign) epilepsies include the petit mal and grand mal epilepsies, whereas the secondary generalized epilepsies include those due to specific and non-specific encephalopathies (Lennox–Gastaut, West and related syndromes). The primary partial epilepsies are exemplified by the benign partial epilepsies of childhood, whereas the secondary partial epilepsies (all due wholly or mainly to identifiable lesions) are, for descriptive purposes, subdivided into those with simple and those with complex semeiology.

During the past few years the current members of the Commission on Classification and Terminology of the International League Against Epilepsy (1985) have been engaged in drawing up proposals for an up-to-date international classification of the epilepsies and epileptic syndromes. The results of their efforts, while underlining the many difficulties posed by their task, have not yet led to the construction of a classification which could command general agreement. Their current proposals preserve the generally accepted subdivision into localized and generalized epilepsies, with the added categories of epilepsies of undetermined origin (focal or generalized) and of special syndromes (febrile convulsions, reflex epilepsies, etc). The differentiation between 'idiopathic' and 'symptomatic' subvarieties of both localized and generalized epilepsies is also recognized. However, attempts to make the classification all-embracing have led to the inclusion of a number of uncommon and sometimes minor entities which tend to make it cumbersome and therefore reduce its usefulness. At the moment it would appear that the whole matter remains *sub judice* and there seems to be little likelihood of any final pronouncements in the immediate future. There are also additional difficulties concerning the classification of epileptic syndromes seen in infancy, childhood and adolescence (Roger et al 1985) and so the work must continue.

REFERENCES

Commission on Classification and Terminology of the International League Against Epilepsy 1981 Proposal for a revised clinical and electroencephalographic classification of epileptic seizures. Epilepsia 22: 489–501

Commission on Classification and Terminology of the International League Against Epilepsy 1985 Proposal for classification of epilepsies and epileptic syndromes. Epilepsia 26: 268–278

Gastaut H 1969a Clinical and Electroencephalographical classification of epileptic Seizures. Epilepsia 10 (suppl): S2–S13

Gastaut H 1969b Classification of the Epilepsies. Proposal for an international classification. Epilepsia 10 (suppl): S14–S21

Gastaut H 1983 A proposed completion of the current international classification of the epilepsies. In: Rose F C (ed) research progress in epilepsy Part I. Pitman, Bath, pp 8–13

Gastaut H, Broughton R 1972 epileptic seizures – clinical and electrographic features, diagnosis and treatment. Thomas, Springfied, pp 125–126

Gloor P, Olivier A, Ives J 1980 Loss of consciousness in temporal lobe seizures: observations obtained with stereotaxic depth electrode recordings and stimulations In: Canger R, Angeleri F, Penry J K (eds) Advances in Epileptology (XI International Epilepsy Symposium) Raven Press, New York, pp 349–353

Gloor P 1986 Personal communication

Jasper H H 1964 some physiological mechanisms involved in epileptic automatisms. Epilepsia 5: 1–20

Parsonage M J 1979 In: Aspects of epilepsy. (Proceedings of the Oxford Scientific Meeting of the International League Against Epilepsy, British Branch). MCS Consultants, Tunbridge Wells, pp 17–25

Penfield W 1969 Epilepsy. Neurophysiology and some brain mechanisms related to consciousness. In: Jasper H H, Ward A A, Pope A (eds) Basic mechanisms of the Epilepsies. Churchill, London, pp 791–805

Penfield W, Jasper H H 1954 In: Epilepsy and the functional anatomy of the human brain. J and A Churchill, London, Ch XIII

Roger J, Dravet C, Bureau M, Dreifuss F E, Wolf P 1985 Epileptic Syndromes in Infancy, Childhood and Adolescence. John Libby, London

Stevens J 1983 Personal communication

PART THREE
R. J. Porter

INTRODUCTION

Efforts to generate an empirical classification of any disorder are, by their very nature, surrounded by controversy. Each expert views the clinical world in a slightly different way, sees patients who differ slightly from those studied by other experts, and formulates a unique understanding of the disorder to be classified. Efforts to classify epileptic seizures afford a case in point: each epileptologist's synthesis of the disorder varies from that of his or her colleagues. When the epileptologist is confronted with a construct (classification) created by someone else, this synthesis is challenged and a resistance to the classification often occurs. The various classifications of epileptic seizures and epileptic syndromes, however – even if less than fully accepted – provide a framework within which we improve our understanding of what we see and what others see, as well as providing a vocabulary for describing what we see. This brief review will consider the classification of epileptic seizures with emphasis on the utility of the 1981 Classification of Epileptic Seizures (Commission on the Classification and Terminology of the International League Against Epilepsy 1981) which was approved by the International League Against Epilepsy (ILAE). Space does not permit a discussion of epileptic syndromes, although a workable classification of syndromes may ultimately prove to be even more useful than the classification of epileptic seizures. A classification of the epilepsies was recently published and provisionally approved by the International League (Commission on the Classification and Terminology of the International League Against Epilepsy 1985).

CLASSIFYING SEIZURES

It is the considered opinion of most United States experts that, of empirical classifications of epileptic seizures and syndromes, the 1981 Classification of Epileptic Seizures is currently the most pragmatic for clinical use. The 1981 classification is extraordinarily empirical, ignoring such factors as anatomic substrate, etiology and age of onset in favour of the videotaped clinical event and its accompanying electroencephalogram. There are several reasons why such a classification is logical. First, the eliminated factors of anatomic substrate, etiology and age of onset are actually the criteria on which a classification of epileptic syndromes must be based, and, indeed, the most recent ILAE effort to classify such syndromes utilizes these data. Secondly, the ability to videotape seizures and record the accompanying EEGs allows these clinical criteria to be available in all classes of patients. Although the seizure is admittedly viewed in isolation, it remains the most complete data set and – apart from the patient's age – is, in some cases, the only useful information available about the patient.

Pragmatic application is a function of any classification. The classification of epileptic seizures assists the physician in determining the seizure diagnosis and may also assist in establishing the etiologic diagnosis in those cases in which etiology can be ascertained. Such determinations will assist directly in planning appropriate therapy for both the patient's seizures and their underlying cause (Porter 1984).

PARTIAL SEIZURES AND GENERALIZED SEIZURES

Epileptic seizures are fundamentally divided into two groups – partial and generalized (Table 1.6). Partial seizures have clinical or electroencephalographic evidence of a localized onset; the word 'partial' is deliberately chosen to avoid the implication that a highly discrete focus exists, as such is often not the case. Arguments against the use of the term 'partial' relate to semantics of the English language rather than to the concept proposed.

Generalized seizures have no evidence of a localized onset. Generalized seizures are, as a group, much more heterogeneous than partial seizures. The inability to localize the onset of generalized attacks, however, may reflect either a multifocal onset or current technical incapability of determining the single locus of onset.

Most seizures can be classified by taking an

Table 1.6 1981 International classification of epileptic seizures

I. PARTIAL SEIZURES (seizures beginning locally)
  A. Simple partial seizures
    (consciousness not impaired)
    1. With motor symptoms
    2. With somatosensory or special sensory symptoms
    3. With autonomic symptoms
    4. With psychic symptoms
  B. Complex partial seizures (with impairment of consciousness)
    1. Beginning as simple partial seizures and progressing to impairment of consciousness
      a. With no other features
      b. With features as in A.1–4
      c. With automatisms
    2. With impairment of consciousness at onset
      a. With no other features
      b. With features as in A.1–4
      c. With automatisms
  C. Partial seizures secondarily generalized

II. GENERALIZED SEIZURES (bilaterally symmetrical and without local onset)
  A. 1. Absence seizures
     2. Atypical absence seizures
  B. Myoclonic seizures
  C. Clonic seizures
  D. Tonic seizures
  E. Tonic-clonic seizures
  F. Atonic seizures

III. UNCLASSIFIED EPILEPTIC SEIZURES (inadequate or incomplete data)

Abstracted from: Commission on Classification and Terminology of the International League Against Epilepsy. This classification was approved by the International League Against Epilepsy in September 1981.

appropriate neurological history from the patient. Only rarely is special monitoring necessary to establish the correct diagnosis.

THE ROLE OF CONSCIOUSNESS IN THE CLASSIFICATION OF EPILEPTIC SEIZURES

Among the more controversial aspects of classifying epileptic seizures is the concept of preserved or altered consciousness. Although consciousness itself is exceedingly difficult to define, a working definition has evolved in which *responsiveness* is the critical factor. If the patients have some decrement in their ability to respond to exogenous stimuli, then responsiveness is considered to be altered. Obviously, the degree of difficulty of the task presented will, in fact, affect the application of this definition to individual patients. Exceptional patients with discrete lesions may be unresponsive but aware (e.g. with aphasia); in these patients, whose recall of ictal events is normal, consciousness is considered to be intact. Although responsiveness clearly represents a limited view of consciousness, this definition has the special advantage of being testable (Porter 1984). Whether alteration of consciousness (defined here as 'responsiveness') necessarily implies bilateral hemispheric involvement is controversial (Gloor et al 1980, Porter 1984).

SEIZURE PROGRESSION AND SEIZURE CLASSIFICATION

Although the concept of seizure progression has long been recognized, the 1981 classification embodied the concept for partial seizures in a way which allows easy classification of this group. If one accepts the tenets that simple partial seizures are associated with preserved consciousness and that complex partial seizures are associated with altered responsiveness, the concept of seizure progression in partial seizures is quickly limited to three fundamental possibilities:

1. a simple partial seizure may occur in isolation;
2. a complex partial seizure may be characterized by alteration of consciousness at onset; and
3. a complex partial seizure may be preceded by a simple partial seizure (often then called an 'aura').

An example of the third possibility would be a foul odour which leads directly to altered responsiveness and fumbling of the hands (an automatism) followed by a gradual return to normal consciousness. The foul odour may occur without progression as in the first possibility, or the complex partial seizure may occur without the aura as in the second possibility. Assuming that partial seizures progress in only one direction (as is most often the case), the possibilities, including secondary generalization, are summarized in Table 1.7.

That seizures in the 'generalized' category may also progress has been documented by Niedermeyer (1976), by Porter & Sato (1982) and by

Table 1.7 Possible progression of partial seizures (from Porter 1984)

Seizure progression	Seizure name
SP	Simple partial seizures
SP→CP	Complex partial seizures (with SP onset)
CP	Complex partial seizures
SP→GTC	Partial seizures secondarily generalized – generalized tonic-clonic seizures
CP→GTC	Partial seizures secondarily generalized – generalized tonic-clonic seizures
SP→CP→GTC	Partial seizures secondarily generalized – generalized tonic-clonic seizures

Stefan (1982). The usual progression observed is from an absence or a clonic seizure to a generalized tonic–clonic attack. The concept of progression in generalized seizures was not included in the 1981 classification, an oversight that will require eventual redress (Wolf 1985). A considerable semantic difficulty arises when a seizure in the 'generalized' category progresses secondarily to a generalized tonic-clonic attack; this problem has been addressed by Porter & Sato (1982) who suggest that the generalized tonic-clonic seizure is the maximal neuronal expression of an epileptic attack and may, in fact, be the only seizure type worthy of being called 'generalized'.

PARTIAL SEIZURES

Simple partial seizures

Simple partial seizures are those attacks which show evidence of a localized onset, but during which consciousness (responsiveness) is preserved. The discharge is usually confined to a single hemisphere, and the symptoms are specific to the affected brain region. Four major groups of simple partial seizures need to be considered:

1. simple partial seizures with motor signs;
2. simple partial seizures with sensory symptoms;
3. simple partial seizures with autonomic symptoms or signs; and
4. simple partial seizures with psychic symptoms.

Most commonly, patients experience either a motor event, such as clonic jerking of an extremity, or a sensory event, such as a bad odour or taste. As noted above, a sensory event also frequently occurs just prior to alteration of consciousness, and is often called an aura; an aura is a simple partial onset to a complex partial or generalized tonic–clonic seizure.

The occurrence of psychic symptoms as the sole manifestation of a simple partial seizure is both uncommon and controversial; most psychic symptoms occur as part of complex – not simple – partial seizures. Video recording has provided evidence that some patients with a seizure involving higher cortical function (e.g. forced thinking) may have preservation of responsiveness during the attack. On the other hand, one must be very cautious in ascribing to epilepsy such psychic phenomena as depersonalization, derealization, jamais vu and déjà vu (Harper & Roth 1962).

Complex partial seizures

Complex partial seizures are those attacks which show evidence of a localized onset and in which consciousness (responsiveness) is altered. In most instances the alteration results from bi-hemispheric involvement (see above). On occasion, a complex partial seizure will be preceded by an aura (a simple partial seizure); the entire ictal event may simply be called a complex partial seizure (see Table 1.6) or more specifically a 'complex partial seizure with simple partial onset'.

It has been argued that by equating 'complex' with 'altered consciousness' the 1981 seizure classification sacrifices some of the intent of the original 1969 classification. This author agrees with Wolf's assessment of the controversy (Wolf 1985). Wolf notes that opponents of the current use of the term 'complex' generally belong to one of two groups: those who hold that the term 'complex' should not be redefined but kept in its old meaning; and those who, while willing to accept a separation between seizures with impaired and seizures with preserved consciousness, are unwilling to accept 'complex' and 'simple' as appropriate labels for this dichotomy. Since, as Wolf points out, the 1969 classification lacked a precise definition of the term 'complex',

it is difficult to know what meaning the first group wishes to retain.

The complex partial seizure has characteristics which have been reviewed in detail using video-tape techniques (Escueta et al 1981, Theodore et al 1983). Automatisms are typical, occurring in 96% of complex partial seizures in one series (Theodore et al 1983): an 'automatism, or automatic behaviour, has been defined as complicated behaviour which requires integration of higher cortical structures and for which the patient has no recollection. A classification of automatisms is helpful and suggests that many such events are not very specific to either the locus of the seizure onset or even to the seizure type. Although a highly detailed classification of automatisms is available (Penry & Dreifuss 1969), most such events can be categorized into one of three fundamental groups (Porter 1984):

1. *De novo automatisms from internal stimuli* (including 'release' phenomena), for example, chewing, lip smacking, swallowing, scratching, rubbing, picking, fumbling, running, and disrobing.
2. *De novo automatisms from external stimuli*, for example, responding to pin-prick, drinking from a cup, chewing gum placed in the mouth, and pushing in response to restraint.
3. *Perseverative automatisms* (the continuation of any complex act initiated prior to loss of consciousness), for example, chewing food, using fork or spoon, drinking, and walking.

Secondarily generalized partial seizures

It is a matter of some debate whether most generalized tonic-clonic (grand mal) seizures are secondary to another seizure type. In the population reviewed by Porter & Sato (1982), most such attacks were preceded by a partial seizure and very few were considered 'primary'; however, this study was based on a referral population and almost certainly does not reflect the large numbers of patients who have infrequent grand mal seizures with no evidence of any other seizure type. On the other hand, many patients do experience a variety of seizure types in conjunction with grand mal attacks; these concomitant attacks often go unrecognized for variable lengths of time. The clinical nature of the secondarily generalized seizure itself does not appear to differ from that of the primary attack.

GENERALIZED SEIZURES

Introduction

The generalized seizures are an exceedingly heterogeneous group. Whether seizures in this group truly arise in both hemispheres simultaneously, or whether our ability to pinpoint the locus of onset is merely deficient is not yet determined. The term 'generalized' has deficiencies as noted earlier in this chapter.

The generalized tonic-clonic (grand mal) seizure

Although the generalized tonic-clonic seizure may progress directly from another seizure as noted above, some such attacks appear to be generalized at onset. The characteristics of the generalized tonic-clonic seizure have been well described by Gastaut & Broughton (1972), whose data have been summarized by Porter (1984).

The absence seizure

The absence (petit mal) seizure begins in childhood or early adolescence and is characterized by unresponsiveness and a variety of associated phenomena. Automatic behaviour is common; as automatisms are frequently observed in both absence and complex partial seizures, such behaviour should not be used to distinguish between the two types of attacks. Some features of the absence seizure may be helpful in establishing the diagnosis: the attacks are short, usually less than 10 seconds and rarely longer than 45 seconds; the onset is paroxysmal and without warning; the cessation is likewise sudden and without post-ictal depression or malaise. Automatisms are more common in longer attacks; clonic motion, usually of the eyelids, is common in shorter seizures

(Penry et al 1975). A patient with absence seizures has a good prognosis if he or she has normal or above average intelligence and a normal neurological examination (Sato et al 1983).

The myoclonias

The myoclonias are very heterogeneous; furthermore, clonic motion is a frequently observed feature of other seizure types. The terms which are commonly used to describe the phenomena (myoclonus, myoclonic, clonus, clonic) have been discussed (Porter 1984), and a volume has been written about epileptic myoclonus (Charleton 1975); classifications of myoclonus continue to evolve (Gastaut 1968, Marsden et al 1982). In general, emphasis should be placed on the clinical observation that clonic jerking is a surprisingly stereotyped movement; it is not a random flailing about. The characteristics of clonic jerking can sometimes be used to distinguish epileptic attacks from pseudoseizures (Porter 1986).

Clonic seizures

Clonic seizures are those generalized convulsive seizures which lack a tonic phase and are, in fact, a fragment of a generalized tonic-clonic seizure. In addition, certain patients with epileptic attacks characterized by repetitive myoclonic jerks must be considered to have 'clonic seizures'. These attacks may progress to generalized tonic-clonic seizures (Porter 1986).

Atonic seizures

Atonic seizures are those often severely incapacitating attacks in which precipitous loss of tone, usually postural, causes the patient to have a sudden nodding of the head or to fall to the floor. Although less sudden losses of tone have been described, the patients are usually at risk for injury, especially to face and head, and may require protective helmets (Porter 1986). Previous terms for atonic seizures include 'akinetic' and 'astatic'; the reasons for the abandonment of these terms have been reviewed (Porter 1984).

SUMMARY

The epilepsies are a heterogeneous symptom complex. Classifications have been designed both for the epileptic seizure and for the epileptic syndromes; the latter classification is currently less well refined. The 1981 Classification of Epileptic Seizures is pragmatic and can be applied to every patient in which epilepsy is in the differential diagnosis. A thorough medical history is necessary if the classification is to be properly utilized. A classification of epileptic syndromes is a classification of patients rather than of seizures; such a classification may eventually prove to be even more effective and of greater benefit to patients and physicians than the classification of epileptic seizures.

REFERENCES

Charleton M H (ed) 1975 Myoclonic seizures. Excerpta Medica, Amsterdam

Commission on Classification and Terminology of the International League Against Epilepsy 1981 Proposal for revised clinical and electroencephalographic classification of epileptic seizures. Epilepsia 22: 489–501

Commission on Classification and Terminology of the International League Against Epilepsy 1985 Proposal for classification of epilepsies and epileptic syndromes. Epilepsia 26: 268–278

Escueta A V, Bacsal F, Treiman D 1981 Complex partial seizures on closed-circuit television and EEG: A study of 691 attacks in 79 patients. Annals of Neurology 11: 292–300

Gastaut H 1968 Sémeiologie des myoclonies et nosologie analytique des syndromes myocloniques. In: Bonduelle M & Gastaut H (eds). Les myoclonies. Masson, Paris, pp. 1–30

Gastaut H, Broughton R 1972 Epileptic seizures: clinical and electrographic features, diagnosis and treatment. Charles C Thomas, Springfield, Ill

Gloor P, Olivier A, Ives J 1980 Loss of consciousness in temporal lobe seizures: observations obtained with stereotaxic depth electrode recordings and stimulations. In: Canger R, Angeleri F & Penry J K (eds) Advances in Epileptology: XIth Epilepsy International Symposium. Raven Press, New York, pp 349–353

Harper M, Roth M 1962 Temporal lobe epilepsy and the phobic anxiety–depersonalization syndrome. Part I: a comparative study. Comprehensive Psychiatry 3: 129–151

Marsden C D, Hallet M, Fahn S 1982 The nosology and pathophysiology of myoclonus. In: Marsden C D & Fahn S (eds) Neurology 2: Movement Disorders. Butterworths, London, pp. 196–248

Niedermyer E 1976 Immediate transition from a petit mal absence into a grand mal seizure: case report. European Neurology 14: 11–16

Penry J K, Dreifuss F E 1969 Automatisms associated with the absence of petit mal epilepsy. Archives of Neurology 21: 142–149

Penry J K, Porter R J, Dreifuss F E 1975 Simultaneous recording of absence seizures with video tape and electroencephalography: a study of 374 seizures in 48 patients. Brain 98: 427–440

Porter R J 1984 Epilepsy: 100 elementary principles. Saunders, London

Porter R J 1986 Recognizing and classifying epileptic seizures and epileptic syndromes. In: Porter R J, Theodore W H (eds) Neurologic clinics: epilepsy. Saunders, Philadelphia

Porter R J & Sato S 1982 Secondary generalization of epileptic seizures. In: Akimoto H, Kazamatsuri H, Seino M, Ward A A Jr (eds) Advances in epileptology: XIIIth Epilepsy International Symposium. Raven Press, New York, pp 47–48

Sato S, Dreifuss F E, Penry J K, Kirby D D, Paleschy 1983 Long-term follow-up of absence seizures. Neurology 33: 1590–1595

Stefan H 1982 Epileptische Absencen: Studien zur Anfallsstruktur, Pathophysiologie und zum klinischen Verlauf. Thieme, Stuttgart

Theodore W H, Porter R J, Penry J K 1983 Complex partial seizures: clinical characteristics and differential diagnosis. Neurology 33: 1115–1121

Wolf P 1985 The classification of seizures and the epilepsies. In Porter R J, Morselli P L (eds) The Epilepsies Butterworths, London, pp 106–124

2

Epidemiology

J. J. Zielinski

INTRODUCTION

Epilepsy is a chronic disorder characterized not only by recurrent seizures, but also by a great variety of medical and psychosocial implications. Its burden to the patients and their families has been recognized, but the impact upon a community is not understood fully. This became apparent as a result of population-based epidemiology studies.

Epidemiology is an academic and an applied discipline concerned not only with the frequency and distribution of various disorders, disabilities and deaths in the human population, but also with identifying biological, clinical, physical and social factors related to the occurrence, course and outcome of a disease.

Over the last 30 years many epidemiological studies of epilepsy have been published. They have significantly increased our knowledge of the condition not only in terms of its frequency, but also its natural course and prognosis.

Epidemiology and clinical medicine

Clinical surveys are based on more or less numerous case series derived from various medical facilities. Unfortunately, mechanisms underlying the formation of these case series have not usually been considered. These mechanisms, however, introduce an unknown and often severe bias which can significantly distort the 'representativeness' of the sample. In turn, conclusions are reached which are limited only to the sample studied. Such conclusions cannot be generalized or extrapolated beyond the group studied or other similarly selected group of patients. The myth of 'unselected case series', or 'consecutive admissions' is still alive and has been frequently considered as sufficient proof of the 'representativeness' of the sample of patients studied. In fact, the precise mechanisms underlying the formation of these case series can be largely unknown to the authors. Generally speaking, case series can be derived from the following sources:

1. general practices (general practitioners, family physicians, pediatricians, etc)
2. insurance companies registers
3. neurological (neuropediatric) out-patient clinics
4. neurological (neuropediatric) hospital departments
5. psychiatric facilities (clinics and/or departments)
6. neurosurgical facilities
7. special centres for epilepsy
8. special centres for mentally retarded or disabled, cerebral palsy, etc
9. death certificates
10. post-mortem series, including forensic medicine departments.

The more benign the epilepsy, the lower the probability the patient will appear beyond the level of general practice or neurological clinics. Many mild cases of epilepsy might remain unknown, even to general practitioners. The only way of finding such cases is through a population-based epidemiological survey. The same applies to files of insurance companies. The records of the medical practitioner provide one of the most easily available sources of information on diagnosed and suspected cases of epilepsy, although its value is limited (see section on prevalence of epilepsy).

The results of epidemiological field surveys, in turn, are useful to the practitioner in many ways. They help to develop and test clinical hypotheses of etiology, to improve the precision of clinical diagnosis, to check accuracy of clinical assessment of long-term prognosis, to recognize the social and environmental implications of disorder, and to improve the organization of treatment and management of patients with epilepsy.

Defining the population under study (denominator)

Knowledge of the population under study (i.e. from which epilepsy cases are collected) constitutes the basic condition in an epidemiological survey. The population should be defined preferably not only in terms of numbers, but also with regard to distribution of basic demographic and possibly socio-economic features (sex, age, marital and professional status, urban versus rural setting, etc.). This data is not always readily available from the census. Special precautions should be undertaken if extrapolation is attempted from the larger area to a smaller one (i.e. for a small city from a county census). Occasionally, additional effort is necessary to obtain information from various sources other than a census (i.e. school or voting registers).

Studies based on a fraction of the general population, unless randomly sampled, often yield less reliable results in terms of magnitude of the epidemiological indices, distribution of basic clinical features and/or prognosis.

Mechanisms of formation of various case series of patients with epilepsy have already been discussed. These mechanisms work irrespective of the disorder, but especially if a disorder is chronic. In 1946, J. Berkson, a physician at the Mayo Clinic, noted that the relative frequency of a disease among hospitalized patients is different when compared to that of a population in a hospital catchment area. Because the risk of hospitalization is higher for those suffering from more than one disease, epidemiological studies based on hospitalized populations will be significantly biased. The same consideration pertains to hospitalized patients entered as controls in any

clinical study. Berkson's hypothesis (or 'paradox') was recently confirmed by Roberts et al (1978) for some internal diseases. There are no known psychiatric or neurological studies on similar topics, but in a random sample of general practices in the UK a positive relationship was found between the occurrence of physical and psychiatric disorders (Eastwood & Trevelyan 1972).

In attempts toward extrapolating results of studies based on patient subpopulations, one has to remember that the value of general practice morbidity studies is limited (Shepherd et al 1981). Only part of the general population might be found in files of general practitioners. Some patients will seek professional care in other specialists' offices, not necessarily in the area in which they reside. This may be particularly so in cases of 'socially labelling' conditions, to which epilepsy belongs. On the other hand, if a physician working within the general practice boundaries is especially interested in a disorder, higher attendance rates of the people from the population covered by the practice can be encountered. Furthermore, medical attitudes can influence medical attendance, especially in chronic disorders. There can be differences between sexes: in the Warsaw survey the percentage of people with epilepsy who had never been treated was slightly higher among males than females (Zielinski 1974a). Among other factors influencing medical attendance, the educational level and socio-economic status should be considered. Finally, bias which is related to different distribution of age groups in the general population and patients' subpopulation can be responsible for erroneous estimations of incidence of epilepsy (high if patients are younger) or mortality (higher, if patients are older than in general population).

Defining 'the case of epilepsy' (numerator)

Although the occurrence of seizures has been considered for centuries as the hallmark of epilepsy, the contemporary criteria of classifying seizures were developed in 1969 (Gastaut 1969) and somewhat modified in recent years. On the other hand, attempts towards developing a widely accepted classification of various types of epilepsy have a long and yet uncertain history.

Epilepsy is primarily a clinical diagnosis based on the presence of recurring seizures. Most physicians, however, rarely have an opportunity to witness personally a seizure and therefore have to rely on the reports of witnesses. This in turn can seriously influence the accuracy of the physician's diagnosis and classification of the patient's seizures. Similarly, the patient's ability to report his own experiences occurring 'before' or during a seizure is very important for arriving at accurate diagnosis and classification, especially in cases of temporal lobe epilepsy. Moreover, diagnosis and classification of some seizures may be difficult, even if they are observed and recorded by the expert. Obtaining such information can be much more problematic, if not impossible, in patients with concomitant mental retardation. Moreover, in many medical files one can find only more or less precise attempts to classify a type of a seizure (i.e. 'grand mal', 'major', 'minor', etc), but no description of its clinical appearance. Interestingly enough, the same trend is observed among laymen reporting the seizures in relatives or persons under their care. This trend of course does not facilitate the diagnosis of 'a case of epilepsy' in surveys based on population or on the records of general practitioners. Furthermore, the major difficulty in comparing the results of various surveys is the use of different diagnostic criteria or even a lack of a precision definition of epilepsy. Gastaut's (1973) definition* is not always applicable to epidemiological field surveys because it may not be possible to carry out medical or EEG examinations.

The term 'chronic disorder' may be ambiguous. During the discussion on the definition and classifications of epilepsy for epidemiological purposes as proposed by Alter et al (1972), it was agreed that cases with a single seizure, including febrile convulsions and those due to an acute cause such as (illness, trauma or intoxication†) should be considered separately in epidemiological studies.

Additionally, there is disagreement about the length of time a patient should be seizure free before being considered 'cured' of epilepsy, or alternatively 'once epileptic, always epileptic' (Lennox 1960). To overcome this difficulty, some authors define the proportions of 'active' and 'non-active' epilepsy in the material of their study. The 'non-active' group includes those who have been free of seizures for usually five, sometimes two, years. Patients who have been in a long remission but who are still on antiepileptic drugs are considered as having 'active epilepsy' (Grudzinska 1974, Gudmundsson 1966, Hauser & Kurland 1975, Nowak 1972, Zielinski 1966, Zielinski 1974a). Some authors exclude cases of symptomatic epilepsy from their estimates (Brewis et al 1966, Leibowitz & Alter 1968); others do not (Goodridge & Shorvon 1983).

Overdiagnosis of epilepsy

Not only are actual cases of epilepsy missed at some levels of care, but individuals are commonly mistakenly diagnosed having epilepsy. Overdiagnosis of epilepsy might be especially frequent among case series derived from general practices, although it occurs occasionally in psychiatric facilities. A diagnosis of epilepsy could not be confirmed during re-examination in approximately 15% of patients diagnosed as 'epileptic' in the Warsaw study. The highest percentage of overdiagnosis was found in paediatric and psychiatric facilities, especially in psychiatry facilities for children (Zielinski 1974a). Similar problems of overdiagnosis were recently encountered in the National Child Developmental Study in Great Britain. Of 103 children reported by their general practitioners or consultants as having epilepsy, the diagnosis could not be substantiated in 39 (Ross & Peckham 1983). 'Inventing' or inducing false seizures in children, although rare, should also be kept in mind (Meadow 1984).

---

* A chronic brain disorder of various etiologies characterized by recurrent seizures due to excessive discharge of cerebral neurones . . . Single or occasional epileptic seizures as well as those occurring during an acute illness should not be classified as epilepsy

† An acute episode is defined as lasting less than 72 hours

BASIC EPIDEMIOLOGICAL MEASUREMENTS

Morbidity rates measure the frequency of the disorder within a defined population and with the time and place specified. *Incidence* (I) is the rate at which new cases of a disease occur. For epilepsy the average annual incidence is usually calculated per 100 000 according to the formula:

$$I = \frac{\text{number of new cases within 1 year}}{\text{population at the mid-year}} \times 100\,000$$

Since the estimate is based on the number of new cases of epilepsy diagnosed, the rate would be described better as the 'first attendance rate' or 'accession rate'. Several years may elapse between the time of first seizure and that of the actual diagnosis of epilepsy (Zielinski 1974a, Hauser & Kurland 1975). There are other patients who never consult a doctor or who remain undiagnosed (Zielinski 1976). It follows that the 'accession rate' may fall well below the real rate, particularly if calculated over a short period.

Prevalence (P) describes the frequency of all current cases of a disease. For epilepsy this rate is usually estimated per 1000 according to the formula:

$$P = \frac{\text{number of epileptic people in population at any given time}}{\text{population at risk}} \times 1000$$

The number of cases in a population on a particular day is the point-prevalence rate and is most often used. Prevalence is the product of time and incidence. With a chronic condition like epilepsy, the number of patients accumulates with time and so the prevalence is high although the incidence rates are low. The so-called 'life-time' or 'total' prevalence can be calculated when the numerator is the number of people who have ever suffered from recurrent seizures. The 'accumulated incidence' (Juul-Jensen & Ipsen 1976, Hauser 1978) can be a better method of estimating the risk of contracting epilepsy during a lifetime. It is calculated by adding the incidence rates for different age groups. For example, if the annual incidence rates for the 0–4 age group and the 5–9 age group are 80 and 50 per 100 000 respectively, then the total number of patients at the end of the first decade would be some 650 per 100 000 or 0.6%.

Mortality rates measure the frequency of deaths within the defined population. The 'cause-specific death rate' is that due to a specific disorder and is calculated per 100 000 according to the formula:

$$\text{Cause-specific death rate} = \frac{\begin{array}{c}\text{number of deaths assigned to a}\\ \text{specific cause in a given time}\\ \text{interval}\end{array}}{\text{mid-interval population}} \times 100\,000$$

The case-fatality ratio (CFR) gives another measure where:

$$\text{CFR} = \frac{\begin{array}{c}\text{number of deaths assigned to a specific}\\ \text{disease during a given time interval}\end{array}}{\begin{array}{c}\text{number of cases of that disease during}\\ \text{the same time interval}\end{array}} \times 100$$

'Standardized mortality ratio' (SMR) measures the proportion of death rates observed in a given sample to that expected; the latter is calculated for the general population from which the sample was derived. All the above rates can be calculated for specific groups defined by age, sex, race, etc.

The estimation and interpretation of death rates and ratios are often difficult in epilepsy. Only a proportion of epileptic patients die of epilepsy. Thus, when estimating the CFR, only deaths due to epilepsy should be entered in the numerator, while the denominator includes cases of 'active' epilepsy or all known cases. Mortality rates are usually calculated as a proportion of all deaths of persons with diagnosed epilepsy to the mid-interval general population.

Case-ascertainment methods

It would be the epidemiologist's dream if every person contracting a disease would immediately consult his doctor and the diagnosis be properly recorded. Unfortunately, just the opposite happens. Many patients do not notice their symptoms or dismiss then as unimportant (Zielinski 1976). In a sample from 17 general practices in Metropolitan London only a fifth of patients with epilepsy had suspected the diagnosis before they decided to consult their doctor (Hopkins & Scambler 1977). Another serious problem is caused by patients who decide to terminate treatment and thus disappear from medical files (Zielinski 1974a). Twenty to 25% of children in Newcastle-upon-Tyne suffering from various types of seizures never sought medical advice (Miller et al 1960). Similar figures were found in Warsaw.

One of the oldest, retrospective methods of case-finding is to review medical and other records in a selected area to find those which mention the diagnosis of epilepsy or of an epileptic seizure. Anderson (1936) reviewed files of epilepsy colonies, mental hospitals, 'county infirmaries' and general practices, along with interviewing 'key-persons' in the area studied. A number of further studies have been based on review of files of general practitioners or their reports (Schleisner 1849, Logan & Cushion 1958, Crombie et al 1960, Pond et al 1960). This method may be supplemented by a medical re-examination of all patients or of a random sample to verify the accuracy of the original diagnosis (Anderson 1936, Gudmundsson 1966, Zielinski 1974a, Goodridge & Shorvon 1983). Another method, combining the retrospective and prospective approach, is to compile a register to which data on new cases of epilepsy in a population are added as they are diagnosed. This method increases the chance of an accurate estimate by bringing together information about the same patient from different sources.* A register of patients for the population of Rochester, with a history of epilepsy, suspected epilepsy and febrile convulsions since 1945 was compiled from the medical files of the Mayo Clinic (Kurland 1959, Hauser & Kurland 1975). A similar register was introduced in Aarhus, Denmark (Juul-Jensen & Ipsen 1976).

Another approach is a specially designed study of chosen general populations or random samples of them. Retrospective, cross-sectional studies of this type have been carried out in Guam, Carlisle, Warsaw and Bogota. In Carlisle and Warsaw medical files were also surveyed.

Some workers limit their surveys to selected groups derived from the population at large

because of a better chance of complete identification of cases. However, results of these studies cannot be extrapolated directly to all people with epilepsy. Examples of such studies are: workers' sick-fund policy holders (Wajsbort et al 1967), mine workers (Bird et al 1962), and army draftees (Bayley et al, Edwards et al, after Lennox 1960).

Reliable results on epilepsy morbidity risk factors and prognosis can be obtained from studies of variously selected cohorts. These studies are prospective in nature and expensive. As with field surveys they are rather difficult to continue and need very careful planning beforehand. Cohorts can be selected from the population according to a specific factor. In epilepsy, most studies of this type have been carried out on newborns and followed for a number of years ('birth-cohort'). Results of these studies will be discussed later (see section on Prevalence in children). An example of another cohort study is a survey by Annegers et al (1980) on seizures in people who suffered from head trauma in a given population.

INCIDENCE OF EPILEPSY

Table 2.1 shows that, despite different methodologies used, most studies give incidence rates from 20 to 50 per 100 000. The British authors (Crombie et al 1960, Pond et al 1960), who had based their estimates on a number of patients in general practice rather than on the general population, reported relatively high incidence. The inclusion of patients with single seizures and febrile convulsions has significantly contributed to high incidence rates, which approach the combined incidence rates of isolated and recurrent seizures in Rochester (Hauser & Kurland 1975). The Guam survey results show that the incidence estimated by the more complete case-finding method of field survey may be twice as high as that based on review of medical records only (Stanhope et al 1972). According to the results of the Rochester study, the combined annual incidence rates for recurrent and single seizures as well as for febrile seizures reach almost 120 per 100 000 (Hauser & Kurland, 1975). Even so, the incidence of the two latter groups still seems

* During the review of medical records in Warsaw it was found that information about 30 per cent of cases was discovered independently in at least two files. This was also found by Gudmundsson 1966, Rutter, Graham & Yule 1970.

Table 2.1 Incidence rates for epilepsy (selected studies)

Country, authors(s)	Case ascertainment method*	Population studied	Annual incidence per 100 000	Comment
Denmark Juul-Jensen & Ipsen 1976	ER	Aarhus	30	Including 'observation for epilepsy'
Great Britain Crombie et al, 1960	GPs	Patients of 67 practices, England & Wales	63	Ss & Fs included
Great Britain Pond et al, 1960	RMR, GPs, Itv	Patients of 14 practices SE England	70	First diagnosis of epilepsy
Great Britain Brewis et al, 1966	RMR, Itv, ME, SP	Carlisle, England	30	Symptomatic, Ss & Fs not included
Guam Stanhope et al, 1972	RMR (N) SP	Guam	23	Fs, Ss not included
Stanhope et al, 1972	Field survey SP, Itv, ME	Guam, same area	46	Fs, Ss not included
Iceland Gudmundsson, 1966	RMR, ME, SP	Iceland	26	Fs, Ss not included
Italy Granieri et al, 1983	RMR, Itv, ME, SP	Copparo	31	Fs, Ss not included
Japan Sato, 1964	RMR	Niigata	17	'Symptomatic' seizures not included
Norway De Graaf 1974	RMR (N & EEG)	Subarctic area	33	Large area, difficult travelling.
Poland Grudzinska, 1974	RMR, ME, SP	Zabrze	22	First attendance, Fs, Ss not included
Zielinski, 1974a	RMR (N & P)	Warsaw	20	As above
USA Kurland 1959	RMR, ER Mayo Clinic	Rochester	30	Fs, Ss not included
Hauser & Kurland, 1975	As above	Rochester 1955–64 1965–67 1935–67	54 46 49	As above

* List of abbreviations:
RMR – Review of medical records in area studied
N, P, EEG – Records of neurological, psychiatric, EEG facilities
ER   – Epilepsy Register
SP   – Study based on general population or sample derived from it
Itv – Interview of inhabitants in population or its sample
ME   – Medical examination or re-examination of people with diagnosed or suspected epilepsy
GPs – General Practitioners
Ss   – cases of single, afebrile seizures
Fs   – cases with febrile seizures only

Table 2.2 Proportions of age-specific incidence rates for epilepsy (average annul incidence rate for all ages = 1.00)

Age	Rochester Minn. 1935–1964	Carlisle England 1955–1961	Iceland 1959–1964	Warsaw Poland 1970–1972	Greater Aarhus Denmark 1960–1972	Copporo Italy 1964–1978
All ages = 1.00	45	28	33	20	30	33
0–9	1.88	2.03	1.87	2.28	2.38	2.91
10–19	0.80	1.71	1.78	1.18	1.62	2.03
20–29	0.51	0.78	0.69	0.64	0.63	
30–39	0.60	0.57	0.54	0.74	0.59	0.61
40–49	0.62	0.78	0.42	0.77	0.60	0.61
50–59	0.82	0.75	0.33	0.69	0.60	0.61
60 and above	1.33	0.42	0.18	0.93	0.52	0.23

to be underestimated. However, these incidence rates make it possible to estimate the number of people who will need medical advice each year because of the occurrence of first seizure.

Sex and age-specific incidence

Most authors have found higher incidence rates in males although Pond's study (Pond et al 1960) showed a higher rate for females. There is a general consensus of opinion concerning age-specific rates (Table 2.2). The rates are higher within the first decade, especially in the first year of life, and somewhat lower in the second decade; thereafter they become low. However, there are obvious differences between the studies, particularly in the figures for those aged 60 and above. In Iceland, Carlisle and Greater Aarhus these rates are lowest, while in the Rochester series and Warsaw field survey there is a marked increase among the oldest age group. This increase may be due to more effective case-finding methods in these two studies. According to Hauser & Kurland (1975), an increased rate in the elderly

does not necessarily reflect a higher incidence of brain tumours or cerebrovascular disease, since in 70% of new cases over 60 no clear etiological factor could be found.

PREVALENCE OF EPILEPSY

The literature contains a considerable number of studies devoted to estimating the prevalence of epilepsy in different countries. Only those which include more or less detailed descriptions of the method employed, definitions of the cases examined and characteristics of the population studied will be considered. The results of selected epidemiological studies are given in Table 2.3.

The overall prevalence rates per 1000 of the general population vary from 1.5 in Niigata, Japan (Sato 1964) to 9.2 in Warsaw (Zielinski 1974a), and as high as 19.5 in Bogota, Colombia (Gomez et al 1978). In over half the studies, the rates lie between 4 and 10 per 1000. In most of the studies where the rate was lower than 4 per 1000, infor-

Table 2.3 Prevalence rates for epilepsy (selected studies)

Country, area studied	Author(s)	Case ascertainment method*	Rate per 1000	Comment*
Chile, Melipilla	Chiofale et al 1979	SP, Itv + ME of selected sample	27.6 Range 21.1–31.9	Children aged 9, method and definition similar to Rose et al (USA)
Colombia, Bogota	Gomez et al 1978	SP, Itv + ME	19.5	Fs, Ss not included

Continued

Table 2.3 (*Cont'd*)

Country, area studied	Author(s)	Case ascertainment method*	Rate per 1000	Comment*
Denmark Aarhus	Juul-Jensen & Ipsen 1976	ER	6.9	Including 1.1 for 'observation of epilepsy'
	Juul-Jensen & Foldspang 1983	ER	4.4	Prevalence rate calculated by this author. Cumulated incidence = 12.7
Great Britain England and Wales	Logan & Cushion 1958	Info GPs from 106 practices	3.3	Epilepsy as diagnosed by GPs, annual attendance 1954/55
England and Wales	Crombie et al 1960	Info from GPs, 67 practices	4.2	Epilepsy as diagnosed by GPs; 'non-active' cases not included
England	Pond et al 1960	RMR in 14 practices + Itv	6.2	Ss included, epilepsy as diagnosed by GPs, prev. per practice ranged 3.0–12.9; prev. of 'chronic' epilepsy – 4.2'
Carlisle	Brewis et al 1966	RMR SP: Itv + ME	5.5 6.0	'Lifetime'; Fs, Ss and symptomatic epilepsy not included
Tonbridge	Goodridge & Shorvon 1983	RMR of 6000 'scrutinized' records of patients of an urban group practice	16.7 total 10.7 males 22.7 females 5.3 'active' 5.0 males 5.7 females	Ss, associated with eclampsia, alcohol withdrawal, stroke, etc included. 'Epilepsy as diagnosed by specialists'
England Scotland Wales	Ross et al 1980	Birth cohort followed by age 11 yrs., Itv	4.1	Follow-up of 15 496 children
Isle of Wight	Rutter et al 1970	ME, cohort of children 5–14 yrs	7.2	5.4 for 'uncomplicated' epilepsy
	Pless & Graham 1970	as above, 10–12 yrs	8.9	6.4 for 'uncomplicated' epilepsy; 4.9 fits in last year
Iceland	Schleisner 1849 (Cit. Gudmundsson 1966)	RMR in 1847	5.8	Cit. Gudmundsson
	Gudmundsson 1966	RMR + ME	3.4 – 'active' 5.2 – 'lifetime'	Fs and Ss not included
Italy	Granieri et al 1983	SP, RMR, Itv + ME	6.2 'active'	Fs and Ss not included
Israel Jerusalem	Leibowitz & Alter 1968	RMR	4.1	Fs and Ss not included, 'idiopathic' only
Japan Niigata City	Sato 1964	RMR	1.5	'Idiopathic' only
Mariana Islands Guam	Lessel, Torres & Kurland 1962	SP, Itv + ME	3.7	Ss included
	Mathai et al 1968	SP, Itv + ME	2.3 – 'active' 4.4 – total	Fs and Ss not included
	Stanhope et al 1972	SP, Itv + ME RMR (N) only	5.3 'active' 3.1 'active'	Fs and Ss not included High proportion of symptomatic epilepsy
Mexico Mexico City	Olivares 1972	RMR	3.5	

Continued

Table 2.3 (*Cont'd*)

Country, area studied	Author(s)	Case ascertainment method*	Rate per 1000	Comment*
Netherlands Zeeland	Bongers et al 1976	GPs	2.9	Epilepsy as diagnosed by interviewed GPs, prevalence per practice ranged 1.0–7.0
Nigeria Lagos	Dada 1968	SP, Itv + ME	3.1	Cit. Dada 1976
Norway Northern	de Graaf 1974	RMR (N + EEG)	3.5	Subarctic area
Poland Pruszkow	Zielinski 1966	RMR (N + P + EEG) + ME	4.3	Urban area, Fs, Ss not included, pop'n aged 16 and above
Kielce	Nowak 1972.	RMR + ME + Itv in rural area	4.9 – urban 2.9 – rural	Fs, Ss not included. Pop'n aged 16 and above
Pruszkow	Kuran 1975	RMR + ME	6.7	School children aged 7–14
Zabrze	Grudzinska 1974	RMR + ME	3.4	Fs, Ss not included, industrialized city
Warsaw	Zielinski 1974a	RMR + ME, SP, Itv + ME	4.3 7.8 'active 9.2 'lifetime'	Fs, Ss not included
Sampled areas all over Poland	Zielinski 1975	Information from medical facilities	2.8	Epilepsy as diagnosed by physician attended in one year
USA Michigan (9 counties)	Anderson 1936	SP, RMR + ME	2.1	81.5% found in the community. No diagnostic definition. Cases not reported by physicians were verified
Rochester Minn.	Kurland 1959	RMR (Mayo Clinic)	3.6	Fs, Ss not included
	Hauser & Kurland 1975	as above	5.3 for 1950 6.2 for 1960 5.7 for 1965	'Active' epilepsy (whether diagnosed or not) on January 1 in previous years
	Annegers & Hauser 1977	as above	6.5 for 1970	As above
Washington County, Md	Rose et al 1973	SP, Itv + ME	18.6 Range 14.1–20.1	School children aged 8–9; included Fs and Ss with EEG changes or positive family history of epilepsy
Multnomah County, Ore	Meighan et al 1976	as above	9.7 Range 7.8–12.8	As above
Maryland	Hirtz et al 1984	Birth cohort followed by age 7 yrs	5.8	54 000 pregnant females, 52 360 live birth, 39,270 followed for up to 7 yrs

*RMR – Review of medical records in area studied
ER – Epilepsy Register, continuous collection of data in area studied
SP – Study based on general population or a sample of it
Itv – Interview of inhabitants in population or its sample
ME – Medical examination or re-examination of epileptic individuals or cases suspected of epilepsy
GPs – General practitioners
Fs – Cases of febrile seizures
Ss – Cases with single afebrile seizure
(N), (P), (EEG) – neurological, psychiatric, EEG facilities

mation has been obtained solely from a review of medical records or from data provided by general practitioners or family physicians. Although their files are the inexpensive and readily available source of information for epidemiological analysis, it should be considered that these records serve practical rather than research purposes. Moreover, practitioners usually do not take into account conditions which are not directly brought to the doctors' attention (Shepherd et al 1981). The same can be said about the Polish survey, which relied upon the total number of medical attendances in randomly sampled geographical areas (Zielinski 1975). Unavoidable incompleteness of such data is shown by the results of the Guam and Warsaw studies (Stanhope et al 1972, Zielinski 1974a). The prevalence rates estimated on the basis of a population survey appeared to be higher by 70% in the former and more than 100% in the latter study. The differences between the rates in the Carlisle study, where they were obtained from medical files and from a house-to-house survey, were minimal. This was probably because only a single question was asked: 'Have you ever suffered from attacks of loss of consciousness?' Moreover, the prevalence in the last year of the Warsaw study, which was based only on cases attending the medical services, was lower by a third at 2.6 per 1000. This shows that the longer the period of study, or the more intensive the case-finding method, the higher the probability of finding a larger number of affected people in the population. It is also worth noting that the prevalence of 'active' cases of epilepsy seems to be quite close in several studies: 2.3 in Guam (Mathai et al 1968), 3.4 in Iceland (Gudmundsson 1966), 5.3 in Tonbridge (Goodridge & Shorvon 1983), 5.7 or 6.5 in Rochester (Hauser et al 1977) and 7.8 in Warsaw (Zielinski 1974a).

'Lifetime' or 'total' prevalence

The estimate of this rate is determined by the number of people within a population who have ever suffered from epileptic seizures. It is difficult, if not virtually impossible, to identify all such cases: because of the varying clinical presentations of seizures, the long-term remissions and the case-finding methods described. The problem

may be illustrated by the Warsaw study, during which two samples of patients were examined: a random sample of epileptic patients based on a review of medical and social services, and those identified in a random sample of the Warsaw population (field survey).

The case-finding method in the field survey occurred in four stages. First, was an interview by questionnaire covering six items about possible epileptic seizures or other forms of paroxysmal events, whether in the present or the past. Secondly, there was an independent evaluation of this information by two neurologists and a psychiatrist. Thirdly, there was a medical interview with those people whose past or present history suggested some form of epileptic seizure. And fourthly, a detailed comprehensive examination was made of those suspected of suffering from epilepsy. Finally, two groups were compared: those known to the medical and social services (group K) and those found in the population survey (group F). According to the distribution of basic clinical variables in these two groups, the following prevalence rates per 1000 population were estimated:

	Group K	Group F
Cases of epilepsy = total	4.3	9.2*
Seizures during past 5 years	4.2	7.8
Ever on medication	3.9	5.2
On medication when examined	3.3	3.2
6 years free of seizures	0.5	1.4

* If the expected number of people with epilepsy among those respondents who refused the questionnaire is included, the rate would rise to 10.4.

It is clear that almost all in the K group are cases of active epilepsy. Over 90% had taken antiepileptic drugs regularly in the past and over 75% were on medication when examined. The prevalence rates of those on medication are almost exactly the same in the two groups, although only some 35% of group F were on drugs. Furthermore, in group F, over 35% of patients had never been on medication and some 25% had never consulted a doctor over their seizure disorder. The percentage of group F patients in the Warsaw study who have never been treated slightly exceeds the 32% found in Iceland. In both these studies, long-term remission is relatively frequent among those never treated. Thus, milder and non-active epilepsy appears to be much more common among undiagnosed and untreated cases. This seems to confirm the opinion of Rodin (1968) that the majority of patients who attend clinics regularly do so because their seizures are not satisfactorily controlled. Juul-Jensen & Ipsen (1976) also point out that a large number of patients become free of seizures and these are not included in the Epilepsy Register. Based on this register, Juul-Jensen & Foldspang (1983) have estimated cumulative incidence rates for all cases with seizures and for epilepsy. The former is 2.4% and reflects the risk of having a seizure during lifetime: for epilepsy the figure is 1.3% and, for febrile convulsions, 0.4%. Prevalence rates were not calculated but, on the basis of data provided by Juul-Jensen & Foldspang, this author estimated prevalence of epilepsy at about 4.4 per 1000 inhabitants of Greater Aarhus. Although Juul-Jensen & Foldspang consider that 'most patients with epilepsy should be registered', they feel that many individuals with milder epilepsy, as well as many of those with febrile seizure, have been missed. This feeling is consistent with the results of the Warsaw field survey (Zielinski 1974b, 1976) and the findings of the National Child Development Study in Great Britain (Ross et al 1980).

In summary, one comes to the conclusion that incidence and prevalence rates based on data from medical records are more or less severely underestimated. The proportion of cases overlooked decreases when a field survey method is used, but even then some patients may refuse to disclose their epilepsy to the interviewer. In the Warsaw field survey, patients whose names were known from medical files refused to complete the questionnaire more often than the rest of the sampled population (8.0% versus 1.4%). The 'accumulated incidence' or 'lifetime risk' of epilepsy differ widely among authors. Whereas Juul-Jensen & Foldspang (1983) came to the figure of about 1.3%, Hauser & Kurland (1975) (assuming that the average life expectancy of a Rochester resident was 70 years), estimated that about 6% of the total population would suffer from at least a single nonfebrile epileptic seizure. This included almost 4% of those who will have had recurrent seizures at some period during their lives.

Sex-and age-specific prevalence rates for epilepsy

In the vast majority of the studies quoted in Table 2.3, males tend to predominate and only in studies by Juul-Jensen, Pond et al and Goodridge & Shorvon were there more females. The last two studies were based on general practices' case-series and no references to general population were made. Moreover, in the Tonbridge study, prevalence rates of 'inactive' epilepsy among female patients seen in general practice are twice as high as in male patients (22.7 and 10.7 per 1000 respectively). For 'active epilepsy', the rates are similar in both sexes (5.7 and 5.0 respectively). The authors did not comment on the striking differences between sex-adjusted prevalence rates of inactive epilepsy. The tendency toward overdiagnosing epilepsy in females in the past is one of the probable explanations of this finding. It is also noteworthy that sex-adjusted prevalence rates of single seizures appeared again twice as high in female patients than in male patients (27.0 and 13.7 per 1000 respectively).

Several authors have suggested that the reason for a high male rate is due, at least in part, to more frequent head injuries. Indeed, in a random sample of the Warsaw population, some 2.2% of children and 4% of adults reported at least one admission to hospital because of a head injury. Furthermore, head injury prior to the onset of seizures was noted nearly twice as often in males (30% versus 16%). The prevalence rates of post-traumatic epilepsy were estimated in the study at 1.0 to 1.5 per thousand (Zielinski 1977).

Age-specific prevalence rates from several studies are shown in Figure 2.1. In most studies the rates, which were based on medical services case-series show a very similar pattern. The lowest rates, which usually occur in the first decade, increase in the older age groups and then show a marked drop after the age of 50. Only in Rochester and Warsaw were there high prevalence rates at greater ages, and in Aarhus (Juul-Jensen & Ipsen 1976) during the sixth decade. This rise in prevalence rates in the elderly is the accumulation of cases discovered by more effective case-finding methods. Prevalence rates of epilepsy appeared to be higher in urban than in rural populations: in

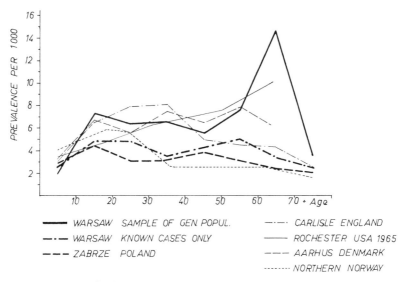

Fig. 2.1 Age-specific prevalence rates of epilepsy per 1000 according to results of selected community surveys

both areas rates were higher in males (Nowak 1972, Nowak et al 1984).

Prevalence in children

Several epidemiological studies covered the youngest age groups in which the chance of seizures occurring is greatest. On follow-up of a cohort of children born in Newcastle-upon-Tyne, Miller et al (1960) found that before the age of 5 one or more seizures occurred in 7% of subjects and 2% had recurrent seizures. Cooper (1965), during a British national survey of 5000 births, estimated that over 2% of children experienced at least one seizure before the age of 2.

An intensive epidemiological survey on children aged 4 to 15 years on the Isle of Wight (Rutter et al 1970) yielded prevalence rate of epilepsy at 7.2 per 1000, including 5.4 for 'uncomplicated epilepsy' (no mental or neurological handicap coexisting with seizure disorder). Similar rates for children aged 10 to 12 years were 8.9 and 6.4 respectively (Pless & Graham 1970). The National Child Development Study included all children born in England, Scotland and Wales in one week of March 1958. Of the 15 496 children with information on seizures gathered at 7 and 11 years, 346 appeared to be suspected of having recurrent seizures. In 64 of them epilepsy was confirmed (prevalence rate of 4.1), whereas in another 39

cases 'epilepsy was reported by doctor, but unsubstantiated' (Ross et al 1980). In addition, in 12 cases convulsions were directly reported by parents, who did not inform the general practitioner. This figure constitutes some 20% of diagnosed cases and shows that a marked proportion of individuals with a history of seizures may be unknown to general practitioners or paediatricians. Febrile convulsions were noted in another 378 children (24.4 per 1000), including 0.8 symptomatic (due to meningitis or encephalitis) and 1.3 in whom afebrile seizures occurred later on (5.3%). Another birth-cohort study was initiated in 1970. This time, 16 004 neonatal survivors born in one week in 1970 were surveyed (a Child Health and Education Study – started as the British Births Survey). Of 13 135 children followed from birth up to the age of 5, 2.3% suffered from febrile convulsions which recurred in one-third on another occasion (Verity et al 1985).

In the USA, Van den Bergh & Yerushalmy (1969) found in a cohort of children born in the San Francisco area that 1% had afebrile seizures before the end of their fifth year, usually early in life. Similarly, according to Gates (1972), 3.4% of a cohort of children born in New York experienced at least one afebrile seizure before the age of 8.

Another extensive birth-cohort study includes

52 360 live births to selected 54 000 pregnant females seen in 12 teaching urban hospitals prior to delivery. Of those born, 39 270 children have been followed up until the age of 7: 2635 of them (67.1 per 1000) reportedly suffered from at least a single seizure (including 502 with febrile seizure), whereas in 218 (5.6 per 1000) recurrent afebrile seizures occurred (Ellenberg et al 1984). The risk of recurring afebrile seizures in this cohort was estimated at some 55% (Hirtz et al 1984). Among the children who had suffered from febrile seizures, the chance of occurrence of non-febrile seizures by the age of 7 was related to the existence of 'risk factors'. These included: abnormal neurological findings, a history of epilepsy in a close relative, and the first febrile seizure of complex type (focal, lasting over 15 minutes or multiple in one day). None of the factors was found in 60% of children, one was found in 34% and two or more in 6%. The occurrence of non-febrile seizures was noted respectively in 2%, 3% and 13% of the above 'risk-groups' (Hirtz & Nelson 1983).

Studies of school children in Poland revealed that 6.7 per 1000, aged 7–8, had repeated seizures, including 5.2 with seizures during the previous two years (Kuran 1975). Studies of Rose et al (1973), Meighan et al (1976) in the United States and Chiofale et al (1979) in Chile used the same methodological approach and included febrile seizures and single seizures with positive EEG findings, or a positive family history of epilepsy. Although in Multnomah County the response rate was lower than in Washington County, the results of these two studies estimate the prevalence of epilepsy among third grade children at about 1–2%, while in the Chilean town of Melipilla it was nearly 3%.

Tsuboi (1984) has studied the prevalence of febrile and afebrile seizures in children up to age 3 in two geographical areas in Japan. Prevalence rates were 83.3 per 1000 in Fuchu City and 99.4 per 1000 in the Pacific island population. The occurrence of afebrile convulsions was in 3% of children with febrile seizures. Analysing data from the literature, the author found that the prevalence rates of febrile and afebrile convulsions in children had a linear correlation, and that ratios of these rates fall into four groups: both moderate, both high, both low, and very high rate of one and low of another. The results of his study can be included in the fourth group, together with results of studies in Guam-Mariana Islands. This may suggest geographic variations.

To summarize, in children followed from birth to 5–11 years of age, the frequency of febrile seizures was relatively low in Great Britain (24 per 1000) compared with the United States (50 per 1000); prevalence of epilepsy appeared more consistent (4.1 and 5.6 respectively). Community-orientated studies on children of school age yielded a somewhat higher prevalence of epilepsy: 7–9 per 1000.

Seizure type

The frequency of various types of seizures has usually been analysed in selected out- and in-patient case-series. Gastaut et al (1975) calculated the relative distribution in a series of 4590 private patients. Unfortunately, only very few epidemiologists have reported comparable data.

Table 2.4 shows that the distribution of patients with primary generalized seizures as contrasted with partial seizures is similar in the Rochester and Warsaw group F studies (field survey). This is close to Gastaut's series but very different from that of Bogota and Tonbridge. The percentage of temporal lobe epilepsy is a great deal higher in the Warsaw group F and Gastaut than in the Rochester and Tonbridge series. The difference in the frequency of partial seizures between Warsaw groups K and F is due to patients with complex partial seizures without secondarily generalization: 12% in group F and 4% in group K, p <0.01. Secondarily generalized temporal lobe seizures at 30% were equally frequent in each group. This shows that some types of seizures, particularly those which do not develop into the tonic–clonic variety, are either ignored by patients or are considered a natural phenomenon of rather minor importance. Most patients do not feel that such problems need medical treatment.

Frequency of chronic institutionalized cases of epilepsy

The percentage of chronic in-patients with epilepsy in mental hospitals and long-stay care

Table 2.4 Relative frequency of generalized and partial seizures in case-series of epileptic patients found during selected epidemiological studies (percentage)

Type of seizure	Rochester[a] (1960)	Warsaw[b] Known cases	Field survey	Bogota[c]	Large epileptic out-patient population (non-epidemiological study)[d]	Tonbridge England patients of a general practice[e],[*]
Generalized	34	48	35	73	38	64
Partial	66	52	65	27	62	29
Including temporal lobe	27	34	43		40	28

a Hauser & Kurland 1975
b Zielinski 1974a
c Gomez et al 1978
d Gastaut et al 1975
e Goodridge & Shorvon 1983
* 'No details' available in 7% of cases

institutions in Poland has been estimated at 3% of all patients with epilepsy known to the medical services. In all these cases, severe mental and/or neurological handicap seemed to be responsible for institutionalization (Zielinski 1972, Zielinski et al 1973). This agrees with Pond & Burden (1963) and Janz (1972) in their estimates for Great Britain and the Federal Republic of Germany. In the USA, the Commission for the Control of Epilepsy (1978) estimates that 5.5% of known cases of epilepsy remain in various long-term facilities and that another 4.8% need such care. The recent trend toward placement of these patients in the community could significantly change the above proportions.

Time trends

Time trends for incidence and prevalence rates have only been given in one study, that of Rochester which covers 40 years. The average annual incidence rates calculated since 1935 for three 10-year periods and for the final three-year period 1965–1967 showed a substantial increase from 35 per 100 000 in 1935–1944 to 54 per 100 000 during the next two periods. In the last three years, however, the rate dropped down to 46. These changes were seen most dramatically for the rates during the first year of life: 111, to 250 and 138 with a drop to 73. Prevalence rates estimated on 1 January of the years 1940, 1950, 1960 and 1970 showed less variation at 3.7, 5.3, 6.2 and 5.7 per 1000 (Hauser & Kurland 1975). Recently Hauser et al (1977) found a further fall in the

annual incidence rate in Rochester during the period 1965–1974 to 33 per 100 000. The fall was particularly marked in the young and was thought to be due to starting treatment more often after a single seizure. This hypothesis should be carefully tested. On the other hand, it should be stressed that the same authors also established a decrease in the incidence rates of single seizures. This might be due to various factors including better pre- and perinatal obstetric care with more effective prevention of brain infections of trauma.

SOCIO-ECONOMIC STATUS

Socio-economic factors, if discussed in epidemiologic or clinical surveys, are usually considered as dependent variables. Only a few authors have considered these factors as independent, i.e. risk factors in the development of a mental and/or neurological disorder (Weissman & Klerman 1978). It might be of interest that low socio-economic status was found to be associated with an increased risk of anencephaly and spina bifida in newborns in Boston hospitals (Naggan & McMahon 1967). National Health Survey (1973) in the US investigated selected chronic conditions. It has shown that epilepsy, diabetes and especially anaemia were reported more often by non-whites and in families with the lowest income level independent of ethnic origin. It is noteworthy that almost 40% of individuals reporting epilepsy were not seen by a doctor during the year preceding the interview. This finding is consistent with the results of Anderson (1936) in the USA, Gudmundsson (1966) in Iceland and Zielinski (1976) in Poland. Another indirect index suggesting a higher prevalence of epilepsy among poor and non-white people was derived from studies on prisoners in Chicago (Whitman et al 1984).

Low socio-economic status can also be responsible for the more severe course of epilepsy. Among patients seen at the Epilepsy Center of Michigan (ECM), only 23% are considered to suffer from 'uncomplicated epilepsy' (Rodin et al 1977). This relatively low percentage of people whose major problem constitutes only epileptic seizures may be attributed, at least in part, to the fact that the ECM patients come primarily from lower socio-economic classes and a considerable proportion of them is unemployed (Zielinski & Rader 1984). The same situation probably applies to case-series seen in various university departments and clinics.

The only population-orientated study on epilepsy that considers race and socio-economic level as the independent variables was conducted in the United States by Shamansky & Glaser (1979) in the New Haven area. The authors reviewed the files of two major EEG laboratories, believing that their case ascertainment bias was minimal. All basic data on children up to 14 years of age referred for routine EEG because of the occurrence of a seizure (or seizures), were derived from routine EEG requisitions and reports. The cases were then classified into three categories: 'definite epilepsy' (557 cases), 'probable epilepsy' (123 cases) and 'neonatal seizures' (53 cases). The last category included cases of perinatal hypoxia, infections and transient biochemical disorders. These three categories were not analysed separately and therefore the authors accepted 'cumulative incidence rates' as a measure of prevalence. Average annual incidence rates were calculated for age, sex and race groups. All in all, rates were higher for blacks than for whites. In both racial groups, rates were lower for females (14.3–15.3 per 1000 in blacks and 8.9–9.3 in whites) than in males (13.2–23.6 and 8.0–10.9, respectively). Among children referred for EEG because of seizures, the authors found an excess of those from lower socio-economic areas. This conclusion, however, does not seem to be sufficiently substan-

tiated. On the other hand, the survey strongly points to the urgent need for further and more detailed studies on socio-economic status as a possible risk factor for epilepsy.

PROGNOSIS

There are numerous studies in the world literature devoted to prognosis in epilepsy. The majority of them, however, are based on shorter or longer follow-ups of selected case-series and therefore the conclusions usually cannot be extrapolated to all the people with epilepsy in a population at large. Neuro-epidemiologists would preferably consider the results of relatively less biased population-orientated studies. Unfortunately, only a few of the latter have been published, most of them within the past decade

There are two indices which can measure two opposite, extreme directions of developments in the natural history of epilepsy: the fraction of people with epilepsy who became seizure-free over a long period (remission rates) and the fraction of those who died (mortality rates). In this chapter only results of population-based studies will be reviewed and discussed.

Remission and relapse rates

The overall prognosis as estimated from relatively unselected, population-based studies on seizure disorder is definitely better than that expected from review of selected case-series. Ellenberg & Nelson (1980), in an extensive review of the world literature on prognosis of febrile fits, have shown that the percentage of children who develop epilepsy after one or more febrile seizures varies from 1.5% to 4.6% (mode–3%) in community-orientated studies; whereas in clinical case-series this percentage varies from 2.6 to 76.9. A review of remission rates in epilepsy, based on studies in hospital and institutional patients and those from two community-orientated studies (including his own), was recently presented by Shorvon (1984).

In the Rochester series (Annegers et al 1979), among 618 patients diagnosed between 1935 and 1974, 93 died within five years of diagnosis and another 50 in under than five years. In 18 cases, information was incomplete and thus final estimates are based on 475 cases, 328 of whom were followed for at least 10 years, and 141 for at least 20 years after diagnosis. Death without remission was treated as withdrawal from observation, and results were based only on patients who survived at 10 or 20 years' follow-up. The total percentage of epileptic individuals seizure-free for at least two years at follow-up are similar in three population-orientated studies – the Warsaw field survey, Rochester and Greater Aarhus – at about 40% (Table 2.5). Only in Tonbridge is this percentage significantly higher. Among 'known cases' in Warsaw, the percentage of patients with remission is relatively low. At least a two-year remission by seizure type is quite similar in the first three studies: probability of remission is lowest for complex partial seizures and relatively highest for 'petit mal' seizures. The follow-up of known cases and people with epilepsy identified during the field survey in Warsaw has yielded more optimistic results: five years after initial examination, 38% in group K and 63% in group F appeared seizure-free for at least two years (Zielinski et al 1978). Remission and relapse rates in the Rochester series (Annegers et al 1979) appear similarly optimistic (Table 2.6). Some 20 years after diagnosis, almost half the patients with idiopathic

Table 2.6 Prognosis in 457 epileptic residents of Rochester, Minnesota. Percentage of patients seizure-free and without medication for at least 5 years at the time of follow-up by etiology of epilepsy (Annegers et al 1979)

| | % of remissions by etiology of epilepsy | | |
| | Idiopathic | Secondary | |
Follow-up period	no known etiological factor	brain lesions acquired post-natally	gross neurological deficit or IQ below 70 (pre- or perinatal brain injury)
10 years	36	18*	14*
20 years	47	54	30

* Approximate percentage

epilepsy became seizure-free for at least five years. For patients with 'secondary epilepsy' (brain trauma, tumour, stroke, i.e. brain injury acquired postnatally), the prognosis is even better. This may be due to marked 'polarization' of the natural course of epilepsy in this group (successfully treated underlying CNS disorder or death). This hypothesis may be supported by a rather poor prognosis in this type of epilepsy at 10-year follow-up (twice as poor as in idiopathic epilepsy). The worst prognosis was encountered in patients with underlying, permanent brain injury acquired very early in life (pre- or perinatal injury to the brain). Nevertheless, even in this group, some

Table 2.5 Prognosis in epileptic residents of Warsaw, Aarhus and Tonbridge by type of seizures

| | Warsaw[a] | | Rochester[b]* | Aarhus[c] | Tonbridge[d] |
| | Known cases | Field survey | | | |
No of cases	313	98	516	1024	100
Patients seizure-free for at least 2 years at follow-up (%)					
Total	26	42	40*	44	68
By seizure type (%)					
Tonic–clonic prim. general.	31	70	44	47	71 ('generalized')
Absence	47	100	55	52	
Partial simple	67	50	24	43	
Partial complex	25	8	41	28	64 ('partial or mixed')
Partial secondarily generalized	19	36	—	49	

a Zielinski 1974a
b Hauser & Kurland 1975
c Juul-Jensen & Foldspang 1983
d Goodridge & Shorvon 1983
* approximate figure

30% of patients have a chance of achieving a remission status at 20 years after diagnosis. In epilepsy of unknown etiology, the prognosis is the best for patients with tonic–clonic seizures: 20 years after diagnosis, half of them remained seizure-free and without antiepileptic drugs (AEDs) for over five years. Prognosis is worse for complex partial seizures, especially after 20 years and without AEDs (Table 2.7). One of the most important findings in the Rochester study is that most patients became seizure-free during the first 5–10 years period after diagnosis. Those still suffering from seizures some 10 to 15 years after diagnosis have a minimal chance of achieving seizure-free status later. Similar results come from the Tonbridge study: 40% of patients entered a two-year seizure-free status shortly after the onset of seizures. Five years later only 21% of those still having seizures achieve a two-year remission compared to 96% of those who were already in remission at that time. Thus, both studies have shown that soon after the onset of seizures the natural course of epilepsy has a tendency toward a 'benign' or 'malignant' spectrum. This polarization can be one of the most potent factors in the

formation of various groups of people with epilepsy. Among these with a 'benign' natural course of the disorder, one can find many untreated and even undiagnosed cases (Zielinski 1974a, 1976), whereas those with poorly controlled epilepsy will form a majority in selected case-series, particularly in special epilepsy centres, university hospitals or institutions (Zielinski 1976, Juul-Jensen & Foldspang 1983, Shorvon 1984). Moreover, it is worth emphasizing that in the Warsaw study, patients who were free of seizures for a long time were unwilling to give information at the follow-up and not infrequently refused to undergo any medical examination. They considered themselves cured and often stated that they did not want to be reminded of their past illness (Zielinski et al 1978). This is yet another factor which contributes to formation of case-series in various medical sources, including the Aarhus epilepsy register (Juul-Jensen & Foldspang 1983).

Actually an observation regarding the various courses of epilepsy in particular cases was made some 24 centuries ago by Hippocrates. He wrote: 'It was of great importance to treat patient before disease [epilepsy] had become chronic . . . inveterate cases are incurable . . .' (cited in Temkin 1971). This statement does not seem to be based on results of treatment, the effectiveness of which would be doubtful, and Hippocrates himself had never disclosed what substances he was using as antiepileptic drugs.

The hypothesis regarding early polarization in the course of epilepsy is also supported by findings on patterns of treatment of people with epilepsy (Table 2.8). In the Warsaw study, the percentage of remissions is the lowest among patients who remain on AEDs at the time of

Table 2.7 Prognosis in 457 epileptic residents of Rochester, Minnesota. Percentage of patients with idiopathic epilepsy seizure-free for at least 5 years at the time of follow-up by type of seizures and medication (Annegers et al 1979)

Follow-up period		Tonic-clonic	Absences	Partial complex
		% of remissions by type of seizures and treatment over last 5 years		
10 years	Total	70	68	63
	No med.	40	38	28
20 years	Total	85	78	65
	No med.	53	60	35

Table 2.8 Prognosis in epilepsy by pattern of medication on follow-up

Medication	*% seizure-free*					
	Warsaw (at least 5 yrs) Known cases N = 100%	%	Field survey N = 100%	%	Tonbridge (at least 2 yrs) N = 100%	%
Never	7	29	36	37	11	55
AEDs discontinued	66	23	28	46	45	80
On AEDs	239	6	34	3	44	59

examination. Thus, patients on AEDs with recurring seizures are most prevalent among 'known' epilepsy case-series. Contrary to that, the majority of people with epilepsy found during the field survey did not take AEDs. Over a third of them had never previously taken AEDs. In Tonbridge, 11% were never treated and 56% did not take AEDs at the time of review. In both the Warsaw and Tonbridge studies, the frequency of two-year remissions was highest among patients in whom AEDs were discontinued, although a significant percentage of those never treated achieved at least a two-year remission.

If one assumes that those never treated form a 'naturally selected' control group, then the above findings may be of importance for interpreting results of medical treatment in newly diagnosed cases of epilepsy. Obviously, the disappearance of seizures may well be due not only to the direct effect of AEDs but also to a natural course of the disorder in an individual. These findings are strongly supportive of the modern approach toward initiation of antiepileptic treatment (see Chapter 12). Finally, they also may be helpful while making a decision about discontinuation of AEDs in cases with long-lasting remission and previously benign course of epilepsy.

The role of epidemiology in the design of clinical trials of anticonvulsants has been extensively reviewed by Hauser (1982).

Discontinuation of AEDs has been thought to increase significantly the patient's risk of relapse, even after achieving a long-term remission. Again, the frequency of relapses is estimated as being higher in selected case-series than in population-orientated studies. During a five-year follow-up of two representative groups of people with epilepsy in Warsaw, recurrence of seizures after at least a two-year remission was noted in 5% among 'known epilepsy' cases and in 3% among those found in the sample of the Warsaw population. The proportion of those who entered remission at the same time was 20% and 26% respectively. Thus, the fraction of those relapsing is four to five times lower than those entering remission (Zielinski et al 1978). In the Rochester study the probability of relapse in the first year after entering remission status is 8%, while by the 20-year follow-up it is 24% (Annegers et al 1979).

The probability of relapse increases with advanced age at diagnosis and for complex partial seizures. In the Tonbridge survey, the proportion of those who achieved remission and then relapsed is lowest at 10% (Shorvon 1984). This seems to be due to a relatively high percentage of cases with benign course of epilepsy among patients studied. Half the subjects were in two-year remission within five years of the onset of seizures (single seizure occurred in 19% of the subjects studied) and 68% of cases had suffered from fewer than 10 seizures altogether.

Early 'polarization' in the natural course of epilepsy has many important clinical implications. In trials of new antiepileptic drugs, patients with recently diagnosed epilepsy and a short history of seizures should not be combined with those who have had epilepsy for years; otherwise, a bias due to case-series selection secondary to the natural course of epilepsy can significantly distort conclusions from the study.

Mortality rates for epilepsy

Studies on mortality and the causes of death are usually based on death certificates and special analyses of selected groups of patients. Some of the methodological difficulties have been discussed already. There is also a difference between the terms 'death due to epilepsy' and 'death of a person with epilepsy'. Even if a patient dies in status epilepticus, then death is not necessarily due to epilepsy, since in many cases status epilepticus can be the first seizure resulting from acute intracranial haemorrhage, trauma, brain tumour, etc. However, in cases of symptomatic epilepsy, the death certificates more often will state the diagnosis of the underlying condition, e.g. head injury or brain tumour. Furthermore, in cases of non-active epilepsy it is unlikely that the diagnosis of seizure disorder will appear on the certificates. On the other hand, even if death is due directly to epilepsy, as from an accident during a seizure, the diagnosis of epilepsy will not appear if the certifying doctor does not happen to know that the victim suffered from epilepsy. Thus, the broader and less specific category 'death of a person with epilepsy' cannot be estimated accurately from an analysis of death certificates.

Mortality statistics based on death certificates

Although only a fraction of all people with epilepsy who die can be identified through death certificates, routine mortality statistics are the only ready source of data with which to compare deaths due to epilepsy in different countries and at different times. Figure 2.2 shows age-adjusted annual death rates for epilepsy in different, mainly European countries. In two-thirds of the selected countries the rates were between 1.1 and 2.0 per 100 000. The rank order of the countries with the highest rates was virtually the same in the years 1951 to 1958 (Goldberg & Kurland 1962) as in the years 1974 to 1976. The differences between countries might result from local methods of filling in death certificates. This hypothesis would be supported by the fact that the countries with the highest rates were also those in which epilepsy was most often certified as the underlying cause of death. This ratio varies between 1.0 and 2.0 per 1000 deaths, except in Chile and Colombia where it is 3.0 and over. It may be noted that recent epidemiological surveys in these countries have shown high prevalence rates for epilepsy (Gomez et al 1978, Chiofale et al 1979), and epilepsy may indeed be a more frequent underlying cause of death. In the USA, the annual death rates for epilepsy tended to decline from 1939 to 1967, whereas in Poland they remained fairly stable between 1960 and 1975 (Kurtzke 1972, Zielinski 1978).

Sex and age-specific death rates

In most countries the death rates are higher for males than for females. Age-specific rates are usually high in the first year of life, and then stay low until they rise again in the fifth and sixth decades.

Death rates according to race, marital status and domicile

A detailed analysis of deaths from epilepsy in the USA (Kurtzke 1972, Kurtzke et al 1973) reveals that the rates are significantly higher for non-whites. This applies particularly to males, for whom the rates are three times as high as those for whites, and five or more times as high between the ages of 25 and 55. This may be due either to fatal cases of epilepsy being more common or a greater chance of epilepsy being listed on the death certificate of a non-white person.

Death rates are significantly higher for single than married persons. Kurtze considers that this reflects a more regular life with more reliable taking of medication among married people with a lesser risk of head injury and alcoholism. However, it seems more probable that factors which have an unfavourable influence on prognosis in epilepsy, like neurological deficit, mental changes, frequent and uncontrollable seizures etc, also tend to lessen a person's chance of getting married.

Some studies, including those conducted in

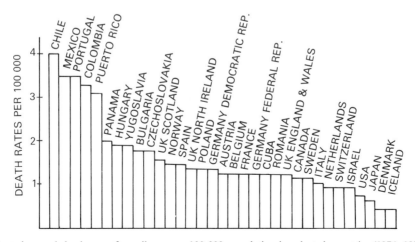

Fig. 2.2 Age-adjusted annual death rates for epilepsy per 100 000 population in selected countries (1974–1976)

Poland, claim that death rates for epilepsy are higher in rural than in urban areas.

Special studies on mortality and survivorship in epilepsy

There are very few studies founded on observation of large and relatively unselected groups of patients. Henriksen et al (1967) carried out a follow-up of Danish epileptic patients aged between 15 and 59, the majority being examined in neurological departments. Those with epilepsy due to tumours or cerebrovascular malformations were excluded. The authors believed that milder cases were only slightly under-represented although they did not try to prove this. Holders of a life insurance policy acted as controls. They found standardized mortality ratios (SMR) for all epileptic patients to be 2.9 for males and 2.2 for females. Excess of deaths was noted particularly in the fourth and fifth decades. If cases with more frequent seizures were excluded, SMR fell to 2.0.

Hauser & Kurland (1975) carried out an analysis of all deaths among Rochester residents with epilepsy followed up to 20 years after the diagnosis was made. These authors claimed that the 'survivorship ratio' – the ratio of survivals among patients to survival among matched controls – seemed to be more useful than the 'mortality ratio' – the ratio of deaths between the two groups. The survivorship ratio for epileptic patients in Rochester was 91% at 5 years, 85% at 10 years and 83% at 15 years after diagnosis. Thus, the greatest difference between the groups occurred during the first few years after the diagnosis. Thereafter the rate of decline of the survivorship is much the same, although the survival curve for the patients is of course lower. The survivorship ratio is better for females and worse for those diagnosed during the first year of life or aged between 20 and 59. It is lower in patients with epilepsy of suspected etiology than in those of unknown origin. No significant difference was found in the ratios for partial and primary generalized epilepsy.

During the Warsaw survey (Zielinski 1974b) an attempt was made to analyse mortality in epileptic patients known to the medical services. Total deaths (TD) during the period of study were 218.

If symptomatic cases with brain tumours or cerebrovascular malformations were excluded – the same criteria as were used by Henriksen et al (1967) – a subgroup (A) had 120 deaths. Only 10% of deaths were of patients within the first three decades, whereas 50% were of patients aged over 60. The average age at death in group TD was 55 years, contrasted with 47 years in group A. For the last year of the study the annual standardized mortality ratio – (i.e. proportion of observed to expected number of deaths) in known epileptic patients reached almost 1.6%. While the total SMR among patients was only 1.8, for those who died before the age of 50 the ratio was as high as 3.5. This would support the hypothesis that younger epileptic patients particularly run a greater than expected risk of death (Table 2.9).

A more recently published analysis of deaths in Rochester cohort (Hauser et al 1980) is based on up to 30 years' follow-up of 618 residents with epilepsy, in addition to 666 children with history of febrile fits and 159 individuals who suffered from a single 'idiopathic' seizure. Standardized mortality ratios are shown in Table 2.10. For all epilepsy cases, the SMR is 2.3: the highest excess of deaths among patients occurred during the first two years after diagnosis, declined subsequently and again became significantly elevated during the last decade of follow-up. A similar trend was noted in cases of idiopathic epilepsy for which SMRs were relatively low. In patients with neurological and/or mental handicap present at birth, SMR showed the highest values, especially over the first five years after diagnosis. Among cases of 'secondary epilepsy' (i.e. due to postnatal brain injury – brain tumour, trauma, cerebrovascular disorder, etc) the SMRs were again the highest in the first two years of follow-up. These findings are consistent with the results of an earlier study dicussed above (Hauser & Kurland 1975). As regards cases with a history of febrile convulsions, 25 patients with underlying permanent neurological disorder were excluded from analysis. Among the remaining cases only four died and the SMR was about 0.7. In other words, no increased mortality has been found in these patients. On the other hand, among 159 cases with a history of a single seizure, the SMR was 2.3 and most of the excess deaths occurred in the first two years after

Table 2.9 Age and sex-specific standardized mortality ratios (SMR) for patients with epilepsy in Warsaw and Rochester

	Standardized mortality ratios			
Age group	Warsaw study (TD)*			Rochester study**
	Males	Females	Total	Total – all cases
0–29	2.5	5.0	3.5	
0–24				8.5
25–44				7.7
30–49	3.6	2.7	3.4	
45–54				3.5
50–59	2.7	1.8	2.5	
55–64				3.0
60–69	1.8	1.5	1.8	
65–74				1.5
70 & over	1.5	1.4	1.5	
75 & over				1.4
Total (TD)	2.0	1.4	1.8	2.3

* TD – total deaths (Zielinski 1974a)
** Hauser et al 1980

Table 2.10 Standardized mortality ratios for patients with epilepsy in the Rochester Study, 1935–74 by etiology of epilepsy and follow-up period (Hauser et al 1980)

	Standardized mortality ratios (observed/expected deaths) by etiology			
Years of follow-up	Total	Idiopathic	Neuro-deficit since birth	Postnatally acquired secondary epilepsy
0–1	3.8	2.5	20.0	4.3
2–4	2.4	1.7	33.3	2.0
5–9	2.0	2.4	2.0	1.6
10–19	1.4	1.1	6.7	1.1
20–29	2.4	2.0	10.0	3.3
Total	2.3	1.8	11.0	2.2

diagnosis. Interestingly enough, among a total of 26 deaths seven were due to neoplasm other than of the brain and no secondary brain lesion was found. As regards seizure type, relatively high SMRs were found for patients suffering from idiopathic, generalized tonic-clonic seizures: 3.5 during the first five years after diagnosis and 2.4 in total. For patients with complex partial seizures (with or without tonic-clonic seizures) excess of deaths was relatively low (SMR 1.5). This difference may be due to various ages of onset. Moreover, among 45 patients with only absence seizures no deaths were noted.

Another interesting but rather pessimistic finding from the Rochester series is that of signifi-cantly elevated SMR in patients in remission (seizure-free for at least five years): 2.0 during the first five years after entering remission. Later there was no excess of deaths and the total SMR for this group was 1.4.

Age-specific SMRs in both the Rochester and Warsaw studies have shown similar trends with the most significant excess of deaths in younger age groups. This tends to decline gradually with age, especially from the fifth decade of life (Table 2.9). SMRs for males are higher than for females both in the Warsaw and Rochester studies: in the latter the SMR for males with idiopathic epilepsy was 2.1 and for females 1.6. It is worth mentioning, however, that in the Warsaw study

SMR is higher for females in the younger age groups. No convincing explanation can be offered about this finding.

Causes of death in epileptic patients

There is a number of papers on causes of death among epileptic out- and, more especially, in-patients. Unfortunately, most of the groups are highly selected. In the highly selected group of patients, including those in mental hospitals and institutions, there were very high percentages of deaths from status epilepticus and pneumonia (Krohn 1963, Neploch 1965, Penning et al 1969, Iivanainen & Lehtinen 1979). Interestingly enough, in the series of the latter authors, chronic intoxication with phenytoin and/or phenobarbitone was a common supplementary factor in patients who died of pneumonia or seizures. This finding significantly contributes to the current discussion on chronic toxicity of antiepileptic drugs.

During the Warsaw survey (Table 2.11), the cause of death in each case was reviewed in the light of information from all available sources, including death certificates, medical and police records, and interviews with the family and general practitioners. Comparable data was obtained on the causes of death for 97 chronic epileptic patients from one of Poland's mental hospitals (Kahl-Kunstetter & Zielinski 1972). It will be seen that in the whole group of 218 (TD) heart disease and brain tumour were the commonest causes of death, with epilepsy coming third. In four out of the nine accidents not related to seizures there was a high blood alcohol level. The miscellaneous causes include 27 strokes and seven acute alcoholic deaths in patients who before death presented severe behavioural problems due to an organic brain syndrome. In group A, epilepsy followed by suicide were the two most common causes of death. In the Rochester series, Hauser & Kurland (1975) found that, apart from an excess due to brain tumour, the rank order by cause of death among Rochester patients with epilepsy was the same as for the general population. More recently, Hauser et al (1980), analysing causes of deaths among patients who died in 29 years' follow-up, found that the highest excess of deaths can be attributed to non-cerebral aneurysm of embolism (SMR 7.1): this cause of death has been encountered in a relatively low percentage of deaths. The most frequent causes of death were: heart diseases (20% of deaths), neoplasms other than of brain (13%) and cerebrovascular lesions (17.3%). SMRs for deaths attributed to these causes were 1.1, 1.8 and 2.6 respectively. Surprisingly, deaths due to epilepsy

Table 2.11 Verified causes of death in epileptic patients known to Warsaw medical services, and in chronic mental hospital patients with epilepsy (percentage; N = 100%)

	% of patients		
	Warsaw known cases		Mental hospital
	Total TD	Group A (symptomatic epilepsy excluded)	MH
Cause of death	N = 218	N = 120	N = 97
Status epilepticus	3.2	5.8	17.5
Death during or after seizure	3.2	5.8	2.1
Sudden unexplained death	4.2	7.5	1.0
Fatal accident due to seizure	3.2	5.0	0
Epilepsy, subtotal	13.8	24.1	20.6
Brain tumour	15.1	0	5.2
Heart disease	16.1	8.3	19.6
Tumour not involving brain	8.7	11.7	2.0
Pneumonia	7.8	9.2	24.7
Suicide	7.3	11.7	3.1
Accident not due to seizure	4.1	7.5	0
Miscellaneous	27.1	27.5	24.8

Table 2.12 Causes of death of epileptic patients – four studies (percentage)

Cause of death	Henriksen et al 1967 Denmark (age 15–59)*	Haltrich (cited by Janz 1969*	Zielinski 1974a (Group A)* Warsaw, Poland	Hauser† et al 1980 Rochester, USA
Status epilepticus	—	10	6	—
Sudden death	—	6	13	—
Accident due to seizure	—	8	5	—
Epilepsy total	26	24	24	3
Suicide	22	10	12	1
Accident not due to seizure	11	3	7	6**
Heart disease	11	9	8	20
Neoplasm*	6	10	12	13
Miscellaneous	17	18	27	29
Not specified	—	—	—	20

* Brain tumours excluded
† Percentage calculated by this author (JJZ): 8% deaths of brain tumours not included
** Relation to seizure not specified

and suicide have been much less frequent than in the Warsaw study and other series reported (Table 2.11 and 2.12). Moreover, deaths due to accidents are not differentiated according to their association with seizures. Finally, in 20% of deaths, the cause has not been specified. Because the authors did not explain the sources from which cause of death was established, it is difficult to compare directly their results to results of the Warsaw study. It should also be pointed out that attempts toward identifying the actual cause of death in every case were far more complete in the Warsaw survey than in any other study yet reported in the world literature.

Annegers et al (1984) confirmed the Rochester findings that no excess of deaths was attributed to heart disease. Sudden cardiac death was significantly increased, but his was primarily limited to those with epilepsy resulting from cerebrovascular disorders.

Because in the Warsaw study group A was selected according to the same criteria as Henricksen's series, and, with the exception of vascular malformations, to Haltrich's (after Janz 1969), the results of the three studies are shown (Table 2.12) along with data from recent Rochester study. The mortality rates for different causes, and particularly for epilepsy, are very similar in the first three series. It would seem, therefore, that the first three studies reviewed

similar epilepsy case-series in which, as in the Warsaw group of 'known' cases, milder cases were greatly under-represented.

Suicides accounted for about 10% of deaths in Poland and West Germany but for twice as many in Denmark. Contrary to these findings, observed frequency of suicide among Rochester patients does not exceed that expected for the total population and counts for around 2% of deaths. In Poland, suicides in epileptic males were five times as high as in the general population and for females twice as high. This excess was particularly marked in group A patients and in the younger age groups. It should be remembered that the frequency of attempted suicide in the general population is highest in the young, and yet among such cases only 2.5% of males and 0.7% of females were diagnosed as having epilepsy (Kostrzewa et al 1972). An extensive review of the literature on suicide in epilepsy has been published by Matthews & Barabas (1981). Robertson & Trimble (1983) have pointed out that the frequencies of both depression and suicides among people with epilepsy are excessive, and thus an increased incidence of suicides can be related to a higher frequency of depressive reactions.

In reviewing the most frequent causes of death among the people with epilepsy, one can ask how often death could be prevented. This question is very important since there is an excess of deaths in younger age groups. Prevention of deaths from epilepsy is associated with early diagnosis and more effective medical treatment. In a series of sudden deaths of 27 children with diagnosed epilepsy treated with phenobarbitone and phenytoin, on autopsy 20 had none or very low serum levels of the medications (Neuspiel & Kuller 1985). On the other hand, fatal status epilepticus can be the first seizure that a person experiences. It is not always possible to prevent the occurrence of accidents associated with epileptic seizures. A relatively high incidence of deaths due to accidents (in the Rochester series SMR = 2.4) raises the question about the extent to which mentally deteriorating side-effects of sedative antiepileptic drugs can contribute to this phenomenon. In addition, the possibility of a carcinogenic action of antiepileptic drugs has been considered, but this association has not yet been substantiated. One of the most preventable causes of death among people with epilepsy is suicide, if the possibility of depression associated with epilepsy is kept in mind. Finally, the high frequency of fatal alcohol abuse should also be considered in the daily management of patients with epilepsy.

Frequency of the diagnosis of epilepsy on death certificates

During the Warsaw study it was found that epilepsy as the underlying cause of death or as an associated condition appeared on 63 (29%) of the 218 certificates of people who for one to four years before their death had attended doctors because of epilepsy.

The data in Tables 2.13 and 2.14 illustrate the probability of finding the diagnosis of epilepsy on death certificates according to where the patient died and the underlying cause of death. It will be seen that these factors influence significantly the estimates of routinely calculated death rates for epilepsy. For instance, the annual mortality rate for known epilepsy in Warsaw in 1969 was 7.8 per 100 000. When the rate was calculated on the basis of death certificates reporting epilepsy as a diagnosis, it dropped to 2.4 and, when based only on death certificates in which epilepsy is given as the underlying cause of death, it fell as low as 1.0 per 100 000, a figure comparable to the epilepsy

Table 2.13 Place of death and diagnosis of epilepsy as underlying or associated disease) in death certificates of 218 epileptic patients*

Place of death	No. of deaths (= 100%)†*	% of death certificates containing diagnosis of epilepsy
Neurological or neurosurgical department	59	37.3
Mental hospital	16	75.0
Other hospital departments	46	15.2
Other places	16	43.8
Total	218	28.9

* From Zielinski 1974b
† In this table as in Table 2.14 the percentage in the right hand column relates to the number in the middle column, e.g. of the 59 patients who died in neurological or neurosurgical departments, 22 or 37.3% had a death certificate containing the diagnosis of epilepsy.

Table 2.14 Verified cause of death and diagnosis of epilepsy (as underlying of associated disease) in death certificates of 218 epileptic patients*

Cause of death(re-evaluated) verified	No. of deaths (= 100%)	% of death certificates containing the diagnosis of epilepsy
Epilepsy	23	73.9
Accident due to seizure	7	42.8
Epilepsy, subtotal	30	66.6
Heart disease	35	28.6
Brain tumour	33	39.4
Stroke	27	14.8
Tumour not involving brain	19	10.5
Pneumonia	19	52.6
Suicide	16	6.3
Accident not due to seizure	9	0
Miscellaneous	30	10.0
Total	218	28.9

* Zielinski 1974b

mortality rate estimated for US population (Kurtzke et al 1973).

Finally, it should be mentioned that, in the Rochester study, the diagnosis of epilepsy was mentioned in less than 10% of death certificates. On the other hand, epilepsy or seizures were recorded on death certificates of five Rochester residents who had no history of epilepsy (Hauser et al 1980). Thus, death certificates are easily obtainable but are an unreliable source of information on both epilepsy mortality and causes of death.

THE NATURE OF POPULATIONS OF PEOPLE WITH EPILEPSY

Because patients conceal their epilepsy and because others ignore certain types of seizures, even the most sophisticated field survey methods are bound to miss some patients. It may be assumed that most of these will be the milder cases. According to the Warsaw study, the variable 'under medication at the time of the examination' correlated highly with frequent major convulsions and lack of remission, as well as with neurological and psychiatric evidence of brain damage. These variables also correlated highly with each other, as well as with variables such as low socio-economic status as evidenced by a low level of education, lack of professional qualifications and a poor work record. It is obvious that this group, which requires special medical and social care, will be over-represented among the population known to the medical and social services as contrasted with their representation in the epileptic population found in a general survey. This must be remembered when trying to generalize from the results of studies on selected case-series. On the other hand, an epidemiological study based on medical records would be likely to give a relatively accurate estimate of the size of the epileptic population which needs special medical and social care.

Personal situation 1
M. S., a 32-year-old female, at questionnaire responded to the question: 'Have you had a feeling of momentary absent-mindedness?' On this basis, two out of three experts rate her as 'slightly suspect of having epilepsy'.

She was the second of a twin delivery and heard from her mother that she was cyanosed at birth and did not breathe spontaneously. Her later physical and intellectual development was normal and after leaving secondary school she worked as a teller. She married and had one healthy child.

Since the age of 20 she has experienced episodes of momentary loss of consciousness, sometimes preceded by brief dizziness. She has never collapsed but occasionally she would drop some object she was holding. Automatic movements of varying complexity had been noticed. After the attack she usually felt slightly confused. She was aware that she had had a blackout. These paroxysmal episodes were always the same and appeared for no apparent reason. They occurred about once a month and they had been less frequent in the year before the interview. She did not think that her symptoms were due to any disease and observed: 'I imagine anyone may feel like that at times'.

No abnormalities were found on neurological or psychiatric examination, and her IQ on the WAIS was 100. On her EEG slow waves at 5 to 6 Hz were seen over both temporal areas and on overbreathing paroxysmal discharges of sharp waves appeared over the same areas with a tendency to generalization.

About five years later, on a follow-up examination, it was found that she had been free of attacks for three years. The patient was never treated for her fits and had refused such an opportunity when she had been first examined

Personal situation 2
J. C. was a 13-year-old secondary school boy. At questionnaire his mother affirmed 'episodes of sudden loss of consciousness' and 'convulsions'. She said that her son had had a single febrile convulsion at the age of four and that since then he had been in good health although he had had infrequent headaches and some difficulties at school. However, there had been no behavioural problems.

On neurological examination the boy admitted that at least once a month he experienced a momentary feeling of confusion when he could not understand what people were talking about and that he was then briefly unconscious. He could not remember for how long he had had these attacks. He thought that they were quite natural and they did not worry him. He never told his mother or anyone else about them. He himself did not know about the febrile convulsion he had had when he was young. Neurological examination was normal. Psychiatric testing showed some evidence of immaturity although his intelligence was normal. His EEG series showed sharp waves and high amplitude theta activity over the right temporal area.

He refused both treatment and further examination. On follow-up five years later, the only information which could be obtained was that he had had no blackouts during the previous two years.

REFERENCES

Alter M, Macland R L, Kurtzke J F et al 1972 Proposed definitions and classifications of epilepsy for epidemiological purposes. In: Hauser W A, Alter M (eds) The epidemiology of epilepsy: a workshop. NINDS Monograph No 14, Washington DC, DHEW, pp 147–148

Anderson C L 1936 Epilepsy in the State of Michigan. Mental Hygiene 20: 441–462

Annegers J F, Hauser W A, Elveback L R 1979 Remission of seizures and relapse in patients with epilepsy. Epilepsia 20: 729–737

Annegers J F, Grabow J D, Groover R V, Laws E R,

Elvesback L R, Kurland L T 1980 Seizures after head trauma: a population study. Neurology 30: 683–689

Annegers J F, Hauser W A, Shirts S B 1984 Heart disease mortality and morbidity in patients with epilepsy. Epilepsia 25: 699–704

Berkson J 1946 Limitations of the application of fourfold table analysis to hospital data. Biomet. Bull. 2: 47–53

Bird A V, Heinz H J, Klintworth G 1962 Convulsive disorders in Bantu mine workers. Epilepsia 3: 175–187

Brewis M, Poskanzer D, Rolland C, Miller H 1966 Neurological disease in an English city. Acta Neurologica Scandinavica 42 (suppl 24): pp 9–89

Bongers E, Coppoolse J, Meinardi H, Posthuma E P S, VanZijl C H W 1986 A survey of epilepsy in Zeeland, the Netherlands. Heemstede Instituut voor Epilepsiebestrijding, Meer en Bosch

Chiofalo N, Kirschbaum A, Fuantes A, Cordero M L, Madsen J 1979 Prevalence of epilepsy in children of Melipilla, Chile. Epilepsia 20: 262–266

Commission for the Control of Epilepsy and its Consequences 1978 Plan for Nationwide Action on Epilepsy. US DHEW, Washington DC

Cooper J E 1965 Epilepsy in a longitudinaal survey of 5000 children. British Medical Journal 1: 1020–1022

Crombie D L, Cross K W, Fry J, Pinsent R J, Watts C A 1960 A survey of the epilepsies in general practice. A report by the Research Committee of College of General Practitioners. British Medical Journal 2: 416–422

Dada T O 1976 The epilepsies: their incidence and causation in Nigeria. In: Janz D (ed) Epileptology (Proceedings of the VIIth International Symposium on Epilepsy, Berlin 1975). Georg Thieme, Stuttgart, p 24

De Graaf A S 1974 Epidemiological aspects of epilepsy in Northern Norway. Epilepsia 15: 291–299

Eastwood M R, Trevelyan M H 1972 Relationship between physical and psychiatric disorder. Psychological Medicine 2: 363–372

Ellenberg J H, Nelson K B 1980 Sample selection and the natural history of disease. Journal of the American Medical Association 243: 1337–1340

Ellenberg J H, Hirtz D G, Nelson K B 1984 The age of onset of seizures in young children. Annals of Neurology 15: 127–134

Gastaut H 1969 Clinical and electroencephalographical classification of epileptic seizures. Epilepsia 19 (suppl): 2–13

Gastaut H 1973 Dictionary of epilepsy. Part I: Definitions. World Health Organization, Geneva

Gastaut H, Gastaut J L, Concalves e Silva G E, Fernandez Sanchez G R 1975 Relative frequency of different types of epilepsy: a study employing the classification of the International League Against Epilepsy. Epilepsia 16: 457–461

Gates M J 1972 Age: risk of seizures in infants. In: Hauser W A, Alter M (eds) The epidemiology of epilepsy: a workshop. NINDS Monograph No 14, DHEW, Washington DC pp 75–81

Goldberg I D, Kurland L T 1962 Mortality in 33 countries from diseases of the nervous system. World Neurology 3: 444–465

Gomez J G, Arciniegas E, Torres J 1978 Pevalence of epilepsy in Bogota, Colombia. Neurology 28: 90–94

Goodridge D M G, Shorvon S D 1983 Epileptic seizures in a population of 6000: I. Demography, diagnosis and classification, role of the hospital services, II. Treatment

and prognosis. British Medical Journal 287: 641–647

Granieri E, Rosati G, Tola R, et al 1983 A descriptive study of epilepsy in the District of Copparo, Italy, 1964–1978. Epilepsia 24: 502–514

Grudzinska B 1974 Epidemiology of epilepsy in population of a large industrial city. Incidence and prevalence (in Polish). Neurologia Neurochirurgia Polska 8: 175–180

Gudmundsson G 1966 Epilepsy in Iceland: a clinical and epidemiological investigation. Acta Neurologica Scandinavica 25 (suppl 43): 1–124

Hauser W A 1982 The role of epidemiology in the design of clinical trials of anticonvulsive drugs. Epilepsia 23 (suppl 1): 43–52

Hauser W A, Kurland L T 1975 The epidemiology of epilepsy in Rochester, Minnesota, 1935 through 1967. Epilepsia 16: 1–66

Hauser W A, Annegers J F, Kurland L T 1977 Is incidence of epilepsy declining? American Journal of Epidemiology 106:146 (abstract)

Hauser W A, Annegers J T, Elveback L R 1980 Mortality in patients with epilepsy. Epilepsia 21: 399–412

Henriksen P B, Juul-Jensen P, Lund M 1967 The mortality of epileptics. Epilepsy and insurance. Social Studies in Epilepsy No. 5, International Bureau for Epilepsy, London

Hirtz D G, Nelson K B 1983 The natural history of febrile seizures. Annual Review of Medicine 34: 453–471

Hirtz D G, Ellenberg J H, Nelson K B 1984 The risk of recurrence of non febrile seizures in children. Neurology 34: 637–641

Hopkins A, Scambler G 1977 How doctors deal with epilepsy. Lancet 1: 183–186

Iivanainen M, Lehtinen J 1979 Causes of death in institutionalized epileptics. Epilepsia 20: 485–492

Janz D 1969 Die Epilepsien. Georg Thieme Verlag, Stuttgart

Janz D 1972 Social prognosis in epilepsy especially in regard to social status and the necessity for institutionalization. Epilepsia 13: 141–147

Juul-Jensen P, Ipsen J 1976 Prevalence and incidence of epilepsy in Greater Aarhus. In: Janz D (ed) Epileptology, Proceedings of the Seventh International Symposium on Epilepsy, Georg Thieme Verlag, Stuttgart, pp 10–17

Juul-Jensen P, Foldspang A 1983 Natural history of epileptic seizures. Epilepsia 24: 297–312

Kahl-Kunstetter J, Zielinski J J 1972 Causes of deaths of epileptic patients-inmates of a mental hospital (in Polish). Neurologia Neurochirurgia Polska 22:847

Kostrzewa T, Mijal K, Pankow T, Pluzek Z, Wilk Z 1972 Attempts of suicide in Krakow, in 1962, 1966, 1967 and 1969 (in Polish). Psychiatrica Polska 6: 299–306

Krohn W 1963 Causes of death among epileptics. Epilepsia 4: 315–321

Kuran W 1975 Epidemiology of epilepsy in school children in two small towns (in Polish). Neurologia Neurochirurgia Polska 9: 57–61

Kurland L T 1959 The incidence and prevalence of convulsive disorders in a small urban community. Epilepsia 1: 143–161

Kurtzke J F 1972 Mortality and morbidity data on epilepsy. In: Hauser W A, Alter M (eds) The Epidemiology of epilepsy: a workshop. NINDS Monograph No. 14, DHEW, Washington DC, p 21

Kurtzke J F, Kurland L T, Goldberg I D, Won Choi N, Reeder F A 1973 Convulsive disorders. In: Kurland L T, Kurtzke J F, Goldberg I D (eds) Epidemiology of neurologic and sense organ disorders. APHA Monographs,

Harvard University Press, Cambridge

Leibowitz M, Alter M 1968 Epilepsy in Jerusalem, Israel. Epilepsia 9: 87–95

Lennox W G 1960 Epilepsy and related disorders. Churchill, London

Lessel S, Torres J M, Kurland L T 1962 Seizure disorders in a Guamanian village. Archives of Neurology 7: 37–44

Logan W P D, Cushion A A 1958 Studies on medical and populattion subjects. No. 14. Morbidity Statistics from General Practice I: 174, HMSO, London

Mathai K V, Dunn D P, Kurland L T, Reeder F A 1968 Convulsive disorders in the Mariana Islands. Epilepsia 9: 77–85

Matthews W S, Barabas G 1981 Suicide and epilepsy: a review of the literature. Psychosomatics 22: 515–524

Meadow R 1984 Fictitious epilepsy. Lancet 2: 25–28

Meighan S S, Queener L, Weitman M 1976 Prevalence of epilepsy in children of Multnomah County, Oregon. Epilepsia 17: 245–256

Miller F J, Court S D, Walton W S et al 1960 Growing up in Newcastle-upon-Tyne. A continuing study of health and illness in young children with their families. Oxford University Press, London

Naggan L, McMahon B 1967 Ethnic differences in the prevalence of anencephaly and spina bifida in Boston, Massachusetts. New England Journal of Medicine 277: 119–123

National Health Survey 1973 Prevalence of chronic conditions of the genitourinary, nervous, endocrine, metabolic and blood and blood-forming systems and of other selected conditions. US:DHEW, Publ. No. (HRA), Washington DC, pp 77–1536

Neploch I 1965 Causes of death in epilepsy (in Russian). Zhurnal Nevropatologii i Psikhiatrii im. Korsakova 65: 1383–1387

Neuspiel D R, Kuller L H 1985 Sudden and unexpected natural death in childhood and adolescence. Journal of the American Medical Association 254: 1321–1325

Nowak S 1972 Epidemiology and social-medical aspects of epilepsy in a rural and city communities (in Polish). Neurologia Neurochirurgia Polska 6: 369–374

Novak S, Olczyk E, Blaszczyk B, Wojcik J, Szmatola S 1984 Late epilepsy in the population of Kielce and selected communities in the Province of Kielce (in Polish). Neurologia Neurochirurgia Polska 18: 313–317

Olivares L 1972 Epilepsy in Mexico: a population study. In: Milton A Hauser W A The epidemiology of epilepsy: a workshop. NINDS Monograph No 14, DHEW, Washington DC

Penning R, Muller C, Ciompi L 1969 Mortality and cause of death in epileptics (in French). Psychiatria Clinica 2: 85–94

Pless B, Graham P 1970 Epidemiology of physical disorders. In: Rutter M, Tizard J, Whitmore K (eds) Education, health and behaviour. Longman, London p 285

Pond D A, Bidwell B H, Stein L 1960 A survey of epilepsy in fourteen general practices. I. Demographic and medical data. Psychiatria Neurologia Neurochirurgia 63: 217–236

Pond D A, Burden G S 1963 Review of the social and medical services for the epileptic patient in England and Wales. Epilepsia 4: 77–89

Roberts R S, Spitzer W O, Delmore T, Sackett D 1978 An empirical demonstration of Berkson's bias. Journal of Chronic Diseases 31: 119–128

Robertson M M, Trimble M R 1983 Depressive illness in patients with epilepsy: a review. Epilepsia 24 (suppl 2): 109–116

Rodin E A 1968 The prognosis of patients with epilepsy. Charles C Thomas, Springfield, Illinois

Rodin E A, Shapiro H L, Lennox K 1977 Epilepsy and life performance. Rehabilitation Literature 38: 34–39

Rose S W, Penry J K, Markush R E, Radloff L A, Putnam P L 1973 Prevalence of epilepsy in children. Epilepsia 14: 133–152

Ross E M, Peckham C S 1983 School children with epilepsy. In: Parsonage M (ed) Advances in epilepsy (XIVth Epilepsy International Symposium). Raven Press, New York

Ross E M, Peckham C S, West P B, Butler N R 1980 Epilepsy in childhood: findings from the National Child Development Study. British Medical Journal I: 207–210

Rutter M, Graham P, Yule W 1970 A neuropsychiatric study in childhood. Spastics International Medical Publishers in association with Heinemann Medical, London

Sato S 1964 An epidemiologic and clinicostatistical study of epilepsy in Niigata City. Epidemiologic study (in Japanese). Clinical Neurology 4: 461–471

Schleisner P A 1849 Doctor's thesis (in Norwegian). Cited by Gudmundsson G, 1966

Shamansky S L, Glaser G H 1979 Socioeconomic characteristics of childhood seizure disorders in New Haven area: an epidemiological study. Epilepsia 20: 457–474

Shepherd M, Cooper B, Brown A C, Kalton G 1981 Psychiatric illness in general practice, 2nd edn. Oxford University Press, Oxford

Shorvon S D 1984 The temporal aspects of prognosis in epilepsy. Journal of Neurology, Neurosurgery and Psychiatry 47: 1157–1165

Stanhope J M, Brody J A, Brink E 1972 Convulsions among the Chamorro people of Guam, Mariana Islands. I. Seizure disorders. American Journal of Epidemiology 95: 292–298

Temkin O 1971 The falling sickness. A history of epilepsy from the Greeks to the beginning of modern neurology, 2nd edn. John Hopkins Press, Baltimore

Tsuboi T 1984 Epidemiology of febrile and afebrile convulsions in children in Japan. Neurology 34: 175–181

Van den Berg B J, Yerushalmy Y 1969 Studies on convulsive disorders in young children. Part I. Incidence of febrile and nonfebrile convulsions by age and other factors. Pediatric Research 3: 298–304

Verity C M, Butler N R, Golding J 1985 Febrile convulsions in a national cohort followed up from birth. I. Prevalence and recurrence in the first five years of life. British Medical Journal 290: 1307–1310

Wajsbort J, Haral N, Alfandary I 1967 A study of the epidemiology of chronic epilepsy in Northern Israel. Epilepsia 8: 105–116

Weissman M M, Klerman G L 1978 Epidemiology of mental disorders. Emerging trends in the United States. Archives of General Psychiatry 35: 705–712

Whitman S, Coleman T E, Patmon C, Desai B T, Cohen R, King L N 1984 Epilepsy in prison: elevated prevalence and no relationship to violence. Neurology 34: 775–782

Zielinski J J 1966 Epileptic patients in the district city population (in Polish). Neurologia Neurochirurgia Polska 16: 511–518

Zielinski J J 1972 Social prognosis in epilepsy. Epilepsia 13: 133–140

Zielinski J J, Okolowicz-Zielinska I, Kuligowski Z W 1973 Long-term epileptic patients of psychiatric hospitals and nursing care institutions (in Polish). Neurologia Neurochirurgia Polska 7: 515–521

Zielinski J J 1974a Epidemiology and medical social problems of epilepsy in Warsaw. Final Report on Research Program No. 19-P-58325-F-01, US:DHEW, Social and Rehabilitation Service, Washington DC

Zielinski J J 1974b Epilepsy and mortality rates and cause of death. Epilepsia 15: 191–201

Zielinski J J 1975 Epidemiology of epilepsy in Poland on the basis of visits to physicians (in Polish). Przeglad Epidemiologiczny 29: 123–132

Zielinski J J 1976 People with epilepsy who do not attend doctors. In: Janz D (ed) Epileptology. Proceedings of the Seventh International Symposium on Epilepsy, Georg Thieme Verlag, Stuttgart, pp 18–23

Zielinski J J 1977 Frequency of head trauma and posttraumatic epilepsy in Warsaw population. In: Posttraumatic epilepsy and pharmacological prophylaxis (Proceedings of First European Regional Conference on Epilepsy). Polish Chapter of the ILAE, Warsaw

Zielinski J J 1978 Neurologic diseases and syndromes in Poland, 1960–1990 (in Polish). In: Kopczynski J, Korzybski T, Sawicki F (eds) Poland 2000: presence and future of frequent diseases in Poland. Zaklad Narodowy im. Ossolinskich, Wroclaw, pp 174–192

Zielinski J J, Kuran W, Witkowska-Olearska K 1978 The course of epilepsy and drug taking in randomly selected groups of patients in the light of five-year follow-up (in Polish). Polski Tygodnik Lekarski 33: 1927–1930

Zielinski J J, Rader B 1984 Employability of persons with epilepsy: difficulties of assessment. In: Porter R J, Mattson R H, Ward Jr A A, Dam M (eds) Advances in epileptology (XVth Epilepsy International Symposium). Raven Press, New York, pp 577–581

3

Genetics

V. E. Anderson
W. A. Hauser

INTRODUCTION

There is convincing evidence that genetic factors are involved in the development of seizures and in EEG variability. The application to clinical practice is not simple, however. The results from various studies show inconsistencies and areas of incompleteness. In dealing with individual patients the relative contribution of genetics (as compared with environmental factors) may be difficult to determine.

Recent developments are clarifying the issues. The genetic studies of epilepsy have been carefully reviewed (Metrakos & Metrakos 1970, Doose 1981, Anderson et al 1982, Hauser et al 1983, Anderson & Hauser 1985, Tsuboi & Okada 1985, Andermann 1985). The clinical features of genetic syndromes which include epilepsy as an outcome are outlined in a neurogenetic directory edited by Myrianthopoulos (1981). Finally, a number of molecular approaches are being applied to nervous system problems (Håkanson & Thorell, 1985; Rosenberg, 1985).

For clinical work with epilepsy patients a basic understanding of genetics along four lines will be useful:

1. Genetic heterogeneity
2. Differential diagnosis
3. Treatment and prognosis and
4. Genetic counselling

Genetic heterogeneity

We cannot expect to find a single mechanism causing seizures. Animal models for epilepsy present firm evidence that genetic factors can influence the hypersensitivity of neurones, but many different etiological pathways appear to be involved. Furthermore, over 140 Mendelian traits in the human carry an increased risk of seizures (Anderson et al, 1986). These conditions include disturbances of amino acids, enzymes and hormones, and vascular changes and neoplasms in the brain. In other syndromes the mechanism of seizure-enhancement is not yet apparent. Obviously, there are many different genetic pathways leading to epilepsy. It is not generally realized that genetics has more to say about individual differences than about family resemblance.

Another argument for genetic heterogeneity in seizure mechanisms comes from the fact that the optimum for neuronal excitability is intermediate between two extremes (hyperexcitability and unresponsiveness). It is generally observed that systems with an intermediate optimum (such as blood clotting and blood glucose) are complex, and involve a number of mechanisms under independent genetic control. Thus, we might expect to find heterogeneity in the epilepsies as well.

Finally, basic research studies show that seizures may result if there are defects in any of the following steps: neuronal inhibition; inactivation of excitatory neurotransmitters; feedback control; and the control of spread of the seizure state. Each of these can be affected by genetic variation, with the result that some individuals may have a reduced ability to handle the effects of environmental insults (such as infections or trauma).

Differential diagnosis

When multiple malformations are encountered in a seizure patient, the possibility of a chromosome problem should be considered. Essentially all of the detectable changes in chromosomes have some effect upon the nervous system, usually in the form of mild to severe mental retardation and, less often, seizures.

The detection of Mendelian (single gene) traits that increase the risk of seizures requires attention to a number of characteristics such as hair form, skin texture, visual or hearing loss, neurological signs and mental retardation.

Only a small proportion of patients with epilepsy (perhaps 1–2%) will have a diagnosable Mendelian trait or chromosomal abnormality, but for these few cases the distinction may be important for treatment and prognosis.

Treatment and prognosis

Family medical history and other genetic information may sometimes influence patient seizure management. In some, but not all, of the Mendelian traits manifesting seizures, the treatment of the underlying genetic problem may also alleviate the seizures.

The family history also may be important in evaluating prognosis. Neonatal convulsions frequently are an indicator of severe dysfunction and a predictor of mortality or subsequent morbidity in terms of epilepsy or mental retardation. In some families, however, multiple members experience neonatal seizures which are benign in outcome. There is no excess of retardation and the risk of subsequent epilepsy is low. The trait is transmitted through a number of generations in a pattern compatible with autosomal dominant inheritance. If a case of neonatal seizures is seen without enquiring about the family background, inappropriate decisions concerning treatment may be made.

In a study of 244 patients who presented for a first unprovoked seizure at any age, the cumulative overall risk of recurrence was 27% by 36 months (Hauser et al 1982). In the subset of idiopathic cases with seizures in siblings, the risk of recurrence in the probands was higher (35%) than in probands with no affected siblings. In addition, the interval between first and second seizure was shorter in the former than in the latter group.

Genetic counselling

The goal of genetic counselling is to provide individuals and families with the information and understanding they need in order to make informed choices about future reproduction (Reed 1980). In the case of epilepsy, close teamwork is required between neurologist and geneticist, with the former evaluating the seizure history and EEG patterns and the latter helping to detect any genetic syndrome and estimating risks for siblings or children.

Whenever a Mendelian or chromosomal syndrome is diagnosed, the sibling risk for the syndrome itself, with or without seizures, is used. In other situations, empiric risks are estimated from family studies, as presented in a later section.

GENETIC APPROACHES

The methods of genetic study range from the level of molecules to that of populations and thus provide a way to integrate the insights from other disciplines. In this section our purpose is to review some of the genetic approaches of particular relevance to epilepsy and to list selected references for any who may wish further details.

The general principles are covered in several recent textbooks on medical genetics (Connor & Ferguson-Smith 1984, Fraser Roberts & Pembrey 1985, Thompson & Thompson 1986, Vogel & Motulsky 1986). More specialized sources address genetics in neurology (Baraitser 1982, Ionasescu & Zellweger 1983), behavioural genetics (Hay 1985, Sakai & Tsuboi 1985) and molecular genetics (Rosenberg et al 1985, Schmitt et al 1982).

Mendelian Traits

In the evaluation of a new patient with seizures, it is essential to consider the possibility of one of the Mendelian traits that increase the risk of seizures. An understanding of these traits is of obvious importance for the clinical evaluation and treatment of seizure patients (Jennings & Bird 1981, Baraitser 1982). Furthermore, it would

Table 3.1 Mendelian traits associated with seizures, with and without mental retardation

	Total number*	Seizures and retardation No.	%	Seizures only No.	%	Total seizures No.	%
Autosomal dominant	1827	9	0.5	16	0.9	25	1.4
Autosomal recessive	1298	65	5.0	31	2.4	96	7.4
X-linked recessive	243	12	4.9	8	3.3	20	8.2
Totals	3368	86	2.6	55	1.6	141	4.2

*From McKusick (1983)

appear that these 'experiments of nature' have much to tell us about etiological pathways which can produce seizures.

Mendelian traits are thus named because each is thought to be controlled by two or more alleles at a single genetic locus. McKusick's sixth edition (1983) provides information on 3368 such traits, and 141 of these increase the risk of seizures (Table 3.1). The three common modes of inheritance are described in the following paragraphs.

Autosomal dominant

In autosomal dominant traits, only one of the pair of alleles at a locus needs to be defective for the disorder to occur. These disorders are often found in several generations, since the defective allele is transmitted from affected persons to offspring with a 50% probability. The genetic basis for such conditions is more easily detected and this fact explains in part why over half of all traits in McKusick's index are inherited in this way.

Dominant traits are usually less severe and have later onset than recessive traits; relatively few lead to seizures. Dominants often affect cell surface phenomena (such as receptors) or structural proteins (such as collagen), rather than enzymes. Furthermore, a dominant gene may sometimes be transmitted through an individual without showing any effect (described as lack of penetrance).

Autosomal recessive

Autosomal recessive traits result when both alleles at a locus are defective. They tend to be more severe and have earlier onset. A large proportion of the traits manifesting seizures (Table 3.1) have this mode of inheritance, particularly those also causing retardation. Often an enzyme defect is involved. In almost all cases, both parents are heterozygous carriers and there is a 25% risk for each sibling of an index case being affected.

If the trait is rare in the population, an individual is unlikely to receive a mutant gene from both parents unless the parents are related. Therefore, when consanguinity is noted, the possibility of autosomal recessive inheritance should be considered. Parents and other presumed carriers also should be examined for clinical signs of heterozygosity (Vogel 1984).

X-linked recessive

Recessive traits carried on the X chromosome are generally seen only in males, since genes on the single X chromosome of the male are readily expressed, while females (with two X chromosomes) are much more likely to be heterozygous. The characteristic pedigree pattern (transmitted through unaffected females and expressed only in males) makes recognition of the genetic basis for such traits relatively easy. In X-linked traits serious enough to limit reproduction, however, the possibility of new mutations must be considered in genetic counselling (Fuhrmann & Vogel 1983).

Genetic mapping of the X chromosome is relatively advanced, with Duchenne muscular dystrophy (Harper 1985) serving as a prototype.

Mendelian disorders involving seizures

Generally, when a Mendelian disorder is diagnosed, medical attention turns to means of treatment for the underlying condition. As a result, the pathways leading to the seizures are seldom explored, and we lose the opportunity to gain more insight into the etiology of seizures. It is likely that genetic mutations may be as useful in discriminating among various physiological explanations for seizures as they have been for the explication of enzyme pathways.

For each of these conditions we need thoughtful attention to these questions:

1. Why do seizures occur at all in this syndrome?
2. Why do seizures occur in some, but not all, of the affected individuals?
3. What variability is observed within families that might be ascribed to environmental variables, modifying genes, sex and age?
4. What is the distribution by age at onset of seizures?
5. What types of seizures are observed?
6. What variations in EEG patterns have been found?
7. Which antiepileptic drugs are most effective and least effective in controlling the seizures associated with this trait?

Comparable population rate

When a family is given an estimate of the risk for seizures in another child, they should have for comparison an estimate of the risk for the general population. Adequate genetic counselling requires both family and population data, such as those provided by studies of Rochester, Minnesota and the surrounding county (Annegers et al 1982). In this situation, neither incidence nor prevalence rates are appropriate. Instead, we need the *cumulative incidence* (or cumulative risk) – the chance that persons of a given age will have been affected by that age. In a study of probands having onset of *idiopathic* epilepsy (recurrent seizures without acute precipitating central nervous system insult) before 15 years of age, 3.6% of the siblings developed epilepsy by the age of 40, as compared with a cumulative incidence rate of 1.7% in the general population (Fig. 3.1). When febrile and other acute symptomatic seizures are added, the rates by the age of 40 are 11.6% for siblings and 5.1% for the population.

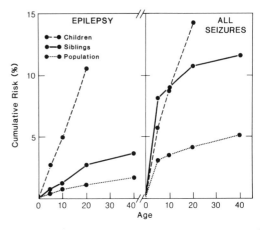

Fig. 3.1 Cumulative risks for epilepsy and for all seizures in the general population of Rochester, Minnesota and in the siblings of probands with initial diagnosis of idiopathic epilepsy before 15 years of age. (Based on data from Annegers et al 1982)

Risk ratios

Epidemiologic studies measure the effect of a particular exposure in terms of *risk ratios* (Annegers & Hauser 1984). This is roughly the ratio of the frequency of the outcome of interest in an exposed group to that of an unexposed group. In genetic studies of epilepsy, 'exposure' may be defined as the presence of seizures or epilepsy in a specific class of relatives. The frequency of epilepsy is then compared with that expected in a non-exposed population which is matched or adjusted for age, sex or other relevant variables. The term *relative risk* may be used in prospective studies which compare the incidence of epilepsy in an exposed and unexposed group. The *standardized morbidity ratio* (SMR) may be a more appropriate statistic for studies such as those in Rochester, Minnesota, which compare the incidence in the exposed group (those with positive family history) to the incidence in the general population including those exposed. This will tend to underestimate slightly the size of the effect. The *odds ratio* approximates the relative risk in retrospective or case control studies.

The use of risk ratios allows comparison of the size of an effect across populations which may have very different base population rates. Thus, in studies of familial risks for febrile seizures (Table 3.2), the 20.7% risk for febrile seizures among siblings of febrile seizure probands in

Table 3.2 Risk of febrile convulsions (FC) among siblings of probands with FC

| Study | Siblings of probands | | | General population | | |
	Total No.	With FC No.	%	Total No.	With FC No.	%
Fukuyama et al (1979)	287	57	(19.9)			
Tsuboi (1982)	1 094	227	(20.7)	16 806	1 123	(6.7)
Schuman & Miller (1966)	213	23	(10.9)	3 953	142	(3.6)
Metrakos & Metrakos (1970)	115	21	(9.8)			
Frantzen et al (1970)	303	33	(10.9)	9 656	292	(3.0)
Van den Berg (1974)	323	29	(9.0)	6 956	144	(2.1)
Hauser et al (1985)	1 046	84	(8.0)	45 304	1 046	(2.3)

Tokyo (Tsuboi 1982) seems much higher than the comparable sibling risk of 8.0% in Rochester, Minnesota (Hauser et al 1985). On the other hand, the population frequency of febrile seizures is also very different in the two populations (6.7% versus 2.3% respectively), so the SMR of 3 is similar in both populations.

Multifactorial (polygenic) inheritance

Many of the more common medical conditions (such as congenital malformations of the heart or central nervous system) do not fit any of the Mendelian inheritance patterns. In such conditions it is assumed that a number of genetic and environmental factors (each with only a small effect) contribute to an underlying liability. In order to facilitate calculations the liability is assumed to take a normal (bell-shaped) distribution. The liability curves for close relatives are assumed to shift to an extent proportional to the heritability (the fraction of liability that is genetically determined).

The relation between population and sibling risks can be expressed in graph form (Fig. 3.2), adapted from Smith (1970) for use with sibling data. Point A represents data for febrile convulsions (FC) in Rochester, Minnesota, (Hauser et al 1985) while point B represents FC data from Tokyo (Table 3.2). Both the population and sibling risks differ sharply between these two populations, but the estimates of the heritability of liability are much more similar (paralleling the similarity in standard morbidity ratios). Thus, if we assume that FC follows multifactorial inheritance, about two-thirds of the variation in liability is genetic.

In contrast, for an autosomal recessive trait the

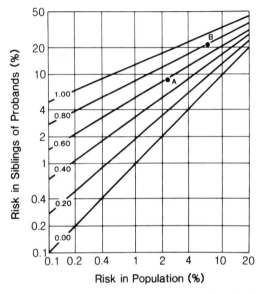

Fig. 3.2 Estimates of the heritability of liability for febrile convulsions in population samples from Minnesota (A) and Japan (B). Based on data from Tsuboi (1982) and Hauser et al (1985). Graph adapted from Smith (1970). (Reproduced with permission from Anderson et al 1986)

line for sibling risk would run straight across the graph at 25%, with little relation to the population rate. It will be noted that for common traits the distinction between single-locus and multifactorial inheritance becomes more difficult since the lines converge.

Segregation analysis

Few of the currently available genetic studies of epilepsy have taken full advantage of the information about the distribution of seizures within and between families. It is now possible to perform complex segregation analysis using computer methods that have been developed to estimate a number of genetic parameters and to test genetic models (Lalouel et al 1983, Moll et al 1983, Williams et al 1983). Several issues should be addressed, however, before attempting such analysis:

1. Relatively large sample sizes are needed. In the case of febrile convulsions, for example, the sample size is now large enough and the category is sufficiently discrete for complex segregation analysis to appear appropriate.
2. The manner in which the sample is collected (the ascertainment criteria) must be specified clearly.
3. It is essential to test several genetic models simultaneously. It is of little interest, for instance to show that epilepsy can be explained by multifactorial inheritance without simultaneous information about the possible exclusion of a simple autosomal pattern.
4. The possibility of aetiological heterogeneity should be considered in the analysis whenever possible.

The epidemiological data from Rochester concerning FC in general are consistent with a polygenic mode of inheritance. More recently Rich et al (1986) used complex segregation analysis on these data and found that all the genetic models involving a single major locus were rejected. The most likely hypothesis was polygenic inheritance with significant heritability of liability (68%).

However, in the small subgroup, in which the proband had three or more FC episodes, the evidence favoured a single major locus. An enlarged sample will be needed to verify this tentative finding, but there are two important implications:

1. Samples of FC may be more heterogeneous than has been suspected.
2. A small subgroup may follow an autosomal dominant pattern of inheritance, while the majority are polygenic, thus suggesting a resolution to former controversies.

Multiplex families

If there is marked heterogeneity, a search for biochemical causes in a routine clinical series of epilepsy cases will be ineffective, since a potentially significant finding in a few individuals will be lost in the data for the total group. On the other hand, the study of multiplex families (each with several affected siblings) will pick out families with a greater likelihood of genetic etiology for their seizures and will permit the detection of biochemical deviations that appear in only one or a few families. This approach has provided interesting data about taurine and haptoglobin and is recommended for wider use (Haines et al 1986).

Taurine

Taurine is a sulphur-containing amino acid that is particularly concentrated in excitable tissues (Fariello et al 1985) and appears to be a neuromodulator. Taurine transport is decreased in the brain and kidney of a genetically seizure-prone rat strain (Bonhaus et al 1983), and taurine content is decreased in the synaptosomal fraction of seizure-susceptible rats (Bonhaus et al 1984). Decreased urinary taurine excretion was noted in a human seizure group, and genetic control of taurine transport in the brain was postulated as one component of a polygenic liability for seizures (Goodman & Connolly 1982). In a study of 18 multiplex families, persons with generalized spike and wave (GSW) patterns on the EEG excreted significantly less taurine than other family members or controls (Haines et al 1986).

Haptoglobin

Low levels of plasma haptoglobin, a protein that binds and facilitates the clearance of free haemoglobin, were detected in 5 out of 14 multiplex families tested (Panter et al 1985). This observation led to a hypothesis that low haptoglobin levels (hypohaptoglobinaemia) reduce an individual's ability to clear free haemoglobin from small bleeds that occur in the brain with modest head injury (or even without apparent injury). As a consequence, the brains of hypohaptoglobinaemic individuals may suffer prolonged exposure to higher concentrations of free haemoglobin, a situation which has been demonstrated to be epileptogenic (Willmore & Triggs 1984).

Twin Studies

The overall concordance rate for epilepsy in six major twin studies was 60% for monozygotic (MZ) pairs and 13% for dizygotic (DZ) pairs (Tsuboi & Okada 1985). In addition, there have been a number of reports of one or a few twin pairs concordant for specific types of epilepsy.

One population-based twin study involved a follow-up of all twins born in Denmark in the years 1870–1910 (Harvald & Hauge 1965). Among the MZ pairs, 10 out of 27 (37%) were concordant for epilepsy. Among the DZ pairs (pooling same-sex and opposite-sex) 10 out of 100 (10%) were concordant.

A series of twins identified through clinical practice was studied carefully by Lennox & Lennox (1960). Where clinical examination suggested a brain lesion in the epilepsy proband, concordance was seen in 4 out of 37 (10.8%) MZ pairs, and in 5 out of 67 (7.5%) DZ pairs. Where there was no evidence of a structural brain lesion in the epileptic proband, however, concordance was 33 out of 47 (70.2%) MZ pairs as contrasted with 3 out of 54 (5.6%) DZ pairs, suggesting a genetic influence.

In a smaller series, Inouye (1960) identified 40 twin pairs from out-patients and in-patients. In re-analysing the data, we excluded a pair with ichthyosis and mental retardation, a pair with phenylketonuria, a pair with tuberous sclerosis, and a pair first identified at 79 years of age. Furthermore, we did not count febrile convulsions alone as epilepsy. Among 24 MZ pairs, 12 were concordant for epilepsy. Among the 12 MZ discordant pairs, the co-twin had abnormal EEG in seven cases; among 12 DZ pairs, none were concordant for epilepsy, although one co-twin had febrile seizures and two showed abnormal EEGs.

Meanwhile, in other conditions, twin methods have been used to explore a number of other clinically interesting questions (Hrubec & Robinette 1984). Eaves (1982), for example, showed how twin studies can be used to study development features and the interaction of multiple variables. Sing (personal communication) has proposed that MZ twin pairs concordant for epilepsy would provide an excellent panel for analysing the effectiveness of antiepileptic drugs. The possible role of genetic factors in idiosyncratic reactions to drugs is suggested by the report of an MZ twin pair, both of whom developed high blood ammonia concentrations following the administration of valproic acid (Campostrini et al 1985).

Association

Association and linkage are distinct phenomena and must not be confused with each other. Individuals with the HLA antigen B27 are at higher risk for ankylosing spondylitis – this is association. The genetic locus for congenital adrenal hyperplasia is very close to the HLA complex – this is linkage.

Smeraldi et al (1975) reported an increased association of HLA–B7 with astatic–myoclonic epilepsy. Cazullo & Canger (1979) found a significant elevation of HLA-B7 (with a relative risk of 4.38) in 22 patients with Lennox–Gastaut syndrome. A significant excess of the A1–B8 haplotype was found in two studies of absence epilepsy (Fichsel & Kessler 1982; Rivas 1983). On the other hand, Eeg-Olofsson et al (1982) found a significant *deficiency* of the A1–B8 haplotype in probands with 'benign epilepsy of childhood' and their parents. Monaghan et al (1982) reported no significant differences in 19 patients with cryptogenic myoclonic epilepsy. Hafez et al (1985) found a significant excess of HLA–A9 in 52 Egyptian children with absence or generalized tonic-clonic seizures. No differences from the expected distributions were found in 19 patients with myoclonic epilepsy (Monaghan et al 1982), in 42 children with febrile seizures (Eeg-Olofsson et al, 1984a) and in 21 patients with primary generalized cortico-reticular epilepsy (Eeg-Olofsson et al, 1984b).

Comparisons among these studies are difficult, since they involved small samples of patients and few reports were based on the same types of seizures. Information about EEG patterns generally was not provided, although most of the syndromes investigated are associated with an increased frequency of generalized spike and wave patterns. Further studies of this type are certainly desirable, although caution in interpretation is advised in view of the statistical difficulties that have been encountered in HLA studies of other conditions.

Linkage

The study of linkage has been greatly enhanced by the identification of DNA restriction fragment length polymorphisms–DNA fragments that vary in length among individuals and thus can be used to mark chromosomes (White 1984; White et al 1985). If the transmission of a specific type of epilepsy within families follows a marker locus on a specific chromosome, there is strong evidence for genetic etiology. This method must be applied first to large pedigrees, since the pooling of data from smaller families assumes homogeneity (i.e. all affected persons have the same disease).

The importance of linkage studies has been demonstrated clearly in the mapping of the gene for Huntington's disease to chromosome 4 (Gusella et al 1983, 1985), although problems remain in the application of this finding to individuals and families (Wexler 1985). The statistical methods are well described (Ott 1985) and have been extended to cover the simultaneous study of multiple markers (Lathrop et al 1984). A systematic investigation of linkage in juvenile myoclonic epilepsy is under way (Delgado-Escueta & Greenberg 1984) and analyses of other selected epilepsy syndromes should be encouraged.

Cellular and molecular mechanisms

Many different mechanisms associated with seizures have been postulated and studied (Wasterlain et al 1985, Delgado-Escueta et al 1986). Pathological changes may be observed in hippocampal structure, intermediate metabolism, the lipid constituents of membranes, calcium levels and protein synthesis. Among the amino acids, glutamate and aspartate are excitatory, while GABA and glycine are generally inhibitory; catecholamines and cyclic nucleotides also are involved. It is difficult, however, to distinguish causes of seizures from their effects and to understand paradoxical findings in different areas of the brain and under varying circumstances.

For the most part, such studies have not yet addressed the problem of genetic variability (except for the animal models discussed below). Tissue slices often are not well identified as to the genotype of the organism from which they are taken. The strategic use of several distinct genotypes to explore variability is seldom considered. It is understandable, of course, that the regularities in any system need to be established first, but it would be helpful to incorporate genetics into the research design as soon as possible thereafter.

Some efforts have been made to study epilepsy patients for evidence of the mechanisms identified through these experimental models. The major barriers have been the complexities of the systems and the fact that most tests of these models would require inaccessible brain tissue. In some cases, the difficulties might be overcome through the use of fibroblast cultures (Breakefield & Pintar 1981). If specific membrane receptors or enzymes can be detected in such cultures, and if mutations affecting the brain also alter fibroblasts (two important but testable qualifications), critical family studies would then become possible.

Another genetic strategy with considerable promise starts with an enzyme or other gene product that is known to be important for nervous system development and function (Kaufman & Tobin 1984). The DNA sequence then can be determined, the specific gene can be isolated and cloned, a search can be made for polymorphisms (individual variation) in the general population and the chromosome location of the gene can be determined. Eventually, a series of neurologically important gene probes will become available for gene mapping and for studying developmental sequences.

Animal models

The evidence for heterogeneity also influences the expectations and interpretations of experimental and animal models of epilepsy. Some models are rejected on the basis that they do not faithfully copy the features of human seizures. In this context Wasterlain et al (1984) stated: 'Since the diversity of the epilepsies must be emphasized, and a unitary mechanism is unlikely, we need models not to imitate a human illness too complex for current methods, but to simplify it and to permit precise testing of specific hypotheses.' Thus, the parallelism should be sought at the level of gene action rather than phenotypic consequences. A model is useful if it permits the careful exploration of a specific mechanism for seizures to the point that the role of that mechanism can be demonstrated or denied in other models and in one or several human epilepsy patients.

Audiogenic seizures (AGS) in the mouse involve severe seizures (often leading to death by respiratory paralysis) in response to a specific sound. These seizures show a number of similarities to certain convulsive disorders in humans (Seyfried & Glaser 1985). AGS appear to involve abnormalities of the brainstem as do absence (petit mal) seizures. There is a characteristic age-dependent incidence pattern with the highest susceptibility at juvenile ages. AGS are sensitive to a number of antiepileptic drugs. The distinct advantage, of course, is that detailed biochemical studies and genetic analyses are possible.

Seyfried & Glaser (1985) used recombinant inbred mouse lines which started with a cross between parents that were resistant and susceptible to AGS, followed by intercrosses which shuffled the chromosome combinations and, later, the establishment of new inbred lines. This strategy has permitted the following conclusions:

1. One gene with a major effect on the difference in susceptibility was detected by its linkage with an enzyme marker locus; other genes are also involved.
2. Juvenile-onset and adult-onset AGS can be caused by different genetic mechanisms.
3. There is a significant association between a low-affinity Ca^{2+} adenosine triphosphatase (ATPase) activity in the brainstem and AGS susceptibility.

Other mouse mutants display seizures in association with ataxia, defective cerebellar development, or myelin disorders (Noebels 1985). A few mutations produce apparently spontaneous seizures, although subtle environmental changes may be involved. Clear genetic variability is also seen in susceptibility to alcohol withdrawal seizures in mice (Crabbe et al 1983).

Genetic susceptibility to seizures in species as diverse as baboons, mice, gerbils, fowl, rats and dogs has been used to analyse the efficacy of antiepileptic drugs (Löscher & Meldrum 1984). At the cellular level of study, benzodiazepine receptor binding was significantly lower in the midbrain but not other brain areas of seizure-susceptible Mongolian gerbils, as compared with seizure-resistant strains. On the other hand, no differences were found in high-affinity GABA (gamma-aminobutyric acid) receptor binding (Olsen et al 1984). Further details about the broader research methods and findings in animal behaviour genetics are provided in a recent review (Wimer & Wimer 1985).

GENETIC EVALUATION OF PATIENTS

The factors involved in the genetic evaluation of epilepsy patients are generally well known to physicians, but some specific details may deserve comment.

Family History

The patient who is the focus of a genetic study is known as the 'proband'. In the absence of information about specific etiological mechanisms, the major source of data about possible genetic factors comes from the reported history of epilepsy and seizures in near relatives. It is important, however, to keep the information about the several types of relatives separate. Siblings of probands, for example, are at increased risk for any of the modes of inheritance, whether autosomal, X-linked or multifactorial. Affected parents or offspring may represent dominant or multifactorial patterns of inheritance, but seldom recessive ones. Therefore, a note in a patient's chart stating only that the family history is negative (or positive) is of little value for patient care or for research.

Specific questions should be directed toward the presence or absence of seizures in parents and siblings, with a more general enquiry about seizures in other relatives. If a relative is reported to have seizures, record should be made of the similarities and differences in seizure history as compared with the features observed in the proband.

If there is a presumed precipitating cause (such as trauma) for the seizures in the index case, but a close relative (such as one parent) also has a seizure history, then the possibility of an under-

Table 3.3 Risk of febrile convulsions (FC) in siblings of FC probands by parental history of FC

Parents with FC	FC in siblings		
	Fukuyama et al (1979)	Tsuboi (1982)	Hauser et al (1985)
Neither	18.0%	17.8%	5.5%
One	23.3%	31.4%	21.7%
Both	66.6%	38.9%	55.6%

lying genetic predisposition should be considered. The importance of enquiring about family history is emphasized by data about febrile convulsions (Table 3.3). It will be noted that there is a steady increase in sibling risk depending upon whether neither, one or both, parents had febrile convulsions.

Age at onset

Seizures involve a number of age-related phenomena. Many of the abnormal EEG patterns in humans show characteristic age patterns rising to a peak at a certain age and falling thereafter.

One of the clearest demonstrations of age-at-onset effects is shown in Figure 3.3. When the onset of major motor seizures in the proband occurred before the age of 4, the cumulative incidence of seizures in siblings rose more sharply than when the onset in the proband was at an

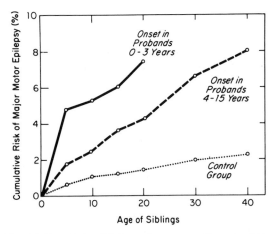

Fig. 3.3 Cumulative risk for major motor epilepsy in siblings of probands with epilepsy, by age at onset in the probands. Based on date from Eisner et al (1959). (Reproduced with permission from Anderson et al 1986)

older age. The control group had a cumulative incidence of 2.3% by the age of 40, a frequency which compares quite closely with the figure of 1.7% for the Rochester study (Fig. 3.1).

This effect of age at onset may result from either of two factors. First, those aetiological subtypes of seizures that have an earlier age at onset may be more influenced by genetic variables (a heterogeneity hypothesis). Secondly, those probands with early onset of seizures may have a higher genetic liability with a corresponding risk for siblings (a multifactorial hypothesis). Under either hypothesis, it is essential to define carefully the age at onset in the proband and in affected relatives. For each sibling the current age (or age at death) should also be noted.

Seizure type

A system for classifying seizure type must meet several different, and sometimes conflicting, functions. For clinical purposes, one needs a system that will help to provide guidance for prescribing treatment and assessing prognosis, but such a system does not necessarily represent discrete aetiological classes. Excellent descriptions of the various seizure types and their relevance for genetic counselling are provided by Blume (1982), and by Delgado-Escueta et al (1982).

It must also be recognized that some of the presumed unique seizure syndromes discussed in the literature are not different entities, but are age-specific variations in the manifestations of seizure predisposition. Thus, a given individual may show distinct seizure syndromes at different ages. Age-related changes in seizure type appear to reflect the complex interaction of:

1. the nature and likelihood of specific antecedent factors;
2. the developmental maturation of the nervous system; and
3. genetic variation influencing the structure and biochemistry of the developing brain.

Classification of the epilepsies

A tentative scheme for the classification of the epilepsies has been proposed by the ILEA (Dreifuss et al 1985). The classification continues to use the clinical seizure type for classification, although epilepsies characterized by partial seizures are termed 'localization related' epilepsies and syndromes, while those characterized by generalized onset seizures are categorized as generalized epilepsies and syndromes. The classification depends heavily upon age-specific syndromatic categorization of cases. Unfortunately, family history is incorporated as part of the definition for some of the syndromes, even though the genetic component is poorly established. A certain degree of circular logic seems unavoidable. The overall usefulness of this classification for the genetic study of family relationships in the epilepsies is uncertain.

EEG Pattern

Some general features of the EEG are of particular importance for genetic considerations. Vogel (1970) reported extensively on a number of characteristics of the EEG, finding a remarkable similarity of EEG frequency spectra among siblings. More recently he has explored the possibility that genetic factors influence the development and maturation of the brain (Vogel et al 1982).

Theta waves

Studies by Doose and his co-workers in Kiel, Germany have shown a strong family occurrence for certain specific EEG patterns. A theta EEG pattern (bilateral, synchronous, monomorphous waves of 4–7 Hz) seen maximally in the parietal area is found most often in children aged 2 to 6 years (Doose & Gundel 1982). Among 3-to-4-year-old siblings of probands with this theta pattern, up to 30% will show the same EEG pattern. Doose & Gundel argue that theta waves may serve as an indicator of a genetic predisposition for seizures.

It is clear that Doose is aware of the similarities between hypnagogic patterns in children and parietal theta rhythms, and he has required that the patients be clearly alert at the time that these patterns occur. No other investigators have systematically searched for this pattern to confirm or refute Doose's observation and his hypothesis of a relationship between these patterns and generalized spike and wave (GSW) patterns.

Photoconvulsive response

Another EEG pattern of interest is the appearance of GSW discharges during stimulation with intermittent light (photoconvulsive response or PCR) (Doose et al 1969). The EEG pattern is essentially similar to the GSW pattern, which occurs spontaneously. PCR has attracted a good deal of attention since it is the most common stimulus-sensitive brain phenomenon thus far identified in the human. (In most other species an auditory stimulus is the most effective in producing such changes.) PCR shows developmental fluctuations with age, with the highest manifestation generally being at 5 to 15 years of age. This, of course, will create difficulty in doing family studies since parents will be in an age range at which a lower percentage of manifestation will be expected.

When PCR declines with increasing age, it may be replaced by some other EEG phenomenon. The photomyoclonic response (PMR) is a muscular response to intermittent light stimuli which seems physiologically different from the PCR. In a combined study of PCR and PMR, Rabending & Klepel (1970) studied relatives of 88 probands with both epilepsy and PCR: among siblings of the probands, 22.0% showed PCR and 1.6% showed PMR; among parents the relative proportions were reversed with 10.3% showing PCR and 19.2% showing PMR. Thus, the two phenomena appeared to behave as age-dependent variations of the same underlying tendency (see also Klingler & Wessely 1977).

Generalized spike and wave

When we come to epilepsy, one of the problems for genetic studies is that generalized spike and wave (GSW) patterns, as well as other epileptiform patterns identified in probands with epilepsy, have rather specific age distributions (Doose 1981, Kellaway 1982). For example, even in individuals with epilepsy, interictal GSW patterns occur in the highest proportion of cases between the ages of 5 to 15 years and are quite uncommon at younger and older ages. Thus, it would be unlikely that parents or younger or older siblings of probands would demonstrate a spike and wave EEG pattern even if one had been expressed at some time in their lives. If, as Doose expects, theta patterns are an equivalent of GSW, it would be important to pay particular attention to these wave forms which might otherwise be treated as normal variations.

There seems little question that GSW discharges aggregate in families. In a recent complex segregation analysis of epilepsy in siblings of probands with epilepsy and a generalized spike and wave EEG pattern (Rich et al 1986), the pattern is consistent with a mixed model, combining an underlying single locus (of low frequency) with a polygenic effect (heritability of 25%). On the other hand, the occurrence of epilepsy among siblings of probands with photoconvulsive response is consistent with a single major locus with nearly dominant gene effects. The apparent independence of the inheritance of these two EEG patterns suggests that different genes may be responsible for the epilepsy in these two conditions.

It is possible that there are major population differences in the frequencies of the GSW pattern. Studies in Sweden (Eeg-Olofsson et al 1970) and in Germany (Doose et al 1977) have revealed base population rates of less than 2%. In contrast, studies in a French Canadian population (Metrakos & Metrakos 1961) and in a Japanese population (Tsuboi 1984) have revealed population rates exceeding 8% and a frequency of GSW in siblings that is concomitantly higher.

Implications

The family studies of epilepsy probands have established the importance of thorough EEG evaluation, not only for diagnostic purposes but also for genetic counselling. Hyperventilation and photic stimulation should be used routinely within those age groups which are potentially responsive (about 4–19 years). Sleep should also be used when possible in order to increase the probability of eliciting a spike-wave pattern. The EEG response under each of these conditions should be recorded separately, since the possibility of heterogeneity has not yet been explored fully.

Antecedent factors

The presence or absence of a history of anoxia, head trauma, cerebrovascular disorder, central nervous system infection, tumour, or drug or alcohol abuse should be explored. There are age-specific changes in the relative contributions of these types of antecedent factors, primarily because of the age-specific patterns of occurrence of each event. Nevertheless, there is little age-related change in the *proportion* of epilepsies which appear idiopathic (i.e. with no antecedent factors apparent).

A distinction can be made between predisposing factors (that tend to increase the general hypersensitivity of neurones without necessarily triggering a seizure) and precipitating factors (that can more directly trigger a seizure episode). Furthermore, the time intervening between the presumed factor and the onset of seizures should be noted. We already have presented evidence (Table 3.3) that the family history of seizures should be explored even if an antecedent factor can be identified.

Estimating sibling risks

In genetic counselling, it has been customary to use the term 'recurrence risk' to identify the estimated risk in siblings of probands. In discussions about seizures, however, the term 'recurrence' generally means the repetition of a seizure event for a given person. Therefore, we find it useful to substitute the phrase 'sibling risk.'

Whenever a Mendelian or chromosomal syndrome is diagnosed, the problem becomes one of estimating the sibling risk for the syndrome (whether or not seizures develop in the sibling).

Estimates of sibling risk in other situations are based on the family studies in the literature and, therefore, are described as 'empiric' risks. The samples are not always defined in a comparable manner, and some types of seizure have not been well studied. A further problem is the failure to report the data separately for epilepsy and for other seizures. Nevertheless, there is enough consistency to permit approximations for counselling purposes.

MENDELIAN DISORDERS INVOLVING SEIZURES

It must be emphasized that there seldom is a one-to-one correspondence between seizures and any Mendelian disorder. In few of these disorders are seizures found in all of the affected individuals; nor is it yet clear whether a comprehensive review of the Mendelian traits will provide insight into the etiological pathways involved for the manifestation of seizures in general. Nevertheless, some points of clinical and genetic interest can be illustrated by reference to a few selected conditions.

Progressive myoclonus epilepsy

Norio & Koskiniemi (1979) reviewed the data for 74 Finnish families with progressive myoclonus epilepsy and calculated the risk for siblings of probands to be 26%, an excellent fit to the hypothesis of autosomal recessive inheritance. Most affected members developed signs in the age range of 8 to 13 years, and there were no Lafora bodies in cases coming to autopsy. The description of this 'Baltic myoclonus epilepsy' in McKusick's (1983) catalogue concludes with an intriguing prediction, not yet realized: 'This appears to be a metabolic disorder with pharmacogenetic implications. Elucidation at a biochemical level may permit fully effective prevention and treatment.'

Benign neonatal familial convulsions

Benign neonatal familial convulsions form another epilepsy syndrome with a clear-cut pattern of inheritance. Bjerre & Corelius (1968) reported 14 family members in five generations who had frequent convulsions within the first few weeks of life. Vitamin B_6 dependency was excluded, and there were no disturbances of electrolyte or glucose balance and no problems with amino acid metabolism. There was no retardation and the

outcome was favourable. Quattlebaum (1979) also reported a family with 15 affected members in four generations. The prognosis in terms of subsequent neurological handicap was excellent and the risk of subsequent epilepsy was low. In these and in other families (Rett & Teubel 1964, Giacoia 1982, Kaplan & Lacey 1983, Zonana et al 1984) the pattern of inheritance is compatible with an autosomal dominant trait.

Tuberous sclerosis and neurofibromatosis

Tuberous sclerosis and neurofibromatosis are autosomal dominant traits that share a number of other interesting features.

1. Series of cases are often identified through hospitals and clinics, and thus tend to miss those with milder manifestations; hence, the population prevalence will be underestimated and the proportion with seizures will be overestimated.
2. The relative severity of the conditions means that reproduction is limited, with the result that a large proportion of cases are isolated (presumably representing new mutations).
3. A careful examination of relatives is essential to identify those with minimal signs.
4. Genetic counselling must take into account the clinical findings and the possibility of new mutations.
5. There is no simple correlation between neurological and other clinical findings, and thus the possibility must be kept open that part of the susceptibility to seizures may result from the direct metabolic consequences of gene action rather than from structural effects of the cerebral lesions.

There are two recent population-based studies of tuberous sclerosis. The prevalence for children under 5 years old was 15.4 per 100 000 for the Oxford, England, area (Hunt & Lindenbaum 1984) and 23.5 per 100 000 in Rochester, Minnesota (Wiederholt et al 1985). The true rates may be higher. In the Oxford series, it was estimated that 50–75% of 68 cases were new mutations, as compared with 70–86% in an earlier review (Bundey & Evans 1969). Four out of eight cases in Rochester developed seizures (all with onset before the age of 2), and two of these were mentally retarded. There were no neurological abnormalities in those free of seizures. Tuberous sclerosis has been identified as an important cause of infantile spasms, in 25 of 195 (13%) in the series investigated by Charlton & Mellinger (1970) and 14 of 54 (26%) in the study by Pampliglione & Pugh (1975). The importance of careful examination of siblings is emphasized by the report of seven cases in which hypopigmented maculae of the skin developed at varying intervals after birth (Oppenheimer et al 1985).

Neurofibromatosis has a population frequency of about one in 3000, and about half of the cases are isolated (presumably new mutations). The genetic counselling is straightforward when the evidence for heterogeneity is recognized (Riccardi 1981, 1984). Seizures are reported in 6–13% of cases (Carey et al 1979). An elevation of nerve growth factor is observed in disseminated neurofibromatosis, but the locus for nerve growth factor on chromosome 1 is not linked to neurofibromatosis (Darby et al 1985).

Homocystinuria

Homocystinuria is an autosomal recessive metabolic disease with interesting features. A deficiency of cystathionine β-synthase leads to increased plasma homocysteine and methionine and decreased cysteine. The major complications are mental retardation, dislocation of the lens, skeletal abnormalities and a tendency to thromboembolic episodes. Mudd et al (1985) reviewed questionnaires and published reports for 629 cases. Among 55 detected on newborn screening and treated, one developed seizures; of those detected at older ages, 21% had seizures, which may have contributed to their recognition as affected. (It is possible that some of the seizures were secondary to cerebrovascular accidents.) Among 19 patients with EEG records, 10 showed mild diffuse non-specific slowing of the background (Del Giudice et al 1983). In nine cases with abnormal EEGs, treatment with pyridoxine was followed by change to a normal EEG in three.

The possibility of a direct biochemical action on seizure threshold is suggested by the observation

that homocysteine induces tonic-clonic seizures and epileptiform EEG activity in rats and mice. Glutamic acid diethyl ester (GDEE) almost completely blocks homocysteine-induced and ethanol withdrawal seizures in mice, but has no effect on audiogenic or pentylenetetrazole-induced seizures (Freed 1985). GDEE is thought to be a selective antagonist of quisqualic acid-sensitive excitatory receptor sites. Further studies show that quisqualate-induced seizures are blocked by valproic acid but not by other antiepileptic drugs (Schwarz & Freed 1985).

Myoclonic epilepsy with mitochondrial myopathy

Finally, myoclonic epilepsy was associated with mitochondrial myopathy in a large pedigree (Rosing et al 1985). Muscle biopsies of affected members showed an increased number of abnormal mitochondria, but the myopathy could not be distinguished from other mitochondrial myopathies (all of which show ragged red fibres). Cerebral dysfunction included prominent photic driving on EEGs and high-amplitude visual and somatosensory evoked responses. Autosomal dominant, autosomal recessive and X-linked recessive inheritance could be excluded. Instead, the family pattern was consistent with maternal inheritance, following the distribution of mitochondrial DNA that has been observed in other traits and should be considered in future studies of epilepsy.

CHROMOSOMAL ABNORMALITIES

Down's syndrome

In a survey of 1654 hospitalized Down's syndrome patients around London and in south-east England, Veall (1974) found a prevalence of epilepsy of 5.8%. In the age group from 0 to 19, the prevalence of epilepsy was 1.9%. In the age groups from 20 to 59 there was some variation, but the average prevalence was 6.5%. In the much smaller sample, from the age of 60, the prevalence was 15.4%.

In a study of 111 patients with Down's syndrome in a hospital serving the city of

Glasgow, there were 11 (8.1%) with epilepsy (MacGillivray 1967). In general, their seizures were milder than those of other retarded patients. In another series of 128 patients in a hospital in Lancaster, England, there were 13 (10.2%) with a history of epilepsy; only five of these had onset of seizures prior to the age of 25 (Tangye 1979).

Alzheimer's disease

A brief note about Alzheimer's disease may be appropriate in view of the similarity of the pathology of this disease with that of older patients with Down's syndrome. In a recent study of patients with autopsy-confirmed Alzheimer's disease, 10% of patients demonstrated unprovoked seizures and 10% demonstrated myoclonus after the onset of Alzheimer's disease symptoms (Hauser et al 1986a). The frequency of seizures was increased ten-fold over that expected based upon the age-specific incidence of seizures in the general population. This observation should not be surprising since disorders of grey matter are in general characterized by seizures. This may explain in part the high frequency of seizures in older Down's syndrome patients, since most will develop pathological brain changes consistent with Alzheimer's disease.

Ring chromosome 14

The diagnosis of tuberous sclerosis was at first entertained for an infant girl with mental retardation and seizures associated with scattered vitiliginous spots and multiple hyperpigmented spots (Schmidt et al 1981). The presence of dysmorphic features of the head and face, however, led to a chromosome study which showed a ring chromosome 14. A review of this and six previously reported cases with a ring 14 showed that seizures occurred in six out of seven. These were generalized tonic-clonic seizures and myoclonic jerks which were fully controlled with antiepileptic treatment.

Inverted duplicated 15

Occasionally, chromosomal changes are found without associated dysmorphology. A high frequency of seizures is found in patients with an extra inverted duplicated chromosome 15 (Schreck et al 1977, Wisniewski et al 1979, Maraschio et al 1981). Of the 28 cases reported in these three papers, 21 (75%) had seizures, but there were no major physical abnormalities.

In the clinical descriptions of patients with various chromosomal problems, most of the attention is given to dysmorphic features. The general level of mental and motor development is usually mentioned, but the presence or absence of seizures may or may not be reported. The data needed for an appropriate epidemiological analysis are almost never available. A comprehensive review of the currently available literature and careful attention in planning new surveys would be helpful.

GENETICS IN SPECIFIC EPILEPSIES

Generalized onset epilepsy

The electroencephalographic hallmark of the generalized epilepsies is the interictal GSW (generalized spike and wave). Thus, studies of the generalized epilepsies are by definition studies of GSW, but GSW may occur also in individuals who have other forms of epilepsy or, for that matter, in asymptomatic individuals. Patients having generalized epilepsies with GSW, therefore, must be considered highly selected groups, and the results from studies of such patients cannot be generalized to all individuals with GSW.

The study carried out by Metrakos & Metrakos (1970) has served as a benchmark for comparison with later studies and deserves an extended discussion. The probands were identified at the Montreal Children's Hospital and thus had onset in childhood. The classification of probands followed the proposal by Penfield & Jasper (1954) which placed seizures into three main groups (localized, unlocalized and centrencephalic) depending upon the presumed origin of the epileptic discharge. Gastaut (1964) suggested that the term 'centrencephalic' be replaced by 'epilepsy of subcortical origin,' while Gloor (1968) preferred the term 'cortico-reticular epilepsy.'

Based on the EEG tracings, the probands were divided into those with typical and atypical patterns (Metrakos & Metrakos 1961). The prevalence rates of convulsions among near relatives of these two categories of probands were not different and thus the data were pooled.

The probands had either recurrent absence (petit mal) seizures or grand mal seizures (presumably 'tonic-clonic' in current terminology) (not tabulated separately) with no obvious neuropathology which would account for their seizures. The EEGs for the probands and relatives were considered positive for a GSW pattern, whether such a pattern occurred during the resting period, during hyperventilation or during photic stimulation. The category of spike-wave abnormalities referred to all types of generalized paroxysmal abnormalities, both epileptiform and nonepileptiform (Andermann 1982).

Control probands were collected by examining every twentieth admission to the same hospital and selecting those who had never had a convulsion, whose illness was not considered to be neuropathologic and whose EEG was within normal or borderline normal limits. The history of seizures among siblings of the probands and controls is shown in Table 3.4.

Table 3.4 Risk of epilepsy or any seizure in siblings of probands with primary generalized epilepsy

Seizure type in proband	Total No. siblings	With epilepsy	Total with seizures
Absence and/or grand mal (GSW*)		%	%
Metrakos & Metrakos (1961, 1966)	519	8.0	12.7
Control	322		4.7
Absence (with or without grand mal) (GSW)			
Matthes (1969)	240	3.7	10.0
Doose et al (1973)	448		6.7
Absence first symptom with onset after 5 yr (GSW)			
Baier & Doose (1985)	131		14.5
Myoclonic-astatic (akinetic)			
Matthes (1969)	131	3.8	6.8
Doose (1985)	154		16.0
Impulsive petit mal (Juvenile myoclonic)			
Tsuboi & Christian (1973)	705		4.4

*GSW = generalized spike and wave EEG pattern

The information about EEG abnormalities among siblings was also evaluated carefully. Follow-up EEG studies were done on 94 of the siblings (Metrakos & Metrakos 1974). At the time of the first EEG, the mean age was 7.6 years and 29% had generalized spike and wave EEGs. The mean age at the time of the second EEG was 15.3 years, and at that time 28% had the EEG trait. However, 45% had the trait in their first and/or second EEG. These data were used to support the hypothesis of an autosomal dominant inheritance for the EEG trait which is thought to underlie the seizures. Recently, Andermann (1982) concluded that the hypothesis of polygenic inheritance (many genes, each with small effect) fits the data better.

Doose et al (1973) found lower sibling risks for seizures among absence probands, than did Metrakos & Metrakos, and they also listed separately the data for probands with GSW occurring spontaneously and the data for those with GSW occurring only during PCR. The results suggest that a GSW in the EEG at rest or during hyperventilation may be genetically different from GSW occurring only during photic stimulation.

Another category of generalized onset epilepsy is seen in the study of juvenile myoclonic epilepsy carried out by Tsuboi & Christian (1973). The majority of the probands were aged 10 to 20 years at onset. In general, the incidence of epilepsy was higher among relatives of female probands than among relatives of male probands. Also, the risk of epilepsy was higher among female relatives than male relatives. This combination of findings (found also for other epilepsy syndromes) does not fit the usual pattern for multifactorial inheritance and thus far has not received a satisfactory explanation (Ottman et al 1985). Among 705 siblings there were 31 (4.4%) who had developed epilepsy (Table 3.4).

Doose et al (1973) studied 252 epileptic children who at some time had shown absences with generalized 3/s spike-waves. Among 448 siblings there were 30 (6.7%) who had one or more seizures (Table 3.4). This rate was higher for sisters than brothers (9.1% versus 3.9%). Among 242 siblings for whom EEG tracings were available there were 54 (22.3%) with GSW and/or PCR. Of these, 15 showed GSW only, 33 PCR only, and 6 showed both.

A later report was restricted to probands whose epilepsy started after the fifth year of life with absences as the first symptom and whose EEGs showed typical 3/sec spikes and waves (Baier & Doose 1985). This limitation was based on evidence that early infantile epilepsies with absences seem to run a worse course and have different sex ratios of affected relatives than diseases of later onset. Nineteen patients from the earlier study (Doose et al 1973) were included in the total of 77 probands. Among 131 siblings, 19 (14.5%) developed seizures and 20 (15.3%) reported migraine (Table 3.4).

Doose (1985) reported studies on probands with myoclonic-astatic petit mal (Table 3.4). The onset is usually in the third and fourth year of life, and the course of the disease is generally unfavourable. Among 154 siblings there were 16% with a history of seizures.

Matthes (1969) carried out similar studies (Table 3.4). Among 240 siblings of probands with absence epilepsy and 3/s GSW there were 9 (3.8%) with epilepsy and 15 (6.3%) with childhood convulsions, for a total of 10.0%. Among 131 siblings of probands with akinetic seizures (but with a slow generalized spike and wave complex) there were 5 (3.8%) with epilepsy and an additional 4 (3%) with childhood convulsions, for a total of 6.9%. While these rates are generally lower, strict comparisons require age adjustments.

Additional information is provided by EEGs on the siblings themselves. Doose et al (1984) studied 294 probands with primary generalized minor seizures (myoclonic-astatic or absence epilepsy with or without tonic-clonic seizures). The highest seizure rate was found in siblings with spikes and waves during rest and hyperventilation (34%), as compared with 9.0% in siblings with only photosensitivity or theta rhythms, and 4.1% in siblings with normal EEGs (Table 3.5).

An interesting parallel comes from the work of Cavazzuti et al (1980). EEGs were recorded in 3726 school children, from 6 to 13 years of age, who were neurologically normal and had no history of epileptic seizures. In 41 (1.1%) there were generalized discharges on the EEG and, upon follow-up over an 8–9 year period, 5 out of 35 (14.3%) developed epileptic seizures. Another 90 (2.3% of the total) showed other epileptiform

Table 3.5 Risk of any seizure by EEG findings in siblings of epilepsy probands with primary generalized minor seizures (Doose et al 1984)

EEG findings in siblings	Siblings No.	With any seizure No. %	
Photosensitivity without other patterns	43	3 7.0	9.0
Theta thythms without spikes and waves	24	3 12.5	
Spike waves without other patterns	20	7 35.0	34.0
Spike waves with photosensitivity and/or theta rhythms	27	9 33.3	
Normal EEG	123	5 4.1	

EEG patterns at the outset, and 2 out of 65 (3.1%) developed epileptic seizures during the follow-up period.

Implications for genetic counselling

As a general figure for genetic counselling we might start with the Rochester, Minnesota study of probands with onset of idiopathic epilepsy at ages up to 15 years (Fig. 3.1). The cumulative risks to the age of 40 for siblings were 3.6% for epilepsy and 4.7% for epilepsy or single idiopathic seizures (not febrile convulsions or seizures due to a presumed acute central nervous system insult). With some rounding, this becomes 4–5%, as compared with 1–2% expected for the general population.

For other questions the estimates from the current literature are inconsistent. Better data already exist in the records of large studies in progress, and we need a collaborative comparison and pooling of the information. Meanwhile, the following estimates of sibling risk for epilepsy when the proband has generalized epilepsy represent our effort to integrate the data presently available:

– 5% when the proband has absence or generalized tonic-clonic seizures and a generalized spike and wave EEG
– 8% when, in addition to the preceding combination, the proband's EEG also shows a photoconvulsive response and/or multifocal spikes (Hauser et al 1986b)

– 8% when both the proband and one parent have idiopathic epilepsy (10% when either or both have an EEG with generalized spike and wave)

– 12–15% for those tested siblings with generalized spike and wave when the proband also has a similar pattern.

It may be noted that the estimates for sibling risks generally will be lower than the families may have feared. With the exception of the rarer genetic syndromes, sibling risks seldom will exceed 10%, as compared with a population base rate of 1–2%.

Partial (localization related) epilepsies

The term 'partial' (or focal) can be applied either to seizure manifestations or to EEG findings. Some of the cases of focal epilepsy may result from a structural epileptogenic focus such as a scar or mass. Others, however, may be more closely related to the primary generalized epilepsies and syndromes, and may share a genetic predisposition (Metrakos & Metrakos 1970).

Bray & Wiser (1964, 1965) studied 40 probands with focal epilepsy whose EEGs showed paroxysmal sharp waves or spikes in the midtemporal area, either unilateral or bilateral. Pedigree analysis was reported to show transmission as an autosomal dominant trait, although the details are not presented (except for a note that in 12 of the families at least one close relative had seizures associated with a focal temporal central spike abnormality on the EEG).

From the clinical EEG descriptions, many of the cases studied by Bray & Wiser appear similar to those studied by Heijbel et al (1975). The probands in the latter study had seizures and also Rolandic discharges on the EEG recording. Among the siblings at each age level, one-third showed Rolandic discharges (Table 3.6). Of those with Rolandic discharges half had seizures. This category of patients often is described as 'benign epilepsy of childhood with centro-temporal EEG foci', and may represent a transition between generalized and partial (localization-related) epilepsies.

A larger series of 203 children with various

Table 3.6 Risk of epilepsy or any seizure in siblings of probands with partial (localization-related) epilepsy

Seizure type in proband	Siblings Total no.	With epilepsy	With any seizure
Benign childhood epilepsy with centro-temporal spikes		%	%
Heijbel et al (1975)	52		15.6
Morikawa et al (1979)	76	1.3	11.8
Partial seizures with focal sharp wave EEG			
Gerken (1977)	157		1.9
Surgically treated partial epilepsy (mostly temporal)			
Jensen (1975)	171	2.9	4.7
Andermann (1982)	229	1.3	4.8
Controls	458		(3.9)

forms of epilepsy were studied by Gerken et al (1977). They were selected for having shown focal sharp waves in the EEG (some in the Rolandic area) at least once. The sibling risk for seizures was considerably lower than in families of probands with spike-wave absences.

One of the most carefully studied series is based on 60 patients with focal cerebral seizures (mostly temporal) who underwent surgical treatment for their epilepsy (Andermann 1982). There was no significant increase in history of seizures among siblings as compared to control relatives (Table 3.6). There was, however, a significant increase in the prevalence of total EEG abnormalities. Upon review of the data, using stricter criteria for EEG classification, the frequency of generalized, but not focal, epileptiform EEG abnormalities was significantly elevated in the relatives of focal probands (Andermann & Straszak 1982).

A larger series of 74 patients who underwent unilateral temporal lobectomy for control of seizures was studied by Jensen (1975). Among 171 siblings there were 5 with epilepsy, and 8 with other convulsions, for a total of 13 (7.6%) with seizure history (Table 3.6). The claim is made that the epilepsy rate among siblings is five to six times higher than expected in the general population, but this most likely results from the improper use of population prevalence values.

Implications

The risk of seizures is about 15% for siblings of probands with benign childhood epilepsy with centro-temporal spikes. For other localization-related epilepsies the risk for siblings by the age of 40 appears to be somewhat higher than population rates, perhaps 3% for epilepsy and 5% for any seizure (excluding febrile). The data base needs considerable strengthening in this area.

Febrile Convulsions (FC)

Convulsions associated with febrile illness are one of the common acute neurological disturbances seen in childhood (Hauser 1981). In the United States one-third of the patients with one FC will experience a recurrence of febrile seizures. Furthermore, patients with febrile seizures have a three- to six-fold increase in the risk of epilepsy when compared with the general population. The detailed studies on FC have provided clear evidence for an increased risk for both FC and epilepsy among siblings of probands (Hauser et al 1985).

Several twin studies also have been reported. Lennox-Buchthal (1971) analysed the data for the twin series collected by W.G. Lennox and found 13 out of 19 pairs (68%) concordant for febrile convulsions. It was noted, however, that these twins had a higher proportion with a severely abnormal birth history and with subsequent epilepsy than did the population-based series studied by Frantzen et al (1970).

Schiøttz-Christiansen (1972) searched the records for twins born in the Copenhagen area from 1950 to 1965. The incidence of febrile convulsions among all twin-born individuals was estimated at 30%. There were 63 participating index pairs with at least one having febrile convulsions. Among the MZ pairs 8 out of 26 (31%) were concordant, while among the DZ pairs 5 out of 37 (14%) were concordant. The case-wise risk of febrile convulsions was 44% for monozygotic co-twins of probands and 20% for dizygotic co-twins. The MZ–DZ differences were not statistically significant, and the results have been cited as evidence against genetic factors. It seems more reasonable to conclude that the results were indefinite (because of the relatively small sample size) and that both genetic and non-genetic factors were involved. This interpretation is strengthened by Tsuboi's (1982) report of concordance rates of 46% (25/54) for MZ pairs and 13% (12/89) for DZ pairs in his study.

Hauser et al (1985) analysed the data for 1046 siblings of 421 FC probands in Rochester, Minnesota. The general population rate for FC was 2.4%; the sibling FC risk was 5.5% when neither parent had a history of FC, 21.7% when one parent had FC and 55.6% with both parents affected (Table 3.3). This effect of parental FC history is seen also in the two Japanese studies.

The Minnesota/Japan contrast for FC risk is sharpest in the families in which neither parent has had a history of FC (Table 3.3). When one or both parents are affected, the sibling risks are similar in the United States and Japan. It is possible that a large proportion of the Japanese cases might represent a dominant mode of inheritance, similar to that hypothesized earlier for the smaller Rochester subgroup.

With this question in mind, a further comparison is reported in Table 3.7 for the Rochester data (Rich, personal communication) and the Tokyo data (Tsuboi, personal communication). If

Table 3.7 Risk of febrile convulsions (FC) among siblings of probands

FC in parents(s)	Number of FCs in probands			Overall Sibling risk	Population rate
	1	2	3+		
Rochester				8.0%	2.4%
Yes	10.8%	22.7%	31.9%		
No	3.1%	8.4%	10.9%		
Tokyo				24.9%	6.7%
Yes	37.6%	36.7%	38.8%		
No	19.4%	21.5%	25.6%		

anything, this analysis tends to intensify the problem rather than to resolve it. If the Rochester/Tokyo differences arose from more Japanese FC probands having affected parents and/or more FC episodes, the sibling risks within comparable cells should have become more alike.

At this point we may consider the possibility that spike-wave EEG abnormalities are indeed more common in Japanese FC probands and that the GSW serves as an indicator of dominant inheritance. There are now reports from at least seven independent groups of investigators suggesting that generalized spike and wave (GSW) patterns occur with a high frequency in children with FC. Tsuboi (1982), Frantzen et al (1968), and Doose et al (1966) have done serial EEG recordings on children following FC. Between 25 and 40% of children have been reported to show GSW in these studies. None reports GSW at the time of FC. Thorn (1981) and Metrakos & Metrakos (1970) did EEG recordings following FC (not serial). They reported GSW in 35% of probands.

The most recent report is from Degen & Degen (1985) who noted GSW almost exclusively during prolonged sleep recording. For some subgroups (older patients, patients with multiple FC, patients with a family history), the frequency of GSW approached 80%. It is possible that such subgroups may represent a distinctive etiological category with a clearer mode of inheritance. The high frequency of GSW in FC probands led the Degens to suggest that FC represents a benign form of generalized epilepsy. It is of interest, however, that GSW has failed to be a predictor of subsequent epilepsy in FC probands thus far in the studies of Tsuboi (1982) and Frantzen et al (1968).

One further observation from the Rochester study deserves comment. The relative risk of epilepsy (Table 3.8) was the same for 967 siblings of probands with FC only (2.4) as for 552 siblings of probands with unprovoked seizures (2.5), but was twice as high for the 79 siblings of those probands who had FC followed by epilepsy (5). These results emphasize the complexity of the familial relationship between epilepsy and FC.

Implications

For the purposes of genetic counselling, the risk estimates in Tables 3.7 and 3.8 should be most helpful. The large sample sizes under study and the relatively high sibling risks make FC a very favourable category for more intensive genetic and epidemiological analysis. Furthermore, it should become possible to select specific subgroups for an evaluation of biochemical hypotheses for the genesis of FC.

Post-traumatic seizures

There is a persistent impression that individuals who have seizures following head trauma may do so because they have a genetic predisposition for seizures (Caveness et al 1979), but data to support this contention are scanty and contradictory. The proportion of cases with post-traumatic seizures was greater in patients with a family history of seizures in the studies of Caveness (1963) and Jennett (1975), but the difference was not significant in either study. Phillips (1954) reported a family history of epilepsy in 12.6% of patients with seizures following closed-head trauma. He concluded that this was no higher than expected among any group of epileptic patients, but

Table 3.8 Risk for febrile convulsions (FC) and unprovoked seizures in siblings of probands (Hauser et al 1985)

Proband seizure type	Total no. siblings	Sibling seizure type			
		Febrile		Unprovoked*	
		Observed	Relative[+] risk	Observed	Relative[+] risk
Febrile only	967	74 (7.7%)	3.5	28 (2.9%)	2.4
Unprovoked* only	552	25 (4.5%)	2.0	16 (2.9%)	2.5
Febrile followed by unprovoked*	79	9 (11.4%)	7.5	5 (6.3%)	5.0

* Single or recurrent unprovoked seizures
+ All relative risks are significantly greater than 1.0 (P <0.05)

presented no comparable information from the general population or from a head trauma cohort. Evans (1962) reported a family history of seizures in 7% of trauma patients with seizures, and in only 2% of trauma patients without seizures. In a follow-up study of 421 Vietnam veterans, a family history of epilepsy had no effect on seizure occurrence (Salazar et al 1985).

Several considerations may help to resolve these conflicting results. In patients with *severe* head injury, diffuse brain injury, and widespread tissue damage (such as that associated with gunshot wounds to the head) any additional risk imparted by genetic factors may be inconsequential. Genetic factors are more likely to be important in epilepsy that develops following *mild* head injury (Majkowski 1980). Furthermore, the mechanisms in early-onset seizures (within one week after trauma) are likely to be quite different from those in later onset (Potter 1978) and genetic factors are probably more important in later-onset seizures. The overall interpretation of the data should take into account the many examples of genetically-controlled responses to environmental stressors (Eaves 1982).

Variables that increase the presence and concentration of free iron in blood or brain may play an important role in the development of post-traumatic epilepsy. A number of studies have demonstrated that iron salts, or iron-containing proteins, cause significant tissue damage and can even be epileptogenic when injected into the brain (Willmore & Triggs 1984). These experiments may provide a model for events following injury, when iron greatly exacerbates central nervous system damage, in part by catalysing chemical reactions that produce and propagate toxic free radicals (Aust et al 1985). In view of this possible role of free iron in brain damage, it may be desirable to consider further experimental study of therapeutics to block this type of damage, e.g. iron chelators and/or calcium blockers (Nayini et al 1985, Deshpande & Wieloch 1986).

Genetic variation could affect plasma and tissue levels of iron (and hence susceptibility to tissue damage following trauma) in several ways (McKusick 1983). Idiopathic haemochromatosis (an autosomal recessive disorder) leads to a moderate elevation of tissue and plasma iron in heterozygous carriers and massive increases in homozygotes. In addition, ferritin (an iron-storage molecule) and transferrin (an iron-transport protein) are both under genetic control. Genetic variation in transferrin is associated with differences in response to toxic substance (Beckman 1985) and in reproductive outcome (Weitkamp & Schacter 1985). More direct evidence about the possible role of genetic variation as a component in seizure susceptibility has been obtained through data on haptoglobin (a haemoglobin-binding plasma protein). This point was discussed earlier as an example of the use of multiplex sibships.

Seizures following hemiplegia

Rimoin & Metrakos (1964) studied two groups of children with hemiplegia: 98 with a history of at least one convulsion and 60 with no history of convulsions. Among the parents of the former group, 2.6% had a history of convulsions and 15% had an epileptiform EEG. The comparable figures for the parents of the latter group were 1.5% and 3%. A similar difference was found for the siblings: in the first group, 5.6% of the siblings had a convulsion and 30% an epileptiform EEG, while in the latter group 3.6% had convulsions and 16% an epileptiform EEG. The results were interpreted as evidence for individual variation in seizure threshold which may be triggered by environmental stimuli, but heterogeneity in the etiological mechanisms leading to hemiplegia would be an alternative explanation.

Risks in offspring

It is difficult to obtain a satisfactory sample of children of probands for analysis. Ideally, the proband should have been identified a generation ago to permit following the offspring to an age reasonably through the risk period.

Tsuboi & Endo (1977) analysed their data about epilepsy and other seizures in children of probands from several points of view (Table 3.9). The results are comparable with those from other studies of children and follow the trends demonstrated for siblings.

1. The risk is higher when the probands had idiopathic (as compared with symptomatic) epilepsy.

Table 3.9 Risk of seizures among offspring of probands with epilepsy (from Tsuboi & Endo 1977)

Category	Offspring No.	Epilepsy %	FC* %	Total %
All Probands	506	2.4	6.7	9.1
Proband with:				
Idiopathic epilepsy	382	2.6	8.4	11.0
Symptomatic epilepsy	124	1.6	1.6	3.2
Sex of proband:				
Male	233	1.7	5.2	6.9
Female	273	2.9	8.1	11.0
Age of proband at onset:				
0–9 years	99	3.0	11.1	14.1
10–29 years	250	2.8	6.4	9.2
30 or older	157	1.3	4.4	5.7
Proband with affected Parent of sibling				
Yes	55			21.8
No	451			7.5
EEG in offspring				
Generalized spike/wave	38			28.9
No specific anomaly	64			4.7

* FC = febrile convulsion

Table 3.10 Risk of epilepsy or febrile convulsions in offspring of probands with epilepsy

Study, seizure type in proband	Total No. offspring	With epilepsy %	With FC %
Tsuboi & Christian (1973)	275	4.4	
Annegers et al (1978)	687	1.9	2.6
Janz & Beck-Mannagetta (1982) Beck-Mannagetta & Janz (1982)	768	3.4	4.7
Tsuboi & Okada (1985)			
Any epilepsy	817	2.4	8.4
Awaking grand mal	208	4.8	11.1
Grand mal during sleep	157	2.0	2.0
Diffuse grand mal	64	6.3	1.6
Myoclonic petit mal	27	14.8	7.4
Absence	30	6.7	10.0
Psychomotor epilepsy	156	0.6	5.1
focal seizure	28	0	3.6

2. The risk is higher for children of affected mothers than for children of affected fathers.
3. The risk is higher when the proband developed epilepsy at younger age.
4. The risk is higher when the proband has an affected parent or sibling.
5. Finally, the risk of seizures is considerably higher for those children who themselves showed a specific EEG abnormality.

An important study in progress in Berlin is beginning to yield information about offspring of epileptic probands (Janz & Beck-Mannagetta 1982, Beck-Mannagetta & Janz 1982). The Rochester, Minnesota, data have also been studied from this perspective (Annegers et al 1978). These studies are compared with more recent data from Tsuboi (1985) in Table 3.10.

The cumulative risks up to the age of 40 for children of probands (with onset of idiopathic epilepsy before the age of 15) in the Rochester, Minnesota, study (Annegers et al 1982) were 10.6% for epilepsy and 14.3% for any seizure (Fig. 3.1). The rates are based on small numbers but they do incorporate an appropriate age adjustment. The restriction to early onset idiopathic epilepsy in the probands also helps to explain these higher rates, as compared with the 1.9% and 2.6% in Table 3.10.

A further point of concern involves those children (of an epileptic proband) who develop febrile convulsions. If we pool the results of two studies (Janz & Beck-Mannagetta 1982, Annegers et al 1978), there were 45 offspring with FC, 7 of which (15.6%) developed epilepsy.

Implications

In most studies, children have not been followed far into adulthood. Hence the available data underestimate the risks, unless appropriate age corrections are used. The risks for children appear to be the same as, or higher than, those for siblings. The data in Tables 3.9 and 3.10 provide reasonable guides for genetic counselling, except that the Japanese risks for febrile convulsions must be reduced for use elsewhere. The risks are sharply higher if the proband has an affected parent or sibling, or if the child has a generalized spike and wave EEG pattern or develops febrile convulsions.

Effects of antiepileptic drugs on the fetus

In the process of providing genetic counselling for women with epilepsy, it is important to consider the possibility that a fetus may be affected by genetic factors associated with the mother's predisposition for seizures or by the antiepileptic drugs that she may be taking. In the Rochester, Minnesota, population-based study the rate of major malformations was 2.4% for children born to mothers with epilepsy not taking antiepileptic drugs during pregnancy, 10.7% for children of mothers who took antiepileptic drugs during pregnancy and 3.8% among the children of men with epilepsy (Annegers et al 1978). In a retrospective study at the Montreal Neurological Hospital, the proportion of viable offspring having major congenital malformations was 15.9% for mothers taking antiepileptic medication, as compared with 6.5% for mothers not taking medication (Dansky et al 1982).

There is evidence that genetic variation in the fetus may affect teratogenic expression. In a dizygotic female pair (Loughnan et al 1973), one twin had a pulmonary atresia with patent ductus arteriosus, while the other was apparently unaffected. In fraternal triplets (one male and two female), all showed malformation, but with considerable variability in extent (Bustamante & Stumpff 1978). In the case of 3-year-old dizygotic twin girls (who may have been fathered by two men of different race), one had a variety of malformations, while the other showed only poor growth and a broad depressed nasal bridge (Phelan et al 1982). Furthermore, fetal genetic variation in epoxide hydralase may affect susceptibility to phenytoin-influenced birth defects (Buehler & Delimont 1985, Strickler et al 1985).

While there seems to be a high correlation between exposure to antiepileptic drugs in utero and malformations, patients taking these drugs during pregnancy may be different from those not

on such medication. Thus, one could not exclude the possibility that the effect could be due in part to the presence of epilepsy in the mother rather than to the antiepileptic drugs (see also Janz 1982, Annegers et al 1983).

Finnell (1981) studied mice of several inbred strains and also an autosomal recessive locus that produces a spontaneous clonic seizure disorder. The occurrence of fetal defects was correlated with maternal serum concentrations of phenytoin, but not with the maternal or fetal genotype or the presence of a seizure disorder. The maternal serum phenytoin level and not the maternal seizure disorder appears to be the agent responsible for the malformations (Finnell & Chernoff 1982).

Implications

It is beyond the scope of this chapter to review the literature about possible teratogenic effects of the various antiepileptic drugs (the subject is dealt with in more detail in Chapter 15, pages 547–551). In general, genetic counselling for epileptic women should consider three points:

1. In most types of epilepsy, the risks for epilepsy or other seizures are higher for offspring of female than of male epilepsy patients (Ottman et al 1985).
2. The possible teratogenic effects of antiepileptic drugs should be discussed, using the best available information.
3. As new evidence emerges, fetal genetic variation in response to tetragenic agents can be considered.

The clinician as researcher

In epilepsy clinics, the research possibilities would be enhanced by attention to certain aspects of the family history.

1. We would urge that such clinics keep a running record of those families in which two or more siblings have seizures. These multisib families would provide an excellent panel for extensive biochemical, clinical or other laboratory studies.
2. A similar record should be maintained for

patients who are twin-born. Both concordant and discordant pairs can be very useful, although for different questions. In the near future we would envisage that twin studies might focus on specific rare clinical patterns. In such an event it would be extremely important and necessary to have a basis for collaboration among various institutions.

3. We would also urge that special note be made of families in which a number of individuals have a seizure history. Kindreds with five or more affected persons can be reviewed to determine which are likely to be informative for linkage studies.

FUTURE PROSPECTS

The many new strategies being developed for analysing brain structure and function will permit a much clearer description of individual variation in underlying pathology among epilepsy patients. With the use of molecular techniques for assessing neurotransmitters and membrane receptors, family studies will become more informative. Specific biochemical genetic hypotheses can be framed and tested more explicitly. To this end it is fortunate that large, carefully documented series of epilepsy families are already available for exploration.

New genetic methods include more sophisticated computer programs for complex segregation analysis and multipoint linkage analysis, a rapidly expanding array of genetic probes for gene mapping and recombinant DNA techniques for studying genetic codes and transcription. This broad range of methodologies will continue to be essential in order to bridge clinical and experimental studies. Finally, all of these efforts will be integrated by pursuing the fundamental questions of genetic heterogeneity, genotype-to-phenotype pathways, genotype–environment interaction and gene structure and function.

REFERENCES

Andermann E 1982 Multifactorial inheritance of generalized and focal epilepsy. In: Anderson V E, Hauser W A, Penry J K, Sing C F (eds) Genetic basis of the epilepsies. Raven Press, New York, pp 355–374

Andermann E 1985 Genetic aspects of the epilepsies. In: Sakai T, Tsuboi T (eds) Genetic aspects of human behavior. Igaku-Shoin, Tokyo, pp 129–145

Andermann E, Straszak M 1982 Family studies of epileptiform EEG abnormalities and photosensitivity in focal epilepsy. In: Akimoto H, Kazamatsuri H, Seino M, Ward A (eds) Advances in epileptology:. XIII Epilepsy International Symposium, pp 105–112

Anderson V E, Hauser W A 1985 The genetics of epilepsy. In: Bearn A G, Motulsky A G, Childs B (eds) Progress in medical genetics. Genetics of Neurological Disorders 6: 9–52

Anderson V E, Hauser W A, Penry J K, Sing C F (eds) 1982 Genetic basis of the epilepsies. Raven Press, New York

Anderson V E, Hauser W A, Rich S S 1986 Genetic heterogeneity in the epilepsies. In: Delgado-Escueta A V, Ward A A Jr, Woodbury D M, Porter R J (eds) Advances in Neurology 44: 59–75

Annegers J F, Hauser W A 1984 Epidemiologic measures of occurrence and association for the study of convulsive disorders. In: Porter R J, Mattson R H, Ward A A Jr, Dam M (eds) Advances in epileptology: XVth Epilepsy International Symposium. Raven Press, New York, pp 521–529

Annegers J F, Hauser W A, Anderson V E 1982 Risk of seizures among relatives of patients with epilepsy: families in a defined population. In: Anderson V E, Hauser W A, Penry J K, Sing C F (eds) Genetic basis of the epilepsies. Raven Press, New York, pp 151–159

Annegers J F, Hauser W A, Elveback L R, Anderson V E, Kurland L T 1978 Congenital malformations and seizure disorders in the offspring of parents with epilepsy. International Journal of Epidemiology 7: 241–247

Annegers J F, Kurland L T, Hauser W A 1983 Teratogenicity of anticonvulsant drugs. In: Ward A A Jr, Penry J K, Purpura D (eds) Epilepsy. Raven Press, New York, pp 239–248

Aust S D, Morehouse L A, Thomas C E 1985 Role of metals in oxygen radical reactions. Journal of Free Radicals in Biology and Medicine 1: 3–25

Baier W K, Doose H 1985 Petit mal-absences of childhood onset: familial prevalences of migraine and seizures. Neuropediatrics 16: 80–83

Baraitser M 1982 The genetics of neurological disorders. Oxford University Press, New York

Beckman L, Beckman G, Cedargren B, Göransson K, Hallqvist E-B, Sikström C 1985 Transferrin C subtypes and occupational photodermatosis of the face. Human Heredity 35: 89–94

Beck-Mannagetta G, Janz D 1982 Febrile convulsions in offspring of epileptic probands. In: Anderson V E, Hauser W A, Penry J K, Sing C F (eds) Genetic basis of the epilepsies. Raven Press, New York, pp 145–150

Bjerre I, Corelius E 1968 Benign familial neonatal convulsions. Acta Paediatrica Scandinavica 57: 557–561

Blume W T 1982 Some seizure disorders affecting neonates and children. In: Anderson V E, Hauser W A, Penry J K, Sing C F (eds) Genetic basis of the epilepsies. Raven Press, New York, pp 35–48

Bonhaus D W, Laird H, Mimaki T, Yamamura H F, Huxtable R J 1983 Possible bases for the anticonvulsant action of taurine. Progress in Clinical and Biological Research 125: 195–209

Bonhaus D W, Lippincott S E, Huxtable R J 1984 Subcellular distribution of neuroactive amino acids in brains of genetically epileptic rats. Epilepsia 25: 564–568

Bray P F, Wiser W C 1964 Evidence for a genetic etiology of temporal-central abnormalities in focal epilepsy. New England Journal of Medicine 271: 926–933

Bray P F, Wiser W C 1965 Hereditary characteristics of familial temporal-central focal epilepsy. Pediatrics 36: 207–211

Breakefield X O, Pintar J E 1981 The use of cell culture to analyze the genetic basis of neurologic disease. In: Gershon E S, Matthysse S, Breakefield X O, Ciaranello R D (eds) Genetic research strategies for psychology and psychiatry. Boxwood Press, New York, pp 407–422

Buehler B A, Delimont D 1985 Epoxide hydralase activity: a direct assay for prediction of potential dilantin teratogenesis (abstract). Proceedings of the Greenwood Genetic Center 4:92–93

Bundey S, Evans K 1969 Tuberous sclerosis: a genetic study. Journal of Neurology, Neurosurgery and Psychiatry 32: 591–603

Bustamante S A, Stumpff L C 1978 Fetal hydantoin syndrome in triplets. American Journal of Diseases of Children 132: 978–979

Campostrini R, Zaccara G, Rossi L, Paganini M, Dorigotti A, Zappoli R 1985 Valproate-induced hyperammonaemia in two epileptic identical twins. Journal of Neurology 232: 167–168.

Carey J C, Laub J M, Hall B D 1979 Penetrance and variability in neurofibromatosis: a genetic study of 60 families. Birth Defects: Original articles series 15 (5B): 271–281.

Cavazzuti G B, Cappella L, Nalin A 1980 Longitudinal study of epileptiform EEG patterns in normal children. Epilepsia 21: 43–55

Caveness W F 1963 Onset and cessation of fits following craniocerebral trauma. Journal of Neurosurgery 20: 570–582

Caveness W F, Meirowsky A M, Rish B L et al 1979 The nature of posttraumatic epilepsy. Journal of Neurosurgery 50: 545–553

Cazzullo C L, Canger R 1979 HLA and epilepsy (abstract). Epilepsia 20:179

Charlton M H, Mellinger J F 1970 Infantile spasms and hypsarrhythmia. Electroencephalography and Clinical Neurophysiology 29:413

Connor J M, Ferguson-Smith M A 1984 Essential medical genetics. Blackwell Scientific, Oxford

Crabbe J C, Kosobud A, Young E R, Janowsky J S 1983 Polygenic and single gene determination of responses to ethanol in BXD/Ty recombinant inbred mouse strains. Neurobehavioral Toxicology and Teratology 5: 181–187

Dansky L, Andermann E, Andermann F 1982 Major congenital malformations in the offspring of epileptic patients: Genetic and environmental risk factors. In: Janz D, Dam M, Richens A, Bossi L, Helge H, Schmidt D (eds) Epilepsy, pregnancy, and the child. Raven Press, New York, pp 223–233

Darby J K, Feder J, Selby M et al 1985 A discordant sibship analysis between β-NGF and neurofibromatosis. American Journal of Human Genetics 37: 52–59

Degen R, Degen H 1985 The sleep EEG in children suffering from febrile seizures: therapeutical and theoretical consequences. Paper presented at the 16th Epilepsy International Congress, Hamburg, September 6–9, 1985

Delgado-Escueta A V, Greenberg D 1984 The search for epilepsies ideal for clinical and molecular genetic studies. Annals of Neurology 16 (suppl): S1–S11

Delgado-Escueta A V, Treiman D M, Enrile-Bacsal F 1982 Phenotypic variations of seizures in adolescents and adults. In: Anderson V E, Hauser W A, Penry J K, Sing C F (eds) Genetic basis of the epilepsies. Raven Press, New York, pp 49–81

Delgado-Escueta A V, Ward A A Jr, Woodbury D M, Porter R J (eds) 1986 Advances in Neurology 44

Del Guidice E, Striano S, Andria G 1983 Electroencephalographic abnormalities in homocystinuria due to cystathionine synthase deficiency. Clinical Neurology and Neurosurgery 85: 165–168

Deshpande J K, Wieloch T 1986 Flunarizine, a calcium entry blocker, ameliorates ischemic brain damage in the rat. Anesthesiology 64: 215–224

Doose H 1981 Genetic aspects of the epilepsies. Folia Psychiatrica et Neurologica Japonica 35: 231–242

Doose H 1985 Myoclonic astatic epilepsy of early childhood. In: Roger J, Dravet C, Bureau M, Dreifuss F E, Wolf P (eds) Epileptic syndromes in infancy, childhood and adolescence. John Libbey Eurotext London, pp 78–88

Doose H, Baier W, Reinsberg E 1984 Genetic heterogeneity of spike-wave epilepsies. In: Porter R J, Mattson R H, Ward A A Jr, Dam M (eds) Advances in epileptology: XVth Epilepsy International Symposium. Raven Press, New York, pp 515–519

Doose H, Gerken H, Hein-Völpel K F, Völzke E 1969 Genetics of photosensitive epilepsy. Neuropädiatrie 1: 56–73

Doose H, Gerken H, Horstmann T, Völzke E 1973 Genetic factors in spike-wave absences. Epilepsia 14: 57–75

Doose H, Gerken H, Kiefer R, Völzke E 1977 Genetic factors in childhood epilepsy with focal sharp waves. II. EEG findings in patients and siblings. Neuropädiatrie 8: 10–20

Doose H, Gundel A 1982 Rhythms of 4 to 7 CPS in the childhood EEG. In: Anderson V E, Hauser W A, Penry J K, Sing C F (eds) Genetic basis of the epilepsies. Raven Press, New York, pp 83–91

Doose H, Völzke E, Peterson C E, Herzberger E 1966 Fieberkrämpfe und epilepsie II. Elektrencephalographische Verlaufsuntersuchungen bei sogenannten Fieber-oder Infektkrämpfen. Archiv für Psychiatrie und Nervenkrankheiten 208: 413–432

Dreifuss F E, Martinez-Lage M, Roger J, Seino M, Wolf P, Dam M 1985 Proposal for classification of epilepsies and epilepsy syndromes. Epilepsia 26: 268–278

Eaves L J 1982 The utility of twins. In: Anderson V E, Hauser W A, Penry J K, Sing C F (eds) Genetic basis of the epilepsies. Raven Press, New York, pp 249–276

Eeg-Olofsson O, Bäckman E, Säfwenberg J 1984a HLA and immunoglobins in children with febrile seizures and their families. In: Porter R J, Mattson R H, Ward A A Jr, Dam M (eds) Advances in epileptology: XVth Epilepsy International Symposium. Raven Press, New York, pp 395–399

Eeg-Olofsson O, Janjua N A, Andermann E, Guttmann R D 1984b Immunoglobulins and HLA in primary generalized corticoreticular epilepsy. In: Porter R J, Mattson R H, Ward A A Jr, Dam M (eds) Advances in epileptology: XVth Epilepsy International Symposium. Raven Press, New York, pp 63–67

Eeg-Olofsson O, Petersen I, Sellden U 1970 The development of the electroencephalogram in normal children from the age of 1 through 15 years. Neuropädiatrie 2: 375–404

Eeg-Olofsson O, Säfwenberg J, Wigertz A 1982 HLA and epilepsy: an investigation of different types of epilepsy in children and their families. Epilepsia 23: 27–34

Eisner V, Pauli L L, Livingston S 1959 Hereditary aspects of epilepsy. Johns Hopkins Hospital Bulletin 105: 245–271

Evans J H 1962 Post traumatic epilepsy. Neurology 12: 665–674

Fariello R G, Golden G T, McNeal R B 1985 Taurine and related amino acids in seizure disorders: current controversies. Progress in Clinical and Biological Research 179: 413–424

Fichsel H, Kessler M 1982 HLA in primary generalized and partial epilepsies. In: Akimoto H, Kazamatsuri H, Seino M, Ward A (eds) Advances in epileptology: XIIIth Epilepsy International Symposium. Raven Press, New York, pp 91–92

Finnell R H 1981 Phenytoin-induced teratogenesis: a mouse model. Science 211: 483–484

Finnell R H, Chernoff G F 1982 Mouse fetal hydantoin syndrome: effects of maternal seizures. Epilepsia 23: 423–429

Frantzen E, Lennox-Buchthal M, Nygaard A 1968 Longitudinal EEG and clinical study of children with febrile convulsions. Electroencephalography and Clinical Neurophysiology 24: 197–212

Frantzen E, Lennox-Buchthal M, Nygaard A, Stene J 1970 A genetic study of febrile convulsions. Neurology 20: 909–917

Fraser Roberts J A, Pembrey M E 1985 An introduction to medical genetics. 8th edn. Oxford University Press, Oxford

Freed W J 1985 Selective inhibition of homocysteine-induced seizures by glutamic acid diethyl ester and other glutamate esters. Epilepsia 26: 30–36

Fuhrmann W, Vogel F 1983 Genetic Counselling. 3rd edn. Springer-Verlag, New York

Fukuyama Y, Kagawa K, Tanaka K 1979 A genetic study of febrile convulsions. European Neurology 18: 166–182

Gastaut H 1964 A proposed international classification of epileptic seizures. Epilepsia 5: 297–306

Gerken H, Kiefer R, Doose H, Völzke E 1977 Genetic factors in childhood epilepsy with focal sharp waves. I: Clinical data and familial morbidity for seizures. Neuropädiatrie 8: 3–9

Giacoia G P 1982 Benign familial neonatal convulsions. Southern Medical Journal 75: 629–630

Gloor P 1968 Generalized cortico-reticular epilepsies. Epilepsia 9:249

Goodman H O, Connolly B M 1982 Taurine transport alleles: dissecting a polygenic complex. In: Anderson V E, Hauser W A, Penry J K, Sing C E (eds) Genetic basis of the epilepsies. Raven Press, New York, pp 171–180

Gusella J F, Tanzi R E, Bader P I et al 1985 Deletion of Huntington's disease-linked G8 (D4S10) locus in Wolf-Hirschhorn Syndrome. Nature 318: 75–78

Gusella J F, Wexler N S, Conneally P M et al 1983 A polymorphic DNA marker genetically linked to Huntington's disease. Nature 306: 234–238

Hafez M, Nagaty M, Saied E 1985 HLA antigens and idiopathic epilepsy. Epilepsia 26: 15–18

Haines J L, Panter S S, Rich S S, Eaton J W, Tsai M Y, Anderson V E 1986 Reduced plasma haptoglobin and urinary taurine in familial seizures identified through the multisib strategy. American Journal of Medical Genetics, 24: 723–734

Håkanson R, Thorell J (eds) 1985 Biogenetics of neurohormonal peptides. Academic Press, London

Harper P S 1985 The genetics of muscular dystrophies. In: Bearn A G, Motulsky A G, Childs B (eds) Genetics of neurological disorders. Progress in Medical Genetics 6: 53–90

Harvald B, Hauge M 1965 Hereditary factors elucidated by twin studies. In: Neel J V, Shaw M W, Schull W J (eds) Genetics and the epidemiology of chronic diseases. Public Health Service Publication No 1163, pp 61–76

Hauser W A 1981 The natural history of febrile seizures. In: Nelson K B, Ellenberg J H (eds) Febrile seizures. Raven Press, New York, pp 5–17

Hauser W A, Anderson V E, Loewenson R B, McRoberts S M 1982 Seizure recurrence after a first unprovoked seizure. New England Journal of Medicine 307: 522–528

Hauser W A, Annegers J F, Anderson V E 1983 Epidemiology and the genetics of epilepsy. In: Ward A A Jr, Penry J K, Purpura D (eds) Epilepsy. Raven Press, New York, pp 267–292

Hauser W A, Annegers J F, Anderson V E, Kurland L T 1985 The risk of seizure disorders among relatives of children with febrile convulsions. Neurology 35: 1268–1273

Hauser W A, Morris M L, Anderson V E, Heston L L 1986a Seizures and myoclonus in patients with Alzheimer Disease. Neurology 36: 1226–1230

Hauser W A, Rich S S, Anderson V E 1986b EEG patterns and sibling risk in epilepsy. Submitted for publication

Hay D A 1985 Essentials of behaviour genetics. Blackwell Scientific, Melbourne

Heijbel J, Blom S, Rasmuson M 1975 Benign epilepsy of childhood with centrotemporal EEG foci: a genetic study. Epilepsia 16: 285–293

Hrubec Z, Robinette C D 1984 The study of human twins in medical research. New England Journal of Medicine 310: 435–441

Hunt A, Lindenbaum R 1984 Tuberous sclerosis: a new estimate of prevalence within the Oxford region. Journal of Medical Genetics 21: 272–277

Inouye E 1960 Observations on forty twin cases with chronic epilepsy and their co-twins. Journal of Nervous and Mental Disease 130: 401–416

Ionasescu V, Zellweger H 1983 Genetics in neurology. Raven Press, New York

Janz D 1982 Antiepileptic drugs and pregnancy: altered utilization patterns and teratogenesis. Epilepsia 23 (suppl 1): S53–S63

Janz D, Beck-Mannagetta G 1982 Epilepsy and neonatal seizures in the offspring of parents with epilepsy. In: Anderson V E, Hauser W A, Penry J K, Sing C E (eds) Genetic basis of the epilepsies. Raven Press, New York, pp 135–143

Jennett B 1975 Epilepsy after non-missile head injuries. Heinemann, Chicago

Jennings M T, Bird J D 1981 Genetic influences in the epilepsies. Review of the literature with practical implications. American Journal of Diseases of Children 135: 450–457

Jensen I 1975 Genetic factors in temporal lobe epilepsy. Acta Neurologica Scandinavica 52: 381–394

Kaplan R E, Lacey D J 1983 Benign familial neonatal-infantile seizures. American Journal of Medical Genetics 16: 595–599

Kaufman D L, Tobin A J 1984 Prospects for the isolation of genes for receptors and other proteins of pharmacological and neurobiological interest. In: Harrison L C, Venter J C (eds) Molecular and chemical characterization of membrane receptors. Alan R. Liss, New York, pp 241–259

Kellaway P 1982 Maturational and biorhythmic changes in the electroencephalogram. In: Anderson V E, Hauser W A, Henry J K, Sing C E (eds) Genetic basis of the epilepsies. Raven Press, New York, pp 21–33

Klingler D, Wessely P 1977 Influence of alcohol on photomyoclonic and photoconvulsive responses. Electroencephalography and Clinical Neurophysiology 43: 272–273

Lalouel J M, Rao D C, Morton N E, Elston R C 1983 A unified model for complex segregation analysis. American Journal of Human Genetics 35: 816–826

Lathrop G M, Lalouel J M, Julier C, Ott J 1984 Strategies for multilocus linkage analysis in humans. Proceedings of the National Academy of Sciences 81: 3443–3446

Lennox W G, Lennox M A 1960 Epilepsy and related disorders. Little Brown, Boston

Lennox-Buchthal M 1971 Febrile and nocturnal convulsions in monozygotic twins. Epilepsia 12: 147–156

Löscher W, Meldrum B S 1984 Evaluation of anticonvulsant drugs in genetic animal models of epilepsy. Federation Proceedings 43: 276–284

Loughnan P M, Gold H, Vance J C 1973 Phenytoin teratogenicity in man. Lancet 1: 70–72

MacGillivray R C 1967 Epilepsy in Down's anomaly. Journal of Mental Deficiency Research 11: 43–48

McKusick V A 1983 Mendelian inheritance in man. 6th edn. Johns Hopkins University Press, Baltimore

Majkowski J 1980 Posttraumatic epilepsy: risk factors, familial susceptibility, and pharmacologic prophylaxis. In: Canger R, Angeleri F, Penry J K (eds) Advances in epileptology: XI Epilepsy International Symposium, pp 323–329

Maraschio P, Zuffardi O, Bernardi F et al 1981 Preferential maternal derivation in inv dup (15). Analysis of eight new cases. Human Genetics 59: 345–350

Matthes A 1969 Genetic studies in epilepsy. In: Gastaut H, Jasper H, Bancaud J, Waltregny A (eds) Charles C. Thomas, Springfield, Illinois, pp 26–35

Metrakos J D, Metrakos K 1966 Childhood epilepsy of subcortical ('centrencephalic') origin. Clinical Pediatrics 5: 536–542

Metrakos J D, Metrakos K 1970 Genetic factors in epilepsy. Modern problems of Pharmacopsychiatry 4: 71–86

Metrakos K, Metrakos J D 1961 Genetics of convulsive disorders II. Genetic and electroencephalographic studies in centrencephalic epilepsy. Neurology 11: 474–483

Metrakos K, Metrakos J D 1974 Genetics of epilepsy. In: Magnus O, Lorentz de Haas A M (eds) Handbook of Clinical Neurology Vol 15. The epilepsies. North-Holland Publishing, Amsterdam, pp 429–439

Moll P P, Berry T D, Weidman W H, Ellefson R, Gordon H, Kottke B A 1983 Detection of genetic heterogeneity among pedigrees through complex segregation analysis: an application to hypercholesterolemia. American Journal of Human Genetics 35: 197–211

Monaghan H P, O'Sullivan M, O'Donohoe N V 1982 HLA antigens and cryptogenic myoclonic epilepsy. Irish Journal of Medical Science 151/6: 188–189

Morikawa T, Osawa T, Ishihara O, Seino M 1979 A reappraisal of 'benign epilepsy of children with centrotemporal EEG foci.' Brain and Development 1: 257–265

Mudd S H, Skovby F, Levy H L et al 1985 The natural history of homocystinuria due to cystathionine β-synthase deficiency. American Journal of Human Genetics 37: 1–31

Myrianthopoulos N C 1981 Neurogenetic directory, Part I. In: Vinken P J, Bruyn G W (eds) Handbook of Clinical Neurology Vol 42. North-Holland Publishing, Amsterdam, pp 667–719

Nayini N R, White B C, Aust S D et al 1985 Post resuscitation iron delocalization and malondialdehyde production in the brain following prolonged cardiac arrest. Journal of Free Radicals in Biology and Medicine 1: 111–116

Noebels J L 1985 Tracing the cellular expression of neuromodulatory genes. Trends in Neurosciences 8: 327–331

Norio R, Koskiniemi M 1979 Progressive myoclonus epilepsy: genetic and nosological aspects with special reference to 107 Finnish patients. Clinical Genetics 15: 382–398

Olsen R W, Wamsley J K, Lee R, Lomax P 1984 Alterations in the benzodiazepine/GABA receptor-chloride ion channel complex in the seizure-sensitive Mongolian gerbil. In: Fariello R G, Lloyd K G, Morselli P L, Quesney L F, Engle J Jr (eds) Neurotransmitters, seizures, and epilepsy, II. Raven Press, New York, pp 201–213

Oppenheimer E Y, Rosman N P, Dooling E C 1985 The late appearance of hypopigmented maculae in tuberous sclerosis. American Journal of Diseases of Children 139: 408–409

Ott J 1985 Analysis of human genetic linkage. The Johns Hopkins University Press, Baltimore.

Ottman R, Hauser W A, Susser M 1985 Genetic and maternal influences on susceptibility seizures. American Journal of Human Genetics 122: 923–939

Pampiglione G, Pugh E 1975 Infantile spasms and subsequent appearance of tuberous sclerosis syndrome. Lancet 2:1046 .

Panter S S, Sadrzadeh S M H, Hallaway P E, Haines J, Anderson V E, Eaton J W 1985 Hypohaptoglobinemia: association with familial epilepsy. Journal of Experimental Medicine 161: 748–754

Penfield W, Jasper H H 1954 Epilepsy and the functional anatomy of the human brain. Little Brown, Boston

Phelan M C, Pellock J M, Nance W E 1982 Discordant expression of fetal hydantoin syndrome in heteropaternal dizygotic twins. New England Journal of Medicine 307: 99–101

Phillips G 1954 Traumatic epilepsy after closed head injury. Journal of Neurology, Neurosurgery, and Psychiatry 17: 1–10

Potter J M 1978 The personal factor in the maturation of epileptogenic brain scars: review and hypothesis. Journal of Neurology, Neurosurgery, and Psychiatry 41: 265–271

Quattlebaum T G 1979 Benign familial convulsions in the neonatal period and early infancy. Journal of Pediatrics 95: 257–259

Rabending G, Klepel H 1970 Fotokonvulsivreaktion und Fotomyoklonus: Altersabhängige genetisch determinierte Varianten der gesteigerten Fotosensibilität. Neuropädiatrie 2: 164–172

Reed S C 1980 Counselling in medical genetics. 3rd edn. Alan R. Liss, New York

Rett A, Teubel R 1964 Neugeborenenkrämpfe im Rahmen einer epileptisch belasteten Familie. Weiner Klinische Wochenschrift 76: 609–613

Riccardi V M 1981 Von Recklinghausen neurofibromatosis. New England Journal of Medicine 305: 1617–1627

Riccardi V M 1984 Neurofibromatosis heterogeneity. Journal of the American Academy of Dermatology 10: 518–519

Rich S S 1985 Personal communication

Rich S S, Annegers J F, Hauser W A, Anderson V E 1986 Complex segregation analysis of febrile convulsions. American Journal of Human Genetics (in press)

Rimoin D L, Metrakos J D 1964 The genetics of convulsive disorders in the families of hemiplegics. Proceedings of the 2nd International Congress of Human Genetics 3: 1655–1658

Rivas M L 1983 Genetic analyses of petit mal epilepsy: I. Evaluation of HLA, blood groups, serum proteins, and red cell enzymes (abstract). Epilepsia 24:115

Rosenberg M B, Hansen C Jr, Breakefield X O 1985 Molecular genetic approaches to neurologic and psychiatric diseases. Progress in Neurobiology 24: 95–140

Rosenberg R N 1985 Neurogenetics: principles and practice. Raven Press, New York

Rosing H S, Hopkins L C, Wallace D C, Epstein C M, Weidenheim K 1985 Maternally inherited mitochondrial myopathy and myoclonic epilepsy. Annals of Neurology 17: 228–237

Sakai T, Tsuboi T (eds) 1985 Genetic aspects of human behavior. Igaku-Shoin, Tokyo

Salazar A M, Bahman J, Vance S C, Grafman J, Amin D, Dillon J D 1985 Epilepsy after penetrating head injury. I. Clinical correlates: a report of the Vietnam Head Injury Study. Neurology 35: 1406–1414

Schiøttz-Christensen E 1972 Genetic factors in febrile convulsions. Acta Neurologica Scandinavica 48:538–546

Schmidt R, Eviatar L, Nitowsky H M, Wong M, Miranda S 1981 Ring chromosome 14: a distinct clinical entity. Journal of Medical Genetics 18: 304–307

Schmitt F O, Bird -S J, Bloom F E (eds) 1982 Molecular genetic neuroscience. Raven Press, New York

Schreck R R, Breg W R, Erlanger B F, Miller O J 1977 Preferential derivation of abnormal human G-group-like chromosomes from chromosome 15. Human Genetics 36: 1–12

Schuman S H, Miller L J 1966 Febrile convulsions in families: findings in an epidemiologic survey. Clinical Pediatrics 5: 604–608

Schwarz S S Freed W J 1985 Inhibition of quisqualate-induced seizures by glutamic acid diethyl ester and antiepileptic drugs (abstract). Epilepsia 26:250

Seyfried T N, Glaser G H 1985 A review of mouse mutants as genetic models of epilepsy. Epilepsia 26: 143–150

Sing C F 1983 Personal communication

Smeraldi E, Smeraldi R, Cazzullo C L, Cazzullo A, Fabio G, Canger R 1975 Immunogenetics of the Lennox-Gastaut syndrome. Frequency of HLA antigens and haplotypes in patients and first-degree relatives. Epilepsia 16: 699–703

Smith C 1970 Heritability of liability and concordance in monozygous twins. Annals of Human Genetics 34: 85–91

Strickler S M, Dansky L V, Miller M A, Seni M-H, Andermann E, Spielberg S P 1985 Genetic predisposition to phenytoin-induced birth defects. Lancet 2: 746–749

Tangye S R 1979 The EEG and incidence of epilepsy in Down's syndrome. Journal of Mental Deficiency Research 23: 17–24

Thompson J S, Thompson M W 1986 Genetics in medicine. 4th edn. W B Saunders, Philadelphia

Thorn I 1981 Prevention of recurrent febrile seizures: intermittent prophylaxis with diazepam compared with continuous treatment with phenobarbital. In: Nelson K B, Ellenberg J H (eds) Febrile seizures. Raven Press, New York, pp 119–126

Tsuboi T 1982 Febrile convulsions. In: Anderson V E, Hauser W A, Penry J K, Sing C E (eds) Genetic basis of the epilepsies. Raven Press, New York, pp 123–134

Tsuboi T 1984 Epidemiology of febrile and afebrile convulsions in children in Japan. Neurology 34: 175–181

Tsuboi T 1985 Personal communication

Tsuboi T, Christian W 1973 On the genetics of the primary generalized epilepsy with sporadic myoclonias of impulsive petit mal type. A clinical and electroencephalographic study of 399 probands. Humangenetik 19: 155–182

Tsuboi T, Endo S 1977 Incidence of seizures and EEG abnormalities among offspring of epileptic patients. Human Genetics 36: 173–189

Tsuboi T, Okada S 1985 The genetics of epilepsy. In: Sakai T, Tsuboi T (eds) Genetic aspects of human behavior. Igaku-Shoin, Tokyo, pp. 113–127

Van den Berg B J 1974 Studies on convulsive disorders in young children. IV: Incidence of convulsions among siblings. Developmental Medicine and Child Neurology 16: 457–464

Veall R M 1974 The prevalence of epilepsy among mongols related to age. Journal of Mental Deficiency Research 18: 99–106

Vogel F 1970 The genetic basis of the normal human electroencephalogram (EEG). Human Genetics 10: 91–114

Vogel F 1984 Clinical consequences of heterozygosity for autosomal recessive diseases. Clinical Genetics 25: 381–415

Vogel F, Motulsky A G 1986 Human genetics: problems and approaches. 2nd edn. Springer-Verlag, Berlin

Vogel F, Schalt E, Krüger J, Klarich G 1982 Relationship between behavioral maturation measured by the 'Baum' test and EEG frequency. A pilot study on monozygotic and dizygotic twins. Human Genetics 62: 60–65

Wasterlain C G, Morin A M, Dwyer B E 1985 The epilepsies. In: Lajtha A (ed) Handbook of Neurochemistry 10: 339–419

Wasterlain C G, Morin A M, Fando J L 1984 Cholinergic kindling, protein phosphorylation, calcium, and epilepsy. In: Fariello R G, Lloyd K G, Morselli P L, Quesney L F, Engle J Jr (eds) Neurotransmitters, seizures, and epilepsy II. Raven Press, New York, pp 23–26

Weitkamp L R, Schacter B Z 1985 Transferrin and HLA: spontaneous abortion, neural tube defects, and natural selection. New England Journal of Medicine 313: 925–932

Wexler N 1985 Genetic jeopardy and the new clairvoyance. In: Bearn A G, Motulsky A G, Childs B (eds) Progress in Medical Genetics: Genetics of Neurological Disorders 6: 277–304

White R 1984 Looking for epilepsy genes. Annals of

Neurology 16 (suppl): S12–S17

White R, Leppert M, Bishop D T et al 1985 Construction of linkage maps with DNA markers for human chromosomes. Nature 313: 101–105

Wiederholt W C, Gomez M R, Kurland L T 1985 Incidence and prevalence of tuberous sclerosis in Rochester, Minnesota, 1950 through 1982. Neurology 35: 600–603

Williams W R, Thompson M W, Morton N E 1983 Complex segregation analysis and computer-assisted genetic risk assessment for Duchenne muscular dystrophy. American Journal of Medical Genetics 14: 315–333

Willmore L J, Triggs W J 1984 Effect of phenytoin and corticosteroids on seizures and lipid peroxidation in experimental posttraumatic epilepsy. Journal of Neurosurgery 60: 467–472

Wimer R E, Wimer C C 1985 Animal behavior genetics: A search for the biological foundations of behavior. Annual Review of Psychology 36: 171–218

Wisniewski L, Hassold T, Heffelfinger J, Higgins J V 1979 Cytogenetic and clinical studies in five cases of inv dup (15). Human Genetics 50: 259–270

Zonana J, Silvey K, Strimling B 1984 Familial neonatal and infantile seizures: an autosomal dominant disorder. American Journal of Medical Genetics 18: 455–459

4

Seizures in children

S. J. Wallace

DEVELOPMENTAL ASPECTS

The clinical features, aetiology and prognosis of childhood seizure disorders are closely related to cerebral maturation. In particular, abnormal cerebral development can increase the risk of seizures and the effects of seizures themselves may vary with the state of cerebral maturation. Drug effects can also differ in relation to age. Thus, it is relevant briefly to review the developmental neuroanatomy and neurophysiology of the infant and young child.

Early neuroanatomy

Dorsal induction of the neural plate is the first major event in the developing nervous system and is followed by ventral induction at 5 to 6 weeks of gestation. Neuronal proliferation, migration, organization and myelination follow in an orderly sequence (Volpe 1981).

Neuronal proliferation

Neuronal proliferation is at its peak in the forebrain at 2 to 4 months gestation and in the cerebellum from 5 months gestation to 1 year or more postnatally. During neuronal proliferation, cells which are destined to be either neuroblasts or glioblasts move from the outer part of the ventricular zone to the inner surface, divide and move out to the periphery again before migrating to form the cortical plate.

Abnormal neuronal proliferation Children with abnormal neuronal proliferation resulting in microcephaly are not usually affected by seizures.

On the other hand, some of the disorders of neuronal proliferation associated with macrocephaly, in particular tuberous sclerosis and unilateral macrocephaly are complicated by seizures which may be intractable (Volpe 1981).

Migration

Migration of the neurones occurs at 3 to 5 months gestation. Radial movement of cells from their site of origin in the subventricular and ventricular zones leads to the formation of the cortex and deep nuclear structures. Some tangential movement of cells over the external surface of the cerebral cortex also occurs. In the cerebellum, the roof nuclei and the Purkinje cells become established following radial migration; tangential migration is responsible for the development of the external granular layer from which the cells later migrate inwards to form the internal granular layer of the cerebellar cortex.

Abnormal neuronal migration Abnormalities of migration are frequently associated with early neurological disorder and in particular with seizures (Volpe 1981). There is failure of normal development of the gyri which at its most severe leads to schizencephaly. Lissencephaly describes the appearance of the brain when virtually no gyri develop. Pachygyria is characterized by a paucity of gyri with those present being broad and associated with abnormal thickness of the cortical plate. Both pachygyria and polymicrogyria, when an excessive number of small gyri are formed, are found in Zellweger's syndrome (or the cerebro-hepato-renal syndrome of Zellweger). Polymicrogyria may be generalized or focal. It is usually associated with seizures, which may be severe and recurrent with a generalized problem or focal if the migratory problem is localized. The least severe form of aberrant migration results in neuronal heterotopias. These may or may not be associated with clinical neurological disorders and seizures. The absolute quantity of heterotopic material is thought to determine the clinical manifestations (Volpe 1981). Agenesis of the corpus callosum is frequently associated with other disorders of neuronal migration.

Organization

In the nervous system, organization occurs maximally from 6 months gestation to the postnatal age of several years. During organization the cortical neurones become aligned, orientated and layered; dendritic and axonal ramifications appear, synaptic contacts are established and there is glial proliferation and differentiation (Volpe 1981).

Abnormal organization It is believed that defective dendritic development may be responsible for a high proportion of those mentally defective children where no specific cause is identified (Volpe 1981). Huttenlocher (1974) has demonstrated such abnormalities in children with severe mental retardation and infantile myoclonic seizures with hypsarrhythmia on the electroencephalogram. In addition, the brains of children with trisomy 21, congenital rubella and phenylketonuria have been shown to have defects of organization. Since birth occurs during the period of maximal organization it is theoretically possible that perinatal insults might also lead to abnormalities in neuronal organization. Definitive confirmation of such an association is lacking in the human.

Myelination

Myelination begins in the phylogenetically oldest parts of the brain at about 3 months gestation and continues at specific times in specific regions of the brain throughout infancy and childhood and into adulthood. Myelination occurs most actively in the greatest number of regions during the first postnatal year (Volpe 1981).

Abnormal myelination Hypoplasia of the cerebral white matter has been found in a group of infants with severe, but apparently non-progressive, neurological deficits in whom seizures were prominent in the neonatal period (Chattha & Richardson 1977). On the other hand, with the exception of Canavan's disease, in the progressive leucodystrophies such as metachromatic leucodystrophy and Alexander's disease, seizures rarely present until the disorder is well advanced. Disturbance of myelination contributes to the neuropathological findings in disorders of amino acid and organic acid metabolism. This could be related to failure of normal synthesis of myelin proteins but, at least with phenylketonuria, it might partly be a consequence of previous abnormal neuronal organization (Volpe 1981). In the human, birth occurs during the period of maximal myelination. Animal studies suggest that both undernutrition in the latter part of pregnancy and early postnatal life, and acute perinatal insults may be important causes of suboptimal myelination (Volpe 1981).

Conclusions

Disorders of neuronal proliferation, migration and organization are important causes of seizure disorders which start early in life and may be intractable.

Developmental neurophysiology

Physiological changes in the developing brain can be reviewed most readily by examining the electroencephalograph (EEG) throughout infancy into childhood. The maturation of conduction in peripheral nerves and evoked responses is of lesser relevance to childhood epilepsy, but awareness of the changing values for these parameters throughout infancy may be helpful in determining whether or not a disorder in which seizures occur is confined to the cerebral hemispheres.

Electroencephalography

Since small infants spend most of the day asleep, the sleep EEG is the one usually examined in premature babies and in those aged up to a few months old.

Before 28 weeks In the very premature infant, the EEG is much the same during sleeping and waking (Dehkharghani 1984). It is characterized by discontinuity of the background activity, which consists of bursts of mixed frequencies lasting for a few seconds, interspersed by periods of almost complete inactivity which may last for several seconds. During the bursts slow delta (0.3 to 1 Hz) activity predominates but scattered sharp waves and spikes can also be identified, even in recordings from a normal preterm infant. These bursts are usually synchronous in right and left hemispheres.

Between 28 and 36 weeks The greater maturity of the infant's brain and the development of recognizable sleep patterns with increasing gestational age is reflected in the EEG. Between 28 and 36 weeks gestation, the periods of relative EEG inactivity gradually decrease and records in various states of alertness and sleep become clearly recognizable. By 36 weeks gestation, the EEG in quiet, non-REM (Rapid Eye Movement) sleep is characterized by 'tracé alternant', i.e. bursts of delta and theta waves lasting about 1 to 5 seconds with associated high frequency low amplitude activity. Between the bursts, relative inactivity persists. In contrast, during active (REM) sleep and when awake, the EEG pattern is continuous and consists of mixed frequencies, though those in the slower frequencies predominate.

The full-term neonate When the full-term infant is awake or in active (REM) sleep, the EEG shows continuous mixed delta and theta activity with possibly more delta during active sleep than in the awake neonate. During quiet (non-REM) sleep tracé alternant is observed but in contrast with younger infants low voltage theta waves are continuous between the bursts of more spectacular activity.

EEG maturation after the perinatal period Tracé alternant disappears at about 44 weeks gestation. After the neonatal period, in keeping with the longer periods of wakefulness, EEGs tend to be recorded with the child awake. There is gradual increase in the dominant frequencies of the background activity throughout childhood. In the first year of life, 3 to 4 Hz rhythms predominate.

Theta activity can be identified at 5 to 9 months and alpha rhythms seen at about 2 years (Pampiglione 1965). At 3 to 5 years the maximal activity is in the 4 to 6 Hz range and at about 8 to 10 years 8 to 10 Hz alpha rhythms start to predominate. There is often slight interhemispheric asymmetry. The young child's EEG is much less stable under provocation by hyperventilation than that of the adult. Decreasing tendencies with age to slowing on overbreathing are further indications of increasing cerebral maturation. The EEG often has features of immaturity until well on into the teens.

Effects of drugs and hormones on the developing brain

Little is known of the cellular pathology of the effects of drugs and hormones on the developing human brain. Experimental work on animals has shown that the changes which these substances may cause can be critically related to the stage of cerebral maturation at the time of exposure, and there is good reason to assume that comparable periods of vulnerability exist also in humans. Such concepts are clearly important in the consideration of both the etiology and the treatment of seizure disorders in childhood.

A review of the literature on the mechanisms of drug action on the developing brain records that cell division is adversely affected by barbiturates, corticosteriods, chlorpromazine, alcohol, reserpine and sex hormones; cell migration is altered by alcohol ingestion; and, the formation of neurones and synapses, i.e. organization, is related to the presence of sex hormones and corticosteroids and may be disturbed by morphine/methadone, antiepileptic drugs and alcohol (Swaab & Mirmiran 1984). In the context of human brain development, since abnormalities of cell migration and organization are those most likely to be associated with later seizure disorders, drug exposure or hormonal imbalance occurring between about 3 and 8 months gestation may be of etiological importance in childhood epilepsy. Since antiepileptic drugs are among those implicated in disorders of cerebral maturation, it is obviously important that they are used in late pregnancy and early infancy only when definite indications exist.

NEONATAL SEIZURES

Seizures in the newborn can take several clinical forms. They are more likely to be symptomatic than in later childhood and the child's outlook is closely related to the underlying cause. There is also evidence from animal experiments that seizure activity can impair brain growth (Wasterlain & Dwyer 1983).

Incidence of seizures

The figures available for the frequency of neonatal seizure disorders usually refer to attacks which have been witnessed clinically. However, with the increasing use of continuous EEG monitoring in infants in the special care baby units, it is becoming apparent that subclinical seizures are common events in the sick newborn (Eyre et al 1983a). Estimates of the incidence of clinically observed seizures vary from as high as 30% (Fenichel 1980) to as low as 0.5% (Mellits et al 1981). Since most neonatal seizures are symptomatic, it has been suggested that the incidence in any newborn unit is a reflection of the standard of perinatal care (Dennis & Chalmers 1982).

Seizure types

In keeping with the immaturities of the anatomy and physiology of the infant brain and the high incidence of recognizable pathological conditions, seizures in the young infant can take a number of clinical forms. Neonatal seizure types are classified as follows:

1. Subtle
2. Clonic: focal, multifocal, hemiconvulsive
3. Tonic
4. Myoclonic
(Tonic-clonic: rare in newborns)

(Volpe 1981, Kellaway & Hrachovy 1983, Lombroso 1983a)

Subtle seizures

Subtle seizures are the most difficult to recognize. Volpe (1981) found that tonic horizontal deviation of the eyes, with or without jerking; eyelid blinking or fluttering; sucking, rowing and pedalling movements; and apnoeic spells were the commonest manifestations of subtle seizures. In addition, limpness and unresponsiveness; thrashing about; smiling; grimacing; capillary dilatation or constriction; nystagmus; flushing; pallor; cyanosis; and salivation have been noted as manifestations of seizures (Kellaway & Hrachovy 1983).

The difficulties in deciding whether or not subtle fits are present are summed up by Dehkharghani & Sarnat (1984). They recognized that any unusual movement which is stereotyped might be a seizure, but emphasized that impairment of cortical function leading to cortical inhibition with release of brain stem and spinal reflexes can be associated with bicycling and chewing movements. It may be necessary to confirm the diagnosis of subtle seizures by simultaneous clinical and EEG observations.

Clonic seizures

Of the 277 infants reported in the American Collaborative Perinatal Project on neonatal seizures, approximately three-quarters had generalized clonic seizures and one-third focal clonic seizures (Holden et al 1982). Concomitant EEG and/or polygraphic recordings of seizures in more than 1000 infants have demonstrated that clonic attacks are always unilateral at the onset and, even if they become clinically bilateral, they are always electrically asynchronous (Kellaway & Hrachovy 1983).

Focal clonic seizures In focal clonic seizures, the jerking is usually well localized and consciousness is usually retained (Volpe 1981). Although Lombroso (1983a) reported that focal clonic seizures are rarely symptomatic of brain lesions, both Volpe (1981) and Dehkharghani & Sarnat (1984) state that persistent clonic movements which are localized to the same part of the body are suggestive of a focal structural abnormality. Volpe (1981) further specified this by recording that such abnormalities are usually focal traumatic lesions such as cerebral contusion in a full-term infant. However, metabolic encephalopathies and other generalized cerebral disturbances can also be associated with focal clonic attacks.

Multifocal clonic seizures In multifocal clonic

seizures, the clonic movements appear in an apparently unrelated manner in different parts of the body. Full-term infants are more likely than preterms to have multifocal clonic seizures (Volpe 1981).

Hemiconvulsive clonic seizures Although Lombroso (1983a) listed this seizure type in the classification of neonatal seizures, he stated that it was rare in the newborn period. Perhaps the only justification for considering these seizures as a separate clinical entity is that they might give rather stronger evidence of a focal structural cerebral abnormality than focal clonic seizures that are not further specified.

Tonic seizures

Tonic seizures are characterized by generalized extension of all limbs so that the infant often takes up an opisthotonic posture. This is the usual seizure type in the premature infant and occurs particularly in association with intraventricular haemorrhage (Volpe 1981). In this circumstance, it is not always easy to distinguish between decerebrate posturing and seizures with increased extensor tone. During predominantly tonic seizures, the infant may take up a decorticate posture with the upper limbs flexed rather than having generalized extension. Seizures are tonic in about 30% to 40% of cases (Holden et al 1982, Kellaway & Hrachovy 1983), when there is a significant relationship to later cerebral palsy, mental retardation and epilepsy (Holden et al 1982).

Myoclonic seizures

Myoclonic seizures are considered to be very rare in the neonatal period (Volpe 1981, Kellaway & Hrachovy, 1983). They may be the forerunners of later infantile spasms (Lombroso 1983b, Volpe 1981). They can be seen in both premature and full term infants and consist of either single or repeated synchronous flexor jerks which involve the upper limbs more than the lower limbs (Volpe 1981). Myoclonic seizures are observed in only 0.5% to 1% of cases (Holden et al 1982, Kellaway & Hrachovy 1983). They are significantly related to mental retardation.

Epileptic syndromes in the newborn

Three epileptic syndromes have been characterized in neonates (Aicardi 1985a, Dulac et al 1985, Plouin 1985).

Benign neonatal convulsions

Two syndromes of benign neonatal convulsions have been identified (Plouin 1985).

Benign idiopathic neonatal convulsions – 'fifth day fits' Details of the 182 cases which appear in the literature have been reviewed by Plouin (1985). About 4% of all neonatal convulsions are examples of this condition; 62% of the infants involved are boys; 95% of the convulsions occur between the ages of 3 and 7 days; and 80% between the fourth and sixth days. The convulsions are usually partial, always clonic and are repeated frequently, leading to status epilepticus over periods of between two hours and three days (mean about 20 hours). At the onset of the seizures the infants are neurologically normal between fits, but they become hypotonic and drowsy as the status progresses. They revert to normality after the status, but may take several days to do so.

In the cases where EEGs have been recorded, bursts of theta rhythms mainly in the Rolandic areas are common interictally, and rhythmic spikes or rhythmic slow waves have been seen during convulsions. However, these changes are not specific for benign idiopathic neonatal convulsions. The condition has a favourable outcome but the diagnosis is largely one of exclusion and may not become unquestionably apparent until after a period of follow-up.

Benign familial neonatal convulsions Details of 14 families in which 87 individuals have had benign neonatal convulsions are reviewed by Plouin (1985). Where the appropriate details have been documented, delivery and birth weight have been normal and convulsions have commenced after an interval, usually of two to three days. The seizures are clonic, brief and repeated frequently for up to seven days. EEG changes are not specific to the condition. Although other seizure types may develop later in infancy or childhood, other aspects of development are unaffected. Inheritance is by autosomal dominant transmission.

Early myoclonic encephalopathy

25 cases of early myoclonic encephalopathy have been reviewed by Aicardi (1985a). This condition is characterized in the neonatal period by fragmentary or partial erratic myoclonus, massive myoclonias and/or partial motor seizures. The EEG is devoid of normal background activity and, in both waking and sleeping, consists of a suppression-burst pattern in which the bursts are complexes of irregularly intermingled spikes, sharp waves and slow waves. The infants are always neurologically very abnormal. Death occurred during the first year of life in more than half the cases reviewed. This condition is considered in more detail in the section on myoclonic epilepsies.

Differential diagnosis in neonatal seizures

Since seizures in the neonate can take so many clinical forms, they may be confused with almost any other type of movement disorder. Jitteriness, i.e. a high-frequency low-amplitude tremor present particularly on stimulation, is the most common alternative diagnosis. It can be distinguished from seizures by the absence of abnormalities of gaze or extra-ocular movement and its cessation on passive flexion (Volpe 1981).

It is possible that not all episodic attacks of extension are epileptic seizures. Kellaway & Hrachovy (1983) reported that in 102 of 400 infants with tonic seizures, the attacks were not accompanied by seizure activity on the EEG. These authors suggest that tonic seizures without EEG epileptiform activity are better explained as 'brain stem release' phenomena and cite evidence which demonstrates that transient anoxic depression of cortical activity, confirmed by the absence of electrical activity, results in hyperextension of the neck, trunk and extremities.

Neonatal tetanus may sometimes be confused with neonatal seizures.

Etiology of convulsions in the neonate

Convulsions in the neonatal period can be symptomatic of any serious central nervous system disorder. The eventual outcome is closely linked to the underlying pathology.

Prenatal causes of seizures

Prenatal causes are rarely remediable unless a biochemical defect that can be corrected is present. Dennis (1978) coined the useful phrase 'fetus with a problem' to embrace the infants whose suboptimal prenatal histories suggested that cerebral development had probably been abnormal prior to delivery.

The prenatal causes of neonatal seizures can be classified as follows:

1. Cerebral dysmorphism – major malformations; abnormalities at a cellular level
2. Prenatal vascular occlusion – porencephalic cysts
3. Prenatal infection
4. Maternal drug ingestion
5. Inborn errors of metabolism – pyridoxine dependency, etc.
6. Heritable disorders of unknown aetiology – benign familial neonatal convulsions

Cerebral dysmorphism Abnormalities of cerebral development account for approximately 10% of neonatal convulsions (Lombroso 1983a).

Major malformations of the cerebrum are often incompatible with survival and seizures are not necessarily the most significant of the neurological signs. Abnormalities at a cellular level are more important. In tuberous sclerosis and some types of macrocephaly, there are disorders of neuronal proliferation (Volpe 1981). In lissencephaly, pachygyria, polymicrogyria and agenesis of corpus callosum abnormalities of neuronal migration are associated with the early development of seizures (Volpe 1981). Defective dendritic development such as can occur in trisomy 21, congenital rubella or maternal hyperphenylalaninaemia, may also be associated with early seizure development (Volpe 1981). Huttenlocher (1974) has described abnormal cerebral organization in infants with severe developmental delay and the early onset of myoclonic seizures. On the whole, abnormalities of myelination are not associated with the early development of convulsions, but Chattha & Richardson (1977) reported a group of infants with seizures in the neonatal period who had hypoplasia of the cerebral white matter.

Prenatal vascular occlusion With the more

frequent use of ultrasound and CT scanning in the investigation of neonatal seizures, there is increasing evidence of prenatal vascular occlusion with the formation of porencephalic cysts. These may act as foci of seizure activity. It is difficult to determine the relative incidence of such abnormalities from the literature, but Holden et al (1982) reported acquired central nervous system abnormalities, i.e. porencephaly and hydrocephaly, in eight of 77 autopsies performed on children who had presented with neonatal seizures.

Prenatal infection Approximately 4% of infants with convulsions in the newborn period have evidence of prenatal infection (Lombroso 1983a). Toxoplasmosis (Couvreur & Desmonts 1962), rubella (Desmond et al 1967) and cytomegalovirus (Holden et al 1982) can cause encephalitis in the fetus, which may lead to abnormalities in cerebral maturation and a subsequent liability to convulse in the neonatal period. Congenital syphillis is now a very unusual cause of fits in the first two weeks of life (Volpe 1981).

Maternal drug ingestion Maternal drug ingestion has the potential to predispose the neonate to seizures by two mechanisms. Firstly, drugs acting on the central nervous system might affect the sequence of normal brain maturation. In a review article, Swaab & Mirmiran (1984) list the possible implications for the developing brain of exposure to hormones and drugs affecting neurotransmission, e.g. alpha-methyldopa, propranolol, chlorpromazine, barbiturates. Although neonatal seizures might be expected to be consequences of the abnormalities of cell division, migration and organization associated with the use of these drugs, Swaab & Mirmiran do not comment on the incidence of fits in the newborn of mothers treated with these substances.

On the other hand, there seems to be no doubt that neonates born to mothers who have been addicted to narcotics can have withdrawal seizures in the first few days of life. Lombroso (1983a) stated that between 4% and 5.5% of neonatal convulsions are related to drug withdrawal. However, since only between 1.2% and 3% of infants with neurological symptoms related to heroin withdrawal have seizures (Herzlinger et al 1977, Zelson et al 1971), this symptom must be a relatively rare indicator of prenatal narcosis.

Withdrawal of barbiturates (Bleyer & Marshall 1972) and of alcohol (Pierog et al 1977) can also precipitate convulsions in the neonate.

Inborn errors of metabolism Inherited biochemical disorders account for 2.5% to 4.5% of neonatal seizure disorders (Lombroso 1983a). Urea cycle defects with hyperammonaemia, maple syrup urine disease, proprionic acidaemia and other organic acidaemias, diseases predisposing to hypoglycaemia (e.g. galactose-l-phosphate-uridyl-transferase deficiency) and disorders of mitochondrial function are those conditions most commonly reported (Dehkharghani & Sarnat 1984).

Abnormal central nervous system gamma-aminobutyric acid (GABA) metabolism can also be associated with neonatal seizures (Jaeken 1985). Pyridoxine-dependent convulsions occur in the presence of a glutamic acid decarboxylase (GAD) defect which prevents normal GABA synthesis (Yoshida et al 1971). Convulsions occur in the first few days of life in GABA-transaminase deficiency (Jaeken 1985).

Although some authors include neurolipidoses and other neurodegenerative disorders among the aetiological possibilities for neonatal seizures, it is virtually unknown for these conditions to present at such an early age.

Maternal illness The infants of mothers who have hyperparathyroidism may present with convulsions associated with hypocalcaemia (Cockburn et al 1973). Where the mother has poorly controlled diabetes the neonate may have convulsions associated with hypoglycaemia.

Heritable causes of unknown aetiology The syndrome of benign familial neonatal convulsions has been discussed above.

Intrapartum causes

Intrapartum causes of neonatal convulsions can be listed as follows:

1. Hypoxic-ischaemic encephalopathy
2. Intracranial haemorrhage
3. Birth trauma
4. Infection
5. Local anaesthetic intoxication

Hypoxic-ischaemic encephalopathy Deficiencies

in oxygen supply to the brain cause impairments of brain energy metabolism which lead to the irreversible structural deficits characteristic of this condition. The pathological changes are preceded by regional alterations in high energy compounds; accumulation of extracellular potassium; intracellular acidosis; and alterations in neurotransmitter metabolism; and can be identified both clinically and electrophysiologically before structural abnormalities are apparent (Volpe 1981).

Fetal hypoxaemia may predate perinatal hypoxic-ischaemic encephalopathy and can be recorded with fetal monitoring equipment. Even when attempts are made to maximise the available oxygen, approximately 10% of infants with prenatal asphyxia and 25% of those who are hypoxic at birth have seizures and other serious neurological deficits (Low et al 1977). Lombroso (1983a) found a significant increase from 11.5% to 24.5% in a proportion of neonates with seizures associated with asphyxia, when comparing data from 1958–68 with those from 1969–79. This is almost certainly related to the survival in the latter period through more intense monitoring and active intervention of infants who would have died in the earlier period.

Intracranial haemorrhage Subdural haemorrhage is virtually always secondary to trauma. It may present acutely with signs of raised intracranial pressure and brain stem compromise rather than seizures. However, if the haemorrhage has localized over the cerebral convexities focal seizures are common and usually associated with dysfunction of muscles innervated by the ipsilateral third nerve (Volpe 1981).

Primary subarachnoid haemorrhage can present with seizures in otherwise apparently well babies. However, on clinical grounds, it may be difficult to distinguish a haemorrhage confined to the subarachnoid space from blood extravasation from other intracranial sources. Intracranial haemorrhages may, in addition, be secondary to coagulation defects, vascular anomalies or haemorrhagic infarction (Volpe 1981).

Periventricular-intraventricular haemorrhage is almost exclusively a condition of premature infants. The incidence increases with decrease in gestational age. In the premature infant, a subependymal germinal matrix is still present;

Heubner's artery, the anterior choroidal artery and the lateral striate arteries are relatively large and appear to carry most of the blood supply to the cerebrum on its way to the basal ganglia and germinal matrix; the capillaries in the periventricular region seem less able to withstand pressure changes; and autoregulation of the vascular bed is immature (Volpe 1981). Intraventricular haemorrhages are precipitated by hypoxia, which increases cerebral blood flow and leads to further inadequacy of vascular autoregulation, increased venous pressure and endothelial injury. In addition, increased fibrinolytic activity has been reported in the periventricular region in the preterm newborn (Gilles et al 1971). Periventricular intraventricular haemorrhage can be catastrophic and associated with generalised tonic-clonic seizures; stupor progressing to coma; respiratory disturbance; decerebrate posturing; brain stem compromise; and flaccid quadriparesis; or can be saltatory when repeated, less severe bleeding occurs and seizures are not a usual clinical feature (Volpe 1981).

Birth trauma Intracranial haemorrhage can be secondary to direct or indirect trauma during delivery. Cerebral contusion may also occur and can be a cause of seizures which are often focal; it is considered an uncommon neonatal problem (Volpe 1981). In keeping with improved obstetric care, the incidence of trauma as the etiological factor in neonatal seizures has fallen significantly from 10% to 4.5% between the 10-year periods up to 1968 and 1979 (Lombroso 1983a).

Infections Both intracranial and extracranial infections may be associated with neonatal seizures. Intracranial infections are present in about 12% of neonatal fits (Volpe 1981). Bacterial meningitis is usually a complication of bacteraemia involving organisms acquired from the mother's birth canal. Thus, *Escherichia coli*, *Listeria monocytogenes* and *Group B β-haemolytic streptococci* are the most common infecting agents. If the onset is early and fulminating, seizures are not a prominent symptom. In cases which present with a more insidious clinical course late in the neonatal period, seizures occur in 75% and are presumed to be related to the effects of infiltration into the cortex of acute inflammation of the arachnoid (Overall 1970). The later complications of bacterial meningitis, i.e. hydrocephalus, subdural effusion and intracerebral abscess, may also be associated with seizures.

Of the non-bacterial intracranial infections, herpes simplex is the most likely to be acquired during passage through an infected birth canal. The incidence of neonatal herpes simplex infection is 1 in 7500 deliveries (Nahmias et al 1970). It presents towards the end of the first week of life with symptoms of general ill health, complicated in about half the cases by stupor, irritability and seizures. Although enteroviruses, particularly Coxsackie B and echoviruses, may cause encephalitic illnesses in the neonatal period, seizures appear to be relatively rare (Volpe 1981).

The classical febrile convulsion is very rare in the neonate, but extracranial infections, acquired during delivery, may also be associated with seizures. In these cases, the seizures are commonly related to electrolyte imbalance or hypoxia secondary to the severity of the illness.

Local anaesthetic intoxication Volpe (1981) emphasized that seizures were a prominent feature of intoxication with local anaesthetics (Mepivacaine, Lidocaine) in the neonate. In such cases, a local anaesthetic had usually been inadvertently injected into the infant's scalp during a maternal paracervical or pudendal block. The seizures were usually tonic, occurred in the first six hours after birth, and were associated with depressed Apgar scores, bradycardia, apnoea, hypertonia, dilated pupils which did not respond to light and absence of the oculocephalic reflex.

Causes of seizures in the early postnatal period

Conditions which are acquired after birth are rather less likely to be the etiological agents in neonatal seizures than those determined pre- or intranatally.

Metabolic disorders Hypoglycaemia is most likely to be complicated by seizures if it is prolonged and treatment delayed (Koivisto et al 1972). Four clinical categories are recognized (Volpe 1981):

1. Early transitional-adaptive hypoglycaemia
2. Secondary hypoglycaemia
3. Transient neonatal hypoglycaemia
4. Severe recurrent hypoglycaemia

Early transitional-adaptive hypoglycaemia is seen in term babies who are large for gestational age such as those born to mothers with diabetes.

Secondary hypoglycaemia occurs in both appropriate-for-gestational-age and small-for-gestational-age infants who are moderately or severely unwell with symptoms largely referrable to the central nervous system, e.g. illness secondary to asphyxia, intracranial haemorrhage or bacteraemia. In this context it is difficult to separate out the effects of the hypoglycaemia.

Classical transient neonatal hypoglycaemia, which used to occur predominantly in small-for-gestation infants who had been undernourished in utero, is now usually avoided by early and appropriate feeding of at risk infants.

Severe recurrent hypoglycaemia can be symptomatic of hormonal deficiencies, hormonal excess and inborn errors of carbohydrate, amino acid or organic acid metabolism and should be regarded as an alerting sign for potentially serious underlying biochemical disorders.

Disturbances of calcium, phosphorus and magnesium are frequently interrelated. In 75 newborns where primary disturbance of mineral metabolism was considered to be the cause of seizures, hypocalcaemia was present in 92%, hypomagnesaemia in 53% and hyperphosphataemia in 64% of cases (Cockburn et al 1973). In almost 80% of these cases the serum level of more than one mineral was abnormal with hypocalcaemia/hypomagnesaemia/hyperphosphataemia; hypocalcaemia/hyperphosphataemia; and hypocalcaemia/hypomagnesaemia being the most common combinations. Isolated hypocalcaemia was present in 19% of cases and isolated hypomagnesaemia in only 3% of cases.

In those newborns with primary disturbance of calcium, phosphorus or magnesium metabolism related to a high dietary intake of phosphate in milk, the peak incidence of the first convulsion was on the sixth day of life and presentation in the first 48 hours or after the tenth day was very rare. The seizures were usually focal or multifocal clonic in type. It was unusual for them to be associated with cyanosis and the infant was usually hyperalert.

Most infants who have seizures in association with primary hypocalcaemia are full term and delivered uneventfully by the vertex. However, there is a tendency for them to be delivered to low social class mothers of relatively high parity towards the end of the winter and to be fed on non-human milk (Roberts et al 1973). In a minority of infants, hypocalcaemia occurring between five and ten days of life may be secondary to, in the mother, hyperparathyroidism or untreated coeliac disease; or, in the infant, congenital hypoparathyroidism, intestinal malabsorption of calcium or magnesium, or renal failure with hyperphosphataemia (Volpe 1981).

Hypocalcaemia in the first two days of life is particularly associated with prematurity, asphyxia and maternal diabetes (Volpe 1981). The affected infant is likely to be stuporous and hypotonic, and seizures are much less common than in late (five to ten-day) onset hypocalcaemia (Roberton et al 1975). Disorders of magnesium absorption can lead to hypomagnesaemia and fits in the neonatal period (Tsang 1972).

Transient hyperammonaemia may complicate respiratory distress in the preterm infant (Ballard et al 1978). Clinically, stupor/coma accompanied by seizures and fixed dilated pupils present between 4 and 48 hours after birth. The pathogenesis of the condition is unknown. It does not appear to be genetically determined.

Hypo- or hypernatraemia may be associated with neonatal seizures, the former is most commonly seen when there is inappropriate antidiuretic hormone (ADH) secretion secondary to bacterial meningitis or intracranial haemorrhage (Volpe 1981).

Infection Although neonatal bacterial meningitis is usually secondary to intrapartum infection, postnatal infections can also occur. In these cases the onset of symptoms is usually later than seven days and the physical signs are likely to be those of meningitis rather than septicaemia or respiratory illness (Volpe 1981).

Of the non-bacterial infections which can be acquired in the early postnatal period, herpes simplex is the one most commonly associated with encephalitis and thus with seizures. If acquired postnatally, the presence of an incubation period means that the neurological illness presents 10 or more days after delivery (Nahmais et al 1970). Although Coxsackie B virus may also cause

meningoencephalitis in the postnatal period, seizures are rare (Eilard et al 1974).

Exogenous toxins The antiseptic hexochlorophane can be absorbed if it comes into contact with the neonate's skin and may cause a toxic encephalopathy with seizures (Brown 1973).

Unknown causes of seizures

In Volpe's series (1981) only 10% of infants with seizures in the neonatal period had neither a definite nor a highly presumptive etiological agent.

Timing of neonatal seizures

Since the various causes of seizures can be effective at different times in the neonatal period, the timing of the onset can be helpful in narrowing down the likely etiology. Onset before birth is recognized only rarely but may be apparent in pyridoxine dependency. If they commence within three days of birth seizures are likely to be associated with:

- perinatal asphyxia
- intracranial haemorrhage
- birth trauma
- cerebral dysmorphism
- prenatal vascular occlusion
- hypoglycaemia
- hypocalcaemia – secondary to perinatal asphyxia etc
- hyperammonaemia – secondary to urea cycle defect and organic acidurias
- amino acid disorders: non-ketotic hyperglycinaemia
- pyridoxine dependency
- maternal ingestion of short-acting drugs
- benign familial neonatal convulsions

Seizures with onset from three to 10 days are usually associated with:

- meningitis
- encephalitis
- hypocalcaemia due to primary disorders of mineral metabolism
- hypoglycaemia secondary to galactosaemia etc

- amino acid disorders – maple syrup urine disease, methionone malabsorption, hyper-beta-alaninaemia etc
- hyperammonaemia secondary to urea cycle defects and organic acidurias
- transient neonatal hyperammonaemia
- cerebral dysmorphism
- prenatal vascular occlusion
- maternal ingestion of long-acting sedative drugs
- benign idiopathic neonatal convulsions (fifth day fits)

Seizures with onset between 10 and 28 days are most likely to be secondary to either infective or metabolic causes.

Pathophysiological aspects

It is reasonable to postulate that hypoxia, ischaemia and hypoglycaemia will interfere with energy production, reduce the available adenosine triphosphate (ATP) and secondarily lead to failure of the sodium-potassium pump; that hypocalcaemia and hypomagnesaemia will alter membrane permeability allowing greater movement of sodium ions; and that pyridoxine dependency will produce a relative excess of excitatory neurotransmitter (Volpe 1981).

There are problems in extrapolating from animal work when considering the special problems of the neonatal brain, since, in many species, the level of cerebral maturity at birth is much greater than in the human neonate. In neonatal rats there is a fall in the brain glucose concentration during sustained seizures even if the plasma glucose is normal or raised; this suggests that the neonatal rat brain has difficulty in maintaining energy supplies during seizures (Wasterlain & Dwyer 1983). Furthermore, rats who had seizures during a critical period between 2 and 11 days postnatally, later had significant reductions in the total brain DNA, RNA and cholesterol. These findings suggest that reduction in cell numbers is related to repeated seizures when these occur at specific stages in cerebral development. In addition, neonatal seizures are probably associated with suboptimal establishment of cell-to-cell connections.

Clinical assessment

The clinical features associated with seizures may assist in identifying the underlying cause.

Family history

A history of previous infants with congenital malformations would lead to the consideration of cerebral dysmorphism. The presence of parental consanguinity, or of death from neurological disease in infancy of siblings, suggests an inborn error of metabolism. Benign syndromes such as that of 'fifth day fits' may be diagnosed if there is a clear history of similar convulsions in parents or prior-born siblings.

Perinatal history

Seizures in premature infants can be associated with any other cause, but those related to intracranial haemorrhage are more common in the preterm than in the full-term infant. It is important to be aware of potentially asphyxiating or traumatic episodes in babies of any gestation. Prolonged rupture of the membranes prior to delivery is a potential precursor of neonatal meningitis.

Neurological examination

Poor feeding, vomiting and/or lethargy progressing to stupor or coma prior to the onset of seizures suggest a metabolic disorder. Extreme irritability and jitteriness may indicate withdrawal from maternal narcotics. The infant who has cerebral dysmorphism is likely to have an abnormally sized or shaped head. When a porencephalic cyst is present, bulging of the cranium overlying the cyst is common. Hemisyndromes suggest focal structural lesions. An alert well-looking baby with jitteriness and seizures commencing towards the end of the first week of life who has very hyperactive tendon reflexes is most likely to be hypocalcaemic.

General features

The small-for-gestational-age infant is liable to

hypoglycaemia, as is the very large infant of the mother who has had poorly controlled diabetes during pregnancy. Specific facies may be present as, for example, in the fetal alcohol syndrome. The presence of an intracranial malformation may be suspected if other dysmorphism is present. In particular, congenital malformations of the optic nerve or other intraorbital structures may be alerting signals for abnormalities of the brain.

It is clearly important to examine the infant in detail so that clues to the etiology of the neonatal seizures can be fully appreciated.

Investigation

General information

In the neonatal period it is particularly important to ensure that the blood pH and gases, urea and electrolytes are normal. The blood glucose, calcium, phosphate and magnesium should also be measured in all newborns who convulse. Unless there is another obvious reason for seizures, lumbar puncture should be performed as a matter of urgency so that meningitis, which may not be clinically apparent, can either be diagnosed with a minimum of delay or be excluded.

Specific investigations

Biochemical If there is any reason to suspect, on clinical grounds, that a serious inborn error of metabolism could be present, specimens of blood for ammonia and quantitative amino acid levels, and of urine for amino and organic acids should be obtained at the time of the seizures. Even if the amino and organic acid levels cannot be estimated immediately, the serum or urine should be obtained and frozen for later estimations. Too often a serious fatal metabolic disorder in a first child remains undiagnosed and appropriate genetic counselling of the parents and management of any subsequently affected siblings are delayed.

Ultrasound scans Ultrasound scans obtained through the fontanelle can demonstrate subependymal and intraventricular haemorrhages and enlargement of the ventricular system. Intracranial

cysts secondary to prenatal vascular occlusions may also be visible but primarily cortical abnormalities, such as lissencephaly and agyria, cannot be readily diagnosed by ultrasound.

Skull X-rays Straightforward skull X-rays rarely demonstrate any pathology since, even in conditions such as cerebral toxoplasmosis, calcification usually develops later.

CT scans Computerized axial tomography (CT scanning) can usefully identify intracranial haemorrhage and will demonstrate subdural collections not visualized by ultrasound. In addition, cortical and other malformations can be delineated by CT scanning.

When normal appearances in infants at different gestational ages have been defined, magnetic resonance imaging will probably provide even more information about the cerebral structural abnormalities associated with seizure disorders.

Electroencephalography The predominant features of the normal neonatal EEG change with increasing gestational age. Normal and abnormal findings have been comprehensively reviewed by Dreyfus-Brissac (1979). Nevertheless, the limits of normality, particularly in the very premature infant, remain imprecisely defined and a number of conditions should be satisfied if maximal information is to be acquired. In particular, the exact gestational age of the infant must be known. Most abnormalities appear during quiet (non-REM) sleep necessitating recordings which are of greater duration than would be usual when recording from older children or adults. Where possible, continuous EEG recording with either compressed spectral analysis or storage on tape, e.g. by using Medilog recording apparatus (Oxford Medical Systems), should be obtained. Such recordings allow subtle seizures to be recognized more readily, and interictal and ictal patterns can be identified over longer periods. (Eyre et al 1983a, 1983b, Aziz et al 1986). Responses to therapy can also be monitored by using continuous EEG recordings.

Harris & Tizard (1960) itemized the abnormalities in the neonatal EEG that are related to seizures as follows: rhythmic slow waves; persistent focal sharp waves; spikes; repeated stereotyped sharp waves or wave complexes; gross asymmetry; small amplitude sharp waves during episodic sleep activity; and fast activity. Dreyfus-Brissac (1979) has reviewed reports on the abnormalities to be found in certain pathological states. In primary or late onset hypocalcaemia the interictal EEG is entirely normal. Conversely, when hypocalcaemia occurs early and is secondary to perinatal asphyxia the interictal EEG is abnormal. Seizure discharges may be seen to commence with the appearance of focal sharp waves which may be mingled with slow waves. The discharge may spread throughout the same hemisphere or become alternately bi- and unilateral. If hypocalcaemia is the major cause of the seizures, normalization of the EEG occurs once the plasma calcium has been restored.

Although abnormalities of the EEG may be found in hypoglycaemia they are non-specific. In other transient metabolic disorders, diffuse or localized spikes and sharp waves or other paroxysmal changes reflect the alterations in electrical activity but are not pathognomonic for any particular condition. Where the disorder is more prominent, e.g. in such conditions as the organic acidurias where convulsions are often associated with interictal coma, the record may be periodic and the bursts characterized by high-voltage sharp waves or sharp complexes followed by slow waves with superimposed rapid rhythms. 'Comb-like rhythms', in association with other EEG abnormalities, are sometimes considered diagnostic of maple syrup urine disease. Complexes of sharp high-voltage slow waves which are mainly frontal and associated with Rolandic, occipital or generalized bursts of alpha rhythms have been described in non-ketotic hyperglycinaemia. Dreyfus-Brissac (1979) has suggested that, when a periodic EEG is seen in a neonate delivered normally after a normal pregnancy, an inborn error of metabolism should be suspected.

The EEG changes in seizures secondary to bacterial infections are non-specific. In herpes meningoencephalitis, a periodic EEG abnormality progresses to inactivity unless the infection can be controlled.

In cerebral dysmorphism, when there is a serious lack of cerebral tissue, such as in hydranencephaly, very low voltage recordings may be obtained with superimposed seizure discharges.

It has been suggested that positive sharp Rolandic waves are particularly associated with intraventricular haemorrhage in the premature infant but, in the most severe cases where seizures are likely to be prominent, slow or rapid spikes, or sharp wave discharges are usually recorded. Subclinical seizure discharges are commonly visible in infants with extensive intracranial haemorrhages.

When the seizures are symptomatic of hypoxic-ischaemic encephalopathy, in the mildest cases the EEG fails to show characteristic sleep patterns. In more severely affected babies seizure discharges, suppression-burst or total inactivity may be observed.

In infants with benign convulsive syndromes the EEG patterns usually consist of a background of low-voltage theta rhythms with bursts of asynchronous or synchronous high-voltage theta activity.

The EEG is an important tool in both the management and prognosis of neonatal seizures. It should be available, preferably as part of the continuous monitoring, for all infants with convulsions.

Treatment

Neonates with seizures should be kept as well oxygenated as possible and their general biochemical status retained in as normal a state as practicable.

Specific management

Where hypoglycaemia, hypocalcaemia, hypomagnesaemia, hypo- or hypernatraemia are the cause of the convulsions, the appropriate treatment is obvious and correction of the metabolic disorder is relatively easy. The more complicated changes associated with disorders of amino or organic acids are much more difficult to rectify and discussion of their treatment is beyond the scope of this text. Transient hyperammonaemia responds to aggressive intervention by exchange transfusion and peritoneal dialysis (Ballard et al 1978). Seizures secondary to pyridoxine dependency respond dramatically to Vitamin B6. It may be better initially to give this intravenously and under EEG control so that the necessity for B6 and confirmation of the diagnosis can be made with greater certainty.

Only in the unusual cases of acute subdural haematoma secondary to birth injury is there a place for surgery in the treatment of neonatal seizures.

Symptomatic management

In the absence of a remediable metabolic disorder, neonatal seizures are treated with antiepileptic drugs. The assessment of their efficacy in the newborn is difficult, since the infants are often generally unwell and frequently paralysed and supported with mechanical ventilation. The recognition of persisting seizures may only be possible by the use of continuous EEG monitoring (Eyre et al, 1983b). Initially, the neonate clears drugs slowly and relatively small doses are likely to be effective but, after the first week, drug clearances increase and higher doses are necessary. Monitoring of drug blood levels is important, so that optimal pharmacological responses may be obtained.

Phenobarbitone Phenobarbitone is the usual first choice. Lockman (1983) has recommended the following regime for the treatment of neonatal seizures using phenobarbitone as the first choice:

1. Give a loading dose of phenobarbitone 20 mg/kg intravenously (or intramuscularly).
2. Monitor seizure activity carefully over the next 6 hours. If seizures do not remit give an additional dose of phenobaritone 10 mg/kg intravenously.
3. If after another 6 hours seizures continue give an initial loading dose of intravenous phenytoin 20 mg/kg.
4. Start phenobarbitone maintenance with 3.5 mg/kg per 24 hours, 24 hours after loading is completed.
5. Determine serum phenobarbitone (and if necessary phenytoin) levels daily so that concentrations can be maintained within the optimal range.

In one carefully monitored study only one-third of the infants had their seizures controlled by phenobarbitone alone (Painter et al 1981).

Phenytoin Phenytoin can be used either as a first choice or when phenobarbitone fails to control seizures. If an adequate serum level is to be obtained the dose of phenytoin is 20 mg/kg given slowly by the intravenous route. This should be followed up by maintenance dosage of 3 to 4 mg/kg/day. Painter et al (1981) did not use phenytoin alone. They found that the number of infants whose seizures were controlled when phenytoin was added to phenobarbitone was twice that when phenobarbitone was used alone. On the other hand, Albani (1983) who used phenytoin as the antiepileptic drug of first choice in 10 newborns, and as a second or third choice in 6 others, reports that 14 of the 16 had their seizures controlled by phenytoin. He emphasized that phenytoin given orally is very poorly absorbed in the neonatal period. Albani gave phenytoin exclusively by the intravenous route and while monitoring serum phenytoin levels, doses as high as 68 mg/kg (mean 54.1 ± 2.6 mg/kg) were given for loading and 14 mg/kg (mean 10.6 ± 2.8 mg/kg) for maintenance therapy. The blood levels were 22.1 ± 4 μg/ml after the first 24 hours, 22.9 ± 7.8 μg/ml after the first 72 hours and 16.4 ± 5.3 μg/ml during the following days. Six of the babies (one-third of the total treated) were unwell in relation to high phenytoin levels; 2 vomited and 6 had urinary retention secondary to atonic bladders. Of 10 babies who survived and were followed up, 6 of those who had responded readily to phenytoin were developing normally at the ages of 9 to 13 months, suggesting that the large doses of phenytoin used to control their seizures had not had any important long-term effects.

Benzodiazepines Intravenous diazepam and intravenous clonazepam are sometimes used for the treatment of recurrent neonatal seizures but their efficacies as first choice treatment remain unexplored. Early concerns that over-sedation might lead to unnecessary complications were probably exaggerated, since most infants with seizures require intensive monitoring and many are electively ventilated. There is a need for a well-conducted study of the use of benzodiazepines in the control of neonatal convulsions.

Other antiepileptic drugs Paraldehyde has been given by some workers but it should be used with caution, if at all. It may be given intravenously as a 10% solution or rectally (Painter 1983). Primidone 20 mg/kg as an oral loading dose has been used with effect as a third antiepileptic drug in difficult cases (Painter 1983).

Duration of therapy There is no satisfactory study of the optimal duration of therapy once treatment with antiepileptic drugs has been started for neonatal seizures. The practice in neonatal follow-up clinics is to withdraw and discontinue them during the first 3 to 6 months of life. However, there is no study showing whether or not this is good practice from the point of view of recurrence of seizures. On theoretical grounds, the first 6 months of life would be a good time to discontinue drug treatment since the seizure threshold appears to be particularly high at this time.

Prognosis

The later outlook for the neonate who has seizures is closely related to the underlying etiology. The overall mortality in a study spanning 15 years was 15% and the incidence of sequelae in survivors was 35% (Volpe 1981).

It is obvious that cerebral dysmorphism will be permanent and that any infant whose seizures are symptomatic of malformations of the brain will be liable to continue to suffer seizures and show mental retardation and clinical neurological deficits.

Where prenatal vascular occlusion with the formation of a porencephalic cyst is associated with seizures, a persistent structural abnormality may be expected to lead to continuing convulsions, mental retardation and clinical neurological abnormalities. However, since children with porencephalic cysts represent a very small percentage of most series of neonatal seizures, it is difficult to estimate the incidence of sequelae in this group.

When prenatal infection is the aetiological agent Lombroso (1983b) estimated that only 10% of children are normal later. On the other hand, withdrawal of drugs, such as occurs when the infant is delivered to a mother who is addicted to sedatives, is reported to have a good prognosis. Almost all such infants subsequently develop normally.

Inborn errors of metabolism which present with seizures in the neonate are often difficult to treat. In Lombroso's series (1983b) only 3 out of 13 (20%) such infants were later normal. Where the seizures appear on the fifth day and are familial the outlook for later normality is good.

When seizures are related to perinatal or intrapartum events there is at least a 50% risk of later abnormality (Lombroso. 1983b, Volpe 1981). Normal development followed seizures associated with hypoxic-ischaemic encephalopathy in 50% of Volpe's series, but in only 20% of that of Lombroso. After intracranial haemorrhage, 30% of infants were normal in Lombroso's study. When those with intraventricular haemorrhage are examined separately from those with primary subarachnoid haemorrhage, Volpe (1981) found that less than 10% of infants with intraventricular haemorrhage were later normal but that if the haemorrhage was primary subarachnoid there was a 90% chance of later normality.

When postnatal infection or bacterial meningitis is the underlying cause of convulsions between 25% and 65% of infants make a good recovery (Volpe 1981, Lombroso 1983b).

Of the metabolic disorders which may present in the neonatal period with seizures, the outcome is good in 36–50% of infants with early onset hypocalcaemia and in 90–100% of those with late onset hypocalcaemia, in 50–70% of neonates with transient hypoglycaemia and in only 28% of those with persistent hypoglycaemia (Lombroso 1983b, Volpe 1981).

In papers which correlated the outcomes in neonatal seizures with prenatal and perinatal events rather than with underlying aetiology, Holden et al (1982) and Mellits et al (1981) found that there was a mortality rate of 34.8% and that, of those followed up to 7 years of age, 70% developed normally. The five-minute Apgar score was significantly related to outcome (Holden et al 1982): 48% of infants with five-minute Apgar scores of less than seven died, and comparable scores were significantly related to later mental retardation and cerebral palsy, but not to epilepsy. Similarly, resuscitation for more than five minutes in infants with subsequent seizures was significantly related to death or later cerebral palsy but not to epilepsy. Of the different seizure types, only tonic and myoclonic seizures appeared prognostically important. Tonic attacks were significantly related to later cerebral palsy, mental retardation and epilepsy, whereas neonatal myoclonic seizures were related only to subsequent mental retardation. With increasing numbers of days on which seizures occurred, the likelihood of later mental retardation, cerebral palsy and epilepsy rose (Holden et al 1982). By use of a multivariate analysis of factors associated with outcome (resuscitation after the first five minutes of life, birth weight, duration of seizures, number of days of seizures, onset time of seizures and five-minute Apgar score), Mellits et al (1981) have shown that the prediction of death, mental retardation, cerebral palsy or epilepsy can be correctly performed in between 64% and 83% of cases.

FEBRILE CONVULSIONS

A febrile convulsion is most suitably defined as any seizure occurring in association with any febrile illness. Once restrictions such as intracranial infection, presence of chronic neurological disorder, or duration or lateralization of convulsion are placed on the definition it becomes extremely difficult to decide whether a convulsion should be characterized as 'febrile' or not. If all seizures which occur in association with a pyrexia are regarded as potentially symptomatic of acute or acute-on-chronic neurological disorders, the possible immediate and long-term consequences fall more readily into place. Febrile seizures occur almost exclusively between 6 months and 5 years of age with most children having their first febrile convulsion between 12 and 24 months.

Incidence

Between 19 and 36 per 1000 children convulse when feverish (Van den Berg & Yerushalmy 1969, Annegers et al 1979, Verity et al 1985a). The incidence in males is greater than in females, both in populations of children with febrile convulsions (Ohtahara 1981) and within sibships where at least one child has had a febrile seizure (Wallace, unpublished data).

Differential diagnosis

Other causes of acute loss of consciousness or rhythmic involuntary movements in early childhood are: breath-holding attacks; reflex anoxic seizures; syncope; rigors; and tetany.

In both breath-holding attacks and reflex anoxic seizures the episodes are acute reactions to noxious stimuli, which are usually unexpected. Syncope is associated with limpness and bradycardia rather than tonic-clonic movements and a tachycardia. Consciousness is not usually lost during rigors or tetany. Benign paroxysmal vertigo, in which sudden acute episodes of unsteadiness occur is not associated with loss of awareness.

Significance of age and sex

Convulsions which occur in association with febrile illnesses are strongly age-related. In a review of 7000 patients reported in the literature, the first seizure occurred before 6 months in 4%, between 6 months and 3 years in 75% and before the age of 5 years in 95% (Millichap 1968). In the British Births Survey 1970 50% of 303 children ascertained had their first febrile convulsion during the second year of life (Verity et al 1985a). Both Taylor (1969) and Wallace (unpublished data) have found that girls tended to have their first convulsions at younger ages than boys. Taylor & Ounsted (1971) suggested that because girls tend to convulse earlier they are more likely than boys to acquire cerebral damage as a result of febrile seizures. Taylor & Ounsted (1971) also showed in their patients that those with positive family histories for convulsive disorders tended to have their first seizures later and thus at a less vulnerable time than those children with negative family histories.

Etiological aspects

In a study conducted when a high proportion of febrile children were admitted to hospital Friderichsen & Melchior (1954) found that only 11.3% had had convulsions. It is therefore relevant to consider the factors which might predispose to convulsions as well as the possible precipitating events.

Pre-conceptual factors

Chronic maternal ill health predating the conceptions of children with febrile convulsions has been found significantly frequently (Wallace 1974a). Parental subfertility is common in families where children, particularly males, have seizures when pyrexial (Van den Berg & Yerushalmy 1974, Wallace 1974a). Thus in some affected children, the prenatal environment may not be conducive to optimal cerebral development.

Prenatal factors

Vaginal bleeding in either early (Wallace 1972) or late pregnancy (Lennox 1949, Wolf et al 1977) is reported more commonly when children later have febrile convulsions. Maternal medication during pregnancy with, in particular, diuretics, antiepileptic drugs, antibiotics, antiemetics and antidepressants was found more frequently during pregnancies resulting in children liable to pyrexial seizures than in their siblings (Wallace 1972). It will be noted that several of these substances might have adverse effects on the developing nervous system.

Perinatal factors

In a study of twins discordant for febrile convulsions Schittz-Christensen (1973) found no significant difference between convulsing and non-convulsing twins for birth first or second, presentation, assisted delivery, or any other unspecified abnormality during the perinatal period. On the other hand Verity et al (1985b) reported an excess of breech presentations. When patients were compared with non-convulsing siblings, fetal distress during labour and delivery by Caesarean section were significantly more common (Wallace 1972). When uncorrected birth weight is taken as a comparative measurement, children with febrile convulsions do not seem particularly disadvantaged (Schiøttz-Christensen 1973, Verity et al 1985b) but, if the birth weights are corrected for gestational age, sex, birth order and maternal height, an excess of infants with later convulsions can be shown to be small for gestational age at birth (Wallace 1972). In one study, 62% of children with febrile convulsions had at least one of a number of pre- and perinatal factors found significantly less commonly in non-convulsing siblings (Wallace 1972).

Later postnatal development

Some authors consider that children with chronic neurological handicaps should be excluded from the possible diagnosis of febrile convulsions. However, since many children who convulse when feverish have difficulties compatible with the description of the minimal cerebral dysfunction syndrome, it is difficult to define a level of severity at which neurological disorder would preclude the use of the term febrile convulsion. Prior to their convulsions in both studies in the general population (unselected) and in hospital patients (selected) children with febrile convulsions have a much higher incidence of delay in motor development or other evidence of neurological suboptimality when compared with the general population or siblings (Nelson & Ellenberg 1976, Wallace 1976, Nelson & Ellenberg 1980).

Family history of seizures

The incidence of convulsive disorders in parents and siblings is significantly higher than in the general population (Harker 1977). In about 30% of children with febrile convulsions, careful enquiry will reveal a positive family history. In one study, first-degree relatives with seizures were apparently more common in the families of affected males (Wallace, unpublished data), but Schiøttz-Christensen (1972) suggested, as a result of his investigation on same-sex twins discordant for febrile convulsions, that genetic factors were more important for females.

Attempts to sort out the genetics of febrile convulsions and to separate them genetically from epilepsy have not been entirely successful. At the time of the first seizure and five to seven years later, Frantzen et al (1970) enquired about a family history of epilepsy and of childhood convulsions in a group of 228 children: epilepsy was present in the relatives of 20% and febrile convulsions in 40%; both epilepsy and febrile convulsions were found in the family histories of 10% of the children. After analysis of their data,

Frantzen et al concluded that febrile convulsions were inherited by a single dominant gene. They noted that the genetic message to convulse when febrile appeared to be strictly age-related and that the pattern for ages at recurrence differed significantly between family history positive and negative cases.

Ounsted (1955) has also shown that febrile convulsions and the epilepsies as a whole are not genetically separate. Ounsted (1971) has further suggested that where children with febrile convulsions subsequently develop epilepsy acute cerebral damage is acquired at the time of the first convulsion. He felt that the genetic message to convulse when febrile is inherited in an autosomal dominant manner. On the other hand Tsuboi (1977a), although agreeing that autosomal dominant inheritance could not be ruled out since incomplete expression is possible, concluded on the basis of a study of 450 children that multifactorial inheritance was probable. However, Tsuboi's arguments are less convincing than those of Ounsted and Frantzen et al.

Regardless of the mode of inheritance there is general agreement that genetic factors are amongst those of aetiological importance in febrile convulsions.

Low serum IgA levels

In a study mainly aimed at examining the frequency and importance of viral infections in children with febrile convulsions Lewis et al (1979, 1980) noted that in some cases the serum IgA levels were low. However, although there may be children who convulse because they are not able adequately to contain viral agents, Lewis et al (1980) did not find that dissemination of viruses was greater in the children with low IgA levels. A further study along the same lines showed that about 1 in 9 children with febrile convulsions have low serum IgA levels (Isaacs et al 1984). However, the significance of this finding remains in doubt.

Summary of factors predisposing to febrile convulsions

In the histories of children who convulse when febrile there are excesses of:

- family history positive for seizure disorders
- chronic maternal ill health
- parental subfertility
- breech presentation
- delivery by Caesarean section
- small birth weight for gestational age
- developmental delay (usually mild and particularly speech)
- minimal cerebral dysfunction
- low serum IgA levels

The precipitating event

Febrile convulsions present in children with predisposing factors only when a feverish illness occurs during the critical age period.

Viral infections

Even before the possibility of identification of actual viruses arose, it was noted that upper respiratory tract infections were most commonly present when a child had a febrile convulsion. The important role of respiratory viruses in the illnesses in which convulsions occur has been demonstrated by Stokes et al (1977). Later Lewis et al (1979), in a very detailed analysis of the evidence for viral infection in a group of 73 children, were able to show that in 86% a viral illness could be held responsible for the fever with which a convulsion occurred. The viruses involved in this latter study were not confined to those considered 'respiratory'. Stokes et al (1977) felt that febrile convulsions related to any particular viral infection were most likely to occur when these infecting agents were present in epidemic concentrations in the community.

Intracranial infection

Although many authors exclude children with intracranial infections, (particularly bacterial meningitis) from their series of febrile convulsions, the long-term outcome no longer seems to be more serious than in those children with clear cerebrospinal fluid (Frantzen 1971). Up to 8% of children who present with febrile convulsions will be found to have bacterial or viral meningitis

(Rutter & Smales 1977, Wallace, unpublished data).

Other causes of fever

Gastrointestinal infections, particularly with shigella or salmonella, have been recorded in between 4% and 13% of cases (Bamberger & Matthes 1959, Degen & Goller 1967, Friderichsen & Melchior 1954, Herlitz 1941, Laplane et al 1958, Zellweger 1948).

With current vaccination schedules, convulsions in association with the consequent fever are reported after 0.09 per 1000 doses of combined diphtheria, tetanus and pertussis antigens, 0.6 per 1000 doses of polio vaccine and 0.93 per 1000 doses of measles vaccine (Harker 1977). Only after measles vaccination is there a significant, but very small, risk of a febrile convulsion.

The concept of predisposition to convulse with fever is emphasized by the wide range of infecting agents and causes of pyrexia which have been identified in children with febrile seizures.

General consequences of infection

Exogenous pyrogens released during viral and bacterial infections cause an upward setting of the thermoregulatory centres in the hypothalamic/preoptic areas. It has been suggested that the associated release of acetylcholine in the caudal hypothalamus, with subsequent activation of nicotinic receptors concerned in thermogenesis, might be directly related to the precipitation of febrile convulsions (Tangri et al 1976). However, recent studies have been unable to confirm that there is a simple relationship between experimental febrile convulsions and the cholinergic system (McCaughran et al 1982, 1984).

There has been considerable interest in whether the rate of rise or the height of temperature is the more important precipitant: both are difficult to monitor. On the whole, height of temperature is more commonly favoured, a view which is supported by simultaneous EEG and temperature monitoring in children who have had febrile convulsions (Minchom & Wallace 1984).

Pathophysiological aspects

The pathophysiology of febrile convulsions can be examined on the basis of:

- cerebral development prior to and at the critical age
- cerebral damage at the time of the convulsion
- pathological sequelae

Cerebral development at the age critical for febrile convulsions

Between the ages of 6 months and 3 years, when febrile convulsions are most common, both organization and myelination are occurring in the child's brain. Since prenatal factors and adverse events in early pregnancy may predispose to febrile convulsions, it is possible that abnormal neuronal proliferation and migration might be contributory events, but there is no pathological evidence to confirm this possibility.

Cerebral damage in association with febrile convulsions

There is a reasonable amount of circumstantial evidence to suggest that single brief (fewer than 15 minutes) generalized convulsions with fever do not cause recognizable cerebral damage. Biochemical evidence of cerebral hypoxia was lacking when the cerebrospinal fluid pyruvate and lactate levels were measured after brief convulsions with fever (Simpson et al 1977a), but prolongation for more than 30 minutes or repetition within a 24-hour period was associated with raised cerebrospinal fluid lactate levels and lactate:pyruvate ratios suggested that cerebral hypoxia had occurred (Simpson et al, 1977b). As correlates to these biochemical studies, Fowler (1957) and Meldrum (1976) have reported on the post-mortem findings in children with febrile convulsions, Aicardi & Chevrie (1983) on the radiological findings in some children with prolonged seizures and Gastaut et al (1960) and Ounsted et al (1966) on the clinical consequences of prolonged unilateral or bilateral seizures with fever.

In five children who died during illnesses in which febrile convulsions occurred, Fowler (1957) described neuronal necrosis throughout the cerebral cortex, but particularly in the frontal and temporal areas, variable changes in the basal ganglia and selective loss of Purkinje cells in the cerebellum. Meldrum (1976) has examined in detail the brain of a 5-month-old infant who died after prolonged seizures with fever. In all areas of the cerebral cortex, ischaemic nerve cell change and reactive astrocytosis were evident. The frontal and occipital horns were more severely affected than the temporal lobes, but bilateral acute Ammon's horn necrosis, characterized by loss of neurones in the H_1 (Sommer) sector and proliferation of glia in this layer and in the subjacent white matter was noted. There was widespread loss of Purkinje cells in the cerebellum. Meldrum commented that this picture was typical of the findings in children who die a few days after prolonged convulsions. The changes are nonspecific in that they are related to severe interference with cerebral energy metabolism such as occurs in arterial hypotension, cardiac arrest, cerebral ischaemia or severe hypoglycaemia. In his studies on adolescent baboons, Meldrum (1976) has further emphasized the importance of the duration of seizures in determining whether or not pathological changes occur. If seizures lasted under 30 minutes there was no correlation with ischaemic neuronal changes, but if the seizure persisted for between 30 and 300 minutes the degree of neuronal damage was related to its duration and to the degree and duration of any pyrexia; the severity and duration of arterial hypotension; and the severity of hypoglycaemia. When the autonomic and motor disturbances of the seizures were eliminated by paralysis and artifical ventilation, the cerebellar pathology was eliminated, but ischaemic neuronal changes still occurred in the neocortex, thalamus and hippocampus, confirming that the increased energy demand of the epileptic discharges themselves was an important factor in the pathological changes.

Pathological sequelae

In children, the gross pathological changes subsequent to prolonged convulsions have been demonstrated radiologically by Aicardi & Chevrie (1983):

cerebral swelling is followed by cerebral atrophy. Aicardi & Chevrie suggest that, in convulsions of lesser duration or greater localization, gross changes may not be demonstrable radiologically but that focal neuronal necrosis may nevertheless occur with resultant sclerosis, such as is found in Ammon's horn (mesiotemporal sclerosis) in those children in whom prolonged unilateral convulsions are followed by temporal lobe epilepsy (Gastaut et al 1960). Ounsted et al (1966) have emphasized the importance of age in determining the cerebral pathology resulting from prolonged seizures. In children aged less than 1 year, febrile convulsions which last for more than 30 minutes have a high risk of subsequent mental retardation. Between the ages of 1 and 3 years there is selective hemispheric vulnerability related to the child's sex. Mesiotemporal sclerosis, with subsequent temporal lobe epilepsy, is the more likely sequel to a prolonged febrile seizure in these somewhat older children (Taylor & Ounsted 1971).

Factors of importance in the first seizure

Since the age at the first seizure, the duration and the number of seizures which occur during any single febrile illness are relevant to the long-term prognosis, it is important that details are recorded as completely as possible. Understandably, since most first febrile seizures occur unexpectedly, there is considerable panic amongst the attendant adults and it is probable that partial features are not recorded as often as they should be. Even if the parents cannot give a figure for the duration of the seizure, it is possible to arrive at a reasonable estimate by asking them what they did during the length of time that the seizure continued. If the child was still convulsing on arrival in hospital the seizure was almost certainly of more than 15 minutes, if not more than 30 minutes, duration.

Prolonged repeated or partial febrile convulsions

In keeping with the findings of Meldrum (1976) most authors define a prolonged convulsion as one of at least 30 minutes duration. The critical time is considered to be 15 minutes by others (Nelson & Ellenberg 1976). It may be preferable to take the shorter period since this is likely to produce a greater sense of urgency in termination of the seizure.

At least 20% of patients in hospital series have febrile convulsions lasting 30 minutes or more (Bamberger & Matthes 1959, Chevrie & Aicardi 1975, Degen & Goller 1967, Harker 1977, Wallace 1975). Before diazepam became readily available, 13–14% of hospital patients were recorded as having febrile seizures of at least one hour's duration (Frantzen et al 1968, Laplane et al 1958). Seizures which are repeated within the same illness have been noted in up to 30% and those which are partial with or without secondary generalization in up to 19% of a hospital series (Wallace 1975). When the convulsions are defined as 'complex' (of at least 15 minutes' duration, repeated within 24 hours and or focal in onset), or 'simple', between one-third and one-fifth of children in population studies have complex initial febrile seizures (Nelson & Ellenberg 1976, Verity et al 1985b). As might be expected, children with complex seizures are more likely to be admitted to hospital (Verity et al 1985a). Thus hospital series tend to overestimate the relative frequency of complex initial febrile convulsions.

Predisposition to complex initial seizures has been explored in a number of studies. In some series, females seemed to be more vulnerable (Herlitz 1941, Aicardi & Chevrie 1970, Taylor & Ounsted 1971). Where both a positive family history and a perinatal abnormality are present and, in females, when previous neurological suboptimality is suspected, the risk of a complex initial seizure rises significantly (Wallace 1975). Younger children, up to 12 to 18 months of age, are at greater risk of an initial complex febrile seizure than those whose first attack occurs after 18 months (Lennox 1949, Aicardi & Chevrie 1970, Wallace 1975).

Neither the rate of rise of temperature nor the duration of the pyrexia appears to be important in determining the duration of the seizure.

Management of the febrile convulsions

The management of febrile convulsions can be considered under the following headings: attention to the effects of the seizure; antiepileptic drugs in the acute stage; identification and treatment of the underlying infection; recognition of parental anxieties.

Attention to the effects of the seizures

In addition to maintaining the airway and giving oxygen and other supportive therapy as necessary, it is particularly important in febrile convulsions actively to normalize the body temperature: tepid sponging, cooling with a fan and paracetamol or other antipyretics given as suppositories can be helpful.

Antiepileptic drugs in the acute stage

After a duration of 10 minutes if the convulsion does not terminate spontaneously it is appropriate to use an antiepileptic drug. Diazepam is the drug of first choice. It acts very rapidly if given in a dose of 0.1 mg/kg body weight intravenously. However, children who are at the peak age for febrile convulsions are often a little plump and intravenous injection may be difficult. Diazepam 0.5 mg/kg body weight given rectally in solution acts almost as rapidly as when the intravenous route is used and is a completely satisfactory alternative. If diazepam is given intramuscularly or in suppositories it is not absorbed sufficiently rapidly to be useful in the acute situation. Should the seizure fail to respond to the first dose of either intravenous or rectal diazepam, after 15 minutes a further comparable dose can be given. If this fails to control the convulsion, the child should be nursed in a unit where intubation and ventilation can be carried out. Further sedation using intravenous phenobarbitone or rectal or intramuscular paraldehyde can then be given under suitable supervision. It is particularly important that facilities for resuscitation are available if phenobarbitone is given after diazepam.

Identification and treatment of the underlying infection

Since a febrile convulsion is always a symptom of a generalized illness, it is clearly important that a good physical examination is performed and that treatment for any remediable condition is instituted. Almost 90% of febrile convulsions are related to viral infections (Lewis et al 1979) and for these children symptomatic therapy will be appropriate. Of the 10% with bacterial infections it is particularly important to consider, and in most cases exclude by lumbar puncture, bacterial meningitis.

Recognition of parental anxieties

The parents of at least 70% of the children believe at the time of the febrile convulsion that their child has died (Clare et al 1978, Baumer et al 1981). The parents are also concerned that their child might have meningitis, become mentally retarded or develop epilepsy (Clare et al 1978). Only by recognizing these anxieties and dealing with them truthfully and realistically will unjustified fears be suitably allayed and the likelihood of long-term sequelae be put into perspective.

Laboratory investigation in the acute stage

Tests on blood, urine or cerebrospinal fluid are relevant to the underlying illness, secondary metabolic changes or the seizure itself.

On the whole, although a neutropenia usually related to a viral illness occurs commonly, blood counts are not helpful in management. Hyponatraemia has been reported (Rutter & O'Callaghan 1978) but seems to be no more than a non-specific response to a febrile illness (Wallace 1975). Calcium and phosphate levels are normal.

Low serum IgA levels are found in some children (Lewis et al 1980, Isaacs et al 1984) and might be of significance in handling the infecting agent but this concept requires further investigation. Active immune responses, which are attributed to the presence of viral antigens within the central nervous system, have been demonstrated by measurement of cerebrospinal fluid immunoglobulins (Ariizumi et al 1981, Eeg-Olofsson & Wigertz 1982).

Lumbar puncture

Lumbar puncture is at best unpleasant and at worst frankly dangerous. It is the most controversial of the investigations appropriate in the child with febrile convulsions. Particularly in younger children it may be impossible to exclude meningitis on clinical grounds (Rutter & Smales 1977, Wolf 1978, Jaffe et al 1981). Although complex seizures are sometimes considered to be indicative of more serious underlying acquired pathology, in a series of 36 children in whom a febrile convulsion was the alerting sign for bacterial meningitis, the convulsions were all under 30 minutes' duration (Ratcliffe & Wolf 1977). It is recommended that, provided there are no signs of raised intracranial pressure, lumbar puncture should be performed as a routine procedure in children aged under 18 months at the time of a febrile seizure and in those aged 18 months or more whose recovery from the convulsion seems to be unexpectedly delayed (Wallace 1985). Where there are signs of raised intracranial pressure or other reasons to suspect that lumbar puncture might be hazardous, before examining the cerebrospinal fluid the child should be transferred to a unit where CT scanning and neurosurgical facilities are available. On very rare occasions it may be justifiable to treat the child empirically for meningitis until such time as the cerebrospinal fluid can be examined under safe conditions.

Radiological examination

Skull X-rays are almost invariably normal (Jaffe et al 1981, Nealis et al 1977, Wolf 1978) and should not be requested routinely. More sophisticated radiological investigation should only be requested when a serious underlying cause is suspected.

Electroencephalography

EEGs recorded during the acute stages of febrile illnesses in which convulsions occur reflect changes related more to the underlying infection than the seizures (Wallace & Zealley 1970). During the first week after a febrile convulsion between 50% and 70% of children have normal EEGs (Lennox 1949, Lerique 1955, Laplane et al 1958, Bamberger & Matthes 1959, Frantzen et al 1968). Up to one-third of patients show some slowing of background rhythms (Laplane et al 1958, Bamberger & Matthes 1959, Frantzen et al 1968). When complex seizures occur in children over 2 years old, the pyrexia exceeds 39°C, the illness lasts more than 36 hours or the underlying infection is gastroenteritis, marked slowing may be found in the background rhythms (Frantzen et al 1968). Lennox (1949) reported marked slowing in association with young age and long duration of fever. However, when EEG changes were related to changes in temperature over a 24-hour period of continuous recording, Minchom & Wallace (1984) were unable to demonstrate any relationship between the frequency of the background rhythm and the height of the pyrexia. During the week following the febrile convulsion, it is unusual to record spikes or other paroxysmal discharges. Even when found, their presence is completely unhelpful in prognosis (Wallace 1977, Matsuo et al 1981). During their continuous recordings for 24 hours after initial convulsions Minchom & Wallace (1984) found that spikes tended to appear during periods of prolonged high fever. However, no child in this study had a further convulsion during the recordings and the exact significance of this finding remains in doubt.

Thus, although EEGs might be expected to give some indication of the likelihood of recurrence of febrile seizures or the later development of epilepsy, to date, all studies have suggested that when recorded in the acute phase they do not provide any useful information for prognosis. Nevertheless, they can be helpful in the acute assessment and management of the child with a febrile seizure.

Recurrence of febrile convulsions

In children who do not receive antiepileptic prophylaxis following their first febrile seizure the overall risk of recurrence is about 50% (Wallace 1974b, Wallace & Aldridge Smith 1981). Approximately one-third of children who have twice had febrile convulsions will have three or more episodes (Hauser 1985). The recurrence rate is related to the presence or absence of risk factors which can be easily defined.

Risk factors for recurrence

Knudsen (1985) has identified five major risk factors:

1. Age less than 15 months
2. Epilepsy in first degree relatives
3. Febrile convulsions in first degree relatives
4. Complex first febrile seizure
5. Day nursery care

If three to five of these factors are present there is an 80% to 100% risk of a recurrence of febrile seizures during the following 18 months. The risk falls to 50% if two factors are present, to 25% if one factor is present and to 12% if none are in evidence.

These factors are similar but not identical to those defined by Wallace & Aldridge Smith (1981):

a. Seizures in first-degree relatives
b. Age less than 20 months
c. Unskilled or unemployed parents

If all three of these risk factors were present the children invariably had a recurrence. Children with two of these factors were significantly more likely to have recurrences than those in whom no risk factor was identified.

Abnormalities of pregnancy and low birth weight and neurological abnormality have also been cited as important in predisposing to recurrent febrile convulsions (Wallace 1974b, Wolf et al 1977, Nelson & Ellenberg 1978, Hauser 1985). On the basis of these studies there should be no difficulty in identifying children at risk of repeated convulsions with fever.

Significance of recurrent febrile convulsions

Hauser (1985) has shown that on long-term follow-up, with increasing numbers of febrile convulsions, the relative risk of subsequent epilepsy rises. In addition, children with recurrent febrile convulsions do not maintain normal intellectual progress (Aldridge Smith & Wallace 1982).

Prevention of recurrent febrile convulsions

Although pyrexia is a necessary precipitant of a febrile convulsion, even detailed antipyretic instruction does not reduce the incidence of further convulsions in subsequent pyrexial illnesses

(Camfield et al 1980). In children with risk factors for recurrence, prophylaxis with an antiepileptic drug should be prescribed.

Intermittent therapy Benzodiazepines are the only group of drugs effective in the control of febrile convulsions when given on an intermittent basis. The intermittent use of phenobarbitone or phenytoin is both irrational and ineffective.

The prophylactic treatment of choice is rectal diazepam in solution: 5 mg in children aged less than 3 years or 7.5 mg in children aged 3 or more years (Knudsen 1985). The diazepam is given when the temperature reaches 38.5°C and is repeated every 12 hours on up to a total of four occasions until the temperature falls below 38.5°C. This regime reduces the incidence of recurrence in children with risk factors to a rate comparable with that in children with no risk factor.

Alternatively, diazepam given in suppositories in a dose of 5 mg every eight hours while the pyrexia lasts has been found to be as effective in preventing recurrences as continuous phenobarbitone (Knudsen & Vestermark 1978).

Both clonazepam and nitrazepam have been used on an intermittent basis during pyrexias. Although effective in prophylaxis, both have tended to cause unacceptable sedation and both have the disadvantage for use in young children with illnesses that oral administration is necessary if either is given at home.

Continuous therapy Some parents find the concept of giving rectal medication unacceptable and in some children there is such a short period of ill health prior to the convulsion that there is no time to give intermittent prophylaxis. In these cases, if risk factors for recurrence are present, either phenobarbitone or sodium valproate should be given until there have been two years' freedom from convulsions (Camfield et al 1980, Ngwane & Bower 1980, Wallace & Aldridge Smith 1980). The dose of phenobarbitone is 4 to 5 mg/kg body weight per day and that of valproate 20 to 30 mg/kg body weight per day. Phenytoin has been found to significantly reduce the recurrence rate only in children aged 3 years or older (Melchior et al 1971) and, in any case, is difficult to use in small children. Carbamazepine has failed to reduce the recurrence risk, either when used as a first choice (Monaco et al 1980) or when given

after phenobarbitone has failed (Camfield et al, 1982).

Problems with prophylactic medication Diazepam may cause some mild drowsiness but this appears to be insufficient to obscure serious underlying infections such as meningitis.

Unacceptable overactivity occurs in 20% of children treated with phenobarbitone for febrile convulsions (Wolf & Forsythe 1978). However, in those children who are not overtly upset, cognitive development has been shown to proceed normally during treatment with phenobarbitone for periods of up to 35 months (Camfield et al 1979, Hellstrom & Barlach-Christoffersen 1980, Wolf et al 1981, Aldridge Smith & Wallace 1982).

Sodium valproate has not been reported to cause serious irreversible side-effects when used as prophylaxis for febrile convulsions. When given over a two-year period it produces significantly fewer behavioural side-effects than phenobarbitone (Wallace 1981) and does not adversely effect cognitive development (Aldridge Smith & Wallace 1982).

Epilepsy after febrile convulsions

There is an increased risk of later epilepsy in children who have had febrile convulsions (Nelson & Ellenberg 1976, Wallace 1977, Hauser 1985).

Incidence of later epilepsy

In a population study children who had not convulsed with fever had a 0.5% risk of epilepsy at the age of 7 whereas 2% of those who had febrile seizures were found to have epilepsy by the same age (Nelson & Ellenberg 1976). Where the follow-up was up to 30 years and actuarial calculations were made to assess the risk of epilepsy in the general population, children who had had febrile convulsions were just over five times more likely to develop epilepsy than those who had not convulsed when febrile (Hauser 1985). When children who have been admitted to hospital for treatment and assessment at the time of their first febrile fit are followed up, the incidence of later epilepsy is higher than that for the general population. In one study, only two-thirds of those with epilepsy when aged 9 to 14 years had had their first non-febrile seizure before the age of 7 (Wallace 1977). Thus figures for the incidence of later epilepsy probably underestimate the problem unless a truly long-term follow-up into adult life is undertaken.

Seizure types subsequent to febrile convulsions

Generalized tonic-clonic seizures are those most commonly reported once epilepsy becomes established (Degen & Goller 1967, Herlitz 1941, Nelson & Ellenberg 1976, Tsuboi & Endo 1977). It is rare for typical absences to be the major seizure type.

When a great deal of care had been taken to characterize the seizure type accurately, the risk for later partial epilepsy was almost twice that for generalized epilepsy in a long-term population study (Hauser 1985). Similarly, when analysing the previous histories of patients with partial epilepsy, Danesi (1985) found that almost a quarter had had febrile convulsions. Although many authors report a high incidence of generalized tonic-clonic seizures, there also appears to be a sizeable risk of later partial seizures in children who have had febrile convulsions.

High incidences of myoclonic or minor seizures have been reported from two centres (Nelson & Ellenberg 1976, Tsuboi & Endo 1977). Complex partial seizures were not mentioned in the Nelson & Ellenberg report. This is surprising since the syndrome of hemiconvulsion (usually febrile), hemiplegia (usually transient) and later complex partial seizures first reported by Gastaut et al (1960) is now well recognized.

It is concluded that any type of epilepsy may be a sequel to convulsions with fever and that, in the past, the categorization of such seizures has not always been optimal.

Risk factors for epilepsy

The important factors for the later development of epilepsy have usually been examined on the assumption that the antecedents of all types of epilepsy are comparable.

In the population study reported by Nelson & Ellenberg (1978) in which children were followed up to the age of 7 years, epilepsy occurred significantly more often in the presence of:

1. Suspect or abnormal development prior to the initial seizure complex.
2. Prolonged, repeated, focal features in the initial seizure
3. Seizures when afebrile in a parent or prior born sibling

In children with one of these factors there was a 1.3% risk of epilepsy at 7 years. If two or three factors were present the risk of epilepsy at age 7 years rose to 9.6%.

When the follow-up period has been up to 30 years, Hauser (1985) found a highly significant correlation between later epilepsy and prior mental retardation and/or cerebral palsy. Prolonged febrile convulsions, age of onset of less than one year and increasing numbers of febrile convulsions also correlated significantly with later epilepsy.

When the factors related to the development of partial epilepsy have been looked at separately from those present in generalized epilepsy, it has been found that persisting generalized tonic-clonic seizures occurred significantly more often in children of unskilled or unemployed parents, where there had been adverse perinatal events and persistent neurological abnormalities; whereas the complex partial seizures occurred significantly more often when the first febrile convulsion had been prolonged and partial (Wallace 1977). When the outcome for children with unilateral febrile convulsions of at least 30 minutes' duration was examined complex partial seizures were found most often in children who were particularly young at the time of their febrile convulsions and in females where the initial seizure was right sided (left hemisphere) (Wallace 1982).

Longitudinal EEG studies

Long-term EEG studies have been conducted with the aims of clarifying genetic trends and of monitoring the progression, or not, to epilepsy.

Doose et al (1983) found bilaterally synchronous spike and wave, photosensitivity and 4 to 7 cycle per second waves, i.e. patterns considered to be genetically determined, in 81% of 89 children with previous febrile convulsions, from whom EEGs had been recorded on 1046 occasions up to the ages of 11 to 13 years. Although these authors concluded that their findings supported their proposal that febrile convulsions occur as a result of a heterogeneous response to polygenetic inheritance, no correlation was found between the EEG characteristics and the family history.

Both Des Termes et al (1977) and Thorn (1982) have reported on the appearance of spikes on EEGs recorded in middle childhood in patients whose earlier EEGs have shown no epileptic activity, and have noted that such appearances bear no relation to clinical events.

On the basis of the information available, it seems that intermittent EEG recording over periods of months or years is unhelpful in clinical management.

Later cognitive development

In children who have been admitted to hospital with their initial febrile seizure between 6% and 18% have been reported to be mentally retarded (IQ less than 70) on subsequent testing (Zellweger 1948, Friderichsen & Melchior 1954, Millichap et al 1960, Aicardi &Chevrie 1976, Wallace & Cull 1979). The absolute incidence of frank mental retardation has not been reported for non-hospital populations. However, in children with febrile convulsions recorded in the British Births Survey 1970, speech problems were significantly more prevalent than expected and tests of design copying and vocabulary at the age of 5 were performed particularly badly by those children whose convulsions had been unilateral or prolonged (Verity et al 1985b).

Although some children are of below average ability, the mean intelligence quotient of any group with febrile convulsions has been invariably reported to be within the average range (Ellenberg & Nelson 1978, Camfield et al 1979, Wallace & Cull 1979, Wolf et al 1981, Aldridge Smith & Wallace 1982). However, specific learning difficulties do seem to be more common than expected. Problems with logical memory, Weschler digit symbol tests, block design, and Part B of the trail-making test were noted in a study where twins discordant for febrile convulsions were compared (Schiøtz-Christensen & Bruhn 1973). Specific reading difficulties have been found in

35% of children whose initial convulsion was right sided (left hemisphere) and either of at least 30 minutes or repeated within the same illness (Wallace 1982). The overall incidence of specific reading retardation was 19% in a hospital-based population who were tested when aged between 8 and 14 years (Cull 1975).

Factors related to suboptimal cognitive ability in children who have had febrile convulsions are:

1. Low social class and perinatal abnormalities (Wallace & Cull 1979)
2. Prior or continuing neurological abnormalities (Ellenberg & Nelson 1978, Wallace & Cull 1979)
3. Recurrence of febrile convulsions (Aldridge Smith & Wallace 1982)
4. Progression to epilepsy (Cull 1975)

MYOCLONIC EPILEPSIES

Myoclonic epilepsies of childhood include a series of seizure disorders which are usually, but not invariably associated with an underlying severe generalized cerebral disturbance. As with all other seizure disorders in childhood, these epilepsies and their implications are most readily understood if the child's age at the time of onset and of assessment are taken into account. As a general rule, the younger the child at the onset of an epilepsy which includes myoclonic seizures the more difficult the seizures are to control and the more serious for the ultimate prognosis.

Three main clinical syndromes can be identified with reasonable ease:

1. Early myoclonic encephalopathy
2. Infantile spasms (West syndrome)
3. Myoclonic-astatic epilepsy of early childhood

However, not all children who have myoclonic seizures can be readily accommodated under one or other of these headings and the following further epileptic syndromes in which myoclonic seizures feature will be considered:

a. Benign myoclonic epilepsy in infants
b. Severe myoclonic epilepsy in infants
c. Epilepsy with myoclonic absences
d. Juvenile myoclonic epilepsy

e. Progressive myoclonic epilepsy of unknown aetiology
f. Lennox–Gastaut syndrome (considered on p. 118)
g. Kojewnikow's syndrome (considered with partial epilepsies)

Early myoclonic encephalopathy

Recognition of epileptic syndromes which include myoclonic seizures and which commence in the neonatal period, or very soon thereafter, is relatively recent and it is not entirely clear from the literature whether early infantile epileptic encephalopathy (Ohtahara 1984) should be considered a separate entity or a variant of the syndrome referred to as early myoclonic encephalopathy (Aicardi 1985a).

Incidence

The incidence of early myoclonic encephalopathy is unknown. Aicardi (1985a) has reviewed the data on 18 cases previously reported in the literature and added information on a further seven infants. In classifying the epilepsies of 1295 patients seen between 1968 and 1971, Ohtahara (1984) does not report any cases of early myoclonic encephalopathy but made the diagnosis of early infantile epileptic encephalopathy on four occasions. If it can be assumed that the conditions are variants of the same epileptic syndrome, these reports suggest that this type of epilepsy is extremely rare.

Seizure types

Erratic fragmentary myoclonus associated with massive myoclonias, partial motor seizures and tonic infantile spasms are characteristic of this syndrome (Aicardi 1985a). In early infantile epileptic encephalopathy, Ohtahara (1984) describes tonic spasms which may or may not occur with series formation and which may be associated with other seizure types. However, myoclonic jerks are not mentioned and it is for this reason that Aicardi (1985a) has been reluctant to assume that early infantile epileptic encephalopathy should be considered another term for early myoclonic encephalopathy.

From his review of published cases, Aicardi (1985a) described the seizures as starting with erratic partial myoclonus, which may be restricted to only one part of a limb or may be generalized but which were usually repetitive to the extent of being more or less continuous during both waking and sleep. The appearance of partial seizures followed closely on the onset of the erratic myoclonus but tonic infantile spasms appeared somewhat later at about 3 to 4 months of age.

Differential diagnosis

The differential diagnosis is largely from other causes of myoclonus in very early infancy and possibly from Ohtahara's syndrome (1984), if this proves to be a separate entity.

Etiology

Both non-ketotic hyperglycinaemia and D-glutaric acidaemia present with early myoclonic encephalopathy (Aicardi 1985b). Other cases have occurred frequently on a familial basis and Aicardi (1985a) noted the following diagnoses or positive findings in seven of the 25 cases he reviewed: poliodystrophy; minor cortical malformations; Menkes' disease in the same family; progressive cerebral atrophy; severe multifocal spongy changes in the cerebral white matter with PAS-positive perivascular concentric bodies; high levels of proprionic acid in the blood and marked poverty of myelin without spongiosis in the cerebral hemispheres; and hemimegalencephaly with astrocytic proliferation but without disturbance of the cortical architecture.

Although in the majority of cases there was no biochemical or pathological confirmation of the underlying problem or problems in early myoclonic encephalopathy, Aicardi (1985a) emphasized the circumstantial evidence that at least some of the cases may have been secondary to autosomal recessive inheritance.

Clinical findings

In all but two of the 25 cases reviewed by Aicardi (1985a), the onset of the myoclonias was in the neonatal period and in all 25 the condition was established by the age of 3 months. Males and females were equally represented. Since the seizures started very early in life neurological deterioration was not readily confirmed. Truncal hypotonia was universally present and sometimes accompanied by hypertonicity of the limbs and later opisthotonic posturing. When measured, head circumferences had been reported to be normal at birth, but failure of head growth with subsequent microcephaly had been noted later. All infants had bilateral pyramidal tract signs and none made any recognizable mental development. In one case involvement of the peripheral nerves was recorded.

Investigations

In the absence of clearly defined causes in most cases of encephalopathy, it is difficult to outline a plan of investigation. Blood lysine and proprionic acid levels should certainly be measured, since non-ketotic hyperglycinaemia and D-glutaric acidaemia can cause clinically indistinguishable pictures and raised blood proprionic acid has been described in a further case. On the whole, the clinical picture suggests an underlying biochemical disorder and a full metabolic work-up seems justifiable in the hope that further aetiological agents will be identified.

So far as neuroradiological investigation is concerned, in most of the patients reviewed, CT scanning was initially normal and in a number it remained normal on repeat examination. In others, progressive cortical and periventricular atrophy was demonstrated (Aicardi 1985a).

Electroencephalography The EEG findings in early myoclonic encephalopathy are among the distinctive features of this syndrome (Aicardi 1985a). Normal background activity is entirely absent. During both waking and sleeping the record is characterized by complex bursts of spikes, sharp waves and slow waves, irregularly intermingled, lasting one to five seconds, and separated by episodes of flattening of the tracing lasting three to 10 seconds. The bursts of activity may occur synchronously or asynchronously over both hemispheres but their individual components are never bilaterally synchronous. Although the paroxysmal bursts on the EEG are not synchron-

ous with the jerks of the erratic myoclonus, they may occur in synchrony with massive myoclonus. During partial seizures, spike discharges remain localized to part of one hemisphere and the suppression-burst pattern may persist unchanged. After the age of 3 to 5 months the pattern may change to atypical hypsarrhythmia or to multifocal paroxysms.

Ohtahara (1984) described a very comparable suppression-burst pattern on the EEGs in his cases of early infantile epileptic encephalopathy. In six of his 10 cases the EEG changed from suppression-burst to a hypsarrhythmic pattern as the infants became older, and in two cases there was further progression to slow spike and wave. On the basis of the EEG findings it is difficult to regard the syndrome of early myoclonic encephalopathy (Aicardi 1985a) as different from early epileptic encephalopathy (Ohtahara 1984).

Treatment

Conventional antiepileptic drugs, ACTH, corticosteroids and pyridoxine are reported to be ineffective in treatment (Aicardi 1985a).

Prognosis

Of the 25 cases reviewed by Aicardi (1985a), 16 had died in early childhood, 9 in the first year of life and 13 before the age of 2 years. All survivors are severely retarded and four are described as vegetative.

Infantile spasms: West syndrome

Infantile spasms were first described by West (1841) when he observed the condition in his own child. The criteria for the diagnosis of West syndrome have been outlined by Jeavons (1985a). Spasms, mental retardation or deterioration and hypsarrhythmia on the EEG constitute typical West syndrome. The presence of atypical cases in which only two of the three components of West syndrome are present, or in which mental retardation and hypsarrhythmia are associated with 'staring seizures' or the Aicardi syndrome, are acknowledged. Jeavons felt that onset after the age of 1 year could not be described as West syndrome.

Incidence

Infantile spasms occur in between 1 in 2400 and 1 in 7800 live births (Lacy & Penry 1976, Riikonen & Donner 1979, Bellman 1983) and are thus a rare form of epilepsy.

Seizure types

Jeavons (1985b) has succinctly categorized the spasms as flexor, extensor or mixed. Flexor spasms may be so brief that, unless the child is under continuous observation, they may not be seen. The neck, trunk and limbs are involved and abduction or adduction of the arms may occur. Extensor spasms involve the neck and trunk with extension, abduction or adduction of the limbs.

Both Kellaway et al (1979) and King et al (1985) have characterized the ictal phenomena in West syndrome by simultaneous EEG and video screening. Kellaway et al (1979) defined a spasm as a brief contraction involving the muscles of the neck, trunk and extremities, bilaterally and symmetrically. The character of the spasm was determined by whether there was maximal involvement of the flexor or extensor muscles and, in an analysis of 5042 seizures, 42% were considered mixed, 34% flexor, 22.5% extensor, 0.6% asymmetrical, with the remaining 1% described as 'arrest'. Most of the 24 patients studied had more than one seizure type. King et al (1985) have examined the characteristics of 1079 spasms which occurred in 10 patients: while the infants were awake, on average 7.7 spasms were observed per hour; the rate fell to 2.5 spasms per hour if the infants were asleep; 46.6% of the spasms occurred in clusters. King et al described the spasms as myoclonic with or without tonic components and/or arrest of activity. Most commonly the spasms were considered to be myoclonic-tonic (40.3%) or myoclonic alone (36.3%) but, when classified by postural motor phenomena, 41.6% were 'flexor', 16.3% 'extensor' 39% 'mixed' and 3.1% were 'arrest' alone. These authors noted that simultaneous EEG monitoring showed that the myoclonic contractions were the initial paroxysmal event and that tonic contractions and arrests were associated with suppression of the EEG with or without rhythmic activity.

On the basis of the clinical descriptions of the seizures, there appears to be no doubt that myoclonic jerks are features of West syndrome and it is not clear why Jeavons (1985b) and Kellaway et al (1979) shy away from this term in their descriptions of the ictal phenomena.

Recognition of the ictal nature of the attacks is sometimes considerably delayed. The correct diagnosis was made by a primary care doctor in only 12% of the cases reported by Bellman (1983).

Differential diagnosis

West syndrome can be differentiated from benign myoclonus of epilepsy on the basis of the EEG (Lombroso & Fejerman 1977). Benign myoclonic epilepsy of infancy and severe myoclonic epilepsy of infancy have distinct and different clinical and EEG patterns. Early myoclonic encephalopathy has a much earlier age on onset and is characterized by suppression burst activity on the EEG (Aicardi 1985a).

Etiology

Jeavons (1985b) divides West syndrome into a primary or cryptogenic group and a secondary or symptomatic group, but admits that, with increasing sophistication and thoroughness of investigation, the relative proportion of symptomatic cases has now reached about 70%. Nevertheless, Bellman (1983) only managed to define an aetiology in 34 of 92 cases he assessed. This is probably a reflection of the variability in the sources and thoroughness of investigation of his cases which were reported to the National Child Encephalopathy Study by paediatricians throughout the British Isles (Miller et al 1981).

Primary or cryptogenic cases Jeavons (1985b) defined the primary or cryptogenic cases as those where the psychomotor development had been normal up to the time of onset of the spasms and in whom there was no evidence of any cerebral disorder.

Secondary/symptomatic cases Early abnormal development with psychomotor retardation or neurological abnormality prior to the onset of spasms has been considered by Jeavons (1985b) to be necessary for inclusion in the secondary or symptomatic group. Infantile spasms are now generally recognized as possible symptoms of a wide variety of conditions which have as their common property an ability to cause gross generalized disturbance of cerebral function. The precipitating factors can be divided into prenatal, perinatal or postnatal.

Of the prenatal causes, tuberous sclerosis and other congenital defects were those most commonly identified in Bellman's series (1983). Aicardi's syndrome (absence of the corpus callosum, choroidoretinitis, infantile spasms, female sex, severe retardation) is but one example of a congenital malformation associated with infantile spasms. Others are immature dendritic development (Huttenlocher 1974), hydranencephaly (Neville 1972) and Down's syndrome (Bellman 1983). Prenatally, i.e. genetically determined, metabolic and degenerative disorders can underly infantile spasms. Bellman (1983) reviewed reports on leucodystrophy, Leigh's disease, Alper's disease, phenylketonuria and abnormalities of glycine metabolism, and Lacy & Penry (1976) noted publications on infantile spasms in histidinaemia and in a patient with hyperornithinaemia, hyperammonaemia and homocitrillinuria.

Clearly, in the investigation of infantile spasms, if no obvious cerebral structural abnormality can be defined, a full metabolic work-up is indicated. Prenatal infections may also be associated with the development of infantile spasms. Publications on congenital cytomegalovirus, toxoplasmosis and syphilis are cited by Lacy & Penry (1976). Prematurity, low birth weight, antepartum haemorrhage and toxaemia of pregnancy have also been considered as etiological agents (Lacy & Penry 1976).

In Bellman's series (1983) and the review of previous literature by Lacy & Penry (1976) adverse perinatal events were the most commonly identified predisposing factors. Of these, hypoxia or anoxia was most frequently reported. Difficult deliveries, intracranial haemorrhage, hypoglycaemia, severe jaundice and septicaemia were also noted to be of etiological importance.

Truly postnatal events rarely cause infantile spasms. However, both Bellman (1983) and Lacy & Penry (1976) record West syndrome after bacterial meningitis or viral meningitis or encephalitis.

Contrary to earlier suggestions there appears to be no causal relationship between immunization or vaccination procedures and the development of West syndrome (Melchior 1977, Bellman 1983).

Pathophysiological considerations

The pathological findings in 66 patients reported in previous publications were reviewed by Lacy & Penry (1976). They divided them into:

1. Perinatal and postnatal encephalopathies
2. Cortical malformations
3. Metabolic disorders
4. Heterodegenerative disorders (tuberous sclerosis)
5. Miscellaneous disorders

In four of the 66 patients the pathological findings were negative.

In the perinatal and postnatal encephalopathies ulegyria, intracortical cysts, sclerosis of the basal ganglia and/or thalamus, cerebellar atrophy and porencephaly feature most commonly. Of the cortical malformations agyria/lissencephaly, pachygyria, micropolygyria, heterotopias and cerebral and cerebellar dysplasias are most often reported. Sudanophilic leucodystrophy, globoid cell leucodystrophy, Leigh's disease and diffuse demyelination secondary to phenylketonuria are amongst the metabolic disorders for which pathological specimens were available. The miscellaneous disorders included meningitis and encephalitis.

With such a diversity of gross pathological findings it is difficult to postulate the physiological consequences which produce the clinical and EEG characteristics of West syndrome. Huttenlocher (1974) has described marked sparsity of dendritic arborization in the neocortex of five patients with mental retardation and myoclonic seizures. The relevance of this finding was discussed in some detail by Lacy & Penry (1976). However, using the criteria of Jeavons (1985a), at the most only two of the five cases described by Huttenlocher (1974) can be diagnosed as having West syndrome.

Clinical features

The peak age of onset is between 4 and 7 months. Males are over-represented. Signs of neurological dysfunction in addition to spasms are common in West syndrome. Microcephaly, various types of cerebral palsy and visual inattention or blindness were reported in more than 50% of the case reports reviewed by Jeavons & Bower (1964). In other publications, despite very full accounts on the nature and frequency of the spasms, there is little information that a thorough search has been made for clues to the underlying etiology. In particular, the skin should be examined both by naked eye and under a Wood's lamp for the ash-leaf-shaped patches of depigmentation most commonly seen on the back of the trunk and legs which would suggest tuberous sclerosis. The shape of the skull may be such as to suggest an underlying malformation, e.g. porencephalic cyst. Stigmata of metabolic disease, such as failure to thrive, vomiting, skin rashes and unusual smelling urine should also be sought. Infantile spasms only rarely are likely to be secondary to an intracranial storage disorder, but the size of the liver and spleen should be checked. When the spasms are symptomatic of a mitochondrial cytopathy the infants are extremely hypotonic (Wallace 1984). Mental retardation is present at the onset in about 95% of cases (Jeavons 1985b).

Investigations

Establishment of the etiology is particularly important from the genetic point of view. Infantile spasms may be symptomatic of any condition which causes a gross generalized cerebral disturbance. So in the absence of a very convincing history of perinatal hypoxia, of definite signs on the CT scan of tuberous sclerosis, or of recognizable abnormalities such as Down's syndrome, a full work-up for possible inherited metabolic disease should be undertaken. Screening for disorders of amino acid, urea, carbohydrate and catecholamine metabolism is particularly important. In addition, the serum titres for cytomegalovirus and toxoplasmosis should be measured.

A CT head scan is mandatory in all infants who have West syndrome. Spasms can present as the first sign of tuberous sclerosis and parents will wish to know as soon as possible whether or not they are carriers of this dominantly inherited condition. Other intracranial pathology of aetiological or genetic importance might also be seen on a CT scan.

Electroencephalography Hypsarrhythmia, the EEG pattern typically found in infantile spasms, is defined by Jeavons (1985b) as a grossly chaotic mixture of very high amplitude (more than 200 μV) slow waves at frequencies of 1 to 7 cycles per second with sharp waves and spikes which vary in amplitude, morphology, duration and site. Jeavons described a modified hypsarrhythmia as having a more organized appearance with some bilaterally synchronous discharges. During actual seizures Kellaway et al (1979) identified 11 different patterns. A total of 5042 seizures were monitored: high-voltage frontal-dominant, generalized slow wave transients were followed by voltage attenuation in 38% of attacks; generalized sharp and slow wave complexes in 17.4%; generalized sharp and slow wave discharges followed by attentuation in 13.2%; attenuation only in 11.9%; generalized slow wave transients only in 10.9%; attenuation with superimposed fast activity in 6.9% of spasms; and four various other combinations of fast activity, attenuation and slow waves in less than 1% of attacks. The significance of these various EEG changes is not entirely obvious, since a close correlation between the EEG and the clinical features of the spasms was not demonstrated. Hrachovy et al (1984) reviewed 290 24-hour polygraphic records of 64 patients with infantile spasms and concluded that features seen in patients in which hypsarrhythmia was recorded depended on the duration of the recording, the clinical state of the patient and the presence of structural cerebral abnormalities. Considerable variations in the records occurred from time to time in the same infants. Hrachovy et al (1984) identified the following variations on the typical hypsarrhythmic pattern: hypsarrhythmia with increased interhemispheric synchronization; asymmetrical hypsarrhythmia; hypsarrhythmia with episodes of attenuation; and hypsarrhythmia comprising primarily high-voltage slow activity with little sharp wave or spike activity. During sleep, particularly REM sleep, there was marked reduction in and sometimes total disappearance of the hypsarrhythmic pattern. There is no discussion in Hrachovy et al's paper of the possible clinical significance of the EEG findings.

Treatment

Infantile spasms do not respond to barbiturates, phenytoin or carbamazepine. Variable success is achieved with ACTH (adrenocorticotrophin) or steroids, sodium valproate or benzodiazepines.

ACTH and steroids Corticotrophin was first used in the treatment of infantile spasms by Sorel & Dusaucy-Bauloye (1958). The success reported by these workers encouraged others to study treatment with oral steroids (Jeavons & Bower 1964). Early reports on the successful control of seizures with subsequent good mental development have not been universally confirmed by subsequent studies. Nevertheless, ACTH or oral steroids retain an important place in the treatment of infantile spasms (Hrachovy et al 1979, 1980, Matsumoto et al 1981, Pentella et al 1982, Riikonen 1982, Willig & Lagenstein 1982, Lombrosco 1983c). Although Lerman & Kivity (1982) advocated high doses of ACTH (80 to 100 IU/day), until the seizures come under control, Riikonen (1982) found that daily doses of ACTH of 120 to 160 IU/ day were no more effective than 20 to 40 IU/day. In a very small number of patients, Hrachovy et al (1980) found that their patients did as well on ACTH 20 IU/day as on 30 to 40 IU/day. All authors agree that ACTH should be given as a course, and if necessary, the course repeated, rather than as a continued long-term medication. There are strong arguments against treating patients with obvious developmental delay or severe neurological abnormalities prior to the onset of infantile spasms with ACTH or steroids. The long-term outlook in these patients is very poor, even if their spasms are controlled, and the side-effects of steroid therapy can be dangerous. On the other hand, there is very good evidence that, where spasms occur on a background of neurodevelopmental normality, rapid control of the seizures by steroids/ACTH is associated with an improved outcome (Lerman & Kivity 1982, Riikonen 1982, Jeavons 1985b). It is suggested

that, in those patients who do not have obvious prior neurodevelopmental abnormalities either ACTH 20 to 40 IU/day or prednisolone 2 mg/kg/day be given for 2 to 4 weeks followed by gradual reduction in dosage over a period of three months. Some studies have found that prednisolone may not be as effective as ACTH in the control of the seizures. (Kellaway et al 1983).

Sodium valproate Jeavons (1985b) has stated that valproate may reduce the frequency of infantile spasms. However, confirmation by controlled trials of the efficacy of valproate in West syndrome is awaited.

Benzodiazepines Both clonazepam and nitrazepam can be effective in the control of infantile spasms. However, tolerance usually develops rapidly. Schmidt (1983a) reported that 22% of children with infantile spasms became seizure-free on clonazepam. An initial dose of clonazepam 0.01 to 0.03 mg/kg/day is suggested, with the subsequent dosage tailored to the individual patient's needs. Rather more than 50% of children with infantile spasms are reported to have responded to nitrazepam (Schmidt 1983a). The dose suggested is initially 0.5 to 1 mg/kg/day, with adjustment related to the seizure control.

Prognosis

The long-term outlook is dependent on the underlying condition. When taken as a whole, without regard to etiology, only about 20% of patients will make a complete recovery (Bellman 1983). Death occurs within seven to 12 years in a further 20% (Friedman & Pampiglione 1971). Approximately one-third of patients have a permanent neurological deficit and two-thirds are mentally retarded. Seizures persist in at least half the children. In some there is progression to the Lennox-Gastaut syndrome and in others generalized tonic-clonic seizures supervene. Factors associated with a more favourable outcome than usual are age at onset of six months or more, 'primary' etiology and short duration of spasms (Bellman 1983). In infants seen very soon after the onset of spasms who are treated immediately with ACTH and whose response is more or less immediate, the likelihood of a good outcome is much greater than for those with preceding neurological abnormality whose spasms have been present for many months prior to treatment.

Benign myoclonic epilepsy in infants

The syndrome of benign myoclonic epilepsy in infants has been characterized by Dravet (1985a). It can be distinguished from the other myoclonic epilepsies of infancy by the normality of the inter-ictal neurological examination and EEG and the readiness with which the seizures respond to treatment.

Incidence

In their discussion of benign myoclonic epilepsy in infants Dravet et al (1985a) were able to review published reports on only 17 cases and observed that the syndrome appeared to have been first recognized in 1981 and seemed to be very uncommon. The incidence was only 7% in a group of 142 patients with various types of myoclonic epilepsy (Dravet et al 1982).

Seizure types

Only one seizure type occurs (Dravet et al 1985a). The attacks are brief, generalized and myoclonic. Initially they may be barely noticeable, but later they may become more intense and, if they are still present when the child is able to stand, they may cause loss of balance. The myoclonus involves the axis of the body and the limbs; the head drops suddenly onto the trunk and there is an upwards-outwards movement of the arms accompanied by flexion of the legs; the eyes may roll up. The attacks usually last from one to three seconds but may persist for as long as 10 seconds. If repeated jerks occur there may be reduction in alertness but loss of consciousness never occurs. These myoclonic seizures can present at any time of day but are never observed during deep sleep.

Although no other seizure type was observed coincidentally with the myoclonus, two of the reported children had had febrile seizures prior to the onset of the myoclonic epilepsy (Dravet et al 1985a).

Differential diagnosis

Benign myoclonic epilepsy in infants can be distinguished from benign myoclonus of early infancy by the absence of EEG changes in the latter condition (Lombroso & Fejerman 1977). Other myoclonic epilepsies are differentiated by the presence of additional seizure types, more severely abnormal EEGs particularly during inter-ictal recording, developmental standstill or regression and their poor response to antiepileptic drug therapy.

Etiology

There is no information in the literature on the possible aetiology of this epileptic syndrome. Dravet et al (1985a) noted that family histories were often positive for other types of seizure disorder and suggested that benign myoclonic epilepsy in infants was a very early expression of primary generalized epilepsy.

Clinical features

In the patients of Dravet et al (1985a) the age of onset was between 6 months and 2 years and there was a male preponderance. Clinical examination was normal.

Investigations

In the one case who had a pneumoencephalograph and the two children who had CT scans the findings were normal (Dravet et al 1985a).

Electroencephalography Video and polygraphic recordings have enabled Dravet et al (1985a) to characterize the attacks in detail. The clinically observed myoclonic seizures were synchronous with a discharge on the EEG of generalized spike-waves or polyspike-waves occurring at 3 cycles per second and of the same duration as a seizure. Between seizures the EEGs were normal for age. In some cases, photic stimulation provoked spike-wave or polyspike-wave but this was always accompanied by myoclonus. Drowsiness and light sleep activated generalized spike-wave but these discharges tended to disappear during slow wave sleep.

Treatment

The treatment of choice is sodium valproate. Barbiturates and benzodiazepines are considered unsuitable (Dravet et al 1985a).

Prognosis

The myoclonic seizures may persist if left untreated and may be replaced by generalized tonic-clonic seizures in later childhood or at puberty. Both types of seizure respond readily to sodium valproate (Dravet et al 1985a). The EEG changes resolve as the clinical seizures disappear.

Four of the seven cases of Dravet et al (1985a) later required special education because of behaviour disturbances or learning problems. These difficulties were attributed to delay in instituting appropriate treatment for the myoclonic seizures, to the early age of their onset and to their frequency, but they leave a question mark over whether this epileptic syndrome is completely benign.

Severe myoclonic epilepsy in infancy

Severe myoclonic epilepsy in infancy has been characterised by Dravet (1985b). As an entity it has been described in the literature in only 82 cases. (Dravet et al 1985b).

Incidence

The overall incidence is unknown. The 42 patients described by Dravet et al (1982) represented 29.5% of a group of 142 children with various types of myoclonic epilepsy in childhood.

Seizure types

Dravet et al (1982) reported that in all but one case, where a generalized tonic-clonic attack occurred, the first seizure for which parents sought advice was clonic. Generalized clonic attacks occurred in seven-eighths of the cases; in the remainder the attacks were unilateral. In at least half the children, the initial seizure was of more than 15 minutes duration and in three-fifths a fever appeared to precipitate the attack. Short

or long myoclonic attacks had been observed before the initial clonic seizures by a small proportion of parents. Frequent recurrences of clonic attacks, usually with fever, were observed before the onset, between one and four years of age, of generalized myoclonic seizures (Dravet et al 1985b). The myoclonic seizures are described as lacking any specific characteristics, recurring several times a day, but not occurring in bouts though they may be very frequent. Severe seizures may cause the child to fall but milder ones may be difficult to discern unless the child is watched during an activity requiring precise movement. Sometimes the myoclonic jerks may be initiated by varying the ambient light intensity. Coincidentally with the appearance of the myoclonic jerks, partial seizures with either autonomic or atonic components and automatisms were observed in one-third of the patients of Dravet et al (1985b). In some children obtunded states were associated with myoclonias.

Differential diagnosis

Severe myoclonic epilepsy of infancy is differentiated from the other myoclonias in this age group by the previous history of clonic seizures with fever, the normality of children at the onset and the absence of a hypsarrhythmic pattern on the EEG. It is not possible to differentiate this condition from recurrent febrile convulsions until the myoclonic seizures begin.

Etiology

The etiology is unknown. A family history of febrile convulsions and/or of epilepsy is present in a quarter of the cases. Dravet et al (1985b) feel that in the absence of known etiological factors and, in the presence of a high percentage of positive family histories, the initial ictal symptomatology and the photosensitivity, a serious form of primary generalized epilepsy is likely.

Clinical features

A slightly higher proportion of males has been noted in the cases reported (Dravet et al 1985b).

In all patients the onset of seizures was in the first year of life with the first convulsion occurring at a mean age of about 6 months. Normal development was universal before the initial seizure. With the appearance of the myoclonic seizures, slowing of language acquisition, ataxia, hyperreflexia and interictal fragmentary and segmental myoclonus appeared (Dravet et al 1985b).

Pathophysiological features

In considering that severe myoclonic epilepsy in infancy was a serious form of primary generalized epilepsy Dravet et al (1985b) hypothesized that the later changes in neurological characteristics could be explained either by the occurrence of repeated prolonged convulsions with fever or the existence of unfavourable genetic factors which might have caused secondary aggravation of a primary epilepsy.

Investigations

A minority of cases have shown dilatation of the cisterna magnum on CT scan (Dravet et al 1985b). Otherwise, with the exception of the EEG, investigation appears to have been unrewarding.

Electroencephalography Comprehensive details of the EEG findings in this syndrome are given by Dravet et al (1985b). The initial records were normal. During the second year paroxysms of generalized spike-waves or polyspike-waves either in isolation or in brief bursts appeared. These eventually became to some extent lateralized, were influenced by intermittent photic stimulation and increased by drowsiness or slow-wave sleep. Photosensitivity was noted before the age of 2 years in up to one-third of patients. In the long term, the EEGs showed considerable variability though spikes, spike-waves and polyspike-waves, usually localized rather than generalized, persisted.

Treatment

Dravet et al (1985b) reported that the seizures are resistant to all forms of treatment but the therapeutic agents which have been given are not enumerated.

Prognosis

The time when seizures are particularly frequent is noted to be very variable from patient to patient (Dravet et al 1985b). Attacks were a continuing problem up to the age of 11 or 12 years in some patients. A reduction in seizure frequency was noted initially during the day with a tendency for nocturnal clonic or tonic-clonic attacks to persist. Coincidentally, the myoclonic jerks appeared as very atypical absence seizures with minor disturbances in consciousness, random myoclonus and a tendency to hypertonia. With these attacks the child may be obtunded and the term 'minor motor status' applicable.

Dravet et al (1985b) felt they had not studied the clinical neurological states of their patients long enough to draw firm conclusions about the long-term motor deficits but noted adults with severe cerebellar and pyramidal syndromes and myoclonus who had histories suggestive of severe myoclonic epilepsy in infancy.

Death in early childhood occurred in approximately one-sixth of the cases of Dravet et al (1985b). All the surviving children required special education and, where the intelligence had been measured, two-thirds were severely subnormal.

Myoclonic-astatic epilepsy

As its name suggests, this epileptic syndrome is characterized by the presence of myoclonic and astatic seizures which may occur either independently or in combination.

Incidence

Myoclonic-astatic epilepsy represents 1% to 2% of all epilepsies in children up to the age of 9 years (Doose 1985a).

Differential diagnosis

The most frequent source of confusion is with the Lennox-Gastaut syndrome. Table 4.1 lists the features which may be used to distinguish myoclonic-astatic epilepsy from the Lennox-Gastaut syndrome.

Table 4.1 Features distinguishing myoclonic astatic epilepsy and the Lennox-Gastaut syndrome.

Distinguishing features	Myoclonic-astatic epilepsy (Doose 1985b)	Lennox-Gastaut syndrome (Beaumanoir 1985a)
Previous neurological history	Normal in 88%	Prior 'encephalopathy'
Inheritance		No familial cases
Family history of seizure disorder	37%	2.5 to 40%
Seizure types:		
Classification	1° generalized	2° generalized
Myoclonic	+	+
Astatic	+	+
Myoclonic: astatic	+	−
Absence with myoclonias and/or atonia	+	−
Generalized tonic-clonic	+	+
Status	36%	common with stupor
Axial tonic	Late only	+
Atypical absence	−	+
Partial	−	+
EEG:		
Background abnormal	Not initially	+
Irregular fast spike-wave and polyspike-wave	+	−
2–3 Hz spike-wave	+ in status	+ diffuse
Focal abnormalities	rare	Multifocal +

Seizure types

The characteristic seizures are myoclonic, astatic or myoclonic-astatic and, by definition, these are present in all children with this syndrome. In addition, absences with myoclonic jerks and irregular myoclonias of the face occur in 62%; febrile convulsions in 28%; generalized tonic-clonic seizures in 75% (in 34% at the onset); and status of minor seizures in 36% (Doose 1985a). Although tonic seizures are more likely to be indicative of the Lennox-Gastaut syndrome than of myoclonic-astatic epilepsy, Doose (1985a) thinks they may be present in this latter syndrome in 30% of cases. A status of minor seizures (minor motor status) produces apathy, stupor and, at worst, an apparent dementia. Irregular twitching of the facial muscles, drooling, aphasia which may or may not be interrupted by more obvious visible, or only palpable, myoclonic jerking may be clinically so non-specific to the uninitiated as to be mistaken for a behaviour disorder.

Etiology

Myoclonic-astatic seizures usually start on a background of normal neuropsychological develop-

ment, but Doose (1985a) was able to identify a history of 'definite higher risk factors' or developmental retardation in 16% of 117 children with this condition. Otherwise Doose felt that the epilepsy could be classified as primary and that genetic predisposition was the most important aetiological factor. He postulated a polygenic type of inheritance.

Pathophysiological aspects

In the absence of a pathologically identified aetiology, the physiological consequences are difficult to define. At 2 to 5 years the peak periods of all aspects of cerebral development have passed, but both organization and myelination are still in progress. This may explain the loss of intellectual skills which occurs in some patients.

Clinical features

The maximal age at onset of the seizures is between 2 and 5 years and boys are more often affected than girls. The children are usually neurologically normal at the onset of the myoclonic-astatic seizures, but in two-thirds of the cases of Doose (1985a) the initial episode was either a febrile or an afebrile generalized tonic-clonic seizure.

There is a family history of seizure disorders, but not necessarily of myoclonic-astatic epilepsy, in just over one-third of the patients.

Investigations

The only investigation for which information is available is electroencephalography.

Electroencephalography Doose (1985a) has given details of the EEGs to be expected as myoclonic-astatic epilepsy evolves. Initially, particularly in those cases where the first seizures are either febrile or afebrile tonic-clonic seizures, monomorphic theta rhythms with parietal accentuation and occipital 4 Hz rhythms blocked by eye opening are the usual EEG findings. Irregular spike and wave activity may also be found exclusively during sleep. Later, bilateral synchronous irregular spikes and waves appear. These may be particularly prominent anteriorly. The EEGs in children whose seizures are mostly myoclonic typically show short paroxysms of irregular spikes and waves and polyspikes. In those whose attacks are astatic or myoclonic-astatic the findings are of 2 to 3 Hz spikes and waves or spike-wave variants on a background of 4 to 7 Hz rhythms or, in the more severe cases, generalized slow activity. Photosensitivity is usual between the ages of 5 and 15 years and spikes and waves are very common during sleep. Occasional records show lateralization of the abnormalities but these are not characteristic of this syndrome.

Treatment

No controlled trial of any individual antiepileptic drug has been performed. Jeavons et al (1977) wrote enthusiastically about the usefulness of sodium valproate, and Doose (1985a) also concluded that valproate was more likely to be helpful in the control of seizures than any other antiepileptic medication. Aicardi (1980) reported that almost half the patients in his series had periods when they were free of seizures for up to one year while still on medication. He does not specify the medication and comments that late

recurrences are not uncommon. Benzodiazepines can be useful, but tolerance develops readily.

Prognosis

The prognosis is to some extent related to seizure frequency. However, the possibility that difficulty with control of the seizures might be indicative of a more serious underlying condition cannot be ignored. Spontaneous remissions occasionally occur, but 50% of those who have had myoclonic-astatic epilepsy continue to have seizures. Neurological abnormalities and dementia then become additional problems. Doose (1985a) stated that the following suggested a poor outcome:

1. Frequent tonic-clonic seizures
2. Nocturnal tonic seizures
3. Minor motor status
4. Onset with tonic-clonic seizures before the age of 2 years
5. Continuance of 4 to 7 Hz rhythms and spike-and-wave during therapy
6. Failure of development of a stable occipital alpha rhythm

For those who do not make a good recovery persistence of generalized tonic-clonic seizures and of nocturnal tonic seizures is usual; mild cerebellar ataxia, gross motor dysfunction, clumsiness and speech disorders become evident; and dementia supervenes.

Epilepsy with myoclonic absences

This syndrome is characterized by frequent seizures in which clonic jerks are associated with 3 Hz spike-waves on the EEG (Tassinari & Bureau 1985).

Incidence

Myoclonic absences are rare. Only 0.5% to 1% of a selected population of children with epilepsy had this seizure type (Tassinari & Bureau 1985).

Seizure types

The onset and offset of myoclonic absences are abrupt. Seizures occur frequently throughout the day and are of 10 to 60 seconds in duration. Consciousness may not be completely lost, though it is thought to be impaired in most instances. The motor component consists of rhythmic jerking of the shoulders, head and arms, and staggering; falls are unusual; arrest or alteration in the respiratory pattern may be observed and some patients are incontinent during the attacks. A tonic contraction may follow the initial myoclonias (Tassinari & Bureau 1985). Some patients also have generalized tonic-clonic seizures. Hyperventilation will precipitate attacks in about two-thirds of the cases and about half the children are photosensitive. Attacks may also be precipitated by wakening from sleep.

Differential diagnosis

Myoclonic absences should be distinguished from other absences by the prominence of the motor symptomatology. In other syndromes with myoclonias the spike-wave discharges on EEG tend to be of 2 Hz rather than 3 Hz frequency.

Etiology

Genetic factors appear important in that a family history of epilepsy is present in 25% of cases; otherwise, nothing is known of the etiology. Tassinari & Bureau (1985) have suggested that myoclonic absences are intermediary between primary generalized and secondary generalized epilepsies, but this suggestion merely highlights uncertainties about the syndrome.

Clinical findings

Males have epilepsy with myoclonic absences more commonly than females. The attacks may commence at almost any age during childhood. In about half the cases of Tassinari & Bureau (1985) mental retardation preceded the onset of seizures.

Investigation

Electroencephalography During seizures, the EEG shows rhythmic 3 Hz spike and wave which is bilateral, synchronous and symmetrical. The spike onset of the spike-wave discharge is strictly and constantly related to the myoclonic jerk (Tassinari & Bureau 1985). Photosensitivity can be demonstrated in about half of the children and attacks provoked by hyperventilation in about three-quarters.

Treatment

Myoclonic absences are relatively resistant to therapy. Indeed, this syndrome should be considered when children who initially appear to have uncomplicated absences fail to respond to treatment. Jeavons et al (1977) found that a combination of sodium valproate and ethosuximide was more likely to control the seizures than other forms of treatment, but Tassinari & Bureau (1985) mention the use of diones and benzodiazepines in addition. No systematic study of treatment of this seizure type is available.

Prognosis

The seizures remit in some cases but in others they become complicated by the appearance of tonic attacks and atypical absences such as occur in the Lennox-Gastaut syndrome. The EEG then shows slow spike-wave discharges rather than 3 Hz paroxysms.

Of the children who are intellectually normal at the onset of the myoclonic absences, about half have later loss of cognitive skills (Tassinari & Bureau 1985). About 75% of this group of patients are finally intellectually impaired.

Progressive myoclonic epilepsy

Progressive myoclonic epilepsy may be symptomatic of recognizable degenerative disorders of the brain or may occur without a definable underlying cause.

The progressive myoclonic epilepsy syndrome is characterized clinically by the presence of:

1. Generalized myoclonus and arrhythmic, asynchronous and asymmetrical, partial or segmental myoclonus
2. Multiple seizure types, usually including generalized tonic-clonic, myoclonic and tonic seizures
3. Progressive mental deterioration with ultimate dementia

4. The development of cerebellar, pyramidal and finally extrapyramidal signs (Roger 1985).

Progressive myoclonic epilepsy associated with identifiable underlying conditions

On reviewing the seizures which occur as symptoms of inborn errors of metabolism Aicardi (1985b) emphasized that a prominent myoclonic component in a seizure disorder should always be an alerting sign for an underlying metabolic disorder.

The following conditions are regularly complicated by myoclonic seizures (Aicardi 1985b):

1. Non-ketotic hyperglycinaemia
2. Early infantile ceroid lipofuscinosis (Santavuori-Hagberg-Haltia)
3. Tay Sachs and Sandhoff diseases
4. Phenylketonuria variant (biopterin deficiency)
5. Late infantile and juvenile ceroid lipofuscinosis
6. Sialosidoses (mucolipidosis 1, cherry red spot with myoclonus syndrome)
7. Juvenile Gaucher's disease
8. Myoclonus epilepsy with ragged red fibres (mitochondrial myopathy)
9. Sub-acute sclerosing panencephalitis

In all these disorders myoclonic seizures are associated with neurological and intellectual deterioration and only in biopterin deficiency is the underlying problem amenable to correction.

Progressive myoclonic epilepsy with no identified underlying cause

Although myoclonias are not necessarily the seizures which are symptomatic of other metabolic disorders, it is justifiable, and indeed desirable, that a full screen for inborn biochemical disorders and a CT head scan be arranged in all infants and children who have myoclonic epilepsies.

Dyssynergia cerebellaris myoclonica with epilepsy (Ramsey-Hunt syndrome) This term has been used to embrace a rather heterogeneous collection of patients, but Roger (1985) considers that a definable disorder can be characterized, the features of which are recessive inheritance with onset between 6 and 20 years and a myoclonic syndrome or epileptic seizures. Typical action and intention

myoclonus may be accompanied by partial myoclonus; the seizures are myoclonic, with or without additional tonic-clonic attacks. They tend to occur less often as the condition evolves and usually respond to antiepileptic drugs. An axial cerebellar syndrome is frequent and may be accompanied by other neurological abnormalities. Intellectual deterioration is common. During evolution of this syndrome the action and intention myoclonus becomes gradually more obvious. The EEG shows a normal background activity and well-organized sleep patterns. Spikes, spike-waves and polyspike-waves are precipitated by intermittent photic stimulation. During REM sleep rapid polyspikes localized to the central and vertex regions are characteristic of this condition.

Baltic myoclonus epilepsy Eldridge et al (1983) have reported their findings in 15 families with this autosomal recessive condition in which seizures commence at about the age of 10 years. Photosensitive, occasionally violent, myoclonus occurs particularly on awakening. It is associated with generalized tonic-clonic seizures and, on occasions, with absences. Some learning difficulties may be present, but dementia is not common unless phenytoin is given. The EEGs show light-sensitive, usually synchronous, spike-and-wave discharges. In the family study, the EEG changes were shown to precede the onset of clinical manifestations. In two patients who died, the autopsy showed marked loss of Purkinje cells of the cerebellum. Inclusion bodies were absent.

It is important to recognize this condition since the patients are made worse by phenytoin and can be greatly improved by sodium valproate.

Juvenile myoclonic epilepsy

The characteristics of juvenile myoclonic epilepsy are myoclonic seizures which commence round about puberty, which are particularly common just after wakening and are often associated with photosensitivity.

Incidence

In a review article, Wolf (1985a) reported that juvenile myoclonic epilepsy occurred in between 3.4% and 5.4% of all patients with epilepsy and that, where video-EEG recordings were obtained from adolescents and adults, this condition accounted for 11.9% of all patients studied and 36% of patients with various forms of generalized minor seizures.

Seizure types

The seizures are bilateral, single or repeated, arrhythmic, irregular myoclonic jerks which predominantly affect the arms; sudden falls with the jerks are unusual; consciousness is usually retained. Generalised tonic-clonic seizures are also present in the majority of cases (Asconapé & Penry 1984, Wolf 1985a). Both seizure types occur almost exclusively on awakening, particularly in the morning. Some patients are aware of precipitation of the seizures by flicker phenomena. Classical absences occur in a minority of patients.

Differential diagnosis

It is important to differentiate juvenile myoclonic epilepsy from other myoclonic syndromes since most others carry a much more serious long-term prognosis. The relatively late age of onset helps to distinguish this condition from both myoclonic-astatic epilepsy and the Lennox-Gastaut syndrome. In myoclonic absences, the jerking is rhythmic and usually symmetrical.

Etiology

No underlying cause has been identified. However, there appears to be a genetic predisposition to this syndrome. The incidence of a positive family history of a seizure disorder has been given as approximately 25% where most of the affected family members had generalized seizure disorders (Tsuboi 1976). It was concluded that the mode of inheritance was probably polygenic. Females were thought to have a lower manifestation threshold.

Pathophysiology

On clinical grounds, no particular underlying lesion or previous event appears consistently to predispose to juvenile myoclonic epilepsy. Microdysgenesis has been reported in the cer-

ebrum of one patient on whom a careful post-mortem examination was performed (Meencke & Janz 1984). Since intellectual deterioration does not occur it seems likely that the seizures do not have serious pathological consequences.

Clinical findings

Males and females are equally represented in groups of patients with juvenile myoclonic epilepsy. The age at onset of the myoclonic jerks is in the early–mid teens. In the series of Asconapé & Penry (1984) myoclonic seizures always preceded any generalized tonic-clonic attacks. Neurological examination and intelligence are normal (Wolf 1985a, Asconapé & Penry 1984). However, Reintoft et al (1976) found there to be a non-significant tendency for patients with this epileptic syndrome to be somewhat immature and socially maladjusted.

Investigation

Electroencephalography The background activity is almost always normal. Ictal changes consist of paroxysmal polyspike and slow wave discharges. These are usually bilaterally synchronous and symmetrical but there may be some interhemispheric asymmetry (Asconapé & Penry 1984). Polyspike-wave complexes also occur interictally but these discharges have fewer spikes prior to the slow waves than when myoclonic jerks are observed. Photosensitivity is demonstrable more commonly in this epileptic syndrome than in any other (Wolf 1985a). Asconapé & Penry (1984) reported that 4 of their 12 patients were photosensitive, a figure in keeping with the 30% reported by Wolf (1985a) after analysis of figures from Goosses (1984); 20% of patients also have polyspike-wave discharges on eye closure (Wolf 1985a). In addition, Asconapé & Penry (1984) reported one patient whose myoclonic seizures were precipitated by loud unexpected noises.

Treatment

Sodium valproate is the treatment of first choice. At least half the patients become seizure-free on valproate alone (Wolf 1985a). Most others will have a useful reduction in seizure frequency with or without the addition of other antiepileptic drugs (Asconapé & Penry 1984). For those who are photosensitive instruction in the avoidance of flicker phenomena is also important.

Prognosis

The outlook for continued neurological and intellectual normality is good. The long-term prognosis for the seizure disorder appears to be less well defined. Both Asconapé & Penry (1984) and Wolf (1985a) give the impression that there is a high risk of recurrence if medication is discontinued even after several years of freedom from seizures.

THE LENNOX-GASTAUT SYNDROME

In a paper entitled 'Clinical correlates of the fast and slow spike-wave electroencephalogram', Lennox & Davies (1950) first drew attention to this clinical syndrome, which was later more clearly defined by Gastaut et al (1966). The cardinal features are the development in children, who are usually neurologically abnormal, of atypical absences, axial tonic seizures and sudden falls (atonic or myoclonic) associated with interictal diffuse slow spike-waves on the waking EEG.

Incidence

Since many authors have included under the heading of the Lennox-Gastaut syndrome children with other epileptic syndromes in which myoclonic seizures occur, it is difficult to be sure how many children strictly have this condition. A minimum estimate is that it is present in 3% of childhood seizure disorders.

Differential diagnosis

When it commences in the first five years of life any serious seizure disorder particularly with associated myoclonias may be confused with the Lennox-Gastaut syndrome. Features distinguishing this syndrome from myoclonic astatic epilepsy are summarized in Table 4.1. Beaumanoir (1985a) has noted that both partial and generalized epilep-sies, during which deterioration in neurological status and intellect occurs, may be erroneously considered to be the Lennox-Gastaut syndrome.

Etiology

There is much emphasis on 'encephalopathy' as a feature which precedes or accompanies the onset of this syndrome. The exact nature of this 'encephalopathy' remains to be determined and the impression given is that a generalized cerebral disorder is being referred to as an encephalopathy for lack of a more specific term. Lagenstein et al (1979) found evidence of cortical atrophy in more than 50% of those cases in their series examined by CT scan and prior neurological abnormality was well documented in 60% of their cases. The roles of viral infection and possible immune deficiency remain incompletely determined.

Seizure type

Tonic seizures are a necessary component of the Lennox-Gastaut syndrome (Beaumanoir 1985b). Such seizures may occur during the day or night and can be axial, axorhizomelic or global; they are brief and loss of consciousness is not necessarily present. If nocturnal, they tend to occur during slow-wave sleep, particularly during the latter part of the night.

Most children also have atypical absences which begin and end gradually. During these, loss of consciousness may be incomplete so that some activities can continue even though the child appears abstracted or obtunded. Loss of tone in the face and neck muscles may cause the child to lean forward with the mouth open and myoclonic twitching of the eyelids and mouth may be observed. Massive myoclonic jerks, myoclonic-atonic attacks and/or atonic seizures are much less frequent manifestations of this epileptic syndrome (Gastaut 1985a). Tonic-clonic, clonic or partial seizures, symptomatic of the underlying, though non-specific, cerebral disorder may also occur (Beaumanoir 1985b). Episodes of status epilepticus characterized by clouding of consciousness and repeat atonic, or less often myoclonic-atonic, seizures can last for days, weeks or even months, are resistant to therapy and are often recurrent.

Pathophysiological aspects

The reason why some children with prior neurological defects should develop the Lennox-Gastaut syndrome is obscure. Similarly, the progressive loss of intellectual skills remains unexplained. Persistent seizure activity may interfere with the child's attention but this fails to explain the severe intellectual and behavioural problems usual in children who have had this condition over a number of years. Reports on post-mortem studies, particularly with sophisticated histological and histochemical examination, appear to be entirely lacking.

Clinical features

The peak age of onset is between 3 and 5 years with extremes of the first year and the tenth year (Beaumanoir 1985b). The syndrome is more common in males than in females. No specific neurological signs are pathognomonic though neurological abnormality is common and usually precedes the onset of seizures. A family history of some sort of epilepsy is common. However, there is no known familial case of the Lennox-Gastaut syndrome (Chevrie & Aicardi 1972).

Investigations

Investigation by CT scanning will help to indicate underlying structural cerebral abnormalities but atrophic lesions are usually non-specific. In the search for an underlying cause of the 'encephalopathy' it is justifiable to undertake a full metabolic screen, to investigate in detail the immunological state of the child and to search as thoroughly as possible for a viral infection. Such continued attention to possible etiologies should eventually lead to a better understanding of this syndrome.

Electroencephalography In brief, the characteristic interictal EEG findings are of diffuse slow (2 to 3 Hz) spike-wave when awake and bursts of 10 Hz rhythms during sleep (Beaumanoir 1985b).

During tonic seizures a discharge of bilateral and mainly frontal or vertical rapid rhythms occurs. Such discharges may be preceded by a short period of flattening of the background rhythms or by a brief discharge of slow spike-waves, but there is no post-ictal depression of activity. When the tonic seizures pass into an automatic stage the rapid rhythms of the tonic phase are followed by diffuse slow spike-wave which corresponds with the automatic phase.

Atypical absences are accompanied by irregular diffuse 2 to 2.5 Hz spike-and-wave occurring more or less symmetrically from the hemispheres. When myoclonic seizures or atonic seizures occur as part of the Lennox-Gastaut syndrome slow polyspike-and-wave, diffuse spike-waves or rapid rhythms with anterior predominance may be recorded (Beaumanoir 1985b).

Treatment

The seizures are very resistant to therapy: responses to phenytoin, carbamazepine or phenobarbitone are usually totally disappointing. Sodium valproate is sometimes helpful, particularly if used in higher than usual dosage (Jeavons et al 1977). Benzodiazepines, particularly nitrazepam or clonazepam, can produce a dramatic cessation of seizures but the effect is usually short-lived, at worst a few days and at best a few months, after which increasing resistance occurs. It is possible temporarily to control the resistance to benzodiazepines by giving intravenous chlormethiazole during a period of seven days of complete benzodiazepine withdrawal. After re-introduction of the benzodiazepine, resistance develops again during the subsequent three to six months, but the parents of many children with this syndrome are grateful for the period of respite which follows chlormethiazole. Some children are dramatically helped by being placed on a ketogenic diet (De Vivo 1983).

Prognosis

A complete recovery with freedom from seizures and normal neurological and psychological development is very unusual (Beaumanoir 1985b). Approximately 5% of children die within 10 years but death is usually due to associated problems. The epilepsy, which initially is so difficult to control, later becomes less prominent, but neurological abnormalities and the progressive psychological problems persist. In children whose seizures have remitted, difficulties with the use of language, organization of movement and with interpersonal relationships often persist and become increasingly important as the child grows older.

GENERALIZED TONIC-CLONIC SEIZURES

Generalized tonic-clonic seizures are a stereotyped expression of maximal involvement of cerebral neurones (Porter 1984). They may be 'primary' or 'secondary'. When primary they are completely generalized from the outset. Partial seizures which later become generalized are referred to as 'secondarily generalized' attacks.

Incidence

Although O'Donohoe (1985) has suggested that between 75% and 80% of childhood seizures are generalized tonic-clonic in type, other authors, notably Cavazzutti (1980), have suggested that partial epilepsies are responsible for about 40% of seizure disorders in childhood. Furthermore, if the less common forms of epilepsy are considered, it is probable that generalized tonic-clonic seizures make up at most 50% of seizures seen in children. Porter (1984) has emphasized that secondary generalized tonic-clonic seizures are probably much more common than primary attacks. However, the exact incidence of each type is unknown, since partial features are often either so brief as to pass unnoticed or relatively inconspicuous when followed by a generalized tonic-clonic convulsion.

Seizure characterisation

In generalized tonic-clonic seizures consciousness is lost. The tonic phase lasts from 10 to 20 seconds. It starts with brief flexion followed by a longer period of extension giving way to a tremor which leads into the clonic phase. The clonic phase lasts about 30 seconds and begins when the muscular relaxation completely interrupts the tonic contraction. It is characterized by brief, violent flexor spasms of the whole body (Porter 1984). Generalized tonic-clonic seizures are followed by post-ictal sleep.

Differential diagnosis

Prolonged vasovagal attacks leading to anoxia associated with clonic jerking are sometimes confused with generalized tonic-clonic seizures. Hysterical seizures are more common in adolescent girls than boys or younger children of either sex. They can be differentiated from epileptic seizures by ambulatory EEG monitoring or by estimation of the serum prolactin, which is raised for up to four hours after a genuine seizure, but remains normal in simulated attacks.

Etiology

Primary generalized tonic-clonic seizures are of unknown etiology; there is a strong genetic predisposition. On the other hand, the etiology is usually known or suspected in secondary generalized tonic-clonic seizures. In these cases, the seizures are symptomatic of an underlying abnormality of the brain. Almost any cerebral lesion due to any pathological process can be responsible, though diffuse or generalized disorders are more likely to be found than well-localized conditions. If generalized tonic-clonic seizures occur secondary to a focal lesion, the lesion is most likely to be in one or other of the frontal lobes. Generalization is then related to synchronization of the cortical discharges by the reticular formation.

Pathophysiology

Gloor (1980) has emphasized the cortical origin of generalized spike-and-wave discharges, i.e. the EEG pattern found in generalized tonic-clonic seizures. Afferent thalamocortical volleys, which would normally lead to the appearance of spindles on the EEG, produce spike discharges when there is a cortical lesion. These activate a recurrent intracortical inhibitory system which intermittently reduces simultaneously the excitability of many pyramidal neurones of the cortex and is characterized on the EEG by the slow-wave component of the spike-and-wave. There is no evidence that brief (under 15 minutes), single, generalized tonic-clonic seizures lead per se to cerebral damage. On the other hand, generalized tonic-clonic status epilepticus is a life-threatening condition. Once such seizures last for 30 minutes or more there is a risk of permanent neurological sequelae. The areas of the brain most vulnerable are, in the cortex, the occipital, frontal and temporal lobes, in particular the amygdala; in the cerebellum, the Purkinje cells; and the thalamus. The histological changes are those of hypoxia/ischaemia. There is considerable evidence that the younger the child and the longer the duration of the seizure, the greater is the likelihood that permanent cerebral damage will result (Aicardi & Chevrie 1983).

Clinical findings

In children who have primary generalized tonic-clonic seizures the neurological examination and intelligence are usually normal. In those where there is underlying neurological abnormality and where the seizures are either secondary generalized tonic-clonic or secondarily generalized after starting as partial attacks, almost any underlying neurological condition can be present. It is clearly important to perform a full examination on all children who have generalized tonic-clonic seizures in order to determine the presence or absence of an accompanying diffuse or localized cerebral disorder. Signs other than those found in the neurological system may give further clues to the aetiology of the seizures. To give just one example – examination of the skin is important in the diagnosis of tuberous sclerosis.

Investigation

The necessity for investigations other than an EEG in children who have generalized tonic-clonic seizures depends entirely on the history surrounding the attack(s) and the physical findings. Where there is good reason to suspect that the child has primary generalized tonic-clonic seizures, biochemical and radiological examinations are not indicated. However, if there are features in the history or examination to suggest that an acquired

structural disorder, such as a space-occupying lesion; or, an underlying biochemical disorder; or, an acute or chronic infection might be present, appropriate neuroradiological, biochemical and/or infection screens should be arranged. Routine examination of the cerebrospinal fluid is not indicated in afebrile children with generalized tonic-clonic seizures.

Electroencephalography In a child who has primary generalized tonic-clonic seizures the interictal EEG may be entirely normal. Since the seizure is associated with considerable muscular activity it is usually difficult to get an artefact-free EEG during a tonic-clonic seizure. The characteristic ictal discharge is bilateral spike-and-wave. However, the synchrony and rhythmicity seen in the absence seizures is not usually present. High-voltage slow waves are seen in the post-ictal period; brief bilateral spike-and-wave discharges may be seen in the interictal record. Photosensitivity is not unusual in children with primary generalized tonic-clonic seizures.

Treatment

Intermittent generalized tonic-clonic seizures In children who have had a single generalized tonic-clonic seizure, continuous antiepileptic medication is not indicated unless the seizure can be demonstrated to be secondary to an underlying neurological disorder in which recurrence appears probable.

After two or more generalized tonic-clonic seizures, serious consideration should be given to regular antiepileptic therapy. No controlled trial of first-line treatment for childhood generalized tonic-clonic epilepsy exists. Sodium valproate 20 to 30 mg/kg/day, carbamazepine 10 to 20 mg/kg/day, phenytoin 5 to 8 mg/kg/day (monitored by serum levels) or primidone 10 to 20 mg/kg/day are probably equally effective in the uncomplicated case.

Generalized tonic-clonic status epilepticus General measures which include maintenance of the airway, administration of oxygen, monitoring and correction of rises or falls in blood pressure and normalization of the body temperature, are as important as specific antiepileptic medication. Diazepam is the drug of first choice. Given intravenously diazepam 0.1 mg/kg is usually effective. This dose can be repeated after 15 to 20 minutes. In the young child, intravenous injection may be difficult. As an alternative, rectal diazepam 0.5 mg/kg acts almost as rapidly as the intravenous injection. Diazepam given in suppositories or intramuscularly is absorbed only very slowly and neither of these routes is suitable for the treatment of status. If diazepam does not rapidly control the status, the child should be nursed in a place where intensive therapy is available. Only then is it safe to give additional antiepileptic drugs, such as slow intravenous phenobarbitone 10 mg/kg or intravenous phenytoin 10 to 15 mg/kg (given very slowly with ECG monitoring). Intramuscular or rectal paraldehyde may also be used, as may intravenous clonazepam, intravenous chlormethiazole or intravenous lignocaine. For the child who has been in prolonged status, dexamethasone or mannitol may be required to reduce cerebral oedema.

Prognosis

On the whole, children with primary generalized tonic-clonic seizures, and who are thus neurologically and intellectually normal, have a good prognosis for later freedom from seizures. This is particularly so if their seizures are readily controlled with medication (Holowach et al 1972). When the seizures are secondary to neurological abnormalities or are refractory to medication, the prognosis is less good. Generalized tonic-clonic seizures are the most obvious form of epilepsy and are those potentially causing most danger if a child is swimming, cycling or climbing trees, etc. Undue restriction of activities may cause resentment and isolation from peer groups making later social integration difficult. It is thus important that physicians aim to render children seizure-free, thereby encouraging the parents of children with major epilepsy to allow their children as much freedom as possible.

Photosensitive epilepsy

Seizures induced by flickering lights are usually generalized tonic-clonic in nature, though they may be preceded by mild clonic jerking (Jeavons

& Harding 1975). Flash frequencies of between 15 and 20 Hz are most likely to be critical for the photosensitive subject. The age at the first seizure is usually in middle childhood with photosensitivity apparently diminishing during the twenties. In more than 90% of patients, stimulation of one eye is less epileptogenic than stimulation of both eyes; 30% of patients with a photoconvulsive response to intermittent photic stimulation are also sensitive to stationary patterns of striped lines (Wilkins & Lindsay 1985). The most epileptogenic patterns are composed of stripes, subtend a large area of the visual fields, have a spacial frequency between 1 and 8 cycles/degree, have a contrast in excess of about 30%, have a high luminance, are vibrating with a temporal frequency between 5 and 30 Hz in a direction orthogonal to that of the stripes and are viewed with both eyes. Television viewed at close quarters has just these characteristics.

Avoidance of seizures induced by intermittent photic stimulation

Television The following steps are recommended to avoid seizures:

1. If possible watch a television with a small screen.
2. If watching a large screen sit as far from it as possible (at lease 2 m distant).
3. Arrange a remote control system for switching on and off and changing the programme.
4. Use 'television glasses' – A sheet of polarizer which enhances the contrast of the picture is placed over the television screen, and the patient wears polaroid spectacles in which one lens has an axis of polarization orthogonal to that of the other, with the result that there is functional monocular occlusion (Wilkins & Lindsay 1985).

Other circumstances Children sensitive to patterns, sunlight on water and visual stimuli other than the television set should be taught to occlude the vision to one eye as soon as a potential epileptogenic circumstance presents itself. However, many find it difficult to comply with this suggestion. Crossed polaroid spectacles may be helpful but are not always acceptable to the child. When physical methods fail, sodium valproate is the drug of first choice for the control of photosensitive epilepsy.

ABSENCE EPILEPSY (PETIT MAL)

Childhood absence epilepsy

Childhood absence epilepsy has been defined as an epilepsy starting before puberty in previously normal children whose initial seizures are absences which are very frequent, are not associated with myoclonus, and are accompanied by synchronous 3 Hz spike-and-wave on the EEG (Loiseau 1985).

Incidence

The incidence of true absence epilepsy is often difficult to determine from figures in the literature since other types of minor seizures are often confused with absences. Cavazzutti (1980) reported that, in school-aged children with epilepsy, 8% had absences.

Seizure types

Absences are usually brief, start and finish abruptly, are associated with loss of awareness, with or without other changes, and occur many times, often more than 100 times per day.

Penry et al (1975) have reported on 374 absence seizures that were analysed after simultaneous video and EEG recordings had been obtained from 48 patients. In 85% of patients the absences were of under 10 seconds duration and in all the patients the duration was 45 seconds or less. Individual patients tended to have absences of more or less the same duration. The absences in this study have been classified according to Gastaut (1970). The patients were significantly likely to have the same type of absence.

Absence simple There is an abrupt onset, with cessation of ongoing activities, complete stillness and loss of awareness, but no loss of posture. The attack ends abruptly and activity is resumed where it left off. Only 9.4% of the attacks recorded by Penry et al (1975) were simple absences.

Absence with mild clonic components The onset is abrupt. During the attack clonic movements may occur in the eyelids, causing 3 per second

blinking or, less frequently, in other muscles, leading to rhythmic jerking which is usually bilaterally symmetrical and does not impair posture. 45.5% of the recorded absences had clonic components.

Absence with increase in postural tone Tonic muscular contraction causing arching of the neck or back, which resolved prior to the end of the seizure, was observed in only 4.5% of absences (Penry et al 1975).

Absence with diminution in postural tone Diminution in postural tone can lead to drooping of the head, rarely slumping of the trunk; dropping of the arms and relaxation of the grip; buckling of the knees; and, rarely, a fall to the ground. Such changes occurred during 22.5% of absences.

Absence with automatisms Automatisms were observed in 63.1% of absences and were significantly related to the duration of the seizure. They were very rare in absences lasting under 3 seconds but occurred in 95% of those of more than 18 seconds duration. Automatisms were of two main types. When perseverative, a patient persisted in activity which was ongoing at the start of the seizure. De novo automatisms commenced after the onset of the seizure and were characterized by licking, swallowing, scratching, 'fiddling' and other small-range, sometimes apparently semipurposeful, movements.

Absence mixed In almost 40% of the absences more than one additional component was noted (Penry et al 1975). However, in the majority of these, two, rather than more, components were observed.

It is usual to refer to absences which are other than simple as complex absences.

Differential diagnosis

Absences with automatisms may be difficult to distinguish clinically from complex partial seizures (temporal lobe epilepsy). If possible, a seizure should be observed. In the untreated patient, absences can almost invariably be precipitated by hyperventilation, whereas complex partial seizures rarely occur under these circumstances. Post-attack confusion is very unusual after an absence, but is invariably present following a complex partial seizure. If the attacks cannot be distinguished clinically, the EEG which is characteristic in absences, should clinch the diagnosis. On occasion, ambulatory EEG monitoring is necessary in order to record a seizure.

Children with emotional difficulties who become withdrawn or inattentive and those who are having problems with school work are sometimes suspected of absence epilepsy. Clinical and EEG observation during hyperventilation should resolve the situation.

It is important to distinguish absence epilepsy from myoclonic absences, in which myoclonic jerking of the proximal upper limbs is associated with loss of awareness, and atypical absences which occur in, for example, the Lennox-Gastaut syndrome. In these latter circumstances both a poor response to therapy and an unfavourable long-term outlook occur.

Etiology

Absences are not usually associated with recognizable focal neurological deficits on clinical examination. However, there is evidence from careful stereo-electroencephalographic work that the convulsive discharges originate in the mesio-orbital gyrus of the frontal cortex and are synchronized in the reticular system (Bancaud & Talairach 1965). There is a family history of seizure disorders in between 15% and 40% of cases (Loiseau 1985). Various modes of inheritance have been suggested, but the exact role of the genetic input has yet to be clarified, particularly in relation to the possible presence of a focal frontal lesion as the primary site of the epileptic discharge.

Pathophysiology

As discussed above it seems probable that a focal disturbance in the mesio-orbital gyrus of the frontal cortex is the basic pathological problem. It is usually assumed that absence seizures themselves cause no additional pathology. However, using (^{18}F) 2-fluoro-2 deoxy-D-glucose (FDG) and positron computed tomography, Engel et al (1982) have demonstrated that glucose metab-

olism is increased by 2 to 3.5 times during a period of 10 minutes in which hyperventilation produced many absences. The increase in glucose metabolism was not related to the frequency or duration of the absences. Hyperventilation alone did not produce comparable changes. The ictal glucose utilization was higher in these patients than in any others with seizures (Mazziotti & Engel 1985). It is suggested that the youth of the patients and the lack of a period of post-ictal suppression may be responsible for this finding. Engel et al (1982) did not demonstrate any area of focal metabolic abnormality, i.e. in the frontal region, but felt that the measurements were not yet sufficiently sophisticated to exclude the presence of such an area. The significance of these acute ictal metabolic changes for long-term cerebral development remains undetermined.

Clinical features

Absence epilepsy is more common in girls than boys in a ratio of about 2:1. The seizures usually start in middle childhood between 5 and 10 years of age, but typical childhood absences may appear as early as 3 years and as late as 13 years. Dalby (1969) considered that almost all children with classical absences were neurologically normal. However, careful examination often reveals minor difficulties with fine movement and co-ordination. Virtually all patients with absences are mentally normal. However, if absences are frequent, attentional defects are likely (Browne et al 1974).

Investigation

Electroencephalography Absences are associated with bilaterally synchronous and symmetrical rhythmic spikes and waves. The discharges commence abruptly but cease over a period of seconds. Spike-wave complexes have a frequency of 3 Hz at the onset but may slow to 2.5 to 2 Hz towards the end of the attack. Irregular spike-wave discharges may also accompany childhood absence seizures (Loiseau 1985). Between attacks, the background activity is usually normal, but single or brief discharges may be found without any recognizable clinical accompaniment. Hyperventilation will usually precipitate an attack if the resting record is non-contributory.

Treatment

Absences are responsive to ethosuximide and to sodium valproate. These drugs are equally efficacious (Callaghan et al 1982, Sato et al 1982b), but ethosuximide is the usual first-choice therapy if absences are uncomplicated by other seizures. If other seizure types are present valproate is indicated.

The starting dose of ethosuximide is 15 mg/kg/day and this can be increased to 40 mg/kg/day if neither the clinical state nor the monitoring of the serum levels suggest that toxicity is occurring. With careful attention to regularity of medication and adjustment of the dosage to ensure optimal serum ethosuximide levels, absences can be controlled for practical purposes in 80% of patients and 60% will become seizure-free (Sherwin 1982).

Sodium valproate 20 to 30 mg/kg/day is indicated if generalized tonic-clonic seizures accompany absences or if the attacks fail to respond to ethosuximide. Where monotherapy with neither ethosuximide nor valproate produces adequate control of absences, the use of both drugs together will be more effective than either alone in some patients (Schmidt 1983b).

For the very small group of patients whose attacks remain clinically uncontrolled by ethosuximide and/or valproate, clonazepam can be helpful, but tolerance is likely to develop (Sato et al 1977).

Prognosis

Seizures It is unusual for absences to persist beyond adolescence. A rapid response to therapy is usually a good prognostic sign. An IQ of at least 90, the absence of generalized tonic-clonic seizures and a negative history for absence status have each been significantly correlated with remission of absences (Sato et al 1982a).

About 40% of children with absences later develop generalized tonic-clonic seizures (Loiseau 1985). Such seizures usually present between five and 10 years after the onset of the absences and are usually infrequent and readily controlled by sodium valproate. The factors predisposing to the development of generalized tonic-clonic seizures are: onset of absences after 8 years of age, male sex, poor initial response of absences to therapy, abnormalities of background activity and/or photosensitivity demonstrable on the EEG (Loiseau 1985).

Other aspects Although intelligence is usually normal, if absences are inadequately controlled the accompanying attentional deficits can be associated with educational under-functioning. One third of the patients studied by Loiseau et al (1983) had behaviour problems. These were attributed to frequent attacks, effects of the parents' attitudes to the absences or to therapy.

Juvenile absence epilepsy

In juvenile absence epilepsy the seizures are clinically similar to those in childhood absence epilepsy, but occur infrequently and often sporadically. The age of onset is about puberty and males and females are equally likely to be affected. If generalized tonic-clonic seizures occur they are most common on awakening. Myoclonic seizures may also be present. Spike-and-wave discharges on the EEG have a frequency greater than 3 Hz (Wolf 1985b).

PARTIAL SEIZURES

By definition, there is clinical or EEG evidence that partial seizures arise from a localized lesion. Nevertheless, it is often difficult to identify the lesion precisely. If the partial seizure spreads to involve neurones throughout both cerebral hemispheres, secondary generalization is deemed to have occurred. Partial seizures account for 40% of childhood seizures (Gastaut et al 1975, Cavazzutti 1980). Childhood partial seizures can be examined in four broad groups:

1. Associated with defined cerebral lesions
2. Complex partial seizures (temporal lobe epilepsy)

3. Epilepsia partialis continua (Kojewnikow's syndrome)
4. Benign partial epilepsies

Partial seizures associated with defined cerebral lesions

Incidence

At least 30% of patients with childhood epilepsy have lesional partial seizures. Since many of the lesions responsible for partial seizures are secondary to perinatal events and head injuries, the incidence is to some extent a reflection of the standard of neonatal care in the population and of the exposure of the child to potentially dangerous situations.

Seizure types

The clinical expression of a partial seizure which occurs in relation to a defined cerebral abnormality clearly depends on the localization of the structural changes, so that partial seizures may be primarily motor, sensory, visual, etc. They may be well localized. i.e. involving only a few muscle groups, or sufficiently extensive as to produce a complete unilateral attack. Virtually any intermittent stereotyped alteration in movement or sensation can be some form of partial seizure.

Differential diagnosis

Partial seizures may be confused with hemiplegic migraine and, when the motor component is well localized, with nervous tics. If visual or auditory seizures occur, psychiatric disturbance may be erroneously diagnosed. A localized EEG disturbance is usually helpful in distinguishing partial seizures from other events, particularly if the EEG can be recorded during an attack with, for example, ambulatory monitoring techniques.

Etiology Any insult which might lead to localized brain disturbance can be associated with partial seizures. Prenatal disorders of neuronal proliferation and organization are probably underdiagnosed. Perinatal abnormalities such as intraventricular haemorrhage in premature infants and hypoxic ischaemic encephalopathy in the full-term infant, as well as more obvious intrapartum cerebral trauma, may cause localized cerebral scarring with later development of partial seizures. Head injuries such as those secondary to non-accidental injury or road traffic accidents are responsible for the epileptogenic lesions in other children. Other causes of brain abnormalities which may be associated with partial seizures are meningitis, encephalitis, cerebral abscess, vascular anomalies, demyelination (multiple sclerosis), hydrocephalus and cerebral tumours. Although for many parents the possibility that a tumour may be the underlying cause of their child's seizures ranks high in their list of anxieties, seizures are only very rarely the presenting event in childhood space-occupying lesions. However, when true Jacksonian seizures with a well-localized distal onset and a recognizable march proximally occur, a very careful search for a slow-growing tumour should be undertaken. Partial epilepsies other than complex partial seizures sometimes follow prolonged unilateral febrile convulsions.

Pathophysiological aspects

Regardless of the initiating process (e.g. head injury, anoxia), neuropathological studies have shown the epileptogenic focus is characterized by neuronal drop-out, gliosis and distortions in neuronal morphology which include loss of dendritic spines, simplification of dendritic arborization patterns and shrinkage of the entire neurone. Such morphological changes may lead to selective loss of GABA-ergic interneurones, with possible attenuation of post-synaptic inhibitory control on dendrites which in turn could allow the emergence of latent burst properties; and, changes in the distribution and density of different ion channels which might affect the relationship between excitatory and inhibitory conductances (Benardo & Pedley 1985). The possible relevance of the subjection of the epileptogenic focus to constantly changing inputs from ascending brain stem projections, the thalamus and other cortical neurones is difficult to quantify and, in practice, a number of pathophysiological routes, may lead to a final common pathway when synchronized cellular bursting occurs. In childhood, and particularly in very young children, the significance of 'acquired' lesions in focal epileptogenesis may be less than disorders of neuronal proliferation or migration.

During the actual seizures, the epileptogenic areas have markedly elevated metabolic rates and blood flow, and associated efflux of potassium and influx of calcium. Reductions in glucose and glycogen content, elevations of lactate, cyclic nucleotides, adenosine, free fatty acids and prostaglandins and inhibition of regional protein synthesis also occur (Chapman 1985). Thus, not only may partial seizures be symptomatic of focal cerebral abnormalities, but the attacks themselves may cause secondary problems if they are sufficiently prolonged.

Clinical features

Since partial seizures are particularly likely to be secondary to a recognizable cerebral lesion it is essential that careful neurological and general systemic examinations are carried out.

Seizures are unusual as the presenting symptoms for space-occupying lesions, but the possibility of an underlying tumour cannot be ignored, particularly when partial seizures occur in association with acquired progressive neurological deficits, headaches, early morning vomiting or other symptoms of raised intracranial pressure. Even in young children, in whom examination of the optic fundi is difficult, it is important to exclude: papilloedema which might be associated with any cause of intracranial hypertension; optic atrophy, which if not related to recognizable perinatal events, might suggest a metabolic cause for the seizures; the scarring of previous choroidoretinitis, such as might follow prenatal toxoplasmosis; retinal pigmentation due to metabolic disorders; and, disorders of the macula such as the cherry red spot characteristically found in GM1 gangliosidosis, Tay Sachs disease and other neurodegenerative disorders.

Other than the central nervous system, the skin is most likely to give clues to an underlying problem. For example, although the typical rash of tuberous sclerosis may not be evident in the young infant, ash-leaf-shaped patches of depigmentation, seen most commonly on the back and the backs of the legs, are early indications of this condition. The facial haemangioma of Sturge-Weber's disease is a much more obvious lesion. When it involves a frontal region it is often associated with seizures affecting the contralateral side of the body. Patients with the café-au-lait spots of neurofibromatosis may have neuronal heterotopias and are at increased risk of intracranial tumours. Enlargement of the liver and spleen may indicate that seizures are symptomatic of a diffuse storage disorder involving the brain.

Investigation

The chief diagnostic aids in the definition of a structural abnormality of the brain are neuro-imaging/radiology and electroencephalography.

Neuro-imaging/radiology Plain X-rays of the skull can show asymmetries of skull size or enlargement of one cranial compartment which may give clues to: the chronicity of the lesion; sutural diastasis, when there is an expanding intracranial lesion present; and, intracranial calcification in tuberous sclerosis, congenital toxoplasmosis and some tumours.

X-ray CT scanning is indicated whenever partial seizures are associated with abnormal neurological signs during interictal periods; when there is a localized slow-wave abnormality on the EEG; when seizures are refractory to medical treatment; and when there is any suspicion that a space-occupying lesion may be present. Localized or generalized cerebral dysgenesis, porencephalic cysts, localized or generalized cortical atrophy or demyelination, tumours, abscesses, localized encephalitis (e.g. herpes) and moderately sized vascular malformations can be identified on a CT scan.

Isotope scanning may be helpful in the early diagnosis of herpes simplex encephalitis and cerebral abscess, both of which are commonly associated with partial seizures.

Ultrasound scanning through the open anterior fontanelle can demonstrate ventricular enlargement, porencephalic cysts and the multiple intracerebral cysts seen following neonatal intraparenchymal haemorrhage, but usually needs to be followed up by CT scanning so that any lesion seen can be more clearly defined.

In future, the roles of computer tomography of the brain using nuclear magnetic resonance

(NMR), positron emission (PET) or single photon emission (SPECT) in the identification of anatomical and physiological abnormalities in childhood seizures will become clearer. It is anticipated that in particular NMR-CT will allow better anatomical definition of the underlying lesions in partial epilepsies.

Angiography is indicated when a vascular abnormality is suspected.

Electroencephalography When there is a definable structural lesion present, standard EEGs are usually abnormal in the interictal period. However, the absence of an interictal abnormality does not totally exclude the possibility of local pathology. Focal or lateralized non-paroxysmal or continuous abnormalities are particularly suggestive of an underlying lesion and may take the form of changes in the background rhythms, focal slow waves, localized depression of activity, asymmetries or local failure of response to activating mechanisms such as sleep or hyperventilation. Of the unifocal spike-waves seen in partial epilepsies, those that are non-repetitive and of varying morphology, of fixed location, whose frequency does not increase with sleep, and are related to focal slow abnormalities are suggestive of a structural lesion, as are the multifocal spike-waves which have a constant localization (Revol 1985). When there is a frontal lesion the EEG abnormality may be bilateral spike-waves which predominate in both frontal regions but may not be totally symmetrical.

Ambulatory monitoring is often helpful in allowing a seizure to be recorded electroencephalographically so that better localization may be obtained. Similarly, sphenoidal or other deeply placed electrodes may give more detailed information on the position of a small lesion.

Other investigations The indications for biochemical investigations, viral serology, examination of the bone marrow for storage disorder etc, vary from case to case and depend on the type of neurological and/or other disorders found on general examination.

Treatment

Partial epilepsy secondary to a defined cerebral lesion may be treated medically or surgically.

When a space-occupying lesion is present the first choice would obviously be surgery, but under almost all other circumstances a trial of antiepileptic drug therapy is indicated. Carbamazepine and phenytoin are both well tried in the treatment of partial seizures. Carbamazepine is preferred since it is less likely to cause side-effects. It should be introduced at a dose of 5 mg/kg/day in two or three divided doses with an increase to 10 mg/kg/day after one week. Subsequent increases up to 20 mg/kg/day may be necessary and in small children, where the elimination rate is high, 30 mg/kg/day given in up to four divided doses may be necessary to acquire constant optimal serum levels throughout 24 hours. If phenytoin is given it can be started at a dose of 5 to 8 mg/kg/day and given in a single daily dose or two divided doses.

The careful serum monitoring essential to the proper use of phenytoin and the gum hypertrophy, hirsutism and possible interference with cognition, are features which make phenytoin less attractive than carbamazepine, but it is undoubtedly effective in many children in whom carbamazepine has failed to control seizures. In a minority of children, the response to combined medication with carbamazepine and phenytoin is better than either drug alone. Recent investigations of the efficacy of valproate suggest that it may also be useful in partial seizures. Primidone sometimes controls such attacks when other antiepileptic drugs have been ineffective.

If the optimal use of drugs fails to control the seizures and there is a clearly localized lesion, surgery should be considered. Very careful assessment should precede surgical intervention and should include realistic consideration of the most appropriate surgical procedure, the possibility of subsequent unacceptable neurological or psychological deficit and the likely benefit (Flanigin et al 1985). Possible procedures are: ablation, i.e. removal of the lesion or its epileptogenic area; disconnection, e.g. cortical undercutting, corpus callosotomy; stereotaxic procedures, e.g. the production of thalamic lesions; stimulation procedures, i.e. cerebellar stimulation; and, cerebral cooling. Of these, ablative and disconnection procedures are those most commonly considered in childhood. The outcome following surgery depends to some extent on the selection of patients but it is probable that between 60% and 90% achieve worthwhile improvement (Flanigin et al 1985).

Prognosis

Partial attacks associated with definite cerebral lesions are amongst the childhood seizures from which remission and cure are unlikely (Rodin 1968, Strobos 1959, Roger et al 1981). Neurological deficits will persist and intellectual problems are common with the exact incidence and type of intellectual defect being dependent on the localisation of the lesion and its etiology. Factors which are associated with a poor prognosis include:

1. Early onset of seizures
2. Associated generalized seizures
3. Frequent seizures
4. Interictal EEG abnormalities and ictal discharges on routine recordings
5. Associated neurological and psychopathological signs (Revol 1985)

Complex partial seizures (temporal lobe epilepsy)

Although complex partial seizures are usually related to discharges arising in one temporal lobe, in some patients the frontal lobe or another area is primarily involved (Porter 1984).

Incidence

Temporal lobe epilepsy accounts for about 25% of the childhood epileptic population (Ounsted et al 1966, Hauser & Kurland 1975).

Seizures

The initial symptom or sign may be loss of consciousness or an aura. The attack may be very brief, as little as under 15 seconds or as long as 8 minutes. Automatisms occur in almost all patients and can be classified as de novo from internal stimuli, de novo from external stimuli and perseverative (Porter 1984). Automatisms which

occur de novo from internal stimuli include chewing, lip-smacking, swallowing, scratching, rubbing, picking, fumbling, running and undressing. Those which occur de novo from external stimuli include response to pin-prick, drinking from a cup and pushing in response to a restraint. In perseverative automatisms, the patient continues to perform any complex act initiated prior to the loss of consciousness. Psychic phenomena such as depersonalization, déjà vu sensations, formed hallucinations, illusions and distortions of perception and ideas of a 'presence' may also occur during complex partial seizures. Secondary generalization may follow.

Differential diagnosis

Complex partial seizures are sometimes confused with absences in which automatisms occur. The distinguishing clinical feature is that awareness returns immediately after an absence, whereas confusion is usual for at least a brief period after a complex partial seizure.

Behavioural aberrations may also cause diagnostic difficulties. On the whole they can be differentiated from complex partial seizures by the retention of awareness, their relationship to situations which cause stress and lack of the stereotyped nature of abnormal behaviour. Although in any one patient the sequence of events observed during a seizure may not be completed each time, the onset is usually the same.

Etiology

Ounsted et al (1966) found that the cause of temporal lobe epilepsy fell into three categories. The first etiological category consisted of organic cerebral insults. These included adverse perinatal events, head injury, tuberous sclerosis, tumours and post-meningitic or encephalitic lesions. In the second category an episode of status epilepticus preceded the development of complex partial seizures usually by some years. There remained a third category in which the etiology never became evident.

The mechanism whereby acute neonatal events may predispose to temporal lobe epilepsy remains obscure. Earlier suggestions related to uncal herniation are now considered untenable. On the other hand there is good evidence that pre- and perinatal events predispose to prolongation and lateralization of febrile seizures (Chevrie & Aicardi 1975, Wallace 1975) and that prolonged unilateral convulsions with fever can be followed by complex partial seizures (Gastaut et al 1960, Wallace 1977, 1982). In a series, not confined to childhood, either a difficult birth, febrile convulsions, or both, preceded complex partial seizures in two-thirds of 63 patients in whom hippocampal sclerosis was found on histology (Mathieson 1975).

Genetic factors are probably not important in the etiology of complex partial seizures as a whole, but for those whose epilepsy follows an episode of status there is a positive history of seizures, usually when feverish, in 30% of siblings (Ounsted et al 1966).

Pathophysiology

Between seizures, local discharges are thought to be initiated in small columnar units in neo- and paleocortical structures located mainly in the temporal lobe, where paroxysmal activity consists of depolarization shifts at the centre of the focus and predominantly inhibitory potentials in the surrounding areas. At the onset of a complex partial seizure there is intensification of the local paroxysmal activity and spread via synapses to other areas, where self- sustained discharges arise. Spread is initially through the ipsilateral hemisphere, during which an aura can occur, and later to the opposite hemisphere when memory and consciousness become disturbed (Goldensohn 1975). The pathology of the lesion cannot be deduced from the clinical features of the seizures.

In a series of 40 children in whom a temporal lobectomy was performed before the age of 15 years mesial temporal sclerosis was found in 24 (associated with a hamartoma in 2), hamartomata alone in 7, tumours in 3, viral encephalitis in 1 and the findings were non-specific in the remaining 7 (Davidson & Falconer 1975).

Clinical features

Of the 100 children with temporal lobe epilepsy examined by Ounsted et al (1966), 63 were males.

In only 9 were gross neurological abnormalities detected, of whom 5 had hemiplegias, and 2 monoplegias; 14 of the children had either visual field defects, optic atrophy or disorders of eye movement. Speech was abnormal in 28 of the 100 children. Complex partial seizures started at a median age of 5 years 4 months for the whole group. For those who had had preceding episodes of status epilepticus, the median age at the first seizure was 1 year 4 months and at the onset of complex partial attacks was 4 years 2 months.

On the whole, children with temporal lobe epilepsy have intelligence levels within the normal range. However, when the epilepsy is a symptom of either a perinatal insult or a sequel of status, the intellectual level is likely to be below average. One-quarter of the children in the group studied by Ounsted (1966) were hyperkinetic and those affected were almost invariably of subnormal intelligence; 36 of the 100 children had catastrophic rage outbursts. Ounsted et al (1966) also reported that social and schooling difficulties were common and that many children with complex partial seizures failed to reach the educational level expected from their intelligence scores. Only half the children whose first seizure occurred before three years completed their education in normal schools. The frequency of complex partial seizures did not influence the outcome for schooling.

Investigation

Biochemical investigation is indicated only when there is evidence from general examination that there is an underlying metabolic disorder.

Neuro-imaging/radiology Skull X-rays will sometimes show asymmetries of the middle cranial fossae, particularly if the underlying lesion is very longstanding. Calcification suggests tuberous sclerosis, a tumour or, occasionally, a vascular malformation which has previously undergone thrombosis.

Even though various scanning devices can give good details of the brain, pneumoencephalography can still add to the delineation of a temporal lesion if atrophy is the major pathological process.

Angiography is indicated when a vascular malformation is suspected and will occasionally demonstrate very small angiomata in temporal lobes which seem to be normal on routine X-ray CT scanning.

X-ray CT scanning is indicated whenever complex partial seizures commence in a child who has had no history of either perinatal problems or status epilepticus, particularly febrile status. It is also indicated in the 'insult' and 'status' groups when medical treatment is apparently ineffective. In these circumstances, an area of atrophy or another definable structural lesion, which might be amenable to surgery, may be outlined.

Preliminary reports on the use of advanced neuro-imaging techniques (PET, SPECT and NMR-CT) suggest that these can be very valuable in the delineation of both the physiological and anatomical characteristics of epileptogenic foci (Mazziotti & Engel 1985). Their usefulness in childhood complex partial seizures remains to be explored.

Electroencephalography In pure temporal lobe epilepsy, abnormalities of the EEG are focal and are recorded predominantly from one or both temporal regions. Spikes, sharp waves or, less frequently, slow waves may be found interictally but are much more likely to be seen if a seizure occurs during the recording. In fact, the record may otherwise be only equivocably abnormal. Repeated standard EEGs are often necessary before a definite focus is seen. When seizures occur several times a week ambulatory monitoring, which can easily incorporate a sleep recording, allows a greater knowledge of the changes during attacks and can produce information about the origin and spread of the seizure discharge. The insertion of sphenoidal and other depth electrodes is rarely justifiable in the establishment of the diagnosis, but may be indicated prior to consideration for surgery. Such depth electrodes can be connected to the Medilog (Oxford Medical Systems) ambulatory EEG monitor, allowing continuous recordings to be collected from intracranial sites over considerable lengths of time.

Treatment

Treatment may be medical or surgical.

In the follow-up of the 100 patients with temporal lobe epilepsy originally reported by Ounsted et al in 1966, Lindsay et al (1984) considered the role neurosurgery played in their biographies. For 42 children surgery was not indicated. Of these 10 had severe intellectual and physical disabilities which were of more serious import than their seizure disorders and, in the other 32, remission of seizures occurred during childhood. Surgery was actually considered in 29 of the other 58 children and performed in 13. However, in only four of the 13 was surgery performed before the age of 16 years, and in three cases the operation was a hemispherectomy rather than a temporal lobectomy. All had periods of freedom from seizures thereafter and Lindsay et al (1984) suggest that surgery might be considered earlier rather than later. However, since in one-third of the cases of Lindsay et al (1984) remission of seizures occurred before adulthood, careful consideration must be given to all aspects of the seizure disorder before submitting the child to surgery.

In the series of Davidson & Falconer (1975) children were selected for temporal lobectomy if they had frequent disabling seizures which were resistant to adequate drug therapy, neuroradiological studies appeared to have ruled out a gross space-occupying lesion and EEGs, including a special study using sphenoidal electrodes under intravenous pentothal narcosis, had shown a spike-discharging focus which was prominent in, or confined to, one temporal lobe. Gross mental retardation was considered a contraindication to surgery. Of the 40 children reported by Davidson & Falconer (1975), surgery produced the most satisfactory results both in terms of seizure control and amelioration of behaviour when the underlying pathology was mesial temporal sclerosis. The least satisfactory results were obtained when non-specific pathological changes were found in the excised temporal lobes. It is clear that surgery can be beneficial, and in some cases curative, but that antiepileptic drugs remain the mainstay of treatment.

There is probably little to choose between the efficacies of phenytoin and carbamazepine in the medical treatment of complex partial seizures, but carbamazepine is the usual first choice since side-effects are less of a problem than with phenytoin.

Valproate or primidone may also be helpful in some cases.

Prognosis

The long-term outcome for children with temporal lobe epilepsy has been reported in considerable detail by Lindsay et al (1979a, b, c). After at least 13 years of follow-up one-third of the patients investigated were free of seizures, on no therapy and self-supporting; one-third were self-supporting, still on antiepileptic drugs but not necessarily seizure-free; rather less than one-third were dependent and 5% were dead (Lindsay et al 1979a). Those whose seizures were secondary to 'birth injury' or to meningitis did poorly. Other adverse factors were an IQ of less than 90, seizures starting before 2 years 4 months, five or more generalized tonic-clonic seizures, complex partial seizures occurring at least once a day, left-sided foci, the hyperkinetic syndrome, catastrophic rage and special schooling. When three or fewer of these adverse factors were present the outcome was on the whole good and when more than five were present no child became seizure-free. A positive family history of seizures appeared to override adverse factors in some cases. In a comparison of the characteristics of children with well-defined right- or left-sided temporal lobe EEG foci, Camfield et al (1984) failed to find any significant right–left differences for intelligence, neuropsychological traits or clinical features, but one-third of the children were shown to be maladjusted on the Personality Inventory for Children. The maladjusted patients did significantly less well on the neuropsychological testing than those who appeared well adjusted, emphasizing the tendency for suboptimality to be present in more than one sphere.

When marriage, parenthood and sexual indifference were considered, slightly less than two-thirds of those deemed marriageable had actually married (Lindsay et al 1979b). Trauma or status was the etiology in most of those who had not married and affected males were much less likely to marry than affected females. Marriage was significantly more common where remission had occurred before puberty and this factor was particularly important for males who, even if they were married, were less likely than females to become parents.

Psychiatric problems had been present during childhood in 85% of the group reported by Lindsay et al (1979c), but by adulthood 70% of those who were not seriously mentally retarded were psychiatrically healthy. Nevertheless, overt schizophreniform psychosis was present in 10%, being most common in males with continuing epilepsy with a left-sided focus, where the incidence was 30%.

Kojewnikow's syndrome

Two types of Kojewnikow's syndrome, or epilepsia partialis continua, have been identified by Bancaud (1985). The first type occurs at any age on the background of a stable neurological deficit and a second, presenting only in children, is associated with progressive neurological and psychological deterioration.

Incidence

Both type I and type II of Kojewnikow's syndrome appear to be rare and figures for the incidence are not available.

Seizure type

Bancaud (1985) used two seizure types as necessary criteria for the diagnosis of this syndrome. The first was semi-continuous or permanent muscle jerks, which were localized and usually confined to a small group of muscles. The second was unilateral somatomotor seizures whether or not they were associated with other seizure types. In type I seizures occurred daily at their most frequent, whereas in type II seizures often occurred very many times per day.

Etiology

There appears to be little argument about the constancy of a definable structural lesion in type I. The etiology of type II remains a matter for discussion.

Type I Although a definable lesion is usually

present its exact nature may be extremely variable (Thomas et al 1977). Infection, vascular abnormalities and tumours have been described (Bancaud 1985).

Type II This subdivision of Kojewnikow's syndrome is a progressive disorder in which 'encephalitis' is said to be the underlying condition (Rasmussen et al 1958). However, no infecting agent has been identified and Bancaud (1985) referred to the 17 patients in his study as all having seizures of unknown aetiology. Although Juul-Jensen & Denny-Brown (1966) suggested that the lesions were often subcortical, Bancaud (1985) claimed unequivocal evidence of the cortical localization of the pathology.

Differential diagnosis

Behavioural tics may be differentiated from both types of Kojewnikow's syndrome by the absence of neurological and EEG abnormalities and, particularly from type II of the syndrome, by the retention of normal intellect.

Clinical features

In a study of 22 patients with this syndrome of whom 5 had the features of type I and 17 the features of type II, Bancaud (1985) found that the onset of the condition could be as early as 8 months and tended to be younger in those patients with type II. In 3 of the 5 children with type I and 14 of the 17 with type II, myoclonic jerks followed unilateral seizures within a year. The interval was less than 4 months in 11 of the 17 patients with type II. Of the 5 patients with type I, 1 had no neurological deficit, 2 had localized abnormalities and 2 had hemiplegias. On the other hand, all 17 patients with type II had hemiplegias which were complicated by other motor deficits in 4 children. All 5 children with type I were mentally unimpaired; whereas of the 17 with type II 13 have severe mental impairment, 2 mild and only 2 no mental impairment.

Investigation

The search for a surgically remediable lesion is clearly important in this group of patients. In the 22 patients of Bancaud (1985) neuroradiology, not further specified, revealed a cortical-subcortical scar in one of five patients with type I. Relatively localized lesions were identified in two, extensive lesions in eight and bilateral or diffuse lesions in the remaining seven of those with type II.

Electroencephalography Bancaud (1985) has investigated his group of patients very extensively, using in addition to more conventional recordings, stereo-EEG.

In patients with type I, the interictal EEG almost invariably showed normal background activity (asymmetry was noted in only one case); delta waves were either absent or localized; spikes and/or spikes-and-waves were localized in four of the five patients; and subclinical paroxysmal discharges were not identified. The ictal discharges were localized to the central region in all type I patients.

In the 17 type II patients, interictally, the EEGs showed background activity which was asymmetrical in 7, and absent or very slow in 10; delta waves which were localized in 3, widespread in 6 and diffuse (or bilateral) in 8; spikes and/or spikes and waves which were widespread in 3 and diffuse (bilateral) in 14; and, subclinical paroxysmal discharges, which were evident in all 17 and bilateral in 13. During seizures, the ictal discharge was confined to the central region in one case only; of the others, the discharge was widespread in 10 and multifocal and/or bilateral in six. Stereo-EEGs allowed identification of the origin of the ictus and it was noted that the end of the intracerebral discharge might not coincide with cessation of the muscle jerks.

Treatment

Since a localized cerebral lesion is usually under consideration, assessment for and subsequent surgical management are the main therapeutic considerations. Bancaud (1985) reported in type I, one patient cured by surgery and one whose seizures were reduced to rare localized nocturnal clonic jerks and; in type II, four of the 17 patients had operations which were initially successful, but were followed by relapse after between one and eight months.

Prognosis

The patients of Bancaud (1985) with type I Kojewnikow's syndrome did not deteriorate during 12 years of follow-up. Those with type II had evidence of a progressive disorder from the EEG and clinical and neuropsychological examination.

Benign partial epilepsies

Following the report by Nayrac & Beaussart (1958) of a benign partial epilepsy with spike-wave discharges in the pre-Rolandic area, the various benign partial epilepsies of childhood have become increasingly well recognized. Benign partial epilepsy with centro-temporal spikes is the variety most commonly reported, but benign epilepsy with occipital paroxysms, benign partial epilepsy with affective symptoms and benign partial epilepsy with extreme somatosensory evoked potentials have also been described.

As a group, the benign partial epilepsies are characterized clinically by absence of neurological or intellectual deficits; a positive family history of epilepsy; onset of seizures after the age of 18 months; seizures which are brief, infrequent, respond readily to treatment, are variable in symptomatology, do not cause prolonged deficits in the post-ictal period; and absence of acquired neurological and psychological deficits throughout the evolution (Dalla Bernardina et al 1985a). The EEGs show normal background activity; normal sleep organization; focal abnormalities such as Rolandic spikes, or sharp waves which increase in frequency during sleep; possibly multifocal abnormalities; possibly brief bursts of generalized spike-wave discharges; and identical ictal patterns during waking and sleep.

Benign partial epilepsy with centro-temporal spikes

Lerman (1985) has stated that 15% to 20% of young people with epilepsy have this form of epilepsy. Seizures usually start in the first decade and cease during the second decade. The age range at onset is 3 to 13 years with a peak at about 9 years (Beaussart 1972, Lerman & Kivity 1975).

Males constitute 60% of cases. The incidence of previous febrile convulsions at 7% to 9% is about twice that in the general population. The children are normal both on neurological and psychological examination. There is a history of seizure disorders or epileptic discharges on the EEG in up to 40% of close relatives and autosomal dominant inheritance with age-dependent penetrance has been suggested (Lerman 1985).

Seizures The seizures are usually infrequent, but can occur as often as many times per day, particularly at the onset. They may occur in clusters, and are usually brief, perhaps 2 minutes at the most. In about two-thirds of cases they occur only during sleep, in about one-sixth during sleep and in the awake state, and in the remaining one-sixth only while the child is awake (Lerman 1985).

The seizures are characterized by a somatosensory onset with unilateral paraesthesias involving the tongue, lips, gums and inner cheeks; followed by unilateral tonic, clonic or tonic-clonic convulsions which involve the face, lips, tongue, pharynx and larynx and lead to speech arrest or anarthria and drooling. Consciousness is preserved (Lombroso 1967). On occasion, the seizure may spread to the arm and more rarely the leg. Diurnal seizures never become generalized, but those occurring during sleep may do so.

Electroencephalography Centro-temporal spikes which may be unifocal or bifocal are seen on the interictal EEG. The spikes are typically slow, diphasic and of high voltage. They may recur at short intervals, appear in clusters and be followed by a slow wave. In the 60% of patients where the spikes are unilateral, they are always synchronous in the central and mid-temporal areas (Lerman 1985). In some patients, occipital spikes occur in addition to, or rather than, centro-temporal discharges and in others generalized spike-wave abnormalities are recorded, but there appear to be no clinical accompaniments. The centro-temporal spikes increase with drowsiness and during sleep.

Treatment Where seizures are infrequent and exclusively nocturnal, antiepileptic treatment is not essential, since the condition is self-limiting. If the seizures are frequent, especially if they occur during waking hours, they should be treated with carbamazepine or phenytoin, either of which usually produces a rapid remission.

Prognosis Even if the seizures are not treated, remission occurs before the age of 20 years. The centro-temporal foci, and any additional occipital ones, disappear from the EEG. Unless a poor prognosis has been erroneously given in the early stages of the condition and the child's activities restricted, the outlook for social integration is also good (Lerman & Kivity 1975).

Benign epilepsy of childhood with occipital paroxysms

This epileptic syndrome has been characterised by Gastaut (1985b). Males and females are equally affected. The age of onset can be up to 17 years but peaks at 7 years. One-third of the patients have a family history of epilepsy, and one-sixth of migraine. Febrile convulsions feature in the previous histories of 14% of cases. Neurological or cognitive abnormalities occur rarely.

Seizures In keeping with the particular involvement of the occipital regions, there is a prominent, but not exclusive, visual component to the seizures. Gastaut (1985b) has listed the visual ictal symptoms in decreasing order of frequency as:

- amaurosis, sometimes preceded by hemianopsia
- elementary visual hallucinations, i.e. phosphenes
- complex visual hallucinations
- visual illusions
- combinations of the individual visual symptoms.

Non-visual symptoms, which may follow the visual disturbances are: hemi-clonic seizures; complex partial seizures with automatisms; generalised tonic-clonic seizures; and, infrequently, other ictal manifestations such as dysaesthesia, adversive seizures, etc. Following the seizures, diffuse headaches occurring in about one-third of the patients, are accompanied by migraine-like nausea and vomiting in about half of those affected.

There are very wide variations in the seizure frequency from patient to patient. Attacks are precipitated in about a quarter of the patients by moving from a dark room to a brightly lit area or vice versa.

Electroencephalography In interictal periods, the background activity is normal. Paroxysmal activity is characterized by spike-waves or, less frequently, sharp-waves, of 200 to 300 μV amplitude, which are recorded over the occipital and postero-temporal regions of one hemisphere, or both hemispheres simultaneously or independently. The paroxysms occur in bursts or trains and are usually rhythmic at 1 to 3 Hz, but may be isolated and appear at irregular intervals. In almost all cases, the paroxysms disappear abruptly on eye opening and reappear within 1 to 20 seconds of eye closure. Hyperventilation and photic stimulation do not usually accentuate the abnormality and slow-wave sleep reinforces the changes in only a minority of cases (Gastaut 1985b).

During seizures the occipital discharge has been recorded over one or both hemispheres.

Treatment No special study of the merits of particular antiepileptic drugs has been conducted for this condition. Carbamazepine, phenobarbitone, valproate or benzodiazepines are reported to control seizures in about 60% of the patients (Gastaut 1985b).

Prognosis The typical seizures associated with benign epilepsy of childhood with occipital paroxysms always disappear during adolescence. Other types of recurring seizures may present in adulthood in about 5% of cases (Gastaut 1985b).

Benign partial epilepsy with affective symptoms

The cardinal feature of this epileptic syndrome is the presence of sudden fright or terror as the ictal phenomenon. In a study of 26 patients, Dalla Bernardina et al (1985b) found males and females to be equally affected. One-third had a family history of seizures and one-fifth had themselves had febrile convulsions of brief duration. The afebrile seizures had started between 2 and 9 years with an early peak up to 5 years and a later one between 6 and 9 years. All 26 patients had normal CT scans.

Seizures The seizures are characterised by sudden fright or terror causing the child to rush to cling to the mother or any other person nearby. Chewing or swallowing movements; distressed laughter; arrest of speech with glottal noises, moans or salivation; or, autonomic phenomena may accompany the periods of terror. Changes in awareness, but not total loss of consciousness, are usual. The seizures last for about 1 to 2 minutes and are not followed by any post-ictal deficit. Brief oro-facial fits may occur nocturnally in a minority of the children, but tonic, clonic, tonic-clonic or atonic seizures do not occur. Seizures are often very frequent soon after the onset and occur in the same form nocturnally as diurnally.

Electroencephalography In all cases the background activity and sleep organization is normal. During interictal periods slow spikes/slow waves are consistently activated by sleep and are recorded from the fronto-temporal or parieto-temporal areas, either uni- or bilaterally. In some children brief bursts of generalized spike-waves are also recorded.

When the EEG is recorded during a seizure, the seizure discharges are usually clearly localized to the fronto-temporal, centro-temporal or parietal areas. Polygraphic studies show that, although movements of various sorts may occur during the seizures, they are never tonic or clonic.

Treatment Carbamazepine is the treatment of choice, but phenobarbitone is probably equally effective in the control of the seizures.

Prognosis Seizures are likely to remit during adolescence and there are no neurological or intellectual sequelae. Although behavioural difficulties can be a problem at times when the seizures are frequent, Dalla Bernardina et al (1985b) found that these resolved on remission of the epilepsy.

Benign partial epilepsy with extreme somato-sensory evoked potentials

This epileptic syndrome has been described by Tassinari & De Marco (1985). Affected children pass through four distinct phases of the syndrome. Initially between the ages of 2.5 to 5.5 years, tapping of the feet during EEG recording produces extreme somato-sensory potentials, manifest as spikes of up to 400 μV in amplitude. Later, spontaneous focal EEG abnormalities appear during sleep, followed by spontaneous focal EEG abnormalities when awake. The spontaneous abnormalities are strikingly similar to those evoked by foot-tapping. In the final stage, five months to two years after the appearance of these spontaneous focal discharges, and at ages between 4.5 and 8 years, clinical seizures appear. These are characterized by head and body version in most cases, but generalized tonic-clonic seizures are also observed. Almost half the patients have personal histories of 'simple' febrile convulsions. Neurological and psychological assessments are normal as are the results of either arteriography or CT scanning. The response of seizures to antiepileptic drugs is unclear but remission is likely within one year.

REFERENCES

Aicardi J 1980 Course and prognosis of certain childhood epilepsies with predominantly myoclonic seizures. In: Wada J A, Penry J K (eds) Advances in epileptology: XIIth Epilepsy International Symposium. Raven Press, New York, pp 159–163

Aicardi J 1985a Early myoclonic encephalopathy. In: Roger J, Dravet C, Bureau M, Dreifuss F E, Wolf P (eds) Epileptic syndromes in infancy, childhood and adolescence. John Libbey Eurotext, London, pp 12–21

Aicardi J 1985b Epileptic seizures in inborn errors of metabolism. In: Roger J, Dravet C, Bureau M, Dreifuss F E, Wolf P (eds) Epileptic syndromes in infancy, childhood and adolescence. John Libbey Eurotext, London. pp 73–77

Aicardi J, Chevrie J-J 1970 Convulsive status epilepticus in infants and children. Epilepsia 11: 187–197

Aicardi J, Chevrie J-J 1976 Febrile convulsions: Neurological sequelae and mental retardation. In: Brazier M A B, Coceani F (eds) Brain dysfunction in infantile febrile convulsions. Raven Press, New York, pp 247–257

Aicardi J, Chevrie J-J 1983 Consequences of status epilepticus in infants and children. In: Delgado-Escueta A V, Wasterlain C G, Treiman D M, Porter R J (eds) Advances in neurology Vol 34: Status epilepticus. Raven Press, New York. pp 115–125

Albani M 1983 Phenytoin in infancy and childhood. In: Delgado-Escueta A V, Wasterlain C G, Treiman D M, Porter R J (eds) Advances in neurology Vol 34: status epilepticus. Raven Press, New York. pp 457–464

Aldridge Smith J, Wallace S J 1982 Intellectual progress in relation to anticonvulsant therapy and to recurrence of fits. Archives of Disease in Childhood 57: 104–107

Annegers J F, Hauser W A, Elveback L R, Kurland L T 1979 The risk of epilepsy following febrile convulsions. Neurology 29: 297–303

Ariizumi M, Kuromori N, Utsumi Y, Shiihara H 1981 Febrile convulsions, childhood epilepsy and csf IgG index. Brain and Development 3:109

Asconapé J, Penry J K 1984 Some clinical and EEG aspects

of benign juvenile myoclonic epilepsy. Epilepsia 25: 108–114

Aziz S S, Wallace S J, Murphy J F, Sainsbury C P Q, Gray O P 1986 Cotside EEG monitoring using computerised spectral analysis. Archives of Disease in Childhood 61: 242–246

Ballard R A, Vinocur B, Reynolds J W et al 1978 Transient hyperammonemia of the preterm infant. New England Journal of Medicine 299: 920–925

Bamberger P, Matthes A 1959 Anfälle im Kindesalter. Karger, Basel

Bancaud J 1985 Kojewnikow's syndrome (Epilepsia partialis continua) in children. In: Roger J, Dravet C, Bureau M, Dreifuss F E, Wolf P (eds) Epileptic syndromes in infancy, childhood and adolescence. John Libbey Eurotext, London, pp 286–298

Bancaud J, Talairach J 1965 Cited by Loiseau 1985

Baumer J H, David T J, Valentine S J, Roberts J E, Hughes B R 1981 Many parents think that their child is dying when having a first febrile convulsion. Developmental Medicine and Child Neurology 23: 462–464

Beaumanoir A 1985a Lennox-Gastaut syndrome. In: Roger J, Dravet C, Bureau M, Dreifuss F E, Wolf P (eds) Epileptic syndromes in infancy, childhood and adolescence. John Libbey Eurotext, London, p 320

Beaumanoir A 1985b The Lennox-Gastaut syndrome. In: Roger J, Dravet C, Bureau M, Dreifuss F E, Wolf P (eds) Epileptic syndromes in infancy, childhood and adolescence. John Libbey Eurotext, London, pp 89–99

Beaussart M 1972 Benign epilepsy of children with rolandic (centro-temporal) paroxysmal foci. Epilepsia 13: 795–811

Bellman M H 1983 Infantile spasms. In: Pedley T A, Meldrum B S (eds) Recent advances in epilepsy No 1. Churchill Livingstone, Edinburgh, pp 113–138

Benardo L S, Pedley T A 1985 Cellular mechanisms of focal epileptogenesis. In: Pedley T A, Meldrum B S (eds) Recent advances in epilepsy No 2. Churchill Livingstone, Edinburgh, pp 1–18

Bleyer W A, Marshall R E 1972 Barbiturate withdrawal syndrome in a passively addicted infant. Journal of the American Medical Association 221: 185–186

Brown J K 1973 Convulsions in the newborn period. Developmental Medicine and Child Neurology 15: 823–846

Browne T R, Penry J K, Porter R J, Dreifuss F E 1974 Responsiveness before, during and after spike-wave paroxysms. Neurology 24: 659–665

Callaghan N, O'Hare J, O'Driscoll D et al 1982 Comparative study of ethosuximide and sodium valproate in the treatment of typical absence seizures (petit mal). Developmental Medicine and Child Neurology 24: 830–836

Camfield C S, Chaplin S, Doyle A-B, Shapiro S H, Cummings C, Camfield P R 1979 Side-effects of phenobarbital in toddlers; behavioural and cognitive aspects. Journal of Pediatrics 95: 361–365

Camfield P R, Camfield C, Shapiro S, Cummings C 1980 The first febrile seizure – antipyretic instruction plus either phenobarbital or placebo to prevent a recurrence. Journal of Pediatrics 97: 16–21

Camfield P R, Camfield C S, Tibbles J 1982 Carbamazepine does not prevent febrile seizures in phenobarbitone failures. Neurology 32: 288–289

Camfield P R, Gates R, Roneu G, Camfield C, Ferguson A, MacDonald G W 1984 Comparison of cognitive ability, personality profile, and school success in epileptic children

with pure right versus left temporal lobe EEG foci. Annals of Neurology 15: 122–126

Cavazzutti G B 1980 Epidemiology of different types of epilepsy in school age children of Modena, Italy. Epilepsia 21: 57–62

Chapman A G 1985 Cerebral energy metabolism and seizures. In: Pedley T A, Meldrum B S (eds) Recent advances in epilepsy No 2. Churchill Livingstone, Edinburgh, pp 19–63

Chattha A S, Richardson E P Jr 1977 Cerebral white-matter hypoplasia. Archives of Neurology 34: 137–141

Chevrie J-J, Aicardi J 1972 Childhood epileptic encephalopathy with slow spike-wave. A statistical study of 80 cases. Epilepsia 13: 259–271

Chevrie J-J, Aicardi J 1975 Duration and lateralisation of febrile convulsions: Relations with etiological factors. Epilepsia 16: 781–789

Clare M, Aldridge Smith J, Wallace S J 1978 A child's first febrile convulsion. Practitioner 221: 775–776

Cockburn F, Brown J K, Belton N R, Forfar J O 1973 Neonatal convulsions associated with primary disturbance of calcium, phosphorus and magnesium metabolism. Archives of Disease in Childhood 48: 99–108

Couvreur J, Desmonts G 1962 Congenital and maternal toxoplasmosis. A review of 300 congenital cases. Developmental Medicine and Child Neurology 4: 519–530

Cull A M 1975 Some psychological aspects of the prognosis of febrile convulsions. M.Phil. thesis, University of Edinburgh

Dalby M A 1969 Epilepsy and 3 per second spike and wave rhythms. A clinical electroencephalographic and prognostic analysis of 346 patients. Acta Neurologica Scandinavica 45: Suppl 40

Dalla Bernardina B, Chiamenti C, Capovilla G, Colamaria V 1985a Benign partial epilepsies in childhood. In: Roger J, Dravet C, Bureau M, Dreifuss F E, Wolf P (eds) Epileptic syndromes in infancy, childhood and adolescence. John Libbey Eurotext, London, pp 137–149

Dalla Bernardina B, Chiarmenti C, Capovilla G, Trevisan E, Tassinari C A 1985b Benign partial epilepsy with affective symptoms ('Benign psychomotor epilepsy'). In: Roger J, Dravet C, Bureau M, Dreifuss F E, Wolf P (eds) Epileptic syndromes in infancy, childhood and adolescence. John Libbey Eurotext, London, pp 171–175

Danesi M A 1985 Classification of the epilepsies: An investigation of 945 patients in a developing country. Epilepsia 26: 131–136

Davidson S, Falconer M A 1975 Outcome of surgery in 40 children with temporal-lobe epilepsy. Lancet i: 1260–1261

De Vivo D C 1983 How to use other drugs (steroids) and the ketogenic diet. In: Morselli P L, Pippenger C E, Penry J K (eds) Antiepileptic drug therapy in pediatrics. Raven Press, New York, pp 283–291

Degen R, Goller K 1967 Die sogenannten Fieberkrämpfe des Kindesalters und ihre Beziehungen zur Epilepsie. Nervenarzt 38: 55–61

Dehkharghani F 1984 Application of electroencephalography and evoked potential studies in the neonatal period. In: Sarnat H B (ed) Topics in Neonatal Neurology. Grune & Stratton, Orlando. p 257–288

Dehkharghani F, Sarnat H B 1984 Neonatal seizures. In: Sarnat H B (ed) Topics in neonatal neurology. Grune & Stratton, Orlando, pp 209–232

Dennis J 1978 Neonatal convulsions. Aetiology, late neonatal status and long-term outcome. Developmental Medicine and Child Neurology 20: 143–148

Dennis J, Chalmers I 1982 Very early neonatal seizure rate: a possible epidemiological indicator of the quality of perinatal care. British Journal of Obstetrics and Gynaecology 89: 418–426

Desmond M M, Wilson G S, Melnick J L et al 1967 Congenital rubella encephalitis. Journal of Pediatrics 71: 311–331

Des Termes H, Mises J, Plouin P, Lerique A, Guyot D 1977 Les 'foyers de pointes' au cours de l'évolution des convulsions hyperpyretiques. Étude eletro-clinique à propos de 35 cas. Revue d'Electroencephalographie et de Neurophysiologie Clinique 7: 455–458

Doose H 1985a Myoclonic astatic epilepsy of early childhood. In: Roger J, Dravet C, Bureau M, Dreifuss F E, Wolf P (eds) Epileptic syndromes in infancy, childhood and adolescence. John Libbey Eurotext, London, pp 78–88

Doose H 1985b Myoclonic astatic epilepsy (cortico-reticular epilepsy with minor seizures and grand mal) of early childhood. In: Roger J, Dravet C, Bureau M, Dreifuss F E, Wolf P (eds) Epileptic syndromes in infancy, childhood and adolescence. John Libbey Eurotext, London, p 319

Doose H, Ritter K, Völzke E 1983 EEG longitudinal studies in febrile convulsions: Genetic aspects. Neuropediatrics 14: 81–87

Dravet C 1985a Infantile myoclonic epilepsy with favourable outcome or benign myoclonic epilepsy in infancy. In: Roger J, Dravet C, Bureau M, Dreifuss F E, Wolf P (eds) Epileptic syndromes in infancy, childhood and adolescence. John Libbey Eurotext, London, p 318

Dravet C 1985b Severe myoclonic epilepsy in infancy. In: Roger J, Dravet C, Bureau M, Dreifuss F E, Wolf P (eds) Epileptic syndromes in infancy, childhood and adolescence. John Libbey Eurotext, London, pp 318

Dravet C, Roger J, Bureau M, Dalla Bernardina B 1982 Myoclonic epilepsies in childhood. In: Akimoto H, Kazamatsuri H, Seino M, Ward A (eds) Advances in epileptology: XIIIth Epilepsy International Symposium. Raven Press, New York, pp 135–140

Dravet C, Bureau M, Roger J 1985a Benign myoclonic epilepsy in infants. In: Roger J, Dravet C, Bureau M, Dreifuss F E, Wolf P (eds) Epileptic syndromes in infancy, childhood and adolescence. John Libbey Eurotext. pp 51–57

Dravet C, Bureau M, Roger J 1985b Severe myoclonic epilepsy in infants. In: Roger J, Dravet C, Bureau M, Dreifuss F E, Wolf P (eds) Epileptic syndromes in infancy, childhood and adolescence. John Libbey Eurotext, London, pp 58–67

Dreyfus-Brissac C 1979 Neonatal electroencephalography. In: Scarpelli E M, Cosmi E V (eds) Reviews in perinatal medicine Vol 3. Raven Press, New York, pp 397–472

Dulac O, Aubourg P, Plouin P 1985 Other epileptic syndromes in neonates. In: Roger J, Dravet C, Bureau M, Dreifuss F E, Wolf P (eds) Epileptic syndromes in infancy, childhood and adolescence. John Libbey Eurotext, London, pp 23–29

Eeg-Olofsson O, Wigertz A 1982 Immunoglobulin abnormalities in cerebrospinal fluid and blood in children with febrile seizures. Neuropediatrics 13: 39–41

Eilard T, Kyllerman M, Wennerblom I, Eeg-Olofsson O, Lycke E 1974 An outbreak of Coxsackie virus type B2 among neonates in an obstetrical ward. Acta Paediatrica Scandinavica 63: 103–107

Eldridge R, Iivanainen M, Stern R, Koerber T, Wilder B J 1983 'Baltic' myoclonus epilepsy: Hereditary disorder of childhood made worse by phenytoin. Lancet 2: 838–842

Ellenberg J H, Nelson K B 1978 Febrile seizures and later intellectual performance. Archives of Neurology 35: 17–21

Engel J Jr, Kuhl D E, Phelps M E 1982 Patterns of human local cerebral glucose metabolism during epileptic seizures. Science 218: 64–66

Eyre J, Oozeer R C, Wilkinson A R 1983a Diagnosis of neonatal seizure by continuous recording and rapid analysis of the electroencephalogram. Archives of Disease in Childhood 58: 785–790

Eyre J, Oozeer R C, Wilkinson A R 1983b Continuous electroencephalographic recording to detect seizures in paralysed newborn babies. British Medical Journal 286: 1017–1018

Fenichel G M 1980 Neonatal neurology. Churchill Livingstone, Edinburgh

Flanigin H, King D, Gallagher B 1985 Surgical treatment of epilepsy. In: Pedley T A, Meldrum B S (eds) Recent advances in epilepsy. Number 2. Churchill Livingstone, Edinburgh, pp 297–339

Fowler M 1957 Brain damage after febrile convulsions. Archives of Disease in Childhood 32: 67–76

Frantzen E 1971 Spinal findings in children with febrile convulsions. Epilepsia 12:192

Frantzen E, Lennox-Buchthal M, Nygaard A 1968 Longitudinal EEG and clinical study of children with febrile convulsions. Electroencephalography and Clinical Neurophysiology 24: 197–212

Frantzen E, Lennox-Buchthal M, Nygaard A, Stene J 1970 A genetic study of febrile convulsions. Neurology 20: 909–917

Friderichsen C, Melchior J 1954 Febrile convulsions in children, their frequency and prognosis. Acta Paediatrica Scandinavica Suppl. 100 43: 307–317

Friedman E, Pampiglione G 1971 Prognostic implications of electroencephalographic findings of hypsarrhythmia in the first year of life. British Medical Journal 4: 323–325

Gastaut H 1970 Clinical and electroencephalographical classification of epileptic seizures. Epilepsia 11: 103–113

Gastaut H 1985a Discussion of myoclonic epilepsies and Lennox-Gastaut syndrome. In: Roger J, Dravet C, Bureau M, Dreifuss F E, Wolf P (eds) Epileptic syndromes in infancy, childhood and adolescence. John Libbey Eurotext, London, pp 100–101

Gastaut H 1985b Benign epilepsy of childhood with occipital paroxysms. In: Roger J, Dravet C, Bureau M, Dreifuss F E, Wolf P (eds) Epileptic syndromes in infancy, childhood and adolescence. John Libbey Eurotext, London, pp 159–170

Gastaut H, Poirier F, Payan H, Salamon G, Toga M, Vigouroux M 1960 H H E syndrome. Hemiconvulsions, hemiplegia, epilepsy. Epilepsia 1: 418–447

Gastaut H, Roger J, Soulayrol R et al 1966 Childhood epileptic encephalopathy with diffuse slow spike-waves (otherwise known as 'petit mal variant') or Lennox syndrome. Epilepsia 7: 139–179

Gastaut H, Gastaut J L, Goncalves de Silva G E, Fernandez Sauchez G R 1975 Relative frequency of different types of epilepsy: a study employing the Classification of International League Against Epilepsy. Epilepsia 16: 457–461

Gilles F H, Price R A, Kevy S V, Berenberg W 1971 Fibrinolytic activity in the ganglionic eminence of the premature human brain. Biology of the Neonate 18: 426–432

Gloor P 1980 Generalized penicillin epilepsy in the cat: The role of excitability changes in cortical neurons in the genesis of spike and wave discharges and their possible relevance as a model for human generalized corticoreticular epilepsy. In: Canger R, Angeleri F, Penry J K (eds) Advances in epileptology: XIth Epilepsy International Symposium. Raven Press, New York, pp 279–284

Goldensohn E S 1975 Initiation and propagation of epileptogenic foci. In: Penry J K, Daly D D (eds) Complex partial seizures and their treatment. Advances in neurology Vol 11. Raven Press, New York, pp 141–162

Goosses R 1984 Die Beziehung der Fotosensibilität zu den verschiedenen epileptischen Syndromen. Thesis, West Berlin, Cited by Wolf P (1985a)

Harker P 1977 Primary immunisation and febrile convulsions in Oxford 1972–5. British Medical Journal 2: 490–493

Harris R, Tizard J P M 1960 The electroencephalogram in neonatal convulsions. Journal of Pediatrics 57: 501–520

Hauser W A 1985 Long-term follow-up of febrile convulsions. Paper delivered at the XVIth Epilepsy International Symposium, Hamburg

Hauser W A, Kurland L T 1975 The epidemiology of epilepsy in Rochester, Minnesota, 1935 through 1967. Epilepsia 16: 1–66

Hellstrom B, Barlach-Christoffersen M 1980 Influence of phenobarbital on the psychomotor development and behaviour in pre-school children with convulsions. Neuropaediatrie 11: 151–160

Herlitz G 1941 Studien uber die sogenannten initialen Fieberkrämpfe bei Kindern. Acta Paediatrica (Suppl 1) 29: S1–S142

Herzlinger R A, Kandall S R, Vaughan H G 1977 Neonatal seizures associated with narcotic withdrawal. Journal of Pediatrics 91: 638–641

Holden K R, Mellits E D, Freeman J M 1982 Neonatal seizures. I. Correlation of prenatal and perinatal events with outcomes. Pediatrics 70: 165–176

Holowach J, Thurston D L, O'Leary J 1972 Prognosis in childhood epilepsy. Follow-up study of 148 cases in which therapy had been suspended after prolonged anticonvulsant control. New England Journal of Medicine 286: 169–174

Hrachovy E A, Frost J D, Kellaway P, Zion T 1979 A controlled study of prednisone therapy in infantile spasms. Epilepsia.20: 403–407

Hrachovy R A, Frost J D, Kellaway P, Zion T 1980 A controlled study of ACTH therapy in infantile spasms. Epilepsia 21: 631–636

Hrachovy R A, Frost J D, Kellaway P 1984 Hypsarrhythmia: Variations on a theme. Epilepsia 25: 317–325

Huttenlocher P R 1974 Dendritic development in neocortex of children with mental defect and infantile spasms. Neurology 24: 203–210

Isaacs D, Webster A D B, Valman H B 1984 Serum immunoglobin concentrations in febrile convulsions. Archives of Disease in Childhood 59: 367–369

Jaeken J 1985 Advances in infantile metabolic brain diseases. Thesis, Catholic University, Leuven

Jaffe M, Bar-Joseph G, Tirosh E 1981 Fever and convulsions - Indications for laboratory investigations. Pediatrics 67: 729–731

Jeavons P M 1985a West syndrome. In: Roger J, Dravet C, Bureau M, Dreifuss F E, Wolf P (eds) Epileptic syndromes in infancy, childhood and adolescence. John Libbey Eurotext, London, p 317

Jeavons P M 1985b West syndrome: Infantile spasms. In: Roger J. Dravet C, Bureau M, Dreifuss F E, Wolf P (eds) Epileptic syndromes in infancy, childhood and adolescence. John Libbey Eurotext, London, pp 42–48

Jeavons P M, Bower B D 1964 Infantile spasms. A review of the literature and a study of 112 cases. Clinics in Developmental Medicine No 15. Heinemann, London.

Jeavons P M, Harding G F A 1975 Photosensitive epilepsy. Clinics in Developmental Medicine No 56. Heinemann, London.

Jeavons P M, Clark J E, Maheshwari M C 1977 Treatment of generalised epilepsies of childhood and adolescence with sodium valproate ('Epilim'). Developmental Medicine and Child Neurology 19: 9–25

Juul-Jensen P, Denny-Brown D 1966 Epilepsia partialis continua. Archives of Neurology 15: 563–578

Kellaway P, Hrachovy R, Frost J D, Zion T 1979 Precise characterisation and quantification of infantile spasms. Annals of Neurology 6: 214–218

Kellaway P, Hrachovy R A 1983 Status epilepticus in newborns: a perspective on neonatal seizures. In: Delgado-Escueta A V, Wasterlain C G, Treiman D M, Porter R J (eds) Advances in neurology Vol 34: status epilepticus. Raven Press, New York, pp 93–99

Kellaway P, Frost J D, Hrachovy R A 1983 Infantile spasms. In: Morselli P, Pippenger C E, Penry J K (eds) Antiepileptic drug therapy in pediatrics. Raven Press, New York, pp 115–136

King D W, Dyken P R, Spinks I L Jr, Murvina A J 1985 Infantile spasms: Ictal phenomena. Pediatric Neurology 1: 213–218

Knudsen F U 1985 Recurrence risk after first febrile seizure and effect of short term diazepam prophylaxis. Archives of Disease in Childhood 60: 1045–1049

Knudsen F U, Vestermark S 1978 Prophylactic diazepam or phenobarbitone in febrile convulsions: a prospective, controlled study. Archives of Disease in Childhood 53: 660–663

Koivisto M, Blanco-Sequeiros M, Krause U 1972 Neonatal symptomatic and asymptomatic hypoglycaemia: A follow-up study of 151 children. Developmental Medicine and Child Neurology 14: 603–614

Lacy J R, Penry J K 1976 Infantile spasms. Raven Press, New York

Lagenstein I, Kuhne D, Sternuwsky H J, Ruthe E 1979 Computerised cranial transverse axial tomography (CTAT) in 145 patients with primary and secondary generalised West syndrome, myoclonic astatic petit mal, absence epilepsy. Neuropädiatrie 10: 15–28

Laplane R, Humbert R, Lager P, Salbreux R, Debray P 1958 Suites immediates et lointaines des convulsions febriles avant quatre ans. Revue Neurologique 99: 26–38

Lennox M A 1949 Febrile convulsions in childhood: a clinical and electroencephalographic study. American Journal of Diseases of Children 78: 868–882

Lennox W G, Davis J P 1950 Clinical correlates of the fast and slow spike wave electroencephalogram. Pediatrics 5: 626–644

Lerique A 1955 Electroencephalograph in febrile convulsions. Electroencephalography and Clinical Neurophysiology 7:451

Lerman P 1985 Benign partial epilepsy with centro-temporal spikes. In: Roger J, Dravet C, Bureau M, Dreifuss F E, Wolf P (eds) Epileptic syndromes in infancy, childhood and adolescence. John Libbey Eurotext, London. pp 150–158

Lerman P, Kivity S 1975 Benign focal epilepsy of childhood. A follow-up study of 100 recovered patients. Archives of Neurology 32: 261–264

Lerman P, Kivity S 1982 The efficacy of corticotrophin in primary infantile spasms. Journal of Pediatrics 101: 294–296

Lewis H M, Parry J V, Parry R P et al 1979 Role of viruses in febrile convulsions. Archives of Disease in Childhood 54: 869–876

Lewis H, Valman H B, Webster D, Tyrrell D A J 1980 Viruses in febrile convulsions. Lancet 2:150

Lindsay J, Ounsted C, Richards P 1979a Long-term outcome in children with temporal lobe seizures. I. Social outcome and childhood factors. Developmental Medicine and Child Neurology 21: 285–298

Lindsay J, Ounsted C, Richards P 1979b Long-term outcome in children with temporal lobe seizures. II. Marriage, parenthood and sexual indifference. Developmental Medicine and Child Neurology 21: 433–440

Lindsay J, Ounsted C, Richards P 1979c Long-term outcome in children with temporal lobe seizures. III. Psychiatric aspects in childhood and adult life. Developmental Medicine and Child Neurology 21: 630–636

Lindsay J, Ounsted C, Richards P 1984 Long-term outcome in children with temporal lobe seizures. V. Indications and contraindications for neurosurgery. Developmental Medicine and Child Neurology 26: 25–32

Lockman L A 1983 Phenobarbital dosage for neonatal seizures. In: Delgado-Escueta A V, Wasterlain C G, Treiman D M, Porter R J (eds) Advances in neurology Vol 34: status epilepticus. Raven Press, New York, pp 505–508

Loiseau P 1985 Childhood absence epilepsy. In: Roger J, Dravet C, Bureau M, Dreifuss F E, Wolf P (eds) Epileptic syndromes in infancy, childhood and adolescence. John Libbey Eurotext, London. pp 106–120

Loiseau P, Pestre M, Dartigues J F, Commenges D, Barberger-Gateau C, Cohadon S 1983 Long-term prognosis in two forms of childhood epilepsy: typical absences and epilepsy with rolandic (centrotemporal) EEG foci: Annals of Neurology 13: 642–648

Lombroso C T 1967 Sylvian seizures and mid-temporal spike foci in children. Archives of Neurology 17: 52–59

Lombroso C T 1983a Differentiation of seizures in newborns and in early infancy. In: Morselli P L, Pippenger C E, Penry J K (eds) Antiepileptic drug therapy in pediatrics. Raven Press, New York, pp 85–102

Lombroso C T 1983b Prognosis in neonatal seizures. In: Delgado-Escueta A V, Wasterlain C G, Treiman D M, Porter R J (eds) Advances in neurology Vol 34: status epilepticus. Raven Press, New York, pp 101–113

Lombroso C T 1983c A prospective study of infantile spasms: clinical and therapeutic considerations. Epilepsia 24: 135–158

Lombroso C T, Fejerman N 1977 Benign myoclonus of early infancy. Annals of Neurology 1: 138–143

Low J A, Pancham S R, Piercy W N, Worthington D, Karchmar J 1977 Intrapartum fetal asphyxia: Clinical characteristics, diagnosis and significance in relation to pattern of development. Americal Journal of Obstetrics and Gynecology 129: 857–870

McCaughran J A, Edwards E, Zito R S, Schecter N 1982 Experimental febrile convulsions: Short and long-term effects on the cholinergic system in the rat. Epilepsia 23:434

McCaughran J A, Edwards E, Schecter N 1984 Experimental febrile convulsions in the developing rat: effects on the cholinergic system. Epilepsia 25: 250–258

Mathieson G 1975 Pathology of temporal lobe foci. In: Penry J K, Daly D D (eds) Complex partial seizures and their treatment. Advances in neurology Vol 11. Raven Press, New York, pp 163–185

Matsumoto A, Watanabe K, Negoro T et al 1981 Long-term prognosis after infantile spasms: a statistical study of prognostic factors in 200 cases. Developmental Medicine and Child Neurology 23: 51–65

Matsuo M, Kurokawa T, Tomita S, Masaki K, Goya N 1981 EEG findings during the period of febrile convulsions and transition to afebrile seizures. Brain and Development 3:104

Mazziotti J C, Engel J Jr 1985 Advanced neuro-imaging techniques in the study of human epilepsy: PET, SPECT and NMR-CT. In: Pedley T A, Meldrum B S (eds) Recent advances in epilepsy No 2. Churchill Livingstone, Edinburgh, pp 65–99

Meencke H J, Janz D 1984 Neuropathological findings in primary generalised epilepsy: a study of eight cases. Epilepsia 25: 8–21

Melchior J C 1977 Infantile spasms and early immunisation against whooping cough. Danish survey from 1970 to 1975. Archives of Disease in Childhood 52: 134–137

Melchior J C, Buchthal F, Lennox-Buchthal M 1971 The ineffectiveness of diphenylhydantoin in preventing febrile convulsions in the age of greatest risk, under three years. Epilepsia 12: 55–62

Meldrum B S 1976 Secondary pathology of febrile and experimental convulsions. In: Brazier M A B, Coceani F (eds) Brain dysfunction in infantile febrile convulsions. Raven Press, New York, pp 213–222

Mellits E D, Holden K R, Freeman J M 1981 Neonatal seizures. II. Multivariate analysis of factors associated with outcome. Pediatrics 70: 177–185

Miller D L, Ross E M, Alderslade R, Bellman M H, Rawson N S B 1981 Pertussis immunisation and serious acute neurological illness in children. British Medical Journal 282: 1595–1599

Millichap J G 1968 Febrile convulsions. Macmillan, New York

Millichap J G, Madsen J A, Aledort L M 1960 Studies in febrile seizures. V. Clinical and electroencephalographic study in unselected patients. Neurology 10: 643–653

Minchom P E, Wallace S J 1984 Febrile convulsions: electroencephalographic changes related to rectal temperature. Archives of Disease in Childhood 59: 371–373

Monaco F, Sechi G P, Mutani R et al 1980 Lack of efficacy of carbamazepine in preventing the recurrence of febrile convulsions. In: Johannessen S I, Morselli P L, Pippenger C E, Richens A, Schmidt D, Meinardi H (eds) Antiepileptic therapy: advances in drug minitoring. Raven Press, New York, pp 75–79

Nahmias A J, Alford C A, Korones S B 1970 Infection of the newborn with herpes virus hominis. In: Schulman I (ed) Advances in pediatrics Vol 17 Year Book. Chicago, pp 185–226

Nayrac P, Beaussart M 1958 Les pointe-ondes pre-rolandiques: expression EEG très particulière. Étude electroclinique de 21 cas. Revue Neurologique 99: 201–206

Nealis J G T, McFadden S W, Asnes R A, Ouellette E M 1977 Routine skull roentgenograms in the management of simple febrile seizures. Journal of Pediatrics 90: 595–596

Nelson K B, Ellenberg J H 1976 Predictors of epilepsy in children who have experienced febrile seizures. New England Journal of Medicine 295: 1029–1033

Nelson K B, Ellenberg J H 1978 Prognosis in children with febrile seizures. Pediatrics 61: 720–727

Nelson K B, Ellenberg J H 1980 They don't do very well. Pediatrics 65:679

Neville B G R 1972 The origin of infantile spasms: evidence from a case of hydrancephaly. Developmental Medicine and Child Neurology 14: 644–656

Ngwane E, Bower B D 1980 Continuous sodium valproate or phenobarbitone in the prevention of 'simple' febrile convulsions. Archives of Disease in Childhood 55: 171–174

O'Donohoe N V 1985 Epilepsies of Childhood. 2nd edn. Butterworths, London.

Ohtahara S 1984 Seizure disorders in infancy and childhood. Brain and Development 6: 509–519

Ohtahara S O, Ishida S, Yamatogi Y, Ishiba T, Ichiba N 1981 Febrile convulsions in Tamano City, Okayama: A neuro-epidemiologic study. Brain and Development 3:103

Oller-Daurella L 1985 Epilepsy with generalised convulsive seizures in childhood. In: Roger J, Dravet C, Bureau M, Dreifuss F E, Wolf P (eds) Epileptic syndromes in infancy, childhood and adolescence. John Libbey Eurotext, London, pp 130–136

Ounsted C 1955 Genetic and social aspects of the epilepsies of childhood. Eugenics Review 47: 33–49

Ounsted C 1971 Some aspects of seizure disorders. In: Gairdner D, Hull D (eds) Recent advances in paediatrics. Churchill, London. pp 363–400

Ounsted C, Lindsay J, Norman R 1966 Biological factors in temporal lobe epilepsy. Clinics in Developmental Medicine 22. Heinemann, London

Overall J C 1970 Neonatal bacterial meningitis. Journal of Pediatrics 76: 499–511

Painter M J 1983 General principles of treatment: Status epilepticus in neonates. In: Delgado-Escueta A V, Wasterlain C G, Treiman D M, Porter R J (eds) Advances in neurology Vol 34: status epilepticus. Raven Press, New York, pp 385–393

Painter M J, Pippenger C, Wasterlain C et al 1981 Phenobarbital and phenytoin in neonatal seizures: Metabolism and tissue distribution. Neurology 31: 1107–1112

Pampiglione G 1965 Brain development and the EEG of normal children of various ethnical groups. British Medical Journal 2: 573–575

Penry J K, Porter R J, Dreifuss F E 1975 Simultaneous recording of absence seizures with videotape and electroencephalography. A study of 374 seizures in 48 patients. Brain 98: 427–440

Pentella K, Bachman D S, Sandman C A 1982 Trial of an ACTH$_{4-9}$ analogue (ORG 2766) in children with intractable seizures. Neuropediatrics 13: 59–62

Pierog S, Chandavasu O, Wexler I 1977 Withdrawal symptoms in infants with fetal alcohol syndrome. Journal of Pediatrics 90: 630–633

Plouin P 1985 Benign neonatal convulsions (familial and non-familial). In: Roger J, Dravet C, Bureau M, Dreifuss F E,

Wolf P (eds) Epileptic syndromes in infancy, childhood and adolescence. John Libbey Eurotext, London, pp 2–9

Porter R J 1984 Epilepsy: 100 elementary principles. W B Saunders, London

Rasmussen T, Olszewski J, Lloyd-Smith D 1958 Focal seizures due to chronic localised encephalitides. Neurology 8: 435–445

Ratcliffe J C, Wolf S M 1977 Febrile convulsions caused by meningitis in young children. Annals of Neurology 1: 285–286

Reintoft H, Simonsen N, Lund M 1976 A controlled sociological study of juvenile myoclonic epilepsy. In: Janz D (ed) Epileptology. Thieme, Stuttgart, pp 48–50

Revol M 1985 Lesional epilepsies with partial seizures. In: Roger J, Dravet C, Bureau M, Dreifuss F E, Wolf P (eds) Epileptic syndromes in infancy, childhood and adolescence. John Libbey Eurotext, London, pp 278–285

Riikonen R 1982 A long-term follow-up study of 214 children with the syndrome of infantile spasms. Neuropediatrics 13: 14–23

Riikonen R, Donner M 1979 Incidence and aetiology of infantile spasms during the period 1960–76. A population study in Finland. Developmental Medicine and Child Neurology 21: 333–343

Roberton N R C, Smith M A 1975 Early neonatal hypocalcaemia. Archives of Disease in Childhood 50: 604–609

Roberts S A, Cohen M D, Forfar J O 1973 Antenatal factors associated with neonatal hypocalcaemic convulsions. Lancet 2: 809–811

Rodin E A 1968 The prognosis of patients with epilepsy. Thomas, Springfield

Roger J 1985 Progressive myoclonic epilepsy in childhood and adolescence. In: Roger J, Dravet C, Bureau M, Dreifuss F E, Wolf P (eds) Epileptic syndromes in infancy, childhood and adolescence. John Libbey Eurotext, London, pp 302–310

Roger J, Dravet C, Menendez P, Bureau M 1981 Les épilepsies partielles de l'enfant. Evolution et facteurs de prognostic. Revue d'Electroencephalographie et de Neurophysiologie Clinique 11: 431–437

Rutter N, O'Callaghan M J 1978 Hyponatraemia in children with febrile convulsions. Archives of Disease in Childhood 53: 85–87

Rutter N, Smales O R C 1977 Role of routine investigations in children presenting with their first febrile convulsion. Archives of Disease in Childhood 52: 188–191

Sato S, Penry J K, Dreifuss F E, Dyken P R 1977 Clonazepam in the treatment of absence seizures: a double-blind clinical trial. Neurology 27:371

Sato S, Dreifuss F E, Penry J K, Kirby D, White B G 1982a Long-term follow-up study of absence seizures. In: Akimoto H, Kazamatsuri H, Seino M, Ward A (eds) Advances in epileptology: XIIIth Epilepsy International Symposium. Raven Press, New York, pp 41–42

Sato S, White B G, Penry J K 1982b Valproic acid versus ethosuximide in the treatment of absence seizures. Neurology 32: 157–163

Schiøtz-Christensen E 1972 Genetic factors in febrile convulsions. Acta Paediatrica Scandinavica 48: 538–546

Schiøtz-Christensen E 1973 Role of birth history in the aetiology and course of febrile convulsions. A twin study. Neuropädiatrie 4: 238–244

Schiøtz-Christensen E, Bruhn P 1973 Intelligence, behaviour and scholastic achievement subsequent to febrile convulsions: an analysis of discordant twin-pairs. Developmental Medicine and Child Neurology 15: 565–575

Schmidt D 1983a How to use benzodiazepines. In: Morselli P L, Pippenger C E, Penry J K (eds) Antiepileptic drug therapy in pediatrics. Raven Press, New York, pp 271–278

Schmidt D 1983b How to use ethosuximide. In: Morselli P L, Pippenger C E, Penry J K (eds) Antiepileptic drug therapy in pediatrics. Raven Press, New York, p 236

Sherwin A L 1982 Ethosuximide: relation of plasma concentration to seizure control. In: Woodbury D M, Penry J K, Pippenger C E (eds) Antiepileptic drugs. Raven Press, New York, pp 637–645

Simpson H, Habel A H, George E L 1977a Cerebrospinal fluid acid-base status and lactate and pyruvate concentrations after short (less than 30 minutes) first febrile convulsions in children. Archives of Disease in Childhood 52: 836–843

Simpson H, Habel A H, George E L 1977b Cerebrospinal fluid acid-base status and lactate and pyruvate concentrations after convulsions of varied duration and aetiology in children. Archives of Disease in Childhood 52: 844–849

Sorel L, Dusaucy-Bauloye 1958 À propos de 21 cas d'hypsarrhythmie de Gibbs: son traitement spectaculaire par l'ACTH. Acta Neurologica et Psychiatrica Belgica 58: 130–141

Stokes M J, Downham M A P S, Webb J K G, McQuillin J, Gardner P S 1977 Virus and febrile convulsions. Archives of Disease in Childhood 52: 129–133

Strobos R J 1959 Prognosis in convulsive disorders. Archives of Neurology 1: 216–225

Swaab D F, Mirmiran M 1984 Possible mechanisms underlying the teratogenic effects of medicines on the developing brain. In: Yanai J (ed) Neurobehavioural Teratology. Elsevier, Amsterdam; pp 55–71

Tangri K K, Misra N, Bhargava K P 1976 Central cholinergic mechanisms of pyrexia. In: Brazier M A B, Coceani F (eds) Brain dysfunction in infantile febrile convulsions. Raven Press, New York, pp 307–317

Tassinari C A, Bureau M 1985 Epilepsy with myoclonic absences. In: Roger J, Dravet C, Bureau M, Dreifuss F E, Wolf P (eds) Epileptic syndromes in infancy, childhood and adolescence. John Libbey Eurotext, London, pp 121–129

Tassinari C A, DeMarco P 1985 Benign partial epilepsy with extreme somato-sensory evoked potentials. In: Roger J, Dravet C, Bureau M, Dreifuss F E, Wolf P (eds) Epileptic syndromes in infancy, childhood and adolescence. John Libbey Eurotext, London, pp 176–180

Taylor D C 1969 Differential rates of cerebral maturation between the sexes and between hemispheres. Evidence from epilepsy. Lancet 2: 140–142

Taylor D C, Ounsted C 1971 Biological mechanisms influencing the outcome of seizures in response to fever. Epilepsia 12: 33–45

Thomas J E, Reagan T J, Klass D W 1977 Epilepsia partialis continua. Archives of Neurology 34: 266–275

Thorn I 1982 The significance of electroencephalography in febrile convulsions. In: Akimoto H, Kazamatsuri H, Seino M, Ward A (eds) Advances in epileptology: XIIIth Epilepsy International Symposium. Raven Press, New York. p 93–95

Tsang R C 1972 Neonatal magnesium disturbances. American Journal of Diseases of Children 124: 282–293

Tsuboi T 1977a Genetic aspects of febrile convulsions. Human Genetics 38: 169–173

Tsuboi T 1977b Primary generalised epilepsy with sporadic myoclonias of myoclonic petit mal type. Thieme, Stuttgart (cited by Wolf P 1985a)

Tsuboi T, Endo S 1977 Febrile convulsions followed by non-febrile convulsions. A clinical, electroencephalographic and follow-up study. Neuropädiatrie 8: 209–223

Van den Berg B J, Yerushalmy J 1969 Studies on convulsive disorders in young children. I. Incidence of febrile and non-febrile convulsions by age and other factors. Pediatric Research 3: 298–304

Van den Berg B J, Yerushalmy J 1974 Studies on convulsive disorders in young children. V. Excess of early fetal deaths among pregnancies preceding the birth of children with febrile or non-febrile convulsions. Journal of Pediatrics 84: 837–840

Verity C M, Butler N R, Golding J 1985a Febrile convulsions in a national cohort followed up from birth. I. Prevalence and recurrence in the first five years of life. British Medical Journal 290: 1307–1310

Verity C M, Butler N R, Golding J 1985b Febrile convulsions in a national cohort followed up from birth. II. Medical history and intellectual ability at 5 years of age. British Medical Journal 290: 1311–1315

Volpe J J 1981 Neurology of the Newborn. Volume XXII in the Series: Major Problems in Clinical Pediatrics. W B Saunders, Philadelphia.

Wallace S J Unpublished data

Wallace S J 1972 Aetiological aspects of febrile convulsions. Pregnancy and perinatal factors. Archives of Disease in Childhood 47: 171–178

Wallace S J 1974a The reproductive efficiency of parents whose children convulse when febrile. Developmental Medicine and Child Neurology 16: 465–474

Wallace S J 1974b Recurrence of febrile convulsions. Archives of Disease in Childhood 49: 763–765

Wallace S J 1975 Factors predisposing to a complicated initial febrile convulsion. Archives of Disease in Childhood 50: 943–947

Wallace S J 1976 Neurological and intellectual deficits: convulsions with fever viewed as acute indications of life-long developmental defects. In: Brazier M A B, Coceani F (eds) Brain dysfunction in infantile febrile convulsions. Raven Press, New York, pp 259–277

Wallace S J 1977 Spontaneous fits after convulsions with fever. Archives of Disease in Childhood 52: 192–196

Wallace S J 1981 Prevention of recurrent febrile seizures using continuous prophylaxis: sodium valproate compared with phenobarbital. In: Nelson K B, Ellenberg J H (eds) Febrile seizures. Raven Press, New York, pp 135–142

Wallace S J 1982 Prognosis after prolonged unilateral febrile convulsions. In: Akimoto H, Kazamatsuri H, Seino M, Ward A (eds) Advances in epileptology: XIIIth Epilepsy International Symposium. Raven Press. New York, pp 97–99

Wallace S J 1984 Infantile spasms: a symptom of mitochondrial cytopathy. Paper presented to the Joint Meeting of the British Dutch & Danish Branches of the International League Against Epilepsy, Denmark

Wallace S J 1985 Convulsions and lumbar puncture. Developmental Medicine and Child Neurology 27: 69–71

Wallace S J, Aldridge Smith J 1980 Successful prophylaxis against febrile convulsions with valproic acid or phenobarbitone. British Medical Journal 280: 353–354

Wallace S J, Aldridge Smith J 1981 Recurrence of convulsions in febrile children on no anticonvulsant. In: Dam M, Gram L, Penry J K (eds) Advances in Epileptology: XIIth Epilepsy International Symposium. Raven Press, New York, pp 499–502

Wallace S J, Cull A M 1979 Long-term psychological outlook for children whose first fit occurs with fever. Development Medicine and Child Neurology 21: 28–40

Wallace S J, Zealley H 1970 Neurological, electroencephalographic and virological findings in febrile children. Archives of Disease in Childhood 45: 611–623

Wasterlain C G, Dwyer B E 1983 Brain metabolism during prolonged seizures in neonates. In: Delgado-Escueta A V, Wasterlain C G, Treiman D M, Porter R J (eds) Advances in neurology Vol 34: status epilepticus. Raven Press, New York, p 241–260

West W J 1841 On a peculiar form of infantile convulsions. Lancet 1: 724–725

Wilkins A, Lindsay J 1985 Common forms of reflex epilepsy: Physiological mechanisms and techniques for treatment. In: Pedley T A, Meldrum B S (eds) Recent advances in epilepsy No 2. Churchill Livingstone, Edinburgh, pp 239–271

Willig R P, Lagenstein I 1982 Use of ACTH fragments in children with infantile spasms. Neuropediatrics 13: 55–58

Wolf P 1985a Juvenile myoclonic epilepsy. In: Roger J, Dravet C, Bureau M, Dreifuss F E, Wolf P (eds) Epileptic syndromes in infancy, childhood and adolescence. John Libbey Eurotext, London, pp 247–258

Wolf P 1985b Juvenile absence epilepsy. In: Roger J, Dravet C, Bureau M, Dreifuss F E, Wolf P (eds) Epileptic syndromes in infancy, childhood and adolescence. John Libbey Eurotext, London, pp 242–246

Wolf S M 1978 Laboratory evaluation of the child with febrile convulsions. Archives of Disease in Childhood 53: 85–87

Wolf S M, Forsythe A 1978 Behavior disturbance, phenobarbital and febrile seizures. Pediatrics 61: 728–731

Wolf S M, Carr A, Davis D C et al 1977 The value of phenobarbital in the child who has had a single febrile seizure: a controlled prospective study. Pediatrics 59: 378–385

Wolf S M, Forsythe A, Stunden A A, Friedman R, Diamond H 1981 Long-term effect of phenobarbital on cognitive function in children with febrile convulsions. Pediatrics 68: 820–823

Yoshida T, Tada K, Arakawa T 1971 Vitamin B_6-dependency of glutamic acid decarboxylase in the kidney from a patient with vitamin B_6-dependent convulsion. Tohoku Journal of Experimental Medicine 104: 195–198 (cited by Jaeken 1985)

Zellweger H 1948 Fieber-oder Infectionskrämpfe. Helvetica Paediatrica Acta (Suppl 5) 3: S58–S140

Zelson C, Rubio E, Wasserman E 1971 Neonatal narcotic addiction. Pediatrics 48: 178–189

5

Seizures in adults

C. D. Marsden
E. H. Reynolds

INTRODUCTION

Neurologists, psychiatrists, paediatricians, general physicians, general practitioners and casualty officers all see and treat patients with epilepsy. But even the most experienced, and perhaps they more than most, have difficulty in defining epilepsy – as is illustrated by the variation in current textbook definitions (Reynolds 1986). A common view is that epilepsy is a tendency to recurrent seizures (fits). This implies that a single seizure is not epilepsy even though some 70–80% of patients with an unprovoked single seizure go on to develop further attacks. To the ancients a single seizure, as well as the recurrent state, constituted the disorder 'epilepsy' (Temkin 1971). Indeed the words 'epilepsy' and 'epileptic', which are of Greek origin, have the same root as the verb 'epilambanein', which means 'to seize' or 'to attack'. Epilepsy therefore means seizure.

The words 'epilepsy', 'epileptic' and 'epileptiform' are widely used by clinical neurophysiologists on EEG reports. To the inexperienced clinician such reports assume great importance in diagnosis. The experienced clinician is more circumspect, aware that so-called epileptic EEG abnormalities are not always synonymous with epilepsy, that they can occur in other clinical conditions and even in otherwise entirely normal individuals. Experimental physiologists also use the word 'epilepsy' and have many different models of the disorder. Although spontaneous seizures can occur throughout the mammalian system, most of the models in use are based on seizures artificially induced by a variety of electrical, pharmacological and chemical means. Single cell physiologists, pharmacologists and

neurochemists all use the word 'epilepsy' and the words 'epileptic neurone' have become fashionable.

The extension of the use of the word 'epilepsy' outside the clinical field can be traced to Jackson (1873), who proposed that the word should be degraded to imply the condition of nerve tissue in sudden and temporary loss of its function. This was crystallized in his famous definition: 'Epilepsy is the name for occasional, sudden, excessive, rapid and local discharges of grey matter'. It is not widely appreciated that Jackson (1890) to some extent retreated from this physiological definition as he began to see epilepsy everywhere. For example, he said that 'a sneeze is a sort of healthy epilepsy'. However, the discovery of the EEG by Berger led a later generation of neurophysiologists to convince themselves that the mysterious electrical discharges that they were observing corresponded to Jackson's intuitive definition.

At the present time, therefore, there is no agreement as to the precise definition of epilepsy or as to whether the term should be restricted, as some have advocated, solely to clinical use (Trimble & Reynolds 1986), where there are difficulties enough in distinguishing the disorder from so-called borderlands (Gowers 1907). One can define a seizure, a disease causing seizures, a precipitating cause of seizures and the consequences of seizures, all of which contribute to the overall picture of epilepsy. A physiologist can define the parameters of abnormal electrical discharge underlying seizures. The biochemist may, in the future, define a local change responsible for generating that electrical discharge. Such events are also part of epilepsy; but epilepsy is also a social distinction: those diagnosed as having epilepsy are, to a greater or lesser extent, penalized both economically and socially.

This chapter is concerned with clinical phenomena, with the etiology, precipitating causes and symptoms of seizures and with the problems of differential diagnosis, investigation and prognosis. Discussion of each of these topics depends on the sort of seizure the patient suffers. To the clinician it is the differences between the various types of seizures that are important, although their similarities are crucial to the research worker hunting for the elusive chemical/physiological event responsible for a seizure. The latter's aim is to discover how a variety of insults may produce the same sign and to identify the proximate cause of the seizure in order to improve preventive therapy. The clinician, however, is committed to dividing seizures into subgroups in order to provide the best advice for the individual patient.

THE CLASSIFICATION OF SEIZURES

The terminology and classification of seizures has evolved over many years, creating a variety of interchangeable and confused descriptive terms. The problem has been, and is, to create a single code to cover three basically incompatible systems of classification, namely: that according to clinical symptoms and signs of the fit; that relating to the anatomical and electrophysiological evidence as to the source of the fit; and that defining the etiology of the fits. An example illustrates the conflict. The symptom complex of an absence seizure prefaced by an abdominal and gustatory aura is often referred to as a temporal lobe seizure (Symonds 1953, Williams 1966), for usually it indicates temporal lobe pathology and electrophysiological evidence of temporal lobe discharges. However, a similar fit occurs on occasion in patients with a frontal lobe abnormality, and to describe such a fit as a temporal lobe seizure is not entirely accurate. Early descriptions of such fits as psychomotor attacks (Gibbs et al 1937) paid attention primarily to the clinical features of the fit, without prejudice to the anatomical source; further experience led to the realization that

psychomotor seizures usually implicated a temporal lobe origin.

It seems necessary to retain a tripartite system of classification and it is not always profitable to force clinical symptomatology, anatomical source and etiology into a single framework, although all three are obviously complementary.

The International League Against Epilepsy, under the chairmanship of Henri Gastaut (1969) attempted the Herculean task of formulating a comprehensive classification of seizures to include the clinical seizure type, EEG seizure type, EEG interictal expression, anatomical substrate, etiology and age. Subsequently, further criteria were added by Gastaut, including the presence or absence of interictal neuropsychiatric changes, the response to therapy and pathophysiology. Others did not accept the original or its modifications and provided alternatives; as Gastaut himself declared, 'Perhaps its chief advantage is that it can serve as an anvil on which critics can hammer out a classification of higher value'. Indeed, the International League's Commission on classification has been attempting to do just this at the present time; this is discussed extensively in Chapter 1.

The crucial problem, for any classification, is who is going to use it. As Whitty (1965) has stated:

> Two broad groups of demand for information arise in epilepsy – the practical or clinical, and the more theoretical or pathophysiological. The two cannot be rigidly separated, but they are likely to give rise to differing approaches to classification. On the clinical side, information is required especially about prognosis with or without treatment . . . From the pathophysiological side, the demand is for information on how the brain works and which parts of it are concerned with which functions . . . Such multiplicity of aims is scarcely compatible with a unitary classification.

While not wishing to denigrate the International Classifications, our aim in this is chapter is to provide a simple, practical classification which is summarized in Table 5.1. This necessarily oversimplifies a very complex topic, but it does highlight some fundamental concepts, based on the clinical features of fits and differences in their pathophysiology. Thus some fits start with electrical discharges in both cerebral hemispheres simultaneously – generalized fits. Others start with a focal discharge in one part of a cerebral hemi-

Table 5.1 Classification of seizures

1. *Generalized*
   a. Tonic-clonic (grand mal)
   b. Tonic
   c. Atonic
   d. Absence (petit mal)
   e. Myoclonic

2. *Partial (FOCAL)*
    i. Without loss of consciousness
   ii. With loss of consciousness
   a. With motor signs (e.g. Jacksonian, versive)
   b. With somato- or special sensory symptoms (e.g. olfactory, visual)
   c. With autonomic features (e.g. epigastric sensations)
   d. With psychic symptoms (e.g. fear, déjà vu)
   e. With automatisms

3. *Partial seizures secondarily generalized*
   i.e. clinical or electrical evidence of focal discharge before, during or after the generalized seizure

4. *Unclassifiable*

Table 5.2 Frequency of fits arising from different sources

Temporal lobe	244
Frontal lobe	35
Parietal lobe	11
Occipital lobe	9
Primary generalized	106
Unlocalized	370
Total number of cases	775

Based on a series of cases referred for EEG examination at Leeds, 1951–1961 (Parsonage 1973)

THE CLINICAL SYMPTOMS OF THE SEIZURE

It is not the purpose of this chapter to describe in detail the clinical phenomena of typical fits; rather, we will concentrate on certain aspects of fits of practical clinical significance.

Generalized seizures

Tonic-clonic (grand mal)

Clinical features A typical major motor seizure or grand mal fit is unmistakable: consisting of a tonic phase, followed by a clonic phase, the whole lasting for up to two minutes, and followed by a further period of five minutes or so of unrousable coma. After this, the patient can be awoken, but is confused and disorientated and usually prefers to sleep for a few hours, to awake often with a headache and sore muscles, but a clear mind. An epileptic cry at the start, cyanosis, frothing at the mouth, emptying the bladder, biting the tongue or other injury are common but not universal. During the fit the pupils dilate, the pulse may slow initially then accelerate, the patient sweats profusely, the plantar responses are extensor and the tendon jerks and corneal reflexes are lost. Inevitably, the patient loses consciousness and falls in a grand mal attack.

Grand mal seizures do not always conform to this classical sequence, but always involve loss of consciousness and convulsion. On some occasions the seizure may cease after the tonic phase, while sometimes only a clonic seizure occurs. Such limited grand mal fits are especially common in children and infants. Grand mal seizures without muscular contractions probably do not occur.

sphere – focal or partial fits. If that part of the brain is eloquent, the patient experiences an aura, a consciously remembered experience that may be a motor, sensory, visceral or psychical event. This aura points to the part of the brain where the fit begins. If the site of origin of the fit is silent, the patient may notice nothing until the electrical discharge spreads to an eloquent area or becomes generalized to involve both hemispheres – focal fits with secondary generalization.

Inevitably, such a classification is not comprehensive. Many patients have seizures which do not fit comfortably into any of the categories. Fits with origin in the temporal lobe may manifest many of the categories of focal symptoms. Some syndromes characterized primarily by fits, such as infantile spasms and progressive myoclonic epilepsy, have generalized seizure discharges with atypical absence attacks, atypical myoclonic seizures, grand mal attacks etc. and cannot be neatly classified. Many infants and children have focal fits which may or may not be associated with a focal abnormality in the EEG; the latter itself may be erratic and change its position. However, this simple scheme serves most of the clinician's needs.

Some indication of the frequency of different types of fits, generalized and focal, in a series of representative patients referred with a diagnosis of epilepsy to one centre, is given in Table 5.2.

True atonic seizures with collapse of muscle tone are closely associated with petit mal absences and myoclonus and with spike and wave discharge in the EEG (see below).

Prodromal symptoms Many patients with grand mal fits are aware of an impending fit or flurry of fits days or hours before the event. Such prodromal symptoms are to be distinguished from the aura to a grand mal fit, which precedes it by seconds or a few minutes. The aura is in itself a focal fit, reflecting an abnormal focal electrical discharge in the brain, while the prodromata are not necessarily signs of seizure activity. Individual patients may complain of prodromal headache, insomnia, irritability, mood change, lethargy, unusual appetite and a variety of other such symptoms. The longer the patient has had fits the more likely is he to be able to recognize such signs. Some of them are due to physiological changes known to precipitate fits, for instance, the water retention preceding menstruation. Others may represent the effects of increasing subclinical seizure discharges, but there is no hard evidence for this. In other patients, it is possible that the prodromata are no more than those changes which precipitate their fits; thus anxiety, whatever its cause, may precipitate seizures and the patient may come to associate fits with a prodroma of anxiety. The incidence and significance of these prodromal changes have not been studied much, but might be a profitable field of investigation.

One form of prodroma that is reasonably common and distinctive is myoclonic jerking. Typically, such patients develop muscle twitching, particularly of arms and trunk, days or hours before a grand mal fit. Such prodromal myoclonus is said to occur in between 10% and 50% of patients with grand mal fits. In our experience, the incidence approximates to the lower figure, but when it occurs it is very distinctive; some patients can accurately predict the day of a fit by the onset of jerks on awakening that morning. The subsequent seizure is not inevitable and a few patients may discover means of preventing it, by rest or extra doses of medication. Whether such premonitory myoclonic jerks represent seizure discharges or not is unclear, but the techniques of continuous EEG monitoring should help to decide.

Focal onset to grand mal. Grand mal fits, either start with bilateral synchronous EEG discharge and abrupt loss of consciousness without aura; may follow an aura indicating a focal origin to the fit, with secondary spread and generalization; or may follow a focal electrical discharge in a silent area of the cerebral cortex unbeknown to the patient but detectable in the EEG. Grand mal with focal onset, be it evident to the patient as an aura or to the doctor as an EEG abnormality prefacing a fit, indicates a high likelihood of a focal structural lesion in the cerebral cortex as the cause of the epilepsy. Other phenomena have a similar, predictive value. Thus while a patient may lose consciousness abruptly without warning, an observer may witness head turning or unilateral muscular contraction prefacing the tonic-clonic phase of a grand mal seizure. Similarly, a focal post-ictal paralysis (Todd's paralysis) or post-ictal speech disturbance indicates the focal origin of some grand mal fits. In all these cases, the fit begins with a local electrical discharge in some part of the cerebral cortex (the focal fit), then the discharge spreads to involve both hemispheres (secondary generalization causing the grand mal seizure). The pathophysiology of this march of events during seizures is discussed at length in Chapter 7; suffice to say that in some way a focal cortical electrical discharge spreads to involve some central structures in the diencephalon and upper brainstem, which then relay bilateral synchronous electrical discharges into both hemispheres to cause the generalized grand mal fit. A focal fit (with local colour and sign) is followed by a generalized seizure.

The nature and location of the neurophysiological events underlying the generalized seizure, be it generalized from onset or focal in origin with secondary generalization, is unknown. Penfield (1952) introduced the concept of a centrencephalic integrating system to explain the origin of generalized seizures. Abnormal electrical discharge in this centren cephalic system in the diencephalon and upper brainstem causes loss of consciousness and a generalized seizure (of either grand mal or petit mal type). Grand mal fits of focal origin occur when the abnormal focal cortical discharge spreads to invade this subcortical centrencephalic system. (Focal fits, whatever their cause, may be followed by grand mal fits, but never by petit mal.) But what happens in patients with generalized epilepsy with no focal origin?

Primary generalized grand mal seizures Here the patient has grand mal seizures, without aura, without focal EEG onset and without focal clinical events either during or after the attack. It has been suggested that such patients, who may be said to have primary (or cryptogenic or idiopathic) generalized epilepsy, have a disorder of function of this hypothetical centrencephalic system. This is an attractive, simple, but unproven, hypothesis. Williams (1965) has marshalled clinical evidence against a centrencephalic origin for primary epilepsy. In particular, he argues that cerebral tumours and other pathological processes which are strongly epileptogenic in cerebral cortex rarely cause fits when located in the thalamus or other subcortical areas, or brainstem. This argument may not be decisive, for recent work implicates the cerebellum in seizure control, yet, by and large, cerebellar disease is not marked by seizures. However, the centrencephalic origin of primary seizures remains a concept and an act of faith.

The alternative proposition is described by Elkington (1950) with particular reference to grand mal:

> There is some reason for believing that every major attack has a local commencement in some region of the brain, and that it is in reality a local fit which rapidly becomes general. When such an attack commences with a local aura there is proof positive of local commencement . . . When the spread of the disturbance is so rapid as to cause instant loss of consciousness there is no memory to retain the initial event of the attack.

This belief that all grand mal is of focal origin is compatible with the centrencephalic concept if it is assumed that primary generalized epilepsy originates in a focal discharge in the centrencephalic system, but there is no certain evidence that this is the case. A more restricted view is that all grand mal is of focal cortical origin. This view is currently expanding along with the belief that structural lesions, such as Ammon's horn sclerosis (hitherto dismissed as the consequences, not the cause of fits) may, in fact, be the focal origin for fits in many cases (see Chapter 7). Again, this is a hypothesis, attractive for its simplicity and practical consequences, but unproven.

The debate remains whether primary grand mal seizures are due to focal cortical lesions undetectable by the patient, the observer or the EEG, or whether they are due to an abnormality of centrencephalic subcortical structures, an abnormality that so far has escaped recognition.

A concept which is relevant to the debate as to the pathophysiological basis of primary generalized or indeed secondary generalized, seizures is that of seizure threshold. Seizure activity can occur in all vertebrate nervous systems and the propensity for seizures increases in parallel with the phylogenetic scale, culminating in the highest incidence in humans, who have the most complex nervous system. Furthermore, it is apparent that all human beings are capable of having a generalized seizure if sufficiently stimulated, as exemplified by convulsive therapy in the treatment of depression. Patients vary, however, in their susceptibility to an induced seizure, perhaps due to variation in seizure threshold, which is presumably set by unknown genetic, neurochemical and other metabolic processes. An unusually low seizure threshold may explain why some patients have spontaneous primary generalized seizures. In others, with a higher threshold, the addition of some insult to the brain, such as a tumour or head injury, may be enough to precipitate seizures. Those with the highest seizure threshold may not experience seizures, even though the nervous system is compromised by some physical disease or metabolic disturbance. Thus the concept of seizure threshold may explain why patients with identical cerebral pathology do not all have seizures. Furthermore, it implies that genetic factors play a role in partial seizures as well as in primary generalized attacks.

Absence (petit mal)

The typical brief staring spells of childhood were earlier called 'pyknolepsy'. One of the most significant contributions of EEG investigation to epilepsy was the delineation by Gibbs et al (1935) of a characteristic paroxysm of three per second bilateral, synchronous, spike and wave discharge accompanying the true petit mal attack. Petit mal is now defined as brief absence attacks occurring almost always in childhood, associated with this classical EEG abnormality. Such attacks, and the associated EEG paroxysm, may be provoked by overbreathing.

For some five to ten seconds the child loses consciousness, his eyes stare, and he may show minor movements such as blinking or twitching of the face and arms, but he does not fall. Suddenly, consciousness is regained, but there is total amnesia for the brief period of the attack. The patient looks around for a moment, but then resumes his previous occupation. If engaged in conversation before the attack, he will have missed a sentence or so. Such classical petit mal attacks may occur very frequently, as often as 100 or more times daily (Lennox 1945, Gibberd 1966a, Dalby 1969).

Not all petit mal attacks are as simple as this. More complex phenomena, akin to those seen in temporal lobe epilepsy, may occur associated with an otherwise typical EEG paroxysm (Penry & Dreifuss 1969). Thus the blank spell may last longer and may be accompanied by lip smacking, chewing or mouthing movements. It may be impossible on clinical grounds to distinguish such episodes from temporal lobe 'absences', indeed such a distinction may not be valid, for some patients with temporal lobe epilepsy may show atypical three per second spike and wave discharge in the EEG. The differential diagnosis of true petit mal from other types of 'absence' attack may, on occasion, be either clinically or electrically impossible. One may sometimes be forced to a therapeutic trial of drugs effective against petit mal in such circumstances.

Head turning or circling phenomena have recently been recognized in association with three per second bilateral spike and wave discharges. Gastaut et al (1986), who describe 28 cases with onset between the ages of 8 and 20 (usually 10–14), emphasize that focal hemispheric discharges were not seen and concluded that the syndrome represents a benign form of primary generalized epilepsy in late childhood.

Associated with classical petit mal in some cases are episodes of myoclonic jerking and drop attacks due to sudden collapse of muscle tone. In the former the arms jerk up, the head nods and the trunk flexes as in an exaggerated startle response. The force of this lightning movement may be

sufficient to throw the patient to the ground, with injury. On occasion, such myoclonic jerks may be asymmetrical or even unilateral. In drop attacks the patient drops, not slumps, to the ground, but can get up immediately.

The association of petit mal, myoclonic jerks and drop attacks was christened the 'petit mal triad' by Lennox (1945), but this concept has been distorted by confusion between classical petit mal with an excellent prognosis and progressive myoclonic epilepsy, which is a disastrous illness with a number of causes. In the latter, absence attacks, grand mal seizures, myoclonus and drop attacks all become increasingly severe and are often associated with a progressive dementia or cerebellar syndrome. Such an illness is most commonly seen in childhood and the many known pathological causes are discussed in more detail in Chapter 6. Confusion with simple petit mal arose because many such patients show atypical spike-wave discharge in addition to other widespread EEG abnormality. This atypical spike-wave discharge (otherwise known as petit mal variant discharge, slow wave and spike, or the two per second spike and wave discharge) is associated with a variety of cerebral pathologies and types of seizure, and a very high incidence of progressive mental deterioration (Blume et al 1973) (Table 5.3). To avoid confusion it is perhaps best to distinguish clearly true petit mal (which may on

Table 5.3 Slow spike and wave abnormality in 84 patients (after Blume et al 1973)

Age at onset of fits*	5 or less	59	
	6–10	16	
	11–20	5	
	No fits	2	
Outcome* (in 68 cases)	Dead or in custodial care	46%	
	Normal intelligence	30%	
	Retarded	24%	
Etiology*	Birth injury	14	
	Immunization	3	27%
	Head injury	4	
	Encephalitis	2	
	Family history of fits	22	26%
	Nil	42	50%

* Information was not available for every patient

occasion be accompanied by myoclonus and drop attacks) with a typical EEG abnormality and excellent prognosis, from the progressive myoclonic epilepsy seen predominantly in childhood due to a variety of cerebral insults which cause progressive brain damage. In practice, this is not a difficult distinction, but the delineation of absence attacks plus myoclonus plus drop attacks as a single syndrome has led to conflict in the literature.

True petit mal is uncommon, and is said to occur only in about 3% of patients (Livingstone et al 1965). Petit mal starts before the age of 15 in nearly all cases and ceases by the age of about 20 in 80% or more of cases (Livingston et al 1965, Gibberd 1966b, Dalby 1969). About 50% of those with petit mal will develop grand mal seizures (Livingston et al 1965, Dalby 1969) and there is some evidence that prophylactic antiepileptic therapy to prevent grand mal attacks will reduce the number of those who continue to have fits in adult life. Intelligence and development is normal in all but the small minority who have additional severe grand mal attacks.

Partial (focal) seizures

Motor fits

Jacksonian seizures The typical focal motor fit recognized by Hughlings Jackson consists of onset of tonic spasm followed soon by repetitive twitching, usually in the angle of the mouth, thumb and index finger or great toe, which then spreads in an orderly manner. The fit is due to a discharge in the opposite motor cortex and the spread or march of the seizure reflects the topography of body representation in the motor strip. Thus, the repetitive movements may begin in a hand, spread to arm and face and then down to leg and foot; or may commence in the foot to spread up the leg then down the arm and into the face. The convulsive movements may remain confined to their site of onset, or may spread to involve one-half of the body and may terminate in a typical grand mal fit with loss of consciousness. If the left hemisphere is the source, speech may be lost during the attack and additional sensory symptoms are common, whichever hemi-

sphere is involved. Whether or not consciousness is lost during such a focal motor seizure seems to depend on the extent of brain involved. Consciousness is usually preserved if the fit remains confined to its site of origin, but is often lost if half the body is affected.

The full-blown typical motor seizure is not seen frequently; more often one encounters partial fragments of the motor fit, such as tonic spasm alone or clonic spasm alone, with or without spread. Very rarely, true inhibition of movement has been described as an epileptic event (Efron 1961). We have never recognized the inhibitory seizure which must be difficult to distinguish from a post-ictal paralysis or transient ischaemic episode. Focal motor fits may be followed by a prolonged period of paralysis of the affected limbs as described by Todd. In some such cases, particularly in adult life, the fits and the hemiplegia are due to stroke, but not all Todd's paralysis can be so explained. In other patients, again adults by and large, a prolonged Todd's paralysis may be due to the tumour causing the fit, and if such paralysis persists for more than 48 hours full investigation is required. In children, however, Todd's paralysis often occurs without any structural lesion and need not be investigated so aggressively.

Adversive seizures Another, not uncommon, form of motor seizure is the adversive attack due to discharge arising in premotor areas of the frontal lobe (Penfield & Welch 1951). Typically, the head and eyes are forced away from the affected hemisphere, usually with preservation of consciousness. Sometimes the head turning is accompanied by abduction of the contralateral arm, external rotation of the shoulder and flexion of the elbow. The patient turns his head and eyes to look at his raised arm, thus adopting the posture of a fencer. The force of turning may be so great as to generate circling movements. Such seizures are sometimes accompanied by an epigastric rising aura and other symptoms that might be confused with epileptic discharge arising in the temporal lobe.

Och et al (1984) have recently questioned the time-honoured assumption that forced lateralized head turning as the initial feature of an epileptic seizure locates the site of origin of the seizure in the opposite frontal lobe. In a study of 106 seizures in 43 patients, with video and EEG telemetry, forced head turning was seen in frontal, temporal and generalized seizures. Ipsilateral head turning was as common as contralateral head turning in all these groups. The authors conclude that initial head turning in a seizure has no localizing or lateralizing significance. Gastaut et al (1986) describe head turning and circling phenomena in association with bilateral three per second spike and wave discharges in late childhood. Although no focal discharges were seen, the adversion was always towards the same side in a given patient.

Speech in fits Further mention must be made about speech and fits. Loss of speech, (speech arrest) or frank dysphasia if the subject retains consciousness, is almost always associated with fits arising in the dominant hemisphere and involving the anterior speech area of Broca, or the parieto-temporal speech area.

Brief stereotyped utterances (speech automatisms) may occur with fits arising in the temporal lobes of either side, most commonly that of the non-dominant hemisphere. The latter must be distinguished from the confused speech that occurs during recovery from fits (Serafetinides & Falconer 1963).

Sensory fits

Somatic sensory seizures As with Jacksonian seizures, somatic sensory seizures characteristically commence in one of the preferred sites, such as thumb or mouth, and show a spread or march. The complaint is usually of numbness or pins and needles. Such fits arise from the contralateral sensory strip which is so close to the motor area that they usually occur with motor phenomena. Very rarely pain or burning has been described, but this may be of subcortical origin.

Visual seizures Two types of visual fits are recognized. Those due to discharge in an occipital pole usually consist of unformed simple visual phenomena such as spots, flashes of light, balls of fire and revolving objects, often throughout the field of vision but sometimes confined to the appropriate homonymous half field. Seizures arising in the temporal lobe may uncommonly cause formed and often vivid coloured visual recall of a particular scenario or event; a visual hallucination that is peculiar to the individual patient and is reported in attack after attack.

Auditory events True epileptic vertigo is uncommon, but rotational or other dysequilibrium may be part of a temporal lobe attack (Behrman & Wyke 1958, Smith 1960). By contrast, many patients with a variety of fits complain of nonspecific dizziness as part of their aura. Temporal lobe attacks may also include auditory hallucinations, such as sensations of buzzing, hissing, whistling, ringing, sea noises or the sound of machinery. All these auditory events suggest involvement of the superior temporal gyrus and adjacent cortex.

Olfactory and gustatory sensations Olfactory hallucinations are frequent in temporal lobe epilepsy, as are the closely related hallucinations of taste. Smells and tastes are characteristically unpleasant, such as burnt onions, excreta, burning rubber or indescribable but horrible (Daly 1958a).

Visceral sensations Visceral sensations are also a common part of the temporal lobe attack, consisting usually of a feeling in the pit of the stomach, often described as a constriction or discomfort, as in fear, which rises into the throat and head. Such an aura may be accompanied by autonomic phenomena, such as tachycardia, sweating, pupillary dilatation and a fall in blood pressure (Van Buren & Ajmone-Marsan 1960). Whether such a sequence of autonomic events occurring briefly and repeatedly, but without any other evidence of epilepsy, is a form of restricted autonomic epilepsy is debatable. However, it has been described with response to antiepileptic drugs (Fox et al 1973).

Involuntary micturition, and much more rarely defaecation, is common in grand mal and temporal lobe epilepsy. It can, however, occur in isolation as possible evidence of seizure discharge in the frontal lobe, often with loss of awareness such that the patient suddenly finds himself wet without any prior knowledge of impending or completed micturition (Maurice-Williams 1974).

Psychic fits

Many of the symptoms of focal seizures described so far may occur together with other complex

Table 5.4 Types of fit in 666 patients with temporal lobe epilepsy (after Currie et al 1971) (percentage)

Grand mal	57
Psychomotor attacks*	51
Minor attacks†	23
Auras	49

* Defined as episodes of confusion or amnesia with or without automatism
† Defined as brief attacks in which there was no profound alteration in consciousness

Table 5.5 Components of temporal lobe fits in 666 patients (after Currie et al 1971) (percentage)

Visceral	40
Motor	14
Adversive	0.5
Masticatory	10
Sensory	18
Visual	16
Auditory	19
Vertigo	12
Olfactory	3
Gustatory	2
Somatic	
Thought disorder	27
Déjà vu	14
Other	3
Speech disorder	22
Dysphasia	16
Speech automatism	3
Emotional disorder	19
Unpleasant	14
Panic	1
Rage	2.5
Violence	0.7

phenomena in temporal lobe epilepsy (Tables 5.4 and 5.5). Thus a fit arising in the temporal lobe may be associated with an aura comprising one or all of the following: an epigastric rising sensation; a foul taste and smell; vertigo and auditory hallucinations; formed visual hallucinations; speech disturbance and autonomic phenomena. In addition, the patient may experience profound and disturbing disorders of thought, perception and emotion during the fit (Williams 1956, Bingley 1958, Mullan & Penfield 1959, Penfield & Peroto 1963).

Thought disturbance The classical feeling of déjà vu that may be experienced during a temporal lobe seizure is often indescribable (Cole & Zangwill 1963). The feeling is an overwhelming sense of familiarity, of it having happened before. Some-

times the experience is linked with a visual and/or auditory hallucination that adds a pictorial image to the familiar scene 'like a re-run of a film'. Sometimes the patient cannot recall the faces, scene, noise, phrase or voice at all, but knows it as familiar. The characteristic feature of such brief ictal events is that the same sequence is usually played each time, that it is repetitively stereotyped and that, like most focal epileptic events, it lasts for a brief period only, usually less than a minute or so, and nearly always under five minutes.

Less common are the phenomena of unreality (jamais vu), in which the patient perceives familiar surroundings as totally unreal 'as if I'd never seen this room before, yet I've lived in it for 20 years', and that of forced thinking in which a recurrent idea intrudes in each aura.

Perceptual disturbance Auditory and visual hallucinations, as well as olfactory and gustatory experiences, have already been commented upon as epileptic events. Other perceptual disturbances may also occur, such as illusions of changes in body size, distortions of time ('my heart and the clock suddenly beat at half pace') or sound receding into the distance.

Emotional experiences These experiences are frequent in temporal lobe seizures. Most common is intense fear (Macrae 1954, Williams 1956), which may drive a person to run in terror (cursive epilepsy) (Chen & Forster 1973) or cower under the bed. Such fear is usually accompanied by an epigastric sensation and often by choking in the throat, such that the patient may fear imminent death. Intense pleasure or ecstasy is much rarer. Sometimes the latter may have sexual connotations – one such patient refused to accept any treatment for his fits as they were so pleasurable. Laughter may also occur during a seizure (gelastic epilepsy) (Daly & Mulder 1957, Druckman & Chao 1957, Gumpert et al 1970), usually of temporal lobe origin. Depression and weeping are uncommon, and rage during a fit, as against during the postictal automatism that may follow, is scarcely if ever reported.

The complexity of the remembered experience in a temporal lobe seizure can only be illustrated by examples:

A thought comes into my mind, which I know I've thought before; then the smell comes, but I black out too quickly to remember what thought it is. I know it's important, and I've tried to catch it, but no . . .

I suddenly see a vivid scene of cowboys and Indians in colour rushing towards me. I'm terrified and try to run away, but I pass out too quickly. Nobody believes me when I tell this story, they just laugh.

Suddenly I'm standing in a church, but I'm so small that I can't see above the pew, only the ceiling miles up in the sky; the organ is playing a piece of music very slowly; I know it, but I can't remember its name or even sing it now.

Such examples abound and one can only marvel at the range and complexity of the experiences as one listens to each individual's peculiar and often unique form of the fit.

The frequency of the components of temporal lobe fits has been studied in 666 patients in whom the clinical features suggested temporal lobe epilepsy and/or the EEG showed a definite temporal lobe focal abnormality (in 92%), either slow waves, or sharp waves and spikes (Currie et al 1971) (Table 5.5). In the 666 cases, epilepsy began under the age of 10 in 12%, between 10 and 15 in 14%, between 15 and 25 in 23%, between 25 and 45 in 32%, and over the age of 45 in 19%. Some 50% of patients did not have their first attack until after the age of 25. Those patients with temporal lobe fits represented 25% of those suffering from epilepsy seen in that department between 1949 and 1967.

Automatisms Periods of automatic, often complex, behaviour may occur during the fit, but usually take place during the post-ictal phase (Liddell 1953). The only certain way of distinguishing ictal from post-ictal automatism is to record EEGs during such events.

Automatisms may be defined as: 'A state of clouding of consciousness which occurs during or immediately after a seizure and during which the individual retains control of posture and muscle tone but performs simple or complex movements and actions without being aware of what is happening' (Fenton 1972). Simple automatisms include lip smacking, chewing, swallowing and fiddling or fumbling with the hands. Complex automatisms consist of semipurposive action, such as undressing, drinking, washing, searching, wandering, running, speech or continuation of prior activity. Such complex stereotyped behaviour is well co-ordinated but inappropriate. Thus a patient during an automatism may make a journey to a pointless destination, may attempt to

cook a meal when none is required, may undress in public, urinate or go to bed. Such complicated behaviour patterns are often repeated from attack to attack in stereotyped form.

Automatisms are of brief duration and last under five minutes in more than 80% of cases (Knox 1968). Uncommonly, they may be of longer duration but, for practical purposes, never longer than an hour. Amnesia for the period of the automatism is usually complete. Aggression during automatism is very rare, apart from a tendency to resist physical interference, and even then dangerous behaviour is almost unknown (Knox 1968). Despite the increased prevalence of epilepsy amongst prisoners, the fits or what may follow them are rarely the cause of offence (Gunn & Fenton 1971).

Most automatisms are associated with epilepsy arising in the temporal lobe and it is estimated that about some 75% of those with temporal lobe epilepsy will have periods of automatism (Feindel & Penfield 1954). Such patients will often be able to recall the aura to their attack prior to the period of automatism. Automatism may arise with other forms of epilepsy, but is uncommon. Automatism as the only manifestation of epilepsy is rare, but can occur.

Special types of fits

Status epilepticus

By definition, status epilepticus consists of recurrent fits without recovery of consciousness between attacks, in contrast to serial fits where recurrent attacks occur frequently but consciousness is regained between episodes. True status epilepticus is a medical emergency, and requires urgent intensive treatment. Serial fits occurring very frequently may herald status, but do not carry the still serious conseqences of status. Nevertheless, serial fits must be controlled rapidly.

Grand mal status Repeated grand mal seizures without recovery of consciousness causes increasing pyrexia, anoxia, hypoglycaemia and other metabolic disturbance, tachycardia and hypotension, which combine to produce brain damage and death unless stopped quickly. Of considerable practical importance is the observation that, in experimental epilepsy, brain damage may occur even if the systemic manifestations are prevented by curarization (see Chapter 7). This indicates that repeated seizure discharge itself may damage the brain, perhaps by local metabolic change, so that even if the patient in status is maintained in good general condition, the continuing cerebral discharges may lead to cerebral necrosis and must be stopped. Even today, grand mal status epilepticus carries an appreciable mortality (10% or so) and an immeasurable morbidity (Table 5.6). Its management is detailed in Chapter 12.

Grand mal status may occur in about 3% of epileptics (Oxbury & Whitty 1971). It may be the first epileptic event in some patients or may be precipitated in a known epileptic by such events as: suddenly stopping anticonvulsant therapy, intercurrent illness, other drugs or alcoholic indulgence (Oxbury & Whitty 1971). Often, however, it occurs without apparent provocation. When grand mal status occurs as the initial episode, it is likely that a recognizable cause will be found. In children, this may be an inflammatory disease such as meningitis or encephalitis, hypoglycaemia, hypocalcaemia or other metabolic change, lead poisoning or the liver disease with encephalopathy known as Reye's syndrome (see Chapter 4 for further details). Most such causes may operate in adult life, but grand mal status as the initial event in an adult is often due to brain tumour, particularly one affecting the frontal lobe, and warrants full investigation (Oxbury & Whitty 1971). Other causes include hypertensive encephalopathy, cortical venous thrombosis or intracranial abscess formation.

Petit mal status Repeated petit mal attacks causing prolonged periods of confused uncooperative behaviour in children is more common than is generally appreciated (Bornstein et al 1956; Niedermeyer & Khalifeh 1965, Brett 1966). The physical appearance of such children often does not arouse a suspicion of epilepsy and the child may be accused of daydreaming or educational backwardness. However, disorientation, repetitive blinking, myoclonus and drooling are frequently seen, and EEG recording will show continuous or repetitive spike-wave activity. Such events, which may last for hours, days or even weeks, may be terminated by intravenous diazepam.

Temporal lobe status Repetitive temporal lobe seizures rarely may produce a prolonged period of automatic behaviour and amnesia, rather similar to petit mal status, and are associated with repetitive atypical spike-wave activity (Schwartz & Scott 1971, Escueta et al 1974). Such events may occur in adults as well as children, but are not common. Their distinction from postepileptic automatisms and other causes of the fugue or twilight state (see below) can only be made with confidence by EEG recording during the attack.

Focal motor status Repetitive continuous focal motor seizures may occur, usually in adults, particularly with acute structural damage due to trauma or vascular disease and less commonly with tumour. A particular form of repetitive focal motor fit is epilepsia partialis continua, which

Table 5.6 Causes and consequences of major status epilepticus in 86 adult patients (after Oxbury & Whitty 1971)

Cause	Number of patients	Number in whom status was initial event	Death in status	Death within follow-up
Tumour	19	10	4	15
Vascular	13	4	0	8
Infection	9	5	1	1
Post-traumatic*	4	1	0	0
Birth injury	4	0	0	3
Other	5	3	1	4
	54	23(43%)	6(11%)	31(57%)
No obvious cause	28	0	1	6
Previous epilepsy	4	1	0	0
Indefinite	32	1(3%)	1(3%)	6(19%)

* Ten other cases of status after severe head trauma were excluded

consists of focal repetitive muscle contractions, usually of the fingers and corner of the mouth, persisting for many days or weeks without loss of consciousness.

Reflex epilepsies

Reflex epilepsy describes fits, most commonly grand mal or focal, which are precipitated by a fixed and clearly recognized sensory stimulus. Although uncommon, reflex epilepsy is of considerable interest, for it gives one of the few clues as to what may trigger fits. A variety of sensory stimuli are recognized as causing reflex epilepsy.

Photosensitive epilepsy Fits provoked by repetitive flashing lights comprise the commonest form of reflex epilepsy. Nowadays the flickering television set is the usual stimulus (Charlton & Hoefer 1964, Binnie et al 1973) but, in a past era, driving down continental highways with their spaced trees lining the route and filtering the sun was a recognized hazard. Children may even learn to provoke their own fits by shaking their hand in front of their eyes while gazing at a light source (Ames 1971). Electroencephalography has harnessed photostimulation as a means of exposing abnormality in the EEG of susceptible subjects.

Auditory epilepsy Sudden noise may be a provocative factor in some patients, while certain music may repeatedly provoke an attack in others (musicogenic epilepsy) (Critchley 1937). We know of one patient whose grand mal seizures were initially provoked by certain types of classical orchestral and church music, who could be induced to have a fit by Beethoven's Fifth Symphony. Interestingly, with time the stimulus became less specific and, over the years, fits could be provoked simply by entering a church and next by thinking of a church scene. Such information suggests that the effective stimulus is not the music itself, at least in this patient, but the atmosphere and emotion it engenders (see below).

Reading epilepsy A very few patients learn that reading silently or aloud may provoke their fits (Bickford et al 1957). In this case it may not be the content of the text that provokes the fit: reading nonsense may produce the attack and other stimuli, such as playing chess or reading a music score, have also been reported as effective. It may be that the passage of vision across the page causes a pattern-evoked visual response, which in susceptible subjects is sufficient to generate epileptic discharges, or that mental decoding of visual information may be responsible. Specific mental effort may be capable of provoking a fit, as in the case of arithmetic epilepsy (Ingvar & Nyman 1962).

Tactile epilepsy Touch or muscle stretch may provoke seizure discharge in some patients, usually focal motor epilepsy or a peculiar form of myoclonus, in which a tap to the hand or foot may cause a spike discharge in the cortex followed by a myoclonic jerk of the stimulated limb, of half the body or of the whole body. Whether this is considered a true epileptic event or not can be argued, but such patients commonly have other forms of fits.

Paroxysmal dystonic seizures An even more debatable epileptic phenomenon is that of paroxysmal involuntary movements. A number of entities have been described, including paroxysmal choreoathetosis, in which tonic spasm, on occasion with superimposed dystonic movements, suddenly affects the limbs of one side or sometimes both, without loss of consciousness, and continues for minutes on end (Lance 1963, Stevens 1966). Such attacks may occur daily without known provocation and the illness may be clearly inherited as an autosomal dominant trait.

In other patients, such dystonic seizures may be provoked by movement (Lishman et al 1962). Sudden action, such as rising from a chair, running or stepping off a kerb, may cause the explosive onset of focal or generalized dystonic writhing movements of limbs or trunk such as are seen in torsion dystonia. Consciousness is not lost, but the patient may fall to the ground. Recovery occurs abruptly within a few minutes. Such seizures may be associated with a sensory aura, but are not usually inherited.

In both conditions, consciousness is preserved, the EEG is not abnormal and other types of fits are most unusual. In these respects such dystonic seizures differ from conventional views of epilepsy due to cerebral cortical discharge, but there seems no reason why they should not be examples of striatal or basal ganglia epilepsy, particularly as they frequently respond to antiepileptic medication.

Other precipitants of seizures

One of the outstanding problems in epilepsy is what triggers a seizure. Mention has already been made of the rare reflex epilepsies and we are aware of many other precipitating factors. However, by far the majority of fits occur without apparent cause; what triggers them is a mystery. It is always useful to enquire closely for any precipitatory cause of fits, for such a discovery may enable the patient to avoid specific dangerous circumstances and learn to control his own seizure pattern to some extent. In addition, some patients may only have fits under certain circumstances and, in this case, there is room for latitude in applying the label 'epilepsy' with its consequent social and financial restrictions.

Fever That a pyrexia may trigger fits in childhood is commonplace and poses a particular problem (see Chapter 4). Fever may also trigger fits in patients who have spontaneous seizures, and the differentiation in early life of banal febrile fits from true epilepsy sometimes triggered by fever, is important for prognosis and management.

Nocturnal seizures Many patients have grand mal seizures only at night or during daytime sleep or drowsiness (Gibberd & Bateson 1974). Sleep enhances epileptic discharges in the EEG and may produce abnormality when daytime recordings while alert are quite normal. Sleep induced by barbiturates is thus used as a provocative test in EEG evaluation of epilepsy, particularly in suspected temporal lobe fits where the resting EEG may be normal.

Menstrual epilepsy and pregnancy The incidence of catamenial exacerbation of fits has varied considerably in different series but has been reported in up to 63% of women (Ansell & Clarke 1956). Cyclical seizures in women unrelated to menstruation have also been documented (Bandler et al 1957). Although it has long been suspected that premenstrual water retention may be a factor, there is no firm evidence for this. There is, however, experimental evidence that oestrogens may reduce seizure threshold. It is of interest, therefore, that Backström (1976), who studied

seven women in detail, found increased tonic-clonic seizures associated with higher oestrogen levels and that Laidlaw (1956) reported a decrease in seizure frequency during the luteal phase.

The effect of pregnancy (and the contraceptive pill) on seizure frequency is unpredictable. Fits may increase, especially in the puerperium, and the risk of toxaemic fits is greater. Indeed, fits appearing during mild toxaemia may be the first indication of recurrent seizures in later life. However, in some patients, fits decrease during pregnancy, particularly in the first trimester. Epilepsy by itself is neither an indication for advice against procreation nor for termination of pregnancy. Such decisions are based more on genetic risks and the ability to discharge the responsibility of parenthood, and are for the patient to make after medical counselling.

The risk of increasing fits by concurrent use of the contraceptive pill does not seem to be great. Indeed, some patients' epilepsy may be improved. One can only discover by trial and we would usually not advise against this form of contraception if it is best suited. However, there is evidence that the contraceptive effect of the pill may fail in the drug-treated epileptic patient (see Chapter 15).

While on the subject of pregnancy, mention must be made of the fact that children of epileptic mothers appear to have a greater than normal risk of bearing a deformed child (Lowe 1973). The risk is not excessive, perhaps 5% against 2% in the normal population. Although fits themselves, by such means as causing anoxia or trauma, may be responsible in part, the major antiepileptic drugs are known to be teratogenic in some animal species (see Chapter 15).

Stress-induced fits and emotional factors A variety of stress factors are known to provoke fits in susceptible individuals (Friis & Lund 1974). Lack of sleep is a common precipitant, often associated with alcohol (see below). Some patients quote physical or mental over-exertion, without emotional background or sleep loss. Intense fear, pain or rage may also be apparent precipitants, and even minor medical manipulations, such as blood-letting, dental treatment or ear syringing, may provoke a fit in a susceptible subject. In many patients with established recurrent seizures, the frequency of fits clearly waxes and wanes with the individual's life circumstances and emotional responses. Emotional stress precipitated fits in 21% of patients with temporal lobe epilepsy (Currie et al 1971). While it is difficult if not impossible, to separate the various potential triggers during a period of misfortune, there is no doubt that such patients' fit frequency is dictated by these events and their consequent effects on mood, happiness and stability. Such a situation may be self-generating, for more fits add to the problems. Some patients will clearly link their fits to their moods, but in such circumstances it is difficult to decide whether the emotional change causes the fits or is due to the same factor that provokes the fits (i.e. menstrual tension and menstrual epilepsy), or whether the emotional change is a prodromal symptom of the fits (i.e. due to increasing but, at that time, still subclinical seizure discharge).

Some patients may even be able to trigger (or to control) their own fits by thought or will. How they achieve this is usually unclear, but as a phenomenon it is of great interest for it may provide a clue as to how patients can be taught to prevent their own disability. Recent experiments with biofeedback of epileptic electrical discharge from the EEG to the patient have been overdramatized as a practical solution, but hold promise as a concept and is worth pursuing for what it tells us about epilepsy (see Chapter 10). Patients who can trigger their own fits, be it by use of a recognized reflex stimulus or by an effort of will, pose particular problems of management since they may learn to use their attacks to manipulate their circumstances. Other patients may feign seizures (hystero-epilepsy is a description not entirely discredited) for the same reasons, often without conscious appreciation of what they are doing. Such patients, often young women, frequently occupy much time and heart-searching in both neurologists and psychiatrists (see Chapter 10 and below).

Drug-induced fits Many drugs are known to provoke fits in susceptible individuals (Dallos & Heathfield 1969, Lancet 1972), including phenothiazines, tricyclic antidepressants, monoamine oxidase inhibitors and isoniazid. Particularly common in this regard is alcohol, often inextricably combined with fatigue, lack of food, and physical and emotional exertion (the hang over fit).

Fits on withdrawal of drugs are well known. Alcohol- and barbiturate-withdrawal fits are common. The risks of status epilepticus developing on sudden withdrawal of antiepileptic drugs has already been commented upon. It is important to emphasize at this point that perhaps the most common cause of recurrence of seizures in epileptic patients is poor compliance with antiepileptic drug therapy, with ensuing withdrawal seizures. Failure to recognize this fact commonly leads to unnecessary polytherapy (Shorvon et al 1978) (see Chapter 12).

In this context, the effect of other drugs on antiepileptic metabolism should be mentioned. Many drugs are now known to interact with antiepileptic drugs, either to increase or decrease their metabolism (see Chapter 12) and fits may be provoked by administration of a drug that lowers blood antiepileptic drug levels.

A practical problem arises when a patient develops an intercurrent illness requiring treatment with a drug known either to provoke fits itself or to interfere with antiepileptic drug activity. Such a situation commonly occurs in patients who develop psychotic illness, either schizophreniform or depressive. Both neuroleptics and antidepressants may cause fits in susceptible individuals but, in practice, if they are required to treat the psychotic illness they generally have to be used. Extra seizures may be prevented by attention to blood levels and by adjustment of medication. In fact, the use of such drugs only infrequently causes major problems in management.

SYMPTOMS BETWEEN FITS

A fit is a signal of a cerebral epileptic discharge but, between attacks, such discharges may continue to be recorded in the EEG without apparent clinical phenomena. An unanswered question in epilepsy is how far do such subclinical seizure discharges cause interictal behavioural phenomena? Undoubtedly there is an increased incidence of psychiatric disability amongst those with epilepsy, particularly in patients with temporal lobe or other focal fits. About a quarter of those with psychomotor attacks in this series had a history of psychiatric disorder or aggression (Table 5.7). Of interest is the observation that a definite cause could be found in only about 25% of these 666 patients with temporal lobe seizures (Table 5.8).

Community surveys in unselected populations have confirmed an increased incidence of psychological disturbance in epileptic patients (Pond & Bidwell 1960, Rutter et al 1960, Gudmundsson 1966). Rutter et al (1960) showed that children with epilepsy had two to three times more psychopathology than children with other chronic physical disorders not involving the brain. Some studies have suggested a particular association between personality and psychiatric disorders and temporal lobe epilepsy, but the evidence is by no means conclusive (Reynolds 1983). Schizophrenic-like psychoses are rare but have aroused great interest, together with a number of conflicting theories, because of the possible implications for the study of schizophrenia (Slater & Beard 1963, Reynolds 1968, Davison & Bagley 1970, Koella & Trimble 1983). Understandably, much more common are depression and anxiety, but these have been little studied (Betts 1981, Robertson & Trimble 1983). The association of epilepsy and decline in intellectual function has been commented on for centuries (Temkin 1971) and Lennox (1942) showed that the longer the history of epilepsy the higher the incidence of impaired intellectual skills. The mechanisms involved in this, as in the other interictal personality disorders referred to above and discussed in detail in Chapter 11, have received little investigation and are poorly understood (Brown & Reynolds 1981). Possible factors are illustrated in Table 5.9. Previously it has proved difficult to separate the relative influence of subclinical seizure activity, brain damage, genetic factors, psychosocial influences and chronic drug therapy. However, with the recent development of more sophisticated techniques for monitoring these different factors some progress has been made (Pond 1981, Reynolds 1981).

Table 5.7 Incidence of psychiatric disability in 666 patients with temporal lobe epilepsy (after Currie et al 1971) (percentage)

Nil	56
Anxious	19
Depressed	11
Aggressive	7
Obsessive	6
Florid-psychiatric disturbance	
Hysteria	3
Schizophreniform psychosis	2
Anxiety neurosis	0.5
Severe depressive illness	0.5

Table 5.8 Causes of temporal lobe epilepsy in 666 patients (after Currie et al 1971) (percentage)

Tumour	9.5
Glioma	7
Meningioma	1
Others	1.5
Trauma	7
Vascular disease[a]	2
Angioma	2
Abscess	1
Meningitis	0.5
Others	3
	25

[a] In another 9% there was a history of cerebrovascular diseases which could have been relevant

Table 5.9 Possible causes of interictal intellectual, personality and psychiatric disturbances

Subclinical seizure activity
Brain damage (causing or resulting from seizures)
Genetic
Psychological
Social
Chronic antiepileptic drug therapy

The management and rehabilitation of such problems require expertise from many disciplines, time and care; this provides one of the strongest reasons for the setting up of special centres for those who suffer from epilepsy.

THE DIFFERENTIAL DIAGNOSIS OF SEIZURES

The wide spectrum of clinical phenomena occurring in fits leads to a variety of diagnostic problems (Parsonage 1973, Gibberd 1973). The most important diagnostic features of seizures are their abrupt onset, brief duration and rapid recovery, and recurring stereotyped symptoms. The best insurance policy against error is a careful complete history and a full interview with a witness to the attacks.

Episodes of unconsciousness

Syncope (Gilliatt 1974)

A simple faint due to a transient drop in blood pressure accompanied by vagal-mediated slowing of the pulse, pallor and sweating nearly always occurs while standing (reflex syncope). Loss of consciousness is gradual, with a premonitory sinking feeling and dizziness; falling is less abrupt than in fits, with rare risk of injury, and incontinence is very uncommon. Recovery with nausea and sweating is usually rapid after the horizontal position is achieved. Such simple syncopal episodes are sometimes called vaso-vagal attacks, but Gowers originally used this term to describe a much more prolonged and complex syndrome. Syncope occurs in adolescents and young adults of either sex, under typically provocative circumstances, such as: rapidly rising from a chair; prolonged periods of standing in uncomfortable circumstances; as a result of pain or emotional shock; and in hot, stuffy surroundings. Similar postural syncopal attacks also occur in the elderly, with some degree of loss of healthy vascular activity, and in patients with autonomic neuropathy such as may occur in diabetes (Sharpey-Schafer & Taylor 1960) and many other neurological conditions (Johnson et al 1966, Bannister 1971). Such postural syncope is the result of a failure of baroreceptor reflexes to adjust heart rate and vascular resistance to abrupt changes in posture (areflexic syncope) (Brigden et al 1950; Barraclough & Sharpey-Schafer 1963).

Syncope can also be provoked by: prolonged coughing (cough syncope) (Sharpey-Schafer 1953) where a sustained Valsalva's manoeuvre prevents venous return to the heart; during micturition in middle-aged or elderly prostatic men who strain to pass water (micturition syncope) (Proudfit & Forteza 1959); and in pregnant women in whom syncope can occur lying flat perhaps by an effect of the gravid uterus on the inferior vena cava (Brigden et al 1950).

A complication that may arise as a consequence of a syncopal attack is that, if the patient's head cannot fall below his or her heart, he or she may go on to have a typical grand mal fit due to cerebral anoxia. Circumstances in which this may occur include a faint on the stairs or in the lavatory, when the head gets caught on the pan. Careful history taking will usually indicate that such fits were provoked by syncope and that the patient is not suffering from epilepsy.

Cardiac dysrhythmias

Abrupt cessation of heart beat or change in rhythm may provoke a faint due to a critical drop in cerebral perfusion. Such Stokes-Adams attacks may be particularly difficult to diagnose unless one has the good fortune to be present at the time. They should be suspected in the elderly with vascular disease, those with known heart disease and those with heart block. The diagnosis is critical in view of the need for cardiac pacemaking to prevent sudden death in selected cases. Clinical clues include an abrupt onset with pallor followed by flushing but, as with simple syncope, a Stokes-Adams attack may cause a fit and the diagnosis can be very difficult. Indeed, some such patients may go on to develop typical spontaneous fits, often temporal lobe in character, perhaps as a result of cerebral ischaemic damage. Whenever such a cardiac dysrhythmia is suspected, a prolonged ECG must be done despite normality between attacks.

Another cardiovascular cause for loss of consciousness is the carotid-sinus syndrome (Hutchinson & Stock 1960), in which elderly patients develop abrupt loss of consciousness on head movement or neck pressure, which may provoke alarming, but transient, cardiac standstill. Patients with aortic stenosis are also prone to sudden episodes of loss of consciousness.

These cardiac causes for syncope are common, especially in the elderly, and are so often difficult to separate from epilepsy that neurologists hold them in great respect.

Other vascular causes

Loss of awareness, amnesia and even unconsciousness may occur in basilar artery migraine in younger patients (Bickerstaff 1961a, b) and vertebrobasilar ischaemic episodes in the more elderly. Similar episodes also occur in the rare situations of rheumatoid arthritis or traumatic damage to the cervical spine. In all these situations loss of consciousness is due to brainstem ischaemia and is therefore usually prefaced by other distinctive symptoms such as diplopia, dysarthria, ataxia and perioral paraesthesiae, while visual symptoms may arise from posterior cerebral ischaemia and headache with or after the attack is common.

Brief loss of consciousness probably does not occur in simple transient ischaemic episodes in carotid territory, but rarely such patients are apparently amnesic for a portion of such an attack, particularly if it involves the dominant hemisphere.

The narcoleptic syndrome

The tetrad of daytime sleep attacks, cataplexy or collapse with emotion, sleep paralysis and hypnagogic hallucinations (Parkes & Marsden 1974) is not usually confused with epilepsy, but has been regarded as a form of seizure disorder. However, other types of fits do not occur, the EEG shows no epileptic activity, and antiepileptic drugs are of no therapeutic value. Confusion may arise on occasion, as when a child falls asleep in class or at table, or when an adult drops off while at the wheel of a car. Cataplexy may be confused with epileptic drop attacks (as may the relatively common but banal drop attacks that occur in middle-aged women for no known reason). However, consciousness is preserved in such events.

Others

Breath-holding attacks in childhood (and masturbation episodes) may be confused with fits. Mention must also be made of the occasional patient with Menière's disease who loses consciousness during an episode of vertigo.

Nocturnal fits (Gibberd & Bateson 1974) may be confused with nightmares or night-terrors. The latter are most common in childhood but can occur in adults. A scream calls the parent who finds the child sitting with staring eyes, recovery is rapid when the child is woken. In adults, nocturnal attacks are usually fits and attacks occurring on waking are also nearly always epileptic.

Hypoglycaemia may cause diagnostic confusion, for it may present with states of altered consciousness and may itself provoke fits. However, clouding of consciousness in hypoglycaemia is gradual and is prefaced by symptoms of sympathetic overactivity, such as faintness, hunger, dryness of the mouth, sweating, fullness of the throat, palpitations and tremor. Such symptoms develop over many minutes, often under characteristic circumstances, such as after a heavy meal in those prone to reactive hypoglycaemia or in those with one of the varieties of dumping syndromes that may follow gastric surgery.

Transient focal cerebral events

Focal fits may be confused with episodes of transient cerebral ischaemia, which in early life may be due to migraine and in later life to embolic or, more rarely, flow disturbance in carotid territory. In such cases, short-lived episodes of paraesthesiae or motor weakness may resemble focal sensory or motor fits, but can usually be distinguished by their longer duration (usually 10 minutes or more), lack of march of events and, in the case of motor phenomena, paralysis rather than tonic or clonic movements. Similarly, the visual symptoms of migraine may be confused with focal fits arising in the occipital lobe, but again last five to 30 minutes or so.

A complication arises when, as sometimes happens, a focal stroke generates focal epilepsy at the onset, but the clinical sequence of events and focal neurological aftermath usually point to the correct diagnosis.

Psychiatric events mimicking epilepsy

While the topic is dealt with at length in Chapter 11, it poses such difficult problems that we will spend some time on it here.

A number of psychiatric syndromes may mimic fits, particularly those of temporal lobe origin. This is not surprising, for many of the symptoms of a temporal lobe attack are those of panic or emotional change, both of which occur as primary events in psychiatrically disturbed patients.

Hyperventilation

Often the result of anxiety, hyperventilation produces symptoms that themselves become the focus of further anxiety. This syndrome is frequently misdiagnosed or dismissed as 'psychological' which only compounds the patients anxieties. The syndrome may mimic neurological, cardiac or gastrointestinal disease. The neurological symptoms may include giddiness or lightheadedness, paraesthesiae, visual disturbance, headache, tremor, ataxia, tinnitus, inability to concentrate and loss of consciousness (Perkin & Joseph 1986). Not infrequently, sensory and motor symptoms may be unilateral, more often left sided (Blau et al 1983). Especially when such unilateral symptoms are combined with autonomic symptoms (such as epigastric discomfort or palpitations) or mood change, a mistaken diagnosis of temporal lobe epilepsy may be entertained.

Panic attacks

The panic attack of a phobic anxiety may closely resemble a temporal lobe seizure (Harper & Roth 1962), with abdominal discomfort often rising into the throat with a choking feeling, fear, autonomic symptoms, sometimes syncope and even micturition in terror. Often, however, the story of the attack is not quite right, consciousness is not disturbed, the event is clearly precipitated by circumstances and is unduly prolonged. There usually is evidence of the underlying phobic anxiety state between attacks on formal psychiatric examination. However, it is often extraordinarily difficult to decide between panic attacks and temporal lobe fits. In these circumstances an EEG may be requested and may show abnormality, but in our experience this is best ignored as far as treatment is concerned. Personal error has been towards calling such attacks epilepsy rather than the other way round. If a therapeutic trial is instigated, a sequence of events follows over many months during which increasing doses of a variety of antiepileptics prove totally ineffective. There is little to be lost by admitting ignorance and deliberately avoiding a diagnosis of epilepsy and antiepileptic therapy. If you are wrong, sooner or later true fits will occur and clinch the matter.

Psychopathic rage outbursts

Outbursts of rage and violence are sometimes suspected of being epileptic, particularly by the law and courts. This question arises when some degree of amnesia is claimed and/or when an EEG is carried out and reveals some minor abnormality. There is less difficulty in distinguishing such events from true epilepsy than is the case with panic attacks. The outburst is usually provoked by external circumstances and a prior motive may be apparent: events during the attack are directed towards an identifiable aim, amnesia is often patchy and no obvious epileptic phenomenon is reported or seen. In such cases, an abnormal EEG is best ignored for true structured violent attack is almost unknown in epilepsy, apart from the tendency to resent and react vigorously to interference during periods of automatic behaviour (see below). Even in these latter circumstances, violence or aggression is poorly directed towards a goal or carried out in a purposeless fashion. However, on occasion, an apparently motiveless crime or attack may be committed for which amnesia is claimed, and in these cases it can be impossible to say with complete conviction that such an event could not be epileptic in origin, although the balance of evidence suggests that this is unlikely to be the case (Walker 1961, Fenton & Udin 1965).

Feigned seizures

Sometimes attacks are seen which clinically resemble epileptic fits, but which are not accompanied by an electrical disturbance in the brain. Whether the patient knowingly feigns such an attack or does so subconsciously is often impossible to discern and often is immaterial. Such attacks may be a signal of psychiatric illness requiring help (see Chapter 11).

Difficulty arises, firstly, because when one has no more than a secondhand account of such events it can be well-nigh impossible to distinguish them from true epilepsy; secondly, because many patients with such attacks also suffer from true fits. In such a situation, to observe a feigned fit on one occasion or to establish a normal EEG during such an episode, does not necessarily mean that all attacks are feigned. It is only by careful and prolonged observation that a balance of evidence may point to such a conclusion, but often with some doubt.

Attacks which are not epileptic can usually be distinguished from true convulsions if witnessed and often are suspected on history. The event occurs to attract attention, i.e. in front of an audience. Attacks at night, alone or in dangerous circumstances are rarely 'hysterical'. The movements in an 'hysterical' convulsion are spectacular and purposeful, without the typical tonic-clonic sequences of a grand mal fit. They are intensified by restraint and mollified by inattention. Consciousness is often preserved and amnesia is frequently patchy. A subject who speaks is not having a major fit. The tendon jerks, blink, corneal and eyelash reflexes are preserved and the plantar responses remain flexor. Incontinence, tongue biting and trauma rarely occur.

Many such patients feign fits because they have epilepsy and know about it, others because they have organic neurological disease and have seen fits. 'Hysterical seizures' occur more commonly than not in patients with organic disease. Again a 'therapeutic trial' of antiepileptic drugs is often doomed to failure in such patients and may itself cause added difficulty by causing drug-toxicity or drug-withdrawal fits. When such a diagnosis is suspected it is often best to admit such patients into units specializing in the management of the problem, where prolonged observation, group therapy, psychiatric treatment and rehabilitation may break what may become a vicious and intractable problem.

Twilight or fugue states

Prolonged periods of altered behaviour with clouding of consciousness or amnesia may be suspected of being epileptic in origin, since a variety of seizure phenomena may induce such a state (see above). Ictal automatisms are brief, lasting a few minutes, but post-ictal automatisms, when frank electrical discharge has ceased in the brain, may last longer. Usually awareness returns and behaviour reverts to normal within minutes, but uncommonly it persists for up to an hour. During such periods of automatic behaviour the patient may undertake complex semipurposive acts, for which he or she is subsequently totally amnesic. An initial aura of a temporal lobe fit may be recalled, but often is not. Similar prolonged periods of semipurposive behaviour with subsequent amnesia may occur during petit mal status or temporal lobe status, in which case an EEG during the episode will reveal the seizure discharges in progress.

Other causes of prolonged fugue are hypoglycaemia, alcoholic intoxication and drugs (Fenton 1972). Stroke and cerebral tumour may cause a prolonged amnesia syndrome and the syndrome of transient global amnesia (Fischer & Adams 1964) is well established.

However, despite the large number of known organic causes for a fugue, many are of psychiatric origin in the form of prolonged loss of memory commonly described in fiction or the press. Provoking circumstances, psychiatric illness and gain can often be identified in such patients. If doubt exists, it is usually best to avoid a label of epilepsy in these circumstances.

Table 5.10 shows the diagnosis established in 31 cases of transient amnesia referred to a group of neurologists over a five-year period (Heathfield et al 1973).

Table 5.10 Causes of transient loss of memory in 31 patients (after Heathfield et al 1973)

Transient global amnesia	19
With associated cerebrovascular disease	9
With no cerebrovascular disease	10
Epilepsy	6
Migraine	1
Temporal lobe encephalitis	2
Psychogenic	3

THE ETIOLOGY OF SEIZURES

The purpose and validity of separating primary or idiopathic epilepsy from symptomatic epilepsy is therapeutic. In the latter we can determine an accepted cause, in the former we cannot. It is likely that many so-called idiopathic epilepsies will become symptomatic as our knowledge advances. The practical aim of this division is to dissect out possible known causes of fits that may be amenable to treatment.

The known causes of fits vary with the age at which they start (Table 5.11). The range of genetic, metabolic, structural and inflammatory causes in infancy and childhood is discussed in detail in Chapter 4. Suffice it to point out that infancy is the time when birth injury, congenital defects, metabolic aberration and infection commonly occur. Between the ages of about 3 and 8 months, the syndrome of infantile spasms presents, while from about 6 months to 5 years is the time of febrile fits. Primary epilepsy usually starts after the age of 3 and is then the commonest form of epilepsy. Throughout adult life structural brain damage dominates the list, in particular brain tumours in early and middle adult life and vascular disease in later years. Head trauma causes fits throughout life.

In this section we propose to discuss in more detail the most common causes of fits in adult life,

Table 5.11 Causes of epilepsy presenting at different ages

Neonatal (first month)
    Birth injury – anoxia or haemorrhage
    Congenital abnormalities
    Metabolic disorders – hypoglycaemia, hypocalcaemia etc
    Meningitis and other infection

Infancy (1–6 months)
    As above
    Infantile spasms

Early childhood (6 months to 3 years)
    Febrile fits
    Birth injury
    Infection
    Trauma
    Poisons and metabolic defects
    Cerebral degenerations

Childhood and adolescence
    Idiopathic or primary epilepsy
    Birth injury
    Trauma
    Infection
    Cerebral degenerations

Early adult life
    Trauma
    Tumour
    Idiopathic or primary epilepsy
    Birth injury
    Infection
    Cerebral degenerations

Late adult life
    Vascular disease
    Trauma
    Tumour
    Cerebral degenerations

Table 5.12 Rarer causes of seizures

Neurological diseases	*Systemic diseases*
Lipid storage diseases	Pulmonary insufficiency
Leucodystrophies	Anoxia
Demyelinating diseases	Hypocalcaemia
Spinocerebellar degenerations	Hypoglycaemia
Tuberous sclerosis	Pyridoxine deficiency
Sturge-Weber syndrome	Amino acid abnormalities
Cysticercosis	Water intoxication
Arteriovenous malformation	Renal failure
Subdural haematoma	Liver failure
Syphilis	Reye's syndrome
	Addison's disease
	Acute intermittent porphyria
	Drug withdrawal
	Drug intoxication
	Lead and other poisoning

namely head injury, brain tumour, cerebral abscess and vascular disease, and to finish with a brief comment on the significance of Ammon's horn sclerosis as a cause of fits. Many other neurological and systemic diseases may be associated with fits (Table 5.12), but are beyond the scope of this chapter. In passing, it is of practical importance to note that multiple sclerosis may cause fits, particularly focal fits (Matthews 1962).

Post-traumatic epilepsy

The reviewer of the literature on post-traumatic epilepsy is confronted by a bewildering array of statistics. However, if due allowance is made for the many factors which influence both the nature and the study of this subject, then a reasonably coherent picture can be constructed. Much of the literature is based on studies of military casualties. American studies stretch from the Civil War through to the Korean and Vietnam Wars, and much European experience is based on the two World Wars (Caveness et al 1979). This can be contrasted with studies of civilian injuries, notably the extensive investigations of Jennett (1962, 1975, 1982). The risk of post-traumatic epilepsy will vary according to the definitions of epilepsy and head injury adopted and the type of population studied.

With regard to epilepsy, there is general agreement that *early* seizures, i.e. within the first week of a head injury, should be distinguished from *late* seizures as they frequently imply a different prognosis. Partial seizures clearly related to the site of the cerebral injury should be distinguished from other partial seizures or generalized seizures. A past or family history of epilepsy, as well as the expected risk of epilepsy in the population under study, should all be taken into consideration.

Head injuries will vary according to whether they are military or civilian, missile or non-missile, open or closed; whether there is a skull fracture, depressed or otherwise, intracranial haemorrhage or wound infection; and according to the duration of unconsciousness or post-traumatic amnesia.

Populations will vary according to whether they are military or civilian, community based or selected, adult or children. Selective factors may include the type of military campaign and the medical facilities for assessment; the severity of head injuries included, the individual practice of a neurosurgeon or the admitting policy for head injuries at the hospital(s) at which he is based. Finally the data may be influenced by whether it is retrospective or prospective, and by the duration of follow up.

Community study

The most unselected civilian study of the magnitude and duration of the risk of post-traumatic epilepsy is the community based investigation of Annegers et al (1980). These authors identified on the records-linkage system of the Mayo Clinic from 1935 to 1974 a cohort of 2747 patients with head injuries from the residents of Olmstead County, Minnesota. The patients were followed for 25 176 person-years. The minimal clinical criterion for eligibility for inclusion in the study was loss of consciousness due to brain injury, post-traumatic amnesia or evidence of skull fracture. Patients were excluded if they died within one month of the injury, had epilepsy before the injury or another head injury before the identifying head injury, or if they came to medical attention as a result of sequelae of the injury rather than the injury itself, e.g. headaches. The head injuries were classified as:

1. Severe, i.e. brain contusion, intracerebral or intracranial haematoma, or 24 hours of unconsciousness or amnesia
2. moderate, i.e. skull fracture or 30 minutes to 24 hours of unconsciousness or amnesia
3. mild, i.e. briefer unconsciousness or amnesia

The overall risk of early seizures (i.e. within the first week) was 2.1%. This was greater in children (2.8%) than adults (1.8%). In severe head injuries the risk rose to 30.5% in children and 10.3% in adults. For *late* seizures the risk in patients with severe injuries was 7.1% at 1 year and 11.5% at 5 years. For moderate injuries the corresponding figures were 0.7% and 1.6%, and for mild injuries 0.1% and 0.6%. The incidence of seizures after mild head injuries was not significantly greater than in the general population. Overall, the risk of late seizures was 3.6 greater than the expected risk. However, this relative risk was 12.7 in the first year, 4.4 in the next 4 years and thereafter 1.4. In contrast to early seizures, the risk for adults was greater than for children. In children there was no relationship between early and late seizures. In adults a relationship between early and late seizures existed but only in the moderate and severe injuries.

Early seizures

These are defined as seizures in the first week (Jennett 1975). In non-missile and missile head injuries, seizures are much more common in the first week than in any subsequent week (Jennet 1982). In half the cases of early epilepsy, the first seizure occurs within 24 hours of injury, and in half of these it is in the first hour. More than 50% of early seizures are focal, at least in onset, and 75% of these are focal motor attacks. Approximately 33% of cases have only a single seizure, but 40% have status, which is more common under the age of 5.

In contrast to the early seizure risk of 2.1% in the community study of Annegers et al (1980), the risk for patients admitted to hospital under the care of neurosurgeons is about 5% (Jennett 1982). However, this figure will vary according to the severity of the head injuries and the admitting policy of the neurosurgical unit. Early epilepsy is more common in patients with intracranial haematoma, depressed skull fracture, prolonged post-traumatic amnesia and in young children. In Scottish neurosurgical units, which accept less than 5% of all head injured patients admitted to hospital, the risk of early epilespy is 13%.

Recurrence of epilepsy is much less common after seizures in the first week than when attacks occur later, and this is especially true of children. However, the occurrence of early seizures does increase the overall risk of later epilepsy by about fourfold, compared with no early attacks, and this is more likely to occur in adults with moderate or severe injuries.

Late post-traumatic epilepsy

This is defined as seizures beginning after the first week of a head injury. As for early epilepsy the risk will vary considerably with the nature and severity of the head injury and the admitting policy of the neurosurgical or other unit, whether military or civilian. According to Jennett (1982)

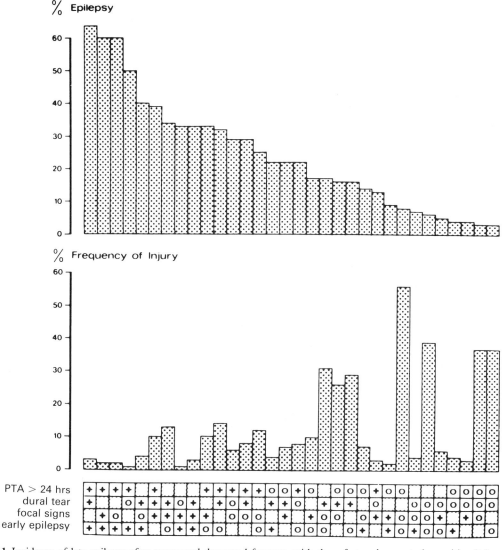

Fig. 5.1 Incidence of late epilepsy after compound depressed fracture, with three factors known to be positive (+) or negative (0) (from Jennett 1982)

the three dominant prognostic factors are the presence of intracranial haematoma, depressed fracture and early epilepsy. The overall incidence in Britain for all hospital admissions where many mildly injured patients are admitted for 24–48 hours is about 3%, For neurosurgical units with a selective admission policy the figure may rise to 16%; for certain severe injuries with several adverse prognostic factors the incidence may rise as high as 60%.

In a civilian neurosurgical population Jennett (1982) has shown how the risk may be calculated in patients with depressed fracture, according to the presence or absence of other prognostic factors, i.e. early epilepsy, focal neurological signs, dural tear or post-traumatic amnesia of more than 24 hours (Fig. 5.1). It is important to stress that the risk of late epilepsy in patients *without* depressed fracture or intracranial haematoma is less than 2%, even when post-traumatic amnesia exceeds 24 hours, unless there has been one early seizure. Civilian and military studies also suggest that genetic predisposition plays some role in the development of post-traumatic epilepsy as, in several series, a family history of epilepsy was more frequently obtained in the epileptic group (Evans 1962, Caveness et al 1979). Improvements in the medical and surgical management of head injuries throughout this century do not appear to

have altered the risk of post-traumatic epilepsy (Caveness et al 1979).

The onset of post-traumatic epilepsy occurs within the first year in some 50–60% of those patients who develop seizures; by 2 years in approximately 85% (e.g. Fig. 5.2). Thereafter the cumulative probability of occurrence is much less with most of the remainder of cases appearing within 5 years. As pointed out by Annegers et al (1980), thereafter the overall risk does not seem to exceed the normal risk in the population. However, in individual cases where the character of the seizures suggest a clear relationship to the site of the cerebral injury, some doubt will remain.

Prolonged follow-up of head injured patients suggests that there is a natural remission rate for some patients with post-traumatic epilepsy, perhaps irrespective of antiepileptic therapy (Earl Walker & Erculei 1970, Caveness et al 1979). Thus, as new cases of post-traumatic epilepsy are appearing, others are going into remission. In one series with prolonged follow-up for at least 15 years, approximately 50% had had no seizures for at least 5 years, approximately 25% were experiencing between 1 and 6 major or 'minor' seizures per year and the other quarter more than 6 seizures per year (Earl Walker & Erculei 1970). The EEG appears to be of little value either in

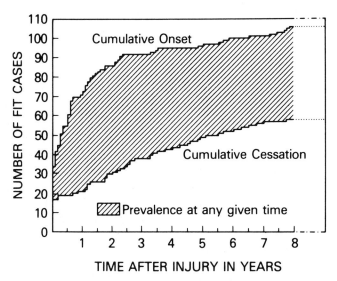

Fig. 5.2 Curves for cumulative onset and cumulative cessation. This graph represents the cases of epilepsy in the Korean campaign (109 cases) as a single group with a common time of injury. The shaded area indicates the number of active seizure cases at any given time after injury. (from Caveness et al 1979)

predicting the occurrence of post-traumatic epilepsy or its subsequent prognosis.

Brain tumour and epilepsy

Brain tumour has gained a notorious reputation as a cause of late-onset epilepsy, because it may be treatable (Parker 1930, Penfield et al 1940). In fact, brain tumours are responsible for late-onset epilepsy in only about 10% or so of all cases (Sheehan 1958, Raynor et al 1959; Hyllested & Pakkenberg 1963; Juul-Jensen 1964a). The incidence of tumour rises steeply in the case of focal fits, where a figure of 30–40% is more appropriate (Raynor et al 1959; Sumi & Teasdall 1963). However, the incidence in focal temporal lobe fits is not that high, about 15% or so (Currie et al 1971) (Table 5.8). In general, these figures are supported by recent studies with the CT scanner in epilepsy (vide infra).

Tumours most likely to cause fits are those affecting the cerebral cortex, and there seems to be an inverse relationship between the malignancy of the tumour and its propensity to cause fits. Meningiomas and benign gliomas characteristically cause seizures, while malignant gliomas do so less frequently. The incidence of fits with different sorts of tumours is in the order of 67% in meningiomas, 70% in astrocytomas and 37% in malignant gliomas (Penfield et al 1940) (Table 5.13). Secondary deposits usually from lung or breast, are also a relatively common cause of symptomatic fits.

Fits are most common with tumours of the fronto-parietal region and very rare with lesions in thalamus, basal ganglia or parapituitary area (Williams 1965) (Table 5.14).

Tumour as a cause of fits in childhood is uncommon, partly because most childhood tumours arise in non-epileptogenic areas, such as the cerebellum, brainstem and diencephalon, also because so many other types of epilepsy appear in childhood.

In general, in about 40% of those with fits due to tumour, the fits are the presenting symptom (Penfield & Jasper 1954). The interval between the onset of fits due to tumour and other symptoms varies considerably. At one extreme is the occurrence of fits almost simultaneously with a

Table 5.13 Incidence of seizures due to different tumours (after Penfield & Jasper 1954)

Number of cases	Tumour types	Presenting with fits %
64	Astrocytoma	70
13	Oligodendroglioma	92
103	Malignant glioma	37
63	Meningioma	67
19	Metastasis	47
32	Pituitary adenoma	9
(54)	(Abscess)	(50)
(71)	(Subdural haematoma)	(25)

Table 5.14 Incidence of seizures due to tumours at different sites (after Penfield & Jasper 1954)

Number of cases	Site	Percentage with fits %
115	Frontal	53
74	Parietal	68
94	Temporal	48
28	Occipital	32
20	Third ventricle	32
12	Thalamic	8
49	Pituitary region	8
Average incidence approximately 37%		

(After Penfield & Jasper, 1954)

rapidly progressive focal deficit due to a malignant glioma. At the other extreme, it may be 20 or more years after the onset of epilepsy before the responsible benign tumour becomes apparent (Douglas 1971). It is partly for this reason that neurological clinics review regularly those with late-onset epilepsy in whom tumour may be the cause in about 1 in 10 of such cases.

The question as to why some patients with brain tumours develop fits and some do not is not fully answered. It is established that successful removal of tumour often does not stop the fits it causes. The presumption must be that it is the remaining damaged cerebral cortex that is the source of the fits, but the nature of the structural, functional or biochemical lesion responsible is not known.

Brain abscess

Epilepsy is a common complication of supratentorial brain abscess. In a recent study (Legg et al

1973), 72% of 70 survivors of supratentorial abscess developed fits in the next month to 15 years, most commonly in the first year after treatment. Generalized grand mal occurred in about 50% of patients, who could have more than one sort of attack. Temporal lobe epilepsy developed in a third, and other focal fits in another third of cases. Prophylactic antiepileptic drugs are recommended.

Vascular disease and seizures

Cerebrovascular disease is an even more common cause of adult-onset fits than tumour (Dodge et al 1954). It may be responsible for about 10–20% of cases of adult-onset epilepsy, but after the age of 50 the figure is 50% or more (Juul-Jensen 1964a, White et al 1953; Woodcock & Cosgrove 1964). It is estimated that as many as 25% of those with cortical infarcts will have fits (Richardson & Dodge 1954), although the incidence of fits in non-embolic cerebral infarcts in general is about 8% (Louis & McDowell 1967). About 50% of such patients develop their fits within a week of the stroke, and early post-stroke epilepsy seems more prone to spontaneous remission than that developing later.

Mention must also be made of arteriovenous malformations, which cause fits, usually focal in nature, in about 40% of cases (Paterson & McKissock 1956). The combination of fits, migraine-like headache, and subarachnoid haemorrhage is diagnostic, as is the tell-tale cranial bruit.

Fits are said to be rare in subdural haematoma, but certainly occur.

Ammon's horn sclerosis

This theme will be discussed and developed in detail elsewhere (Chapter 7), but its practical importance and potential significance are such as to merit further mention.

Stated simply, the facts are that this pathological lesion, Ammon's horn sclerosis, is found commonly in the brain of patients with epilepsy of no apparent cause (Sano & Malamud 1953, Corsellis 1957, Margerison & Corsellis 1966) and in temporal lobes removed for successful surgical treatment of temporal lobe epilepsy (Falconer et al 1964). It is commonly unilateral (Margerison & Corsellis 1966).

Is this lesion therefore the source of such epilepsy (Falconer 1974)? Some of the patients give a history of a prior episode of prolonged seizures in childhood, often febrile status epilepticus. Experimental status epilepticus in primates can produce a histological mimic of Ammon's horn sclerosis, often unilaterally (see Chapter 7). The question arises as to whether Ammon's horn sclerosis is caused by severe febrile fits in childhood and then itself ripens into an epileptogenic scar producing recurrent seizures in adult life. The hypothesis can be, and is, under experimental test. If established, the consequences are profound. The genetic background to idiopathic epilepsy may be that of febrile fits, which may cause Ammon's horn sclerosis and thereby generate recurrent seizures in a proportion of cases. Aggressive treatment of febrile fits may have the greatest prophylactic impact on epilepsy (along with measures to prevent head injury). Methods will have to be devised to detect the lesion in those with idiopathic epilepsy during life, in order to assess its contribution to the incidence of unexplained fits and to assess a wider range of cases for possible surgical treatment. These, and many other notions, stem from the development of the hypothesis that Ammon's horn sclerosis, itself a product of epilepsy, may be a frequent cause of fits – a cause open both to prevention and to treatment.

In assessing the possible role of Ammon's horn sclerosis as a cause of temporal lobe epilepsy, the series of Currie et al (1971) is of interest. A definite cause for the temporal lobe fits was found in 25% of the 666 patients they studied (Table 5.8). An additional 5% of cases gave a history of seizures in infancy and another 7% had had an isolated fit in childhood; 7% gave a history of an abnormal birth and 11% had a family history of fits. These data do not suggest that fits in childhood are a common cause of temporal lobe epilepsy in later life, but the information was obtained retrospectively.

THE INVESTIGATION OF SEIZURES

Having recognized epilepsy, the next step in management is to decide how far to press investigation for a cause. This will depend initially on the age of the patient. Epilepsy in infants under the age of 6 months is of sinister import, as it may well be in those aged under a year. By this time, however, febrile fits are beginning to appear and require less intensive investigation. The management of children with epilepsy is described in detail in Chapter 4 and the following discussion will be confined to epilepsy in late childhood, adolescence and adult life.

Needless to say, the initial step in investigating a case of epilepsy is a full history, from both the patient and a witness, and clinical examination. A number of causes of epilepsy may be recognized in the clinic. A history of birth trauma or anoxia combined with body asymmetry, such as a small thumb or toe, will point to cerebral damage in early life. Tuberous sclerosis and Sturge-Weber syndrome will be indicated by the appropriate skin lesions and congenital or genetically determined syndromes may be suggested by a characteristic facial appearance or other signs as, for example, in mongolism. General medical examination may point to an extracerebral cause of the fits. Usually, however, no such clues are apparent. In such cases examination is directly concerned with detecting signs of focal brain damage or raised intracranial pressure. Particularly important are the optic discs and visual fields. The only sign of a temporal lobe lesion may be an upper quadrantanopia. Mild facial weakness, a hemiparesis and extensor plantar response point to a unilateral hemisphere lesion.

Initial out-patient investigation

At this stage simple tests will be required. In older children and adolescents these should include a plain X-ray of the skull and an EEG. Now that multiple haematological and biochemical investigation is automated, we arrange routinely for a full blood count, WR or TPHA test for syphilis and SMA 12 biochemical screen, which includes a blood sugar and calcium. We have rarely detected a cause for fits by such blood tests, but do them to provide baselines for subsequent monitoring of chronic effects of drug treatment (see Chapter 12). In adults presenting with epilepsy for the first time, an X-ray of the chest is also necessary and may reveal a bronchogenic carcinoma. In those who have spent time abroad, an X-ray of the thighs may show the calcified cysts of cysticercosis, but this illness is very rare today in the UK.

The value of routine X-rays of the skull and EEGs require further comment.

Skull X-ray

Although a routine skull X-ray is usually normal in patients with fits, it can establish the diagnosis of the cause: evidence of raised intracranial pressure, intracranial calcifications in tumour or other lesions and the bony changes of meningiomas may be detected; pineal shift may indicate a mass lesion. Asymmetry, particularly of the middle cranial fossae, may point to a longstanding atrophic lesion. Such information is crucial in a few cases and a skull X-ray should be undertaken in every epileptic patient.

EEG

Much has been written about the EEG in epilepsy. While it provides much interesting information for the doctor, it is not always helpful to the patient. During political unrest or staff shortage it is possible to practice the neurology of epilepsy without EEG data. However, there are certain circumstances in which it is invaluable, provided it is realized that an abnormal EEG does not indicate epilepsy, which is a clinical diagnosis; a number of normal people have abnormal EEGs; and that a normal EEG does not exclude epilepsy (or brain tumour).

The situations in which an EEG may be expected to help are:

1. In the definitive diagnosis of petit mal, in particular to separate petit mal and temporal lobe fits as a cause of absence attacks

2. To detect a focal as against a generalized abnormality
3. To examine certain regions of the brain that are clinically silent, for example, the frontal lobes.

An initial EEG may also prove of value later in the course of the illness as, for example, in assessing the possibility of drug toxicity, the progression of the underlying disease or in deciding when to stop treatment in those rendered free of fits. In these situations comparison of a recent EEG with the initial record may provide helpful information. The same is true when surgery for epilepsy is contemplated. Since one cannot be sure of the future of any individual with epilepsy, we regard an initial EEG examination as essential in each case of epilepsy.

Telemetric EEG monitoring

Regrettably, the routine EEG is almost always an *interictal* recording, with all the limitations that this implies. The desirability and advantages of recording the EEG during a seizure are obvious and if this can be combined with video monitoring of the clinical seizure so much the better. There have been considerable technological developments in the last decade, reviewed by Binnie (1983) and discussed in Chapter 8, which have resulted in increasingly sophisticated in-patient and out-patient (ambulatory) monitoring. These expensive techniques are not generally available but are now essential in any special department or centre concerned with the more difficult and intractable diagnostic and management problems, including evaluation for surgery.

CT scan

Two other harmless means of detecting intracranial structural abnormality now are available: radio-isotope brain scanning and computerized axial tomography (the CT scan). Both can be undertaken as an out-patient and neither involve more than an intravenous injection. Of the two, the CT scan is the most powerful, for it detects not only tumours, but also atrophy, ventricular dilatation, infarct and haemorrhage.

Gastaut (1976) has summarized the CT scan findings in 1702 epileptic patients of all ages combined from seven research groups. Overall, the proportion of abnormalities varied from 34% to 51%, with a mean of 46%. Amongst these lesions, 56% were atrophic in character. Tumours were found in 8% to 11% of patients, but this figure rose to 16% in patients over the age of 20 and to 22% when only partial seizures were considered.

The relationship of CT abnormalities to various seizure types is well illustrated by the study of Gastaut & Gastaut (1976) in 401 patients (Table 5.15). A clear difference emerges between the relatively low incidence (11%) associated with primary generalized seizures and the much higher proportion (60–80%) in relation to other seizure types. These authors also estimate that CT scan detects 20% more cerebral lesions than the combination of long-established techniques (skull X-ray, EEG, angiography etc).

Table 5.15 Abnormalities on CT scan in relation to seizure type (after Gastaut & Gastaut 1976) (percentage)

Seizure type	Abnormal CT
Primary generalized	11
Secondary generalized	61
Partial	63
Lennox-Gastaut syndrome	60
Post-traumatic	80

These observations have been extended by Yang et al (1979) who scanned 256 children between the ages of a few days and 17 years (mean 4 years). Abnormalities of the type classified in Table 5.16 were seen overall in 33%. They were able to distinguish a low yield group (2.5% to 8%) with

Table 5.16 Classification of CT findings (after Yang et al 1979)

1. Normal
2. Bilateral atrophy
   Central atrophy: dilation of lateral ventricles only
   Cortical atrophy: dilation of sulci, lateral ventricles normal
   Generalized atrophy: dilation of sulci and lateral ventricles
3. Focal findings
   Atrophy
   Hemiatrophy
   Porencephalic cysts
   Tumours
4. Other findings
   Pathological calcifications
   Congenital abnormalities of brain
   Evidence of intracranial bleeding

idiopathic generalized seizures on normal neurological examination or focal slowing (but not focal spiking) on the EEG (Table 5.17). The highest incidence was seen in neonatal seizures or a history of seizures beginning in the neonatal period. Amongst children with mental retardation, 45% had abnormal scans. Only 2% of the series had tumours. If the initial scan was normal, contrast enhancement added no new information but, if it was initially abnormal, enhancement gave more information in 10%.

It is possible that the above studies overestimate the prevalence of CT scan abnormalities, since they are mostly based on retrospective analyses from specialized centres. Prospective studies in less selected or community based populations are needed. However, Ramirez-Lassepas et al (1984) found CT abnormalities in 37% of 148 adult neurological out-patients scanned within 30 days of their first seizure. They noted that structural lesions were detected in 15% of patients with normal neurological examination and in 22% of patients with generalized EEG disturbances, emphasizing that CT scanning should not be confined to those with focal neurological or EEG abnormalities. On the other hand Young et al (1982), who found CT abnormalities in 24% of 220 adult patients with newly diagnosed (including single seizures) or *established* epilepsy, recommend that CT scanning should be reserved for patients with focal seizures, focal signs or focal EEG abnormalities. In fact, in both studies CT abnormalities were found in only 6% of patients who had no focal features of any sort. MacArdle et al (1987) found a lower yield of only 16% abnormal scans in a series of 124 children with newly diagnosed untreated epilepsy. There were significant associations between scan abnormality and (a) focal seizures, (b) neurological abnormality, (c) mental handicap and (d) poor response to antiepileptic therapy.

Although Gastaut & Gastaut (1976) argue that all epileptic patients should have a CT scan, the economics of the UK would preclude such a course. It is clear, in any case, that patients with primary generalized seizures and with no focal signs on clinical or EEG examination would yield few abnormalities. Although the remote possibility of a tumour may exist in a few such patients it is questionable whether early detection is a great advantage when the only symptoms are seizures. This view would be reversed if it were clear that early surgery for brain tumours carried little risk and was necessary. At present, there is little to be lost in observing the low yield group regularly in out-patients. If, however, the seizures fail to respond to optimum therapy with one or two drugs there is an increased likelihood of a detectable brain lesion on the scan (Dellaportas et al 1982, MacArdle et al 1987).

Table 5.17 CT scan findings in children with epilepsy (after Yang et al 1979) (percentage)

Low Yield Groups	Abnormal CT
1. Idiopathic generalized seizure	8
2. Neurologic examination and EEG normal (neonates not included)	5
3. Generalized seizure (idiopathic or known aetiology with normal neurologic examination and normal EEG)	2.5

High Yield Group	Abnormal CT
1. Partial seizures with elementary symptomatology	52
2. Partial seizures with complex symptomatology	30
3. Generalized seizures (known aetiology)	40
4. Neonates with seizures	68
5. Children whose seizures began as neonates	100
6. Focal slowing on EEG	63
7. Abnormal neurologic examination	64

Psychometry

Standard psychometric techniques may be useful in documenting the more gross evidence of intellectual decline and/or focal brain lesions in children or adults with mental retardation, dementia or apparent focal cognitive abnormality. They have proved disappointing in assessing the more subtle but undoubted adverse effects of subclinical seizure activity and chronic drug therapy. Utilizing specially developed verbal and non-verbal short-term memory tasks presented in the form of television games Aarts et al (1984) have reported that 50% of 46 patients with 'subclinical' generalized or focal EEG discharges exhibited transient cognitive impairment (TCI). A significant association was found between left-sided discharges and errors in verbal tasks and right-sided discharges with impairment of non-verbal tasks. Newly developed batteries of tasks, some of them computer based, have demonstrated that most antiepileptic drugs have subtle effects on cognitive function in epileptic patients, especially involving attention, concentration, memory and psychomotor speed (Trimble & Reynolds 1984). Differences between the individual drugs in these adverse effects are important in the choice of drug for seizure control.

In-patient investigation

From what has already been said, it is apparent that only those with symptoms or signs (clinical or EEG) of a focal cerebral lesion require further investigation. Even this simple summary requires amplification.

Focal epilepsy in childhood is unlikely to be due to tumour, for reasons stated earlier. Focal fits in children are therefore not in themselves an indication to submit the child to full neuroradiological study. However, it is here that the simple CT scan may be expected to help and may delineate the common atrophic lesion causing the focal fits.

Temporal lobe epilepsy in adults is also much less likely to be due to tumour than other focal fits. Unless it is accompanied by signs or EEG evidence suggesting tumour, it is not in itself an indication for full neuroradiological study. Again, CT scanning will help in this problem.

Focal fits in the elderly are just as likely to be due to vascular disease as tumour and, again, the decision as to whether to carry out the more dangerous neuroradiological studies may be resolved by CT scanning.

However, if there is strong indication from clinical, EEG and skull X-ray information that a tumour may be present, CT scanning, and sometimes carotid angiography and air encephalography, will be required. Angiography also is necessary to delineate fully arteriovenous malformations (although epilepsy alone is not always an indication for surgery). However, such full neuroradiological investigation is now only occasionally required in those presenting with epilepsy, and the type and timing of the tests required is usually fairly obvious from the clinical and EEG picture. In passing, it must also be mentioned that lumbar puncture gives no useful information in a case of epilepsy alone. Lumbar puncture is only required when it is suspected that the epilepsy may be due to infection or encephalitis, to stroke or other intracranial vascular disaster.

Special problems

Provoked seizures

Some patients may only have an occasional seizure under specific circumstances as, for example, while watching television or while taking a provocative drug. Such people are best not labelled as having epilepsy and, if the provoking factor can be avoided, further investigation and therapy may not be required. In these cases, judgement has to be exercised on each individual case as to what course to pursue.

Status epilepticus

Status in a known person with epilepsy requires no further investigation other than that required to manage the problem, or unless otherwise indicated.

Patients whose epilepsy presents as status epilepticus require full investigation; in children directed particularly towards infection or metabolic error as the cause, and in adults towards tumour.

Twilight states

An EEG is the only way to distinguish petit mal or psychomotor status and may help to point to metabolic or structural causes. Blood sugar estimation is mandatory and other metabolic tests may be required if the situation still exists when the patient is seen. If, however, the patient has fully recovered by the time he or she reaches medical care, only simple out-patient tests are warranted.

Todd's paralysis

A post-ictal paralysis lasting more than 48 hours justifies full investigation, the extent of which will depend on the age of the patient and the likely cause.

Assessment for surgery This topic is discussed fully in Chapter 13. Extensive clinical, psychometric, EEG and neuroradiological investigation is required to establish suitability for surgery.

PROGNOSIS OF EPILEPSY

Our views of the prognosis of patients with epilepsy have been gradually changing in the last few years in the light of new evidence from studies of epilepsy in the community and at the time of first referral to hospital. The older pessimistic concepts of prognosis based on studies of chronic patients in institutions or attending hospital clinics are giving way to a more optimistic perspective.

The traditional and rather gloomy view of prognosis was summarized in the detailed, authoritative and classic review by Rodin in 1968 which spanned the period from Gowers, who first applied a statistical approach to prognosis in the late nineteenth century, to Rodin's own valuable studies. Rodin concluded:

1. Although different types of epilepsy have a varying outcome the overall prognosis is unsatisfactory with only approximately one-third of patients achieving even a two-year remission. This is illustrated by several studies summarized in Table 5.18.
2. Patients with tonic-clonic seizures have a better prognosis than those with psychomotor seizures or mixed seizure types.
3. An abnormal neurological or mental status examination or low IQ adversely affect prognosis.

Table 5.18 Studies of the prognosis for seizure control in patients with epilepsy

Study	Number of patients	Seizure-free Period Years	Seizure-Free %
Alström (1950)	897	3	22
Strobos (1959)	228	2	38
Kiørboe (1960)	130	4	32
Trolle (1960)	799	2	37
Juul-Jensen (1963)	969	2	32
Rodin (1968)	90	2	32

4. The more seizures that have occurred and the longer the illness, the worse the prognosis.
5. The interictal EEG is of limited value for prognosis.
6. The longer patients are followed up the more likely is relapse to occur.

Thus, 80% of all patients with epilepsy are likely to have a chronic seizure disorder. Although the latter does not rule out short-term remissions it emphasizes that epilepsy should be regarded as a chronic condition with remissions and exacerbations.

Rodin recognized that his review was based almost wholly on studies of chronic patients in institutions or those attending special out-patient clinics. At the time of his review there had been no systematic study of epilepsy at its onset. As Shorvon (1984) has pointed out, a weakness or source of misunderstanding in the studies reviewed was a failure to appreciate certain temporal aspects of the development of epilepsy, arising from the retrospective, cross-sectional nature of the investigations which were based on heterogeneous populations of patients with a very variable duration of epilepsy. Another interesting feature of the period reviewed by Rodin, which covered about a century, was the introduction and use of many major antiepileptic drugs of undoubted efficacy, from bromides, through barbiturates, to hydantoins, succinamides and carbamazepine, most of which are still widely prescribed today. Rodin questioned whether there had been any improvement in overall prognosis throughout this time. A factor which was and still is missing in our understanding of prognosis is any information about the prognosis of *untreated* epilepsy. Practice was, and still is perhaps, influenced by Gowers (1881) view that the spontaneous cessation of the disease was an event too rare to be reasonably anticipated in any given case. But even Gowers may have been misled by the selection of patients who consulted him.

In the last decade new studies have focused attention on epilepsy as viewed and followed from the *onset* of the disorder, both in the community and the hospital clinic. This has given some new insights into the temporal evolution of epilepsy, dispelled some of the gloomier views of prognosis based on studies of chronic patients and raised some fundamental questions about the nature and treatment of epilepsy.

Community-based studies

Prevalence rates for active epilepsy vary from 4 to 10 per 1000, depending on definitions and methods of study (see Chapter 2). If, however, up to 5% of the general population may at some time experience a non-febrile seizure, as has been reported (Research Committee of the College of General Practitioners 1960) this suggests that most of them do *not* go on to develop *chronic* epilepsy. In keeping with this, Goodridge & Shorvon (1983) found that the *lifetime* prevalence of epilepsy (excluding febrile convulsions but including single seizures) was 20.2 per 1000, whereas the point prevalence of continuing 'active' epilepsy was 5.3 per 1000.

Annegers et al (1979) retrospectively reviewed the prognosis of 475 patients who had an initial diagnosis of epilepsy recorded on the Mayo Clinic record linkage system between 1935 and 1974. In contrast to Rodin's (1968) observations, remission rates improved with duration of follow up; and in those followed for 20 years as many as 70% were in five-year remission and 50% had withdrawn medication. Goodridge & Shorvon (1983) reviewed the general practice records of a population of

6000 in Kent, UK: of 122 patients identified with at least one non-febrile seizure (82% of which were recurrent) 69% were in four-year remission at 15 years of follow-up.

The much more favourable picture of prognosis emerging from these retrospective community-based studies is also supported by recent hospital-based studies of patients followed *prospectively* from the onset of their epilepsy.

Prospective studies of newly diagnosed epilepsy

Elwes et al (1984) studied 106 newly diagnosed, previously untreated patients referred to the neurology department of a district general hospital with at least two tonic-clonic and/or partial seizures in a year. They were treated with carefully monitored monotherapy (phenytoin or carbamazepine) and followed for up to 8 years, median 66 months. The overall prognosis was very good (Fig. 5.3): 73% were in 1-year remission by 2 years of follow up, 88% by 4 years and 92% by 8 years; the pattern for 2-year remission rates was similar with 73% in 2-year remission by 4 years of follow up and 82% by 8 years. As in the studies of chronic patients, reviewed by Rodin (1968), it was found that adverse prognostic factors included partial seizures as compared with tonic-clonic seizures, and the presence of additional neuro-

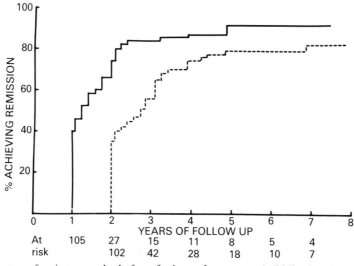

Fig. 5.3 Actuarial percentage of patients completely free of seizures for one year (solid lines) and two years (broken lines) (from Elwes et al 1984)

logical, psychiatric or social handicaps. Only 21 patients (20%) failed to enter remission on monotherapy and all went on to develop chronic epilepsy. When compared to 21 carefully matched patients, from the original 106 who had achieved remission, the two most important factors to emerge in relation to failure of treatment were poor compliance and the presence of a cerebral lesion (Chesterman et al 1987).

Shorvon (1984) has summarized other recent studies of prospective treatment with monotherapy in newly diagnosed patients followed for up to two years at the most. As shown in Table 5.19, between 58% and 95% were reported to be 'completely controlled'. So far, such studies have been reported in adolescent or adult patients, but similar results are beginning to emerge in children (McGowan et al 1983).

At the present time there is no evidence that for a particular seizure type any one major antiepileptic drug is superior in efficacy to any other, although careful comparative trials are rather few and further large scale studies are needed (Elwes et al 1984, Chadwick & Turnbull 1985, Mattson et al 1985).

Early treatment: the prevention of chronic epilepsy

The newer view of prognosis emerging from the recent community-based and hospital-based studies of epilepsy from its onset is that, for most patients, the outlook for seizure control is very good with high remission rates in the early years of treatment. However, about a quarter of patients do go on to develop chronic epilepsy. The first two years of treatment appear to be crucial as the pattern of chronicity is usually established within this period (Shorvon & Reynolds 1982, Elwes et al 1984). It is also apparent that the treatment of chronic epilepsy is very difficult. In most Western countries special multidisciplinary centres or clinics have been established, or at least recommended, for such patients, who accordingly utilize most of the limited resources available for epilepsy.

Two important questions therefore are: how does epilepsy become chronic? And, can chronic epilepsy be prevented? (Reynolds et al 1983). In the retrospective studies of chronic patients (Rodin 1968) and the prospective studies of newly diagnosed patients (Elwes et al 1984), it has been noted that the longer seizures continue the more difficult they are to control. This is illustrated in Figure 5.4 which shows that if seizures are still continuing after two years of treatment the subsequent one-year remission rate is halved. One view of such patients who fail to go into remission and therefore develop chronic epilepsy is that they have more 'severe' epilepsy; so 'severe' that they are unresponsive to currently available drugs. An alternative view is that there is a process of escalation of epilepsy by a mechanism which was proposed by Gowers (1881) a century ago, who commented:

When one attack has occurred, whether in apparent consequence of an immediate excitant or not, others usually follow without any immediate traceable cause. The effect of a convulsion on the nerve centres is such as to render the occurrence of another more easy, to intensify the predisposition that already exists. Thus every fit may be said to be, in part, the result of those which have preceded it, the cause of those which follow it.

Table 5.19 Seizure control in newly diagnosed patients on monotherapy (from Shorvon 1984)

Author	Number	Drugs used	Follow up on treatment	Complete control %
Cork Group*	47	DPH, Pb, CBZ Sul.	2–22 mns	81
Strandjord & Johannessen (1979)	24	CBZ	Mean 24 mns	83
Shakir et al (1981)	21	SVP, DPH	Mean 26 mns	95
Hakkarainen (1981)	100	DPH, CBZ	24 mns	67
Turnbull et al (1982)	88	SVP, DPH	< 12 mns	58

DPH = phenytoin; CBZ = carbamazepine; SVP = sodium valproate; Pb = phenobarbitone; Sul = sulthiame
* See Shorvon 1984

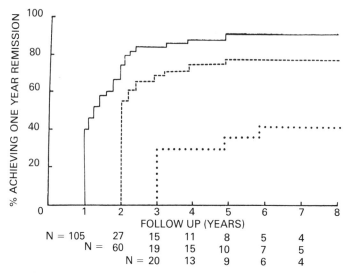

Fig. 5.4 Influence of duration of seizures on actuarial percentage of patients completely free of seizures for one year. Solid lines represent all patients from start of treatment, broken lines patients with seizures in the first year of follow-up, and dots patients with seizures in the first two years of follow-up (from Elwes et al 1984)

The implication of this hypothesis is that early effective treatment for epilepsy may prevent the later development of chronic epilepsy which is increasingly drug resistant (Reynolds et al 1983). It is notable that the main cause of failure of monotherapy in newly diagnosed epilepsy is poor compliance (Chesterman et al 1982) and this is clearly an area that can be improved upon (Reynolds 1985).

The natural history of untreated epilepsy

One difficulty in evaluating the results of treatment in epilepsy is the lack of data about the natural history of untreated epilepsy. For ethical reasons no one has compared drug treatment with placebo in newly referred, previously untreated patients. It is possible to obtain a brief retrospective view of natural history in such patients and this has been attempted by Elwes et al (1987) in 183 patients with two or more untreated tonic-clonic seizures in whom it was possible accurately to date the attacks. As shown in Table 5.20 there is a tendency for the inter-seizure interval to fall progressively in many, but not all, patients. This is in keeping with Gowers' hypothesis (above) and supports the view that early effective treatment may be important in preventing an increasingly intractable process of epilepsy (Reynolds et al

Table 5.20 Untreated tonic-clonic seizures median inter-seizure interval (weeks) (from Elwes et al 1986)

Number of seizures	2	3	4	5	All
Number of patients	101	53	18	11	183
Seizure 1–2	12	12	22	24	12
Seizure 2–3		8	16	4	8
Seizure 3–4			6	4	4
Seizure 4–5				3	3

1983, Shorvon & Reynolds 1986). Whether drug treatment increases the prospect of natural remission is unknown. That remission in epilepsy is not simply a matter of drug treatment is illustrated, for example, by the natural tendency to remission of petit mal or benign Rolandic epilepsy of childhood.

PROGNOSIS OF A SINGLE SEIZURE

As already noted, this is a common clinical problem. However studies of prognosis have appeared contradictory with several reporting low recurrence rates (Table 5.21). One reason for the differences in prognosis in published studies is the interval between the occurrence of the seizure and the time of first referral to a neurological or other clinic where such studies have been undertaken. There is likely to be a high recurrence rate in the weeks immediately after a first seizure, as was

Table 5.21 Studies of prognosis after first tonic-clonic seizure

Study	Number	Recurrence %	Mean (range) Follow-up (months)
Thomas (1959)	48	27	NK (42–102)
Johnson et al (1972)	77	64	36
Saunders & Marshall (1975)	39	33	26 (10–48)
Blom et al (1978)	74	56	36
Cleland et al (1981)	70	39	57 (36–120)
Hauser et al (1982)	244	27	22 (6–55)
Elwes et al (1985)	133	71	15 (6–36)

NK = not known

recognized by Gowers (1881). If several weeks elapse before referral to a clinic, many will already have developed epilepsy and therefore be excluded from studies of prognosis of a first seizure.

Elwes et al (1985) examined the prognosis for seizure recurrence in 133 patients who presented to their GP or Casualty Officer at a median of one day after a first ever tonic-clonic seizure. Seizures related to fever, alcohol, drugs or acute metabolic disturbance were excluded. None of the patients was treated. The cumulative probability of recurrence was 20% by 1 month, 28% by 2 months, 32% by 3 months, 46% by 6 months, 62% by 1 year and 71% by 3–4 years (Fig. 5.5). In a retrospective survey of lifetime general practice records of 6000 patients Goodridge & Shorvon (1983) also found that of those patients with seizures only 20% had a single attack. It is therefore apparent that, as described by Gowers (1881), epilepsy is likely to develop in the majority of patients after a single tonic-clonic seizure, where no obvious precipitating cause can be identified.

It appears to be the practice of most neurologists, at least in the UK, not to treat a single seizure (Reynolds 1985). If most go on to develop

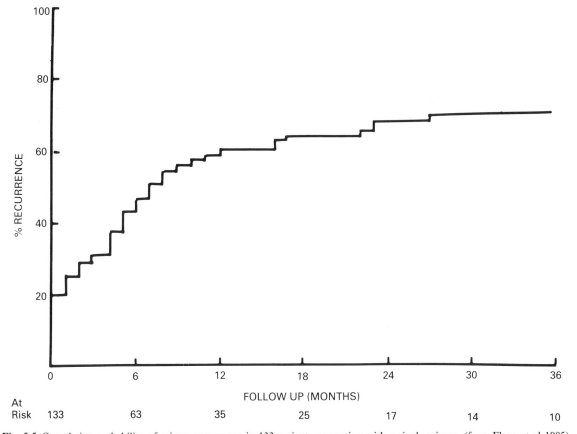

Fig. 5.5 Cumulative probability of seizure recurrence in 133 patients presenting with a single seizure. (from Elwes et al 1985)

epilepsy and early treatment is important, should more be treated? There has been no investigation of the value or otherwise of treating single seizures and such studies are clearly needed.

CONCLUSION

The information discussed in this chapter forms the background essential to the neurologist, or other physician, responsible for evaluating a new patient presenting with a history suggestive of epilepsy. Such initial evaluation, diagnosis and investigation, and therapeutic decision usually occupies no more than the first few months or so of a patient's epileptic life. It seems curious that the chapter stops here for, over the following 20 or more years, that patient and his or her doctor may have to engage in continual combat against fits and their consequences. The success or failure of that battle is one of the major tasks and pleasures of neurology.

The additional knowledge and experience required to help such patients deserves a chapter equally long, if not longer, than that already written. Such matters are dealt with elsewhere in this volume, but it is worth asking who should look after epileptic patients. There is no easy answer, for each section of the medical and social community has different fields of expertise to offer the patient. The general practitioner has the considerable benefit of knowing the patient as an individual, his or her family and life circumstances. Yet the GP must nearly always suffer from relative inexperience of the medical vagaries of the illness. With an incidence of about 1 in 200

of the population, the practitioner with an average list may have some 20 epileptics in his or her care at any one time. Many of these may not require the expertise of those with greater experience, but some undoubtedly do.

The neurologist may see as many as 200 or more new patients a year, and may have many hundreds of established epileptic patients attending the clinic. His or her experience becomes great, but time is limited. Unless the neurologist has a special interest in epilepsy, it is almost inevitable that such patients, after initial evaluation, will fall into the routine of a brief visit on increasingly rare occasions, often to be seen by a member of the junior staff. The neurologist, with his or her clinical neurophysiological and neuroradiological colleagues is best equipped to undertake the initial evaluation of patients suspected of epilepsy, and from experience can offer useful advice on specific topics in later years, particularly on treatment. But there are those who also require the help of psychiatrists and others such as social workers, industrial rehabilitation officers and lay organizations. For those requiring such help, the concept of centres for epilepsy has been advanced and in certain places instituted. Such centres should provide the full range of expertise required to help those patients with epilepsy whose problems exceed the capacity of their local services. This may not be a large proportion of all those with fits, but patients in this category undoubtedly benefit from such concentrated exposure to all possible therapeutic disciplines. The establishment and adequate continuing finance of such centres must improve the lot of those with the misfortune to suffer from epilepsy.

REFERENCES

Aarts J H P, Binnie C D, Smit A M, Wilkins A J 1984 Selective cognitive impairment during focal and generalized epileptiform EEG activity. Brain 107:293

Alström C H 1950 A study of epilepsy in its clinical, social and genetic aspects. Acta Psychiatrica et Neurologica Scandinavica 63 (Suppl):1

Ames F R 1971 'Self-induction' in photosensitive epilepsy. Brain 94:781

Annegers J F, Hauser W A, Elveback L R 1979 Remission of seizures and relapse in patients with epilepsy. Epilepsia 20: 729

Annegers J F, Grahow J D, Groover R V, Laws E R,

Elveback L R, Kurland L T 1980 Seizures after head trauma: a population study. Neurology 30:683

Ansell B, Blarke J 1956 The role of water retention in menstruating epileptics. Lancet ii:7232

Backstrom T 1976 Epileptic seizures in women related to plasma oestrogen and progesterone during the menstrual cycle. Acta Neurologica Scandinavica 54:321

Bandler B, Kaufmann I C, Dyken J W, Schleifer N, Shapiro L N 1957 Seizures and the menstrual cycle. American Journal of Psychiatry 113:704

Bannister R G 1971 Degeneration of the autonomic nervous system. Lancet 2:175

Barraclough M A, Sharpey-Schafer E P 1963 Hypotension from absent circulatory reflexes: Effect of alcohol, barbiturates, psychotherapeutic drugs, and other mechanisms. Lancet 1:1121

Behrman S & Wyke B D 1958 Vestibular seizures. Brain 81:529

Betts T A 1981 Depression, anxiety and epilepsy. In: Reynolds E H, Trimble M R(eds) Epilepsy and psychiatry. Raven Press, Edinburgh, pp 60–71

Bickerstaff E R 1961a Basilar artery migraine. Lancet 1:15

Bickerstaff E R 1961b Impairment of consciousness in migraine. Lancet 2:1057

Bickford R G, Whelan J L, Klass D W, Corbin K B 1957 Reading epilepsy. Transaction of the American Neurological Association 81:100

Bingley T 1958 Mental symptoms in temporal lobe epilepsy and temporal lobe gliomas. Acta Psychiatrica et Neurologica Scandinavica 33 (suppl 120): S1–S151

Binnie C D, Darby C E, Hindley A T 1973 Electroencephalographic changes in epileptics while viewing television. British Medical Journal 4:378

Binnie C D 1983 Telemetric EEG monitoring in epilepsy. In: Pedley T A, Meldrum B S. (eds) Recent advances in epilepsy. Churchill Livingstone, Edinburgh, pp 155–178

Blau J N, Wiles C M, Solomon F S 1983 Unilateral somatic symptoms due to hyperventilation. British Medical Journal 286:1108

Blom S, Heijbel J, Bergfors P G 1978 Incidence of epilepsy in children: a follow-up study three years after the first seizure. Epilepsia 19: 343–350

Blume W T, David R B, Gomez M R 1973 Generalized sharp and slow wave complexes. Association clinical features and long-term follow up. Brain 96:289

Bornstein M, Codden D, Song S 1956 Prolonged alterations in behaviour associated with a continuous electroencephalographic (spike and dome) abnormality. Neurology 6:444

Brett E M 1966 Minor epileptic status. Journal of Neurological Sciences 3:52

Brigden W, Howarth S, Sharpey-Schafer E P 1950 Postural changes in the peripheral blood-flow of normal subjects with observations on vasovagal fainting reactions as a result of tilting, the lordotic posture, pregnancy and spinal anaesthesia. Clinical Science 9:79

Caveness W F, Meirowsky A M, Rish B L et al 1979 The nature of posttraumatic epilepsy. Journal of Neurosurgery 50:545

Chadwick D, Turnbull D M 1985 The comparative efficacy of antiepileptic drugs for partial and tonic clonic seizures. Journal of Neurology, Neurosurgery and Psychiatry 48:1073

Charlton M H, Hoefer P F A 1964 Television and epilepsy. Archives of Neurology 11:239

Chen R C, Forster F M 1973 Cursive epilepsy and gelastic epilepsy. Neurology (Minneapolis) 23:1019

Chesterman P, Elwes R D C, Reynolds E H 1987 Failure of monotherapy in newly diagnosed epilepsy. In: Wolf P, Dam M, Janz D, Dreifuss F E (eds) Proceedings of the XVIth Epilepsy International Congress, Hamburg. Advances in Epileptology 16

Cleland P J, Mosquera I, Steward W P, Foster J B 1981 Prognosis of isolated seizures in adult life. British Medical Journal 283:1364

Cole M, Zangwill O L 1963 Déjà vu in temporal lobe

epilepsy. Journal of Neurology, Neurosurgery and Psychiatry 26:37

Corsellis J A N 1957 The incidence of Ammon's horn sclerosis. Brain 80:193

Critchley M 1937 Musicogenic epilepsy. Brain 60:13

Currie S, Heathfield K W G, Henson R A, Scott D F 1971 Clinical course and prognosis of temporal lobe epilepsy. A survey of 666 patients. Brain 94:173

Dalby M A 1969 Epilepsy and 3 per second spike and wave rhythms. Acta Neurologica Scandinavica 45 (suppl 40):1–183

Dallos V, Heathfield K (1969) Iatrogenic epilepsy due to antidepressant drugs. British Medical Journal 4:80

Daly D D 1958a Uncinate fits. Neurology 8:250

Daly D D 1958b Ictal affect. American Journal of Psychiatry 115:97

Daly D D, Mulder D W 1957 Gelastic epilepsy. Neurology 7:189

Davison K, Bagley C 1969 Schizophrenia-like psychoses associated with organic disorders of the nervous system. In: Current problems in psychiatry. British Journal of Psychiatry: Special Publication No 4

Dellaportas C I, Galbraith A W, Reynolds E H, Dawson J, Hoare R D

Dillon J D, Weiss G H 1979 The nature of posttraumatic epilepsy. Journal of Neurosurgery 50: 545–553

Dodge P R, Richardson E P Jr, Victor M 1954 Recurrent convulsive seizures as a sequel to cerebral infarction; a clinical and pathological study. Brain 77:610

Douglas D B 1971 Interval between first seizure and diagnosis of brain tumour. Diseases of the Nervous System 32:255

Druckman R, Chao D 1957 Laughter in epilepsy. Neurology 7:26

Earl Walker A, Erculei 1970 Post-traumatic epilepsy 15 years later. Epilepsia 11:17

Efron R 1961 Post-epileptic paralysis: theoretical critique and report of a case. Brain 84:381

Elwes R D C, Johnson A L, Shorvon S D, Reynolds E H 1984 The prognosis for seizure control in newly diagnosed epilepsy. New England Journal of Medicine 311:944

Elwes R D C, Chesterman P, Reynolds E H 1985 Prognosis after a first untreated tonic-clonic seizure. Lancet 2:752

Elwes R D C, Johnson A L, Reynolds E H 1987 The natural history of untreated epilepsy. To be published.

Escueta A V, Boxley J, Stubbs N, Waddell G, Wilson W A 1974 Prolonged twilight state and automatisms. Neurology 24:331

Evans J H 1962 Post-traumatic epilepsy. Neurology 12: 665–674

Falconer M A 1974 Mesial temporal sclerosis (Ammon's horn sclerosis) as a common cause of epilepsy. Lancet 2:767

Falconer M A, Serafetinides E A, Corsellis J A N 1964 Etiology and pathogenesis of temporal lobe epilepsy. Archives of Neurology 10: 233

Feindel W, Penfield W 1954 Localization of discharge in temporal lobe automatism. Archives of Neurology and Psychiatry 72:605

Fenton G W 1972 Epilepsy and automatisms. British Journal of Hospital Medicine 7:57

Fenton G W, Udwin E L 1965 Homocide, temporal lobe epilepsy and depression: a case report. British Journal of Psychiatry 111:304

Fischer C M, Adams R D 1964 Transient global amnesia.

Acta Neurological Scandinavica 40 (suppl 9): 1–83

Fox R H, Wilkins D C, Bell J A et al 1973 Spontaneous periodic hypothermia; diencephalic epilepsy. British Medical Journal 2:693

Friis M L, Lund M 1974 Stress convulsions. Archives of Neurology (Chicago) 31:155

Gastaut H 1969 Clinical and electroencephalographical classification of epileptic seizures. Epilepsia 10 (Suppl): S1–S28

Gastaut H 1976 Conclusions: Computerized trasnverse axial tomography in epilepsy. Epilepsia 17:337

Gastaut H, Gastaut J L 1976 Computerised transverse axial tomography in epilepsy. Epilepsia 17:325

Gastaut H, Aguglia U, Tinuper P 1986 Benign versive or circling epilepsy with bilateral 3-cps spike-and-wave discharges in late childhood. Annals of Neurology 19:301

Gibberd F 1966a The clinical features of petit mal. Acta Neurologica Scandinavica 42:176

Gibberd F 1966b the prognosis of petit mal. Brain 89:531

Gibberd F 1973 The diagnosis and investigation of epilepsy. British Journal of Hospital Medicine 9:152

Gibberd F B, Bateson M C 1974 Sleep epilepsy: its pattern and prognosis. British Medical Journal 2:403

Gibbs F A, Davies H, Lennox W G 1935 The electroencephalogram in epilepsy and in conditions of impaired consciousness. Archives of Neurology and Psychiatry 34:1133

Gibbs F A, Gibbs E L, Lennox W 1937 Epilepsy: a paroxysmal cerebral dysrhythmia. Brain 60:377

Gilliatt R W 1974 Syncope. Medicine 31:1823

Goodridge D M G, Shorvon S D 1983 Epileptic seizures in a population of 6000. 1. Demography, diagnosis and classification, and the role of the hospital services. 2. Treatment and prognosis. British Medical Journal 287:641

Gowers W R 1881 Epilepsy and other chronic convulsive diseases. Churchill, London

Gowers W R 1907 The borderland of epilepsy. Churchill, London

Gudmundsson G 1966 Epilepsy in Iceland. Acta Neurological Scandinavica suppl 25

Gumpert J, Hanisota P Upton A 1970 Gelastic epilepsy. Journal of Neurology, Neurosurgery and Psychiatry 33:479

Gunn T, Fenton G 1971 Epilepsy, automatism and crime. Lancet 1:1173

Hakkarainen H 1981 Carbamazepine and diphenylhydantoin as monotherapy or in combination in the treatment of adult epilepsy. Presented at the XIIIth Epilepsy International Symposium, Kyoto

Harper M, Roth M 1962 Temporal lobe epilepsy and the phobic anxiety-depersonalization syndrome. Part 1. A comparative study. Comprehensive Psychiatry 3:129

Hauser W A, Anderson V E, Lowenson R B, McRoberts S M 1982 Seizure recurrence after a first unprovoked seizure. New England Journal of Medicine 307: 522–528

Heathfield K W G, Croft P B, Swash M 1973 The syndrome of transient global amnesia. Brain 96:729

Hutchinson E C, Stock J P P 1960 The carotid-sinus syndrome. Lancet 2:445

Hyllested K, Pakkenberg H 1963 Prognosis in epilepsy of late onset. Neurology 13:641

Ingvar D H, Nyman G E 1962 Epilepticus arithmetices. A new psychologic trigger mechanism in a case of epilepsy. Neurology 12:282

Jackson J H 1873 On the anatomical, physiological, and pathological investigation of epilepsies. West Riding Lunatic Asylum Medical Reports 3:315

Jackson J H 1890 On convulsive seizures. British Medical Journal 1: 703–821

Jennett W B 1962 Epilepsy after blunt head injuries. Heinemann, London

Jennett W B 1975 Epilepsy after non-missile head injuries. 2nd edn. Heinemann, London

Jennett W B 1982 Post-traumatic epilepsy In: Laidlaw J, Richens A (eds) A textbook on epilepsy. 2nd edn. Churchill Livingstone, Edinburgh pp 146–154

Johnson L C, DeBolt W L, Long et al 1972 Diagnostic factors in adult males following initial seizures. Archives of Neurology 27:193

Johnson R H, Lee G de J, Oppenheimer D R, Spalding J M K 1966 Autonomic failure with orthostatic hypotension due to intermediolateral column degeneration. Quarerely Journal of Medicine 35:276

Juul-Jensen P 1963 Epilepsy: a clinical and social analysis of 1020 adult patients with epileptic seizures. Munksgaard, Copenhagen

Juul-Jensen P 1964 Epilepsy. A clinical and social analysis of 1020 adult patients with epileptic seizures. Acta Neurologica Scandinavica 40 (suppl 5): 1–285

Kiørboe E 1961 the prognosis of epilepsy. Acta Psychiatrica Neurologica Scandinavica 150 (suppl): 166–178

Koella W P, Trimble M R (eds) 1982 Advances in biological psychiatry Vol 8. Temporal lobe epilepsy, mania, and schizophrenia and the limbic system. Karger, Basle

Knox S J 1968 Epileptic automatism and violence. Medical Science and Law 8:96

Laidlaw J 1956 Catamenial epilepsy. Lancet ii 71:1235

Lance J W 1963 Sporadic and familial varieties of tonic seizures. Journal of Neurology, Neurosurgery and Psychiatry 26:51

Lancet 1972 Report from Boston Collaborative Drug Surveillance Program. Drug-induced convulsions. Lancet 2:677

Legg N J, Gupta P C, Scott D F 1973 Epilepsy following cerebral abscess. A clinical and EEG study of 70 patients. Brain 96:259

Lennox W G 1942 Brain injury, drugs and environment as causes of mental decay in epilepsy. American Journal of Psychiatry Suppl 18:201

Lennox W G 1945 The petit mal epilepsies. Their treatment with tridione. Journal of the American Medical Association 129:1069

Liddell D W 1953 Observations on epileptic automatism in a mental hospital population. Journal of Mental Science 99:732

Lishman W A, Symonds P, Whitty C W M, Willison R G 1962 Seizures induced by movement. Brain 85:93

Livingston S, Torres I, Pauli L L, Rider R V 1965 Petit mal epilepsy. Results of a prolonged follow-up study of 117 patients. Journal of the American Medical Association 194:227

Louis S, McDowell F 1967 Epileptic seizures in non-embolic cerebral infarction. Archives of Neurology 17:414

Lowe C R 1973 Congenital malformations among infants born to epileptic women. Lancet 1:9

MacArdle B M, Cox T C S, Binnie C D, Reynolds E H 1987 Computerized tomography (CT) scanning in newly diagnosed children with epilepsy. To be published

Macrae D 1954 Isolated fear: A temporal lobe aura. Neurology 4:497

Margerison J H, Corsellis J A N 1966 Epilepsy and the temporal lobes: A clinical electroencephalographic and neuropathological study of the brain in epilepsy, with particular reference to the temporal lobes. Brain 89:499

Matthews W B 1962 Epilepsy and disseminated sclerosis. Quarterly Journal of Medicine 31:141

Mattson R H, Cramer J A, Collins J F et al 1985 Comparison of carbamazepine, phenobarbital, phenytoin, and primidone in partial and secondarily generalized tonic-clonic seizures. New England Journal of Medicine 313:145

Maurice-Williams R M 1974 Micturition symptoms in frontal tumours. Journal of Neurology, Neurosurgery and Psychiatry 37:431

McGowan M E L, Neville B G R, ReynoldsE H 1983 Monotherapy in children with epilepsy. A preliminary report. In: Parsonage M, Grant R H E, Craig A G, Ward Jr A A (eds) Advances in epileptology. XIVth Epilepsy International Symposium. New York, Raven Press, p 283–290

Mullan S, Penfield W 1959 Illusions of comparative interpretation and emotion; production by epileptic discharge and by electrical stimulation in the temporal cortex. Archives of Neurology and Psychiatry 81:269

Neidermeyer E, Khalifeh R 1965 Petit mal status (spike-wave stupor). Epilepsia 6:250

Ochs R, Gloor P, Quesney F, Ives J, Olivier A 1984 Does head-turning during a seizure have lateralizing or localizing significance? Neurology 34:884

Oxbury J M, Whitty C W M 1971 Causes and consequences of status epilepticus in adults. A survey of 86 cases. Brain 94:733

Parker H L 1930 Epileptiform convulsions. The incidence of attacks in cases of intracranial tumour. Archives of Neurology and Psychiatry 23:1032

Parkes J D, Marsden C D 1974 Narcolepsy. British Journal of Hospital Medicine 12:325

Parsonage M 1973 The differential diagnosis of seizures. Journal of the Royal College of Physicians 7:213

Paterson J H, McKissock W 1956 A clinical survey of intracranial angiomas with special reference to their mode of prognosis and surgical treatment: a report of 110 cases. Brain 79:233

Penfield W 1952 Epileptic automatism and the centrencephalic integrating system. Research Publications of the Association for Research into Nervous and Mental Diseases 30:513

Penfield W, Welch K 1951 The supplementary motor area of the cerebral cortex. Archives of Neurology and Psychiatry 66:289

Penfield W, Jasper H 1954 Epilepsy and the Functional Anatomy of the Human Brain. Little Brown, Boston

Penfield W, Perot P 1963 The brain's record of auditory and visual experience. Brain 86:595

Penfield W, Erickson T C, Tarlov I 1940 Relation of intracranial tumours and symptomatic epilepsy. Archives of Neurology and Psychiatry 44:300

Penry J K, Dreifuss F E 1969 Automatisms associated with absence of petit mal epilepsy. Archives of Neurology 21:142

Perkin G D, Joseph R 1986 Neurological manifestations of the hyperventilation syndrome. Journal of the Royal Society of Medicine 79:448

Pond D 1981 Psychosocial aspects of epilepsy – the family. In: Reynolds E H, Trimble M R (eds) Epilepsy and psychiatry. Churchill Livingstone, Edinburgh, pp 60–71

Pond D, Bidwell D 1960 A survey of epilepsy in fourteen general practices. Epilepsia 1:285

Proudfit W L, Forteza M E 1959 Micturition syncope. New England Journal of Medicine 260:328

Ramirez-Lassepas M, Cipolle R J, Morillo L R, Gumnit R J 1984 Value of computed tomographic scan in the evaluation of adult patients after their first seizure. Annals of Neurology 15:536

Raynor R B, Paine R S, Carmichael E A 1959 Epilepsy of late onset. Neurology 9:111

Research Committee of the College of General Practitioners 1960 A study of the epilepsies in general practice. British Medical Journal ii:416

Reynolds E H 1968 Epilepsy and schizophrenia: relationship and biochemistry. Lancet 1:398

Reynolds E H 1981 Biological factors in psychological disorders associated with epilepsy. In: Reynolds E H, Trimble M R (eds) Epilepsy and psychiatry. Churchill Livingstone, Edinburgh, pp 60–71

Reynolds E H 1983 Interictal behaviour in temporal lobe epilepsy. British Medical Journal 286:918

Reynolds E H 1985 The initiation of anticonvulsant drug therapy. Implications for prognosis. In: Pedley T A, Meldrum B S (eds) Recent Advances in Epilepsy Vol 2. Churchill Livingstone, Edinburgh, pp 101–110

Reynolds E H 1986 The clinical concept of epilepsy: an historical perspective. In: Trimble M R, Reynolds E H (eds) What is epilepsy? Churchill Livingstone, Edinburgh, pp 1–7

Reynolds E H, Elwes R D C, Shorvon S D 1983 Why does epilepsy become intractable? Prevention of chronic epilepsy. Lancet 2:952

Richardson E P, Dodge P R 1954 Epilepsy in cerebral vascular disease. Epilepsia 3:49

Robertson M M, Trimble M R 1983 Depressive illness in patients with epilepsy: A review. Epilepsia 24 (Suppl 2):S109

Rodin E A 1968 The prognosis of patients with epilepsy. Thomas, Springfield

Rodin E A, Katz M, Lennox K 1976 Differences between patients with temporal lobe seizures and those with other forms of epileptic attacks. Epilepsia 17:313

Rutter M, Graham P, Yule W 1960 A Neuropsychiatric Study in Childhood. In: Clinics in developmental medicine No 35. Spastics International Press, Heinemann, London

Sano K, Malamud N 1953 Clinical significance of sclerosis of the cornu ammonis. Archives of Neurology and Psychiatry (Chicago) 70:40

Saunders M, Marshall C 1975 Isolated seizures: an EEG and clinical assessment. Epilepsia 16: 731–733

Schwartz M S, Scott R 1971 Isolated petit mal status presenting de novo in middle age. Lancet 2:1399

Serafetinides E A, Falconer M A 1963 Speech disturbances in temporal lobe seizures: A study in 100 epileptic patients submitted to anterior temporal lobectomy. Brain 86:333

Shakir R, Johnson R, Lambie D, Melville I, Nanda R 1981 Comparison of sodium valproate and phenytoin as single drug treatment in epilepsy. Epilepsia 22: 27–33

Sharpey-Schafer E P 1953 The mechanism of syncope after coughing. British Medical Journal 2:860

Sharpey-Schafer E P, Taylor P J 1960 Absent circulatory reflexes in diabetic neuritis. Lancet 1:559

Sheehan S 1958 One thousand cases of late onset epilepsy. Irish Journal of Medical Science 6:261

Shorvon S D 1984 The temporal aspects of prognosis in epilepsy. Journal of Neurology, Neurosurgery and Psychiatry 47:1157

Shorvon S D, Reynolds E H 1982 Early prognosis of epilepsy. British Medical Journal 285: 1699–1701

Shorvon S D, Chadwick D, Galbraith A W, Reynolds E H 1978 One drug for epilepsy. British Medical Journal 1:474

Shorvon S D, Reynolds E H 1986 The nature of epilepsy: evidence from studies of epidemiology, temporal patterns of seizures, prognosis and treatment. In: Trimble M R, Reynolds E H (eds) What is epilepsy? Churchill Livingstone, Edinburgh, pp 36–45

Slater E, Beard A W 1963 The schizophrenia-like psychoses of epilepsy. British Journal of Psychiatry 109:95

Smith B H 1960 Vestibular disturbance in epilepsy. Neurology 10:475

Stevens H 1966 Paroxysmal choreo-athetosis. A form of reflex epilepsy. Archives of Neurology 14:415

Strobos R R J 1959 Prognosis in convulsive disorders. Archives of Neurology 1: 216–225

Sumi S M, Teasdall R D 1963 Focal seizures. A review of 150 cases. Neurology 13:582

Strandjord R, Johannessen S 1980 Carbamazepine as the only drug in patients with epilepsy: Serum level and clinical effect. In: Johannessen S et al (eds) Antiepileptic therapy: advances in drug monitoring. New York, Raven Press, pp 299–301

Symonds C P 1954 Classification of the epilepsies with particular references to psychomotor seizures. Archives of Neurology and Psychiatry 72: 631

Temkin O 1971 The falling sickness. Johns Hopkins Press, Baltimore

Thomas M H 1959 The single seizure: its study and management. Journal of the American Medical Association 169: 457–459

Trimble M R, Reynolds E H 1984 Neuropsychiatric toxicity of anticonvulsant drugs. In: Matthews G B, Glaser G H (eds) Recent advances in clinical neurology 4. Churchill Livingstone, Edinburgh, pp 261–280

Trimble M R, Reynolds E H 1986 (eds) What is epilepsy? Churchill Livingstone, Edinburgh

Trolle E 1960 Drug therapy of epilepsy. Acta Psychiatrica Neurologica Scandinavica (suppl) 150: 187–199

Turnbull D M, Rawlins M D, Weightman D, Chadwick D W 1982 A comparison of phenytoin and valproate in previously untreated adult epileptic patients. Journal of Neurology, Neurosurgery and Psychiatry 45: 55–59

Van Buren J M, Ajmone-Marsen C 1960 Correlation of autonomic and EEG components in temporal lobe epilepsy. Archives of Neurology 3:683

Walker A 1961 Murder or epilepsy. Journal of Nervous and Mental Disease 133:430

White P J, Bailey A A, Bickford R G 1953 Epileptic disorders in the aged. Neurology 3:674

Whitty C W M 1965 A note on the classification of epilepsy. Lancet 1:99

Williams D 1956 The structure of emotions reflected in epileptic experiences. Brain 79:29

Williams D 1965 The thalamus and epilepsy. Brain 88:539

Williams D 1966 Temporal lobe epilepsy. British Medical Journal 1:1439

Woodcock S, Cosgrove J B R 1964 Epilepsy after the age of 50. A five-year follow-up study. Neurology 14:34

Yang P J, Berger P E, Cohen M E, Duffner P K 1979 Computed tomography and childhood seizure disorders. Neurology 29:1084

Young A C, Mohr P D, Costanzi J B, Forbes W St C 1982 Is routine computerized axial tomography in epilepsy worth while? Lancet II:1446

Zielinski J J 1986 Epidemiology. In: Laidlaw J, Richens A (eds) A textbook of epilepsy. 3rd edn. Churchill Livingstone, Edinburgh

6

Pathology

G. Mathieson

INTRODUCTION

Morphological studies have made a modest but well-defined contribution to our knowledge of the dynamic disorder of epilepsy in humans. With increasing awareness of the focal origin of seizures in many patients and the efficacy of surgical therapy in some, there has been a growing need and opportunity to study the tissue changes associated with seizures of focal onset. In contrast, pathological studies of patients with corticoreticular epilepsy have been rather barren. In a third broad group of patients, those with endogenous metabolic encephalopathies, histopathological investigation has delineated some distinct diseases which are almost invariably associated with some form of epilepsy.

Since there are no specific histopathological criteria to determine definitively whether or not any particular pattern of cerebral lesion will give rise to seizure discharges, our knowledge depends in large part on implication by association. We must therefore distinguish:

1. Lesions which, directly or indirectly, cause epileptic neuronal discharges
2. Lesions which result from repeated seizures, i.e. ictal brain damage. These secondary lesions may in their turn be potentially epileptogenic
3. Lesions sharing an etiology with epileptogenic lesions but not themselves epileptogenic
4. Incidental lesions in the brains of habitual epileptics not causally related to the seizure tendency

The concept of epileptic threshold, applying to the brain as a whole, and to various structures and cortical regions in the brain, clearly implies that the patient's morphological lesion is only one factor in determining if and when cerebral seizures will occur. Brain lesions may therefore be regarded as predisposing to epilepsy and determining the site of origin of abnormal discharges in susceptible subjects.

By common consent, the proximate cause of an epileptic event is an abnormal pattern of discharge in a neuronal pool. Structural abnormalities of individual neurones or, more frequently, an alteration in their number and arrangement are observed in some epileptic lesions but, in many patients, non-neural elements dominate the morphological picture – for example, vascular malformations, scars, glial neoplasms. These obscure the neuronal component of the lesion, but indicate, to a first approximation, its pathogenesis. Thus many of the lesions described in this chapter are at least once removed from the essential predisposing mechanism of the patient's epilepsy. Their demonstration, however, is essential in elucidating intermediary pathogenetic steps; they may also provide valuable clues in the clinical and laboratory investigation of patients with epilepsy.

CATEGORIES OF EPILEPTOGENIC LESIONS

A systematic etiological classification is the ultimate aim of an account of the pathology of epilepsy. Our present knowledge does not as yet allow this. The range of response of the brain to injury is limited so that, in the long term, the results of various noxious processes may be very similar (pathogenetic convergence). The state of maturation of the brain at the time of initial insult is important. In retrospective assessment of an adult epileptic patient, the age at which the presumed causal event occurred is often more reliably ascertained than the exact nature of the event.

The classification of lesions offered here (Table 6.1) is heterogeneous, being based partly on the stage of development at which the initial cerebral insult occurred, and partly on standard pathological concepts of etiology.

Table 6.1 Outline classification of epileptogenic lesions

Lesions originating during intrauterine life
Lesions associated with childbirth
Lesions resulting from febrile convulsions of childhood
Inflammatory lesions and their residua
Lesions resulting from head injury
Acquired vascular lesions of adults
Neoplasms
Subtle dendritic lesions
Endogenous metabolic encephalopathies
Metabolic encephalopathies of extra-cerebral origin.

Epileptogenic lesions originating during intrauterine life

Disturbances of the complex sequence of events by which the embryonic neural tube becomes the neonate brain give rise to a wide spectrum of neurological abnormalities. Some are incompatible with extrauterine survival; others, e.g. dysraphic states, do not concern us here. Lilienfeld & Pasamanick (1954) and Pasamanick & Lilienfeld (1955), in a retrospective survey with controls matched for age, and for maternal age, showed that mothers of epileptic patients had a significantly ($p < 0.05$) higher incidence of complications of pregnancy and delivery in general. In particular, the incidence of maternal bleeding and toxaemia of pregnancy was increased over controls. Their epileptic patient records were clinical, and histopathological evidence was not available to them.

The formal origin of some of these developmental abnormalities is known in general terms. Clues to etiology may be available in the maternal history: placental abnormality, anoxic episodes, radiation, viral infection and undernutrition have all been implicated. An appropriate gestational age at the time of the noxious event appears to be essential for the development of certain anomalies, e.g. polymicrogyria. Diffuse and morphologically more subtle abnormalities may occur with undernutrition during the brain growth spurt (Dobbing & Sands 1973, Dobbing & Smart 1974), but it is speculative whether these increase the liability to the development of life-long epilepsy, as distinct from impaired motor skills and mentation. Our main concern here is with certain distinctive patterns of anomalous development readily recognized histologically and known to be associated with habitual epilepsy. They are listed in Table 6.2.

Table 6.2 Epileptogenic lesions originating during intrauterine life

A. *Disorders of cellular migration and differentiation*
   Heterotopias
   Polymicrogyria
   Megalencephaly
   Focal cortical dysplasia
   Tuberous sclerosis and formes frustes
   Hamartomas
   Meningio-angiomatosis
   Neuro-cutaneous melanosis
   Dermoid and epidermoid cysts
B. *Disorders of vascular organisation*
   Cavernous haemangioma
   Arterio-venous malformation
   Sturge-Weber disease

Heterotopias

Occasional neurones scattered in the subcortical white matter are a common finding of no significance. Large ectopic clusters of neurones and glia forming grey masses occur in two patterns: laminar within the centrum ovale and nodular at the angles of the lateral ventricles (Fig. 6.1). Some people with heterotopias are free from any neurological disability; others have seizures and some degree of mental retardation. The lesions are commonly bilateral and roughly symmetrical. In the unilateral case reported by Layton (1962), there was close correlation between the site of the lesion and its clinical and electrographic manifestations. Cortical gyral pattern and lamination are usually normal. However, cases also occur in which heterotopias are but one component of a complex cerebral maldevelopment. Crome (1952) has reported occipital heterotopia in a case of

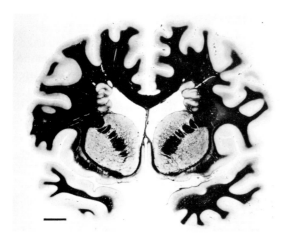

Fig. 6.1 Nodular heterotopias at the angles of the lateral ventricles. From a mildly retarded girl; seizures of varying pattern began in early adolescence; death at 19 years in status epilepticus. Heidenhain's method for myelin. Scale marker 1 cm.

extensive polymicrogyria, and Kirschbaum (1947) and Norman (1958) in association with agenesis of the corpus callosum and megalencephaly.

Polymicrogyria

This distinctive lesion is characterized by many small gyrus-like formations without formed sulci. The surface of the involved brain presents rather wide gyri with wrinkled surfaces. The lesion may be fairly extensive and bilateral but, in adults, isolated patches of this malformed cortex are more

commonly encountered. The opercula of the insula are frequent sites of predilection (Fig. 6.2). Cortical lamination is typically four-layered (Fig. 6.3). Small foci of this lesion may be quite inconspicuous in surgically excised specimens (Fig. 6.4).

Neonates succumbing to cytomegalovirus infection frequently show polymicrogyria in extreme degree (Crome & France 1959, Crome 1961, Bignami & Appicciutoli 1964). It is reasonable to suppose that less severe brain involvement with survival into adult life may result from intra-

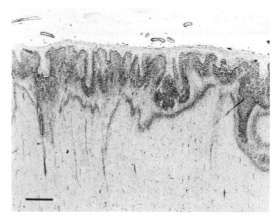

Fig. 6.3 Polymicrogyria. Four-layered cortex in a neonate with disseminated cytomegalovirus infection. Haematoxylin and eosin. Scale marker 1 mm.

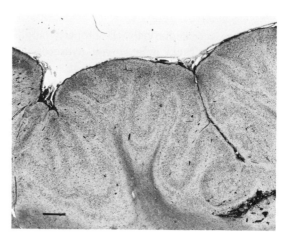

Fig. 6.4 Polymicrogyria. Patient began having seizures characterized by an aura of 'buzzing' followed by automatism at 12 years of age. Left temporal lobectomy at 23 years. Focal polymicrogyria is readily apparent histologically but was inconspicuous on naked eye examination. Luxol fast blue-cresyl violet. Scale marker 1 mm.

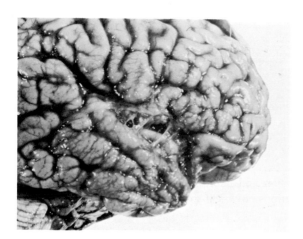

Fig. 6.2 Polymicrogyria. Right frontal and temporal gyri adjacent to the Sylvian fissure are involved.

uterine infection by this and possibly other viruses. A range of nonspecific noxious events, e.g. coal gas poisoning, occurring at a critical stage of cortical maturation, usually in the fifth month of intrauterine life, can produce an identical lesion. Polymicrogyria is, then, generally regarded as resulting from a disturbance of the orderly pattern of differentiation and migration of neuroblasts into the cerebral mantle. An alternative point of view is that the four-layered cortical lamination is due to post-migratory destruction. This has received support from a serial section study (Richman et al 1974) of a 27 week fetus in whom the cell sparse zone of the polymicrogyric cortex was shown to be in continuity with layer V of the intact cortex. The outer cellular layer may thus be formed by layers II, III and IV and the inner cellular layer by layer VI. However, this post-migrational encephaloclastic concept does not account for the abnormality of convolutional pattern. Polymicrogyria may accompany other major malformations. Extensive, usually bilateral, porencephaly was recorded by Dekaban (1965) in 11 patients with profound neurological deficits, including epilepsy; fields of polymicrogyric cortex lay adjacent to these pallial defects. Peach (1965) observed a four-layered cortex type of microgyria in 11 of 20 cases of Arnold-Chiari malformation.

Megalencephaly

The term 'megalencephaly' is properly applied only when the brain is large, not hydrocephalic, and storage diseases such as lipidosis have been rigorously excluded. It is not to be equated with the clinical descriptive term 'macrocephaly'. Essentially, the cerebral cortex is unduly thick and heterotopias are absent. Laurence (1946a) reported a patient with unilateral involvement and persistent seizures leading to death at $5\frac{1}{2}$ months of age; both neurones and glia contributed to the enlarged hemisphere. In another unilateral example, Bignami et al (1968) using quantitative histochemical techniques showed a three-fold increase in neuronal nuclear volume and suggested heteroploidy as the basic disorder. Laurence (1964b) in a brief review stressed the frequency of seizures in children with this lesion.

Focal cortical dysplasia

This lesion, while often inconspicuous on naked eye examination, presents prominent histopathological features. Lamination of the involved cortex is lost. Abnormally large neurones are scattered throughout the cortex in a disorderly fashion (Fig. 6.5) and may extend in small clusters into the subjacent white matter (Fig. 6.6). There is an overall reduction in neuronal population in the affected cortex, which is sharply demarcated from adjoining normal cortex. Astrocytes with abundant cytoplasm, lobulated or multiple nuclei, and

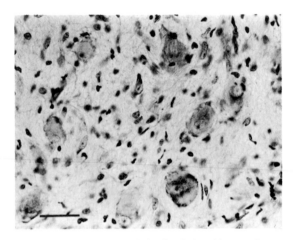

Fig. 6.5 Focal cortical dysplasia. Cortical architecture is disorganized by scattered large neurones and glial proliferation. Luxol fast blue-cresyl violet. Scale marker 50 m.

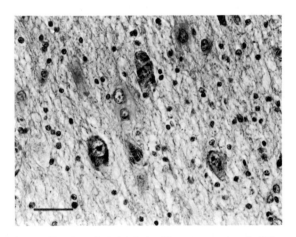

Fig. 6.6 Focal cortical dysplasia. Large neurones and glial cells are clustered in the subcortical white matter. Haematoxylin and eosin. Scale marker 50 μm.

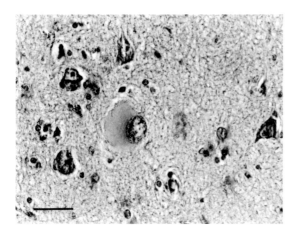

Fig. 6.7 Focal cortical dysplasia. A large astrocyte with voluminous cytoplasm is in the centre of the field. Several small binucleate astrocytes are also present. Haematoxylin and eosin. Scale marker 50 μm.

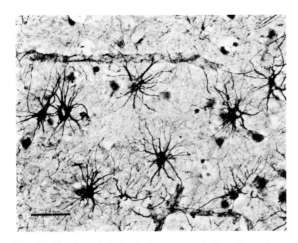

Fig. 6.8 Focal cortical dysplasia. Astrocytic fibre formation in dysplastic cortex. Cajal's gold sublimate impregnation. Scale marker 50 μm.
6.5 to 6.8 are from the second temporal gyrus of a 26-year-old woman whose complex partial seizures began at the age of 15. Her birth and early life were normal and she had no features suggesting tuberous sclerosis.

fibre formation are frequent (Figs. 6.7, 6.8). These features are reminiscent of tuberous sclerosis, but cortical nodularity, calcification, subependymal lesions and the cutaneous and visceral manifestations of tuberous sclerosis do not occur in patients with focal cortical dysplasia.

One of the three cases described by Crome (1957) had an extensive, although unilateral,

lesion accompanied by cortico-spinal tract degeneration. His patients were under 3 years of age, and had intractable focal seizures, retarded development and motor deficits. Two were siblings. The patient reported by Cravioto & Feigin (1960), a 21-year-old woman, had seizures with focal onset beginning at 6 months of age. She had permanent interictal neurological deficits but these are not invariable.

The status of this entity was firmly established by Taylor et al (1971) in a detailed account of ten patients operated upon for intractable seizures; one subsequently died in status epilepticus. These authors give convincing reasons for regarding this disease as distinct from tuberous sclerosis and its formes frustes. A remarkable clinical feature reported by them is the range of age at first seizure of from 2 to 31 years. This latency is interesting in view of the undoubtedly intrauterine developmental origin of the lesion.

Tuberous sclerosis and formes frustes

The pathology of tuberous sclerosis is systematically described by Urich (1976). Our present concern is with patients whose disease is limited, in whom mental retardation and/or cutaneous manifestations are lacking, so that diagnosis is uncertain in the absence of histopathological evidence. Such partial forms of tuberous sclerosis are being increasingly recognized. The three patients reported in detail by Duvoisin & Vinson (1961) were of superior intelligence, although all had radiological evidence of cerebral involvement as well as lesions of tuberous sclerosis elsewhere. Lagos & Gomez (1967) reviewed the records of 71 patients with tuberous sclerosis studied at the Mayo Clinic: 26 of the 69 patients on whom there were records of intellectual capacity had normal intelligence; 18 of these 26 had seizures. Surgical excision of cortical lesions for the relief of seizures in such patients, as carried out by Perot et al (1966), allows histopathological confirmation of the diagnosis. The essential pathological features distinguishing oligosymptomatic tuberous sclerosis from focal cortical dysplasia, which undoubtedly resemble each other, are given in the section above.

Hamartomas

These lesions are tumour-like malformations. On microscopic examination, many bear a strong resemblance to neoplasms but they lack the property of progressive growth and expansion. Penfield & Ward (1948) directed attention to this lesion as a rare anatomical substrate of temporal lobe seizures. Twenty years later, hamartomas (and closely related lesions) were reported as the essential pathological finding in 22 and 100 consecutive epileptic patients treated by anterior temporal lobectomy (Falconer & Taylor 1968). In the Penfield–Rasmussen–Feindel series from Montreal (reported by Mathieson 1975a), a diagnosis of hamartoma was made in 14 of 202 discrete focal lesions, in a series of 857 patients undergoing surgical excision for epilepsy. This three-fold discrepancy of incidence in the two series may be a consequence of lack of uniform histopathological criteria and terminology, as well as patient selection.

The exact nature of these lesions is thoroughly discussed by Cavanagh (1958), whose paper remains the definitive account and should be consulted for detailed histopathology. Most such hamartomas occur in the amygdaloid nucleus, medial occipito-temporal (fusiform) gyrus or less frequently in the hippocampus. Occurrence in the frontal and parietal lobes has been recorded (Mathieson 1975b, Table 5, p. 114). Any combination of astrocytes, oligodendrocytes and neurones may occur. Calcification is frequent.

An interesting clinical correlation of hamartomatous lesions has emerged from Falconer's (1973) review of patients operated on by him. Patients with a psychosis accompanying their epilepsy were statistically more likely to have a hamartoma than an atrophic temporal lobe lesion. Furthermore, although relief of seizures occurred in patients with both types of lesions, aggressive behaviour or a schizophrenia-like illness were more likely to persist in patients who had a pathological diagnosis of hamartoma. The reason for this rather surprising finding remains speculative (Geschwind 1973).

Meningio-angiomatosis

Strictly this lesion should be considered under the above heading of hamartoma, for such it is. However, it is non-glial and predominantly composed of cellular elements which normally lie outside the pia mater. Meningio-angiomatosis is not to be confused with examples of multiple meningiomas such as sometimes occur in Von Recklinghausen's disease, nor with meningioma-en-plaque. In meningio-angiomatosis a portion of cerebral cortex is replaced by tissue having the structure of meningioma but lacking its propensity to grow. Large neurones are scattered within the lesion (Fig. 6.9). These were present in case 1 of Worster-Drought et al (1937) who gave the first clear account of the lesion and established its association with central neurofibromatosis. This disease probably belongs to that large group of conditions referred to as neurocristopathies by Bolande (1974).

Neurocutaneous melanosis

This striking complex comprises a 'garment type' pigmented lesion of the skin and an excessive accumulation of melanocytes in the leptomeninges. Additionally, in some cases, melanin of both cutaneous and neuronal type is found in neurones, melanocytes and macrophages within certain brain structures. These include the amygdaloid nuclei and dentate nuclei of the cerebellum (Fox et al 1964, Slaughter et al 1969). The devel-

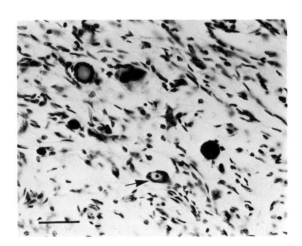

Fig. 6.9 Meningio-angiomatosis. The meningioma-like structure contains psammoma bodies and occasional neurones (arrow). From the insular cortex of an adolescent girl with focal cerebral seizures. Haematoxylin and van Gieson. Scale marker 50 µm.

opment of primary malignant intracranial melanomata bring these patients to the attention of pathologists. In some, however, focal seizures clearly arise from causes other than intracranial neoplasm. In a patient studied personally in conjunction with Dr F. Andermann, seizures began at 3 years of age, had a consistent stereotyped pattern and occurred infrequently. Electrophysiological evidence indicated an origin in one amygdaloid nucleus. The appropriate temporal lobe, resected at 26 years of age, showed intense melanosis of the amygdala. There has been no seizure recurrence or evidence of tumour during a three year follow up.

Dermoid and epidermoid cysts

The features of dermoid and epidermoid cysts are too well known to require detailed description here. Most are basally situated. Intracerebral examples are most likely to have epilepsy as a prominent, or occasionally the sole clinical feature (Tytus & Pennybacker 1956).

Disorders of vascular organization

The extensive remodelling that the cerebral vasculature undergoes during embryogenesis occasionally results in malformations. Those that concern us here are cavernous haemangioma, arteriovenous malformation and Sturge-Weber disease.

Cavernous haemangiomas are usually static lesions and are certainly not neoplastic despite their terminology. Composed essentially of endothelial lined channels with thick collagenous walls, they often have a surrounding zone of gliosed brain and scattered haemosiderin pigment. Calcification is common. The lesions reported as haemangioma calcificans by Penfield & Ward (1948) in the temporal lobes of five patients with longstanding seizures belongs in this category. The frequent incidence of focal motor seizures associated with cavernous haemangiomata in the region of the central fissure is stressed by Russell and Rubinstein (1977). Familial occurrence has been reported by Clark (1970).

In contrast, the shunting of arterial blood into much altered venous channels in arteriovenous malformations produces a dynamic lesion with profound local, and occasionally systemic, alterations in cerebral blood flow. Widespread zones of anomalous patterns of epicerebral blood flow and regional cortical blood flow have been demonstrated by Feindel et al (1971). Regional autoregulation of cerebral blood flow is lost. Fluctuating hypoxia of nearby cortex may play a role in the genesis of seizures which occur so commonly in patients with this lesion. An overview of these and related lesions is given by McCormick (1966).

The well-known triad of facial naevus flammeus, seizures and intracerebral calcification which forms Sturge-Weber disease or encephalofacial angiomatosis is the subject of an extensive literature. The monograph by Alexander & Norman (1960) and the systematic account by Urich (1976) should be consulted. The extent of the pial venous angioma varies considerably; cortical atrophy is often more extensive than the vascular abnormality. The site or sites of most active epileptic cortical discharge may be some distance away from the mossy carpet of abnormal pial blood vessels as displayed at operation. Surgical aspects of therapy and the light they shed on pathology are considered by Falconer & Rushworth (1960) and by Rasmussen et al (1972).

Lesions associated with childbirth

By long tradition, birth injury is believed to give rise to lesions causing habitual epilepsy. That prematurity, excessive moulding, precipitate delivery and neonatal asphyxia may give rise to intracranial lesions is not in dispute. Some lesions, such as subependymal cell-plate haemorrhages with secondary ventricular rupture are not compatible with prolonged survival. Others, such as periventricular leukomalacia and basal ganglia lesions are not associated with epilepsy. Lesions identified as being related to habitual epilepsy are listed in Table 6.3.

The early stages of laminar cortical necrosis in neonatal asphyxia are illustrated by Banker (1967) and Friede (1975). The selective involvement of the depths of sulci compared with the crowns of gyri is clear and consistent, but why this pattern should occur remains unknown.

Ulegyria, often in the boundary zones of major cerebral arteries, can readily be visualized as

Table 6.3 Lesions associated with childbirth

Neonatal asphyxia
   Laminar cortical necrosis
   Ulegyria
   Lobular cerebellar sclerosis
Perinatal arterial occlusion
   Cerebral infarct
Excessive moulding
   Medial temporal lobe lesions ('incisural sclerosis')
   Inferior temporal and medial occipital lobe infarction

evolving from these earlier stages by resorption of necrotic tissue and gliosis to form the unmistakable mushroom-like gyri. Hypotension complicating hypoxia is believed to determine the distribution of ulegyria in these cases (Norman et al 1957). In some early accounts of the surgical treatment of epilepsy (e.g. Penfield & Humphries 1940, Penfield & Jasper 1954) these lesions are referred to as focal microgyria, although it is clear from their illustrations that they are entirely different from the lesion termed microgyria by Crome (1952) and described above under the now more customary term of polymicrogyria.

Circumscribed lobular cerebellar sclerosis is discussed and illustrated in a later section of this chapter.

Large, well-defined, destructive lesions occurring in recognized arterial territories in the brains of patients with seizures and often with fixed neurological deficits are readily recognized as old infarcts. Clinical data in some of these patients indicate that the lesion occurred in the perinatal period. The patients with temporal lobe epilepsy and homonymous hemianopia reported by Remillard et al (1974) undoubtedly belong in this category; some of the 85 patients reviewed by Rasmussen & Gossman (1963) under the term 'gross destructive brain lesions' probably had neonatal infarcts; a case is illustrated by Mathieson (1975a). Autopsy accounts in neonates by Clark & Linell (1954) and by Banker (1961) confirmed the occurrence of perinatal arterial cerebral infarcts. In the infantile cases reported by Cocker et al (1965) there was excellent correlation between the regions of brain infarcted and the sites of arterial lesions; these occurred at arterial bifurcations, suggesting lodgement of an embolus. The cause of arterial occlusion is often obscure although in some cases there is evidence of embol-

ism from the placenta, fetal placental veins or mural cardiac thrombus. In patients who develop epilepsy in later infancy or childhood and are found to have a cerebral infarct, the etiology of the perinatal arterial occlusion usually remains tentative and dependent on analogy with cases studied carefully at an earlier stage of their evolution.

Increasing recognition of the frequency of a temporal lobe origin of habitual seizures and the demonstration of atrophic lesions in therapeutic excisions led Earle et al (1953) to formulate a hypothesis about their origin. In essence, they postulated that transtentorial herniation of medial temporal structures, resulting from excessive moulding of the skull vault during delivery, might compress the anterior choroidal and posterior cerebral arteries with resultant ischaemic lesions in their territories; hence their term 'incisural sclerosis'. With our increasing knowledge of temporal lobe pathology, this mechanicovascular hypothesis has proved to be untenable in the many cases of sclerotic temporal atrophy which are now attributed to other cases. The term 'incisural sclerosis' has thus generally lapsed. The distribution of the temporal atrophy, which could not be mapped in the earlier limited therapeutic excisions, is not consistent with anterior choroidal or posterior cerebral occlusion (Falconer et al 1964, Falconer & Taylor 1968). However, some unusual cases with extensive inferior temporal and medial occipital infarction may be a consequence of posterior cerebral artery compression at the incisura tentorii.

Lesions resulting from febrile illness of childhood

Convulsions due to pyrexial illness, not primarily involving the brain, are reported to occur in from 19 to 48 per 1000 children, mostly between the ages of 6 months and 5 years (Miller et al 1960, Costeff 1965, Schuman & Miller 1966, Van den Berg & Yerushalmy 1969, Rose et al 1973). The tendency for a child to convulse when febrile appears to be genetically determined (Lennox 1949a, Ounsted 1952, Schuman & Miller 1966, Ounsted 1955). Furthermore the evidence indicates that this tendency is inherited in an autosomal dominant fashion (Ounsted, Lindsay & Norman, 1966, Frantzen et al 1970). The tendency becomes manifest only when febrile provocation occurs within the appropriate age range in childhood (Ounsted 1971). The whole subject of febrile convulsions is discussed in detail by Lennox-Buchthal (1973), and in Chapter 4 of this book.

During the age of susceptibility to febrile convulsions, the brain is in a phase of active growth and maturation. On general grounds, therefore, it might be supposed that excessive neuronal discharge and hypoxia occurring during prolonged and/or recurrent convulsions might be particularly likely to cause brain damage. The evidence is that this is so. Zimmerman (1938) described cortical neuronal necrosis, sometimes widespread, occasionally laminar, and often most evident in the walls and depths of sulci in 11 children (age range 5 months to 6 years) who died within 1 to 13 days of the onset of severe febrile convulsions. This type of lesion is illustrated in Figure 6.10. Destruction of neurones of Sommer's sector of the hippocampus was prominent in Zimmerman's cases. Cerebellar lesions occurred in some patients. The five patients under 3 years of age reported by Fowler (1957) were previously healthy but, following convulsions associated with fever, had extensive brain lesions with neuronal necrosis and loss. The distribution of lesions included cerebral cortex, hippocampus, amygdaloid nucleus, thalamus and basal ganglia. In one case the hippocampi were normal. Cortical lesions,

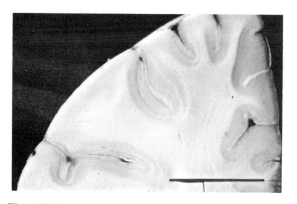

Fig. 6.10 Laminar cortical necrosis. U-shaped involvement of walls and depths of sulci of convexity. From an 18-month-old male infant whose persistent febrile convulsions terminated in death on the 3rd day. Scale marker 2 cm.

where not complete, tended to be laminar, with layer III most frequently involved. Inflammatory lesions of meninges or brain were not present.

Necropsy studies such as these and others in the literature necessarily describe lethal, and therefore exceptionally severe, instances of insult to the brain. Their relevance to longlasting habitual epilepsy is by extrapolation to patients with lesser degrees of cerebral damage. Thom (1942) quotes figures to indicate that children with a history of febrile convulsions are twelve times more likely to have epilepsy than children without such a history. This theme has been further developed with examples by Lennox (1949b).

Viewed retrospectively, patients with established temporal lobe epilepsy have a greater than normal probability of having had febrile convulsion in early life (Ounsted et al 1966, Ounsted 1967, Mathieson 1975b). Furthermore, patients with temporal lobe epilepsy and a preceding history of febrile convulsions are more likely (at a high degree of statistical significance) to have siblings who have also had febrile convulsions (Ounsted 1967). Of 100 patients treated by temporal lobectomy, those shown histologically to have gliosis of medial temporal structures had a significantly ($p < 0.01$) more frequent onset with status epilepticus than those with other lesions such as hamartomas or cryptic tumours (Falconer & Taylor 1968).

The pathogenetic sequence of events, for which the evidence has been given above, is summarized in Figure 6.11. This is probably not the only etiology of sclerotic atrophy of the temporal lobe, nor are the lesions resulting from febrile status invariably temporal in distribution. An example of widespread destruction with ulegyria and accentuation in arterial watershed zones is shown in Figure 6.12. The tendency for less severe lesions, especially those in the temporal lobe, to be predominantly unilateral is not yet fully understood; possible operative factors include greater seizure discharge on one side (Aicardi & Chevrie 1970) and a hypothesis regarding differential maturation rates of the cerebral hemispheres (Taylor 1969, Taylor & Ounsted 1971).

Evidence derived from animal experimentation relevant to this problem is discussed in a subsequent section of this chapter.

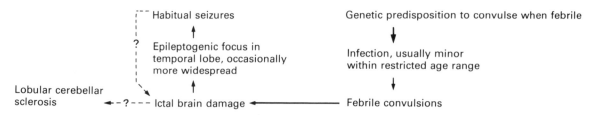

Fig. 6.11 Suggested sequence of events in some patients following prolonged or repeated febrile convulsions. See text for evidence.

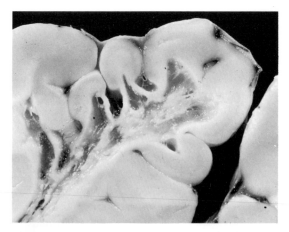

Fig. 6.12 Ulegyria. Birth and early development entirely normal. Severe febrile convulsions at two years. Frequent seizures of variable pattern, resistent to medication. Death following epileptic fit at 10 years. Autopsy showed widespread ulegyria mainly in arterial watershed distribution.

Inflammatory lesions and their residua

Established and essentially static epileptogenic lesions may follow bacterial meningitis and cerebral abscess. In some patients with epilepsia partialis continua and progressive neurological deficit and encephalitic histopathology has been found.

In patients with pyogenic meningitis, several pathogenetic mechanisms may be operative. Although fibrinopurulent exudate is usually confined to the leptomeninges, microscopic changes are observed in the superficial cortical layers even in the early stages. These comprise microglial infiltration and astrocytic hypertrophy which may be surmised to affect dendritic arborisations in these layers. Selective neuronal necrosis occurs in some patients (Smith & Landing 1960). More obvious ischaemic lesions, taking the form of patchy infarcts, result from endarteritis obli-

terans, with or without supervening thrombosis of leptomeningeal vessels, especially in patients who have received inappropriate or delayed antibiotic therapy and have passed into a subacute phase. A third pathogenetic mechanism, that of convulsions consequent upon fever, may operate in genetically susceptible children of appropriate age. Dodge and Swartz (1965) reported four of 99 patients as having seizures as a late sequel of pyogenic meningitis.

Cerebral abscesses with their attendant granulation tissue, fibrosis and progressive surrounding zone of gliosed brain form potent epileptogenic foci, as a voluminous literature attests. Legg et al (1973) recorded epilepsy as occurring in 51 of 70 patients with supratentorial abscesses, with a mean latency of 3.3 years; latency was shorter in patients with a temporal site than in those with a frontal site. Carey et al (1971) reported a 32% incidence of seizures in 40 patients surviving surgical therapy; seizures in children were more frequent and more resistent to antiepileptic drug therapy than in adults. Morgan et al (1973) found a 55 % incidence of seizures in 31 patients with supratentorial abscesses; onset was within two years of operation in all but one patient. Other published series confirm that one-third to one-half of patients surviving cerebral abscess develop epilepsy, no matter how treated. These figures bear eloquent witness to the potent epileptogenicity of this lesion.

Seizures are a prominent clinical feature of various forms of encephalitis of known or suspected viral etiology. Of special interest are those patients in whom epilepsia partialis continua or recurrent seizures with focal onset are accompanied by a slowly progressive neurological deficit. A histopathological picture of encephalitis, still apparently active many months after onset, has been described in some such patients by Rasmussen et al (1958) and by Aguilar & Rasmussen (1960). The syndrome occurs mainly in the first decade of life (Mathieson 1975a). While inflammatory features are impressive, inclusion bodies are rarely found. Serological evidence of viral infection is lacking and attempts to demonstrate virus by electronmicroscopy and culture have not as yet yielded convincing results, despite a number of preliminary published reports, unfortunately unconfirmed. Clinically there is some resemblance to the syndrome of hemiconvulsions, hemiplegia and epilepsy discussed by Gastaut et al (1959) but this latter usually has an abrupt onset and is believed to result from vascular occlusion in most instances, although Coxsackie A9 viral infection causing focal vasculitis or encephalitis has been described (Roden et al 1975, Chalhub et al 1977).

Parasitic infestation of the brain in the form of cysticercosis cerebri is generally limited to certain geographical regions.

Lesions resulting from head injury

Convulsions occurring contralateral to severe head injury have been observed since early times (Hippocrates, cited by Temkin 1971). More recent accounts of post-traumatic epilepsy have been concerned, inter alia, with the probability of its occurrence following varying degrees and types of injury (see Ch. 5). Caveness & Liss (1961) and Caveness (1963) in studies of Korean war veterans found an incidence ranging from 8.5% after mild closed injury to over 50% after dural and brain penetration. Jennet (1975) in a long-term statistical study of epilepsy following non-missile injuries reported an overall incidence of 5%. This risk was greatly increased by acute intracranial haematoma, by early epilepsy and by depressed skull fracture. In pathological terms, these factors reflect laceration of the brain, as occurs inevitably in penetrating injury. Breach of the pial barrier and mechanical damage to the cortex are therefore important determinants of post-traumatic epilepsy.

Morphologically, the focal residual lesions of trauma comprise saucer-shaped defects with smoothly scalloped borders, occurring most frequently on the crests of the orbital frontal and lateral temporal gyri. Lesions extending into the depths of sulci may result from transient interference with the epicerebral circulation and consequent infarction. Histopathologically, the superficial or all cortical layers are destroyed; a variable amount of collagenous fibrosis intermingled with glial proliferation forms a meningocerebral cicatrix. A narrow bordering zone of partially depopulated cortex is usual.

The more obvious lesions may not be the only important ones. Microscopic lesions, widely scattered throughout the cerebral hemispheres and brain stem, were recorded by Oppenheimer (1968) as occurring in about three-quarters of fatal head injuries; not all brain injuries were severe in the conventional sense, as death in some patients was due to non-neurological causes. Essentially, these lesions seem to stem from stretching and tearing of axons and subsequent cellular reaction. They are considered to be the precursors of the more extensive lesions described by Strich (1956, 1961) in patients with profound neurological deficits following closed head injury. It may be postulated that these predominantly subcortical abnormalities cause partial deafferentation of the cortex and predispose to the development of post-traumatic epilepsy. The evidence from therapeutic cortical resection, however, at least in selected cases of post-traumatic epilepsy (Rasmussen 1969) suggests that the local cortical lesion is of paramount importance in the genesis of seizures; the role of possible subcortical damage in the 33% of patients whose seizures were not ameliorated by cortical excision remains speculative.

Another factor possibly contributing to seizures in head injured patients is anoxic encephalopathy consequent upon systemic hypoxia from thoracic and other injuries.

Acquired vascular lesions of adults

Some patients develop epilepsy following a stroke. Louis & McDowell (167) recorded seizures in 77 of 1000 patients surviving a cerebral infarct; 29 patients had long term seizures as a sequel of their infarcts. Richardson & Dodge (1954) reported a 12.5% incidence of seizures in a consecutive series of 104 stroke patients. The importance of occlusive cerebrovascular disease in the genesis of epilepsy in the population as a whole is heavily age dependent. In a study of 1008 adult epileptic patients, roughly representative of the population at risk, seizures were attributed to cerebrovascular disease in 8.7%. In patients with onset of seizures after age 40, the proportion attributed to cerebrovascular disease rose to 44.5% (Juul-Jensen 1963).

What determines whether or not a stroke patient develops seizures is unclear. Involvement of the cerebral cortex appears to be essential (Dodge et al 1954). The responsible infarcts are often small and consequent upon small branch occlusion in the epicerebral circulation (Richardson 1958, Waddington 1970). Nevertheless, patients with medium to large infarcts and associated fixed neurological deficits do occasionally have recurrent seizures. The infarcts and the morphological changes in the brain surrounding them differ in no discernible way from those seen in non-convulsing patients. Patients surviving massive stroke rarely have persistent seizures.

Neoplasms

Brain tumours as a cause of adult onset epilepsy are so well known as to require little description here. Some general conclusions can be drawn from the large published series of cases, for example those of White et al (1948), Penfield & Jasper (1954) and Wyke (1959). Almost any supratentorial intracranial tumour can cause brain changes giving rise to seizures. The tendency of different tumours to do so depends partly on their site, but also to a considerable degree on their growth rate as determined by their histopathology. Whether the tumour impinges on the cerebral cortex from without (e.g. meningioma) or infiltrates the brain substance from within (e.g. astrocytoma) appears to make little difference to epileptogenicity. Proximity to the Rolandic motor strip or, more generally, a frontal situation increases the probability of seizures. Chronicity of the lesion is a major factor in epileptogenicity. Thus well-differentiated tumours with low biological growth potential and a course running for several years rather than months are more likely to be associated with epilepsy. Small indolent gliomas with seizures as

their sole clinical manifestation are sometimes distinguished with difficulty, if at all, from glial hamartomas (Cavanagh 1958, Mathieson 1975b).

In the case of extrinsic tumours, the essential morphological change appears to be an area of pressure atrophy of the cortex characterised by neuronal loss and gliosis. Intrinsic tumours produce a peripheral zone of infiltrated, but incompletely destroyed, brain tissue. This zone, with engulfed but viable neurones, is characteristically prominent in oligodendrogliomas and well differentiated astrocytomas; these lesions are associated with a high incidence of seizures.

For detailed pathological descriptions of nervous system tumours, the reader is referred to standard monographs such as those of Russell & Rubinstein (1977) and Rubinstein (1972).

Subtle dendritic lesions

The arrangement and structure of dendrites are poorly displayed by the staining methods customarily used in light microscopy. Electron microscopy presents difficulties in sampling and the availability of adequately fixed tissue. Morphological observations on dendrites in naturally occurring epileptogenic foci in humans are therefore regrettably sparse, despite the importance of the dendritic tree in the electrophysiological status of neurones. This is in sharp contrast to extensive accounts of dendritic changes in experimental models of epileptogenic foci.

Using Golgi techniques, the Scheibels have described a constellation of dendritic changes in the hippocampal neurones of patients with temporal lobe epilepsy (Scheibel et al 1974, Scheibel & Scheibel 1973). Loss of dendritic spines, nodularity of the dendritic shaft and fusiform swellings of apical dendrites occurred in a patchy fashion in neurones of the pyramidal cell layer. Changes in the neurones of the gyrus dentatus were less consistent but included a 'windswept' appearance of dendrites and narrowing of the dendritic field giving a 'closed parasol' appearance. These changes were not thought to result from deafferentation or remote anoxic injury: in only 50% of the patients reported was there a history of difficult birth or febrile convulsions in childhood. Paucity of dendritic spines has been corroborated by electron microscopic studies, but the fine structure of dendritic nodularity has not been observed (Brown 1973). It is not clear whether the changes described by these investigators form a part of the customary hippocampal sclerosis or are a distinct abnormality selectively involving dendritic spines such as has been described by Marin-Padilla (1972) in infants with established chromosomal anomalies. The authors considered that they constituted a continuing process of neuronal destruction.

Endogeneous metabolic encephalopathies

A host of diseases due to endogenous metabolic abnormality (inborn errors of metabolism) give rise to seizures. They defy brief description. Reference should be made to standard texts, such as that of Blackwood & Corsellis (1976), which give access to primary sources. Some of these diseases are readily recognized clinically and have a chemically characterized storage product and enzymatic deficiency, for example Tay-Sachs disease, GM2 gangliosidosis and hexosaminidase deficiency. Others, such as neuronal ceroid-lipofuscinosis (Zeman et al 1970, Boehme et al 1971) await full biochemical elucidation. Yet others remain to be segregated from the so-called degenerative diseases.

Clinical manifestations of many endogenous metabolic encephalopathies begin in childhood, but some are asymptomatic until well into adult life, for example adult ceroid-lipofuscinosis or Kufs' disease. Some of the non-gangliosidotic storage diseases may be diagnosed by histochemical and electronmicroscopic examination of sweat glands obtained by skin biopsy (Carpenter et al 1972, Carpenter et al 1973) or of lymphocytes (Noonan et al 1978). Lafora's disease, in which myoclonic and generalized seizures are prominent clinical features, may be diagnosed by cerebral biopsy and demonstration of characteristic neuronal inclusions; a detailed description is given by Van Heycop ten Ham (1974). Increasing knowledge of the biochemical abnormalities in the endogenous metabolic encephalopathies should lead to their more precise diagnosis by non-invasive methods.

Metabolic encephalopathies of extracerebral origin

Foremost in frequency and importance amongst these is anoxic encephalopathy which is increasingly encountered among general hospital patients following cardiopulmonary resuscitation. Persistent myoclonic jerks and occasional generalized seizures occur in some patients. Typically at autopsy there is laminar cortical necrosis with accentuation in sulcal depths. An arterial watershed distribution is sometimes encountered or superimposed on a more widespread abnormality.

A morphologically similar encephalopathy may follow profound hypoglycaemia.

ATROPHIC LESIONS OF THE TEMPORAL LOBE

Alike from their frequency, amenability to surgical therapy, and possible prevention, atrophic lesions of the temporal lobe merit our special attention. Sano & Malamud (1953) observed hippocampal sclerosis in 29 of 50 long-term epileptics at autopsy; 16 of the 18 with normal mentation had what we would now term complex partial seizures. Corsellis (1957) reported Ammon's horn sclerosis in 15 of 32 patients. Margerison & Corsellis (1966) found hippocampal sclerosis at autopsy in 36 of 55 unselected epileptic patients. Most early descriptions of temporal lobe pathology stressed hippocampal lesions (see Falconer 1970 for a historical review) but other temporal lobe structures are involved in patients with temporal lobe epilepsy. Neuronal loss and gliosis in the amygdaloid nucleus and uncus of the parahippocampal gyrus occur in a substantial proportion of cases (Meyer & Beck 1955, Margerison & Corsellis 1966). In tabulating severe and often widespread lesions in the temporal lobe, Cavanagh & Meyer (1956) recorded involvement of the fusiform gyrus and the inferior and middle temporal gyri in about half the cases with hippocampal sclerosis. These considerations led Falconer et al (1964) to introduce the term 'mesial temporal sclerosis' as descriptive of the diffuse lesion found in a large proportion of their patients operated upon for temporal lobe epilepsy. In view of the laterally situated lesions in some cases, and the pantemporal atrophy in severe examples, sclerotic temporal atrophy has been suggested as a synonym (Mathieson 1975b).

Niceties of terminology aside, the important fact is that atrophic lesions extend beyond the hippocampus and other mesial structures to involve both cortex and white matter of the temporal convolutions. They lie beyond the territories of irrigation of both choroidal and posterior cerebral arteries and we must look to mechanisms other than impaired circulation in any single vessel for their genesis. Indeed, the laminar cortical cell loss involving mainly the second and third layers with accentuation in the depths of sulci (Meyer et al 1954) is unlikely to be the result of infarction, either arterial or venous. While opinions remain to some extent open, there is a general trend towards the view that most cases of sclerotic temporal atrophy result from severe and/or recurrent febrile convulsions in early childhood; that pre-existing cerebral damage from perinatal asphyxia increases the risk; and that some patients develop this lesion solely as a consequence of birth anoxia. The magnitude of the problem is indicated by the study of Nelson & Ellenberger (1976): 2% of 1706 children who had had one or more febrile convulsions developed epilepsy by the seventh year of life. Children known or suspected of having some neurological abnormality before the febrile convulsive episode had a higher than average incidence of subsequent afebrile seizures. The prophylactic measures indicated are, in principle, clear (Mathieson 1975b, Meldrum 1975). Whether the maturing lesion can be influenced in respect of its potential epileptogenicity following the initiating events is another matter.

The range of severity of lesions found and their histopathological pattern, is illustrated in Figures 6.13 to 6.18.

Lesser degrees of presumed abnormality in resected temporal lobes sometimes make it difficult for the surgical pathologist to give a clear opinion. In patients operated upon in middle life some degree of subpial (Chaslun's) gliosis and perivascular atrophy of the white matter are not unexpected. The gyral pattern of the temporal lobe is variable. Studies by Geschwind & Levitsky

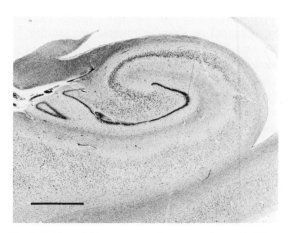

Fig. 6.13 Normal hippocampus. For comparison with Figure 6.14. Cresyl violet. Scale marker 2 mm.

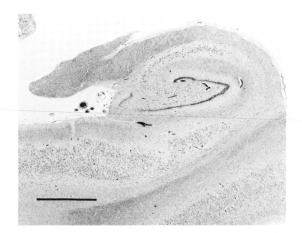

Fig. 6.14 Hippocampal sclerosis. Neuronal loss in Hl Sommer's sector and in end plate. The hippocampus is shrunken. Cresyl violet. Scale marker 2 mm.

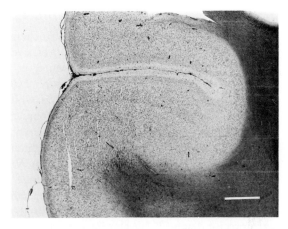

Fig. 6.15 Normal temporal neocortex. For comparison with Fig. 6.16. Luxol fast blue-cresyl violet. Scale marker 2 mm.

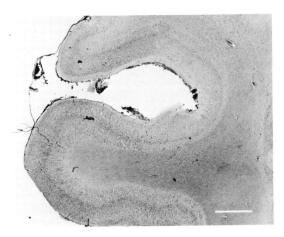

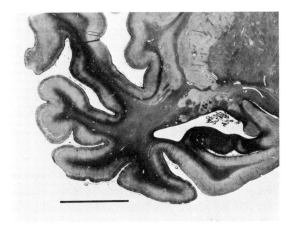

Fig. 6.16 Temporal neocortex. Cortical atrophy especially in depth of sulcus. The flask-shaped dilatation of the sulcus is the most readily apparent feature. From a 42-year-old man who had had focal seizures since 20 years of age. Early history not available. Luxol fast blue-PAS. Scale marker 2 mm.

Fig. 6.17 Sclerotic temporal atrophy. There is intense gliosis of the pes hippocampi and diffuse gliosis of gyral white matter. Cortex of all gyri shows patchy thinning and gliosis, especially in walls and depths of sulci. Long history of temporal lobe epilepsy. Holzer's method for glial fibres. Scale marker 1 cm.

(1968), Witelson & Pallie (1973) and Yeni-Komshian & Benson (1976) indicate that there are systematic anatomical differences between right and left temporal lobes. There are thus formidable difficulties in the path of morphometric investigation of resected temporal lobes. Additionally, Crome (1955) has pointed out that many of the

histopathological features seen in temporal lobe epilepsy occur in non-epileptic subjects including some of normal intelligence. Equally disturbing are the approximately 20% of therapeutically excised temporal lobes which show little or no morphological abnormality (Mathieson 1975a). Increasing experience suggests that recognition of

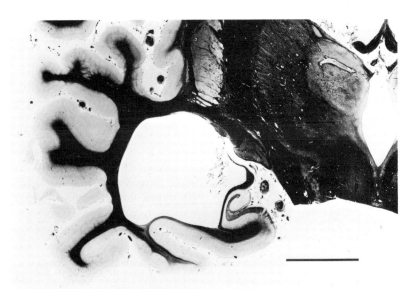

Fig. 6.18 Sclerotic temporal atrophy. Ulegyria of lateral and basal temporal gyri, extending to floor of insula. Hippocampal atrophy. Dilatation of temporal horn of lateral ventricle. Patient had a history of difficult birth and convulsions in infancy. Habitual seizures of varying pattern began at nine years; episodes of status epilepticus; death from unrelated causes at 50 years of age. Heidenhain's method for myelin. Scale marker 1 cm.

flask-shaped dilatation of sulci indicating local cortical atrophy will reduce this percentage. Those remaining emphasize the need for studies of dendritic and synaptic morphology and for biochemical collaboration.

CEREBELLAR LESIONS IN PATIENTS WITH EPILEPSY

These take the form of either a diffuse cortical atrophy with Purkinje cell loss, gliosis of the molecular layer and sometimes granular cell layer involvement, or a rather well-circumscribed lobular cerebellar sclerosis. This latter lesion (Fig. 6.19) is commonly bilateral and in the posterolateral cerebellar hemispheres suggesting a border zone hypoxia-ischaemic pathogenesis. Lobular cerebellar sclerosis is most often observed in institutionalized patients with severe seizures, making it tempting to assume that the lesion is the cumulative effect of ictal brain damage. While this may be so in some cases, the alternative view that the cerebral epileptogenic foci and the cerebellar lesions both stem from a common episode of perinatal anoxia or febrile convulsions (such as cause ulegyria of watershed distribution) is more attractive. The concepts are not mutually exclusive. The Purkinje and basket cells are known to be selectively vulnerable to hypoxia; boundary zone lesions occur either when there is

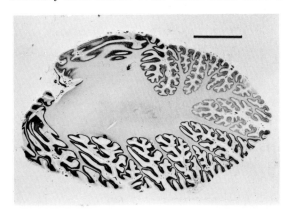

Fig. 6.19 Cerebellum. Lobular cerebellar sclerosis involving posterolateral parts of hemispheres bilaterally. Frequent generalized seizures began at 11 years; early history uncertain; erratic and antisocial behaviour. Death at 25 years due to aspiration pneumonia following seizure. Cresyl violet stain. Scale marker 1 cm.

an abrupt fall in blood pressure or sudden severe hypoxaemia (Brierly et al 1973). Cerebellar lesions in epileptic patients were recognized before the introduction of phenytoin and are probably not attributable to its use.

IATROGENIC LESIONS IN PATIENTS WITH EPILEPSY

The lesions include gingival hyperplasia, a peculiar form of lymphadenopathy and, arguably, cerebellar cortical abnormalities, all relating to phenytoin therapy.

The gum changes, histologically, consist of proliferation of the submucosal connective tissue with plasma cell infiltration and acanthosis of the epithelium (Van der Kwast 1956). Symmers (1978) regards the essential change as hyperplasia of connective tissue, but secondary inflammatory features are usually present.

Hydantoin lymphadenopathy most frequently involves cervical nodes which become enlarged but not matted. Histologically, there is proliferation of reticulum cells, formation of binucleate cells, some loss of nodal architecture, and variable degrees of eosinophilic infiltration and necrosis (Saltzstein & Ackerman, 1959, Krasznai & Györy 1968, Symmers 1978). The major differential diagnosis is that of Hodgkin's disease. Regression of nodal enlargement on withdrawal of the drug is the best demonstration of a benign reactive process. In very rare cases, the lymphadenopathy progresses to malignant lymphoma, even following initial regression (Gams et al 1968).

While an ataxic syndrome is well recognized clinically following phenytoin intoxication, its morphological basis, if any, has proved to be something of a mirage. Purkinje cell loss following phenytoin administration to experimental animals has been described (Utterback 1958 and other investigators) but morphometric studies by Dam (1972) do not confirm any such cell loss in rats, pigs or monkeys. Furthermore, Dam (1970) has shown that a diminished Purkinje cell population in patients with major seizures is related to the frequency of seizures rather than prolonged large doses of phenytoin. Fine structural changes in Purkinje cell dendrites in rats subjected to near lethal doses of phenytoin were described by Del Cerro & Snider (1967), but Nielsen et al (1971) found normal Purkinje cell ultrastructure in rats subject to intoxicating but sublethal doses of this drug.

CONCLUSION

The outstanding feature of any review of the pathology of epilepsy is the range and diversity of lesions which can give rise to seizures. It is clear that the obvious and readily categorized lesions are several steps removed from the essential local abnormality which is causative of seizures. Our inability to find consistent changes in patients with corticoreticular seizures emphasizes this problem. Whether the lesions are discrete and focal, or diffuse and subtle, the abnormal discharges take place in remaining viable neurones. Their environment has been changed not only in structure but also physiologically and biochemically. These aspects are considered in the ensuing section of this book.

REFERENCES

Aguilar M J, Rasmussen T 1960 Role of encephalitis in pathogenesis of epilepsy. Archives of Neurology 2:663

Aicardi J, Chevrie J J 1970 Convulsive status epilepticus in infants and children. A study of 239 cases. Epilepsia 11:187

Alexander G L, Norman R M 1960 The Sturge-Weber syndrome. Wright, Bristol

Banker B Q 1961 Cerebral vascular disease in infancy and childhood. I. Occlusive vascular disease. Journal of Neuropathology and Experimental Neurology 20:127

Banker B Q 1967 The neuropathological effects of anoxia and hypoglycaemia in the newborn. Developmental Medicine and Child Neurology 9:544

Bignami A, Appicciutoli L 1964 Micropolygyria and cerebral calcification in cytomegalic inclusion disease. Acta Neuropathologica 4:127

Bignami A, Palladini G, Zappella M 1968 Unilateral megalencephaly with nerve cell hypertrophy. An anatomical and quantitative histochemical study. Brain Research 9:103

Blackwood W, Corsellis J A N 1976 (eds) Greenfield's neuropathology. 3rd end. Edward Arnold, Edinburgh

Boehme D H, Cottrell J C, Leonberg S C, Zeman W 1971 A dominant form of neuronal ceroid-lipofuscinosis. Brain 94:745

Bolande R P 1974 The neurocristopathies. A unifying concept of disease arising in neural crest maldevelopment. Human Pathology 5:409

Brierly J B, Meldrum B S, Brown A W 1973 The threshold and neuropathology of cerebral 'anoxic-ischemic' cell change. Archives of Neurology 29:367

Brown W J 1973 In: Brazier M A B (ed) Epilepsy. Its phenomena in man. Academic Press, New York

Carey M E, Chou S N, French L A 1971 Long-term neurological residua in patients surviving brain abscess with surgery. Journal of Neurosurgery 34:652

Carpenter S, Karpati G, Andermann F 1972 Specific involvement of muscle, nerve and skin in late infantile and juvenile amaurotic idiocy. Neurology 22:170

Carpenter S, Karpati G, Wolfe L S, Andermann F (1973) A type of juvenile cerebromacular degeneration characterized by granular osmiophilic deposits. Journal of the Neurological Sciences 18:67

Cavanagh J B 1958 On certain small tumours encountered in the temporal lobe. Brain 81:389

Cavanagh J B, Meyer A 1956 Aetiological aspects of Ammon's horn sclerosis associated with temporal lobe epilepsy. British Medical Journal 2:1403

Caveness W F 1963 Onset and cessation of fits following craniocerebral trauma. Journal of Neurosurgery 20:570

Caveness W F, Liss H R 1961 Incidence of post-traumatic epilepsy. Epilepsia 2:123

Chalhub E G, Devivo D C, Siegal B A, Gado M H, Feigin R D 1977 Coxsackie A9 focal encephalitis associated with acute infantile hemiplegia and porencephaly. Neurology 27:574

Clark J V 1970 Familial occurrence of cavernous angiomata of the brain. Journal of Neurology, Neurosurgery and Psychiatry 33:871

Clark R M, Linell E A 1954 Case report: prenatal occlusion of the internal carotid artery. Journal of Neurology, Neurosurgery and Psychiatry 17:295

Cocker J, George S W, Yates P O 1965 Perinatal occlusion of the middle cerebral artery. Developmental Medicine and Child Neurology 7:235

Corsellis J A N 1957 the incidence of Ammon's horn sclerosis. Brain 80:193

Costeff N 1965 Convulsions in childhood. Their natural history and indications for treatment. New England Journal of Medicine 273:1410

Cravioto H, Feigin I 1960 Localized cerebral gliosis with giant neurons histologically resembling tuberous sclerosis. Journal of Neuropathology and Experimental Neurology 19:572

Crome L 1952 Microgyria. Journal of Pathology and Bacteriology 64:479

Crome L 1955 A morphological critique of temporal lobectomy. Lancet 1:882

Crome L 1957 Infantile cerebral gliosis with giant nerve cells. Journal of Neurology, Neurosurgery and Psychiatry 20:117

Crome L 1961 Cytomegalic inclusion – body disease. World Neurology 2:447

Crome L, France N E 1959 Microgyria and cytomegalic inclusion disease in infancy. Journal of Clinical Pathology 12:427

Dam M 1970 Number of Purkinje cells in patients with

grand mal epilepsy treated with diphenylhydantoin. Epilepsia 11:313

Dam M 1972 The density and ultrastructure of the Purkinje cells following diphenylhydantoin treatment in animals and man. Acta Neurolgica Scandinavica 48 (suppl 49):3

Dekaban A 1965 Large defects in cerebral hemispheres associated with cortical dysgenesis. Journal of Neuropathology and Experimental Neurology 24:512

Del Cerro M P, Snider R S 1967 Studies on Dilantin intoxication. Neurology 17:452

Dobbing J, Sands J 1973 Quantitative growth and development of human brain. Archives of Diseases in Childhood 48:757

Dobbing J, Smart J L 1974 Vulnerability of developing brain and behaviour. British Medical Bulletin 30:164

Dodge P R, Richardson E P, Victor M 1954 Recurrent convulsive seizures as a sequal to cerebral infarction: a clinical and pathological study. Brain 77:610

Dodge P R, Swartz M N 1965 Bacterial meningitis – a review of selected aspects. II. Special neurological problems, postmeningitic complications and clinicopathological correlations. New England Journal of Medicine 272:1003

Duvoisin R C, Vinson W M 1961 Tuberous sclerosis. Report of three cases without mental defect. Journal of the American Medical Association 175:869

Earle K M, Baldwin M, Penfield W 1953 Incisural sclerosis and temporal lobe seizures produced by hippocampal herniation at birth. Archives of Neurology and Psychiatry 69:27

Falconer M A 1970 Historical review. The pathological substrate of temporal lobe epilepsy. Guy's Hospital Reports 119:47

Falconer M A 1973 Reversibility by temporal-lobe resection of the behavioural abnormalities of temporal-lobe epilepsy. New England Journal of Medicine 289:451

Falconer M A, Rushworth R G 1960 Treatment of encephalotrigeminal angiomatosis (Sturge-Weber disease) by hemispherectomy. Archives of Disease in Childhood 35:433

Falconer M A, Taylor D C 1968 Surgical treatment of drug-resistant epilepsy due to mesial temporal sclerosis. Archives of Neurology 19:353

Falconer M A, Serafetinides E A, Corsellis J A N 1964 Etiology and pathogenesis of temporal lobe epilepsy. Archives of Neurology 10:233

Feindel W, Yamamoto Y L, Hodge C L 1971 Red cerebral veins and the cerebral steal syndrome. Evidence from fluorescein angiography and microregional blood flow by radioisotopes during excision of an angioma. Journal of Neurosurgery 35:167

Fowler M 1957 Brain damage after febrile convulsions. Archives of Diseases in Childhood 32:67

Fox H, Emery J L, Goodbody R A, Yates P O 1964 Neuro-cutaneous melanosis. Archives of Disease in Childhood 39:508

Frantzen E, Lennox-Buchthal M, Nygaard A, Stene J 1970 A genetic study of febrile convulsions. Neurology 20:909

Friede R L 1975 Developmental Neuropathology. New York – Springer-Verlag, Wien

Gams R A, Neal J A, Conrad F G 1968 Hydantoin induce pseudo-pseudolymphoma. Annals of Internal Medicine 69:557

Gastaut H, Poirier F, Payan H, Salamon G, Toga M,

Vigouroux M 1959 HHE syndrome. Hemiconvulsions, hemiplegia, epilepsy. Epilepsia 1:418

Geschwind N 1973 Effects of temporal lobe surgery on behaviour. New England Journal of Medicine 289:480

Geschwind N, Levitsky W 1968 Human brain: left–right asymmetries in temporal speech region. Science 161:186

Jennett B 1975 Epilepsy After Non-missile Head Injuries. 2nd edn. Heinemann, London

Juul-Jensen P 1963 Epilepsy. A clinical and social analysis of 1020 adult patients with epileptic seizures. Acta Neurologica Scandinavica 40 (suppl 5):1

Kirschbaum W 1947 Agenesis of the corpus callosum and associated malformations. Journal of Neuropathology and Experimental Neurology 6:78

Krasznai G, Györy Gy 1968 Hydantoin lymphadenopathy. Journal of Pathology and Bacteriology 95:314

Lagos J C, Gomez M R 1967 Tuberous sclerosis; reappraisal of a clinical entity. Mayo Clinic Proceedings 42:26

Laurence K M 1964a A case of unilateral megalencephaly. Developmental Medicine and Child Neurology 6:585

Laurence K M 1964b Megalencephaly (Annotation) Developmental Medicine and Child Neurology 6:638

Layton D D 1962 Heterotopic cerebral gray matter as an epileptogenic focus. Journal of Neuropathology and Experimental Neurology 21:244

Legg N J, Gupta P C, Scott D F 1973 Epilepsy following cerebral abscess. A clinical and EEG study of 70 patients. Brain 96:259

Lennox M A 1949a Febrile convulsions in childhood. A clinical and electroencephalographic study. American Journal of Diseases of Children 78:868

Lennox M A 1949b Febrile convulsions in childhood: their relationship to adult epilepsy. Journal of Pediatrics 35:427

Lennox-Buchthal M A 1973 Febrile convulsions. A reappraisal. Electroencephalography and clinical neurophysiology supplement no 32. Elsevier, Amsterdam

Lilienfeld A M. Pasamanick B 1954 Association of maternal and fetal factors with the development of epilepsy. I. Abnormalities of the prenatal and paranatal periods. Journal of the American Medical Association 155:719

Louis S, McDowell F 1967 Epileptic seizures in nonembolic cerebral infarction. Archives of Neurology 17:414

Margerison J H, Corsellis J A N 1966 epilepsy and the temporal lobes. A clinical, electroencephalographic and neuropathological study of the brain in epilepsy with particular reference to the temporal lobes. Brain 89:499

Marin-Padilla M 1972 Structural abnormalities of the cerebral cortex in human chromosomal aberrations: a Golgi study. Brain Research 44:625

Mathieson G 1975a Pathologic aspects of epilepsy with special reference to the surgical pathology of focal cerebral seizures. In: Purpura D P, Penry J K, Walter R D (eds) Advances in neurology Vol 8. Neurosurgical management of the epilepsies. Raven Press, New York

Mathieson G 1975b Pathology of temporal lobe foci. In: Penry J K, Daly D D (eds) Advances in neurology Vol II. Complex partial seizures and their treatment. Raven Press, New York

McCormick W F 1966 the pathology of vascular ('arteriovenous') malformations. Journal of Neurosurgery 24:807

Meldrum B S 1975 Present views on hippocampal sclerosis and epilepsy. In: Williams D (ed) Modern trends in neurology Vol 6. Butterworths, London

Meyer A, Beck E 1955 The hippocampal formation in

temporal lobe epilepsy. Proceedings of the Royal Society of Medicine 48:457

Meyer A, Falconer M A, Beck E 1954 Pathological findings in temporal lobe epilepsy. Journal of Neurology, Neurosurgery and Psychiatry 17:276

Miller F J W, Court S D M, Walton W S, Knox E J 1960 Growing up in Newcastle upon Tyne: a continuing study of health and illness in young children within their families. Oxford University Press, London

Morgan H, Wood M W, Murphy F 1973 Experience with 88 consecutive cases of brain abscess. Journal of Neurosurgery 38:698

Nelson K B, Ellenberger J H 1976 Predictors of epilepsy in children who have experienced febrile seizures. New England Journal of Medicine 295:1029

Nielsen M H, Dam M, Klinken L 1971 The ultrastructure of Purkinje cells in diphenylhydantoin intoxicated rats. Experimental Brain Research 12:447

Noonan S M, Desousa J, Riddle J M 1978 Lymphocyte ultrastructures in two cases of neuronal ceroid-lipofuscinosis. Neurology 28:472

Norman R M 1958 Malformations of the nervous system, birth injury and diseases of early life. In: Greenfield J G (ed) Neuropathology, Arnold, London

Norman R M, Urich H, McMenemey W H 1957 Vascular mechanisms of birth injury. Brain 80:49

Oppenheimer D R 1968 Microscopic lesions in the brain following head injury. Journal of Neurology, Neurosurgery and Psychiatry 31:299

Ounsted C 1952 The factor of inheritance in convulsive disorders in childhood. Proceedings of the Royal Society of Medicine 45:865

Ounsted C 1955 Genetic and social aspect of the epilepsies of childhood. Eugenics Review 47:33

Ounsted C 1967 Temporal lobe epilepsy: the problem of aetiology and prophylaxis. Journal of the Royal College of Physicians of London 1:273

Ounsted C 1971 In: Gairdner D, Hull D (eds) Recent advances in paediatrics. 4th edn. Churchill, London

Ounsted C, Lindsay J, Norman R 1966 Biological factors in temporal lobe epilepsy. Clinics in developmental medicine no 22. Heinemann, London

Pasamanick B, Lilienfeld A M 1955 Maternal and fetal factors in the development of epilepsy. 2. Relationship to some clinical features of epilepsy. Neurology 5:77

Peach B 1965 Arnold-Chiari malformation. Anatomic features of 20 cases. Archives of Neurology 12:613

Penfield W, Humphreys S 1940 Epileptogenic lesions of the brain. A histologic study. Archives of Neurology and Psychiatry 43:240

Penfield W, Jasper H 1954 Epilepsy and the functional anatomy of the human brain. Little Brown, Boston

Penfield W, Ward A 1948 Calcifying epileptogenic lesions. Haemangioma calcificans; report of a case. Archives of Neurology and Psychiatry 60:20

Perot P, Weir B, Rasmussen T 1966 Tuberous sclerosis. Surgical therapy for seizures. Archives of Neurology 15:498

Rasmussen T 1969 Surgical therapy of post traumatic epilepsy. In: Walker A E, Caveness W F, Critchley M (eds) The late effects of head injury. Thomas, Springfield

Rasmussen T, Gossman H 1963 Epilepsy due to gross destructive brain lesions. Neurology 13:659

Rasmussen T, Mathieson G, LeBlanc F 1972 Surgical therapy of typical and a forme fruste variety of the Sturge-Weber Syndrome. Schweizer Archiv für Neurologie, Neurochirurgie und Psychiatrie 111:393

Rasmussen T, Olszewski J, Lloyd-Smith D 1958 Focal seizures due to chronic localized encephalitis. Neurology 8:435

Remillard G M, Ethier R, Andermann F 1974 Temporal lobe epilepsy and perinatal occlusion of the posterior cerebral artery. Neurology 24:1001

Richardson E P 1958 Late life epilepsy. Medical Clinics of North America 42:349

Richardson E P, Dodge P R 1954 Epilepsy in cerebral vascular disease. Epilepsia (3rd series) 3:49

Richman D P, Stewart R M, Caviness V S Jr 1974 Cerebral microgyria in a 27-week fetus. An architectonic and topographic analysis. Journal of Neuropathology and Experimental Neurology 33:374

Roden V J, Cantor H E, O'Connor D M, Schmidt R R, Cherry J D 1975 Acute hemiplegia of childhood associated with Coxsackie A9 viral infection. Journal of Pediatrics 86:56

Rose S W, Penry J K, Markush R E, Radloff L A, Putnam P L 1973 Prevalence of epilepsy in children. Epilepsia 14:133

Rubinstein L J 1972 Tumours of the central nervous system. Atlas of Tumor Pathology, 2nd Series, Fasicle 6. Armed Forces Institute of Pathology, Washington DC

Russell D S, Rubinstein L J 1977 Pathology of tumours of the nervous system. Arnold, London

Saltzstein S L, Ackerman L V 1959 Lymphadenopathy induced by anti-convulsant drugs and mimicking clinically and pathologically malignant lymphomas. Cancer 12:164

Sano K, Malamud N 1953 Clinical significance of sclerosis of the cornu Ammonis. Archives of Neurology and Psychiatry 70:40

Scheibel M E, Crandall P H, Scheibel A B 1974 The hippocampaldentate complex in temporal lobe epilepsy. A Golgi study. Epilepsia 15:55

Scheibel M E, Scheibel A B 1973 In: Brazier M A B (ed) Epilepsy. Its phenomena in man. Academic Press, New York

Schuman S H, Miller L J 1966 Febrile convulsions in families: findings in an epidemiological survey. Clinical Pediatrics 5:604

Slaughter J C, Hardman J M, Kempe L G, Earle K M 1969 Neurocutaneous melanosis and leptomeningeal melanomatosis in children. Archives of Pathology 88:298

Smith J F, Landing B H 1960 Mechanisms of brain damage in H. influenzae meningitis. Journal of Neuropathology and Experimental Neurology 19:248

Strich S J 1956 Diffuse degeneration of the cerebral white matter in severe dementia following head injury. Journal of Neurology, Neurosurgery and Psychiatry 19:163

Strich S J 1961 Shearing of nerve fibres as a cause of brain damage due to head injury. Lancet 2:443

Symmers W StC 1978 In: Symmers, W StC (ed) Systemic Pathology, Vol 2. 2nd end. Churchill Livingstone, Edinburgh

Taylor D C 1969 Differential rates of cerebral maturation between sexes and between hemispheres. Evidence from epilepsy. Lancet 2:140

Taylor D C, Ounsted C 1971 Biological mechanisms influencing the outcome of seizures in response to fever. Epilepsia 12:33

Taylor D C, Falconer M A, Bruton C T, Corsellis J A N 1971 Focal dysplasia of the cerebral cortex in epilepsy.

Journal of Neurology, Neurosurgery and Psychiatry 34:369

Temkin O 1971 The falling sickness. 2nd ed. Johns Hopkins Press, Baltimore, p 35

Thom D A 1942 Convulsions of early life and their relation to the chronic convulsive disorders and mental defect. American Journal of Psychiatry 98:574

Tytus J S, Pennybacker J 1956 Pearly tumours in relation to the central nervous system. Journal of Neurology, Neurosurgery and Psychiatry 19:241

Urich H 1976 In: Blackwood W, Corsellis J A N (eds) Greenfield's neuropathology. Arnold, London

Utterback R A 1958 parenchymatous cerebellar degeneration complicating diphenylhydantoin (Dilantin) therapy. Archives of Neurology and Psychiatry 80:180

Van den Berg B J, Yerushalmy J 1969 Studies on convulsive disorders in young children. 1. Incidence of febrile and nonfebrile convulsions by age and other factors. Pediatric Research 3:298

Van der Kwast W A M 1956 Speculations regarding the nature of gingival hyperplasia due to diphenylhydantoin-sodium. Acta Medica Scandinavica 153:399

Van Heycop ten Ham 1974 Lafora disease. A form of progressive myoclonus epilepsy. In: Vinken P J, Bruyn G W (eds) Handbook of clinical neurology Vol 15. North Holland Publishing, Amsterdam

Waddington M W 1970 Angiographic changes in focal motor epilepsy. Neurology 20:879

White J C, Liu C T, Mixter W J 1948 Focal epilepsy. A statistical study of its causes and the results of surgical treatment. I. Epilepsy secondary to intracranial tumours. New England Journal of Medicine 238:891

Witelson S F, Pallie W 1973 Left hemisphere specialisation for language in the newborn. Neuroanatomical evidence of asymmetry. Brain 96:641

Worster-Drought C, Dickson W E C, McMenemy W H, (1937) Multiple meningeal and perineural tumours with analogous tumours in the glia and ependyma (neurofibroblastomatosis). Brain 60:85

Wyke B D 1959 The cortical control of movement. A contribution to the surgical physiology of seizures. Epilepsia (4th series) 1:4

Yeni-Komshian G H, Benson D A 1976 Anatomical study of cerebral asymmetry in the temporal lobe of humans, chimpanzees and rhesus monkeys. Science 192:387

Zeman W, Donahue S, Dyken P, Green J 1970 The neuronal ceroidlipofuscinoses (Batten-Vogt Syndrome). In: Vinken P J, Bruyn G W (eds) Handbook of clinical neurology Vol 10. North Holland Publishing, Amsterdam

Zimmerman H M 1938 The histopathology of convulsive disorders in children. Journal of Pediatrics 13:859

7

Pathophysiology

B. S. Meldrum

An ideal account of the pathophysiology of epilepsy would provide an explanation for the clinical phenomena of epilepsy in terms of events described at the cellular or molecular level. A great deal is known about abnormal patterns of electrical activity that can be recorded at the cellular level during ictal or interictal activity, in both focal and generalized epilepsy. Some of this information is summarized in Chapter 8. A recent volume provides up-to-date reviews (Delgado-Escueta et al 1986). However, most of the clinical phenomena of epilepsy cannot yet be described in terms of molecular or cellular events.

In this chapter the action of physiological and pathological processes in epileptic phenomena will be described under four headings:

1. Systemic factors, physiological and pathological, that influence the occurrence of seizures
2. Epileptogenesis at the cellular level
3. Physiological events that occur as a result of seizures
4. Pathological changes that occur in the brain as a result of seizures.

SYSTEMIC FACTORS

That physiological or pathological changes involving the whole body can increase the excitability of the brain, and thus favour the occurrence of fits in predisposed subjects, has been appreciated since the time of Galen. Fits occurring subsequent to systemic disturbances can be considered in three categories. First, patients with epilepsy sometimes find that their usual type of seizure is apt to occur under certain physiological circumstances (e.g. on awakening, premenstrually, during overbreathing or hypoglycaemia). Secondly, fits may occur in subjects with an appropriate predisposition only during a specific stress (e.g. febrile convulsions in a genetically predisposed child). Thirdly, in subjects with no neurological abnormality, and no special predisposition to seizures, certain severe stresses (including profound hypoglycaemia and a wide range of poisonings) may induce focal or generalized seizures.

The factors discussed below are all quantifiable and their effects on seizures have been demonstrated in both clinical and experimental studies. Many patients and their physicians believe that emotional stress can favour the occurrence of fits and there is evidence for a clinical group where seizures occur only after stress (Friis & Lund 1974). Emotional stress is often accompanied by some of the physiological changes discussed below, such as overbreathing and, most important, the lack of sleep. However, it is possible that psychological factors can modify cerebral excitability irrespective of systemic changes.

Water and electrolyte disturbances

If the quantity of water, sodium, calcium or magnesium in the extracellular or intracellular compartments of the body is abnormal, seizures may be facilitated in epileptic and non-epileptic subjects. Table 7.1 summarizes data on critical variations in plasma composition. Systemic disturbances of potassium balance tend not to alter susceptibility to seizures. Reviews of disturbances of hydration and electrolytes in relation to epilepsy are provided by Teglbjaerg (1936), Reynolds (1970) and Millichap (1974).

Table 7.1 Deviations in plasma composition and seizure activity

	Normal range	Deviation	'Epileptogenicity' in humans		Seizures in animals	References
			No epilepsy	With epilepsy		
Arterial PO₂:	11–14 kPa (85–105 mm Hg)	<4kPa (30mm Hg)	+ gm (++ ts)	+ pm	++	Luft & Noell (1956); Passouant et al (1967)
		>300kPa	++		+++	Wood (1972)
Arterial PCO₂	4.7–6.0 kPa (35–45 mm Hg)	<4 kPa (30 mm Hg)	0	++ pm / + gm		Lennox et al (1936); Toman & Davis (1949)
		>32 kPa (240 mm Hg)	0		++	Woodbury et al (1958)
Glucose	2.5–10 mmol/l (45–180 mg/100 ml)	<1.2 mmol/l (22 mg/100 ml)	+++ my / + gm	+		Poiré (1969)
		>40 mmol/l (720 mg/100 ml)	+		+	Maccario (1968)
Sodium	132–142 mmol/l	<125 mmol/l	+	+	+++	Rymer & Fishman (1973); Funck-Brentano et al (1960)
		150 mmol/l	++	+		Morris-Jones et al (1967)
Calcium	2.25–2.65 mmol/l (9–10.6 mg/100 ml)	<1.7 mmol/l (6.5 mg/100 ml)	++ my or ts / + gm	++ my or ts	+++	Frame & Carter (1955); Corriol et al (1969); Glaser & Levy (1960)
Magnesium	0.7–0.9 mmol/l (1.4–1.8 mEq/l)	<0.6mmol/l (1.2 mEq/l)	+		++	Suter & Klingman (1955); Kruse et al (1932)
Urea	2.5–7.5 mmol/l	>25 mmol/l	+		++	Prill et al (1969); Zuckerman & Glaser (1972)
Ammonia	23–41 μmol/l	>500 μmol/l	+		+ or ++	Hindfelt & Siesjö (1971); Gastaut et al (1968)
Osmolarity	285–295 mosmol/kg	>340 mosmol/kg	+		+	Kurtz et al (1971); Singh (1973)

Values are given in SI Units (with traditional units in parenthesis).
'Epileptogenicity' is graded as:

+	=	0–33%
++	=	33–67%
+++	=	67–100%

pm = petit mal; gm = grand mal
f   = focal seizure; my = myoclonus
hs = habitual pattern of seizure; ts = tonic spasm.

Overhydration, hyponatraemia

The experimental induction of seizures by over-hydration was described by Rowntree (1923, 1926). Subsequently, a pitressin water load test was devised (McQuarrie & Peeler 1931) to confirm or eliminate the diagnosis of epilepsy. The habitual type of attack was reliably induced in epileptic children given pitressin and an oral water load (2–5 ml/kg each hour). Seizures did not occur in non-epileptic children. This test was used to screen military recruits in the 1939–45 war (see Garland et al 1943) but is no longer in routine use.

Children with no neurological abnormality may experience generalized seizures during the course of rehydration following a severe dehydrating illness or after hypernatraemia (Melekian et al 1962, Friis-Hansen & Buchthal 1965).

Overhydration is usually associated with a reduction in the osmolarity of plasma and with hyponatraemia, i.e. a plasma sodium concentration below 125 mEq/l. Hyponatraemia with coma, or more rarely convulsions, can occur in anterior hypopituitarism and in Addison's disease; it is more commonly the result of inadequate management of an acute illness. Hyponatraemia seizures are not uncommon in psychiatric patients as a result of self-induced water intoxication (Jose et al 1979).

Seizures due to overhydration or to hyponatraemia respond poorly to antiepileptic drugs. The slow administration of hypertonic saline (e.g. 3% NaCl) is the usual treatment. The successful use of rapid IV administration of 50 ml of 29.2% saline has recently been described (Worthley & Thomas 1986). Potassium or calcium depletion may also require correction.

Experimentally, generalized seizures can be induced by administering a massive water load to normal rats, rabbits or cats (Funck-Brentano et al 1960, Waltregny & Mesdjian 1969). Such seizures can be prevented if sodium chloride is given with the water load. During a rapid reduction in plasma osmolarity the brain swells, because of an increase in intracellular water. This so-called *vasogenic* cerebral oedema occurs also after local ischaemia (Klatzo 1967) and favours the initiation of epileptic activity. In water-intoxicated rats, the potassium content of the brain (on a dry weight basis) is reduced by 20%. This ion shift probably serves to limit brain swelling. Coma and convulsions appear to arise from the increase in intra-cellular water rather than the decrease in potassium content (Rymer & Fishman 1973).

Dehydration, hypernatraemia, hyperosmolal coma

Illnesses associated with severe dehydration are not uncommonly complicated by seizures. Melekian et al (1962) saw convulsions in 48 out of 324 children with acute dehydration, an incidence of 15%. However, a high proportion of the children with convulsions were pyrexial and in two-thirds of the cases convulsions occurred during rehydration. The incidence of convulsions during rehydration can be reduced by infusing saline and calcium as well as glucose. Hypernatraemia (i.e. plasma sodium concentration above 150 mEq/l) usually accompanies dehydration, but it may also occur in the absence of dehydration, sometimes as a complication of focal cerebral disorders involving the hypothalamus or frontal lobe (Lascelles & Lewis 1972). Seizures may accompany hypernatraemia. They are very apt to occur during its correction even when this is performed cautiously so as to avoid overhydration or hyponatraemia.

Hyperosmolal coma may occur when the combined osmotic effect of plasma electrolytes and glucose exceeds 340 mosmol/kg. It usually takes the form of non-ketotic diabetic coma, in which blood glucose concentrations of 33–66 mmol/l (600–1200 mg/100 ml) are found. Generalized or focal convulsions sometimes complicate such comas, indeed epilepsia partialis continua is the presenting symptom in 6% of cases (Singh et al 1973). That convulsions are a direct consequence of the hyperosmolality is suggested by the high incidence of convulsions in hyperosmolal coma induced in experimental animals by loading glucose, saline, mannitol or urea (Maccario 1968, Zuckerman & Glaser 1972).

In rats, perfusion with hypertonic mannitol leads to focal opening of the blood–brain barrier associated with a marked increase in local glucose utilization, which probably indicates focal seizure activity (Pappius et al 1979). Osmotically induced shrinkage of the brain can modify the blood–brain barrier and permit more ready access to the brain of substances normally partially, or totally, excluded. It can also cause subdural haemorrhages through venous ruptures (Luttrell et al 1959).

It has frequently been claimed that cellular dehydration or plasma hyperosmolality has a protective action against seizures. Clearly, in cases where generalized or focal cerebral oedema is a contributory cause of the seizures, cellular dehydration might well diminish the probability of seizure activity.

Several American authors had difficulty repeating the initial successful results with dehydration therapy described by Fay (1929, 1931). Teglbjaerg (1936), in two relatively large trials of epileptic inpatients, found that a dehydrating diet reduced the incidence of generalized seizures in 68% of men and 80% of women. However, most of the patients were receiving barbiturates and dehydration might have been effective through an elevation of the plasma barbiturate content.

Experiments originally considered to show that cerebral dehydration protects rodents against chemically induced convulsions (Defeudis & Elliott 1967) should probably be explained by a different mechanism (Meldrum & Stephenson 1975).

Hypocalcaemia

Ionized calcium 'stabilizes' nerve and muscle cell membranes, preventing spontaneous or mechanically triggered oscillations in membrane potential. Movement of calcium ions across the nerve cell membrane plays an important role in synaptic transmission. Approximately half the 2.25–2.65 mmol calcium/litre serum is protein-bound, the proportion depending on the serum protein concentration. Tetany and seizures are not unusual when the ionized calcium concentration falls below 0.6 mmol/l (2.4 mg/100 ml). Such hypocalcaemia may be seen following parathyroidectomy, in rickets and neonatal tetany, in steatorrhoea or in the therapy of severe dehydration. Tetany and seizures due to hypocalcaemia respond promptly to the administration of calcium gluconate.

Hypomagnesaemia

In some cases of tetany and seizures, the serum levels of both magnesium and calcium are low and a clear therapeutic response is obtained following the administration of magnesium sulphate. Such treatment raises plasma ionized calcium concentration (Zimmet 1968). Magnesium depletion has been described in the course of various nutritional and metabolic disorders and is sometimes associated with seizures (Suter & Klingman 1955).

Hypoglycaemia

We can distinguish three types of seizure which occur during hypoglycaemia. First, in a minority of patients with epilepsy, mild to moderate hypoglycaemia sometimes precipitates their habitual type of seizure, which may therefore be an absence or a focal Jacksonian fit, a temporal lobe seizure or a generalized seizure. Fits triggered in this way occur well before the stage of hypoglycaemic coma is reached; usually only mild signs and symptoms of hypoglycaemia are present (increased pulse pressure, sweating, hunger).

The second type of seizure is seen most clearly in patients at or after the transition from pre-coma to coma in the course of profound insulin-induced hypoglycaemia (as in insulin therapy for schizophrenia, but also in brittle diabetics and the newborn). Initially, there is irregular and fragmentary myoclonus, commonly involving the muscles of the face or of one limb. It becomes progressively more rhythmic, generalized and sustained, and is associated with rhythmic spikes and waves on the EEG. This generalized myoclonus may lead to a tonic seizure associated with the usual EEG picture of fast rhythmic activity of augmenting amplitude, followed by a phase of slow generalized myoclonus, and then post-ictal depression with an isoelectric EEG record. In a series of over 20 000 insulin comas in schizophrenic patients (Poire 1969), myoclonus was seen in 90% of comas, but generalized tonic-clonic seizures in only 3%. Although patients responding to hypoglycaemia with tonic-clonic seizures were not known to suffer from epilepsy, most of them showed EEG signs of epilepsy during stroboscopic stimulation. Myoclonus, or seizures following myoclonus, can be aborted within seconds by the intravenous administration of glucose. The mechanism linking cerebral glucose metabolism with seizure activity is uncertain; brain energy state is unchanged at this stage in experimental hypoglycaemia (Lewis et al 1974a) but the concentration of amino acids and tricarboxylic acid cycle intermediates is altered (Lewis et al 1974b).

Thirdly, during profound hypoglycaemic coma, tonic spasms sometimes appear while the EEG shows generalized high amplitude delta activity. This phenomenon occurs irrespective of any epileptic predisposition and is apparently a release phenomenon arising in subcortical centres and thus comparable to anoxic spasms. Experimentally, it occurs when derangement of cerebral energy metabolism is demonstrable. The brain is undoubtedly at risk of hypoglycaemic brain damage.

Clinical significance

Except in petit mal, hypoglycaemia is only rarely a cause of fits. There is experimental evidence that moderately severe hypoglycaemia makes some types of epileptic activity less likely (Naquet et al 1970). This may explain the observation that patients with epilepsy are not more likely than non epileptics to show generalized convulsions during therapeutic insulin coma.

The weak focal myoclonus that may be the only sign of sustained epileptic activity during profound hypoglycaemia in the newborn, is not always recognized as the urgent signal for therapy that it is. Hypoglycaemia in the absence of seizure activity can produce brain damage (Ingram et al 1967, Meldrum et al 1971, Brierley et al 1971a, b) and the presence of seizure activity exacerbates the crisis by augmenting the energy demand, but sometimes also leads to an increase in blood glucose (see p. 223).

Blood gases and pH

That a reduction in atmospheric pressure can induce seizures in animals was demonstrated by Boyle (1660). The use of overbreathing to reduce the partial pressure of carbon dioxide and trigger epileptic activity is routine in electroencephalography. However, seizure susceptibility is often unchanged during severe changes in plasma pH occurring during metabolic acidosis or alkalosis.

As with the disturbances of water, electrolytes and glucose, we must consider both the possibility of triggering seizures in patients with epilepsy and of convulsions in patients with no chronic neurological disorder.

Cerebral oxygenation

Moderate cerebral hypoxia may occasionally facilitate epileptic activity in patients with epilepsy, especially petit mal. With sudden severe hypoxia, as in sudden atmospheric decompression, a small number of susceptible subjects (not necessarily having epilepsy) show grand mal seizures at the moment of transition to unconsciousness. During profound unconsciousness, when scalp EEG records indicate that cortical activity is suppressed, tonic spasms may be observed. Oxygen is essential for the energy metabolism that sustains epileptic activity. In experimental drug-induced convulsions, the cortical epileptic discharges can be suppressed by systemic hypoxia (Gellhorn & Ballin 1950, Caspers & Speckmann 1972).

The seizures directly related to impaired cerebral oxygenation that provide the most important clinical problem are those which occur during the course of recovery. After severe cerebral anoxia, however caused (e.g. asphyxia, cardiac arrest, cerebral air embolism, vascular obstruction, head injury, atmospheric decompression), restoration of cerebral blood flow and oxygenation is commonly complicated by seizures. These first appear one to four hours after the anoxic episode, at the time that cerebral oedema is also first evident and when ischaemic cell change becomes histologically apparent. Status epilepticus carries a particularly bad prognosis: it is common when the stress has led to brain damage and it may itself damage the brain. Lesions that result from cerebral hypoxia or ischaemia may become the focal source of seizures later in life (see below).

Hyperbaric oxygen Partial pressures of oxygen in the blood produced by breathing pure oxygen at 3–6 atmospheres pressure (300–600 kPa) induce generalized tonic-clonic seizures in animals and humans. Although diving accidents of this kind are now rare, the situation is of considerable theoretical and experimental interest. Oxidation occurs in SH groups that play a critical role in certain enzymes (either in the active centre or by maintaining the tertiary structure of the enzyme). Among the enzymes affected is glutamic acid decarboxylase which synthesises gamma-amino-butyric acid (GABA), a major inhibitory neuro-transmitter within the brain. A correlation has been demonstrated between the fall in brain GABA content and the onset of seizures during hyperbaric oxygenation (Wood 1972).

Carbon dioxide

Changes in the partial pressure of carbon dioxide in the arterial blood dramatically modify cerebral blood flow (reviewed by Purves 1972). The reduction in $PaCO_2$ following hyperventilation reduces cerebral blood flow to 40% of normal; breathing air containing 7% of carbon dioxide doubles cerebral blood flow (Kety & Schmidt 1948). The reduced availability of oxygen to the brain during hyperventilation can be demonstrated by polarographic measurements (Cooper 1974). This cerebral hypoxia is thought to be partially responsible for the diffuse frontal slow waves and for the activation of epileptic activity (especially of bursts of spikes and waves associated with motor signs of petit mal) seen during hyperventilation. There is also evidence from clinical and experimental studies that the $PaCO_2$ modifies cerebral activity and excitability independently of any effect on cerebral oxygenation (Wyke 1963). Thus, when the activating effect of hyperventilation on EEG signs of epilepsy was first reported (Lennox et al 1936), suppression of such signs by raised respiratory carbon dioxide was also described. Experimentally, the threshold for electroconvulsive shock rises in animals breathing carbon dioxide mixtures containing up to 15% CO_2. However, very high concentrations of CO_2 (30–40%) may facilitate convulsions and coma (Brodie & Woodbury 1958, Woodbury et al 1958). Convulsions induced in monkeys or small mammals can be suppressed by the inhalation of 9–40% CO_2 (Meyer et al 1961; Caspers & Speckmann 1972). In rats, inhalation of 25–35% CO_2 induces seizures (Woodbury et al 1958, Withrow 1972).

Activation of epilepsy by respiratory alkalosis and inhibition by acidosis is probably related to changes in intracellular pH. Acidosis favours the synthesis of the inhibitory transmitter GABA; alkalosis favours its further metabolism by GABA-transaminase (Meldrum 1975b).

Temperature

Febrile convulsions (seizures associated with pyrexia, believed to result from infection not involving the brain) are common in infants and young children, affecting 29–72 per 1000 (Lennox-Buchthal 1973). The incidence is maximal between 9 and 20 months of age. There is a strong genetic element controlling susceptibility to febrile convulsions. In general, the severity of the pyrexia, not the nature of the illness, determines the occurrence of a fit; in 75% of children the temperature is above 39.2° C (Herlitz 1941). Hyperthermia induced artificially in the absence of infection in rats, rabbits and kittens leads to generalized convulsions (Millichap 1968).

The clinical features of febrile convulsions are described in Chapter 4. Seizures are usually isolated or brief. Prolonged or repetitive seizures are sometimes followed by behavioural disorders, neurological deficits and later established epilepsy (Ounsted et al 1966, Aicardi & Chevrie 1970; Lennox-Buchthal 1973). This commonly takes the form of temporal lobe seizures, but petit mal is seen in 10–20% of children developing epilepsy after febrile convulsions (Lennox-Buchthal 1973). The occurrence of a unilateral Ammon's horn sclerosis as a result of prolonged febrile convulsions is discussed below.

A separate phenomenon is that of pyrexia secondary to seizures. This may arise as a result of the increased energy consumption by the brain, heart and muscles during the seizure, or because of disturbance in the temperature regulating mechanisms. The effect of sustained myoclonic activity is evident in experimental studies (Meldrum & Horton 1973a, Meldrum et al 1973).

The raised cerebral temperature increases the likelihood of epileptic brain damage (Meldrum & Brierley 1973).

Aminoff & Simon (1980) found rectal temperatures elevated in 79 of 90 adult patients in status. Temperatures of 107° F in 2 patients with prolonged status, were associated with severe neurological sequelae.

Sleep

The complex and important relationships between seizures and the sleeping – waking cycle have been reviewed by Janz (1974), Kellaway (1985) and Baldy-Moulinier (1986). Four phenomena can be differentiated:

1. The traditional observation that in many patients seizures occur predominantly at a particular time of day was analysed quantitatively by Langdon-Down & Brain (1929), and a synthesis of more recent studies is given by Janz (1974). Adults with major seizures can be classified as: *random epilepsies*, not contingent upon the phase of the sleeping-waking cycle (23%); *sleep epilepsies*, generalized, often originating in the temporal lobe, occurring predominantly just after falling asleep or in the early morning sleep period (44%); and *waking epilepsies*, grand mal seizures occurring after waking or during the late afternoon (30%). Over the years, some waking epilepsies and some sleep epilepsies become random epilepsies. The majority of random epilepsies are symptomatic whereas waking epilepsies are only about 10%. The shift towards sleeping and random epilepsies during the course of the illness probably reflects the development or progression of brain damage related to the seizures (see Section 4 of this chapter).

2. Interictal EEG signs of epilepsy appear preferentially in certain phases of sleep and wakefulness; the distribution between the phases is different according to the kind of seizure (this is discussed in Ch. 8). Not surprisingly, background slowing and dysrhythmias are more common during waking in waking epilepsy than in sleeping epilepsy (Christian 1960).

3. Abnormalities of sleep patterns are found in patients with epilepsy. An excess of the deeper phases of sleep is found in patients with sleep epilepsy, particularly in patients with generalized seizures that originate in the temporal lobe. An excess of light sleep occurs in patients with waking epilepsy (Jovanovic 1967).

4. Perhaps related to the above, sleep deprivation increases the likelihood of certain types of seizure, especially waking epilepsy (grand mal) and pykno-epilepsy (very frequent absences). Sleep deprivation can be used as a specific precipitant for diagnostic purposes in the latter two syndromes (Christian 1960, Bennett 1963). Deprivation of rapid-eye movement (REM) sleep in rats or cats leads to lowering of the electroshock seizure threshold (Owen & Bliss 1970, Cohen et al 1970).

In the pathophysiology of epilepsy, the phenomena relating to the sleep-waking cycle have a two-fold significance. First, they indicate an important biological difference between sleeping and waking epilepsies. Secondly, they challenge the research worker to identify the physiological features of sleep and wakefulness that are responsible for the changes in seizure susceptibility: these may include endocrine or metabolic factors as numerous hormones show circadian rhythms, most notably cortisol (Dixon et al 1974) but also growth hormone (Sassin et al 1969). There are changes in body temperature, water and electrolyte excretion. Wakefulness and the different phases of sleep are associated with altered activity in the serotoninergic and catecholaminergic systems that ascend from the brain stem (Jouvet 1972) and there is much experimental evidence linking changes in seizure threshold to changes in activity in aminergic systems (Meldrum et al 1975). Changes in background EEG rhythms are associated with altered seizure susceptibility and incidence of EEG signs of epilepsy.

Nutrition

Food intake can modify the tendency to seizures either because of a specific deficiency (e.g. vitamin B, magnesium) or an excess (e.g. water, lipids).

An intake of lipids that is very high relative to protein and carbohydrate forms the basis of the 'ketogenic diet' which has some therapeutic action in childhood epilepsy (Wilder 1921, Huttenlocher et al 1971, Livingston 1972). The mechanism of this is not understood. The metabolic acidosis itself is probably not antiepileptic; there may be some degree of cerebral dehydration involved. It has recently been shown that the brain in young animals and in starving people is capable of utilizing ketone bodies (acetoacetate and β-hydroxybutyrate) for energy metabolism (Owen et al 1967, Hawkins et al 1971) and this metabolic shift might change seizure susceptibility.

The plasma concentrations of acetoacetate and β-hydroxybutyrate rise in rats fed on a high-fat diet. The cerebral sodium content also increases and the electroconvulsive shock threshold is elevated (Appleton & DeVivo 1974).

The possibility is currently being explored that the concentration of inhibitory transmitter substances in the brain can be raised by dietary treatments. GABA (gamma-aminobutyric acid) glycine and taurine are putative central inhibitory neurotransmitter compounds (Curtis & Johnston 1974, Meldrum 1985). Experimental studies indicate that they enter the brain only to a very limited extent following systemic administration. However, it is possible to raise the cerebral concentration of serotonin and noradrenaline by administration of the precursors L-tryptophan and tyrosine. The effect on seizures in humans of changes in brain amine content has yet to be defined (Chadwick et al 1978).

Dietary deficiency of vitamin B_6 can give rise to seizures in infants fed deficient milk preparations (Coursin 1954). Vitamin B_6 forms pyridoxal phosphate, a coenzyme essential for numerous cerebral enzymes, including glutamic acid decarboxylase, which synthesizes the inhibitory transmitter GABA (reviewed by Meldrum 1975b).

Endocrine changes

As already indicated, hormones influencing plasma osmolarity or content of glucose ionized calcium can modify seizure susceptibility. Hormones with other primary actions that have been shown clinically and experimentally to influence the course of fits include glucocorticoids, thyroxine, oestrogen and progesterone. Pituitary dysfunction, because of its influence on the other systems, may also be a factor affecting seizure susceptibility. A

review of experimental studies on the role of hormones is given by Timiras (1969).

As well as the effect of primary disorders of endocrine function on the occurrence of seizures, there is also evidence for altered endocrine function occurring secondarily to epilepsy or to antiepileptic drug therapy. Thus, plasma levels of sex-hormone binding globulins are commonly raised in patients on antiepileptic drug therapy (see Toone 1986). In males, this may be associated with a decrease in plasma free testosterone and reduced sexual activity.

Hormonal changes that directly follow seizures are discussed below.

Adrenal steroids and ACTH

Mineralocorticoids have an antiepileptic action in several test systems. An anaesthetic-like action of desoxycorticosterone acetate was described by Selye (1941), and it was subsequently reported to give therapeutic benefit to some patients with grand mal seizures (Aird & Gordan 1951). Woodbury and numerous colleagues (reviewed Woodbury 1958) demonstrated a raised threshold for electroshock seizures in animals treated with desoxycorticosterone.

Glucocorticoids (cortisol and related eleven-oxosteroids) when given to rats increase brain excitability and lower the electroshock seizure threshold (Woodbury & Vernadakis 1966). An acute seizure-enhancing effect of the administration of cortisone has been demonstrated in baboons with photosensitive epilepsy (Ehlers & Killam 1979). That a similar effect may operate in humans is suggested by the occurrence of convulsions in Cushings's syndrome (Starr 1952). The mechanism is unknown.

Although petit mal may be benefited by ACTH or steroids (Miribel & Poirier 1961), the syndrome that responds most decisively to ACTH or adrenal steroids is hypsarrhythmia – infantile spasms (Sorel & Dusaucy-Bauloye, 1958, Jeavons & Bower 1964). This effect is probably by mineralocorticoids. It is independent of cortisol stimulation (Farwell et al 1984). Commonly, the brain shows diffuse pathological changes in hypsarrhythmia and the adrenal steroids may act directly on the pathological process. Alternatively, they could be modifying the rate of synthesis of cortical enzymes such as glycerolphosphate dehydrogenase (De Vellis & Inglish 1968).

The CSF concentration of ACTH is reduced in children with infantile spasms and hypsarrythmia (Nalin et al 1985), suggesting that ACTH therapy may be compensating for a deficit. In contrast, in patients with temporal lobe epilepsy plasma ACTH concentration (and ACTH secretory rate) are elevated in comparison with antiepileptic drug-treated patients with pseudoseizures or with normal controls (Gallagher et al 1984). Temporal lobectomy restores ACTH secretion to normal.

Thyroid disorders

Both myxoedema and thyrotoxicosis can be complicated by epilepsy and a return to a euthyroid state may cure the epilepsy (Evans 1960, Skanse & Nyman 1956). Acute thyrotoxicosis not uncommonly (perhaps 9% of cases) presents with seizures (Jabbari & Huott, 1980). There is animal experimental evidence for a therapeutic action of thyroxine administration in photosensitive epilepsy (Serbanescu & Balzamo 1974) and for increased cerebral excitability (reduced threshold for electroshock seizures) following thyroxine (Timiras & Woodbury 1956). Sound-induced seizures in DBA/2 mice are associated with high serum thyroxine levels and can be suppressed by antithyroid drugs (Seyfried et al 1979). The mechanism of these effects is not clear, but thyroxine modifies ionic distribution as well as altering metabolic rate.

Oestrogens and progesterone

Oestrogens have been shown to be epileptogenic by systemic administration to rats and rabbits, by local cortical application in animals and by systemic injection in humans (Woolley & Timiras 1962ab, Marcus et al 1966, Marcus 1972) They are proconvulsant for limbic seizures induced in rats by kainate and kindling (Nicoletti et al 1985, Horr & Buterbaugh 1986). This is probably because oestrogens reduce glutamic acid decarboxylase activity and hence produce a fall in GABA synthesis in the brain (Wallis & Luttge 1980, Nicoletti et al 1982).

Progesterone can, like desoxycorticosterone, act as a general anaesthetic (Seyle 1941). It has a protective action against convulsions in some animal test systems (Costa & Bonnycastle 1952, Woolley & Timiras, 1962a). For kainate seizures this is more marked in female than in male rats (Nicoletti et al 1985).

In rats, the phase of the oestrus cycle influences both the threshold to electroshock seizures (Woolley & Timiras 1962b) and the local seizure susceptibility within the limbic system (Timiras 1969).

These effects of sex hormones may explain the phenomenon of catemenial epilepsy. Among 50 women in a hospital for epileptics, analysing 33 468 fits in 939 patient years, Laidlaw (1956) found that the fits occurred in relation to the phase of the menstrual cycle in 72% of cases. There was a reduction in fit frequency during the luteal phase and an exacerbation the day before menstruation, and subsequently up to the sixth day of the cycle. More recent studies have been reviewed by Newmark & Penry (1980).

Hormonal effects on sleep

As well as the potential mechanisms of action already mentioned, endocrine changes may modify seizure susceptibility by altering sleep patterns or by acting on protein synthesis in the brain. Specifically, a decrease in adrenal steroids is associated with reduction in sleep phases III and IV (Gillin et al 1974) and an increase in sleep stages III and IV is associated with hyperthyroidism (Dunleavy et al 1974). Adrenal steroids can induce enzymes involved in the metabolism of neurotransmitters (Moore & Phillipson 1975).

Endogenous toxic states

Endogenously derived toxic compounds may accumulate in relation to liver failure, renal failure or certain inborn errors of metabolism. The mechanism leading to seizures in these situations may not, however, be different from some already discussed under previous headings.

Liver failure

Hepatic coma is not usually associated with

Table 7.2 Exogenous toxins producing seizures

Source or 'category'	Action	Convulsant dose (mg/kg) IV in animals	Type of seizures	References
Strychnine, Brucine — Plant alkaloids	Block inhibition due to glycine	2–3	'Spinal', tonic extension	Everett & Richards (1944), Pylkko & Woodbury (1961)
Picrotoxin, Bicuculline — Plant toxins	Block GABA-mediated inhibition	1–2, 0.2–80	Sustain Generalised	Meldrum & Horton (1974), Meldrum & Horton (1971)
Benzyl-penicillin — Antibiotic; Pentylene tetrazol — Synthetic	—	400 000 units/kg, 20–80	'Myoclonic', Tonic-clonic	Gloor & Testa (1974), Goodman et al (1953), Chusid & Kopeloff (1969)
Isoniazid, Thiosemicarbazide — Tuberculostatic hydrazides; Allylglycine — Amino acid; 3-mercaptopropionic acid; 4-deoxypyridoxine — Pyridoxine analogue	Inhibits GABA synthesis	100–150, 7–10, 200–400, 25–70, 100–150	Tonic-clonic	Meldrum et al (1970), Meldrum et al (1970), Horton & Meldrum (1973), Horton & Meldrum (1973), Meldrum & Horton (1971)
Fluorothyl — Volatile ether; Bemegride — Analeptic; Thujone, Catechol — Absinthe	— —	(Vapour), 5–9, 5–7, 8	Myoclonus	Krantz (1963), Chusid & Kopeloff (1969), Opper (1939), Angel & Lemon (1974)
Imipramine, Amitriptyline, Desmethylimipramine — Tricyclic anti-depressants	—	25–50	Clonic-tonic	Wallach et al (1969), Trimble (1977)
Cocaine, Lignocaine — Local anaesthetic		50, 7–14	Limbic seizures, Tonic-clonic	Eidelberg et al (1963), Munson & Wagman (1969), Wagman et al (1968)
Diphenhydramine — Antihistamine		20	Tonic-clonic	Chusid et al (1956)
Methionine, dl-sulphoximine — Agenized flour	Alters amino acid metabolism	300	Long latency	Folbergrova et al (1969)
Homocysteine — Amino acid	Alters ammonia metabolism	700–1400 i.p.	Repetitive	Folbergrova (1975)
Dieldrin, Lindane — Chlorinated hydrocarbon insecticides		6, 12	Tonic or tonic-clonic	St Omer (1971)

		Dose	Seizure type	References
Di-isopropylfluoro-phosphate *Tetra-ethylpyro-phosphate parathion*	Organophosphorous insecticides	Irreversible inhibitors of cholinesterase	1–2 i.m. 6 i.m.		Grob (1963) Stone (1957)
Fluoroacetate *Iodoacetate*	Metabolic poisons	Inhibits aconitase Inhibits glycolysis at phosphoglycer-aldehyde dehydrogenase	2 180 i.p.	Tonic-clonic	Peters (1963) Samson & Dahl (1957)
Cyanide		Inhibits cytochrome oxidase	2–4	Myoclonus	Wheatley et al (1947)
2-deoxyglucose		Impairs glycolysis	1000–30 000		Meldrum & Horton (1973a)

seizures in spite of the high blood ammonia levels. Comparable blood and brain ammonia levels induced acutely by the administration of ammonium salts may be associated with generalized seizures (Gastaut et al 1968).

Renal failure

Seizures are relatively common in the various syndromes of renal insufficiency (chronic renal failure following glomerulonephritis, eclampsia of pregnancy etc). They are usually primarily generalized grand mal seizures and, in most cases, there is evidence of some antecedent cerebral pathology. Correlative EEG and metabolic studies have been decribed by Prill et al (1969). These authors and Gastaut et al (1971), considered that the severity of uraemia was not a critical determinant of seizure onset. Urea infusions given to cats produce initially facial then generalized myoclonus, associated with reticular spikes, and ultimately status epilepticus (Zuckerman & Glaser 1972). Hypocalcaemia and overhydration probably play a role in some cases of renal failure. A common finding is a primary metabolic acidosis leading to a compensatory reduction in arterial pCO_2 (which increases cerebral excitability) and, when corrected, a reduction in ionized calcium.

During dialysis, grand mal seizures and sometimes status epilepticus occur because of the *disequilibrium syndrome*. Brain and plasma share hyperosmolarity (urea, creatinine, electrolytes) during renal failure and rapid correction of the plasma composition may lead to intracellular overhydration. This is usually prevented by dialysis with a hyperosmolar fluid.

Inborn errors of metabolism

Seizures are a major feature in a number of these syndromes and, in some, the accumulation of an unusual metabolite appears to be responsible. Most common among the aminoacidurias is phenylketonuria, in which the inability to hydroxylate phenylalanine to tyrosine leads to the accumulation of metabolites of phenylalanine not usually detectable in blood or urine. It is not certain whether it is deficiency of the compounds normally derived from tyrosine (such as the catecholamine transmitter substances) or the excess of abnormal metabolites (such as phenylacetic acid which is known to inhibit the enzyme synthesizing GABA) that is primarily responsible for the seizure tendency. Other inborn errors associated with seizures are described by Crome & Stern (1972).

Exogenous toxins

It is not possible here even to classify the vast range of toxic substances that can produce seizures. A restricted list is given in Table 7.2. Of great theoretical interest are the compounds that compete with inhibitory transmitter substances for receptor sites. The best established experimentally is the competition between strychnine, or related alkaloids, and glycine for sites on spinal motoneurones. Two toxins of plant origin, bicuculline and picrotoxin, block inhibition due to GABA in many parts of the brain including the cerebral cortex, and benzyl penicillin probably acts in the same way (Curtis & Johnston 1974). A vast range of enzyme inhibitors produce generalized seizures. These include anticholinesterases such as 'nerve gases' and organophosphorus insecticides, and pyridoxal phosphate antagonists that inhibit glutamic acid decarboxylase (Meldrum 1975b). Compounds that interfere with cerebral energy metabolism (such as cyanide or 2-deoxyglucose) also produce seizures (Meldrum & Horton 1973a).

Clinically, the most significant exogenous toxins are drug overdoses, particularly of drugs used in psychiatry, including the tricyclic antidepressants (Wallach et al 1969). Many drugs given therapeutically, not necessarily in an overdose, can precipitate seizures. Thus, generalized fits occurring during status asthmaticus are commonly due to aminophylline (Holmgren & Kraeplin 1953, Schwartz & Scott 1974). Seizures due to the administration of penicillin directly into the CSF have long been recognized, but high doses of penicillin given intravenously can also be epileptogenic.

Seizures due to withdrawal of barbiturates or drugs of addiction may take the form of status epilepticus. Such seizures may follow the emergency hospitalization of a patient whose intake of addictive drugs is not known to the medical staff.

Summary

When a patient suffers his or her first fit, it is necessary for the physician to consider the possible role of systemic factors. The physician must distinguish between factors that might be precipitants in a subject likely to have further seizures and factors which are causal and, if prevented, would remove the likelihood of further fits. The distinction is not absolute. Seizures triggered by sleep deprivation, overbreathing, overhydration or mild hypoglycaemia, are often the forerunners of seizures occurring without evident contributory factors, whereas a drug overdose or severe hypoglycaemia will provoke fits in subjects who are unlikely to experience seizures in the absence of such severe insults.

EPILEPTOGENESIS AT THE CELLULAR LEVEL

The gross cerebral pathology giving rise to epilepsy is described in this chapter. It is natural to look for common cellular mechanisms that may provide links between different primary lesions and epilepsy (Table 7.3). Several features in the clinical history (e.g. latent period and family history of epilepsy) are common to focal or generalized seizures following a tumour, cerebral abscess or penetrating head injury. This suggests that all three pathologies induce similar critical cellular changes. Similarly, one looks for a single

Table 7.3 'Unifying' hypotheses of the basic pathology of epilepsy

1. Meningocerebral cicatrix
   Vascular abnormality leading to focal ischaemia
2. Blood or iron as epileptiogens
3. Cytological mechanisms
   a. Loss of inhibitory interneurones
   b. 'Deafferentation'
      i. Supersensitivity
      ii. Loss of dendritic spines
   c. Enhanced activity at excitatory synapses
   d. Proliferation of fibrous astrocytes
      (? inadequate regulation of extracellular potassium concentration)
4. Enzymic defects
   a. Synthesis of inhibitory transmitter substances
   b. Membrane ATPase deficiency
      i. Sodium potassium activated
      ii. Calcium activated

cellular or focal neuropathology that is common to the diffuse disorders producing myoclonic syndromes. Infantile spasms, or West's syndrome (Jeavons & Bower 1964) also provide a very distinctive clinical syndrome suggesting there must be specific changes in the brain that can follow numerous primary pathologies.

Meningocerebral cicatrix

Penfield & Jasper (1954) have claimed that scar tissue vascularized by both cerebral and meningeal arteries plays a critical role in focal epileptogenesis following purulent meningitis, cerebral abscess and penetrating brain injury. They suggested that the vessels of extracerebral origin might show abnormal or inappropriate vasoconstrictive responses; that, within and around the scar, capillaries were abnormal or deficient; and that, with progressive shrinkage of the scar, the surrounding capillaries could become obstructed, thus creating new ischaemic lesions. Following Penfield's advocacy many neurosurgeons selected operative procedures designed to minimize the formation of meningocerebral anastomotic vessels. Proof that this practice has significantly altered the post-operative incidence of epilepsy is lacking.

The cellular changes around a scar include loss of neurones and proliferation of glial elements – initially, microglial (rod) cells; subsequently, reactive astrocytes and fat-laden phagocytes. Such changes are not confined to meningocerebral scars but are found in almost all the disorders discussed in this section.

Blood, haemoglobin and iron

Experimental studies provide strong evidence for blood or iron as factors causing focal epileptogenesis. This indicates a probable mechanism for induction of post-traumatic epilepsy, but could also be relevant to seizures after cerebrovascular accidents, vascular malformations or invasive tumours.

Haemolysed blood applied to the cat cortex was initially shown to produce spike discharges (Levitt et al 1971). Subsequently, the injection of ferrous or ferric chloride into the cortex was shown to have both an acute and a chronic epileptogenic effect (Willmore et al 1978). Studies of the time course of the development of focal discharges after blood or haemoglobin application suggest that release of iron during the course of haemoglobin breakdown could be the critical step in epileptogenesis (Rosen & Frumin 1979, Hammond et al 1980).

Selective loss of neurones

The normal functioning of the nervous system depends on the interplay of inhibitory and excitatory activity (see Eccles 1964, 1969, Tebecis 1974). Although the action of some transmitter substances varies according to the specificity of the post-synaptic receptor site, some compounds, such as glycine and gamma-aminobutyric acid (GABA) have an important inhibitory action almost everywhere they are found in the vertebrate brain or spinal cord (Curtis & Johnston 1974). Reduction in the efficiency of such inhibitory tranmission leads to seizures in many experimental situations (Meldrum 1975b). Thus, if ischaemic or other pathological processes can produce a destruction of neurones that is at least partially selective for inhibitory interneurones, their epileptogenicity can be explained. The selective vulnerability to hypoxia of different areas of grey matter and of different neuronal populations within those areas is well established (Schade & McMenemy 1963, Brierley et al 1973) and there is substantial evidence for a relatively greater involvement of neurones that can be identified on biochemical or physiological criteria as inhibitory interneurones.

Arterial occlusion producing spinal cord ischaemia for one hour can be shown by chemical measurements to destroy, with partial selectiveness, neurones containing the inhibitory transmitter glycine (Werman et al 1968). This lesion produces spasticity and sometimes myoclonic limb jerks, but not epileptic seizures.

In the cerebellum, hypoxia, arterial hypertension or hypoglycaemia selectively destroy the Purkinje cells and basket cells (Brierley et al 1973); these neurones are inhibitory in function and contain high concentrations of GABA (Curtis & Johnston 1974, Tebecis 1974). Other regions showing selective vulnerability (third and fifth

layers of neocortex; hippocampus, basal ganglia and thalamus) have a relatively high content of GABA and of glutamic acid decarboxylase, the enzyme synthesizing GABA (Fahn & Cote, 1968, Perry et al 1971). In the motor cortex, the large pyramidal neurones which initiate motor activity are relatively insensitive, whereas the small interneurones are highly sensitive to hypoxia or ischaemia. Thus, in infant monkeys, after 30 minutes of moderate hypoxia there is a selective loss of GABAergic aspinous stellate neurones (Sloper et al 1980).

Using an immunocytochemical method that stains terminals containing glutamic acid decarboxylase, Ribak et al (1979) have demonstrated a reduction in the number of such inhibitory endings in the cortex adjacent to an epileptic focus (induced in monkeys by alumina gel). Biochemical determinations show a reduced glutamic acid decarboxylase activity in focal epileptic tissue from a proportion of patients with temporal lobe epilepsy (Lloyd et al 1981).

The action myoclonus appearing in some patients after cardiac arrest or asphyxia responds therapeutically to oral or intravenous administration of 5-hydroxytryptophan, the precursor of serotonin (Lhermitte et al 1972). Experimental studies with lesions or biochemical manipulations suggest that there is an interaction of GABA and serotonin mediated transmission in the brain stem and basal ganglia (Hassler 1972) so that a therapeutic action of 5-hydroxytryptophan is not incompatible with a deficit in availability of GABA being responsible for the myoclonus. However, it does raise the possibility that a selective destruction of the serotoninergic systems originating in the brain stem might be responsible for the syndrome. Changes in seizures and myoclonic responses following manipulation of serotoninergic transmission have been extensively described in animal models of epilepsy (Meldrum et al 1975). Additionally, measurement of the concentration of serotonin and of 5-hydroxyindoleacetic acid (a metabolite of serotonin) in the cerebrospinal fluid of children and adults with epilepsy has suggested that the synthesis and turnover of serotonin are reduced (Papeschi et al 1972, Shaywitz et al 1975).

A very marked regional deficiency in the concentration of glutamic acid decarboxylase and of GABA has been demonstrated in the basal ganglia of brains from patients with Huntington's chorea (Perry et al 1973, Bird & Iversen 1974). Generalized seizures occur in up to 50% of cases of Huntington's chorea. A small but significant fall in the GABA content of occipital cortex was measured (Perry et al 1973). The selective loss of GABA-containing neurones in the basal ganglia probably contributes to the chorea, and the smaller changes elsewhere in the brain may contribute to the occasional generalized seizures.

Deafferentation and loss of dendritic spines

Physiological and morphological studies suggest that there are mechanisms by which neuronal loss could favour epileptogenesis without being selective for inhibitory neurones. Thus, when neocortex which has been 'deafferented' by undercutting (Halpern 1972) is given a brief electrical stimulus it shows a sustained *after-discharge* which has many properties resembling those of a focal cortical discharge. The mechanism of this change is not understood, but the time course of its development suggests that a process occurs which resembles the denervation supersensitivity that can be demonstrated in skeletal muscle or autonomic effector organs when peripheral nerves are cut (Sharpless 1969).

Morphological studies employing Golgi impregnations (Globus & Scheibel 1966) reveal a structural correlate of deafferentation of cortical neurones, namely, a loss of dendritic spines.

A similar loss of dendritic spines has been seen in temporal lobectomy specimens removed from patients undergoing neurosurgery for temporal lobe epilepsy (Scheibel & Scheibel 1973, Scheibel et al 1974). The hippocampal pyramidal neurones and dentate granular cells also showed shrinkage or simplification of the apical dendritic system and the appearance of nodular deformities on the dendritic extremities. Such appearances in Golgi preparations are not confined to the hippocampus and temporal lobe epilepsy. They were, in fact, first described in epileptic neocortex by DeMoor in 1898. They can also be found in and around epileptogenic foci created in the neocortex of monkeys by the application of alumina cream (Westrum et al 1965, Ward 1969). Electrophys-

iological studies of the behaviour of single neurones in such experimental foci have led to the identification of so-called *epileptic neurones* which show firing activity of an abnormal pattern with repetitive bursts. The abnormal neurones identified in Golgi preparations may provide the structural correlate of these *epileptic neurones* (Ward 1969).

The primary loss of neurones can occur in brain areas anatomically distant from the area in which the deafferentation and loss of dendritic spines occurs provided there are sufficient afferent connections. Such a mechanism operating on subcortical centres could lead to seizures of generalized onset following focal cortical lesions.

Enhanced activity at excitatory synapses

In two experimental models of epilepsy, an abnormal pattern of electrical activity apparently contributes to the creation of an epileptic focus. In the *mirror focus* phenomenon (Wilder 1969), a primary focus created by a destructive neocortical lesion (e.g. from cobalt, penicillin, freezing or alumina cream) gives rise to a secondary focus in the contralateral hemisphere. In the *kindling* phenomenon, repeated *subthreshold* focal electrical stimulation of the amygdala or other nuclei modifies the threshold for seizure induction so that ultimately spontaneous seizures may occur (Goddard et al 1969, Wada et al 1974). In neither of these phenomena can degenerative phenomena be excluded (Westmoreland et al 1972). However, electronmicrographic studies of projected foci in the rat and measurement of the localization and density of synaptic vesicles in somatosensory cortex suggest that there is a concentration of such vesicles close to the presynaptic membrane (Fischer 1973) which would have the effect of enhancing transmission.

Enhanced excitatory activity could also arise from an increase in the number or efficacy of postsynaptic excitatory receptor sites. This could arise from 'up-regulation' following deafferentation. One subtype of receptor – that responds specifically to N-methyl-D-aspartate, quinolinate and related compounds, with a paroxysmal depolarising shift and burst firing – is of particular relevance in epilepsy (Meldrum 1986). It appears to be upregulated in the rat hippocampus during kindling (Wadman & Heinemann 1985).

Proliferation of fibrous astrocytes

One cytological change that is almost universally identifiable in the brains of patients dying with epilepsy is the proliferation of fibrous astrocytes. Such gliosis is seen in and around all chronic focal lesions and it occurs incidentally in a large number of the diffuse *degenerative* pathologies that may lead to epilepsy. It also occurs patchily or diffusely in the most superficial layer of the cortex (subpial or marginal gliosis) as first described by Chaslin (1891). Gliosis is also seen in the hippocampus, amygdala and temporal gyrus in *mesial temporal sclerosis* the most characteristic pathology of temporal lobe epilepsy (see below). Fibrous or reactive astrocytes differ in morphology and staining reactions from normal astrocytes. The latter have end-feet that terminate in relation to capillaries or to neurones. They are believed to transport metabolic substrates and other materials to and from neurones, and to regulate the composition of extracellular fluid (Trachtenberg & Pollen 1970, Henn et al 1972). Changes in the ionic composition of extracellular fluid modify the excitability of neurones – particularly an increase in the extracellular content of potassium – can induce epileptic discharges, especially in the hippocampus (Zuckerman & Glaser 1970).

These observations have led to the hypothesis that faulty regulation of extracellular potassium concentration by reactive astrocytes could be responsible for epileptogenesis in gliotic lesions (Pollen & Trachtenberg 1970). However, direct measurements of intracellular potentials and membrane properties in reactive glial cells in a focus created by injury show high resting potentials and a high *glial safety factor*, and thus fail to confirm the presence of impaired regulation of extracellular potassium concentration in gliosis (Grossman & Rosman 1971, Glotzner 1973).

Enzyme defects

It is possible that the final common path by which various pathological processes create the tendency to seizures is to be found, not at the level of the cell, but at that of the protein molecule. The activity of particular enzymes could be impaired by diverse mechanisms, ranging from genetically determined deficiency to lack of a co-factor or trace metal or the presence of toxic factors.

It is natural to consider first the enzymes involved in the synthesis of transmitter substances. Early reports suggested that there was an alteration in the metabolism of acetylcholine in the epileptogenic focus (Tower & Elliott 1952). More recently, interest has centred on the metabolism of glycine, GABA, taurine, serotonin, dopamine and noradrenaline, as these compounds are believed to act as inhibitory transmitters. A reduction in the brain GABA content due to dietary deficiency of pyridoxine (required as the co-factor of glutamate decarboxylase) is associated with seizures (Coursin 1964). There is also a rare genetically determined epileptic syndrome (pyridoxine dependency) that responds dramatically to sustained administration of high doses of vitamin B (Hunt et al 1954, Tower 1969). A reduction in the concentration of GABA in CSF (cerobrospinal fluid) of patients with epilepsy (receiving drug therapy) has been reported (Wood et al 1979).

The possible involvement of taurine in epilepsy is discussed by Barbeau and Donaldson (1974). In some animal experimental models of epilepsy depletion of brain amines (as by reserpine or by inhibition of tyrosine hydroxylase) is associated with a lowered threshold for seizures (Meldrum et al 1975). Measurements of amines and their metabolites in CSF (mentioned above under 'loss of inhibitory interneurones') suggest that there may be an abnormality of amine metabolism in epilepsy; however, enzyme studies are lacking.

The possibility also exists of an abnormality in receptor molecules (for inhibitory or excitory transmitters).

Using 3H ligands to study GABA and benzodiazepine binding sites, a deficit in the GABA/benzodiazepine receptor system has been observed in the midbrain and brain stem of Mongolian gerbils and of DBA/2 mice which show genetically determined syndromes of epilepsy. (Olsen et al 1985a,b).

The intracellular–extracellular concentration ratios of sodium and potassium critically determine resting, action and synaptic potential (Eccles

1964), and the maintenance of these ratios depends on a magnesium-dependent, sodium potassium-activated ATPase found in neuronal and glial membranes. Evidence of various kinds suggests that abnormalities in the functioning of this enzyme may be important in seizures. Compounds known to inhibit the membrane ATPase, such as ouabain, induce seizure discharges when applied locally to the cortex of hippocampus (Bignami & Palladini 1966, Baldy-Moulinier et al 1973). A diminished cerebral ATPase activity was described by Abood & Gerard (1955) in the genetically determined syndrome of audiogenic seizures found in DBA/2 mice.

More recent studies show that the deficiency is in a membrane calcium dependent ATPase (Rosenblatt et al 1976). Recombinant genetic studies show that this enzymic defect is closely linked to inheritance of the enhanced seizure susceptibility in DBA/2 mice (Palayoor & Seyfried 1984).

Epilepsy occurs incidentally in numerous inborn errors of metabolism, such as phenylketonuria, maple syrup urine disease and homocystinuria. There are over 140 Mendelian traits that increase the risk of seizures (Anderson et al 1986). Genetic studies of epilepsy (reviewed by Metrakos & Metrakos 1974) show a familial incidence of *centrencephalic epilepsy* (with 3 per second spike and wave discharges on the EEG) that is consistent with autosomal dominant transmission. Simple febrile convulsions show a similar pattern of transmission but with an even more pronounced age dependence in the expression of disorder (Lennox-Buchthal 1973). Non-epileptic subjects may show spikes or spikes and waves on

the EEG in response to stroboscopic stimulation. This syndrome is age and sex dependent and also shows a familial incidence consistent with autosomal dominant transmission. Genetic linkage studies are currently in progress to determine the chromosomal sites responsible for benign juvenile myoclonic epilepsy. At a subsequent stage, recombinant DNA technology could elucidate the inherited defect (Delgado-Escueta et al 1986).

PHYSIOLOGICAL CHANGES ASSOCIATED WITH SEIZURES

Changes that are secondary to seizures include metabolic changes in the brain that are a direct result of normal activity and systemic changes. The former are reviewed by Chapman (1985). The latter are reviewed by Simon (1985) and are summarized in Table 7.4.

Systemic changes arise in two ways. First, there are physiological and metabolic changes secondary to the motor component of the seizure (i.e. changes in blood gases and pH, a rise in body temperature). Their dependence on the motor activity can be demonstrated in experiments employing peripheral muscular paralysis (by curare-like agents) and artificial respiration. Secondly, there are autonomic and endocrine changes which, although they may be influenced by the motor activity, appear to arise primarily through the direct effect of neuronal discharges impinging on the hypothalamus and other controlling centres.

The significance of the physiological changes accompanying seizures is best understood when

Table 7.4 Physiological changes in generalized seizures (tonic-clonic or status epilepticus)

Transient or early (0–30 minutes)	'Late' (after 30 minutes)
Arterial hypertension	Arterial hypotension
Cerebral venous pressure (CVP) raised	CVP raised or normal
Arterial PO_2 low or normal	Arterial PO_2 low or normal
Arterial PCO_2 high	Arterial PCO_2 normal
CV PO_2 normal (or low or high)	CV PO_2 normal or low
CV PCO_2 high	CV PCO_2 normal (or high)
Cerebral blood flow (CBF) increased	CBF increased normal or decreased
Hyperglycaemia	Normoglycaemia, hypoglycaemia
Hyperkalaemia	Hyperkalaemia
Hemoconcentration	
Lactacidosis	Hyperpyrexia (secondary)

they are considered in relation to data summarised elsewhere in this chapter. Thus, some changes will tend to prolong seizure activity, whereas others will facilitate its termination. Epileptic brain damage (described later) is the result of the interaction of systemic factors and local metabolic changes, and may be diminished or prevented if these are appropriately manipulated. A more obscure problem is the refractory period, or increase in seizure threshold, that follows a generalized seizure. This is presumably the result of metabolic or physiological changes that accompany and follow the seizure.

Cardiovascular changes

Blood pressure

A dramatic increase in systolic and diastolic blood pressure is usually seen at the onset of a generalized tonic seizure, whether it occurs spontaneously or is induced by electroshock or drugs in humans or animals (White et al 1961, Magnaes & Nornes 1974, Meldrum & Horton 1973b, Meyer et al 1966, Posner et al 1969, Plum et al 1968). There is initially a marked tachycardia but sometimes when the pressure reaches its peak the heart slows. With brief seizures the mean arterial pressure remains elevated throughout the seizure and returns to normal in the first few minutes of the post-ictal period.

The arterial hypertension and tachycardia are the results of enhanced sympathetic activity. They can be abolished by ganglionic blockade (or a spinal section in animals).

Several factors interact to produce the phenomena associated with more prolonged seizures. Comparison of the blood pressure changes in experimental primates with and without peripheral muscular paralysis (Meldrum & Horton 1973b, Meldrum et al 1973) shows that the initial rise in blood pressure is similar. However, in the paralysed, ventilated animal, this increase is transient and the blood pressure returns to normal levels and remains relatively stable even when cerebral seizure activity continues for many hours. In the non-paralysed animal, the initial rise in blood pressure is sometimes more sustained (up to 20–30 minutes) indicating that the excessive

motor activity is raising the blood pressure, perhaps partially through the improved venous return but more probably reflexly through changes in blood gases and pH acting on the chemoreceptors in the aortic arch and carotid body. Late in status epilepticus, both experimentally and in humans, there is commonly a drop in the mean arterial blood pressure below normal, and this arterial hypotension may persist in the post-ictal period (Meldrum & Horton 1973b). The peripheral vascular resistance drops in muscle, skin and brain and the heart is unable to sustain the increase in output necessary to maintain mean arterial pressure.

The massive sympathetic and vagal discharges reaching the heart early in a seizure are probably responsible for a significant proportion of unexpected deaths in young epileptic patients (Hirsch & Martin 1971). Ventricular tachycardia, conduction block or asystole apparently result from the sudden excessive autonomic bombardment early in the seizure.

Another consequence of excessive motor activity that affects the heart is hyperkalaemia. This initially produces characteristic disturbances of the cardiac rhythm and electrocardiogram. If untreated, the blood pressure may suddenly collapse and cardiac arrest and death follow.

Cerebral blood flow

A marked increase in cerebral blood flow (up to three or even five times normal) occurs within one to two seconds of the onset of generalized seizure activity, and a comparable focal increase in blood flow accompanies focal seizures (Penfield et al 1939, White et al 1961, Meyer et al 1966, Ingvar 1973, Magnaes & Nornes 1974, Meldrum & Nilsson 1976). This focal or general increase in blood flow arises as much or more from the decrease in cerebral vascular resistance as from the increase in arterial pressure. It is still seen in the absence of any change in arterial pressure.

The decrease in cerebral vascular resistance is attributed by many authors (Brodersen et al 1973, Kety 1964; Meyer et al 1966, Plum & Duffy 1975) to a direct effect on the vessels of a local increase in PCO_2 and lactic acid or hydrogen ion concentration. It is evident that this explanation is not quantitatively adequate. The increase in blood flow is often more than sufficient to compensate for the increased metabolic demand of the brain during the seizure. Thus the oxygen tension in the cerebral venous blood often rises during seizures (Plum et al 1968, Meldrum & Horton 1973b), and the rise in cerebral venous PCO_2 is often small and slow. Yet the cerebral blood flow increases at, or slightly before, the onset of the tonic seizure (Plum et al 1968). The possibility of direct neuronally mediated vasodilatation deserves consideration. The existence of a cerebral vasodilator mechanism that runs in the VIIth cranial nerve can be reflexly activated, and is more powerful than the sympathetic vasoconstrictor mechanism demonstrated by Ponte & Purves (1974). Thus the early dilatation of the peripheral resistance vessels in the brain could be a consequence of the autonomic discharge triggered by the seizure. Rises in arterial PCO_2 might, at a later stage, sustain the cerebral vasodilatation through an action on the normal reflex mechanism, i.e. chemoreceptors in the aortic arch and carotid sinus, vagal afferents and outflow via the VIIth nerve (James 1975).

Clearly, the normal mechanisms for autoregulation that ensure a uniform cerebral blood flow, despite variations in cerebral perfusion pressure, cease to be effective during a generalized seizure. The presence of dilated cerebral vessels in the presence of a normal or reduced arterial pressure can lead to focally or generally inadequate cerebral perfusion.

Cerebral venous pressure

During a tonic seizure the cerebral venous pressure rises dramatically; values above 10 kPa (1000 mm H_2O) are seen in experimental animals (Hendley et al 1965, Meldrum & Horton 1973b). The increase in muscle tone and intrathoracic pressure makes an important contribution to this. Thus transient rises accompany whole body jerks during a myoclonic seizure. That the cerebral vasodilatation is also an important factor is shown by the reduced but still substantial rise in cerebral venous pressure seen in paralysed, artificially ventilated animals.

In paralysed, ventilated volunteers receiving pentylenetetrazol, cerebrospinal fluid pressure rose on average by 5.5 kPa (549 mm H_2O) during the seizure (White et al 1961).

The small haemorrhages occurring subpially and elsewhere (see final section) may result from the excessive venous pressure.

Haemoconcentration

Early in generalized seizures haemoconcentration, as shown by a rise in haemotocrit or haemoglobin content of the blood of about 5%, is seen. This is part of the autonomic response. Release of splenic reserves of red cells may play a part, but a sudden increase in the rate of fluid secretion is probably more important.

Respiratory changes

The effects of seizures on respiration are complex and vary with the type of seizure and the phase of the individual fit. Tachypnoea and/or a transient apnoea are nearly always seen in relation to a tonic seizure. A change in respiratory rate or pattern is sometimes the most notable motor sign in a petit mal attack.

There are three mechanisms by which cerebral seizure activity leads to respiratory embarrassment:

1. Brain stem centres regulating respiration may be directly influenced by the cerebral seizure activity. There is evidence for this not only in most types of generalized seizure, but also in some partial seizures such as temporal lobe epilepsy.

2. Abnormal motor activity may directly impair normal mechanical respiration and additionally, by greatly increasing whole body oxygen consumption and carbon dioxide production, may overload the respiratory exchange capacity of the lungs.

3. Peripheral autonomic components of the seizure may have a dramatic influence on gas exchange in the lungs. This is the explanation for the drop in arterial PO_2 and rise in PCO_2 seen during drug-induced seizures in paralysed, artificially ventilated animals (Meldrum et al 1973). The excessive glandular outpouring, not only of the salivary glands but, more importantly, of the tracheobronchial secretions, is the most evident

factor and gives rise to the classical *foaming at the mouth*. However, parasympathetically mediated bronchial constriction and haemodynamic factors leading to less efficient alveolar gas exchange may also be important. In experimental animals haemorrhagic consolidation of the lungs has been described after pentylenetetrazol or high-pressure oxygen convulsions (Bean et al 1966, Harris & Van den Brenk 1968).

The net effect of these three factors during generalized tonic or clonic seizures can be a severe impairment of respiratory function. It is usually only transient; a severe degree of hypoxia rarely lasts more than two or three minutes.

Autonomic events

Reference has been made to the autonomic components of seizures in the discussion of cardiovascular and respiratory changes. A massive activation of both the sympathetic and parasympathetic systems occurs in generalized tonic seizures (see Table 7.5). One sign of this is the rise in serum dopamine-β-hydroxylase activity that is seen one to five minutes after electroconvulsive shock in humans and experimental animals (Lamprecht et al 1974). Some of the autonomic manifestations are reflexly operated, but it is likely that local spread of abnormal activity to diencephalic and brain stem centres is the critical factor in most cases. It is through the connections of the amygdala and hippocampus with hypothalamic and other centres controlling autonomic function that temporal lobe seizures provoke autonomic changes. However, the greater emphasis on autonomic changes in clinical descriptions of temporal lobe seizures compared with generalized seizures

Table 7.5 Autonomic components of seizures

Sympathetic	Parasympathetic
Tachycardia	Bradycardia
Arterial hypertension	Cerebral vasodilation
Skin vasoconstriction	Bronchial constriction
	Exocrine secretion
Mydriasis	Miosis
Galvanic skin response	Bladder detrusor contraction
Sweating	
Adrenaline release	
Glucagon release	

should not lead to the conclusion that such changes are greater or occur more frequently in temporal lobe seizures. The reverse is the case but, subjectively, autonomic symptoms are important in temporal lobe epilepsy because they occur while consciousness is preserved. Events corresponding to the epigastric aura appear variable, but oesophageal peristalses and inhibition of gastric contraction have been recorded (Van Buren & Ajmone-Marsan 1960). In petit mal, changes in heart rate and a galvanic skin response are sometimes seen about two seconds after the clinical signs of an attack (Johnson & Davidoff 1964). They are probably the result of awareness of an attack.

The autonomic events may pursue a characteristic sequence of parasympathetic and sympathetic components, as in some cases of temporal lobe epilepsy, some pure tonic seizures and some experimental models (Van Buren & Ajmone-Marsan 1960, Huot et al 1973). In some seizures they may be the only or the predominant signs. However, in most generalized tonic-clonic seizures, a variety of sympathetic and parasympathetic responses occur more or less simultaneously and, where the two systems act in opposition, it appears that the most powerful system predominates. Sympathetic activity produces tachycardia, arterial hypertension, mydriasis, a falling skin resistance, sweating and adrenaline release. Parasympathetic activity produces exocrine secretion (sialorrhoea, tracheobronchial and gastrointestinal secretion), bladder contraction, miosis (which sometimes precedes or follows mydriasis) and cerebrovascular vasodilation.

Cerebral arterioles receive an adrenergic innervation via the superior cervical ganglion, which has a vasoconstrictor action (James 1975, Owman & Edvinsson 1978). This system is potently activated during seizures (Mueller et al 1979). It produces a marked reduction in blood volume in the face at the onset of seizures (Ancri et al 1979). Denervation experiments indicate that sympathetic activity diminishes the increase in cerebral cortical blood flow during seizures by about 10% (Mueller et al 1979).

The parasympathetic vasodilator mechanism is poorly understood in anatomical and pharmacological terms. Cholinergic nerves have been identified in extracerebral vessels, but not significantly in the vertebral artery system (Owman & Edvinsson 1978). There is immunocytochemical evidence for a peptidergic, vasodilator system, utilizing vasoactive intestinal peptide (Owman & Edvinsson 1978). This has a higher density in the forebrain than in the hindbrain. Prostaglandins may also play a role.

There is no experimental evidence that allows a quantitative assessment of the relative importance of parasympathetically induced vasodilation compared with that of local factors (PCO_2, pH, [K^+]) in the increased cerebral blood flow during seizures.

Endocrine events

Seizure activity within the limbic system is thought to activate the hypothalamic nuclei controlling pituitary hormone secretion, leading directly to changes in plasma hormone concentration. There are also effects secondary to peripheral autonomic activation. In support of the first mechanism, staining the hypothalamus of cats and baboons to reveal neurosecretory granules shows activation of neurosecretion following pentylenetetrazol seizures in cats (Seite et al 1964) or photically induced myoclonus in *Papio papio* (Luciani et al 1969, Riche 1973).

In support of the second mechanism, the hyperglycaemia that follows generalized seizures induced by electroshock or pentylenetetrazol (Georgi & Strauss 1938) is associated with an increased concentration of adrenaline in the blood (Weil-Malherbe 1955).

A comparable hyperglycaemia is observed in a wide variety of animal test systems (Feldman 1940, Kessler & Gellhorn 1941, Belton et al 1965, Naquet et al 1970, Meldrum & Horton 1973b, Chapman et al 1977). Cutting the splanchnic nerves or removing adrenal glands (Feldman et al 1940) markedly reduces the hyperglycaemia in rats and rabbits, suggesting adrenaline release of glucagon from the pancreas also contributes (Meldrum et al 1979).

The peak blood glucose can be moderately high (over 200 mg/100 ml) 15–30 minutes after seizure onset (Meldrum & Horton 1973b). In humans and experimental primates, the hyperglycaemia is sometimes followed by hypoglycaemia, which is primarily due to the action of insulin but increased glucose consumption may play a part (Meldrum & Horton 1973b, Meldrum et al 1979).

In adrenalectomized rats, pentylenetetrazol seizures evoke a hypoglycaemia which can be prevented by prior vagotomy (Feldman et al 1940); presumably, parasympathetic activity leads to insulin release. In bicuculline-induced seizures in baboons, the major increase in plasma insulin occurs in response to the early increase in blood glucose (Meldrum et al 1979).

Following generalized seizures, there is an immediate increase in plasma ACTH concentration (and in plasma beta endorphin and beta lipotropin) and a secondary rise (after 60–120 minutes) in plasma cortisol (Aminoff et al 1984).

Plasma prolactin levels increase a few minutes after ECT in depressed patients (Ohman et al 1976) or drug-induced seizures in baboons (Meldrum et al 1979). Blood samples taken 20 minutes after spontaneous generalized or complex partial seizures show an increased plasma prolactin, which returns to normal at 1–2 hours after the seizure (Aminoff et al 1984, Dana-Haeri et al 1983). Plasma luteinizing hormone and follicle stimulating hormone also show elevation in some patients after 20–60 minutes (Dana-Haeri et al 1983). Growth hormone is not consistently elevated (Aminoff et al 1984).

Metabolic changes in the brain

Changes in the brain occur during seizures, (a) as a consequence of the other physiological changes described in this section, and (b) as a direct result of the abnormal neuronal activity. Such changes may influence the continuation, or cessation, of seizure activity. They are also a critical factor in the inception of ischaemic neuronal damage (see next Section).

Cerebral metabolic rate

The usual procedure for estimating cerebral metabolic rate is to determine the cerebral blood flow (in ml blood/100 g brain/min) and the arterial and cerebral venous oxygen content and from these values to derive the oxygen consumption, CMR O_2. It is remarkably constant in humans at 3.3 ml $O_2/100$ g brain/min (147 μmol/100 g/min). Quantitative studies in humans of the change in metabolic rate during seizures are not available.

In monkeys, Schmidt et al (1945) found cerebral metabolic rate was increased by 0–80% during pictrotoxin or pentylenetetrazol seizures. A 60% increase in CMR O_2 was reported for dogs receiving pentylenetetrazol (Plum et al 1968). Gilboe & Betz (1973) found no increase in CMR O_2 for the isolated canine brain during pentylenetetrazol seizures. For various technical reasons, these three studies have probably underestimated the maximum increases occurring during seizures. In rats a sustained two- to three-fold increase in cerebral oxygen consumption has been demonstrated (Chapman et al 1975, Meldrum & Nilsson 1976) throughout two hours of status epilepticus (induced by bicuculline).

By measuring the rate of change in the concentration of energy metabolites (see below) in mouse brain in the first few seconds of seizures induced by electroshock or pentylenetetrazol, King et al (1967) and Collins et al (1970) were able to show a three- to four-fold increase in the rate of energy utilization.

Energy metabolites

The energy derived from the oxidation of glucose and required for the active transport of sodium and potassium is stored in the form of adenosine triphosphate and creatine phosphate. The concentrations of these *high-energy* phosphate compounds in the brain are remarkably stable in normal physiological circumstances. They decline progressively in total anoxia or ischaemia. They decline as fast, or faster, in the first few seconds of a generalized seizure in mice (Sacktor et al 1966, King et al 1967). If the mice are paralysed and ventilated with air the decline in high-energy phosphates is smaller and, if they are ventilated on oxygen, it is absent (Collins et al 1970). Thus, in the presence of adequate oxygenation, the brain is able to increase the rate of oxidative metabolism to compensate for the increased energy requirement.

When the oxygen supply is insufficient, the rate of glycolysis is speeded up, but lactate accumu-lates instead of being further metabolized. This and the increase in PCO_2 produce a marked acid shift in the intracellular pH.

The most marked changes in concentration of energy metabolites occur within the first 30 seconds of generalized seizures. After 60–90 seconds stable levels are reached and, even if seizure activity continues, further changes in creatine phosphate, adenosine triphosphate and glucose concentrations occur extremely slowly (Sacktor et al 1966, King et al 1970, Chapman et al 1977). It is probable that in prolonged seizures or status epilepticus further falls in concentration occur, but exact data are not available.

Other metabolic changes

Changes in the cerebral concentrations of a wide variety of other compounds can be detected during or after seizures. Ionic shifts between extracellular and intracellular compartments are a direct consequence of the neuronal activity. Evidence from arteriovenous differences in humans suggests that the brain gains sodium and loses potassium during generalized seizures (Meyer et al 1966). An increased brain sodium content has been observed in rats following electroconvulsive shock (Woodbury 1955). By utilizing ion-specific microelectrodes, it is possible to measure the extracellular concentration of potassium in the cerebral cortex (Prince et al 1973). During seizure activity or local after-discharges potassium concentration rises to 8–10 mmol/l but falls during prolonged activity, and shows an underswing to below normal values post-ictally (Lux 1974, Sypert & Ward 1974). The membrane ATPase is apparently activated by the change in ionic distribution. The onset of discharges showed no relation to extracellular potassium concentration in acute penicillin foci (Futamachi et al 1974), but a threshold elevation of potassium concentration is required for propagated seizure activity (Sypert & Ward 1974).

Brain ammonia concentration is raised following convulsions induced by electroshock, pentylene-tetrazol (Richter & Dawson 1948) or bicuculline. Complex changes in the concentrations of amino acids and tricarboxylic acid cycle intermediates include increases in alanine and glutamine and decreases in glutamate and aspartate concentration (Chapman et al 1977).

A variety of effects on amine metabolism follow electroshock (reviewed by Essman 1973). Thus there is a sustained increase in the rate of synthesis of noradrenaline in the rat brain (Kety et al 1967). The activity of the enzyme tyrosine hydroxylase is enhanced (Musacchio et al 1969). Electroshock also increases the forebrain concentration of serotonin in the rat, rabbit and other animals (Garattini et al 1960, Bertaccini 1959, Essman 1973).

Changes in brain amine metabolism could be responsible for a wide range of post-ictal phenomena, such as the resistance to fits (Herberg & Watkins 1966), alterations in sleep, feeding behaviour and mood.

PATHOLOGICAL CHANGES IN BRAIN RESULTING FROM SEIZURES

The apparently clear, logical distinction between (a) cerebral pathology, which is a direct or indirect consequence of fits; (b) cerebral pathology which is a cause of fits; and (c) pathology which occurs coincidentally in the brains of epileptic patients, is not easily made in practice (Meldrum 1975a). Some of the problems posed by the differentiation between (b) and (c) are presented in the section above. The difficulty in distinguishing group (a) is that pathology arising as a direct consequence of seizures is of an anoxic-ischaemic kind and may therefore be indistinguishable from pathology arising from, say, perinatal asphyxia or later cardiac or cerebrovascular disorders. This problem is most severe for chronic lesions in the brains of patients who have had epilepsy for the greater part of their lives. It is less severe in patients dying a few hours or days after an episode of status epilepticus and showing only acute lesions in the brain.

Physiological changes during seizures as causes of epileptic brain damage

Evidently, lesions found in the brains of patients dying after status epilepticus or chronic epilepsy may be a cause of the seizures or indeed be unrelated to the seizures. However, in the case of *ischaemic* or hypoxic brain damage of the type described under *Status Epilepticus* there are reasons for thinking that the lesions are the result of events occurring during or directly after the episode of status. In individual cases viral infections may contribute directly to the pathology, as suggested by Wallace & Zealley (1970). However, the similarity of the lesions in the presence of diverse primary factors (such as abrupt drug withdrawal, a frontal tumour or an acute febrile dehydrating illness) implicates events directly related to the prolonged seizure. The similarity of the cerebral lesions after status epilepticus, after chronic epilepsy and after known episodes of cerebral hypoxia or ischaemia (e.g. cardiac arrest) led Spielmeyer (1927) and Scholz (1951) to conclude that the epileptic brain damage was the result of cerebral hypoxia or ischaemia occurring immediately before, during, or after the seizure. Because *vasospasm* or *angiospasm* was then believed to play a role in the initiation of seizures, they thought it likely that arterial constriction might also be important in the aetiology of brain damage. This hypothesis was abandoned when it became clear from studies in humans and animals that vasodilatation was the predominant vascular reaction during seizures.

Lindenberg (1955) drew attention to the occurrence of ischaemic lesions in the inferior and medial aspect of the temporal lobe, resulting from compression of branches of the posterior cerebral artery at the tentorial edge, in patients with severe elevation of supratentorial pressure, as in acute intracranial haemorrhage. Scholz (1959) and Gastaut et al (1960) subsequently suggested that cerebral oedema resulting from a prolonged seizure could lead to a similar compression of cerebral arteries and secondary ischaemic lesions. The moderate or severe systemic hypoxia occurring during the tonic phase of a generalized seizure is commonly presumed to lead to cerebral hypoxia. Similarly, post-ictal electrical silence or depression has been widely (but erroneously) supposed to be a manifestation of cerebral hypoxia developing during the course of a seizure. It has not been possible in humans to demonstrate quantitative correlations between physiological changes during seizures and subsequent brain damage.

Animal experiments have led to some conclusions about the causes of epileptic brain damage (Meldrum 1978). In adolescent baboons, physiological changes can be closely monitored during status epilepticus induced with bicuculline, and then correlated with the focal incidence and severity of ischaemic neuronal changes in the brain (Meldrum & Horton 1973b, Meldrum & Brierley 1973). The total duration of seizure activity is important in determining brain damage: less than 90 minutes of sustained epileptic activity did not cause brain damage in the baboons. Several other animal studies have also shown an absence of pathological changes after up to 90 minutes of seizure activity (Schwartz et al 1970, Brennan et al 1972). The possible greater vulnerability of very young animals has not yet been investigated. Among systemic changes, the events occurring after 30 minutes of seizure activity correlate most clearly with brain damage. These include arterial hypotension, hyperpyrexia secondary to the motor activity and hypoglycaemia (see Table 7.4). These changes are themselves capable of producing ischaemic neuronal changes under experimental conditions.

Cerebral metabolic rate is greatly increased during a seizure; hyperpyrexia further increases it (Nemoto & Frankel 1970) and the effects of hypoglycaemia or oligaemia would be additive in producing a failure of cerebral energy metabolism. Secondary systemic changes are much reduced in paralysed, ventilated animals, thus permitting an evaluation of their importance (Meldrum et al 1973). Their contributory role is shown by the longer duration of seizure activity required to produce neocortical, thalamic or hippocampal damage in paralysed animals. Hyperpyrexia and arterial hypotension appear to be significant causes of cerebellar damage (which fails to occur in baboons when these changes are absent).

Marked transient rises in cerebral venous pressure are probably responsible for the small subarachnoid haemorrhages seen after experimental seizures (Krushinsky 1962, Meldrum & Horton 1973). More sustained rises in cerebral venous pressure, focal venous obstruction or venous thrombosis could contribute to the development of focal or more generalized cerebral oedema (Gastaut et al 1960, McLardy 1974).

Experimentally, epileptic brain damage can occur when oedema is not macroscopically evident. Radiological studies in children show that focal or hemispheric oedema can be severe a few days after generalized or unilateral status epilepticus (Isler 1971). Evidence has been presented showing that such oedema can cause herniation of the medial aspect of the temporal lobe (parahippocampal gyrus) over the tentorial edge, compressing the branches of the anterior choroidal and posterior cerebral arteries and producing a secondary cerebral ischaemia (Gastaut et al 1960).

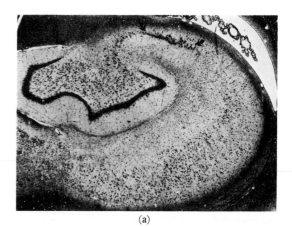

(a)

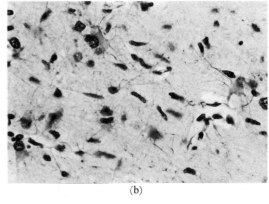

(b)

Fig. 7.1 Microscopical appearance of right hippocampus in an adolescent baboon whose brain was fixed by perfusion 3 weeks after an 8-hour long sequence of 34 brief seizures induced by the intravenous injection of allylglycine. (For experimental details see Meldrum et al 1974) (a) the h_2 zone lies between the arrows. A loss of pyramidal neurones is evident in the Sommer sector and is most severe at its junction with the h_2 zone. There is also loss of neurones in the h_3 Sommer sector, showing loss of neurones and dense gliosis, comprising microglia and fibrous (reactive) astrocytes. (Paraffin section stained with phosphotungstic acid haematoxylin × 600)

Experimentally, pathological changes confined to or predominating in the hippocampus can follow a sequence of brief generalized seizures, not associated with severe systemic changes (Meldrum, Horton & Brierley 1974) or sustained seizures involving only the limbic system (Baldy-Moulinier et al 1973). Such lesions, examined one to six weeks after a seizure sequence (see Fig. 7.1), show a striking resemblance to lesions found in the hippocampi of patients with chronic epilepsy. The marked loss of neurones within the Sommer sector tends to be unilateral, whereas the changes in the endfolium occur symmetrically, thus conforming to the pattern described by Margerison & Corsellis (1966). A microglial response with neuronophagia is evident after one week; subsequently, the proliferation of fibrous astrocytes predominates.

A swelling of astrocytic end-feet within the vulnerable areas of the hippocampus can be identified during seizure activity (De Robertis et al 1969, Meldrum et al 1973). Presumably, the uptake function of astrocytes is overloaded by the excessive local release of potassium and amino acids. The changes within the astrocytes will impair the exchange and transport of metabolites for neurones and will also lead to an impaired capillary circulation. Thus intraneuronal metabolism will be unable to meet the energy demand of seizure activity, and ischaemic neuronal changes will follow.

CONCLUSIONS

In considering the pathophysiology of epilepsy we are constantly seeking, with variable success, to separate causes and effects. It is not difficult to demonstrate that changes in blood gases, plasma glucose, electrolyte or hormone levels can influence the occurrence of seizures, or that seizures themselves can modify all these factors. However, we do not know what factors lead to the spontaneous termination of a seizure, or cause a prolonged seizure to become self sustaining. In a high proportion of patients we cannot even give an account of the seizures that explains why the patient is epileptic and why seizures occur at some times and not at others. The same problems occur in relation to the pathological changes in the brain: we can describe the diverse lesions within the brain that may cause epilepsy, but why one such lesion is epileptogenic and another similar one is not remains unknown.

Undoubtedly, more could be done on the basis of existing knowledge to reduce the incidence of epilepsy in Europe and North America, and vastly more could be achieved in the tropical countries. However, additional basic knowledge is required before we can specify the medical and social measures that will reduce the incidence of epilepsy substantially below its current prevalence of 1 in 200 in the Western world.

REFERENCES

Abood L G, Gerard R W 1955 A phosphorylation defect in the brains of mice susceptible to audiogenic seizure. In: Biochemistry of the developing nervous system. Academic Press, New York, p 467

Aicardi J, Chevrie J J 1970 Convulsive status epilepticus in infants and children. A study of 239 cases. Epilepsia 11:187

Aird R B, Gordan G S 1951 Anticonvulsive properties of desoxycorticosterone. Journal of the American Medical Association 145:715

Aminoff M J, Simon R P 1980 Status epilepticus. Causes, clinical features and consequences in 98 patients. American Journal of Medicine 69:657

Aminoff M J, Simon R P, Wiedemann E 1984 The hormonal responses to generalized tonic-clonic seizures. Brain 107:569

Ancri D, Naquet R, Basset J Y et al 1979 Correlation entre volume sanguin regional et crise d'epilepsie chezz le Papio Papio. Bulletin d'Académie Sciences 3:343

Anderson V E, Hauser W A, Rich S S 1986 Genetic heterogeneity in the epilepsies. In: Delgado-Escueta A V , Eward A A, Woodbury D M, Porter R J (eds) Advances in neurology 44, 59. New York, Raven Press

Angel A, Lemon R N 1974 An experimental model of sensory myoclonus produced by 1,2-dihydroxybenzene in the anaesthetized rat. In: Harris P, Mawdsley C (eds) Epilepsy. Churchill Livingstone, Edinburgh, p 37

Appleton D B, DeVivo D C 1974 An animal model for the ketogenic diet. Epilepsia 15:211

Baldy-Moulinier M 1986 Inter-relationships between epilepsy. In: Pedley T A, Meldrum B S, Recent advances in epilepsy 3, 37. Churchill Livingstone, Edinburgh

Baldy-Moulinier M, Arias L P, Passouant P 1973 Hippocampal epilepsy produced by ouabain. European Neurology 9:333

Barbeau A, Donaldson J 1974 Zinc, taurine and epilepsy. Archives of Neurology 30:52

Bean J W, Zee D, Thom D 1966 Pulmonary changes with convulsions induced by drugs and oxygen at high pressure. Journal of Applied Physiology 21:865

Belton N R, Etheridge J E, Millichap J G 1965 Effects of convulsions and anticonvulsants on blood sugar in rabbits. Epilepsia 6:243

Bennett D R 1963 Sleep deprivation and major motor seizures. Neurology 13:953

Bertaccini G 1959 Effect of convulsant treatment on the 5-hydroxytryptamine content of brain and other tissues of the rat. Journal of Neurochemistry 4:217

Bignami A, Palladini G 1966 Experimentally produced cerebral status spongiosus and continuous pseudorhythmic electroencephalographic discharges with a membrane-ATPase inhibitor in the rat. Nature 209:413

Bird E D, Iversen L L 1974 Huntington's chorea. Post-mortem measurement of glutamic acid decarboxylase, choline acetyltransferase and dopamine in basal ganglia. Brain 97:457

Boyle R 1660 New experiments: Physico-mechanical. Touching the spring of air and its effects. Hall, Oxford

Brennan R W, Petito C K, Porro R S 1972 Single seizures cause no ultrastructural change in brain. Brain Research 45:574

Brierley J B 1971 The neuropathological sequelae of profound hypoxia. In: Brierley J B, Meldrum B S (eds) Brain hypoxia. Heinemann, London, p 147

Brierley J B, Brown A W, Meldrum B S 1971a The neuropathology of insulin-induced hypoglycaemia in the primate: topography and cellular nature. In: Brierley J B, Meldrum B S (eds) Brain hypoxia. Clinics in developmental medicine No 39/40. William Heinemann, London, p 255 Medical Books.

Brierley J B, Brown A W, Meldrum B S 1971b The nature and time course of the neuronal alterations resulting from oligaemia and hypoglycaemia in the brain of Macaca mulatta. Brain Research 25:483

Brierley J B, Meldrum B S, Brown A W 1973 The threshold and neuropathology of cerebal 'naoxic-ischaemic' cell change. Archives of Neurology 29:367

Brodersen P, Paulson O B, Bolwig T G, Rogon Z E, Rafaelsen O J, Lassen N A 1973 On the mechanism of cerebral hyperaemia in electrically-induced epileptic seizures in man. Stroke 4:359

Brodie D A, Woodbury D M 1958 Acid-base changes in brain and blood of rats exposed to high concentrations of carbon dioxide. American Journal of Physiology 192:91

Caspers H, Speckmann E J 1972 Cerebral pO_2, pCO_2 and pH. Changes during convulsive activity and their significance for spontaneous arrest of seizures. Epilepsia 13:699

Chadwick D, Trimble M, Jenner P, Driver M V, Reynolds E H 1978 Manipulation of cerebral monoamines in the treatment of human epilepsy. A pilot study. Epilepsia 19:3

Chapman A G 1985 Cerebral energy metabolism and seizures. In: Pedley T A, Meldrum B S (eds) Recent advances in epilepsy 2, 19. Churchill Livingstone, Edinburgh

Chapman A G, Meldrum B S, Siesjö B K 1975 Cerebral blood flow and cerebral metabolic rate during prolonged epileptic seizures in rats. Journal of Physiology 254:61

Chapman A G, Meldrum B S, Siesjo B K 1977 Cerebral metabolic changes during prolonged epileptic seizures in rats. Journal of Neurochemistry 28:1025

Chaslin P 1891 Contribution à l'étude de la sclérose cerebrale. Archives Med. Exp. Anat. Pathol. 3:305

Christian W 1960 Biolektrische Charakteristik tages-periodisch gebundener Verlaufsformen epileptischer Erkrankungen. Deutsch Zeit Nervenheilk 181:413

Chusid J G, Kopeloff L M 1969 Use of chronic irritative foci in laboratory evaluation of antiepileptic drugs. Epilepsia 10:239

Chusid J G, Kopeloff L M, Kopeloff N 1956 Convulsant action of antihistamines in monkeys. Journal of Applied Physiology 9:271

Cohen H, Thomas J, Dement W C 1970 Sleep stages. REM deprivation and electroconvulsive threshold in the cat. Brain Research 19:317

Collins R C, Posner J B, Plum F 1970 Cerebral energy metabolism during electroshock seizures in mice. American Journal of Physiology 218:943

Cooper R 1974 Influence on the EEG of certain physiological states and other parameters. In: Rémond A (ed) Handbook of Electroencephalography and Clinical Neurophysiology Part B 7:1

Corriol J, Papy J-J, Rhoner J J, Joanny P 1969 Electroclinical correlations established during tetanic manifestations induced by parathyroid removal in the dog. In: Gastaut H, Jasper H H, Bancaud J, Waltregny A (eds) Physiopathogenesis of the epilepsies. Thomas, Springfield, p 128

Costa P J, Bonnycastle D D 1952 The effect of DCA, compound E, testosterone, progesterone and ACTH in modifying 'agene induced' convulsions in dogs. Archives Internationales Pharmacodynamie 91:330

Coursin D B 1954 Convulsive seizures in infants with pyridoxine-deficient diet. Journal of the American Medical Association 154:406

Coursin D B 1964 Vitamin B metabolism in infants and children. Vitamins and Hormones 22:755

Crome L C, Stern J 1972 The pathology of mental retardation. 2nd edn. Churchill Livingstone, London

Curtis D R, Johnston G A R 1974 Amino acid transmitters in the mammalian central nervous system. Ergebnisse der Physiologie 69:97

Dana-Haeri J, Trimble M R, Daley J 1983 Prolactin and gonadotrophin changes following generalized and partial seizures. Journal of Neurology, Neurosurgery and Psychiatry 46: 331–335

De-Feudis F V, Elliott K A C 1967 Delay or inhibition of convulsions by intraperitoneal injections of diverse substances. Canadian Journal of Physiological and Pharmacology 45:857

Delgado-Escueta A V, Ward A A, Woodbury D M, Porter R J 1986 (eds) Basic mechanisms of the epilepsies: molecular and cellular approaches. Advances in neurology 44. Raven Press, New York

Delgado-Escueta A V, White R, Greenberg D A, Treiman L J 1986 Looking for epilepsy genes: clinical and molecular genetic studies. In: Delgado-Escueta A V, Ward A A, Woodbury D M, Porter R J (eds) Advances in neurology 44, 77. Raven Press, New York

Demoor J 1898 Le mécanisme et la signification de l'état monifornie des neurones. Annales de la Société Royale des Sciences Médicales et Naturelles de Bruxelles 7:205

De Robertis E, Alberici M, De Lores Arnaiz G R 1969 Astroglial swelling and phosphohydrolases in cerebral cortex of metrazol convulsant rats. Brain Research 12:461

De Vellis I, Inglish D 1968 Hormonal control of glycerolphosphate dehydrogenase in the rat brain. Journal of Neurochemistry 15:1061

Dixon P F, Booth M, Butler J 1914 The corticosteroids. In:

Gray C H, Bacharach A L (eds) Hormones in blood 2,305. Academic Press, London & New

Dunicavy D L F, Oswald I, Brows P, Strong J A 1974 Hyperthyroidism, sleep and growth hormone. Electroencephalography and Clinical Neurophysiology 36:259

Eccles J C 1964 The physiology of synopsies. Springer-Verlag, Berlin, p 316

Eccles J C 1969 The inhibitory pathways of the central nervous system. Thomas, Springfield

Ehlers C L, Killiam E K 1979 The influence of cortisone on EEG and seizure activity in the baboon, Papio Papio. Electroencephalography and Clinical Neurophysiology 47:404

Eidelberg E, Lesse H, Gault F P 1963 An experimental model of temporal lobe epilepsy. Studies of the convulsant properties of cocaine. In: Glaser G H (ed) EEG and behaviour. Basic Books, New York, p 272

Essman W B 1973 Neurochemistry of cerebral electroshock. Spectrum Publications, New York, p 181

Evans E C 1960 Neurologic complications of myxoedema convulsions. Annals of Internal Medicine 52:434

Everett G M, Richards R K 1944 Comparative anticonvulsive action of 3, 5, 5-trimethyl-oxazolidine-2, 4-dione (Triadone), Dilantin and phenobarbital. Journal of Pharmacology and Experimental Therapeutics 81:402

Fahn S, Côté L J 1968 Regional distribution of γ-aminobutyric acid (GABA) in brain of the rhesus monkey. Journal of Neurochemistry 15:209

Farwell J, Milstein J, Opheim K, Smith E, Glass S 1984 Adrenocorticotropic hormone controls infantile spasms independently of cortisol stimulation. Epilepsia 25: 605–608

Fay T 1929 Factors in 'mechanical theory of epilepsy' with especial reference to influence of fluid, and its control, in treatment of certain cases. American Journal of Psychiatry 8:783

Fay T 1931 Convulsive seizures, their production and control, with especial reference to the probable mechanism of the seizure itself. American Journal of Psychiatry 10:551

Feldman J, Cortell R, Gellhorn E 1940 On the vago-insulin and sympathetico-adrenal system and their mutual relationship under conditions of central excitation induced by anoxia and convulsant drugs. American Journal of Physiology 131:281

Fischer J 1973 Change in the number of vesicles in synapses of a projected epileptic cortical focus in rats. Physiologia Bohemoslovaca 22:537

Folbergrova J 1975 Changes in glycogen phosphorylase activity and glycogen levels of mouse cerebral cortex during convulsions induced by homocysteine. Journal of Neurochemistry 24:15

Folbergrova J, Passonneau J V, Lowry O H, Schulz D W 1969 Glycogen, ammonia and related metabolites in the brain during seizures evoked by methionine sulphoximine. Journal of Neurochemistry 16:191

Frame B, Carter S 1955 Pseudohypoparathyroidism. Clinical picture and relation to clinical seizures. Neurology 5:295

Friis M L, Lund M 1974 Stress convulsions. Archives of Neurology 31:155

Friis-Hansen B, Buchthal F 1965 EEG findings in an infant with intoxication and convulsions incident to hypernatraema. Electroencephalography and Clinical Neurophysiology 19:387

Funck-Brentano J L, Lossky-Nekhorocheff I, Altman J 1960 Étude expérimentale des manifestations cérébrales de l'intoxication par l'eau. Electroencephalography and Clinical Neurophysiology 12:185

Futamachi K J, Mutani R, Prince D A 1974 Potassium activity in rabbit cortex. Britain Research 75:5

Gallagher B B, Murvin A, Flanigin H F, King D W, Luney D 1984 Pituitary and adrenal function in epileptic patients. Epilepsia 25: 683–689

Garattini S, Kato R, Valzelli L 1960 Biochemical and pharmacological effects induced by electroshock. Psychiatrica Neurologica 140:190

Garland H G, Dick A P, Whitty C W M 1943 Water-pitressin test in the diagnosis of epilepsy. Lancet ii:566

Gastaut H, Papy J J, Toga M, Murisasco A, Dubois D 1971 Epilepsie de l'insuffisance rénale et crises épileptiques accidentales au cours de l'épuration extra-rénale (rein artificiel). Revue EEG Neurophysiologie 1:151

Gastaut H, Saier J, Mano T, Santos D, Lyagoubi S 1968 Generalized epileptic seizures, induced by 'non-convulsant' substances. Part 2. Experimental study with special reference to ammonium chloride. Epilepsia 9:317

Gastaut H, Poirier F, Payan H, Salamon G, Toga M, Vigouroux M 1960 HHE Syndrome. Hemiconvulsions, hemiplegia, epilepsy. Epilepsia 1:418

Gellhorn E, Ballin H M 1950 Further investigations on effect of anoxia on convulsions. American Journal of Physiology 162:503

Georgi F, Strauss R 1938 The problem of convulsions and insulin therapy. II. Special comment on the method described by Meduna. American Journal of Psychiatry 94: suppl 76

Gilboe D D, Betz A 1973 Oxygen uptake in the isolated canine brain. American Journal of Physiology 224:588

Gillin J C, Jacobs L S, Snyder F, Henkin R I 1974 Effects of decreased adrenal corticosteroids: changes in sleep in normal subjects and patients with adrenal cortical insufficiency. Electroencephalography and Clinical Neurophysiology 36:282

Glaser G H, Levy L L 1960 Seizures and idiopathic hypoparathyroidism. Epilepsia I:454

Globus A, Scheibel A B 1966 Loss of dendritic spines as an index of presynaptic terminal patterns. Nature 212:463

Gloor P, Testa G 1974 Generalized penicillin epilepsy in the cat: effects of intracarotid and intravertebal pentylenetetrazol and amobarbital injections. Electroncephalography and Clinical Neurophysiology 36:499

Glotzner F L 1973 Membrane properties of neuroglia in epileptogenic gliosis. Brain Research 55:159

Goddard G V, McIntyre D, Leech C 1969 A permanent change in brain function resulting from daily electrical stimulation. Experimental Neurology, 25:295

Goodman L S, Grewal M S, Brown W C, Swinyard E A 1953 Comparison of maximal seizures evoked by pentylenetetrazol (Metrazol) and electroshock in mice, and their modification by anticonvulsants. Journal of Pharmacology and Experimental Therapeutics 108:168

Grob D 1963 Anticholinesterase intoxication in man and its treatment. In: Handbuch der experimentellen Pharmakologie (Supplement 15:989). Cholinesterases and Anticholinesterase Agents. Springer-Verlag, Berlin

Grossman R G, Rosman L J 1971 Intracellular potentials of inexcitable cells in epileptogenic cortex undergoing fibrillary gliosis after a local injury. Brain Research 28:181

Halpern L M 1972 Chronically isolated aggregates of

mammalian cerebral cortical neurons studied in situ. In: Purpura D P, Penry J K, Tower D B, Woodbury D M, Walter R D (eds) Experimental models of epilepsy. Raven Press, New York p 197

Hammond E J, Ramsay R E, Villarreal H J, Wilder B J 1980 Effects of intracortical injection of blood and blood components on the electrocorticogram. Epilepsia 21:3

Harris J W, van den Brenk H A S 1968 Comparative effects of hyperbaric oxygen and pentylenetetrazol on lung weight and non-protein sulfhydryl content of experimental animals. Biochemical Pharmacology 17:1181

Hassler R 1972 Physiopathology of rigidity. In: Siegfried J, Hawkins R A, Williamson D H, Krebs H A (eds) 1971 Parkinson's Disease. Hans Huber, Vienna p 20

Hawkins R A, Williamson D H, Krebs H A 1971 Ketone body utilization by adult and suckling rat brain in vivo. Biochemical Journal 122:13

Hendley C D, Spudis E V, De la Torre E 1965 Intracranial pressure during electroshock convulsions in the dog. Neurology 15:351

Henn F A, Haljamae H, Hamberger A 1972 Glial cell function: Active control of extracellular K+ concentration. Brain Research 43:437

Herberg L J, Watkins P J 1966 Epileptiform seizures induced by hypothalamic stimulation in the rat: Resistance to fits. Nature 209:515

Herlitz G 1941 Studien uber die sogenannten initialen Fieberkrampfe bei Kinden. Acta Paediatrica Scandinavica 29 (suppl 1):142

Heuser G, Eidelberg E 1961 Steroid-induced convulsions in experimental animals. Endocrinology 69:915

Hindfelt B, Siesjo B K 1971 Cerebral effects of acute ammonia intoxication. The influence on intracellular and extracellular acid-base parameters. Scandinavian Journal of Clinical and Laboratory Investigation 28:353

Hirsch C S, Martin D L 1971 Unexpected deaths in young epileptics. Neurology 21:682

Holmgren B, Kraeplin S 1953 Electroencephalographic study of asthmatic children. Acta Pediatrica 42:432

Hom A C, Buterbaugh G G 1986 Estrogen alters the acquisition of seizures kindled by repeated amygdala stimulation or pentylenetetrazol administration in ovariectomized female rats. Epilepsia 27: 103–108

Horton R W, Meldrum B S 1973 Seizures induced by allylglycine, 3-mercaptopropionic acid and 4-deoxypyridoxine in mice and photosensitive baboons, and different modes of inhibition of cerebral glutomic acid decarboxylase. British Journal of Pharmacology 49:52

Hunt A D, Stokes J, McCrory W W, Stround H H 1954 Pyridoxine dependency: report of a case of intractable convulsions in an infant controlled by pyridoxine. Pediatrics 13:140

Huot J, Radouco-Thomas S, Radouco-Thomas C 1973 Qualitative and quantitative evaluation of experimentally-induced seizures. In: Mercier J (ed.) Anticonvulsant drugs. Pergamon Press, Oxford, p 123

Huttenlocher P R, Wilbourn A J, Signore J M 1971 Medium chain triglycerides as a therapy for intractable childhood epilepsy. Neurology 21:1097

Ingram T T S, Stark G D, Blackburn I 1967 Ataxia and other neurological disorders as sequels of severe hypoglycaemia in childhood. Brain 90 851

Ingvar D H 1973 rCBF in focal cortical epilepsy. Stroke 4:359

Isler W 1971 Acute hemiplegia and hemisyndromes in childhood. Clinics in developmental medicine nos 41–42. Heinemann, London, p 314

Jabbari B, Huott A D 1980 Seizures in thyrotoxicosis. Epilepsia 21:91

James I M 1975 Autonomic control of the cerebral circulation. In: Meldrum B S, Marsden C D (eds) Primate models of neurological disorders, Raven Press, New York, p 167

Janz D 1974 Epilepsy and the sleeping-waking cycle. In: Vinken P J, Bruyn G W (eds) Handbook of clinical neurology. The epilepsies. North Holland Publishing, Amsterdam, p 311

Jeavons P M, Bower B D 1964 Infantile spasms. A review of the literature and a study of 112 cases. Clinics in development medicine no 15. Heinemann, London

Jeavons P M, Bower B D, Dimitrakoudi M 1973 Long-term prognosis of 150 cases of 'West syndrome'. Epilepsiaa 14:153

Johnson L C, Davidoff R A 1964 Autonomic changes during paroxysmal EEG activity. Electroencephalography and Clinical Neurophysiology 17:25

Jose C J, Barton J L, Perex-Cruet J 1979 Hyponatraemic seizures in psychiatric patients. Biological Psychiatry 14:839

Jouvet M 1972 The role of monoamines and acetylcholine-containing neurons in the regulation of the sleep-waking cycle. Ergebnisse Physiologie 64:166

Jovanovic U J 1967 Das schlafverhalten der epileptiker. I. Schlafdauer, schlaftiefe und bensonderheiten der schlafperiodik. Deutsche Zeitschrift fur Nervenheilkunde 190:159

Kellaway P 1985 Sleep and epilepsy. Epilepsia 26: S15–S30

Kessler M, Gellhorn E 1941 Effect of electrically-induced convulsions on vago-insulin and sympathetico-adrenal system. Proceedings of the Society for Experimental Biology and Medicine 46:64

Kety S S, Schmidt C F 1948 The effects of altered arterial tensions of carbon dioxide and oxygen on cerebral blood flow and cerebral oxygen consumption of normal young men. Journal of Clinical Investigation 27:484

Kety S S 1964 The cerebral circulation. In: Field V (ed.) Handbook of physiology. I. Neurophysiology. American Physiological Society, Washington DC, p 1751

Kety S S, Javoy F, Thierry A M, Julou I, Glowinski J A 1967 A sustained effect of electroconvulsive shock on the turnover of norepinephrine in the central nervous system of the rat. Proceedings of the National Academy of Science 58:1249

King L J, Lowry O H, Passoneau J V, Venson V 1967 Effects of convulsants on energy reserves in the cerebral cortex. Journal of Neurochemistry 14:599

King L J, Webb O L, Carl J 1970 Effects of duration of convulsions on energy reserves of the brain. Journal of Neurochemistry 17:13

Klatzo I 1967 Neuropathological aspects of brain oedema. Journal of Neuropathology and Experimental Neurology 26:1

Krantz J C 1963 Volatile anaesthetics and Indoklon. Journal of Neuropsychiatry 4:157

Kruse H D, Orent E R, McCollum E V 1932 Studies on magnesium deficiency in animals. I. Symptomatology resulting from magnesium deprivation. Journal of Biological Chemistry 96:519

Krushinsky L V 1962 A study of pathophysiological mechanisms of cerebral haemorrhage provoked by reflex epileptic seizures in rats. Epilepsia 3:363

Kurtz D, Micheletti G, Tempe J D, Brogard J M, Girardel M, Fletto R 1971 Etude électroclinique des comas hyperodmolsitrd. Revue EEG et Neurophysiologie, 1:353

Laidlaw J 1956 Catamenial epilepsy. Lancet, 2, 1235

Lamprecht F, Ebert M H, Turek I, Kopin I J 1974 Serum dopamaaine-Beta hydroxylase in depressed patients and the effect of electroconvulsive shock treatment. Psychopharmacologia 40:241

Langdon-Down M, Brain W R 1929 Times of day in relation to convulsions in epilepsy. Lancet I:1029

Lascelles P T, Lewis P D 1972 Hypodipsia and hypernatraemia associated with hypothalamic and suprasellar lesions. Brain 95:249

Lennox W G, Gibbs F A, Gibbs E L 1936 Effect on the electroencephalogram of drugs and conditions which influence seizures. Archives of Neurology and Psychiatry 36:1236

Lennox-Buchthal M A 1973 Febrile convulsions. Electroencephalography and Clinical Neurophysiology (suppl. 32) 1

Levitt P, Wilson W, Wilkins R 1971 The effects of subarachnoid blood on the electrocorticogram of the cat. Journal of Neurosurgery 35: 185–191

Lewis L D, Ljunggren B, Norberg K, Siesjo B K (1974a) Changes in carbohydrate substrates, amino acids and ammonia in the brain during insulin-induced hypoglycaemia. Journal of Neurosurgery 23:659

Lewis L D, Ljunggren B, Ratcheson R A, Siesjo B K 1974b Cerebral energy state in insulin-induced hypoglycaemia, related to blood glucose and to EEG. Journal of Neurochemistry 23:673

Lbermitte F, Marteau R, Degos C F 1972 Analyse pharmacologique d'un nouveau cas de myoclonies d'intentioh et d'action post-anoxiques. Revue Neurologique 126:107

Lindenberg R 1955 Compression of brain arteries as pathogenetic factor for tissue necroses and their areas of predilection. Journal of Neuropathology and Experimental Neurology 14:223

Livingston S 1972 Comprehensive management of epilepsy in infancy and childhood. Thomas, Springfield

Lloyd K G, Munari C, Bossi L, Bancaud J, Talairach J, Morselli P L 1981 Biochemical evidence for the alterations of GABA-mediated synaptic transmission in pathological brain tissue (stereo EEG or morphological definition) from epileptic patients. In: Morsellie P L, Lloyd K G, Loscher W, Meldrum B, Reynolds E H (eds) Neurotransmitters, seizures and epilepsy. Raven Press, New York, p 331

Luciani J, Riche D, Lanoir J, Seite R 1969 Modifications de la neurosecretion hypothalamique sous l'influence de manifestations épileptiformes par photo stimulation chez le Papio papio. Comptes Rendues du Societes Biologiques 163:1167

Luft V C, Noell W K 1956 Manifestations of brief instantaneous anoxia in man. Journal of Applied Physiology 8:444

Luttrell C M, Finberg L, Drawdy L P 1959 Hemorrhagic encephalopathy induced by hypernatraemia. II. Experimental observations on hyperosmolarity in cats. Archives of Neurology 1:153

Lux H D 1974 The kinetics of extracellular potassium: relation to epileptogenesis. Epilepsia 15:375

Maccario M 1968 Neurological dysfunction associated with non-ketotic hyperglycaemia. Archives of Neurology 19:525

Magnaes B, Nornes H 1974 Circulatory and respiratory changes in spontaneous epileptic seizures in man. European Neurology 12:104

Marcus E M, Watson C W, Goldman P L 1966 Effects of steroids on cerebral electrical activity: epileptogenic effects of conjugated oestrogens and related compounds in the cat and rabbit. Archives of Neurology 15:521

Marcus E M 1972 Experimental models of petit mal epilepsy. In: Purpura D P, Penry J K, Tower D, Woodbury D M, Walter R (eds) Experimental models of epilepsy. Raven Press, New York, p 113

Margerison J H, Corsellis J A N 1966 Epilepsy and the temporal lobes – a clinical, electroencephalographic and neuropathological study of the brain in epilepsy, with particular references to the temporal lobes. Brain 89:499

McLardy T 1974 Pathogenesis of epileptic-hypoxic Ammon's horn sclerosis: contribution of basal vein constriction by looped posterior cerebral artery. IRCS Anatomy: Neurology 2:1574

McQuarrie I, Peeler D B 1931 The effects of sustained pituitary antidiuresis and forced water drinking in epileptic children. A diagnostic and etiologic study. Journal of Clinical Investigation 10:915

Meldrum B S 1974a Present views on hippocampal sclerosis and epilepsy. In: Williams D (ed.) Modern trends in neurology 6. Butterworths, London, p 223

Meldrum B S 1975b Epilepsy and γ-amino butyric acid-medited inhibition. International Review of Neurobiology 17

Meldrum B S 1978 Physiological changes during prolonged seizures and epileptic brain damage. Neuropadiatrie 9:203

Meldrum B S 1985 GABA and other amino acids. In: Frey H H, Janz D (eds) Antiepileptic drugs. Handbook of Experimental Pharmacology 74:153

Meldrum B 1986 Is epilepsy a disorder of excitatory transmission? In: Trimble M, Reynolds E H (eds) What is epilepsy? Churchill Livingstone, Edinburgh, p 293

Meldrum B S, Brierley J B 1973 Prolonged epileptic seizures in primates: ischaemic cell change and its relation to ictal physiological events. Archives of Neurology 28:10

Meldrum B S, Horton R W 1971 Convulsive effects of 4-deoxypyridoxine and of bicuculline in photosensitive baboons (Papio papio) and in rhesus monkeys (Macaca mulatta). Brain Research 35:419

Meldrum B S, Horton R W 1973a Cerebral functional effects of 2-deoxy-D-glucose and 3-O-methylglucose in rhesus monkeys. Electroencephalography and Clinical Neurophysiology 35:59

Meldrum B S, Horton R W 1973b Physiology of status epilepticus in primates. Archives of Neurology 28:1

Meldrum B S, Horton R W 1974 Neuronal inhibition mediated by Gaba, and patterns of convulsions in photosensitive baboons and epilepsy (Papio papio). In: Harris P, Mawdsley C (eds) The natural history and management of epilepsy. Churchill Livingstone, Edinburgh, p 54

Meldrum B S, Nilsson B 1976 Cerebral blood flow and metabolic rate early and late in prolonged epileptic seizures induced in rats by bicuculline. Brain 99: 523–542

Meldrum B S, Stephenson J D 1975 Enhancement of picrotoxin convulsions in chicks and mice by the prior intraperitoneal injection of hypertonic GABAa or mannitol. European Journal of Pharmacology 30:368

Meldrum B S, Anlezark G, Trimble M 1975 Drugs

modifying dopaminergic activity and behaviour, the EEG and epilepsy in Papio papio.

Meldrum B S, Horton R W, Brierley J B 1971 Insulin-induced hypoglycaemia in the primate: relationship between physiological changes and ultimate neuropathology. In: Brierley J B, Meldrum B S (eds) Brain Hypoxia. Edited by Clinics in developmental medicine No 39/40. Heinemann, London p 207

Meldrum B S, Horton R W, Brierley J B 1974 Epileptic brain damage in adolescent baboons following seizures induced by allyglycine. Brain 97:407

Meldrum B S, Vigouroux R A, Brierley J B 1973 Systemic factors and epileptic brain damage. Prolonged seizures in paralysed artificially ventilated baboons. Archives of Neurology 29:82

Meldrum B S, Balzano E, Gadea M, Naquet R 1970 Photic and drug-induced epilepsy in the baboon (Papio papio). The effects of isoniazid, thiosemicarbazide, pyridoxine and amino-oxyacetic acid. Electroencephalography and Clinical Neurophysiology 29:333

Meldrum B S, Balzano E, Horton R W Lee G, Trimble M 1975 Photically-induced epilepsy in Papio papio as a model for drug studies. In: Meldrum B S, Marsden C D (eds) Primate models of neurological disorders. Advances in neurology 10. Raven Press, New York

Meldrum B S, Horton R W, Bloom S R, Butler J, Keenan J 1979 Endocrine factors and glucose metabolism during prolonged seizures in baboons. Epilepsia 20:527

Melekian B, Labplane R, Debray P 1962 Considerations cliniques et statistiques sur les convulsions au cours des deshydrations aigues. Annales de Pediatrie 34:1494

Metrakos K, Metrakos J D 1974 Genetics of epilepsy. In: Vinken P J Bruyn G W (eds) Handbook of clinical neurology 15, 429. North Holland Publishing, Amsterdam

Meyer J S, Gotoh F, Tazaki Y 1961 Inhibitory action of carbon dioxide and acetazolamide in seizure activity. Electroencephalography and Clinical Neurophysiology 13:762

Meyer J S, Gotoh F, Favale E 1966 Cerebral metabolism during epileptic seizures in man. Electroencephalography and Clinical Neurophysiology 21:10

Millichap J G 1968 Febrile convulsions. Macmillan, New York

Millichap J G 1974 Metabolic and endocrine factors. In: Vinken P J, Bruyn G W (eds) Handbook of clinical neurology. The epilepsies 15/311 North Holland Publishing, Amsterdam

Miribel J, Poirier F 1961 Effects of ACTH and adrenocortical hormones in juvenile epilepsy. Epilepsia 2:345

Moore K E, Phillipson O T 1975 Effects of dexamethasone on phenylethamolamine N-methyltransferase (PNMT) and adrenaline (A) in the brains of adult and neonatal rats. British Journal of Pharmacology 53:453

Morris-Jones P H, Houston I B, Evans R C 1967 Prognosis of the neurological complications of acute hypernatraemia. Lancet 2:13852

Mueller S M, Heistad D D, Marcus M L 1979 Effect of sympathetic nerves on cerebral vessels during seizures. American Journal of Physiology 237: H178–H184

Munson E S, Wagman I H 1969 Acid-base changes during lidocaine-induced seizures in Macaca mulatta. Archives of Neurology 20:406

Musacchio J M, Julou L, Kety S S, Glowinski J 1969 Increase in rat tyrosine hydroxylase activity produced by electroconvulsive shock. Proceedings of the National Academy of Sciences 63:1117

Nalin A, Facchinetti F, Galli V, Petraglia F, Storchi R, Genazzani A R 1985 Reduced ACTH content in cerebrospinal fluid of children affected by cryptogenic infantile spasms with hypsarryhthmia. Epilepsia 26: 446–449

Naquet R, Meldrum B S, Balzano E, Charrier J P 1970 Phoeically-induced epilepsy and glucose metabolism in the adolescent baboon (Papio papio). Brain Research 18:503

Newark M E, Penry J K 1980 Catamenial epilepsy: a review. Epilepsia 21: 281–300

Nicoletti F, Patti F, Ferrara N et al (1982) Comparative effects of estrogens and prolactin on nigral and striatal GAD activity. Brain Research 232: 238–241

Nicoletti F, Speciale C, Sortino M A 1985 Comparative effects of estradiol benzoate, the antiestrogen clomiphene citrate, and the progestin medroxyprogesterone acetate on kainic acid-induced seizures in male and female rats. Epilepsia 26: 252–257

Ohman R, Walinder J, Balldin J, Wallin L, Abrahamsson L 1976 Prolactin response to electroconvulsive therapy. Lancet 2:936

Olsen R W, Wamsley J K, McCabe R T, Lee R J, Lomax P 1985a Benzodiazepine/γ-aminobutyric acid receptor deficit in the midbrain of the seizure-susceptibe gerbil. Proceedings of the National Academy of Science 82:6701

Olsen R W, Jones I, Seyfried T N, McCabe R T, Wamsley J K 1985b Benzodiazepine receptor binding deficit in audiogenic seizure-susceptible mice. Federation Proceedings 44:1106

Opper L 1939 Pathologic picture of thujone and monobromated camphor convulsions. Archives of Neurology and Psychiatry 41:460

Ounted C, Lindsay J, Norman R 1966 Biological factors in temporal lobe epilepsy. Clinics in developmental medicine no 22. Heinemann, London

Owen O E, Morgan A P, Kemp H G, Sullivan J M, Herrera M G, Cahill G F 1967 Brain metabolism during fasting. Journal of Clinical Investigation 46:1589

Owen M, Bliss E L 1970 Sleep loss and cerebral excitability. American Journal of Physiology 218:171

Owman C, Edvinsson L 1978 Histochemical and pharmacological approach to the investigation of neurotransmitters, with particular regard to the cerebrovascular bed. In: Cerebral vascular smooth muscle and its control. CIBA Foundation Symposium 56: 275–304

Palayoor S T, Seyfried T N 1984 Genetic association between Ca_2^+ ATPase activity and audiogenic seizures in mice. Journal of Neurochemistry 42:1771

Papeschi R, Molina-Negro P, Sourkes T L, Erba G 1972 The concentration of homovanillic and 5-hydroxyindoleacetic acids in ventricular and lumbar CSF: Studies in patients with extrapyramidal disorders, epilepsy and other diseases. Neurology 22:1151

Pappius H M, Savaki H E, Fieschi C, Rapoport S I, Sokoloff L 1979 Osmotic opening of the blood-brain barrier and local cerebral glucose utilisation. Annals of Neurology 5:211

Passouant P, Cadilhac J, Pternitis C, Baldy-Moulinier M 1967 Epilepsie temporale et decharges ammoniques provoquees par l'anoxie exprive. Revue Neurologique 117:65

Penfield W, Jasper H 1954 Epilepsy and the functional anatomy of the human brain. Little, Brown, Boston

Penfield W, Von Santha K, Cipriani A 1939 Cerebral blood flow during induced epileptiform seizures in animals and man. Journal of Neurophysiology 2:257

Perry T L, Berry K, Hansen S, Diamond S, Mok C 1971 Regional distribution of amino acids in human brain obtained at autopsy. Journal of Neurochemistry 18:513

Perry T L, Hansen S, Kloster M 1973 Huntington's chorea: deficiency of γ-aminobutyric acid in brain. New England Journal of Medicine 288:337

Peters R A 1963 Biochemical lesions and lethal synthesis. Pergamon Press, Oxford

Plum F, Duffy T E 1975 The couple between cerebral metabolism and blood flow during seizures. In: Alfred Benzon Symposium 8: The working brain. Munksgaard, Copenhagen

Plum F, Posner J B, Troy B 1968 Cerebral metabolic and circulatory responses to induced convulsions in animals. Archives of Neurology 18:1

Poire 1969 Hypoglycaemic epilepsy: Clinical electrographic and biological study during induced hypoglycaemia in man. In: Gastaut H, Jasper H, Bancaud J (eds) Archives of Neurology 20:388

Pollen D A, Trachtenberg M C 1970 Neuroglia: gliosis and focal epilepsy. Science 167:1252

Ponte J, Purves M J 1974 The role of the carotid body chemoreceptors and carotid sinus baroreceptors in the control of cerebral blood vessels. Journal of Physiology 237:315

Posner J B, Plum F, Poznak A V 1969 Cerebral metabolism during electrically-induced seizures in man. Archives of Neurology 20:388

Prill A, Quellhorst E, Scheler F 1969 Epilepsy: Clinical and electroencephalographic findings in patients with renal insufficiency. In: Gastaut H, Jasper H, Bancaud H, Waltregny A (eds) The physiopathogenesis of the epilepsies. Thomas, Springfield, p 60

Prince D A, Lux H D, Neher E 1973 Measurement of extracellular potassium activity in cat cortex. Brain Research 50:489

Purves M J 1972 The physiology of the cerebral circulation. Cambridge University Press, Cambridge

Pylkko O O, Woodbury D M 1961 The effect of maturation on chemically-induced seizures in rats. Journal of Pharmacology and Experimental Therapeutics 131:185

Reynolds E H 1970 Water, electrolytes and epilepsy. Journal of the Neurological Sciences 11:327

Ribak C E, Harris A B, Vaughn J E, Roberts 1979 Inhibitory GABAergic nerve terminals decrease at sites of focal epilepsy. Science 205:211

Riche D 1973 L'hypothalamus du singe Papio papio (Desm): stereotaxi, cytologie et modifications neurosecretoires liees aux crises d'épilepsie induites par la lumiere. Journal fur Hirnforschung 14:527

Richter D, Dawson R M C 1948 The ammonia and glutamine content of the brain. Journal of Biological Chemistry 176:1199

Rosen A D, Frumin N V 1979 Focal epileptogenesis after intracortical hemoglobin injection. Experimental Neurology 66:277

Rosenblatt D E, Lauter C J, Trams E G 1976 Deficiency of a $Ca_2 +$ ATPase in brains of seizure prone mice. Journal of Neurochemistry 27:1299

Rowntree L G 1923 Water intoxication. Archives of Internal Medicine 32:157

Rowntree L G 1926 The effects on mammals of the administration of excessive quantities of water. Journal of Pharmacology and Experimental Therapeutics 29:135

Rymer M M, Fishman R A 1973 Protective adaptation of brain to water intoxication. Archives of Neurology 28:49

Sacktor B, Wilson J E, Tiekert C G 1966 Regulation of glycolysis in brain, in situ, during convulsions. Journal of Biological Chemistry 241:5071

Samson F E, Dahl N A 1957 Cerebral energy requirement of neonatal rats. American Journal of Physiology 188:277

Sassin J F, Parker D C, Mace J W, Gotlin R W, Johnson L C, Rossman L G 1969 Human growth hormone release: relation to slow-wave sleep-waking cycles. Science 165:513

Schade J P, McMenemy W H 1963 Selective vulnerability of the brain in hypoxaemia. Blackwell Scientific, Oxford

Scheibel M E, Scheibel A B 1973 Hippocampal pathology in temporal lobe epilepsy. A Golgi survey. In: Epilepsy: its phenomena in man. UCLA Forum in Medical Sciences 17:311

Scheibel M E, Crandall P H, Scheibel A B 1974 The hippocampala-dentate complex in temporal lobe epilepsy. Epilepsia 15:55

Schmidt C F, Kety S A, Pennes H H 1945 the gaseous metabolism of the brain of the monkey. American Journal of Physiology 143:33

Scholz W 1951 Die Krampfschadigungen des Gehirns. Monographien aus dem Gesamtegebiete der Neurologie und Psychiatri. Heft 75. Springer-Verlag, Berlin

Scholz W 1959 The contribution of patho-anatomical research to the problem of epilepsy. Epilepsia 1:36

Schwartz I R, Broggi G, Pappas G D 1970 Fine structure of cat hippocampus during sustained seizures. Brain Research 18:176

Schwartz M S, Scott D F 1974 Aminophylline-induced seizures. Epilepsia 15:501

Seite R, Picard D, Luciani J 1964 In: Bargmann, Schade (eds) Progress in brain research. Elsevier, Amsterdam p 171

Selye H 1941 Anaesthetic effect of steroid hormones. Proceedings of the Society of Experimental Biology and Medicine 46:116

Serbanescu T, Balzano E 1974 The influence of thyroxine in photosensitive baboons, Papio papio. Electroencephalography and Clinical Neurophysiology 36:253

Seyfried T N, Glaser G H, Yu R K 1979 Thyroid hormone influence on the susceptibility of mice to audiogenic seizures. Science 205:598

Sharpless S K 1969 Isolated and deafferented neurons: disuse supersensitivity In: Jasper H H, Ward A A, Pope A (eds) Basic mechanisms of the epilepsies. Churchill, London p 299

Shaywitz B A, Cohen D J, Bowers N B 1975 Reduced cerebrospinal fluid 5-hydroxyindoleacetic acid and homovanillic acid in children with epilepsy. Neurology 25:72

Simon R P 1985 Management of status epilepticus In: Pedley T A, Meldrum B S (eds) Recent advances in epilepsy 2. Churchill Livingstone, Edinburgh, p 137

Singh B M, Gupta D R, Strobos R J 1973 Non-ketonic rhesus monkeys. Electroencephalography and Clinical Neurophysiology 35:59

Skanse B, Nyman G E 1956 Thyrotoxicosis as a cause of cerebral dysrhythmia and convulsive seizures. Acta Endocrinologica 22:246

Sloper J J, Johnson P, Powell T R S 1980 Selective

degeneration of interneurons in the motor cortex of infant monkeys following controlled hypoxia: a possible cause of epilepsy. Brain Research 198:204

Sorel L, Dusaucy-Bauloye A 1958 A propos de 21 cas d'hypsarhythmia de Gibbs. Traitement spectaculaire par l'ACTH. Revue Neurologique 99:136

Spielmeyer W 1927 Die pathogenese des epileptischen krampfes. Zeitschrift fur die gesarnt. Neurologie und Psychiatrie 109:501

St Omer V 1971 Investigatiaons into mechanisms responsible for seizures induced by chlorinated hydrocarbon insecticides: The role of brain ammonia and glutamine in convulsions in the rat and cockerel. Journal of Neurochemistry 18:365

Starr A M 1952 Personality change in Cushing's syndrome. Journal of Clinical Endocrinology 12:502

Stone W E 1957 The role of acetylcholine in brain metabolism and function. American Journal of Physical Medicine 36:222

Suter C, Klingman W O 1955 Neurologic manifestations of magnesium depletion states. Neurology 5:691

Sypert G W, Ward A A 1974 Changes in extracellular potassium activity during neocortical propagated seizures. Experimental Neurology 45:19

Tebecis A K 1974 Transmitters and identified neurons in the mammalian central nervous system. Scientechnica Publishers, Bristol

Teglbjaerg H P S 1936 Investigations in epilepsy and water metabolism. Acta Pyschiatrica et Neurologica: suppl 9

Timiras P S, Woodbury D M 1956 Effect of thyroid activity on brain function and brain electrolyte distribution in rats. Endocrinology 58:191

Timiras P S 1969 Role of hormones in development of seizures. In: Jasper H H, Ward A S, Pope A (eds) Basic mechanisms of the epilepsies. Churchill, London, p 727

Toman J E P, Davis J P 1949 The effects of drugs upon the electrical activity of the brain. Journal of Pharmacology & Experimental Therapeutics 97:425

Toone B 1986 Sexual disorders in epilepsy. In: Pedley T A, Meldrum B S (eds) Recent advances in epilepsy 3,233. Churchill Livingstone, Edinburgh

Tower D B, Elliott K A C 1952 Activity of acetylcholine system in human epileptogenic focus. Journal of Applied Physiology 4:669

Tower D B 1969 Neurochemical Mechanisms. In: Jasper H H, Ward A A, Pope A (eds) Basic mechanisms of the epilepsies. Little Brown, Boston, p 611

Trachtenberg M C, Pollen D A 1970 Neuroglia: Biophysical properties and physiologic function. Science 167:1248

Trimble M R 1978 Serum prolactin in epilepsy and hysteria. British Medical Journal 2:1682

Trimble M, Anlezark G, Meldrum B S 1977 Seizure activity in photosensitive baboons following antidepressant drugs and the role of serotoninergic mechanisms. Psychopharmacologia 51:159

Van Buren J M, Ajmone-Marsan C 1960 A correlation of autonomic and EEG components in temporal lobe epilepsy. Archives of Neurology 3:683

Wada J A, Sato M, Corcoran M E 1974 Persistent seizure susceptibility and recurrent spontaneous seizures in kindled cats. Epilepsia 15:465

Wadman W J, Heinemann U 1985 Laminar profiles of $[K^+]o$ and $[Ca^+]o$ in region CA1 of the hippocampus of kindled rats. In: Kessler M et al (eds) Physiology and Medicine. Springer-Verlag, Berlin, p 221

Wagman I H, DeJong R H, Prince D A 1968 Effects of lidocaine on spontaneous cortical and subcortical electrical activity. Archives of Neurology 18:277

Wallace S J, Zealley H 1970 Neurological, electroencephalographic and virological findings in febrile children. Archives of Disease in Childhood 45:611

Wallach M B, Winters W D, Mandell A J, Spooner C E 1969 A correlation of EEG, reticular multiple unit activity and gross behaviour following various antidepressant agents in the cat. IV. Electroencephalography and Clinical Neurophysiology 27:563

Wallis C J, Luttge W G 1980 Influence of estrogen and progesterone on glutamic acid decarboxylase activity in discrete regions of rat brain. Journal of Neurochemistry 34:609

Waltregny A, Mesdijan E 1969 Convulse seizure and water intoxication. A polygraphic study. In: Gastaut H, Jasper H, Bancaud J, Waltregny A (eds) The physiopathogenesis of the epilepsies. Thomas, Springfield, p 69

Ward A A 1969 The epileptic neurone: Chronic foci in animals and man. In: Jasper H H, Ward A A, Pope A (eds) Basic mechanisms of the epilepsies. Churchill, London, p 263

Weil-Malherbe H 1955 The concentration of adrenaline in human plasma and its relation to mental activity. Journal of Mental Science 101:733

Werman R, Davidoff R A, Aprison M H 1968 Inhibitory action of glycine on spinal neurons in the cat. Journal of Neurophysiology 31:82

Westmoreland B F, Hanna G R, Bass N H 1972 Cortical alterations in zones of secondary epileptogenesis: a neurophysiologic, morphologic and microchemical correlation study in the albino rat. Brain Research 43:485

Westrum L E, White L E, Ward A A 1965 Morphology of the experimental epileptic focus. Journal of Neurosurgery 21:1033

Wheatley M D, Lipton B, Ward A A 1947 Repeated cyanide convulsions without central nervous pathology. Journal of Neuropathology & Experimental Neurology 6:408

White P T, Grant P, Mosier J, Craig A 1961 Changes in cerebral dynamics associated with seizures. Neurology 11:354

Wilder B J 1969 Projection phenomena and secondary epileptogenesis-mirror foci. In: Purpura D P, Penry J K, Tower D, Woodbury D M, Walter R (eds) Experimental models of epilepsy. Raven Press, New York, p 85

Wilder R M 1921 The effect of ketonuria on course of epilepsy. Mayo Clinic Proceedings 2:307

Willmore L J, Sypert G W, Munson J B, Hurd R W 1978 Chronic focal epileptiform discharges induced by injection of iron into rat and cat cortex. Science 200:1501

Withrow C D 1972 Systemic carbon dioxide derangements. In: Purpura D P, Penry J K, Woodbury D M, Walter R (eds) Experimental models of epilepsy. Raven Press, New York, p 477

Wood J D 1972 Systemic carbon dioxide derangements. In: Purpura D P, Penry J K, Woodbury D M, Water R (eds) Experimental models of epilepsy. Raven Press, New York, p 459

Wood J H, Hare T A Glaeser B S, Ballenger J C, Post R M 1979 Cerebrospinal fluid GABA reductions in seizure patients. Neurology 29:1203

Woodbury D M 1955 Effects of diphenylhydantoin on electrolytes and radiosodium turnover in brain and other tissues of normal, hyponatraemic, and post-ictal rates. Journal of Pharmacology 74:115

Woodbury D M 1958 Relation between the adrenal cortex and the central nervous system. Pharmacological Reviews 10:275

Woodbury D M, Vernadakis A 1966 Effects of steroids on the central nervous system. In: Dorfman R J (ed) Methods in Hormone research vol 5, Academic Press, New York p 1

Woodbury D M, Rollins L T, Gardner M D 1958 Effects of carbon dioxide on brain excitability and electrolytes. American Journal of Physiology 192:79

Woolley D E, Timiras P S 1962a The gonad–brain relationship: effects of female sex hormones on electroshock convulsions in the rat. Endocrinology 70:196

Woolley D E, Timiras P S 1962b Estrous and circadian periodicity and electroshock convulsions in rats. American Journal of Physiology 202:379

Worthley L I G, Thomas P D 1986 Treatment of hyponatraemic seizures with intravenous 29.2% saline. British Medical Journal 292:168

Wyke B 1963 Brain function and metabolic disorders. Butterworths, London

Zimmett P, Breidahl H D, Nayler W G 1968 Plasma ionized calcium in hypomagnesaemia. British Medical Journal 1:622

Zuckerman E C, Glaser G H 1970 Slow potential shifts in dorsal hippocampus during epileptogenic perfusion of the inferior horn with high-potassium CSF. Electroencephalagraphy and Clinical Neurophysiology 18:236

Zuckerman E G, Glaser G H 1972 Urea-induced myoclonic seizures. Archives of Neurology 27:14

8

Electroencephalography

C. D. Binnie

INTRODUCTION

It may have been as much good fortune as prophetic insight which led Hughlings Jackson in 1873 to define the epileptic seizure as 'an occasional sudden, excessive, rapid and local discharge of grey matter of some part of the brain', for half a century was to elapse before it became possible to record such discharges in the electroencephalogram. Nevertheless, episodic dysfunction of cerebral neurones, particularly increased and synchronous activity, remains central to current concepts of epilepsy.

PRINCIPLES OF ELECTROENCEPHALOGRAPHY

It is beyond the scope of the present text to explain at length how the electroencephalogram (EEG) is generated, recorded or interpreted. For the reader wishing to pursue these questions a good starting-point would be '*Electroencephalography*' by Niedermeyer and Lopes da Silva (1982). There follows a brief summary which may help to elucidate later sections of this chapter.

Physiological basis of the electroencephalogram

The EEG is a record of cerebral electrical activity made typically with some 20 electrodes of roughly 1 cm^2 surface area applied to the scalp. The electrocorticogram (ECoG) is registered directly from the surface of the cerebral cortex by somewhat smaller electrodes inserted at operation. A depth recording, or stereo-electroencephalogram (SEEG), is obtained by means of generally more numerous and much smaller electrodes, with a surface area of about 1 mm^2, inserted into the brain. All three techniques involve recording from millions of neurones by means of electrodes which are relatively few and large. Consequently, the signals obtained represent only a very crude average of neuronal activity in a relatively large volume of brain tissue.

Neurones undergo two main types of electrical change: slow postsynaptic potentials on a time scale of 5–50 msec and much briefer action potentials lasting only of the order of 1 msec. These last do not generate fields recordable far from their site of origin and thus it is virtually only postsynaptic potentials which contribute to the EEG. The fact that the electrodes record the summated signals from many neurones implies that only synchronous activity displayed by many cells simultaneously will be registered. An analogy may be found in the experience of someone listening outside a football stadium. He hears but cannot understand the confused shouts of the crowd; however, the general applause when the home team scores a goal and the universal gasp when one is missed are easily recognized. Similarly, electrophysiological recordings with large electrodes reflect only the synchronous activity of cerebral neurones.

Synchronous neuronal activity is, from the point of view of information processing, highly redundant and occurs most readily in drowsiness, sleep and in pathological conditions in which cerebral function is impaired. Conversely attention is associated with desynchronization of neurones and a reduced amplitude of the EEG. The philosophical implications of a test of cerebral function,

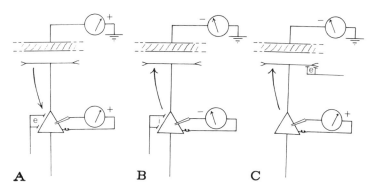

Fig. 8.1 Schematic representation of relationship between surface EEG and activity of cortical neurones. **A.** excitatory post-synaptic potential on cell body (positive-going change inside the cell) produces positive change on the surface; **B.** inhibitory post synaptic potential on the cell body (negative-going change inside the cell) produces negative surface change; **C.** excitation of dendrites in contrast to **a**, produces negative surface change. Large arrow shows direction of current flow

which reflects the resting behaviour of neuronal populations not engaged in information processing need not concern us here; abnormal synchronous discharge is the hallmark of the pathophysiology of epilepsy and its manifestations in the EEG are the subject of this chapter.

Although scalp electrodes can in some circumstances pick up widespread electrical fields arising at a distance in the brain, more usually they record the summated activity of the underlying cerebral cortex over an area of about 6 cm² (Cooper et al 1965). The cerebral cortex is a laminar structure and the neurones which contribute most to the EEG are orientated vertically. Changes occurring in membrane potential are usually localized, either to the cell body deep in the cortex or to the dendrites lying more superficially (Fig. 8.1). This will result in the production of a dipole, a potential difference between deep and superficial layers of cortex. The extent to which this electrical field can be registered in the EEG will depend upon the orientation of the dipole with respect to the overlying electrode (more strictly, it depends on the solid angle subtended at the electrode by the generator surface). If the affected cortex is in the wall of a sulcus and the dipole thus orientated tangenterally to the surface of the brain it may not be detected.

The relations between EEG waves and activity of cerebral neurones are complex and depend on:

1. The parts of the neurone where changes in membrane potential are occurring (the soma deep in the cortex or the dendrites more superficially)

2. The nature of the change (increased negativity inside the cell with inhibitory, and decreased negativity with excitatory, postsynaptic potentials)

3. The rate of spread from one part of the cell to another (during slow changes the surface EEG changes with a polarity opposite to that inside the cell body whereas with more rapid changes the two tend to be in phase (Fig. 8.2)).

Thus fast negative spikes in the EEG may reflect cellular excitation and depolarization and

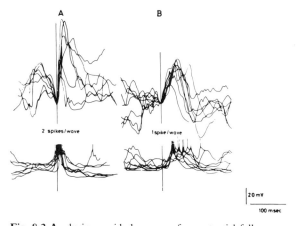

Fig. 8.2 A. during rapid changes surface potential follows that inside body of cortical neurone; **B.** during slower changes surface potential is out of phase with inside of cell body (N.B. Recording convention is negative upwards for EEG and downwards for intracellular tracing). (Reprinted with permission from Creutzfeldt et al (1966).)

surface negative slow waves may occur during hyperpolarization due to inhibition.

The clinical EEG

As previously noted, accounts of EEG phenomenology and technology should be sought elsewhere. Suffice it that, for the present purpose, when describing EEGs a division is made between more or less continuous 'background' activity and episodic transients, and between those phenomena which are generalized or involve large areas of the scalp bilaterally and those which are more localized or 'focal'. Background activity is normally symmetrical and is classified into four frequency bands: delta up to 4 waves per second, theta 4–8/s, alpha 8–14/s and beta above 14/s.

An EEG machine has typically 8–20 channels, each of which writes out on a paper chart a continuous tracing of the potential difference between two points. There are essentially two ways of recording the EEG. One, 'common reference derivation', displays on each channel the potential difference between one electrode on the scalp and a common reference point which is the same for all channels. The reference may itself be either a particular electrode or an electrical connection inside the EEG machine which corresponds to the average potential of all the electrodes in use. If the reference is appropriately chosen, a localized EEG phenomenon will produce waves on the write out which are largest on the channel recording from the overlying electrode. An alternative method, which is generally preferred in Europe, is so-called 'bipolar' derivation. This involves connecting rows of electrodes to the EEG machine so that the channels record from consecutive pairs (channel 1 – electrodes A and B; channel 2 – electrodes B and C; channel 3 – electrodes C and D . . .). This has the effect of highlighting any localized phenomenon, which will produce deflections in opposite directions on the two channels connected to the affected electrode, so-called 'phase reversal' (Fig. 8.3).

The appearance of the term 'phase reversal' in an EEG report thus merely signifies that a particular method of recording has been used to demonstrate a localized EEG event. Examples of both common reference and bipolar derivation will be found in various illustrations to this chapter.

THE ICTAL EEG

Depth recording

Intracranial electrodes provide a clearer picture of the electrophysiological events during a seizure than does the scalp EEG. In humans, the occasion to insert intracranial electrodes arises only where

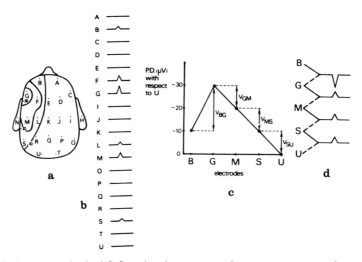

Fig. 8.3 A localized EEG phenomenon in the left frontal region represented **a.** as a contour map; **b.** on common reference derivation referred to an electrode, H, at a point on the scalp remote from the physiological event in question; **c.** as a graph of potential against distance along the line of electrodes B, G, M, S and U on bipolar derivation from the same line of electrodes showing phase-reversal at electrode G. (Reprinted, with permission, from Binnie et al 1982).

there is thought to be a possibility of neurosurgical treatment, i.e. in partial epilepsies. An electrode at the site where the seizure commences will typically show at the onset of the attack a high frequency discharge, perhaps of 60/s or faster, reflecting highly synchronized activity within a very restricted volume of surrounding brain. This may sometimes be preceded by a transient event, a DC shift, an isolated sharp wave of 100 to 200 ms duration or a spike followed by a slower wave (Fig. 8.4).

Sometimes, the initial change appears to be a reduction in amplitude of the ongoing background activity or even a cessation of interictal spiky transients which were previously present. There follows a gradual evolution in both time and space. The picture is very varied, but typically the discharges decrease in frequency and progressively increase in amplitude, changing as they do to discrete spikes falling progressively from a frequency of 20/s to 10/s. The spikes generally give way to spike-wave activity – short spiky transients alternating with slower waves of some hundreds of ms duration – and the frequency continues to fall progressively over the course of the seizure. The discharges may become irregular before they finally cease, leaving a post-ictal picture, either of slowing or of a very low amplitude record which gradually gives way to high-voltage slow activity. This post-ictal record in turn shows a progressive rise in frequency and fall in amplitude until the previous interictal pattern of background activity is restored.

The evolution in space of the ictal disturbance will determine the clinical manifestations. The discharge may remain confined within a small volume of tissue close to its site of onset, for instance the amygdala-hippocampus complex on one side. Alternatively, it may spread to involve adjacent cortex within the same hemisphere or, usually abruptly, generalize through the commisural systems to involve the contralateral hemisphere also. Gradual spread through cortex adjacent to the focus will give rise to the classical Jacksonian march; bilateral limbic involvement will produce the impairment of consciousness characteristic of a complex partial seizure; and generalization, involving cortex, thalamus and possibly brain stem structures, will produce a secondarily generalized tonic-clonic convulsion. Depending on the site of onset and the anatomical spread, various subtly different ictal patterns may be distinguished, as documented by Wieser (1983a). With bilateral hemispheric involvement discharges will generally be synchronous. Residual post-ictal disturbance may produce focal neurological deficit, if focal (Todd's palsy), or confusion, if generalized.

Intracerebral ictal recordings in human primary generalized epilepsy have understandably rarely been reported. However, Williams (1953) described rhythmic spike-wave activity during petit mal absences which was synchronous in thalamus and cortex. Depth electrode studies of experimental generalized epilepsies have usually employed chemical models with varying results. Systemic administration of massive doses of penicillin produces seizures with a diffuse corticothalamic onset with generalized spike-wave activity. By contrast, bicuculline and pentalenetetrazol produce changes which are first apparent in the brain stem reticular formation or the lateral geniculate body consisting of high-frequency multi-unit activity sometimes reaching frequencies of several hundred Hz (Rodin et al 1971, Binnie et al 1985c).

Scalp EEG

Scalp EEG recording involves further loss of information as compared with depth registration and, in particular, sharply localized ictal events may be undetectable in the conventional EEG. During partial seizures, the EEG presents a picture which may be regarded as a simplification of that obtainable with depth recording. Typically, a similar evolution will be seen from rapid, spiky discharges to spike-wave activity of greater amplitude and lower frequency with eventual post-ictal reduction of amplitude and/or slowing. Again, typically, the onset of such changes will be focal, roughly overlying the deep focus, and generalization may occur to a greater or lesser degree. However, simultaneous depth and scalp recording show that the initial events found at the depth electrodes may not appear at all on the surface, and the scalp EEG changes may appear only some tens of seconds after the onset of the seizure. High-frequency seizure activity in particular is often lacking in a

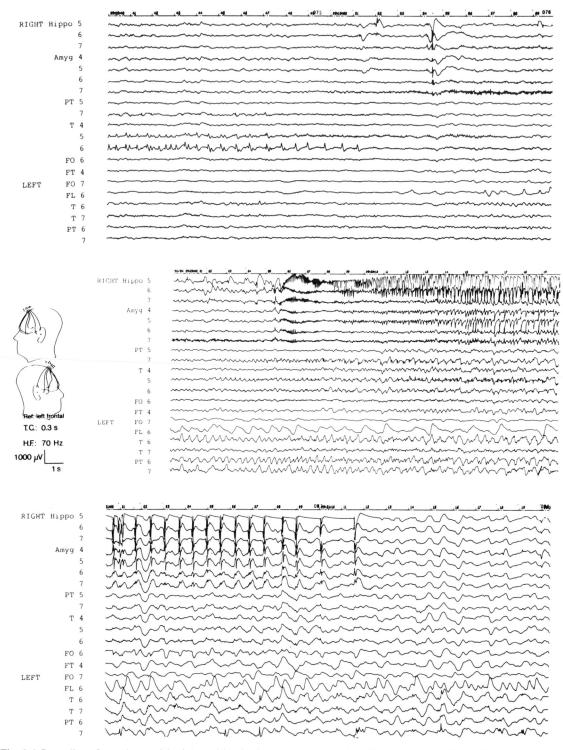

Fig. 8.4 Recording of complex partial seizure arising in the right temporal lobe with depth and subdural electrodes.

scalp recording and the ictal changes in the scalp EEG may commence with spikes, sharp waves or spike-wave activity. Although spiky waveforms due to intense synchronous discharge are probably an invariable finding in depth recording in partial seizures (assuming that an electrode is placed at the appropriate site), ictal changes in the scalp EEG are not necessarily spiky. Seizure onset may be heralded by the appearance of an activity not previously present, within the theta, alpha or beta range (Fig. 8.5).

The initial, or indeed the only, EEG change may be a reduction in amplitude of ongoing activity (an 'electrodecremental event'). The physiological basis of this is uncertain, but is most probably desynchronization of cortical activity due to corticopetal inputs from the epileptic focus. Ictal changes in the scalp EEG in partial epilepsy are not necessarily focal or even unilateral. Rhythmic, non-spiky activities or an electrodecremental event are particularly likely to be generalized and often symmetrical, but even frank spikes or spike-wave discharges may be generalized or show a localization or lateralization which does not reflect the topography of the seizure onset in deep structures. This may be understandable when the evolution of a partial seizure is followed with a combination of depth and subdural electrodes as illustrated in Figure 8.4. This shows a clearly focal ictal onset in a patient with partial complex seizures due to a right mesial temporal sclerotic lesion. The electrographic pattern was consistent

during ten seizures registered with intracranial electrodes. The initial discharge remained localized to deep right temporal structures for some five to ten seconds. Once the spread to more remote cortical structures occurred, the discharges were bilateral and initially more prominent over the contralateral hemisphere. This gave rise to misleading lateralization of the focus in ictal scalp EEGs.

Some partial seizures produce no apparent change in the scalp EEG (Ives & Woods (1980). An absence of ictal change in the scalp EEG in partial epilepsies is most common during simple partial seizures and, indeed, is the usual finding in those with psychic symptomatology (Wieser 1979), or in attacks consisting only of a viscerosensory aura.

The evolution of electrical activity in the EEG during a tonic-clonic convulsion of generalized onset closely parallels that of many partial seizures but without localizing features (Fig. 8.6). Possibly after a brief electrodecremental event, a rapid build-up of spikes is typically seen followed by generalized spike-wave activity. In the clonic phase, the muscle jerks appear synchronous with the spike-wave complexes and, as the seizure ends, both become less frequent and irregular. A marked, generalized post-ictal slowing is seen, possibly preceded by a period of flattening. The generalized convulsive seizures most conveniently studied in humans are those produced by bilateral ECT, and here the duration of post-ictal flattening

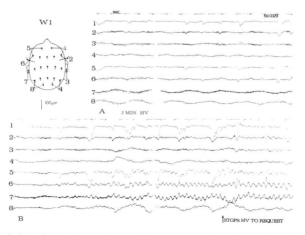

Fig. 8.5 Ictal EEG change consisting of left-sided rhythmic delta activity without 'epileptiform' or spiky phenomena. This picture consistently accompanied the patient's complex partial seizures, induced in this case by overbreathing.

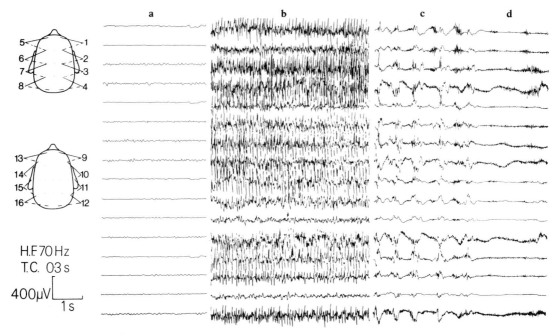

H.F. 70 Hz
T.C. 0.3 s
400 μV
1 s

Fig. 8.6 Evolution of EEG during tonic-clonic seizure. **a.** pre-ictal pattern; **b.** high-frequency spiking intermixed with muscle artefact at seizure onset; **c.** generalized spike-wave activity **d.** post-ictal slowing.

is inversely related to the duration of the convulsive phase (Robin et al 1985). In general, the more severe and prolonged the post-ictal disturbance in the EEG, the more marked is the clinical symptomatology. However, some patients may show residual slowing and bursts of delta waves, often rhythmic, 24 hours after apparent clinical recovery.

The classical absence seizure of primary generalized epilepsy is accompanied by generalized, fairly symmetrical, regular spike-wave activity of about three per second which commences abruptly, usually one or two seconds before the onset of apparent clinical manifestations, and which may continue briefly after consciousness has started to return. In absence seizures, spike-wave discharges of under three seconds duration are not usually accompanied by obvious clinical change, although transitory impairment of cognitive function is often demonstrable during shorter discharges (see p. 267). The phenomenology of the absence seizure is in fact very varied. Those attacks in which myoclonic phenomena are prominent are often accompanied by multiple spike and wave activity. As has been pointed out by Binnie

& Van der Wens (1986) there is some considerable overlap in clinical and electrical phenomena between absence seizures, which may include involuntary movements and automatisms, and brief complex partial seizures with loss of consciousness at onset. The overlapping clinical pattern probably reflects a common pathophysiology, for both are accompanied by generalized spike-wave activity. It has been claimed that differentiation by the ictal EEG between a complex absence and a brief complex partial seizure may rest on the demonstration of a focal onset of the latter. However, some authors have suggested that the distinction may be somewhat artificial and find that in those patients where this differential diagnosis is difficult, satisfactory therapeutic response is generally obtained only by a combination of drugs usually effective in partial seizures and in absences (Binnie & Van der Wens 1986, Hendrickson 1986, Stefan, 1986).

A lack of apparent ictal EEG change is far less common in generalized than in partial seizures. However, pure atonic seizures without other ictal manifestations may be accompanied only by an electrodecremental event in the scalp EEG (Egli et al 1985). This may be difficult to detect if the EEG is contaminated by artefact as the patient falls.

'EPILEPTIFORM ACTIVITY'

Definitions

A feature of the ictal EEG as described above, whether recorded from the scalp or with intra-cranial electrodes, is the occurrence of spiky waveforms due to abnormal, synchronous cerebral neuronal activity. Similar discharges, spikes, spike-wave complexes and sharp waves, are also seen in the interictal EEGs of most people with epilepsy. It might therefore seem useful to have a generic term for discharges of this kind, but the question of agreeing a suitable terminology has led to a semantic debate, which in turn has to some extent confused the clinical interpretation of these phenomena.

Such terms as 'epileptic discharge' are not acceptable, as these waveforms are sometimes seen in the EEGs of people who do not apparently have epilepsy. Yet less satisfactory is the American usage 'seizure discharge' as, even in people who do have epilepsy, the discharges are not necess-arily ictal. The term 'paroxysmal activity' has been widely used but, strictly speaking, describes any episodic phenomenon as, for instance, a K-complex. Other euphemisms which are used in some European countries include 'irritative activity'. It is not clear whether this implies that the activity is irritating the brain or that it is a manifestation of cerebral irritation, in either case there remains the implication of epileptogenesis. In reality, what is at issue is not the name but the underlying concept; namely, that these phenomena are typical of, but not specific to, epilepsy. Throughout this text the term 'epileptiform activity' will be used, both recognizing the stat-istical association with epilepsy and stressing that, as a descriptive EEG term, it refers only to a waveform and not an interpretation.

Numerous terms are listed by the terminology committee of the International Federation of Societies of Electroencephalography and Clinical Neurophysiology (Chatrian et al 1974) to describe the various types of epileptiform activity and many more non-approved expressions are in use. The essential quality of these discharges is their spiky aspect, the steep gradients seen in the EEG tracing and particularly the abrupt change in direction of pen deflection which gives each wave a sharp peak. Those spiky transients which are of less than 80 ms duration are called spikes, those lasting from 80–120 ms are sharp waves. Waves of longer duration than 120 ms and of sharp appearance may also represent epileptiform activity, but there is no official term used to describe them. Published definitions beg the ques-tion of how sharp a wave has to be to qualify as a spike or a sharp wave. The identification of these waveforms depends in part on the background EEG activity. Continuing rhythmic beta activity may, for instance, be made up of waves every one of which would be regarded as a spike if it occurred against a background from which high frequency components were absent (Fig. 8.7).

Spikes may occur as continuous bursts of activity, the most extreme examples of which are the multi-unit discharges recorded with depth electrodes close to the site of orgin of a seizure. Discrete spikes and sharp waves are usually

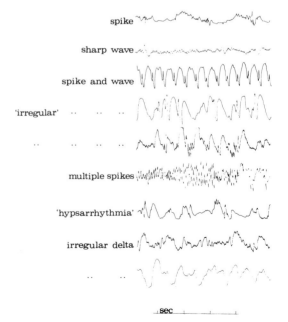

Fig. 8.7 Examples of more or less obvious epileptiform activity.

followed by a slower wave and, if this is prominent, the two together are described as a spike-wave complex or sharp and slow-wave complex. Often multiple spikes occur with a single slow wave. Spike-wave complexes themselves may be isolated or occur as more or less rhythmic activity. Focal spikes are often polyphasic, but the most prominent component is usually negative, reflecting current flow towards the underlying cortical surface. Positive spikes at 6 or 14/s occur as a normal phenomenon (see below). Otherwise, positive focal spikes are rare, occur mostly in children and are also seen where a gross cortical defect allows the electrode to record from the deep surface of the cortex in the wall of an adjacent sulcus (Matsuo & Knott, 1977). The writer has seen one corticographically proven instance of positive spikes arising from the surface of intact, if slightly gliotic, cortex in an adult.

Normal epileptiform phenomena

A discussion of definitions and description of the typical waveforms by no means ends the confusion surrounding epileptiform activity. Some spiky waveforms conforming these descriptions are normal phenomena frequently found in EEGs of healthy subjects and having no significance in relation to epilepsy. They are recognizable, however, by characteristic morphology and topography, and by occurring under specific circumstances. Some instances will be considered here; for a fuller review see Naquet (1983) and Riley (1983). A good example is provided by so-called '6 and 14 per second positive spikes' (Fig. 8.8).

As the name suggests, these are rhythmic spiky discharges at 6 or 14/s, the most conspicuous component being positive at the surface of the scalp and generally focal towards the posterior

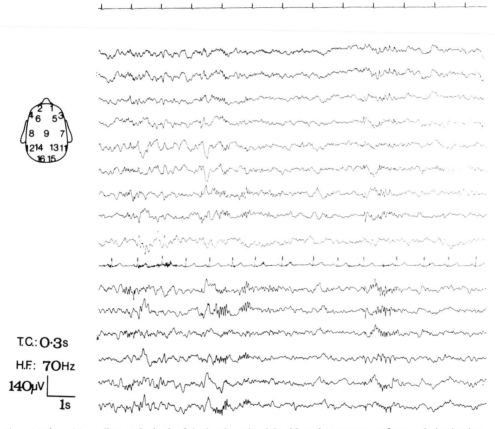

T.C.: 0·3s

H.F.: 70Hz

140μV

1s

Fig. 8.8 6/s and 14/s positive spikes at the back of the head on the right. Note that common reference derivation has been used to display this phenomenon.

temporal region on one or both sides of the head. This is itself an unusual feature as other kinds of focal spikes are predominantly surface negative. This activity occurs in drowsiness and light sleep, and is most often seen in adolescents and young adults where the incidence may be 20% or more. The spikes are of low amplitude and produce widespread electrical fields over the scalp without steep potential gradients and, consequently, are more readily detected when common reference methods of EEG derivation are employed than in bipolar montages. It is probably for this technical reason that positive spikes are reported more commonly in North America than in Europe, as in most European countries bipolar methods of recording are used more than common reference. Controlled studies of particular groups of patients, most notably with psychiatric disorders and allergic conditions, show some increase in incidence of positive spikes. However, the association is too weak to be of any clinical significance and any event epilepsy is not one of those conditions associated with an increased incidence of this phenomenon.

Another example of a spiky waveform without clinical significance is provided by benign epileptiform transients of sleep (BETS). These are spikes or spike-wave complexes of very short duration and stereotyped waveform occurring in the anterior temporal regions during sleep. These, too, are seen frequently in normal subjects, possibly in as many as 50% when appropriate electrode placements are used (White et al 1977). BETS also appear to occur more often in some groups of patients than in normal subjects and their clinical significance is disputed (Hughes & Grunener 1984). In any event, the finding of BETS does not contribute to the diagnosis of epilepsy and, indeed, depth recordings in patients with partial seizures of temporal lobe origin clearly show the BETS to be independent of the epileptogenic foci from which the seizures arise (Westmoreland et al 1979).

Mid-temporal rhythmic discharge consists of rhythmic sharp-waves at about six per second over the temporal regions. This activity may occur for a few seconds or for hours at a time and may be present in repeated EEGs over many years. It appears to be unaffected by vigilance, attention or overbreathing, and is unresponsive to antiepileptic drugs. During the discharge, no ictal clinical manifestations are seen and no cognitive disturbance is demonstrable. Despite formerly being termed 'psychomotor variant' because of a supposed relationship with temporal lobe epilepsy (Gibbs & Gibbs 1953), it is often seen in patients without evident cerebral disorder and the association with epilepsy is weak (Lipman & Hughes 1969, Hugnes & Cayaffa 1973). A similar phenomenon, 'sub-clinical rhythmic epileptiform discharge of adults' (or SREDA), occurs further posteriorly in the parieto-temporal-occipital region and is virtually confined to adults of more than 50 years of age (Naquet et al 1961, Westmoreland & Klass 1981). Again, it appears to have no clinical significance.

To the catalogue of EEG phenomena which may mistakenly be interpreted as evidence for epilepsy, must be added various responses to 'activation procedures' (see below). Hyperventilation is routinely carried out for some 3 min during clinical EEG examination and may induce epileptiform discharges, most dramatically generalized 3/s spike-wave activity in patients with absence seizures. However, young normal subjects respond to this procedure by a slowing of the EEG and, in anyone under the age of 30 who overbreathes vigorously for 3 min, rhythmic bifrontal delta activity at about 3/s may be expected. This normal physiological response is often misinterpreted as evidence of 'cortical instability' and wrongly supposed to support a diagnosis of epilepsy. Amazingly, it is not uncommon for healthy children to receive antiepileptic medication for years because of a normal slow-wave response to overbreathing.

Intermittent photic stimulation (IPS) is also used for EEG activation. The normal response consists of rhythmic activity at the back of the head following the frequency of the flicker. Some patients with epilepsy respond with clear, generalized epileptiform discharges. However, between these extremes a variety of unusual or atypical responses may occur. These include occipital spikes at the frequency of the stimulus, following at sub- or supraharmonics of the flash rate, and the occurrence of theta or delta activity at the back of the head. These various atypical responses are largely genetically determined (Doose & Gerken 1973) and occur in some 15% of normal children. Some indeed have a weak association with epilepsy: nearly half of those exhibiting occipital spikes suffer from seizures and, when the photoconvulsive response is suppressed by effective medication, IPS may continue to elicit occipital spikes or marked harmonic following. It would, however, be misleading to regard any response short of a generalized epileptiform discharge as supportive of epilepsy.

Clinical significance of epileptiform activity

From the above it should be clear that any statement concerning the clinical predictive significance of finding 'epileptiform activity' in the EEG depends firstly on how this term is used. Epileptiform phenomena in the widest sense of spiky waveforms are common in normal people, particularly in the young and during drowsiness or sleep. Any author using the term in this sense may rightly state that epileptiform discharges are common in healthy subjects and are not reliably predictive of epilepsy, nor indeed of any other cerebral disorder. If, however, the term is used more narrowly to exclude those spiky waveforms which are known to be normal or unrelated to epilepsy, a different picture emerges. It is necessary, moreover, to distinguish between the significance of epileptiform activity as evidence of cerebral dysfunction and its specificity to epilepsy.

When EEG abnormalities are found in supposedly healthy volunteers, further enquiry usually reveals that the subjects suffer from, or have a history of, a cerebral disorder (Roubicek et al 1967, Binnie et al 1978). One of the largest studies of normal subjects was performed by Robin et al (1978) in 7400 airmen: 140 exhibited epileptiform EEG activity following stringent criteria. However, of those who were followed up, it transpired that more than half had a history of epilepsy and most of the remainder had been declared unfit for flying duties on neuropsychiatric grounds. In this series, the eventual incidence of epileptiform EEG activity in subjects without evidence of brain dysfunction was of the order of 2 per 1000.

A different picture emerges when patient populations are considered, not suffering from epilepsy but undergoing EEG examination because of other complaints. Here the incidence of epileptiform EEG activity is considerably higher and may be as high as 20% in those with migraine and 40% in patients with diffuse brain damage manifest by mental subnormality (Ajmone Marsan & Zivin 1970). The presence of epileptiform activity is thus of much more value for distinguishing between a person with epilepsy and a healthy volunteer or a patient whose symptoms are of psychiatric origin, than for deciding whether or not known brain disease is likely to give rise to seizures.

Variability of the EEG in Epilepsy

Epilepsy, although a chronic disorder, is not a static condition. Long, seizure-free, interictal periods are interspersed with brief seizures, which may vary substantially from one attack to the next and which may be preceded by a prodromal phase or followed by a post-ictal state with residual sensory, motor or cognitive deficits, lasting from seconds to days. Outside centres with special facilities for prolonged monitoring, the EEG investigation of epilepsy is concerned chiefly with interictal recording. Occasionally, a seizure occurs by chance during EEG registration, or an emergency record can be obtained from a patient still in a post-ictal state.

Even the interictal EEG is highly variable, and, under apparently constant conditions, epileptiform discharges may be absent in one half-hour period and profuse in the next. It is no wonder then that the findings in 'routine' EEGs of 30–40 min duration in centres which conform to accepted standards (and less than 10 min in many others) are so inconsistent. Some of the variability is apparently random but the most important single factor is sleep and waking (see section below and p. 291).

EFFECTS OF SLEEP

During sleep the EEG changes dramatically, showing first a loss of the alpha rhythm, and then, with increasing depth of sleep, progressively greater amounts of slow activity. Sleep depth is conventionally classified into four levels according to criteria proposed by Dement & Kleitmann in 1957. There is a further stage of sleep characterized by rapid eye movements (REM) and associated with dreaming. Interictal epileptiform discharges are often very sensitive to changes in the state of awareness.

With the onset of drowsiness and stage I sleep, generalized spike-wave activity may either disappear or increase, but focal discharges will generally become more frequent or may appear if absent in the alert state. In light (stage II) sleep the focal epileptiform activity is generally most prominent, whereas generalized discharges may attain a maximum in stage III. REM sleep is usually associated with a reduction in rate of both generalized (Gastaut et al 1965, Ross et al 1966, Passouant 1967, Billiard 1982) and focal discharges (Batini et al 1963, Perria et al 1966, Angelieri 1974, Daskalov 1975). However, some authors claim an increase of focal temporal discharges in REM sleep (Passouant et al 1965, Epstein & Hill 1966, Mayersdorf & Wilder 1974). Bursts of generalized spike-wave activity may become longer although less numerous during REM (Stevens et al 1971). The increase in discharges during sleep may be dramatic and Tassinari et al (1982) described a group of children who exhibited continuous epileptiform discharges during sleep, although these were generally absent in the waking state.

During all-night sleep recording some patients may show a characteristic distribution of discharges, with maxima shortly after falling asleep, in the middle of the night or towards morning (Kellaway & Frost 1983). Many patients show a circadian pattern of seizure incidence related to sleep and wake which may provide a basis for classifying epilepsy into sleeping, awakening and diffuse forms (Janz 1962). Janz suggested that diffuse epilepsy most often had a lesional basis, whereas wakening epilepsy was usually of the primary generalized type. Others, as Billiard (1982), do not confirm this. In general, the time of occurrence of the maximum EEG discharge rate corresponds to that of seizure frequency (Martins da Silva et al 1984). Thus, patients with awakening epilepsy tend to show the maximum EEG discharge rates at about the time of wakening from spontaneous, nocturnal sleep.

Conversely, epilepsy and epileptiform discharges affect sleep patterns: REM sleep may occur earlier than in control subjects, the amount of time spent in light sleep (stages I and II) may increase, and there may be more frequent shifts between sleep stages (Jovanovic 1967, Halász and Dévéyi 1974, Chemburkar et al 1976, Baldy-Moulinier 1982). Sleep EEG patterns may themselves be so disrupted that sleep staging by the normal criteria is impossible (Bordas-Ferrer et al 1966, Besset 1982). However, some authors have been unable to confirm any abnormalities of sleep pattern in epilepsy, provided no attack occurred during the night (Delange et al 1962, Angelieri et al 1967, Kazamatsuri et al 1970, Sato et al 1973). The picture is complicated by the effects of antiepileptic drugs. However, Röder-Wanner et al (1985) reported a series of nocturnal sleep studies in untreated patients. Their main finding was an increase of deep sleep in the first part of the night in photosensitive patients with generalized epilepsy. Wolf et al (1985) found specific effects of different antiepileptic drugs on the sleep of previously untreated subjects, but the pattern was complicated by interactions between drugs and various epilepsy syndromes.

THE DIAGNOSTIC EEG SERIES IN EPILEPSY

Ajmone Marsan & Zivin (1970) performed repeated routine waking EEG examinations in a large series of patients with epilepsy. Some 35% showed interictal epileptiform discharges in all recordings; 15%, by contrast, were never shown to have interictal discharges even when the EEG was repeated ten times or more. The remaining 50% exhibited epileptiform activity in some tracings and not in others. From these figures it would be expected that, in a group of patients with epilepsy, a single waking EEG will demonstrate epileptiform activity in approximately 50% and that, with repeated recordings, discharges will be found sooner or later in 85%. The yield of diagnostically useful information can, however, be increased by recording during sleep, as this increases the incidence of interictal epileptiform

Table 8.1 Diagnosis EEG investigation of epilepsy (after Binnie 1968b)

	Patients with epilepsy to be investigated 100			
	never	sometimes	always	E.A found* (cumulative)
Interictal epileptiform activity (E.A.) in waking	15	50	35	
Wake EEG recorded	15	50	35	
E.A. present	0	15	35	50
absent	15	35	0	
Sleep EEG recorded	15	35	—	
E.A. present	5	25	—	80
absent	10	10		
Repeated wake & sleep EEGs recorded	10	10	0	
E.A. found	2	10	—	92
absent	8			

* EEG investigation of these patients is not necessarily complete: some may require further studies, for instance, for localization of a focus.

activity. A suitable diagnostic strategy is illustrated in Table 8.1.

In a typical sample of patients with epilepsy referred for diagnostic EEG investigation, the initial recording will demonstrate epileptiform activity in 50%. In some of these, it may be considered that the EEG has provided as much diagnostic information as is required to support the clinical findings, in others, further studies may be needed to address specific problems, for instance to determine whether a focus can be demonstrated during sleep or whether frequent EEG discharges are accompanied by clinical manifestations which have been overlooked. In the 50% in whom the initial EEG failed to demonstrate epileptiform activity, a further recording should be obtained, including a period of sleep. This will increase the yield of diagnostically useful information, partly as a result simply of repeating the EEG and partly because of the emergence of new phenomena, including epileptiform discharges, during sleep. If the findings remain negative and there is a degree of diagnostic uncertainty

requiring further investigation, the sleep EEG may be repeated, and many workers would prefer on this occasion to induce sleep by a method which may itself have some activating effect; for instance by previous deprivation of sleep or by drugs which may themselves have some proconvulsive action. Sleep and methods of sleep induction are considered further elsewhere. There will remain some 10% of the original patients with epilepsy in whom no interictal epileptiform discharges have been demonstrated. This group will consist chiefly of patients with infrequent generalized seizures or simple partial seizures, particularly with sensorimotor symptoms only. In many of these patients, the diagnosis of epilepsy appears certain on clinical grounds and further investigation is not justified. However, in perhaps 5% of the original sample a confident clinical diagnosis is not possible and here an attempt may usefully be made by long-term monitoring of the EEG to obtain an ictal recording (see below).

ACTIVATION PROCEDURES

The yield of epileptiform EEG activity and of other abnormalities may be increased by the use of various so-called 'activation procedures'. Of these, hyperventilation and intermittent photic stimulation are performed routinely in clinical EEG examination in most departments, irrespective of the reason for referral. Sleep is widely used to increase the yield of diagnostically useful information in epilepsy; and other techniques, mostly using chemical convulsant agents, are employed less frequently.

HYPERVENTILATION

The hypocapnia produced by voluntary hyperventilation results in cerebral vasoconstriction and reduced cerebral blood flow. It is probably by this mechanism that the EEG changes on overbreathing are elicited. The degree of response is closely related to the vigour with which overbreathing is performed or, more exactly, to the fall in end-tidal pCO_2. Binnie et al (1969) suggested that the progressive reduction in EEG responses to overbreathing with increasing age could be attributed to a smaller fall in pCO_2 in older subjects. The effects are enhanced by hypoglycaemia (Heppenstall 1944).

In the older literature, it was suggested that in various groups of patients, including those with epilepsy, the changes in background activity on overbreathing were enhanced. It may be questioned whether this was in any way attributable to the seizure disorder or merely to the familiarity with the procedure of patients who had undergone many previous EEG investigations. In any event, it is unwise to suppose that a marked but qualitatively normal response to overbreathing is supportive of epilepsy (see p. 245 above). In many patients with epilepsy, discharges appear or occur more frequently during overbreathing. Both generalized and focal activities may be affected, but those most consistently increased are the generalized spike-wave discharges of about 3/s seen in patients with absence seizures. Indeed 3 min of vigorous overbreathing in such a patient will usually elicit not only a discharge but also an attack. The absence of spike-wave activity after 3 min of overbreathing, performed sufficiently vigorously to produce marked changes in background activity, must cast considerable doubt on a diagnosis of absence seizures; it does not, of course, exclude the possibility that a patient's episodes of unconsciousness are seizures of some other type, such as complex partial.

Photic stimulation

Intermittent photic stimulation (IPS) normally elicits discrete visual evoked responses at low flash rates and rhythmic 'photic following' at frequencies from 4/s up to 10/s and sometimes higher, to 20/s or more. These responses are of greatest amplitude at the back of the head and are fairly symmetrical. Gross asymmetry (more than 50% right-left amplitude difference) may reflect cerebral pathology (Kooi et al 1960) and is generally paralleled by a corresponding asymmetry of the alpha rhythm. As noted above, a variety of atypical responses may also occur. At the back of the head occipital spikes may be seen. These are large, atypical visual evoked responses (Panayiotopoulos et al 1970, 1972, Dimitrakoudi et al 1973) and have a one-to-one relationship to the flashes. They do have a weak association with epilepsy which is present in half the patients showing occipital spikes (Maheshwari & Jeavons 1975). They may be seen in some photosensitive subjects during stimulation at frequencies too low to elicit a PCR, and may persist as a residual abnormality after photosensitivity has been abolished by medication (Harding et al 1978). Other anomalous posterior responses to IPS include runs of theta or delta activity; these are genetically determined but of no clinical significance. Another normal but potentially confusing response consists of spikes synchronous with the flashes and recorded at the front of the head. This is photomyoclonus (Bickford et al 1952) and consists of myogenic potentials due to rhythmic contraction of scalp muscles in time with the flashes. It is a normal finding which can be demonstrated in 50% of volunteers if a sufficiently bright flash is used and if they voluntarily increase their facial muscle tone by grimacing. It has no apparent connection with the photomyoclonus seen in the Senegalese baboon, which is a form of visually induced myoclonic epileptic seizure.

Most important in the context of epilepsy is the so-called 'photoconvulsive response' (PCR). This comprises generalized epileptiform activity (spikes or spike-wave discharges), which are not phase-locked to the flash train and continue for some hundreds of milliseconds or longer after stimulation has ceased. A response having these characteristics is rarely found in a person who does not suffer from epilepsy or have a family history of seizures. The distinction, therefore, between the PCR and other atypical responses to photic stimulation is clinically important, and has been confused by the use by some authors of the term 'photosensitivity' to describe both the PCR and normal variants of the photic response. A majority of photosensitive patients are subject to seizures induced by environmental visual stimuli, and the recognition of photosensitivity is therefore often critical to their management. Because of the importance of EEG investigation in this particular group of patients, photosensitive epilepsy is the subject of a later section of this chapter.

Reliable assessment of responses to photic

stimulation requires careful technique (Binnie et al 1982a). The methods used vary greatly between laboratories and are rarely optimal for demonstrating a PCR. In patients with a history of seizures precipitated by viewing television or by visual patterns, it may be appropriate to assess the EEG responses to these provocative stimuli, using methods similar in principal to those employed for flicker stimulation (Wilkins et al 1979b, Darby et al 1980a).

Sleep induction

The effects of sleep on the EEG in epilepsy and the importance of sleep in diagnostic EEG investigation were noted above. For clinical purposes, it is not often convenient to record during nocturnal sleep and various methods may be used to induce sleep during the working hours of the EEG laboratory. The ideal is probably a restful environment and a relaxed approach to recording which will encourage the patient to sleep spontaneously. The artificial method most often used is administration of sedative drugs, notably quinalbarbitone and chloral hydrate (or its derivatives as such dichloralphenazone). In addition to activating epileptiform discharges, these drugs may provide further diagnostically useful information by virtue of the beta activity which they induce in the EEG. The appearance of beta activity is a normal response to barbiturates in particular and an asymmetry may reflect underlying cerebral pathology.

Other drugs used to induce sleep may have some proconvulsive action in their own right. This is probably the case with methohexitone and possibly with promethazine. Methohexitone has the feature of being administered intravenously, giving a rapid response, saving time and allowing the dose to be titrated accurately. It has the disadvantage that the patient passes rapidly into deep sleep, whereas it is during drowsiness and light sleep in particular that information of diagnostic value in partial epilepsies is most likely to be obtained. Promethazine may be particularly suitable for inducing sleep in children and is available as a syrup which may be more acceptable than sleeping tablets. Diazepam, given intravenously or by mouth, may seem ill suited as a sleep-inducing agent for investigating epilepsy in view of its antiepileptic action. However, as diazepam selectively suppresses generalized rather than focal discharges, it may be useful for inducing sleep in suspected partial epilepsy where the purpose of the investigation is specifically to attempt to demonstrate a focus (Gotman et al 1982). Thus, where it is suspected that bilateral discharges seen in the waking EEG represent secondary generalization, slow intravenous injection of diazepam may first suppress the generalized activity, unmasking the focus, and then cause the focal discharges to increase as the patient lapses into sleep. A similar result may be obtained with thiopentone, given in a small intravenous dose (0.5–1 mg/kg) so that the patient does not fall asleep too rapidly (Lombroso & Erba 1970). In light drowsiness, generalized spike-wave discharges are suppressed and focal epileptiform activity may appear. If there is also a depression of barbiturate-induced fast activity at the same site, confidence in localization of the focus is reinforced.

One highly effective method of obtaining sleep during the normal working hours of an EEG laboratory is to arrange for the patient to remain awake all or part of the previous night. This not only produces a fairly natural sleep pattern, uncomplicated by the effects of hypnotic drugs, but also has been claimed to have some activating effect in its own right. This not unreasonable belief is based on the finding that prolonged sleep deprivation can induce seizures even in persons not ordinarily suffering from epilepsy (Bennett 1962, Bennett et al 1969). However, a difficulty in assessing the yield of diagnostically useful information, both from sleep recording in general and from recording after sleep deprivation in particular, is that the available evidence is mostly derived from uncontrolled studies under conditions of routine clinical practice. The decision to proceed to sleep recording, either drug induced or after sleep deprivation, generally follows from the failure of the initial EEG to provide the information required. The findings therefore confound the effects of the activation procedures as such with those of simply repeating the EEG. Only one study (Veldhuizen et al 1983) overcomes this problem: in a group of patients with refractory epilepsy, wake, drug induced sleep and sleep deprivation records were obtained in random sequence and regardless of the previous findings. There was no evidence of an increased incidence of epileptiform activity in the waking state after sleep deprivation nor was the yield of new information during sleep any greater when this was induced by deprivation rather than by drugs. A limitation, however, of this study was that it included no children and no patients with primary generalized epilepsy: both groups in which the earlier literature, notwithstanding its methodological deficiencies, claims the greatest yield of activation by sleep deprivation.

A too rigid distinction should perhaps not be made between wake and sleep recordings for diagnostic investigation of epilepsy. In partial epilepsies in particular, the yield of new information is likely to be greatest in the early stages of drowsiness, which may be attained during a 'routine' recording if the environment is restful and the approach of the EEG technologist unhurried. This may account for the surprising conclusion, from a major centre for the preoperative assessment of patients with partial epilepsies, that the contribution of recording during drug-induced sleep for diagnostic assessment was minimal (Gloor et al 1957).

Antiepileptic drug withdrawal

When the diagnosis of epilepsy is in doubt, clinical considerations will often dictate a trial of antiepileptic drug (AED) withdrawal, to determine the effect, if any, on the seizure frequency. This will also provide the opportunity to reassess the EEG in the absence of medication. It is, however, important to distinguish the results, both clinical and electroencephalographic, of removing the antiepileptic action of the drugs from the proconvulsant effects of acute AED withdrawal. Epileptiform activity not previously present is more likely to be significant if focal or recorded a week or more after the last reduction of medication; whereas generalized discharges, photosensitivity and abnormalities seen in the acute phase of AED withdrawal do not represent evidence of epilepsy (Ludwig & Ajmone Marsan 1975).

Convulsant drugs

Administration of such convulsant drugs as pentylenetetrazol (Metrazol) in normal subjects will induce photosensitivity, spontaneous epileptiform discharges and, eventually, seizures. However, in patients with epilepsy, the dose required to produce these effects may be less and this formed the basis of the 'photometrazol test' (Gastaut 1950), which in clinical practice proved unreliable. Convulsants may also be used in an attempt to activate a focus in a patient undergoing assessment for possible surgical treatment of epilepsy (Kaufman et al 1947). However, comparison of convulsant-induced and spontaneous seizures, with recording from both scalp and depth electrodes, shows that the drug-induced seizures are often generalized and, even if focal, are different both clinically and electrographically from those occurring spontaneously (Bancaud et al 1968, Wieser et al 1979). The localizing value of convulsant-induced focal EEG abnormalities is therefore highly questionable and convulsant activation of the EEG has fallen into disuse, except in some specialized centres for neurosurgical treatment of epilepsy where, it may be assumed, the limitations of the method are appreciated.

Tests of vasomotor lability

As an aid to differential diagnosis between epilepsy and syncope, various manoeuvres may be used to induce postural hypotension by means of a tilt table, or to induce a vasovagal attack by carotid sinus massage or ocular compression. As these manoeuvres often produce hypotensive attacks in normal subjects and negative results in patients who suffer from syncope, their diagnostic reliability is questionable and does not appear to justify the undoubted risks of embolism resulting from massaging a diseased carotid artery or retinal detachment due to eyeball pressure.

THE EEG AND CLASSIFICATION OF EPILEPSY

At the time of writing, international conventions on the classification of epilepsy are in some disarray. The current two-dimensional international classification (partial or generalized, primary or secondary) was intended to be only provisional (Merlis 1970). The terminology committee of the International League Against Epilepsy has drafted a system which combines a revised version of the present classification with a list of epilepsy syndromes which are not mutually exclusive (Dreifuss et al 1985). However, this system is still undergoing evaluation and has not yet been accepted (see Ch. 1). The present text will list the typical EEG features of the groups described in the 1970 classification, noting at the same time some particular syndromes which show special electrographic characteristics.

Although the distinction between generalized and partial (focal) seizures has proved useful for descriptive purposes, as an aid to communication and in selecting therapy, its physiological basis is suspect. The striking appearance of generalized, bilaterally symmetrical and synchronous discharges led, from the early 1940s, to the concept of a central diencephalic pacemaker (Jasper & Kershman 1941, Jasper & Droogleever-Fortuyn 1947) and hence to the concept of centrencephalic epilepsy formulated by Penfield & Jasper (1954). Experimental data supported this theory: during absence seizures 3/sec spike-wave activity had been recorded in the thalamus (Williams 1953) and spike-wave activity or absence-like seizures could be induced by stimulation of the thalamus (Jasper & Kershman 1941, Hunter & Jasper 1949a, Pollen et al 1963, Jasper & Droogleever-Fortuyn 1947) or of the midbrain reticular formation (Weir 1964). Thalamic lesions in kittens are also considered to provide an experimental model of absence seizures (Guerreo-Figueroa et al 1963). Some workers never accepted the centrencephalic concept, notably Gibbs & Lennox (Gibbs et al 1937) who regarded generalized epilepsy as a cortical disorder. An experiment by Bennett (1958) in the Gibbs' laboratory, which was subsequently repeated and extended by the Montreal School of Gloor and colleagues (Gloor 1968, 1972) began to undermine this model. The effects of injecting convulsant or anticonvulsant agents into the carotid and vertebrobasilar circulations were studied in humans, in the course of preoperative assessment (p. 283). From the hypothesis of a diencephalic pacemaker for generalized epileptiform discharges, it would be expected that injection of convulsant drugs into the vertebrobasilar system (the principal blood supply of the diencephalon) should induce generalized discharges, whereas injection of anticonvulsants should inhibit them. This was not found.

Conversely, although it might be expected that carotid injections of convulsants or anticonvulsants should have little effect if the primary source of epileptogenesis were diencephalic, the reverse was the case: unilateral carotid amytal injection abolished generalized discharges, and unilateral injection of the convulsant pentylenetetrazol induced generalized discharges and seizures. Clearly, the cortex was at least as important as the diencephalon for the generation of generalized spike-wave activity.

Marcus & Watson (Marcus & Watson 1966, Marcus et al 1968) showed that bilateral topical application to the frontal cortex of metrazol or premarine elicited absence-like seizures and generalized spike-wave activity. These effects persisted after destruction of subcortical grey matter but were abolished by callosal section. Prince & Farrell (1969) showed that parenteral injection of penicillin in the cat would produce generalized spike wave activity and absence-like seizures; and systemic or topical application of penicillin has formed the experimental model on which much of the subsequent work by the Montreal group has been based. Topical application of penicillin to the cortex, but not to subcortical structures, produces generalized spike-wave activity (Gloor et al 1977). The spike-wave appears first in the cortex and only later in subcortical structures (Fisher & Prince 1977). The initiation of spike-wave activity is closely related to that of spindle formations of the normal EEG (Quesney et al 1977, Kostopoulos & Gloor 1982), and reduction of cortical excitability causes the spike-wave to be replaced by spindles (Gloor et al 1979). The model which thus emerges for 'generalized corticoreticular epilepsies' is thus of a bilaterally hyperexcitable cerebral cortex which responds abnormally with spike-wave activity to afferent impulses from the diencephalon, which are themselves normal and would ordinarily give rise to spindles. This model also helps to explain the marked influence of state of awareness (i.e the activity of the reticular activating system) on seizures and EEG discharges.

The model, however, leaves many observations unexplained. If generalized spike-wave activity and seizures are of cortical origin and can be provoked by unilateral carotid injection of a convulsant, then the distinction between generalized discharges and focal discharges with secondary generalization appears to be blurred. Tükel & Jasper (1952) showed that parasaggital lesions could produce bilateral discharges and Bancaud (1972), using depth recording, found that seemingly symmetrical generalized discharges could arise from a mesial frontal focus. Huck et al (1980) reported the emergence of unilateral foci after callosal section in patients with generalized discharges. Conversely, mesial frontal stimulation can produce bilaterally synchronous spike-wave activity (Bancaud et al 1974). A study by Wilkins et al (1981), using hemifield pattern stimulation in photosensitive subjects, showed that the threshold for inducing spike-wave activity could be markedly asymmetrical between the two hemispheres, implying an asymmetry of the postulated cortical hyper-excitability. There is also some difficulty in extrapolating from experiments on feline penicillin epilepsy to generalized seizures in humans. Penicillin does not ordinarily cross the blood–brain barrier. Reported experiments on feline penicillin epilepsy have all apparently employed acutely or subacutely implanted electrodes which presumably compromised the blood–brain barrier. Binnie et al (1985c) found in dogs that, if upwards of three months were allowed for recovery from electrode insertion, no convulsant effect was obtained with massive parenteral doses of penicillin. Feline penicillin epilepsy is thus a model, not of generalized, but rather of multifocal epilepsy, the brain being exposed to the convulsant drug wherever electrodes have been placed. Using other chemical models (bicuculline and pentylenetetrazol) Rodin et al (1971, 1975, 1977) found the initial ictal event to be very high-frequency multi-unit activity in brainstem structures preceding onset of spike-wave discharges in cortex and thalamus, whereas penicillin did indeed induce corticothalamic discharges from the start. Binnie et al (1985c) confirmed these findings in

respect of pentylenetetrazol and bicuculline in dogs and, moreover, found the most frequent site at which the first ictal changes were found to be the lateral geniculate body. Other models implicate the substantia nigra as a site of chemical epileptogenesis and as a specific target organ for some antiepileptic drugs (Gale 1985, Turski et al 1986). Which of these models is most relevant to generalized seizures in humans remains uncertain.

The following didactic account will employ the conventional distinction between generalized and partial epilepsies and seizures, but it should be recognized that these concepts are at best oversimplifications and the physiological models on which they are based are disputed.

Primary generalized epilepsy

The EEG in primary generalized epilepsy is characterized by generalized discharges, most often spike-wave activity, arising against a normal background. In patients with absence seizures, this is rhythmic and has a frequency of 2.5–4/s. If the discharge is of less than 2 or 3 s duration, no clinical manifestations may be seen, although psychological testing may reveal transitory cognitive impairment (see p. 267). During longer discharges, an overt absence may be observed, consciousness being lost within the first 2 s and gradually beginning to return some 3 s before the end of the discharge. The phenomenon of cognitive impairment during the shorter discharges has led some authors to suggest that all the generalized spike-wave activity is ictal or that 'in absence seizures interictal discharges probably do not occur' (Delgado-Escueta 1979). The generalized spike-wave activity is of greatest amplitude at the front of the head and may show bifrontal maxima or a single maximum in the midline. It has been suggested by Dondey (1983) that the absence seizures in patients with a single midline maximum are atypical and have a poor prognosis. Minor asymmetries are often present and there appear to be no accepted criteria for determining what degree of asymmetry is acceptable before the question of possible secondary generalization arises. Suspicion will be heightened if the discharges are irregular in form or frequency, or are slower than 2.5/s and if the asymmetry is consistent. Onset and termination of the discharge are abrupt but, during a long run of spike-wave activity, the frequency may gradually decrease. Post-ictal changes are not seen. In those patients whose absence seizures are accompanied by a prominent myoclonus, and most notably in the juvenile myoclonic epilepsy, the spike components are generally multiple. Less regular generalized spike-wave occurs in the interictal EEGs of patients with tonic-clonic convulsions, as may generalized polyspike discharges. These are often activated by sleep, appearing maximally in Stage III. The ictal EEG during a tonic-clonic seizure is characterized by an initial burst of generalized spiking, a tonic phase in which the tracing is usually obscured by muscle artefact and then rhythmic polyspike-wave discharges occurring synchronously with the clonic jerks. As these become irregular and less frequent so also do the spike-wave complexes and, in the post-ictal state, the EEG is characterized by generalized slowing, possibly preceded by a period of low amplitude. Photosensitivity is most common in patients with primary generalized epilepsy, having an incidence of some 20% in a typical EEG practice, rising to some 40% in children.

Partial epilepsy

Ictal findings during a partial epileptic seizure have been described above. The interictal EEG may contain normal background activity or exhibit abnormalities reflecting the underlying pathology. These may range from an asymmetry of background activity in a patient with a unilateral chronic lesion such as mesial temporal sclerosis, to a gross delta focus with generalized slowing in a patient with a tumour. For further discussion of the EEG in cerebral lesions the reader is referred to such standard texts as Niedermeyer & Lopes da Silva (1982).

Focal epileptiform activity may vary very much in its incidence, both within and between subjects, and is often markedly influenced by state of awareness. It is common for a patient to exhibit no epileptiform activity when tense and apprehensive at the start of a recording, but to show progressively increasing discharges if encouraged to relax as the investigation proceeds. Focal epileptiform activity occurs most regularly over the temporal regions. This is seen most typically, of course, in patients with seizures of temporal lobe origin; however, central and frontal lesions may also produce focal discharges in the anterior or superior temporal region. In addition to typical spikes, sharp waves and spike-wave complexes, some patients exhibit runs of focal slow activity in the theta or delta range which appear to be related to the 'epileptogenic activity'. Interictal focal epileptiform discharges in partial epilepsy are generally isolated transients or bursts of less than 1 s duration. Sometimes longer discharges occur, lasting some tens of seconds, often with a progressive change in morphology and frequency and without any apparent clinical events. It is tempting to describe those loosely as 'subclinical electrical seizures'. However, it is difficult to establish the absence of clinical manifestations, and one study, using psychological testing during the EEG, showed cognitive disturbances even during extremely brief focal discharges (Aarts et al 1984) (see also p. 267).

Many patients with partial epilepsy and focal EEG discharges exhibit more than one focus. In most instances the foci appear functionally independent and, indeed, the patient may even exhibit various seizure types which can be shown by ictal recording to arise from different foci. Most often the foci occur over homologous regions of the right and left hemispheres, most typically anterior temporal, and sometimes they may occur synchronously or rather with a small delay between one side and the other. The pathophysiological basis of this EEG picture has not been established and the synchronous foci could reflect either transmission from one hemisphere to the other or simultaneous activation of two independent foci by a common subcortical input. Ralston (1958) found that spikes recorded in the vicinity of an acute experimental lesion tended to be associated with spiky after-discharges and those at a distance did not. Ralston & Papatheodorou (1960) made similar observations in humans, but such discharges are rarely found in human clinical EEGs and do not appear to be of value for locating epileptogenic lesions (Engel et al 1975). Micro-electrode studies show discharge rates of neurones in the focus from which seizures arise to be higher than in other foci, with a tendency to firing in bursts (Babb & Crandall 1976). Larger depth electrodes also record higher and more regular discharge rates at the site of seizure onset (Lieb et al 1978).

One possible explanation of multiple foci over homologous areas of both hemispheres is offered by experimental work on the so-called 'mirror focus' (Morrell 1960). An experimental lesion is created which gives rise to focal EEG spikes and seizures. After an interval ranging from hours to weeks (depending on the site of the focus and the age and species of the animal) a 'mirror focus' of spikes appears over the homologous area of the contralateral hemisphere. At first the foci are functionally interrelated, the mirror spikes following those in the primary focus, with a delay presumably due to interhemispheric transmission. Later, the secondary focus becomes independent of the primary spiking. Development of a mirror focus can be prevented by section of interhemispheric connections and by administration of antiepileptic drugs. Removal of the primary focus, or its temporary inactivation by intracarotid barbiturates abolishes the mirror focus if this has not yet become functionally independent. When the firing of the mirror and primary foci is no longer time related, there is an intermediate phase during which ablation of the primary focus will result in a gradual disappearance of the secondary. Finally, the mirror focus achieves full independence, may itself give rise to seizures and will persist, even if the primary is removed; biochemical and micro-electrode studies then show local abnormalities of cortical neurones.

Morrell & Whisler (1980) report a study of patients with well-documented unilateral epileptogenic lesions with bilateral foci. In those patients where intravenous methohexitone suppressed the focus contralateral to the lesion, removal of the latter resulted in relief of seizures. A secondary focus resistant to barbiturate was considered to have attained the stage of independence and operation did not abolish the seizures. In a long-term study, Hughes (1985) found that 40% of unilateral foci eventually became bilateral, particularly where the original focus was left-sided or frontal. Other authors contend that it has not yet been reliably established whether or not the phenomenon of the mirror focus seen in experimental animals actually occurs in humans (Goldensohn 1984). Whatever the physiological basis of interdependence of bilateral foci the second focus often disappears gradually after removal of an epileptogenic lesion (Falconer & Kennedy 1961). In Morrell's terms such foci must presumably have reached the intermediate phase of secondary epileptogenesis.

Focal discharges may spread to a greater or lesser degree not only within one hemisphere or to the homologous region on the other side, but also to produce generalized epileptiform activity (Fig. 8.9). This phenomenon of 'secondary generalization' is seen both in the interictal recording and in the ictal EEG, where it is often associated with the onset of complex symptomatology. Indeed, it is implicit in the 1981 revision of the International Classification of Epileptic Seizures (Dreifuss 1981) that complex symptomatology (i.e. impairment of consciousness) in partial seizures is due to secondary generalization. The term 'secondary generalization' invites confusion with 'secondary generalized epilepsy'. It should be stressed that secondary generalization is a physiological phenomenon reflected in the spread of an initially focal EEG and/or clinical disturbance. In the term 'secondary generalized epilepsy' the word 'secondary', indicates that the epilepsy is considered to be symptomatic, or secondary to cerebral pathology.

Secondary generalization occurs more readily in children with partial epilepsy than in adults. However, when a patient in whom only generalized discharges have been found exhibits a clear focus with increasing age, it may be impossible to determine whether the focus has always been present but unrecognized due to the generalized activity, or has developed de novo. If this latter were the case, it would suggest that primary generalized epilepsy could evolve to partial, as a result of ictal brain damage. In children with a clear focus, migration from the posterior to the anterior temporal regions may be seen as a function of age (Gibbs & Gibbs 1960).

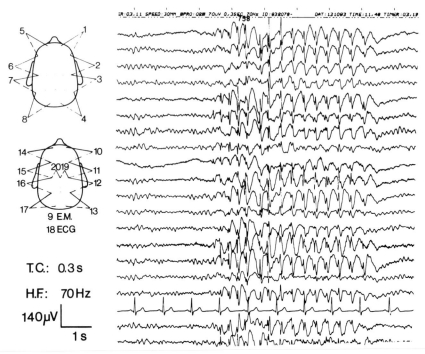

Fig. 8.9 Secondary generalization of an initially focal discharge in the left frontal region. The patient's seizures commenced with jerking of the right hand sometimes followed by loss of consciousness.

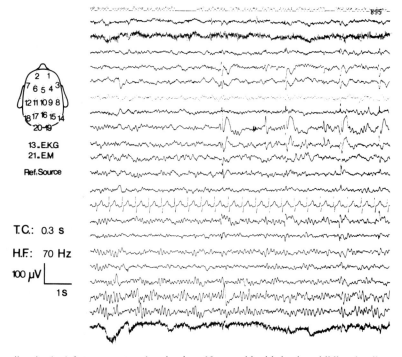

Fig. 8.10 Rolandic spikes in the left centrotemporal region in a 10-year-old with benign childhood epilepsy.

Primary partial epilepsy

Although the bidimensional classification of epilepsy has been in use for many years, it was pointed out only comparatively recently by Gastaut (1982) that the niche for primary partial epilepsy is occupied by the benign epilepsy of childhood. This has not only a very characteristic clinical picture of predominantly nocturnal partial seizures in a child between the ages of 4 and 14, but also produces a striking EEG pattern. Spikes, or spike-wave complexes, of amplitudes often greater than 100 μv are seen, sharply localized, typically over the central region of one or both hemispheres, or sometimes lower in the central coronal plane at a superior or midtemporal site (Fig. 8.10).

The discharges may occur many times a minute and, if not correctly identified, may cause some alarm. However, the type of epilepsy associated with these characteristic 'pointes Rolandiques' is highly sensitive to antiepileptic drugs and disappears by the age of 14. Despite the profuse discharges, some children with benign childhood epilepsy may have suffered only one seizure in their lives and 'pointes Rolandiques' may be asymptomatic, particularly in siblings of children with overt benign childhood epilepsy. An atypical distribution of the focal discharges is, however, often associated with a different clinical picture and a less favourable prognosis (Wong 1985).

Far less common than the typical benign childhood epilepsy of Rolandic origin are temporal and occipital forms. This last is characterized by occipital spike-wave bursts and visual ictal symptoms, including scotomata. Many cases of the occipital form of benign childhood epilepsy are probably misdiagnosed as basilar migraine (Gastaut 1982).

Secondary generalized epilepsy

As secondary generalized epilepsy is by definition due to proven or presumed widespread cerebral pathology, an abnormal background activity may be expected in the EEG. This may range from a

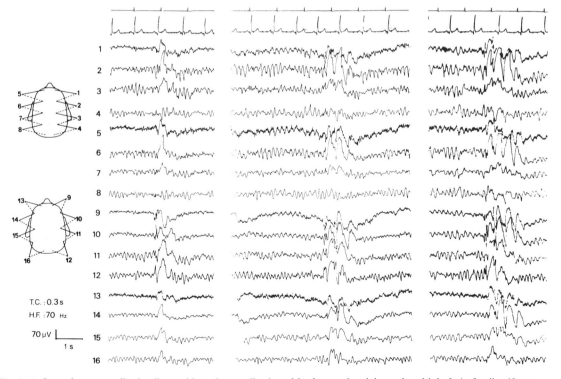

Fig. 8.11 Secondary generalized epilepsy. Note abnormally slowed background activity and multiple foci of epileptiform discharges, showing a tendency to generalize.

slight excess of theta activity to a grossly disturbed picture from which normal rhythms are totally absent. Multiple foci of epileptiform activity are often seen (Fig. 8.11) and this may reflect the multiple seizure patterns often seen in this condition. The discharges may become secondarily generalized (but note that this has nothing to do with the reasons for calling this condition 'secondary generalized epilepsy'). The discharges may be very frequent and may indeed occupy more than 50% of the entire recording. In secondary generalized epilepsy there is often little correlation between the seizure frequency and the discharge rate, the EEG remaining unimproved even when the patient's attacks are well controlled.

Although patients with secondary generalized epilepsy often exhibit multiple seizure types, two particular patterns may be noted. Atonic seizures are very characteristic of this form of epilepsy, often causing the patient to fall and suffer injury. The ictal EEG changes are varied but, if the attack consists merely of a loss of muscle tone, the EEG may show only an electrodecremental event (Egli et al 1985). Episodes of impaired awareness, atypical absences, also occur in secondary generalized epilepsy and are typically associated with the very slow spike-wave activity at only one per second or less (Fig. 8.12) characteristic of the Lennox-Gastaut syndrome. It is rarely necessary to resort to sleep recording to detect epileptiform activity in secondary generalized epilepsy. Often the sleeping EEG is characterized by the appear-

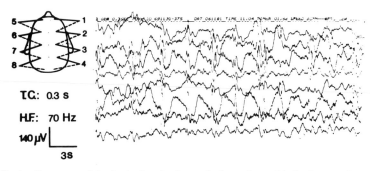

Fig. 8.12 Slow generalized spike-wave activity in the interictal record of a patient with the Lennox-Gastaut syndrome.

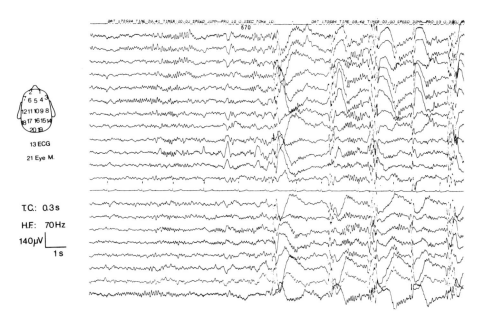

Fig. 8.13 Polyspike wave activity during sleep in a patient with secondary generalized epilepsy.

ance of profuse, generalized polyspike-wave discharges in stages III and IV (Fig. 8.13)

A particular form of secondary generalised epilepsy, West's syndrome, is usually associated with a striking EEG picture known as 'hypsarrhythmia' (Fig. 8.14). The record contains multiple epileptiform discharges, both focal and generalized, and displays a grossly disturbed background dominated by slow activity, often interspersed with episodes of reduced amplitude. However, the most striking feature is the chaotic quality, the lack of any consistent organization in either topography or timing of the events. In some patients, the infantile spasms may accompany high voltage generalized epileptiform discharges and the intervening sections of the record are of relatively low amplitude. Often even this degree of consistency is lacking. For further details of the EEG investigation of West's syndrome see Jeavons & Bower (1964) and Harris (1972).

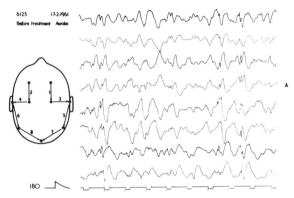

Fig. 8.14 Hypsarrhythmia in a 6-month-old baby with West's syndrome. Note the chaotic high-amplitude slow activity and epileptiform discharges without any consistent distributions.

Unclassifiable epilepsy

The electroencephalographer asked to classify patients' epilepsy on the basis of the EEG rapidly finds himself in difficulties. Although the typical clinical and electrographic pictures of partial and secondary generalized epilepsy are readily distinguished, the boundary between them is ill defined. Some patients with diffuse brain disease may nevertheless have a single EEG focus and a single seizure type; some patients have more than one EEG focus, several seizure types and, possibly, multiple cerebral lesions. In both these instances – partial seizures in the context of generalized cerebral disease on the one hand, and multifocal epilepsy on the other – it is difficult to determine whether the appropriate designation is partial or secondary generalized epilepsy. The difficulty lies, of course, not with interpretation of the EEG findings but with the classification itself.

STATUS EPILEPTICUS

In the early stages of status epilepticus, ictal discharges appropriate to the seizure type are repeatedly seen with incomplete recovery of the post-ictal disturbance between seizures. With prolonged status involving partial or tonic-clonic seizures the ictal patterns may become progressively less dramatic and the interictal disturbance more severe. Thus, in a prolonged partial status, the EEG may be grossly slowed and asymmetrical, being lower of amplitude on the side of the causative focus. Ictal discharges may be confined to brief runs of spikes and, indeed, where there is marked reduction of amplitude on the side of the original focus, ictal spiking may eventually be seen only over the contralateral hemisphere.

Although status epilepticus with tonic-clonic or simple partial motor seizures may readily be recognized on clinical grounds, status with complex partial or absence seizures may present with psychiatric symptomatology or a fluctuating confusional state. Here the EEG findings may be crucial to diagnosis. Absence status in particular is characterized by irregular spike-wave activity, less well formed than that typical in absence seizures and often waxing and waning in amount rather than showing a clear distinction between ictal and interictal periods.

Drug treatment of status epilepticus has been much improved since the introduction of benzodiazepines, and intractable status is seen less often in epileptological practice than amongst terminally brain-damaged patients in the intensive care unit. Where status does not respond rapidly to treatment, and particularly where it is necessary to resort to anaesthesia and the use of muscle relaxants and artificial ventilation, clinical observation of the attacks becomes difficult and EEG monitoring may be the only satisfactory way of following progress. In this context it may be noted that the conventional multichannel EEGs may usefully be supplemented by continuous registration of ictal events on a slowly moving chart by such devices as the cerebral function monitor (Prior & Maynard 1976).

EPILEPSY MONITORING

One of the great fascinations of epilepsy is the intermittent nature both of the disease and of its electrophysiological manifestations. The full picture can never be grasped by examining the patient at one moment in time or recording the electrical activity of the brain for a few minutes only. The condition is, moreover, profoundly influenced by sleep and waking, vigilance, cognitive function and biorhythms. These considerations led various workers in the 1960s to undertake long-term observation of patients with epilepsy engaged in a variety of everyday activities in, so far as possible, a normal environment. Clinical manifestations were registered first on cine film (Hunter & Jasper 1949b, Schwab et al 1954, Ajmone Marsan & Abraham 1960). However, the advent of video recording provided a far more cost-effective means of recording behaviour over hours or days in order to capture infrequent clinical events of a few minutes' duration (Penin 1968).

This technology was combined with EEG registration by radio telemetry, in order to allow the patient greater freedom of movement and a wider range of physical activities than was possible under the conditions of conventional EEG recording. These early studies were concerned chiefly with the effects of psychological tasks on EEG discharges and seizures (Vidart & Geier 1967, Guey et al 1969) or with documentation of unusual seizure types (Harrison-Covello & De Barros-Ferreira 1975, Dreyer & Wehmeyer 1978). The development of these techniques in a research context led only gradually to the realization of their potential as an aid to the clinical assessment of patients with known or suspected epilepsy. The number of units worldwide routinely employing such facilities has expanded from some dozens in the late 1970s to several hundreds at the present time, and epilepsy monitoring can be counted one of the most important recent developments of epileptology (So & Penry 1981).

Monitoring technologies

For short, comprehensive reviews of the technologies employed for epilepsy monitoring see Binnie (1983b) and Ebersole (1986); a multi–author monograph describing the techniques and experience of many of the world's leading centres is provided by Gotman et al (1985).

EEG monitoring

The possibility of recording the EEG for some hours continuously on a conventional electroencephalograph is often overlooked, and the development of elaborate telemetry systems seems to have created a myth that an ictal EEG cannot properly be recorded without this technology. The advent of head box preamplifiers, connected to the EEG machine by a cable of 3–5 m, has made it possible to obtain satisfactory recordings from a patient who, while not free to indulge in strenuous activity, can at least sit up and move about within the radius of the cable. This restriction on movement is less than that imposed by many other standard medical procedures, and, indeed, if satisfactory video recordings are to be obtained without multiple cameras and personnel to direct them, it is generally necessary for the patient to be confined within a fairly small area. In practice, monitoring by means of a conventional EEG machine, possibly with some minor modifications such as a miniaturized electrode input box is very acceptable for periods of up to 24 hours, and has proved very suitable for seizure documentation (Penin 1968, Penry et al 1975, Stefan et al 1981).

A logical extension of this technique, involving further miniaturization of head box and preamplifiers so that they can be carried on the patient's person, leads to cable telemetry (Ives et al 1976). The signals from the various channels are usually multiplexed (mixed) so that they can be transmitted down a single pair of flexible wires, typically through a cable up to 50 m long which also provides the power supply (Kamp et al 1979). The patient can move freely within this radius, which gives him the run of a typical hospital ward

(Binnie et al 1981). If the data acquisition system is located in an EEG laboratory at a distance from the recording area, the signals can with further amplification be transmitted by cable over distances of hundreds of metres around a hospital site (Ives et al 1976). The technology employed for cable telemetry is not appreciably more costly than that used in conventional EEG machines and the technical specification can be as high or better in terms of bandwidth, dynamic range, number of channels etc. The inconvenience to the patient of having to trail a cable about proves, in the event, to be minimal and it is usually the need for close observation and video recording rather than the cable which limits activity.

Greater freedom of movement may, however, be achieved by providing a radio link between the miniaturized amplifiers on the patient and the data acquisition system (Breakell et al 1949, Kamp 1963). The price paid for this increased freedom of movement is considerable, and not only in economic terms. The reliability of radio telemetry is generally lower than that of cable and, while commercially available systems may have a range of 100 m or more in free field, within a steel-and-concrete-framed building reception may be erratic, unless multiple antennae are provided (Porter et al 1971). Telecommunications regulations in many countries limit the range of frequencies which may be used (Manson 1974), which in turn limits the dynamic range, bandwidth and number of channels of the system. Power is supplied by batteries, which add to the size and weight of the pack carried by the patient. When EEG monitoring was first introduced, radio transmission was viewed with enthusiasm by most workers and the use of cable derided as not being true telemetry. The position is now reversed: many users prefer cable and manufacturers have found it necessary to provide the options of radio or a hard-wired linkage. Radio telemetry remains the ideal technology for EEG monitoring during physical activity requiring freedom of movement, an application which is more likely to be useful in research than for clinical investigation of epilepsy.

Ambulatory monitoring employs a completely portable data acquisition system carried on the patient's person. This is currently achieved by the use of small cassette recorders which may run either at conventional tape speeds providing up to 15 hours continuous recording (Kaiser 1976, Ives 1982a) or with a reduced tape speed for up to 24 hours (Ives & Woods 1975). A normal tape speed provides a bandwidth sufficient for recordings of excellent technical quality but, if continuous registration for 24 hours is required, the systems presently available offer a very limited bandwidth and dynamic range, with a maximum of 8 channels. Ambulatory monitoring is usually, although not necessarily, performed without simultaneous video registration and most systems provide no means of synchronizing the EEG with video images (see below). The technique comes into its own for investigating the patient in his own natural environment; for instance, to determine how frequently a child suffers absence seizures at school or to test the claim that a patient has seizures at home which cease on admission for observation in hospital.

Because of the considerable capital costs of monitoring equipment, until recently few workers had experience of more than one system and tended therefore to be very partisan in their advocacy of a particular method. Ambulatory monitoring in particular has been overused for applications for which it was not very suitable, chiefly because it was the first technique to become widely available commercially. Conversely, the possibilities for monitoring with a conventional EEG machine are often undervalued. An increasing number of workers now have access to all the techniques described above and advocate the selective use of different technologies for various applications (Ives 1982b, O'Kane et al 1982, Gotman et al 1985, Ebersole 1986) (see Table 8.2).

Data acquisition

In ambulatory monitoring, facilities for data acquisition onto magnetic tape form an integral part of the system. When other methods of monitoring are used, EEG data may be collected either directly on to a paper chart or on to magnetic media. The advantage of continuous chart recording is that it is continuously visible so that immediate action can be taken to correct tech-

Table 8.2 Advantages limitations and uses of available monitoring technologies (after Binnie 1983b)

Conventional EEG recorders

Advantages	high quality recording of many channels; ease of selecting filters, montage etc.
Disadvantage	lack of patient mobility
Application	seizure monitoring for up to 24 hrs

Cable telemetry

Advantages	high quality recording of many channels at low cost; less susceptible to artefact than most EEG machines
Disadvantage	limited mobility range of up to 50 m
Application	all forms of intensive monitoring in hospital except during physical exercise

Radio telemetry

Advantages	excellent mobility particularly out of doors
Disadvantage	highcost; limited range within buildings; limited bandwidth, number of channels and dynamic range
Application	all forms of intensive monitoring close to laboratory including sporting activities etc

Cassette recorders (normal tape speed)

Advantages	as cable but with greater mobility
Disadvantage	recording duration limited to 90 min between tape changes; cannot easily be time indexed to video record
Applications	EEG monitoring during tasks of short duration; seizure recording (if combined with buffer memory)

Cassette recorders (low tape speed)

Advantages	excellent mobility, 24 hrs recording between cassette changes
Disadvantages	few channels, poor dynamic range and high frequency response; cannot be time indexed to video record; high cost; more expensive than telemetry
Applications	prolonged monitoring, remote from laboratory, of known preferably generalized, EEG phenomena. Rarely suitable except as preliminary screening procedure for differential diagnosis of epileptic and pseudoseizures; unsuitable for focus localization

nical problems or to respond to clinical events; and the chart itself may easily be annotated with information about behaviour, administration of drugs etc. Moreover, a permanent, easily readable record is provided directly without the need for off-line transcription of magnetic media. The obvious disadvantages are in terms of cost, both of paper (1 km/24 h at reasonable chart speeds), storage of the records and the requirement for the continuous presence of personnel to check the chart transport and the paper and ink supplies. Magnetic recording may use reel-to-reel instrumentation recorders but, if simultaneous video registration is also undertaken, there may be considerable advantages in storing the EEG signals on video tape, together with the images of the patient. This may be done in three ways: as a split-screen video picture (see below); on to the standard audio channels of the video recorder; or into the upper margin of the video frame (which modern video cassette recorders use for hi-fi registration). This last method gives the best-quality recording and permits recovery of the original electrical signals for subsequent write-out on chart, computer analysis etc.

All the above methods of magnetic registration (with the exception of the use of the hi-fi channel of a video recorder) permit rapid replay for scanning the recorded signals to find particular events of interest. Split-screen video images can simply be scanned in fast picture search mode. Both ambulatory monitoring and the reel-to-reel tape systems provide options for fast replay either as an image which pans continuously across the screen, or in page-turning mode where some 10 s of EEG are momentarily presented for about 1 s each.

In many applications, only a small section of the registration encompassing a particular clinical event is of interest. Here it may be possible to economize on recording media by storing only those few minutes of the record which are required. As the initial EEG events in a seizure are of particular importance, it is too late to commence registration only after clinical changes have been detected. Some form of buffer memory is therefore needed so that, when an event of interest is detected, a permanent registration can be made of the signals, commencing some seconds or minutes before the detection and continuing until after the event of interest. This was achieved by Ives et al (1976) using a computer disc as a buffer memory. Other technological possibilities include an extended tape path to introduce a time delay between the record and playback heads of a tape deck, or the use of solid state digital memory. Such a system may be usefully combined with automatic detection of epileptiform discharges (Gotman et al 1979) or of seizures (Gotman 1981, 1982). Standalone systems for recognizing and counting epileptiform events have been used for data reduction (Quy et al 1980, De Vries et al 1981, Zetterlund 1982) but, except in the case of spike-wave activity (Principe et al 1985), have not yet achieved any high level of reliability in distinguishing epileptiform events from the artefacts which are invariably present in telemetric records from active subjects.

Documentation of behaviour

Fully to document the clinical events of any but the simplest seizure requires a permanent record which can be replayed repeatedly and preferably at reduced speed. For this purpose, video recording is ideal. Depending on the application and the funds available, the system used may range from a single camera with a wide-angle lens and a home video recorder, to multiple cameras covering an entire hospital ward with remote control facilities and broadcast quality video tape equipment. For many purposes it is essential to be able accurately to relate clinical events to the EEG at the same moment in time, and for this purpose some method of synchronizing the video image with the EEG is required. The simplest and most widely used method is to record EEG and the image of the patient together, either as a split-screen display or by superimposing the EEG on the video picture. If the video registration is time indexed by a standard time–date generator, this latter can be linked to a microcomputer to write out time indexing simultaneously on the EEG chart (Ives 1982c).

The sensitivity of clinical observation may be further enhanced by engaging the subject in structured, continuous activity, the performance of which can be measured. This may permit detection of momentary lapses of cognitive function during subclinical EEG discharges (see below).

Applications

The distinction between the clinical and research applications of monitoring is often blurred, as a routine service generally yields data of scientific value. However, the principle indications proposed in various evaluation studies of epilepsy monitoring are summarized in Table 8.3.

Table 8.3 Suggested indications for epilepsy monitoring and yield of useful information in 9 evaluation reports (after Binnie 1987)

Indications for epilepsy monitoring	Refs,*
Differential diagnosis	123456789
Subjective Complaints	3 5 7
Pseudoseizures?	2 456 8
Enuresis	45
Nocturnal Restlessness/Apnoea	345
Cardiac Disorder/Syncope?	23 6
Diurnal Sleepiness	3
Episodic Behavioural Disturbances	4 789
Hyperventilation?	8
EEG correlates of known seizures	123456
Classification	1 3 56
Focus Localisation	3 5
Clinical correlates of EEG discharge	2 45
Transitory Cognitive Impairment	2 45
Seizure frequency	2345 9
Seizure precipitants	1 3 5 8
Reflex Epilepsy	5
Self-induction	5
Situational Factors	3

* *Authors and Yield of Clinically useful Information*

1 Bowden et al (1975)	88%	6 Sindrup (1980)		50%
2 Stålberg (1976)	65%	7 Holmes et al (1982)		89%
3 Vignaendra et al (1979)	47%	8 Smith (1982)		?
4 Bruens & Knijff (1980)	?	9 Ramsay (1982)		11%
5 Binnie et al (1981)	72%			

Differential diagnosis

As noted earlier, in some 5% of persons with epilepsy, conventional clinical and EEG assessment fail to establish the diagnosis with any certainty. To this figure must be added a substantial number of patients, typically some 15% of new referrals to specialist epileptological practice, who eventually prove to be suffering from episodic events which are not epileptic in origin. In both groups of patients, prolonged observation by means of monitoring may offer the most effective means of establishing the true diagnosis. The differential diagnosis of epilepsy is considered elsewhere in Chapter 5 but, in the present context, it should be noted that monitoring of the EEG, together with other appropriate physiological variables, may assist the identification of syncope, cardiac dysrhythmias, sleep apnoea, narcolepsy and the parasomnias. However, the chief differential diagnosis for which EEG and video monitoring are required is to distinguish between epileptic and pseudoseizures.

Clinical studies of pseudoseizures (Gross 1983, Riley & Roy 1982) tend to concentrate on background psychiatric and psychological factors and accounts of the ictal phenomenology are mostly confined to emphasizing the more bizarre and histrionic features. However, many patients with pseudoseizures also suffer from epilepsy and their fictitious attacks may closely mimic their habitual epileptic seizure pattern (Roy 1977). Moreover, it has only recently been realized that partial epilepsies of mesial frontal origin in particular can give rise to a florid symptomatology previously thought to typify pseudoseizures, including bilaterally symmetrical flapping movements, arc de circle, and obscene or aggressive utterances. Binnie & Van der Wens (1986) attempted to classify the clinical manifestations of 105 video-recorded pseudoseizures, as if they were true epileptic attacks according to the international classification of Dreifuss (1981). Most of the attacks fell well within the range of known epileptic phenomenology. The pseudoseizures in patients who also had epilepsy differed little from those of the patients who did not. However, there was a tendency for pseudoseizures in non-epileptic patients to be more bizarre, whilst attacks resembling absences or complex partial seizures occurred mostly in people with epilepsy. It has been pointed out, for instance by Pedley (1983), that some details of clinical seizure pattern may distinguish pseudo from epileptic seizures. For instance, a true absence is of abrupt onset and an attack with a prodromal phase of gradual loss of consciousness cannot be an absence. Conversely,

any but the shortest complex partial seizure ends with a fairly gradual return of consciousness and, if the patient abruptly awakens and demands to know what has happened, it is unlikely to have been a complex partial seizure. Monitoring attacks thus assists the differential diagnosis of epileptic and pseudoseizures, not only by providing EEG information, but also by permitting accurate documentation of the clinical events.

However, obtaining an ictal EEG by no means invariably provides a solution to the differential diagnosis of pseudo and epileptic seizures. The occurrence of ictal EEG changes appropriate to the seizure type is, of course, conclusive in establishing at least that the observed attack was epileptic in nature. The conclusion sometimes comes as a considerable surprise to those concerned with the patient's management; and, particularly in the case of partial complex seizures of mesial frontal origin, the attacks may be so grotesque as to invite a psychiatric interpretation. Indeed, patients presenting this problem often have also psychosocial difficulties which have not been helped by the insistence of their medical advisers that their attacks were psychogenic.

The problem of the negative ictal EEG has been noted previously and interpreting the findings in the context of the differential diagnosis of pseudoseizures it is essential to consider the EEG in relation to the clinical manifestations. If the seizure is of a type which invariably, if epileptic, produces ictal EEG change and the recording is of sufficient technical quality to establish that no change occurred, one may confidently conclude that the seizure was not epileptic. If the clinical manifestations fall, however, within the range of those seizure types which do not usually produce changes in the scalp EEG, the only possible conclusion is that the findings do not resolve the differential diagnosis but are certainly compatible with an epileptic origin. This problem arises more often than might perhaps be expected, as pseudoseizures are often seen in patients with refractory partial epilepsy when, after many years of failure, effective drug control is achieved. The patient, whose habitual epileptic seizures commenced with a prodromal event, such as a rising epigastric sensation or feeling of derealization, continues to report such episodes which no longer proceed to a fully developed complex partial seizure. Such attacks fall within the classification of simple partial seizures with special sensory or psychic symptomatology and these are types which usually fail to produce changes in the scalp EEG. In undertaking monitoring of such a patient, the most one can hope is that epileptiform activity will nevertheless be found in some of the attacks, establishing an epileptic basis, or conversely that the patient may sometimes display impaired consciousness (complex symptomatology) without ictal EEG change, proving that the attack was not epileptic.

Evaluation of the ictal EEG

In patients where the diagnosis of epilepsy is not in doubt, an ictal EEG may be required, either as an aid to classification of the seizures or for purposes of focus localization prior to possible surgical treatment. This latter application will be considered further in a later section on the EEG in operative treatment of epilepsy. Seizure classification is claimed as a valuable clinical application of monitoring (Porter et al 1977, Sutula et al 1981). Typically, the argument runs that therapy resistance may be due to the use of inappropriate medication and that correct classification of the seizures is essential to determine the appropriate drugs. In support of this claim, the differential diagnosis of brief partial complex seizures and absence attacks is cited. An analysis of 273 monitored seizures from therapy-resistant patients presenting this problem showed the issue to be more complex than had been suggested (Binnie & Van der Wens 1986). There was a considerable overlap in both clinical and EEG phenomenology between absence seizures and brief complex partial seizures presenting as transitory impairment of awareness. Where the clinical manifestations (complex automatism etc) clearly fell outside the range of absence symptomatology or where the ictal EEG changes were predominantly focal, the diagnosis could readily be determined. However, in the remainder, more than half of this group of patients, there was no consistent association between EEG and clinical features which could form a basis for classifying these absence-like attacks. In practice, patients showing these features do not respond satisfactorily to monoth-

erapy, either with drugs used for absence seizures (sodium valproate, ethosuximide) nor with those appropriate to partial seizures (phenytoin, carbamazepine) and a combination of drugs from both categories is often required (Binnie & Van der Wens 1986, Hendrickson 1986, Stefan & Burr 1986).

In conclusion, while monitoring to determine seizure type may provide useful insights into a patient's problems, it is over-optimistic to suppose that it will usually lead to the choice of appropriate medication in a patient who is therapy resistant.

Seizure frequency

It is often important to establish seizure frequency, notably in assessing the effects of medication (Penry et al 1971; Dreifuss et al 1975, Stefan et al 1980). Such studies may usefully be combined with monitoring of AED levels (Rowan et al 1979). It may also sometimes be important to establish how often seizures occur under particular circumstances; for instance, the frequency of absence attacks at school in a child with learning difficulties. Absences can occur several hundred times per day, and estimates of their frequency by patients and other observers are often unreliable (Browne et al 1974a). Less commonly, brief partial seizures may be difficult to identify or may be reported by the patient more frequently than they are observed by relatives or nursing staff. In these circumstances, monitoring provides a valuable means of assessing seizure frequency. Clearly, it is applicable only where the suspected seizure frequency is so high that a reasonable number of attacks may be expected within an acceptable period of monitoring. It will be noted that this is an application for which ambulatory cassette recorders are particularly suitable and are indeed the only means of monitoring seizure frequency in the patient's own natural environment outside the hospital.

Clinical correlates of known EEG phenomena

The first and second applications above largely concern the study of the EEG during recognizable clinical events. The converse may also be of interest; namely, to establish whether or not improved behavioural observation allows clinical change to be detected during discharges which are known to occur in the EEG. Often this is possible: for instance, in a study by Overweg et al (1986) of patients who were supposed to have been seizure-free for more than three years, monitoring for only five to six hours showed that in more than 10% of the subjects EEG discharges were accompanied by brief seizures of which they and their relatives were unaware. Sometimes the difficulty in detecting seizures arises from their brevity and the lack of subjective events detected or remembered by the patient. On occasion, the clinical ictal manifestations fall within the patient's normal behavioural repertoire and it is only the simultaneous EEG registration which enables them to be identified as epileptic. For instance, a momentary hesitation in speech, a blink, a glance to one side, a brief smile without obvious cause, may all pass as normal behaviour, until it is shown that these events are consistently accompanied by an epileptiform discharge. For addressing this problem, the importance of synchronizing the EEG with the video recording of behaviour will be appreciated and split-screen video recording will generally be the most appropriate technology.

Where passive observation of behaviour during subclinical discharges fails to show any change, the possibility exists of increasing the sensitivity of observation by requiring the patient to carry out a task, the performance of which can be continually monitored. The discovery of the 3/s spike-wave discharge of the absence seizure was rapidly followed by the realization that these discharges could occur without evident clinical change (Gibbs et al 1936). However, it was then soon found that continuous psychological testing might reveal brief episodes of impaired functioning, even during apparently subclinical discharges (Schwab 1939). Some 50 subsequent published studies have, with only two exceptions (Milstein & Stevens 1961, Prechtl et al 1961), succeeded in confirming the occurrence of transitory cognitive impairment during subclinical generalized EEG discharges (for a review, see Binnie 1980). The findings are similar even in patients not considered to suffer from epilepsy (Ishihara & Yoshii 1967).

On several aspects there is general agreement. The probability of demonstrating transitory cognitive impairment (TCI), is dependent on task

difficulty (Tizard & Margerison 1963a, Mirsky & Van Buren 1965): simple, repetitious motor acts such as tapping or following a pursuit rotor (Browne et al 1974b) are relatively insensitive to the effects of subclinical discharges, whereas more complex tasks, particularly those involving signal detection, language or memory, are much more likely to be disrupted (Shimazano et al 1953, Tizard & Margerison, 1963a, Mirsky & Van Buren 1965, Geller & Geller 1970, Hutt et al 1976, Hutt & Gilbert 1980). Generalized, symmetrical, regular discharges, particularly 3/s spike-wave activity, are most likely to produce demonstrable TCI. The effects gradually increase in the course of the discharge and then diminish towards the end (the so-called 'trough of consciousness') and discharges of at least 3 s duration are more likely to produce apparent effects than are shorter episodes. Despite differences in the patient populations studied and in the sensitivity of the tasks employed, most authors were able to demonstrate TCI in approximately half of the patients investigated.

Until recently, TCI appears to have been regarded chiefly as an interesting research topic rather than a problem of possible practical importance for the individual patient. One reason may be the difficulty of investigating TCI routinely as a clinical service. To demonstrate convincingly that TCI occurs during subclinical discharges, the patient must exhibit epileptiform activity with sufficient frequency to allow a substantial number of discharges to be captured within a period acceptable for psychological testing. The tests employed for research purposes have generally been so tedious that patients could not reasonably be required to perform them for more than a few minutes at a time and, moreover, the attention involved tended to suppress spontaneous discharges. Research studies were therefore restricted to highly selected subjects with exceptionally large amounts of epileptiform activity. To test patients with subclinical discharges for TCI as a routine service, it is necessary to devise tasks which can acceptably be used over long periods and which are sufficiently sensitive, yet do not demand such concentration that the discharges are suppressed. Aarts et al (1984) reported the use of a short-term memory task, presented as an entertaining television game, which appeared to meet these requirements. This task also proved to be so sensitive to disruption by EEG discharges, that effects were demonstrable not only during generalized epileptiform activity but also when very brief focal spiking occurred. Moreover, it was found that left-sided discharges selectively impaired performance of a task using verbal stimuli, whereas right-sided discharges had a greater effect when the material to be recalled was topographic.

The phenomenon of TCI itself calls into question the definition of an epileptic seizure, and it may be considered that an EEG discharge accompanied by cognitive changes cannot properly be called 'subclinical'. Whether or not one accepts the view of Tizard & Margerison (1963b) that TCI 'should be considered evidence of a seizure', the phenomenon is of undoubted practical importance for some patients whose everyday psychosocial function is adversely affected by episodes of impaired cognition related to EEG discharges. Some such people have been helped by administration of antiepileptic drugs. Whether they are few, or represent a large proportion of those with subclinical EEG discharge, is unclear. In any event, monitoring of EEG and behaviour, preferably under the constraints of psychological testing, is a useful approach to determining whether known epileptiform activity has clinical correlates in a particular patient.

Precipitating factors

In a large proportion of patients, seizures may be precipitated by environmental, biological or psychological factors. These range from the general (stress, sleep or lack of it, biorhythms) to the highly particular as in reflex epilepsies triggered by specific cognitive activities (Forster 1977). Estimates vary concerning the importance of such factors but, in any event, one easily recognized group, patients with visually precipitated seizures, make up 3% of all people with epilepsy.

Recognition of precipitating factors may be of importance in the management of the individual patient who may be helped more by avoiding the trigger than by medication. Where the alleged precipitant is not a simple sensory stimulus, such as flicker or pattern, which can be investigated

during a routine EEG investigation, monitoring may be required. Seizures precipitated, for instance, by reading, playing chess or playing music may occur only after the activity in question has been practised for an hour or more; here, particularly if some physical activity is involved, monitoring is the appropriate technology for investigating the problem. It should also be noted that some patients deliberately induced seizures or EEG discharges in themselves, most often making use of photosensitivity for the purpose. This problem may be recognized only during monitoring in a natural environment, and it is suggested that monitoring is for this reason probably indicated in all photosensitive subjects, 25% of whom self-induce (see later section).

Evaluation studies

Epilepsy monitoring has proved a useful research tool and has brought valuable new insights into the phenomenology of epileptic seizures. It is, therefore, perhaps unsurprising that this development has been accepted with general, but often uncritical, enthusiasm. Data collection by telemetry with simultaneous video monitoring is extremely labour intensive, as is the subsequent analysis of the results; particularly when this involves visual searching of cassettes obtained by ambulatory monitoring for events the precise timing of which is unknown.

The cost-effectiveness of monitoring as a routine clinical procedure has been considered by few authors. Several (Table 8.3) have listed indications for monitoring but the earliest evaluation study appears to be that of Stalberg (1976). He found that telemetry and video monitoring, undertaken for about half a day at a time chiefly for purposes of differential diagnosis or determining seizure frequency, yielded useful information in some 65% of instances. Penry, Porter and colleagues (Penry & Porter 1977, Porter et al 1977) stressed the benefits of comprehensive reassessment of epilepsy in a unit which offered a wide range of facilities including monitoring. Sutula et al (1981) suggested that reclassification of the seizures in 43% of patients represented a major contribution of monitoring to the patients' overall clinical improvement. Evidence in support of such claims is hard to find, although one group (Binnie et al 1981, Binnie 1983b) assessed the results of monitoring in terms of practical consequences. At the simplest level of answering the questions of the referring physicians, the success rate increased from 67% over the period 1979–1980 to over 80% by 1981–1982. The clinicians were required to commit themselves to a diagnosis and management plan prior to monitoring and to decide how far these had to be changed in the light of new evidence. The importance of the findings was reflected in the fact that they were considered to have influenced management in 56% of the original referrals. At long-term follow-up, management decisions based on monitoring were considered to have benefited 23% of the original series of over 324 patients. This apparently modest result compares favourably with the use of other diagnostic aids in neurology (Derouesne et al 1979) but does perhaps serve to emphasize that this costly method of investigation must be employed selectively and for appropriate indications.

Case histories

Two case histories will be given. This first illustrates the use of monitoring to establish the diagnosis of epilepsy in a patient thought to have pseudoseizures only, and to plan successful surgical removal of a focus which could not have been located without monitoring.

A 22-year-old woman with many personal problems had undergone repeated admissions to mental hospitals since the age of 10, on account of attacks which occurred up to 10 times daily. These were characterized by screaming, dropping to the floor without injuring herself, and assuming a classical arc-de-cercle posture, often with rhythmic pelvic thrusting. Numerous interictal EEGs had been normal and other investigations were negative. She attracted some interest as the seizures resembled those of classical 'hystero-epilepsy' as described by Charcot (1887), rarely seen in modern epileptological practice. During video and EEG monitoring by cable telemetry 10 seizures were registered which followed the pattern described above. At seizure onset the EEG was generally obscured by muscle and movement artefact, however on three occasions a run of spikes was recorded at the right superior frontal electrode at the start of the seizure. This finding led to a revision of the provisional diagnosis and it appeared that the patient's attacks were epileptic and arising from a frontal epileptic focus. Nuclear magnetic resource scanning (NMR) showed a localized abnormality in the wall of a sulcus in the right frontal region directly underlying the superior frontal electrode. On the strength of these findings, subdural electrodes were inserted, together with an intracerebral bundle passing through the site of the NMR abnormality. Further monitoring captured another ten seizures, all of which were characterized by onset with high-frequency spikes in the right frontal cortex (Fig. 8.15). The affected area was resected and the patient is now seizure-free. Histological examination of the tissue removed showed patchy gliosis.

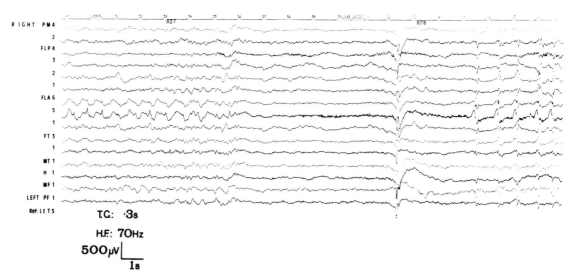

Fig. 8.15 Ictal recording with depth and subdural electrodes from patient with bizarre attacks supposed to be pseudoseizures. Onset of seizure with high-frequency discharge in right frontolateral electrode bundle, FLA 5).

The second case illustrates the detection of unsuspected but socially disabling TCI which was then successfully treated.

A 28-year-old man complained of difficulty in concentration at work. This problem had caused him to abandon his studies of law at university, after which he had become a librarian. However, he was greatly hampered in his work by difficulty in concentration when cataloguing. This was attributed by various psychiatrists and psychologists to his obsessional personality and perfectionism. However, he had occasion to write a letter to an ENT surgeon who, noting very astutely that his writing intermittently trailed away, suggested that he might have epilepsy. Routine electroencephalography including sleep recording and five hours' monitoring in a relaxing environment was negative; however, when the patient was required to perform a continuous psychological task, repeated generalized spike-wave discharges occurred and these were associated with marked impairment of performance. No other ictal symptoms were detected. The patient was put on sodium valproate, the discharges seen on monitoring during an intellectually demanding task were greatly reduced, and he no longer has any difficulty in cataloguing.

PHOTOSENSITIVE EPILEPSY

As indicated in previous sections, intermittent photic stimulation (IPS) can elicit, besides photic following, a wide range of atypical responses, which some authors loosely describe as 'photosensitivity', causing some terminological confusion (Newmark & Penry 1979). Many of these variants are genetically determined, occur most frequently in children and adolescents, and are more common in females than males (Doose et al 1969). Interestingly, similar phenomena are found in other primates. Atypical photic responses are often found in normal subjects, although some types have a weak statistical association with epilepsy. However, the photoconvulsive response (PCR) as described by Bickford et al (1952) is of much greater clinical significance. The PCR consists of generalized spikes or multiple spike-wave activity with a frontal maximum (Fig. 8.16). The discharge, once initiated, is self-sustaining, has a frequency independent of that of the flashes and continues for some hundreds of milliseconds after the stimulus train has ceased. Discharges meeting this last criterion are virtually confined to people with epilepsy or their close relatives (Reilly & Peters 1973). For the present purpose the term 'photosensitivity' will be used to describe a liability to produce a PCR in this narrow sense.

G. F. A. Harding (cited by Jeavons 1982) estimates the prevalence of photosensitivity in a population aged 5–24 years to be slightly less than 1 in 4000. As the prevalence of active epilepsy is of the order of 0.5% (Pond et al 1960, Gudmundsson 1966, Hauser & Kurland 1975, Goodridge & Shorvon 1983), this figure agrees closely with the finding that some 5% of people with epilepsy are photosensitive, provided most photosensitive subjects also have epilepsy. The 5% prevalence among persons with epilepsy is a general finding in Caucasians and Japanese (Seino, personal communication) in epileptological practice. A lower incidence is found in Nigerians (Danesi & Oni 1983) and in black, but not white, South Africans (De Graaf et al 1980). Danesi (1985) found a reduced incidence of photosensitivity in the summer in London and concluded that the low incidence in Nigeria was attributable to climatic factors. This observation is, however, contrary to the findings of Scott et al (1985) in London and of the author (in the Netherlands): both found a slightly increased prevalence in patients tested during the summer. Danesi's hypothesis also fails to explain De Graaf's observation of differences between whites and blacks in the same country, supporting a genetic basis.

Two-thirds of photosensitive subjects are female and the peak prevalence is in early adolescence. Photosensitivity is rare, but not unknown, in infants and the elderly, but is chiefly found between the ages of 4 and 20 years. Age of onset is difficult to determine. The diagnosis is typically made at about the age of 12, but this largely reflects a delay in referral for EEG. Some photosensitive subjects are observed from infancy to have been attracted by bright lights. Being to a considerable extent genetically determined, photosensitivity is most common in the primary generalized form of epilepsy, where the prevalence may

Table 8.4 Incidence of photosensitivity in 6500 referrals for EEG investigation of epilepsy (Instituut voor Epilepsiebestijding, Netherlands 1978–1983

Primary generalized epilepsy	21.2%
Secondary generalized epilepsy	5.1%
Partial	2.8%
Unclassified	2.9%
Overall	5.5%

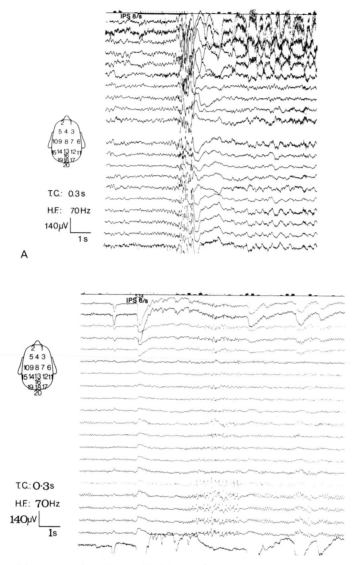

Fig. 8.16 A. Photoconvulsive response in a 10-year-old girl. Note discharge consists of multiple spikes and slow-waves; although arguably of posterior onset it rapidly becomes generalized with a frontal maximum; the spikes are not phase-locked to the flashes; discharge continues after stimulation has ceased. **B.** Occipital spikes; high-amplitude steady state flash-evoked response of maximum amplitude at the back of the head and phase-locked to the stimulus. This is not a photoconvulsive response and is only weakly associated with epilepsy.

be of the order of 25% (Table 8.4).

In 70% of photosensitive patients with epilepsy, there is a history of seizures precipitated by environmental stimuli and, indeed, photic stimulation may also trigger seizures in the EEG laboratory. Numerous environmental stimuli may be implicated – including the sun seen through trees or reflected on moving water, discotheque lighting and arcade games – but in western Europe, television is most often the precipitant (in some 50% of patients, Table 8.5). Some patients report seizures on entering a brightly lit environment, even in the absence of flicker. In about 50% of photosensitive subjects no spontaneous seizures occur, all the attacks being apparently triggered by visual stimuli (Jeavons & Harding 1975).

Table 8.5 Clinical features of 358 photosensitive patients with epilepsy

Sex ratio F/M	2.5%
Age (mean)	19 yrs
Type of epilepsy	
1° Generalized	43%
2° Generalized	23%
Partial	29%
Unclassified	5%
Sensitive to static pattern	45%
* Sensitive to moving pattern	60%
Sensitive to TV	45%
** Photogenic seizures	
TV induced	46%
Disco-induced	34%
Pattern-induced	18%
All types	61%
** Symptoms during IPS	42%
** Visually-induced ocular discomfort	39%
Self-induction	26%

 * Not always tested
** Smaller sample (N=250) personally interviewed by the author or by Dr D.G.A. Kasteleijn-Nolst-Trenité

Jeavons & Harding (1975) classify photosensitive subjects into three types:

1. Those with 'pure photosensitive epilepsy', i.e. with visually induced seizures only (40%)
2. Epileptic patients with photosensitivity and spontaneous seizures, with or without known visually-induced seizures (the majority)
3. Photosensitive people without epilepsy.

This last group appears (when a strict definition of EEG photosensitivity is used) to be very small and was later discarded (Jeavons 1982).

Most visually-induced seizures reported by patients are tonic-clonic convulsions. However, the PCR elicited in the EEG laboratory is usually accompanied by myoclonus or by strange subjective feelings (in over 70% of subjects). On direct questioning, patients admit to similar sensations when exposed to epileptogenic environmental stimuli; these experiences too should probably be regarded as seizures. Absences, usually with myoclonus, are rarely reported, but are often observed during IPS or in patients with self-induced attacks (see below). Photosensitivity is found in 50% of patients with juvenile myoclonic epilepsy (Janz syndrome) (see Ch. 116). Both the spontaneous discharges (chiefly seen soon after waking) and those induced by IPS consist of spike-wave activity with multiple spikes.

Photic stimulation

Demonstration of photosensitivity in the EEG laboratory depends on adequate apparatus and technique. For detailed recommendations see Jeavons (1969), Jeavons & Harding (1975) and Binnie et al. (1982a). The stimulus intensity should if possible be at least 100 nit-s/flash. The stroboscope lamp must be centrally fixated; if the patient looks at the edge of the lamp housing, a PCR will rarely be obtained. The probability of eliciting a PCR is probably greater if the flash stimulus is patterned (Jeavons et al 1972), although some authors could not confirm this (Engel 1974, Kirstein & Nilsson 1977). Some lamps are patterned, having wire grids in or behind the glass, for reasons of electrical screening or safety; if the glass is clear, pattern can be introduced by inserting a plastic sheet bearing a grid or grating with a spatial frequency of about 2 cycles per degree (i.e. black and white stripes each 1.2 mm wide if the pattern is to be viewed at 30 cm). This measure can increase the likelihood of finding a PCR on routine examination by as much as 50% (assuming that the lamp intensity is adjusted to compensate for light absorption by the pattern). It may be less suitable for use in a research context, as this stimulus confounds the effects of flicker with those of pattern.

Red light is reputed to be more epileptogenic than other colours or white. Early studies on which this claim was based, failed to consider whether the eyes were open or closed during stimulation (the closed eyelids will selectively transmit red light) or to use adequate photometric calibration of the stimuli used (Walter & Walter 1949, Livingston 1952, Carterette & Symmes 1952, Marshall et al 1953, Pantelakis et al 1962, Brausch & Ferguson 1965, Capron 1966). Harding et al (1975), taking account of these factors, found no effect of the colour of illumination. By contrast Takahashi, in a series of meticulous experiments (Takahashi et al 1980, 1981) demonstrated red light to be most effective, and to produce a PCR at extremely low levels of intensity (25 candella/m²

or less). Binnie et al (1984a) confirmed the findings of Takahashi but demonstrated that this
effect was obtainable only with monochromatic,
deep-red light at the extreme limit of the visible
spectrum, and was probably due to inhibitory
interactions between systems subserving different
colours when light was used which was capable of
stimulating populations of cones with different
spectral sensitivities. It appeared that the extreme
epileptogenicity of monochromatic long wave-
length flicker (which is difficult to generate with
conventional light sources using filters etc) would
not present an environmental hazard unless new
sources appeared, such as instrumentation using
deep-red light-emitting diodes or laser shows.

Photic stimulation is often performed in dark-
ness in the reasonable expectation that the flashes
should appear relatively brighter and therefore be
more effective. However, Van Egmond et al
(1980) found no consistent effect of environmental
lighting on photosensitivity and suggested that
photic stimulation should be performed under
conditions of normal or subdued room lighting so
that the technician could observe the patient,
controlling ocular fixation and noting any clinical
ictal manifestations.

Eye opening and closure have a marked effect
on photosensitivity, most patients are more sensitive with the eyes open than closed, but the
majority exhibit the greatest sensitivity if stimulation commences at the moment of eye closure.
The flash rate is important in determining the
occurrence of a PCR. A patient is sensitive over
a continuous range between upper and lower
threshold frequencies, but outside these limits
exhibits normal photic following or often an
atypical response not meeting the criteria for a
PCR. The 'photosensitivity range' may be used as
a measure of the severity of sensitivity and is
reduced by effective medication (Jeavons &
Harding 1975, Binnie et al 1986a). The flash rate
most likely to elicit a PCR is of the order of
15–18/s; only 10% of photosensitive patients
respond at 6/s or at 60/s (Fig. 8.17).

Once it is established that a patient is photosensitive, the photosensitivity range can be determined by approaching the lower frequency
threshold from below and the upper threshold
from above. There should thus be no need to

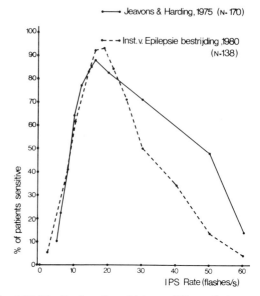

Fig. 8.17 Distribution of sensitivity to different flash-rates in
two studies of photosensitivity. The difference in incidence
of sensitivity to higher frequencies probably reflects the fact
that sodium valproate was not available in the United
Kingdom during most of the period covered by the study of
Jeavons & Harding (1975)

employ stimuli at frequencies between these
limits, which may induce a convulsive seizure. If
a given stimulus frequency is effective in a
particular patient, a PCR will develop rapidly,
usually within two seconds and almost always
within four seconds. No useful purpose is therefore served by prolonged IPS.

Monocular stimulation is usually much less
epileptogenic than binocular. During routine
examination of a photosensitive patient, it is worth
checking the effect of covering one eye with the
hand, as, if effective, this manoeuvre may be
recommended to protect against environmental
epileptogenic stimuli.

Pattern sensitivity

Viewing static linear patterns elicits epileptiform
discharges in over 30% of photosensitive subjects
(Stefannson et al 1977, Porter 1985) but, if the
pattern oscillates in a direction orthogonal to the
line orientation, 70% of patients exhibit discharges.
A history of seizures induced by pattern is volunteered by only a small proportion of these patients
(Table 8.5), probably because the causal relation-

ship is not recognized as readily as in the case of environmental flicker. However, close questioning reveals that attacks may be precipitated by stimuli as varied as venetian blinds, railings, stainless steel escalator treads, striped domestic furnishings and clothing (nurses' uniforms!), and when ironing striped shirts.

Pattern sensitive epilepsy was first described by Bickford et al (1953) and was occasionally reported as an interesting rarity up to the mid-1970s (Bickford & Klass 1962, 1969, Gastaut & Tassinari 1966, Chatrian et al 1970a, b). A key study by Wilkins et al (1975) showed that the physical characteristics of the pattern were crucial in determining its epileptogenicity and that checkerboards, widely used for eliciting evoked responses, were particularly ineffective. Thus Stefannson et al (1977), using stimuli more appropriate than those employed by previous investigators, were able to demonstrate pattern sensitivity in a majority of photosensitive subjects. This finding in turn encouraged more detailed enquiry after possible pattern-induced seizures.

Pattern stimuli lend themselves to physiological studies of photosensitivity (Wilkins et al 1979a) as much is already known from experimental work of pattern vision and of the influence of the physical characteristics of the stimulus on events in neurones within the visual system. To be epileptogenic, a pattern requires a high contrast (usually at least 0.4) and an illumination generally greater than 50 lux. Gratings (stripes) are most effective, whereas grids and checkerboards are not so epileptogenic. The optimal spatial frequency is 2–4 cycles/degree (i.e. each pair of stripes should subtend an angle of 15 to 30 min of arc). The orientation of the grating is usually unimportant (unless the patient is astigmatic). Binocular stimuli are more effective than monocular but, under conditions of binocular rivalry, e.g. gratings of different orientations exposed to each eye, the patterns become much less epileptogenic. The probability of eliciting a discharge is related to the size of the stimulus or, more precisely, to the area of visual cortex stimulated having regard to the site of the retinal image and the cortical magnification factor. Thus, a small central stimulus may be as effective as a much larger one in peripheral vision. The effects of discrete patterned areas are additive if they fall in the same visual field (i.e. project to the same hemisphere) but there is no spatial summation between right and left fields.

From these detailed findings, which are reviewed more fully by Wilkins et al (1980) various physiological conclusions follow.

Physiology of photosensitivity

Patterns which are optimally epileptogenic are closely similar in their physical characteristics to those which produce the maximum discharge rate in visual cortical neurones in experimental animals, and also to those which are experienced by normal subjects as being most disagreeable to look at. This may amount to the somewhat trivial statement that physiologically potent stimuli are most effective in inducing seizures and inducing peculiar sensations. However, the physiological data on pattern sensitivity also show that epileptogenicity is abolished by presentation of images with different spatial orientations in the two eyes. Binocularly innervated orientation selective units are not, apparently, found lower in the visual pathway than the complex cells of the visual cortex. This finding therefore implies a central role for the visual cortex in the triggering of EEG discharges by pattern. Presentation of pattern stimuli within the right or left visual field elicits, in sensitive subjects, focal discharges over the contralateral posterior temporal occipital region (Soso et al 1980, Wilkins et al 1981). This finding implies not only that the visual or previsual cortex is involved in the triggering of the epileptiform discharge but, indeed, that epileptiform activity arises at this site. Flicker stimulation provides less evidence concerning physiological mechanisms but it is of interest to note that, as the generalized photoconvulsive response is suppressed by effective medication, the discharges may become confined to the posterior regions (Binnie et al 1980a) and eventually the only residual abnormality may be the presence of occipital spikes (Harding et al 1978). Together, these observations suggest that photosensitivity, although seen most often in patients with primary generalized epilepsy, is in a sense a model of partial epilepsy with secondary generalization; epileptogenesis thus appears to commence in the occipital regions, giving rise to secondarily generalized discharges which can be suppressed by drugs such as sodium valproate.

A striking characteristic of flicker stimulation is its temporal rhythmicity, which is not obviously shared by pattern stimuli and the question arises to what extent entrainment of cortical discharges by the rhythmic stimulus gives rise to synchronous discharges and how far this is important to the triggering of epileptiform activity. Binnie et al (1985a) report an experiment comparing three types of pattern stimulation: drifting gratings, oscillating gratings and static gratings. It was argued that the contours of drifting gratings should enter and leave the receptive field of different cortical units asynchronously, producing no synchronization of cortical activity. Oscillating gratings, by contrast, should elicit synchronous activity alternately in populations of neurones sensitive to movement in one direction or the other. Static gratings might give rise to some synchronization because of oscillation of the retinal image secondary to ocular tremor. The hypothesis that synchronization by the stimulus contributed to epileptogenesis therefore led to the predication that the oscillating gratings should be most epileptogenic, the static gratings less so and the drifting gratings virtually without effect. This prediction proved correct.

In conclusion, it appears that triggering of EEG discharges by visual stimuli, particularly pattern, takes place in striate or prestriate cortex; depends on the efficacy of the stimulus in eliciting action potentials in cortical neurones and the size of the neuronal population activated within one hemisphere; and is promoted by synchronizing effects of the stimulus itself. It may be noted that the mechanisms involved in photosensitivity in some other species, notably the Senegalese baboon, are almost certainly different: discharges arising in the frontal cortex under the influence of diffuse subcortical projections; corticocortical pathways from other areas including the visual cortex; and proprioceptive inputs to the frontal eye fields (Menini 1976).

Television epilepsy

As many people spend hours daily watching television, it is not surprising that seizures often occur in front of the television set. However, where a causal relationship to television viewing is demonstrable, the patient can almost invariably be shown to be photosensitive. Early reports stressed the role of malfunction of the television set (Lange 1961, Mawdsley 1961, Charlton & Hoefer 1964), but the crucial factor may in fact be that the patient had approached the set to adjust it or to change channels. Many patients undoubtedly have seizures induced by a normally functioning television (Pantelakis et al 1962) and Stefannson et al (1977) demonstrated that a normal television induced EEG discharges in 70% of photosensitive patients, although curiously Gastaut et al (1960a) could not. Black and white television is said to be more likely to induce seizures (Connell et al 1975). This may reflect the greater clarity of the raster pattern of a black and white set (see below). However, the difference in epileptogenicity is not great (Wilkins et al 1979b) and for the patient to invest in a colour set is no solution to television epilepsy.

The television screen flickers at mains frequency, i.e. 50 Hz in Western Europe, 60 Hz in North America. In Europe, almost 90% of patients with 'pure photosensitive epilepsy' have suffered television-induced seizures.

Television epilepsy was recognized later in the USA (Charlton & Hoefer 1964) than in Europe (Klapatek 1959, Richter 1960, Lange 1961, Dumermuth 1961) and is reported less often, possibly because of the higher mains frequency. However, the majority of patients with television epilepsy are not photosensitive at frequencies even as high as 50 Hz and some alternative explanation must be found for the triggering of their seizures.

Wilkins et al (1979b) showed two mechanisms to be involved. Patients who are photosensitive at 50 Hz often exhibit EEG discharges whilst viewing at several metres from the television screen. Patients with television epilepsy who are not sensitive to 50 Hz flicker are pattern sensitive and discharges can be elicited only when the viewing distance is so small that the raster pattern of the screen can be resolved. Television pictures are presented at half mains frequency (25 frames/s in Europe) but are actually scanned as two half-frames, the odd and even-numbered lines being traced alternately. Thus at several metres distance the only epileptogenic stimulus is the mains frequency flicker of the whole screen, but close up the patient is confronted by a grating pattern, apparently oscillating (actually alternating) at 25 Hz. The distinction between these two different mechanisms is of some practical importance. Those 50 Hz sensitive patients who respond at distances of several metres from the screen are less sensitive when viewing in a well-lit environment. By contrast, the pattern-sensitive subjects responding only at close viewing become more sensitive when the background is brightly lit (Binnie et al (1980b).

The first group of patients may be protected from adverse effects of television by viewing in a well-lit room whilst the second group must adopt other measures; they should avoid close proximity to the screen (which has become easier since the advent of remote control units), should cover one eye if it is necessary to approach the television, or should obtain a set so small (e.g. less than 30 cm diagonally) that the spatial frequency of the raster, even at the near point of vision, is too high to be epileptogenic. A more elaborate way of avoiding binocular television stimulation is to cover the screen with a polarizing sheet and for the patient to wear spectacles, one lens of which is polarized in an axis orthogonal to that of the screen (Wilkins et al 1977, Wilkins & Lindsay 1985). The patient can thus see the television with only one eye, but vision for the rest of the environment is binocular. This method is effective but acceptable to only a minority of patients, because of eye strain or cosmetic considerations.

In view of the undoubted epileptogenicity of television for many photosensitive patients, it has been suggested that visual display units (VDUs) could represent a hazard to people with epilepsy. However, the physical characteristics of a VDU differ from those of a domestic television in ways that, on theoretical grounds, make them unlikely to be epileptogenic. EEG recording from photosensitive subjects whilst viewing VDUs of various types with both static and scrolling displays fails to demonstrate any activating effect (Binnie et al 1985b). A similar procedure elicits discharges in 40% of photosensitive subjects if a black and white television is used. There is no evidence, theoretical, experimental or clinical, that textual computer displays on a VDU represent a hazard to photosensitive patients. However, a domestic television set employed as a computer display device may prove even more epileptogenic than when it is used for watching programs, as the viewing distance will be less. Arcade games often use flashing effects which are themselves epileptogenic, whatever the method of display.

Treatment of photosensitive epilepsy

As indicated in the previous section in the context of television epilepsy, simple practical measures to avoid epileptogenic stimulation may provide protection against visually induced seizures and, in patients with no spontaneous attacks, medication may not be necessary. Other practical measures include the use of dark glasses when exposed to potentially epileptogenic stimuli out of doors. To provide effective protection, these must absorb some 90% of the incident light, which means that the lenses should be considerably darker than those normally worn, other than for winter sport, and may be cosmetically unacceptable. The belief that polaroid glasses confer particular benefit appears to have no basis except where there is a source of plane polarized flicker (at sea or when the ground is snow-covered?). Patients should not be encouraged to obtain expensive photochromatic lenses, as these generally respond too slowly to prevent seizures that may be induced, for instance, on suddenly entering a brightly lit environment. Every patient with photosensitive epilepsy should be taught to cover one eye as an emergency measure, when suddenly confronted with an epileptogenic stimulus. Complete occlusion with the palm is required, not just shading the eye with the radial side of the hand against the forehead.

Where medication is necessary, sodium valproate, ethosuximide and the benzodiazepines are most effective, but tolerance usually develops to the latter. Dosage should be adjusted to abolish photosensitivity if possible. This can be achieved with sodium valproate in a little over 50% of patients (Harding et al 1978) and nearly 80% show a substantial reduction. If it is decided after some years' freedom from seizures to withdraw this drug, at least 6 months' follow-up is required, as the suppressant effect on photosensitivity continues for weeks or months after valproate is withdrawn. Various methods of deconditioning have been attempted (Forster et al 1964, Braham 1967, Jeavons & Harding 1975) but with little success.

On acute administration, representatives of all major groups of antiepileptic drugs suppress photosensitivity. This response is not predictive of their chronic effects in photosensitive epilepsy, but may provide a useful means of assessing efficacy of new experimental AEDs, (Binnie et al 1986a).

Self-induced seizures

The first descriptions of photosensitive epilepsy date from before the clinical use of EEG and concern patients who induced attacks in themselves by staring at the sun and waving the outspread fingers of one hand in front of the eyes to produce flicker (Radovici et al 1932). Patients displaying this behaviour are often mentally subnormal (Andermann et al 1962). More recently, however, it has been realized that many more photosensitive subjects employ a manoeuvre involving extreme upward deviation of the eyes with slow eyelid closure to induce seizures or epileptiform discharges in themselves (Green 1966). The eye movements may themselves be misinterpreted as an ictal phenomenon, eyelid myoclonia, and indeed some authors have regarded the hand waving in the same way (Ames 1971, 1974, Livingstone & Torres 1964). There is, however, compelling evidence against this view.

1. When placed in a poorly-lit environment patients continue to exhibit the slow eye closures, at least for some minutes, but no discharges occur.

2. The oculographic artefact accompanying the inducing movements shows them to be different from those seen on normal blinking, eye closure to command, or during spontaneous absence seizures. The syndrome of visual self-induction can indeed be recognized from clinical observation alone: since drawing the attention of colleagues to the phenomenon the writer has received referrals of self-inducing patients who were correctly identified before an EEG had been recorded and before photosensitivity was suspected.

3. Despite a reluctance to discuss the subject, some patients admit to deliberately practising self-induction and describe the sensations produced. Some report using other methods in addition to eye closure and hand waving, viewing patterns or television for instance.

4. Many other photosensitive patients who do not habitually self-induce have discovered the slow eye closure manoeuvre and can describe the subjective effects.

Some patients learn a technique of initiating a discharge by eye closure and prolonging or enhancing it by hand waving. This is well illustrated in the series of cine stills published by Ames (1974). Some photosensitive patients exhibit epileptiform discharges, either generalized or at the back of the head, on normal eye closure. This appears to be a phenomenon different from self-induction: the oculographic artefact is normal and no pleasurable experience is reported; but obviously the mechanism involved could be related to that used in self-induction. Studies employing telemetric monitoring of photosensitive subjects suggest that some 25% of susceptible patients indulge in self-induction, if not of seizures at least of discharges (Darby et al 1980b, Binnie et al 1980c). Patients are usually embarrassed to discuss this habit but may admit to experiencing a pleasurable sensation or a relief of tension when self-inducing. The rate of self-induction usually increases under stress and frequencies of 100 episodes per hour are not unusual. The self-induced seizures range from pleasurable subjective experiences, through sexual arousal (including orgasm) and absence seizures, to tonic-clonic convulsions.

Some patients with television epilepsy are compulsively attracted to the screen. Most are children, with a small preponderance of adult males. Some of these patients, particularly the adults, admit to using television as a method of self-induction (Harley et al 1967, Andermann 1971). One freely admitted to inducing tonic-clonic seizures with television as a 'do it yourself' convulsive therapy, which relieved the severe bouts of depression from which she suffered. Others insist that the compulsion is distressing to them but irresistible, and it is uncertain whether or not some instances of compulsive attraction to television are to be regarded as self-inducing behaviour or as ictal phenomena. Wilkins & Lindsay (1985) argue from the rapid abolition of compulsive attraction when polarized glasses are issued (see above) that the behaviour is usually not learned but is ictal. However, these patients are often attracted to a television seen across a large room from distances at which no epileptogenic effect is demonstrable.

Self-induced epilepsy is notoriously resistant to therapy (Andermann et al 1962, Hutchinson et al 1958, Rabending et al 1969, Rail 1973, Ames & Enderstein 1976). This may in part be due to reluctance to take medication, but even compliant patients appear refractory to AEDs. A few patients have responded to psychotherapy (Libo et al 1971) or can be persuaded to wear dark glasses. Overweg & Binnie (1980) noted an analogy between this behaviour and electrical self-stimulation of the brain in experimental animals, a phenomenon which is suppressed by dopamine antagonists. They therefore attempted therapy with chlorpromazine or haloperidol and reported an improvement in six out of seven patients. Kasteleijn-Nolst-Trenite et al (1983) also obtained a reduced incidence of self-stimulation in a controlled trial of pimozide.

Reading epilepsy

Photosensitive epilepsy is by far the most common of the reflex epilepsies. Patients with seizures induced by other stimuli than flicker or pattern, such as eating, are often also photosensitive. One of the less rare forms of reflex epilepsy is characterized by seizures induced by prolonged reading. If a patient with reading epilepsy is also photosensitive, the question arises of whether or not the seizures are induced by sensitivity to the pattern formed by the lines of text (Mayersdorf & Marshall 1970). If this mechanism is ever involved, it is probably rare: very few pattern-sensitive patients have reading epilepsy or exhibit EEG discharges on viewing text; content and context are usually important determinants of epileptogenicity in reading epilepsy. Perhaps the most striking difference between reading epilepsy and pattern sensitivity is that reading induces EEG discharges or seizures only after many

minutes, whereas pattern sensitivity is demonstrable within seconds of exposure.

Conclusion

Photosensitive epilepsy is of special interest to the electroencephalographer as, even though careful enquiry will usually establish a history of visually induced seizures, in practice the diagnosis is usually made after finding a PCR in the EEG laboratory. Although photosensitive subjects represent only 5% of patients with epilepsy, the condition is of some considerable interest representing, apart from ECT, the only human experimental model of epilepsy, and can be used both to investigate physiological mechanisms of epileptogenesis and for preliminary assessment of antiepileptic drugs. Moreover, the finding of photosensitivity is important to those patients whose seizures are all visually precipitated, as they may often be effectively treated by simple practical measures to avoid visual triggers and may not need medication. Finally, it is important to identify the 25% of photosensitive subjects who practise self-induction. If the problem is not recognized, they may be regarded simply as having therapy-resistant epilepsy and treated unsuccessfully to the point of intoxication with antiepileptic drugs.

APPENDIX: TECHNIQUES OF VISUAL STIMULATION IN THE EEG LABORATORY

Standardized method for photic stimulation (Jeavons & Harding 1975)

1. The procedure is explained to the patient.
2. The same photostimulator is used in all repeat tests as was used initially.
3. Illumination of the room is standardized by drawing blinds and using artificial light.
4. The lowest intensity light is used initially, increased if there is no abnormality and standardized in subsequent tests.
5. A pattern of small squares with narrow black lines (0.3 mm), with spacing of 2 mm × 2 mm, or a pattern of parallel lines (1 mm) spaced 1.5 mm apart, is placed behind the glass of the lamp (dry print transfers are cheap and easily available).

6. A circle of 3 cm diameter is drawn in the centre of the glass and the patient looks at this circle.
7. The lamp is placed at 30 cm from the eyes.
8. Testing is carried out with eyes kept open or kept closed, and only if no PCR is evoked is the effect of eye closure tested.
9. 16 Hz can be used as an initial test frequency to identify the photosensitive patient. If no PCR is elicited, testing starts at 1 Hz and rates up to 25 Hz are used, followed by 30, 40, 50 Hz.
10. In the photosensitive patient the duration of the stimulus should not usually exceed 2 s.
11. In the photosensitive patient, testing starts at 1 Hz and increases in steps of 1 Hz until a PCR is evoked. The upper limit is then established by starting at 60 Hz and reducing in steps of 10 Hz.
12. The sensitivity limit is defined as the lowest or highest flash rate which consistently evokes a PCR. The sensitivity range is obtained by substracting the lower from the upper limit.

Four further comments or suggestions may be added (Binnie et al 1986a)
13. In a known photosensitive patient, it is necessary only to find the upper and lower frequency thresholds for producing a PCR in order to determine the photosensitivity range. No useful purpose will be served by performing IPS at frequencies between these limits, and this carries moreover a risk of inducing a convulsive seizure.
14. As the probability of eliciting a discharge increases by only 6%/Hz over the range of flash rates 1–18/s, it may not be cost-effective to increase the stimulus frequency in steps of only 1 Hz. The standard frequencies – 18, 6, 8, 10, 15, 20, 30, 40, 50, 60 – are recommended, corresponding to the optimum for eliciting a PCR (18/s) and those above and below this, to which 10, 20, 40, 60 or 80% of photosensitive subjects respond.
15. Also, in the interests of saving time, if the stimulator is turned on for 8 s as the eyes are closed and the patient is asked to open the eyes 4 s later, all three eye conditions, closure, closed and open, can be tested at a single stimulus presentation. If a PCR occurs the stimulus train should immediately be terminated.
16. Many commercially available photic stimulators are unsatisfactory. The maximum flash rate available should be at least 50 Hz (60 Hz in North America) for assessing patients with television epilepsy. The maximum flash intensity (which is rarely specified in photometric units by the manufacturer) should be at least 100 nit-s/flash.

Summary of method of testing pattern sensitivity (Darby et al 1980a)
1. The pattern is circular, diameter 48 cm with stripes of 2.5 mm.
2. The black and white stripes should be parallel and of equal size.
3. The optimal width is 2 cs/degree of visual angle (15 min of arc) subtending more than 16 degrees.
4. The contrast should be high and brightness above 200 cd/m².
5. The patient stares at a spot in the centre of the pattern.

6. Viewing is at arm's length (57 cm) and the pattern is illuminated by a spotlight behind the patient*.
7. The pattern is held steady for 30 s and is vibrated if no paroxysmal activity is evoked.
8. The optimal frequency of vibration at right angles is 20 Hz, although vibration by hand cannot exceed 10 Hz.

PREOPERATIVE ASSESSMENT

There is probably no other clinical decision in which the EEG plays such a pivotal role as in the selection of patients for surgical treatment of epilepsy. Preoperative assessment is, however, an area to which that modish and overworked term, 'a multidisciplinary approach', is truly applicable. EEG is but one aspect of preoperative assessment and for a full, balanced account of the wider context of the EEG investigations the reader is referred to Chapter 13 on the neurosurgical treatment of epilepsy. Very few patients with epilepsy qualify for consideration as possible candidates for surgery and very few centres can call upon the range of skills and experience required for successful assessment and operation. This section therefore describes an application of electroencephalography which, although interesting, will be of practical importance to very few readers.

Amongst other requirements listed in Chapter 13, two electrophysiological criteria must be satisfied. First, a focus of abnormal cerebral electrical activity must be demonstrable; secondly, there must be reasonable evidence that this represents the site of onset of the patient's seizures. The second of these criteria is generally more difficult to satisfy than the first, and may be approached by phased investigations of increasing complexity.

Phase Ia: interictal EEG studies

Routine diagnostic EEG investigation should have been completed long before any question of neurosurgical referral arises. However, as necessary, preoperative assessment may include further recordings of the EEG in waking and in sleep in order to demonstrate and locate accurately any focus of epileptiform activity. Additional elec-

---

* At this viewing distance 1 cm subtends 1°, so the spatial frequency of the pattern described is 2 cycles/degree.

trodes may be employed, either non-standard scalp placements particularly for recording from the anterior temporal region, or basal electrodes inserted in the nasopharynx, the naso-ethmoid recess or under the skull close to the foramen ovale.

To some extent, the need for additional electrodes arises from the deficiencies of the International 10/20 System of electrode placement (Jasper 1958) promoted by the International Federation of Societies for Electroencephalography and Clinical Neurophysiology. However commendable the striving after an international convention, the standard 10/20 placements fail to cover one-third of the temporal convexity, including the entire anterior temporal region. Systems providing better coverage have been described (Pampiglione 1956, Margerison et al 1970) but are not widely used except in Great Britain. The anterior temporal placement of Silverman (1960) has been more generally accepted and has proved useful. A more comprehensive approach is that of Lueders et al (1982), using an array of additional electrodes between and below the standard 10/20 sites. They found that, in scalp recordings from patients with complex partial seizures, the spike focus was most often maximal immediately superficial to the temporal pole (Morris et al 1983). They stressed, however, the importance of using the entire array to locate the focus, not merely a single anterior temporal electrode to capture spikes.

Basal placements include nasopharyngeal electrodes (Gastaut 1948, Maclean 1949) inserted through the nostrils. They are susceptible to artefact and rarely provide information not obtainable from an anterior temporal placement (Binnie et al 1982b). A naso-ethmoid electrode (Lehtinen & Bergstrom 1970) is less widely used, but Quesney et al (1981) find it useful for recording from inferomesial frontal foci. Morris & Lueders (1985) confirm this, but report that very similar results are obtained with electrodes on the side of the bridge of the nose or below the eye. Sphenoidal electrodes (Jones 1951, Pampiglione & Kerridge 1956, Rovit et al 1960) are flexible wires inserted with a needle to lie under the foramen ovale. They certainly provide information not obtainable with the standard 10/20 placements

(Christodoulou 1967), but the yield of new data is less if they are compared with anterior temporal placements. Nevertheless, they do sometimes identify a focus not readily detected with superficial electrodes (Sperling et al 1986). At the present time, the optimal extracranial placement for recording from mesial temporal structures remains in doubt: Wilkus & Thompson (1984) have, for instance, demonstrated that spontaneous or deliberate displacement of the sphenoidal electrode from below the foramen ovale to a more superficial position has no apparent effect on the activity recorded. Investigations with basal electrodes will usually include sleep registrations and possibly the intravenous thiopentone test of Lombroso & Erba (1970) (see section 'Sleep induction' above).

Confidence in EEG localization will be increased if other abnormalities, focal slow activity and reduction in amplitude of barbiturate-induced fast activity are found at the same site as the spike focus. The lateralizing value of decreased fast activity was questioned by Margerison & Corsellis (1966), but their study concerned severely handicapped patients with extensive brain damage. In the type of patients considered for surgery, reduction of barbiturate-induced fast activity appears to be a reliable lateralizing sign (Kennedy & Hill 1958, Engel et al 1975).

In some patients, conventional EEG recording with, as necessary, sleep and the use of additional or special electrode placements, will have demonstrated a single, stable focus of epileptiform discharges, possibly together with a local abnormality of background activity, at a site amenable to surgery, and concordant with clinical, neuroradiological and neuropsychological evidence concerning the origin of the seizures. In such patients, preoperative EEG work-up may be considered complete and some teams would at this point be prepared to proceed with surgery, particularly if the focus were thought to be anterior or mesial temporal (Bloom et al 1959, Polkey 1981).

Phase Ib: ictal EEG studies

In some patients no stable focus may have been demonstrated; multiple EEG abnormalities may have been detected at different sites; the localization may cast doubt on the practicability of surgery (midtemporal involvement or a frontal or parietal focus) or EEG localization may not be concordant with clinical, radiological or neuropsychological findings. Indeed, in some patients interictal, superficial EEG recording may have failed to locate any focus at all.

In some centres it would be usual at this point to abandon the assessment and to regard the patient as unsuitable for surgery. Otherwise, the following step is to attempt to obtain an ictal recording using scalp electrodes, possibly with the addition of flexible sphenoidal wires (Ives & Gloor 1977). Recordings of high technical quality are required, with a minimum of 16 channels to ensure reliable localization and with careful documentation of the relationship between EEG and clinical events. For this purpose video and EEG monitoring are used, the latter employing either a hard-wired EEG machine, radio, or preferably cable, telemetry (see earlier section). It is important to determine whether the site of onset of electrical ictal change is constant; therefore recordings of upwards of five seizures are desirable and some workers prefer to obtain 20 or more (Olivier et al 1983). Patients undergoing preoperative assessment typically have about one seizure a week and to capture five or more attacks requires an unacceptably long period of registration. Seizure frequency may, however, be increased by antiepileptic drug reduction or withdrawal, or use may be made of any observed pattern in the patient's seizure liability, for instance, a tendency for the attacks to occur in clusters. As seizures provoked by chemical means often differ both clinically and electrographically from the patient's habitual pattern (see p. 251), it may be questioned whether attacks provoked by a drop in blood AED levels may also exhibit misleading localization (Spencer et al 1981). Although Engel & Crandall (1983) have documented one such instance, in general, seizures released by AED reduction appear to conform to the patient's habitual pattern. Most seizures provoked by acute AED withdrawal are secondarily generalized, whereas those occurring more than four half-lives after the most recent drug reduction are likely to be non-generalized

(Marciani et al 1985). In selecting the drug to be withdrawn first in a patient on polypharmacy, reduction of carbamazepine appears most effective in producing withdrawal seizures, probably because of the combination of efficacy in partial epilepsy and a short half-life. Valproate withdrawal is unlikely to be useful.

Reassessment after ictal scalp recordings may show that a consistent focal onset has now been demonstrated corresponding with the site of maximum interictal discharge, attenuation of fast activity and interictal slow-wave abnormalities (if any), and that the findings are concordant with clinical, neuroradiological and neuropsychological evidence. On this basis, it may now be possible to proceed to operation. However, there remain patients in whom ictal scalp recordings will have shown no epileptiform activity, or will have demonstrated an unstable or ill-defined localization. If only minimal seizures, or auras, have been recorded, this will usually be the case. With fully developed complex partial seizures, 50% or more of scalp EEG recordings may show no epileptiform activity or, more commonly, bilateral discharges only (Lieb et al 1976). Few authors (Spencer et al 1985) have commented on the difficulty of interpreting ictal scalp EEGs. Interrater agreement even on lateralization is less than 75% (Spencer et al 1985). Estimates of reliability of EEG against depth recording must depend on how conservatively the findings are interpreted. Thus, Lieb et al (1976) found no instance of incorrect lateralization, but could not lateralize at all in 50%. Spencer et al (1985) predicted laterality in two-thirds of cases, but agreement with depth recordings was little better than chance. When unclassified records were excluded, lateralization of temporal foci was about 80% reliable, but that of frontal foci remained random.

A detailed study by Delgado Escueta et al (1982) compared surface EEG, including sphenoidal or nasopharyngeal electrode placements, with clinical events documented by video recording, with similar conclusions. Over half the patients showed non-lateralizing ictal EEG changes. However, those attacks commencing with a motionless stare, which the authors considered on clinical grounds to be of temporal lobe origin, were accompanied in 70% of instances by focal or lateralizing EEG signs, whereas other seizure types, presumed to arise outside the temporal lobes, produced symmetrical or diffuse EEG changes. It was suggested that depth recording would be required only in the patients without staring and a lateralized EEG seizure onset. However, depth studies in such patients also failed in most cases to offer clear evidence of localization and surgical outcome was poor (Delgado-Escueta & Walsh 1983); an alternative conclusion from their findings would be that patients without an ictal EEG focus and staring at seizure onset should be regarded as unsuitable for surgery.

Occasionally, the EEG localization may seem to conflict with other evidence. False lateralization, even in ictal EEGs, may result from damage so severe on the affected side that surface discharges can be recorded only from the intact contralateral temporal lobe after propagation has occurred beyond the primary focus. Conflict between EEG and other localizing evidence should lead to this possibility being considered (Engel et al 1980). Here the decision must be made between abandoning preoperative work-up or proceeding to intracranial recording. This may be acute, lasting up to 12 hours; or subacute, continuing from a few days to several weeks.

Phase II: subacute corticography

Subacute intracranial recording, may use epidural, subdural or depth electrodes, or a combination of both superficial and deep placements; although this last option appears rarely to be adopted. Extracerebral electrodes include small plastic strips bearing 4–8 contacts inserted through a burr hole or craniectomy (Ajmone Marsan & Van Buren 1958, Wyler et al 1984); long flexible monopolar electrodes (Broseta et al 1980) or multipolar bundles (Storm van Leeuwen 1982) manipulated under fluoroscopy through a burr hole; and large subdural or epidural electrode matrices on plastic sheets introduced through an extensive craniotomy (Goldring 1978, Lesser et al 1984). Electrodes mounted on mats or plastic strips can cover much of the convexity but cannot readily be placed below the temporal lobes. Attempting to obtain a subtemporal location through a lateral burr hole carries a risk of haemorrhage from damage to veins in the middle fossa. Flexible bundles provide considerably more extensive cover and can be manipulated through a central burr hole to reach the entire convexity and to orbital and frontal and subtemporal sites, but have not been widely used (Storm van Leeuwen, 1982). The technique of stereotactic placement of multiple depth electrodes, developed by Bancaud & Talairach (Bancaud et al 1965) (Fig. 8.18), has been exploited in particular by Wieser (1983a) who has studied clinical and electrographic ictal patterns, documenting meticulously the onset and spread of the ictal discharge and the concomitant clinical manifestations.

For the more pragmatic purpose of, for instance, determining which of two known mesial temporal foci is the site of onset of a patient's seizures, simpler methods may suffice; with the insertion of one or two bundles into the mesial temporal structures of both sides from bilateral central burr holes. In some patients, a less invasive approach of inserting electrodes into the subdural space through the foramen ovale (Wieser et al 1985) may provide the information required and obviate the need for conventional intracranial recording. There do not appear to have been any substantial comparative studies of the diagnostic reliability of depth and subdural electrodes.

It is difficult to sample efficiently the electrical activity of cortical grey matter with radially inserted multipolar depth electrodes. Many contacts may be located uselessly in white matter or may be so positioned that they fail to register any activity from nearby cortical electrical dipoles (Gloor 1987). This difficulty can to some extent be overcome by the use of depth electrodes with large cylindrical contacts (Maxwell et al 1983), but to obtain an adequate picture of the onset and evolution of the seizure with depth electrodes alone, a large number of insertion tracks will generally be needed. Complications of inserting depth electrodes, haemorrhage and infection, are rare but have been fatal (Ajmone Marsan 1980, Spencer 1981), and Rasmussen (1976) has also questioned whether inserting electrodes into the healthy parts of a brain, which has demonstrated its potential to generate seizures, could itself cause epileptogenic lesions.

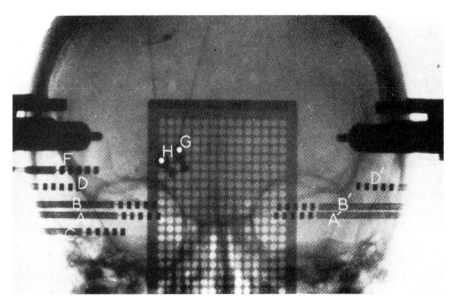

Fig. 8.18 System of depth electrode placement pioneered by Bancaud & Talairach. Note multicontact electrodes A–F inserted transversely. The grid is used to control electrode placement and is now positioned for insertion in an anteroposterior direction. (Reproduced with permission from Bancaud et al 1965)

The present writer would advocate using as few depth electrodes as is necessary to monitor the suspected site of ictal onset, supplemented by flexible subdural electrode bundles. These can all be inserted through the same bilateral central burr holes. If few intracerebral placements are employed, these need to be augmented by a more extensive subdural coverage to exclude the possibility that the ictal events detected at the limited deep placements have spread from elsewhere. Subdural electrodes without any depth placements may simply present the same ambiguities as were found in the scalp recordings as, once a mesial temporal discharge, for instance, has spread to the convexity, it may on occasion be more prominent on the contralateral than on the ipsilateral side (Fig. 8.4). Viral infections as Jakob-Creutzfeldt disease can be transmitted by intracranial electrodes (Bernoulli et al 1977) and some workers would not therefore be prepared to re-use electrodes, despite their considerable cost (Wyler et al 1984).

Although the main purpose of subacute corticography is to obtain ictal records, it might be expected that the interictal activity would contain some relevant information. In general, if multiple foci are present, the rate of spiking will be greater and the variability of interspike intervals less on the side of the epileptogenic focus (Lieb et al 1978). The responsible focus in particular is less likely to show changes in discharge rate with different sleep stages and yet is more readily activated with thiopentone (Engel et al 1981). Various writers continue to investigate methods of demonstrating the time relations and patterns of spread between functionally interdependent foci (Brazier 1973, Rossi 1973, Mars & Lopez da Silva 1983, Lange et al 1983). It is hoped this will provide a means of identifying the site of origin of seizures on the basis of interictal records.

In those patients who prove amenable to surgery, the electrographic pattern at seizure onset is usually very stereotyped, far more so than in the scalp EEG. In addition to episodes recognized as the patient's habitual attacks, electrographic seizures occur, with minimal or no overt clinical change. These will generally have the same site of onset as the full, typical seizures. In the type of patient usually considered for surgery, it is usually possible to capture ten or more overt seizures within a few days, with reduction of medication if necessary, and in the same period dozens of electrographic seizures may be seen.

Spencer (1981) estimated that the use of depth recording increased by 36% the population of patients amenable to surgical treatment of epilepsy, whilst preventing unsuccessful operations in another 18% of patients who prove to have multiple foci. The procedure could thus alter the decision whether or not to operate in half the patients. Olivier et al (1983) interestingly report the experience of increasing the use of routine depth recording in a unit with a vast experience of selecting patients for surgery on conservative criteria using only interictal or ictal scalp EEGs. Their conclusions were similar to those of Spencer.

Discussions of interictal versus ictal recording, or of EEG versus depth registration, generally appear to consider these as alternatives, with the ictal depth recorded data representing the 'correct' findings. Lieb and colleagues (Lieb et al 1981a, b), stress rather that the purpose of electrophysiological assessment is prediction of outcome or identification of operable epileptogenic lesions. By these criteria, ictal, interictal, surface and depth findings contain non-redundant information, and all were used by a non-linear pattern-recognition algorithm for predicting outcome. Specifically, the following were predictive of a poor outcome and negative pathology: interictal bilaterally synchronous surface spikes; interictal independent surface spikes on the side selected for operation; ictal onset with bilateral or unilateral surface involvement (with or without deep spikes); multiple onset sites; and suppression at onset. The outcomes considered above related to removal of abnormal tissue and seizure relief. However, some of the adverse findings listed, notably bilaterally synchronous ictal onset and interictal discharges, were also predictive of postoperative psychological deterioration (Lieb et al 1982).

The proportion of patients considered amenable to surgery after depth recording must depend on the selection criteria for performing this investigation. Half the patients of Spencer et al (1982) exhibited multiple or unlocalizable sites of ictal onset in depth recording and, if the most active focus was excised, results were poor. Unlocalized depth recordings were obtained in 80% of patients with non-localizing ictal scalp recordings. From the studies of Lieb and Spencer and their

colleagues it seems that depth recording may often be required to confirm the finding of a focal onset in the scalp EEG but, where the EEG is non-localizing, depth recording is unlikely to offer a basis for successful surgery. The findings of Delgado-Escueta and colleagues (Delgado-Escueta et al 1982, Delgado-Escueta & Walsh 1983) may be considered to lead to the same conclusion, although this is not the view of the authors themselves.

Localization of cerebral functions

Where a decision in principle has been taken to perform surgical resection for treatment of epilepsy, it is essential to determine what neurological or psychological deficit may result. This is the more difficult as the majority of resections for epilepsy involve the temporal lobes and a patient with temporal damage may have abnormal lateralization of speech and memory.

When subacute corticography is performed, the opportunity may also be taken of performing leisurely electrical mapping, if necessary over several days, determining location of cerebral functions by electrical stimulation and by evoked responses (Gregorie & Goldring 1984). Electrical stimulation is also used to find the threshold for eliciting an after-discharge, which should in theory be elevated in a region of neuronal loss. However, once an after-discharge has been elicited, the threshold may be markedly changed. After-discharge threshold is probably not a reliable guide to localizing an epileptogenic focus (Ajmone Marsan 1973). An attempt may also be made to evoke an attack corresponding to the patient's habitual seizure pattern from stimulation at the site of the presumed focus. This is less reliable as evidence of localization if an after-discharge occurs, as this may spread to involve structures at a distance from the site of stimulation (Gloor 1975). For functional mapping large electrode matrices are ideal, whereas narrow flexible bundles are unsuitable as attempts at electrical stimulation generally elicit pain from the dura.

Where there is any uncertainty concerning lateralization of cerebral functions, the carotid amytal test (Wada & Rasmussen 1960) is performed and this is carried out under EEG control. EEG electrodes are applied, an arterial catheter is inserted into each internal carotid artery in turn and angiography performed to confirm the location of the catheter and to determine whether or not any cross-flow occurs from one internal carotid to the contralateral cerebral vessels. The patient is instructed in the performance of several simple neuropsychological tests, chiefly concerned with speech and verbal and non-verbal memory, and baseline values are established. The patient is then asked to elevate both hands and sodium amytal is injected into the carotid artery, typically in a dose of 100 mg. A falling away of the contralateral hand signals onset of hemiparesis and anaesthesia of the hemisphere. Psychological tests are repeated during the period of unilateral suppression of cerebral function, which usually lasts only 2–5 min. The chief role of the EEG is to determine the onset and duration of anaesthesia and to establish that the effects are, in fact, unilateral. Typically, high-voltage beta activity appears on the affected side within some 20 s, rapidly followed by the onset of delta activity. As the effects wear off, the delta activity becomes intermittent and, for a brief period, is intermixed with a returning alpha rhythm. Spontaneous epileptiform discharges are usually suppressed. Occurrence of substantial changes over the contralateral hemisphere (with the exception of suppression of bilateral epileptiform discharges) indicates significant cross-flow of amytal. Ideally the investigation should demonstrate preservation of speech and memory functions during anaesthesia of the hemisphere on which it is proposed to operate, and abolition of these functions when the contralateral hemisphere is anaesthetised. Often some function is preserved when either side is anaesthetized, suggesting incomplete lateralization.

A further use claimed for EEG recording during the carotid amytal test is identification of the side of origin of secondarily generalized discharges. Bilateral suppression of generalized spike-wave activity by injection of amytal into one carotid artery and not the other, may indicate secondary generalization from a focus on the side giving suppression. For obvious reasons, well-controlled data to support this claim do not appear to be available and, given current views on the corticocortical mechanisms of generation of generalized

discharges (see earlier section) the fact that secondary bilateral synchrony is often of mesial frontal origin and that cross-flow often occurs into the contralateral anterior communicating artery, the findings should probably be interpreted with caution. Moreover, surgical outcome in patients with bilateral discharges is generally poor (Lieb et al 1981a, Spencer et al 1982). Similarly, care is necessary in interpreting effects of intracarotid metrazol, which has been suggested as a means of determining seizure threshold on the two sides and hence possibly deciding which of two foci is the source of the patient's seizures (Garretson et al 1966). Gloor (1975), whilst advocating both carotid amytal and metrazol tests for identification of secondary bilateral synchrony, concedes that they often fail to give an unequivocal result and suggests this may be due to diffuse or multifocal brain disease.

Phase III: acute corticography

Acute electrocorticography has been a standard procedure in epilepsy surgery since the work of Penfield & Jasper (1954). It will usually be performed through a craniotomy and will therefore rarely be undertaken unless a decision has already been made concerning the site of a possible resection. In patients with seizures thought to be of temporal lobe origin, this implies that a focal EEG abnormality will already have been found and the role of corticography will be limited to confirming previous findings. The chances of recording a spontaneous seizure at acute corticography are poor, and the only new evidence this procedure can usually offer is more precise localization of the site and extent of the interictal EEG disturbances. If little or no epileptiform activity occurs, this can be activated by intravenous thiopentone or methohexitone (Wilder 1971). Seizures may be induced by electrical stimulation at the site of the focus; although it is gratifying if these resemble the patient's habitual seizure pattern, this finding does not have any value for predicting the therapeutic outcome (Engel et al 1975). Both surface and depth electrodes may be used, the latter ranging in sophistication from one or two needles placed manually in such structures as the amygdala or hippocampus to stereotactic placement of 100 contacts or more (Bancaud et al 1965, Talairach & Bancaud 1973, 1974).

Where possible, acute corticography is conducted under local anaesthesia, both to permit mapping of cortical functions by electrical stimulation, and because general anaesthetics may suppress epileptiform activity. On completion of the pre-resection corticography, intravenous thiopentone or methohexitone may be given to activate the discharges.

In patients with simple partial seizures with sensorimotor symptoms, suggesting a focal origin in the Rolandic area, the interictal EEG is often normal and even ictal records may fail to show a focus. Here there may often be a case for explor-atory corticography at a site determined by the clinical findings. This is usually successful and, if the focal discharges occur over an area of visibly abnormal tissue, resection is likely to be followed by seizure reduction. Again, electrical stimulation can be employed. This will of course elicit sensori-motor seizures in normal subjects, but a progressive spread of the discharge and 'march' of the clinical manifestations reinforces the view that the site of origin of the patient's habitual seizure has been found. Finally, it is important to note the possibility of artefact in corticographic recordings, as the surgery itself may give rise to epileptiform discharges. Thus Engel et al (1975) report positive spikes in the hippocampus occurring only in those patients without a lesion at this site. The absence of this phenomenon in mesial temporal sclerosis suggested that it was an injury after-discharge due to insertion of the needle electrode into an intact hippocampus. Where it is anticipated that cortico-graphic findings may be crucial to the operative procedure, a preliminary record should be obtained through the intact dura before the cortex is exposed.

Particularly where electrical mapping of cerebral functions is required, acute corticography may be undertaken even when subacute ictal recordings are available, and will at least provide additional information concerning the extent and location of the interictal discharges. If acute corticography is being performed, then it is usual also to obtain a further registration following the resection. Only in exceptional circumstances will the finding of residual, or new, epileptiform activity at the margin of the resection justify removal of additional tissue. However, the persist-ence of substantial amounts of epileptiform activity is generally regarded as an unfavourable prognostic sign by the Montreal school (Jasper et al 1951, Bengzon et al 1968), but this is disputed by others (Ajmone Marsan & Baldwin 1958, Walker et al 1960).

Postoperative EEG follow-up

Assessment of EEG findings after operation is hampered by the fact that preoperative assess ment is generally much more intensive than subsequent follow-up. It is unrealistic to compare short, waking postoperative records with prolonged recordings using additional electrodes and various activation techniques prior to surgery. However, Van Buren et al (1975) showed a marked reduc-tion in epileptiform discharges in most patients postoperatively and, more importantly, a strong association between EEG improvement and seizure remission. The predictive reliability of the EEG increases in the second postoperative year. Van Buren et al (1975) found that, of those patients with epileptiform EEG discharges after two years, only 7% remained seizure-free; whereas an absence of epileptiform discharges at two years was accompanied by clinical improvement in 87%. Taking EEG and clinical findings together, the presence of persisting EEG abnormality in a patient with early seizures confirms a poor prog-nosis, whereas a negative EEG carries a possibility of subsequent clinical improvement (in about 50% of patients).

Conclusion

The above may give the impression of an alarming divergence of opinion and variation in practice between centres undertaking epilepsy surgery. However, this is more a reflection of the different patient populations seen than of fundamental theoretical disagreement. The writer has been privileged to work with two teams representing the extremes of practice. In one centre, the majority of patients treated had mesial temporal sclerosis, which was reliably located by interictal

Table 8.6 Preoperative assessment

Criteria for admission to preoperative assessment programme
1. Partial seizures of such a frequency, having regard to their nature and to the patient's life style, as to be a serious disability
2. Failure of seizure control with appropriate medication (at least phenytoin and carbamazepine) given to the limits of tolerance
3. Patient has the emotional resources to withstand the procedure, including the possibility of being found unsuitable for surgery after lengthy investigations
4. IQ not less than 70
5. No other medical contra-indication, e.g. coagulation defect

Phase Ia
1. Interictal EEG; wake, sleep, barbiturate activation with sphenoidal and possibly other non-standard electrodes
2. Neuroradiology; CT scan, pneumo-encephalography, possibly PET scan and MRI
3. Neuropsychology and possibly psychiatric assessment

Assessment

Is there a single temporal EEG focus concordant with:
  background EEG abnormalities, if any
  seizure pattern
  neuroradiological abnormalities
  neuropsychological findings

		↓ NO	↓ YES		
Abandon	YES ←	Are there generalized interictal discharges ↓ NO proceed to *Phase Ib*	Is the site operable ↓ NO *Abandon* or proceed to *Phase Ib*	YES →	Some teams will *operate*, others proceed to *Phase Ib*

Phase Ib
1. EEG telemetry with sphenoidal electrodes and possible AED reduction to obtain ictal records.
2. Possible carotid amytal test.

Reassessment

Is there a single ictal focus concordant with:
  background EEG abnormalities, if any
  seizure pattern
  neuroradiological abnormalities
  neuropsychological findings

		↓ NO	↓ YES		
Abandon	YES ←	Are there generalized EEG changes at seizure onset? ↓ NO Are ictal symptoms mainly sensorimotor? ↓ NO Proceed to *Phase II*	Is the site operable ↓ NO *Abandon* → YES →	YES → Proceed to *Phase III* or possibly *Phase II*	Most teams will *operate* some proceed to *Phase II*

Phase II
1. Intracranial recording of seizures with possible AED reduction.
2. Possible functional mapping, evoked responses, electrical stimulation to elicit seizures and determine after-discharge thresholds.
3. Assess interictal discharge, spike frequency at different sites, autonomy during nocturnal sleep stages, thiopentone activation.

Reassessment   Consistent ictal onset→YES→*operate* if site is operable
                   ↓ NO
                   Do most seizures start at a site which:
                     Is operable
                     Is most active in interictal record
                     Is autonomous during sleep
                     Is activated by thiopentone
                     Shows ongoing abnormality (slow activity, reduced barbiturate-induced fast activity)
                     Has elevated after-discharge threshold
                     Gives rise to habitual seizure pattern on electrical stimulation
                       ↓ YES to most of above   ↓ NO
                       Possibly operate   *Abandon*

EEG recording with confirmation if required by acute corticography. In the other, mesial temporal sclerosis was rarely seen, many patients had non-temporal lesions, multiple EEG foci and the pathologies included penetrating injuries, old brain abscesses and hamartomata. Here ictal recordings with depth electrodes were almost always necessary. The different approaches were dictated by the patient population, not by any theoretical position adopted by the investigators.

Table 8.6 attempts to summarize the sequence of electrophysiological investigations which may be required for preoperative assessment. In some patients Phase Ia alone provides an adequate basis for surgery, in others a difficult decision remains to be made even after Phase II.

MISCELLANEOUS DIAGNOSTIC PROBLEMS

Febrile convulsions

As the incidence of febrile convulsions is about 3% (Lennox-Buchtal 1973), the electroencephalographer is often asked to investigate a child who has recently suffered a seizure while pyrexial. Questions which may be asked concern: possible acute cerebral disease underlying both the fever and the seizure; the risk of recurrence of febrile convulsions; and the prognosis for developing epilepsy. Within 24 hours following a febrile convulsion, nearly 90% of children will show an abnormal EEG (Laplane & Salbreux 1963) and after three to five days about one-third of the records are still abnormal (Frantzen et al 1968). Slowing of background rhythms is generally seen, which may be symmetrical or asymmetrical; the latter particularly if the seizure itself was asymmetrical or unilateral.

The more severe abnormalities may be difficult to distinguish from the effects of acute encephalopathy and serial EEG recording may be required to resolve this issue. Reviewing several previous series, Lennox-Buchtal (1973) found that extreme or focal slowing of the EEG was significantly associated with severity of the convulsion, duration of the fever, height of the fever, and past history of brain injury. There was a non-significant association with a subsequent liability to afebrile convulsions. However, as under 10% of children with extreme or focal slowing subsequently developed epilepsy, this finding was of little predictive value in any individual. Epileptiform discharges, in the immediate post-ictal phase are of little significance in relation to subsequent epilepsy but, particularly if focal, may reflect acute underlying pathology. Gastaut et al (1960b) described a syndrome of a severe unilateral febrile convulsion and an EEG showing contralateral reduction in amplitude of background activity with focal abnormalities, slow waves, spikes or spike-wave complexes, in children who subsequently developed hemiconvulsions, hemiplegia and epilepsy. In the absence of cerebral pathology, the initial EEG does not usually contain epileptiform activity except in the older children and its presence is in any event of no prognostic significance (Frantzen et al 1968). At follow-up, generalized spike-wave activity shows an association with a family history of convulsions (Frantzen et al 1970) but does not increase the likelihood of further seizures. Serial studies show development of epileptiform EEG discharges in those children who develop epilepsy. However, the first EEG record containing epileptiform activity may follow the first afebrile seizure (Laplane & Salbreux 1963).

In summary, the EEG offers less evidence than might be hoped concerning prognosis following febrile convulsions, and its chief value in the first few days after the seizure is for detecting acute underlying cerebral disease.

Psychiatric problems in epilepsy

There is a recognized association between epilepsy, particularly with partial seizures of temporal lobe origin, and psychosis. Most authors find this chiefly in patients with focal discharges over the dominant hemisphere (Slater et al 1963, Flor-Henry 1969, 1972, 1976, Taylor 1977). Kristensen & Sindrup (1978), by contrast, found bilateral spike foci to be most strongly associated with psychosis. Lateralisation of the discharges also appears to influence the nature of the psychotic syndrome. Thus Flor-Henry (1969) found schizophreniform features in patients with left-sided or bilateral foci, and manic-depressive symptoms with right-sided discharges. The effects of laterality are complex, however: a schizophreniform picture is associated with left-handedness in subjects with either left-sided (Sherwin 1981) or right-sided foci (Trimble & Perez 1981).

There appears to be an inverse relationship between seizure occurrence and liability to psychosis. Thus Flor-Henry (1972, 1976) and Kristensen & Sindrup (1978) found a reduced incidence of complex partial seizures when patients became psychotic. Similarly, following successful operative treatment of temporal lobe epilepsy, psychosis may develop (Jensen & Larsen 1979, Taylor 1972, Stevens 1966) or deteriorate (Sherwin 1981). These changes are often accompanied by the disappearance of EEG abnormalities, leading to the concept of forced normalization of the EEG (Landolt 1958). A speculative neurochemical basis for this relationship is offered by the observation that dopamine antagonists, effective in schizophrenia, are epileptogenic and that some antiepileptic drugs have a secondary dopaminergic action.

In children too a relationship exists between lateralization of focal EEG discharges and psychosocial dysfunction. Thus Stores (1978) found that left-temporal discharges in boys, but not in girls, were associated with educational and behavioural problems. Surprisingly perhaps, generalized epileptiform activity, which might have been expected to cause inattention, was less likely to be associated with school difficulties.

Epilepsy, aggression and crime

Despite a widespread belief in the liability of persons with complex partial seizures to display aggressive and/or criminal behaviour during their attacks, convincing evidence of ictal aggression is exceedingly difficult to find. In this context, it is important to distinguish directed ictal aggression from the random, confused, resistive behaviour seen during seizures and particularly in the postictal state. Delgado-Escueta et al (1981) attempted to collect reports documented by telemetric ictal EEG studies of patients who became aggressive during seizures, but found no convincing evidence of directed aggression against persons.

The question of ictal aggression is, however, confused by other electrophysiological evidence. Spiking has been recorded from the mesial part of the amygdala during spontaneous aggressive behaviour in monkeys and in humans (Heath 1954, 1972, 1975, Heath & Mickle 1960). Both psychotic and epileptic patients exhibited 12–18/s spindles in the hypocampus and amygdala during episodes of dyscontrol but, in those with epilepsy, these were intermixed with spike-wave activity. Stevens (1977a, b) suggests that neural spiking, so far from being only a pathological phenomenon, is a means of transmitting information of imperative biological importance and can be found in various species, including humans during aggression, suckling and orgasm (Heath, 1975). Current views of the ethics of human experimentation preclude further systematic investigation of these phenomena in humans but observations incidental to preoperative assessment of people with epilepsy confirm the finding of deep spike discharges, not detectable in the scalp EEG, during aggressive behaviour in humans (Wieser 1983b). If, however, deep temporal discharges can be a correlate of normal, adaptive, aggressive behaviour, it could be argued that all aggression is ictal; in any event, these observations beg the question of what is epilepsy, and make it almost impossible to claim with certainty that an otherwise inexplicable aggressive act did not have an epileptic basis.

There is, however, no evidence to support the proposition that EEG abnormalities in a person without epilepsy reflect an 'epileptic tendency' which can cause criminal behaviour when activated by alcohol. Unfortunately this claim, has been established as a precedent by English case law (Regina v. Coster 1959) and persons without epilepsy charged with violent criminal acts (particularly under the influence of alcohol) are regularly referred for EEG investigation in the hope that some anomaly can be found and used as a basis for a plea of insanity or of diminished responsibility. There is an increased incidence of sociopathy, criminality and cerebral disease, including epilepsy, amongst socially disadvantaged groups, and a raised incidence of epilepsy amongst convicted criminals (Gunn & Fenton 1971). There is, moreover, an association between criminality in general and aggressive crimes in particular, and non-epileptiform EEG anomalies (Williams 1969). However, no association exists between violence and epileptiform EEG disturbances (Driver et al 1974).

In summary, psychoses, behavioural disorders and social dysfunction in people with epilepsy are not only of practical importance but also of theoretical interest, and in this latter context EEG findings are highly relevant. However, diagnostic EEG investigation of a psychiatrically disturbed or socially malfunctioning person, with the intention of detecting previously unidentified epilepsy, is rarely useful and often indeed simply misleading. Schizophrenics receiving neuroleptics will often exhibit bitemporal sharp waves, which may either be misinterpreted as evidence of epilepsy or at least lead to a series of further fruitless investigations, including sleep records or repeat EEGs after withdrawal of medication. Aggressive criminals and psychopaths are often victims as well as instigators of violence, and may have suffered multiple head injuries in fights and road traffic accidents by the time they undergo EEG investigation. In the absence of known epilepsy, the clinical or forensic significance of minor EEG abnormalities under such circumstances is uncertain.

EEG and driving licences

Most societies refuse people with epilepsy the right to drive a motor vehicle; however, there is considerable variation in the regulations governing the restoration of a driving licence to a person who has become seizure-free. In some countries, such as the Netherlands, regular neurological follow-up of people who have regained their licence after remission of epilepsy is mandatory, and includes an EEG recording. The use to be made of the EEG information is not further specified. It would appear unreasonable to refuse anyone a driving licence on the basis of interictal EEG anomalies alone. It is, however, established that seemingly subclinical discharges may be accompanied by transitory cognitive impairment (p. 267) and EEG telemetry during prolonged driving of a

suitably instrumented dual-control vehicle, has shown that such impairment may include a disturbance of driving skills (Kasteleijn-Nolst Trenité & Binnie, in preparation). It would seem a reasonable policy to attempt to demonstrate by simultaneous video recording, and preferably psychological testing, whether or not subclinical EEG discharges are accompanied by demonstrable cognitive impairment and to withold a driving licence only where this is the case.

THE USES AND LIMITATIONS OF ELECTROENCEPHALOGRAPHY IN EPILEPSY

Misconceptions

It should be apparent from this and previous chapters that EEG findings are fundamental to present concepts concerning both the nature of epilepsy and the classification of its various manifestations. This has led to some expectations concerning the value of the EEG for clinical investigation of epilepsy which are either false or subject to important qualifications;

1. That the ictal EEG invariably exhibits epileptiform discharges and the absence of such phenomena during a seizure excludes an epileptic basis for the attack
2. That the interictal EEG can be used to establish or refute the diagnosis of epilepsy
3. That the degree of EEG abnormality, especially the frequency of epileptiform discharge, closely reflects the severity of epilepsy, particularly the seizure frequency, and is reduced by effective antiepileptic medication
4. That the interictal EEG is predictive of prognosis in epilepsy and specifically that patients with interictal discharges are less likely to become, or to remain, seizure-free than those with normal EEGs

Non-fulfilment of these expectations has led some authors to question the clinical value of electroencephalography in epilepsy, or indeed for any other purpose (Matthews 1964, Hopkins & Scambler 1977).

The negative ictal EEG

As indicated above (first section), an epileptic seizure is by definition accompanied by a cerebral electrophysiological disturbance. With appropriately placed intracranial electrodes, this must always be detectable. Ictal changes in the scalp EEG are not necessarily present, however. Some seizure types, it would appear, are invariably associated with ictal EEG change: a convulsive attack without spikes in the EEG (assuming, of course, a technically acceptable tracing has been obtained) is not epileptic; nor probably is an episode of unconsciousness resembling an absence seizure, but without epileptiform EEG activity. Other seizure types sometimes produce ictal EEG changes and sometimes do not, notably simple partial seizures with motor symptomatology. Some kinds of seizures never or rarely produce ictal change in the scalp EEG, particularly simple partial seizures with psychic symptomatology or consisting only of viscerosensory hallucinosis. Finally, it must be noted that ictal EEG change does not necessarily consist of spikes or spike-wave complexes and subtle alterations, such as an electrodecremental event, may be undetectable in the presence of muscle and movement artefact or if the technical specification of the recording system used is not adequate (see section on monitoring).

Proof and disproof of epilepsy

The request for an EEG 'to exclude epilepsy' may be only an abbreviated way for the referring physician to indicate his wishes for diagnostic assessment, but certainly implies a serious misconception. A single interictal EEG will fail to detect epileptiform activity in 50% of people with epilepsy. It is difficult to justify, on economic or any other grounds, referring a patient with suspected epilepsy for a waking EEG and then declining the offer of a sleep recording if this first investigation is negative. Even if a full diagnostic series is performed as suggested earlier some 10% of patients will consistently fail to exhibit interictal epileptiform discharges, in which event the only possibility of obtaining electrophysiological evidence in favour of, or against, the diagnosis of epilepsy is by an ictal recording, probably during monitoring.

The confusion concerning the incidence of epileptiform activity in persons without seizure disorders was noted earlier. Where there is a differential diagnosis between epilepsy and a psychiatric cause for a patient's attacks, the presence of interictal epileptiform discharges must (not taking into account other clinical considerations) greatly increase the statistical probability of epilepsy. By contrast, where there is already evidence of cerebral disease, for instance after severe head injury or in the presence of a cerebral tumour or mental subnormality, the presence of epileptiform activity may contribute little to the clinical decision of whether or not a patient's attacks are epileptic.

If only to discourage misguided treatment of abnormal EEGs rather than patients, it must be clearly stated that epilepsy is a clinical diagnosis and that epileptiform EEG discharges without seizures do not constitute epilepsy. However, in interpreting this incontrovertible proposition, it must be also noted that clinical ictal manifestations include subtle cognitive changes which may not be recognized either by the patient or other observers without the help of some form of psychological testing (see p. 267). The incidence and clinical importance of such unrecognized transitory cognitive impairment in patients with subclinical discharges is, at the present time, unknown.

Severity of epilepsy and effects of antiepileptic drugs (AEDs)

The reasonable assumption that the frequency of EEG discharge should relate to seizure incidence does hold good in the case of patients with absence seizures. In this particular instance, however, it could be argued that all the discharges are in fact ictal and that there is therefore inevitably a one-to-one relationship between generalized spike-wave activity and absences. Certainly it is the case that drugs effective in absence seizures dramatically reduce the incidence of generalized 3/s spike-wave activity and that patients who appear to be seizure-free show a 95–100% reduction of their discharges. At the other extreme, in secondary generalized epilepsy there may be a complete dissociation between seizure frequency and EEG abnormality so that the record may be dominated by generalized discharges, even in a patient who appears to be seizure-free.

In routine epileptological EEG practice covering a wide spectrum of types of epilepsy, Binnie (1986b) found a positive association between changes in discharge rate in serial EEGs and changes in seizure frequency (Table 8.7), but the association, although statistically significant, was extremely weak.

Table 8.7 Weak association of change in discharge rate in 'routine' EEG with reported seizure frequency.

Change in epileptiform activity	Reported change in seizure frequency	
	Increase	Decrease
Increase	75	84
No change	441	507
Decrease	40	97

Gotman & Marciani (1985) found no clear relationship in more detailed serial EEG investigations and seizure frequency in patients with partial epilepsy. In general, the spiking rate did not change before seizures but increased, sometimes for several days after them (Gotman & Marciani 1985). A small series of patients with partial or secondary generalized epilepsy, studied with twice-weekly standardized EEGs over many months, was briefly reported by Binnie (1983a). The subjects fell into two distinct groups: those who showed a strong, highly significant association between seizure frequency and spike counts; and others who showed no such relationship. There were no other apparent clinical differences between the groups. A tendency to a higher discharge rate following seizures as reported by Gotman & Marciani (1985) was not found.

A follow-up EEG to assess progress is clearly of value in absence seizures which are, moreover, often reported unreliably by patients and relatives. In other forms of epilepsy it is of marginal clinical value, except possibly in postoperative assessment where a successful outcome is usually associated with marked EEG improvement (Falconer & Serafetinides 1963) and relapse is often heralded by the return of interictal discharges.

Gram et al (1982) noted that the majority of controlled trials of AEDs included EEG studies, but that in over a half the findings were of so little interest that the authors had not apparently considered them worth analysing. Excluding studies of absence seizures, only a handful of controlled trials show that the preferred drug treatment was accompanied by a reduction in EEG discharges (Wilkus & Green 1974, Kellaway et al 1978, Binnie et al 1986b). Carbamazepine in particular produces an increase in EEG abnormalities, notably disturbances in background activity. Van Wieringen et al (1987) comparing the findings of six AED trials, found that only one drug (Lamotrigine) produced both clinical improvement and reduction in EEG discharges, and that one other (an experimental benzodiazepine prodrug), on withdrawal, gave rise both to an exacerbation of seizures and to an increase in EEG abnormality.

Short-term fluctuation in levels of AEDs in patients with partial epilepsy on chronic therapy have little or no effect on the rate of EEG or depth discharges in telemetric records over 24 to 48 hours (Martins da Silva et al 1984, Gotman & Marciani 1985).

The failure to find an association between seizure frequency and drug effects on the one hand and EEG discharge rate on the other may arise from two sources: first, the statistical sampling problem created by the inherent variability of EEG discharge rate; and, secondly, a possible lack of the expected relationship between discharges and seizures. Spontaneous interictal discharges change systematically with waking and sleep and under the influence of various circadian, ultradian, or infradian biorhythms (Stevens et al 1971, Martins da Silva et al 1984, Binnie et al 1984b, Broughton et al 1985). They also fluctuate in association with uncontrolled and generally undocumented factors as attention, vigilance and cognitive activity (Guey et al 1969). Finally, there are many unexplained fluctuations which, for all practical purposes, must be regarded as random. A typical half-hour 'routine' waking EEG therefore generally represents a statistically unreliable sample of a changing process. More reliable estimates of discharge rate may be obtained by recording for long periods, by telemetry or otherwise, or by short periods of registration under standardized conditions of vigilance, psychological tasks etc. Where these measures are adopted it may be possible to show a relationship between seizure frequency and discharge rate (Binnie 1983a) or drug effects (Milligan & Richens 1981, 1982, Milligan et al 1982, 1983, Binnie 1986).

The theoretical basis of the presumed relationship of interictal discharge rate to seizure liability merits critical examination. The genesis of a clinical seizure involves a hierarchy of events, from the virtually continuous dysfunction of individual neurones, manifest, for instance, in paroxysmal depolarisation shifts, through the intermittent synchronous discharges in neuronal populations giving rise to spikes which may be detected with depth or even scalp electrodes, to the occasional recruitment of larger, or specific, populations of neurones required for the clinical expression of a seizure. Rodin (1968) distinguishes 'seizure threshold', a liability to abnormal neuronal discharge, and 'seizure propensity', the tendency for such discharges to find' clinical expression. These speculations are underpinned by some physiological evidence. At the core of an experimental epileptic focus are 'Group 1' neurones, which display continuous autonomous abnormal activity uninfluenced by afferent stimuli. Surrounding neurones ('Group 2') also have an abnormal tendency to fire in bursts, but remain under normal afferent control. Recruitment of Group 2 neurones produces a partial seizure (Lockard & Ward 1981). Because Group 2 neurones are subject to normal afferent influences, their liability to recruitment (i.e. seizure propensity) depends on such various extrinsic factors as attention, wake and sleep, stress etc. An interictal discharge is, by definition, one which fails to give rise to a seizure, and thus a heightened seizure propensity should give rise, not to an increased, but to a reduced interictal discharge rate. In theory, an effective antiepileptic drug could work at the level of primary neuronal dysfunction, increasing seizure threshold and reducing both epileptiform discharges and seizures. Another agent might act rather at the level of ictal propagation, reducing seizure propensity and thus producing a dissociation between frequency of seizures and discharges. Further investigation of

these relationships might provide valuable insights both into the physiology of epilepsy and into the different modes of action of various antiepileptic drugs.

The clinical interpretation of interictal discharges, and indeed the whole concept of epileptiform activity, is coloured by the EEG phenomenology of epileptic seizures. Yet apart from 3/s generalized spike-wave activity (which arguably is always ictal) the morphology of interictal epileptiform activity is generally different from that seen during seizures, particularly at the onset of the attack. Indeed, seizure onset is usually heralded by attenuation of continuing interictal discharges, which are replaced by regular activity 'rhythmic ictal transformation' (Geiger & Harner 1978). In a patient whose seizures are characterized by an electrodecremental event, rhythmic theta activity or high frequency multi-unit activity, it is perhaps naive to expect any close relationship of the attacks to interictal slow spike-wave complexes or sharp waves. Interictal discharges often resemble most closely the phenomena seen in the later stages of a seizure and it may be worth considering the possibility that some types at least of epileptiform activity are related to inhibitory mechanisms which limit or prevent seizures, rather than to those which precipitate them. Such an interpretation would explain many of the paradoxes of the EEG in epilepsy.

In addition to showing effects, or sometimes a singular lack of effect, on spontaneous epileptiform discharges, AEDs may also change background activity. The effects range from minimal or absent in the case of sodium valproate (Benninger et al 1985), to marked with carbamazepine, which produces a deterioration of background activity, typically an increase in the slower components. Most other antiepileptic drugs in routine use give an increase in beta and theta activity. The beta activity is most prominent and usually fairly fast (20/s and above) in the case of the barbiturates; whereas benzodiazepines produce a large amount of slower beta activity, often taking the form of a fast alpha variant. The appearance of a slowed EEG with an excess of fast activity in a drowsy patient with epilepsy will generally give rise to a suspicion of AED intoxication. It should, however, rarely fall to the electroencephalographer to detect this problem, which should already have been identified on the basis of clinical findings and/or serum level monitoring by the referring physician. EEG investigation may, however, make a useful contribution in patients with such symptoms as apathy, which could be due either to medication or to depression, and with levels of (usually several) antiepileptic drugs, which are highly therapeutic but not individually toxic. Here the finding of a slowed EEG with an excess of beta activity will suggest that a reduction of the dosage or of the number of drugs is desirable.

Prognosis

Gross EEG abnormality in a patient with epilepsy generally implies a poor prognosis for becoming seizure-free (Rodin 1968, Rowan et al 1980). However, background abnormalities are as important in this respect as epileptiform activity and this relationship probably simply reflects an association of severe cerebral pathology, both with continued seizure liability and with EEG abnormality. By contrast, two specific and striking EEG patterns, 3/s spike-wave activity with absence seizures and Rolandic spikes, both support the diagnosis of particular epilepsy syndromes which have a good prognosis for seizure control on medication and for terminal remission.

After a single non-febrile seizure, focal epileptiform discharge is reported to be significantly predictive of recurrence in children, the recurrence rate being 68% with focal discharge against 22% without (Camfield et al 1985). This finding is surprising as the authors did not apparently consider Rolandic spikes as a special category. In adults, by contrast, generalized spike-wave activity is associated with recurrence after a first seizure (Hauser et al 1982).

In patients who have remained seizure-free on medication for two years or more, the possibility arises of withdrawing antiepileptic drugs. However, a substantial proportion of patients, as high as 60% in some series, relapse when this is attempted. It is generally regarded as self-evident that the continued presence of epileptiform EEG activity or its recurrence when AEDs are reduced is predictive of relapse. Indeed, many investigators have considered it ethically unacceptable to

put this proposition to the test, and have excluded from studies of AED withdrawal any patients exhibiting epileptiform discharges (Zenker et al 1957, Juul-Jensen 1964, van Heycop ten Ham 1980, Holowach et al 1972, Rodin & John 1980). The claim that epileptiform EEG activity is predictive of relapse on drug withdrawal has therefore become a self-fulfilling prophecy. The few studies of the use of EEG in predicting outcome of AED withdrawal have confirmed that this is indeed the case in children (Emerson et al 1981, Todt 1981, 1984, Shinnar et al 1985, Le Pestre et al 1985). Only two investigations appear to have addressed this question in adults (Overweg 1985, Overweg et al 1987, Wallis 1985) and neither found any evidence that the presence of epileptiform discharges was predictive of relapse. Overweg, indeed, found a significant positive association between the presence of sharp waves and continued remission.

These findings too can be explained by the concepts put forward in the previous section. Terminal remission may not necessarily indicate a disappearance of the original underlying neuronal dysfunction reflected in the presence of spikes and sharp waves, but rather a reduced seizure propensity, so that the patient's discharges are now self-limiting and no longer give rise to clinical manifestations. The decision whether or not to withdraw AEDs in a patient who is seizure-free is again clearly a matter which should be determined by clinical considerations, without misguided concern for the cosmetic appearance of the EEG.

Applications of the EEG in epilepsy

Although the previous section has stressed the limitations of electroencephalography in epilepsy, the useful applications are not inconsiderable. Where the clinical diagnosis of epilepsy is in doubt and the patient is not suffering from other obvious cerebral disease, the finding of interictal epileptiform activity, either in a single routine EEG or in the course of a full diagnostic series, must importantly reinforce that diagnosis. Negative findings will be of less diagnostic value, although a normal resting EEG with a normal response to adequate hyperventilation must cast considerable suspicion on any claim that a patient has uncontrolled absence seizures. Where clinical assessment and interictal EEGs have not permitted a confident diagnosis an ictal recording should be obtained, assuming that the attacks occur sufficiently frequently, so that there is a reasonable chance of capturing a seizure during an acceptable period of registration. If necessary medication, if already instituted, can be reduced in the hope of increasing the seizure frequency. Usually, the appropriate technology will be telemetric monitoring with simultaneous video registration. Ambulatory monitoring provides an alternative but its limitations for this application have been noted above. Ictal EEG change during a seizure proves its epileptic nature, provided a cardiac cause is excluded by simultaneous ECG registration. The interpretation of negative ictal EEG findings depends on the seizure pattern.

Establishing the diagnosis of epilepsy on clinical grounds may be less difficult than determining the classification. Here both interictal and ictal EEGs make an important contribution. Where there is an inadequate history of episodes of impaired consciousness, the finding of generalized spike-wave activity on the one hand or of a focal abnormality on the other may be critical to distinguishing primary generalized epilepsy with absence seizures from partial epilepsy with complex partial seizures. In a patient with partial seizures where the possibility of surgical treatment is being considered, the finding of an EEG picture typical of secondary generalized epilepsy will cause this programme to be reconsidered. In the recognition of various epileptic syndromes, the role of the EEG ranges from supportive (as in the Lennox-Gastaut and West's syndromes) to virtually diagnostic (benign childhood epilepsy, photosensitive epilepsy).

In following the progress of persons with epilepsy and in predicting prognosis, the role of the EEG is limited and often overvalued. In patients with frequent, brief seizures which are difficult to recognize, notably absences, both conventional recordings and ambulatory monitoring can be valuable for following progress. As a routine means of follow-up in other types of epilepsy, electroencephalography is of very limited value, although EEG recording may provide the opportunity of detecting unrecognized minor seizures or identifying possible episodes of transitory cognitive impairment. In status epilepticus, particularly in refractory cases where the patient is anaesthetized and artificially ventilated, the EEG may provide the only means of monitoring response to treatment.

The surgery of epilepsy is a highly specialized field which concerns few clinicians and offers help to only a small proportion of people with epilepsy. Nevertheless, both for the preoperative assessment and during operation, detailed, complex electrophysiological assessment is indispensible.

CONCLUSION

As a functional disorder, epilepsy would appear an ideal application of electroencephalography. Certainly the use of the EEG in investigation of persons with epilepsy is illustrative of various general principles of electroencephalography. Perhaps the most important of these, which this chapter demonstrates, is that the recording of 'routine' EEGs for no clear indication is a misuse of resources which can better be applied to detailed and, if necessary prolonged, investigation of the specific problems of individual patients, an activity which can prove extremely rewarding.

REFERENCES

Aarts J H P, Binnie C D, Smit A M, Wilkins A J 1984 Selective cognitive impairment during focal and generalized epileptiform EEG activity. Brain 107: 293–308

Ajmone Marsan C 1973 Electrocorticography. In: Rémond A (ed) Handbook of electroencephalography and clinical neurophysiology Vol 10 Part C. Elsevier, Amsterdam

Ajmone Marsan C 1980 Depth electrography and electrocorticography. In: Aminoff M J (ed) Electrodiagnosis in clinical neurology. Churchill-Livingstone, New York pp 167–196

Ajmone Marsan C, Baldwin M 1958 Electroencephalography. In: Baldwin M, Bailey P (eds) Temporal lobe epilepsy. Thomas, Springfield

Ajmone Marsan C A, Van Buren J M 1958 Epileptiform activity in cortical and subcortical structures in the temporal lobe of man. In: Baldwin M, Bailey P (eds)

Temporal lobe epilepsy. Thomas, Springfield pp 78–108

Ajmone Marsan C, Abraham K 1960 A seizure atlas. Electroencephalography and Clinical Neurophysiology (suppl) 15

Ajmone Marsan C, Zivin L S 1970 Factors related to the occurrence of typical paroxysmal abnormalities in the EEG records of epileptic patients. Epilepsia 11: 361–381

Ames F R 1971 'Self-induction' in photosensitive epilepsy. Brain 94: 781–798

Ames F R 1974 Cinefilm and EEG recording during 'hand-waving' attacks of an epileptic, photosensitive child. Electroencephalography and Clinical Neurophysiology 37: 301–304

Ames F R, Enderstein O 1976 Clinical and EEG response to clonazepam in four patients with self-induced photosensitive epilepsy. South African Medical Journal 50:1423

Andermann F 1971 Self-induced television epilepsy. Epilepsia 12: 269–275

Andermann K, Berman S, Cooke P M et al 1962 Self-induced epilepsy. A collection of self-induced epilepsy cases compared with some other photoconvulsive cases. Archives of Neurology 6: 49–65

Angelieri F 1974 Partial epilepsies and nocturnal sleep. In: Levin P, Koella W P (eds) Sleep. Karger, Basel, pp 196–203

Angelieri F, Bergonzi P, Ferroni A 1967 Le fasi ed i cidi del sonno notturno negli epilettici. Rivista di Patalogia Nervosa e Mentale 88: 107–148

Babb T L, Crandall P H 1976 Epileptogenesis of human limbic neurons in psychomotor epileptics. Electroencephalography and Clinical Neurophysiology 40: 225–243

Baldy-Moulinier M 1982 Temporal lobe epilepsy and sleep organization. In: Sterman M B, Passouant P (eds) Sleep and epilepsy. Academic Press, New York, pp 347–359

Bancaud J 1972 Mechanisms of cortical discharges in 'generalized' epilepsies in man. In: Petsche H, Brazier M A B (eds) Synchronisation of EEG activity in epilepsies. Springer Verlag, New York, pp 368–380

Bancaud J, Talairach J, Bonis A et al 1965 La Stéréo-électroencéphalographie dans l'épilepsie. Informations neurophysiopathologiques apportées par l'investigation fonctionelle stéréotaxique. Masson, Paris

Bancaud J, Talairach J, Waltregny A, Bresson M, Morel P 1968 L'activation par le mégimide dans le diagnostic topographique des épilepsies corticales focales (étude clinique et EEG et SEEG). Revue Neurologique (Paris) 119: 320–325

Bancaud J, Talairach J, Morel P et al 1974 'Generalised' epileptic seizures elicited by electrical stimulation of the frontal lobe in man. Electroencephalography and Clinical Neurophysiology 37: 275–282

Batini C, Fressy J, Naquet R, Orfanos A, Saint-Laurent J 1963 Étude du sommeil nocturne chez 20 sujets présentant des décharges imitatives focalisées. Revue Neurologique (Paris) 108: 172–173

Bengzon A R A, Rasmussen T, Gloor P, Dussault J, Stephens M 1968 Prognostic factors in the surgical treatment of temporal lobe epileptics. Neurology 18: 717–731

Bennett D R 1962 Sleep deprivation and major motor convulsions. Neurology 13: 953–958

Bennett D R, Ziter F A, Liske E A 1969

Electroencephalographic study of sleep deprivation in flying personnel. Neurology 19: 375–377

Bennett F E 1953 Intracarotid and intravertebral Metrazol in petit mal epilepsy. Neurology 3: 668–673

Benninger C, Matthis P, Scheffner D 1985 Spectral analysis of the EEG in children during the introduction of antiepileptic therapy with valproic acid. Neuropsychobiology 13: 93–96

Bernoulli C, Siegfried J, Baumgartner G et al 1977 Danger of accidental person-to-person transmission by Creutzfeldt-Jakob disease by surgery. Lancet 1: 478–479

Besset A 1982 Influence of generalized seizures on sleep organization. In: Sterman M B, Shouse M N, Passouant P (eds) Sleep and epilepsy. Academic Press, New York, pp 339–346

Bickford R G, Klass D W 1962 Stimulus factors in the mechanism of television-induced seizures. Transactions of the American Neurological Association 87: 176–178

Bickford R G, Klass D W 1969 Sensory precipitation and reflex mechanisms. In: Jasper H H, Ward A A, Pope A (eds) Basic mechanisms of the epilepsies. Little, Brown pp 543–564

Bickford R G, Sem-Jacobsen C W, White P T, Daly D 1952 Some observations on the mechanism of photic and photo-metrazol activation. Electroencephalography and Clinical Neurophysiology 4: 275–282

Bickford R G, Daly D, Keith H M 1953 Convulsive effects of light stimulation in children. American Journal of Diseases in Children 86: 170–183

Billiard M 1982 Epilepsies and the sleep-wake cycle. In: Sterman M B, Shouse M N, Passouant P (eds) Sleep and epilepsy. Academic Press, New York, pp 269–286

Binnie C D 1980 Detection of transitory cognitive impairment during epileptiform EEG discharges: problems in clinical practice. In: Kulig B M, Meinardi H, Stores G (eds) Epilepsy and behavior 1979. Swets and Zeitlinger, Lisse pp 91–97

Binnie C D 1983a EEG and blood levels of antiepileptic drugs. In: Buser P, Cobb W A, Okuma T (eds) Proceedings 10th International Congress of Electroencephalography and Clinical Neurophysiology, Kyoto. Electroencephalography and Clinical Neurophysiology (suppl) 36: 504–512

Binnie C D 1983b Telemetric EEG monitoring in epilepsy. In: Pedley T A Meldrum B S (eds) Recent Advances in epilepsy I. Churchill Livingstone, Edinburgh, pp 155–178

Binnie C D 1986 The interictal EEG. In: Trimble M R, Reynolds E H (eds) What is epilepsy? Churchill Livingstone, Edinburgh, 16–125

Binnie C D 1987 Ambulatory diagnostic monitoring of seizures in the adult. In: Gumnit R J (ed) Advances in neurology: International Conference on Neurodiagnostic Monitoring. Raven Press, New York, pp 169–182

Binnie C D, Van der Wens P 1986 Diagnostic re-evaluation by intensive monitoring of intractable absence seizures. In: Schmidt D, Morselli P (eds) Intractable epilepsy: experimental and clinical aspects. Raven Press, New York, pp 99–107

Binnie C D, Coles P A, Margerison J H 1969 The influence of end-tidal carbon dioxide tension on EEG changes during routine hyperventilation in different age groups. Electroencephalography and Clinical Neurophysiology 27: 304–306

Binnie C D, Batchelor B G, Bowring P A et al 1978 Computer-assisted interpretation of clinical EEGs.

Electroencephalograpy and Clinical Neurophysiology 44: 575–585

Binnie C D, De Korte J W A, Meijer A J, Rowan A J, Warfield C 1980a Acute effects of sodium valproate on the photoconvulsive response in man. Journal of the Royal Society of Medicine International Congress Series 30: 103–113

Binnie C D, Darby C E, De Korte R A, Veldhuizen R, Wilkins A J 1980b EEG sensitivity to television: effects of ambient lighting. Electroencephalography and Clinical Neurophysiology 50: 329–331

Binnie C D, Darby C E, De Korte R A, Wilkins A J 1980c Self-induction of epileptic seizures by eyeclosure: incidence and recognition. Journal of Neurology, Neurosurgery and Psychiatry 43: 386–389

Binnie C D, Rowan A J, Overweg J et al 1981 Telemetric EEG and video monitoring in epilepsy. Neurology 31: 298–303

Binnie C D, Rowan A J, Gutter T 1982a A Manual of EEG technology. Cambridge University Press, Cambridge

Binnie C D, Dekker E, Smit A, Van der Linden G 1982b Practical considerations in the positioning of EEG electrodes. Electroencephalography and Clinical Neurophysiology 53: 453–458

Binnie C D, Estevez O, Kasteleijn-Nolst Trenité D G A, Peters A 1984a Colour and photosensitive epilepsy. Electroencephalography and Clinical Neurophysiology 58: 387–391

Binnie C D, Aarts J H P, Houtkooper M A et al 1984b Temporal characteristics of seizures and epileptiform discharges. Electroencephalography and Clinical Neurophysiology 58: 498–505

Binnie C D, Findlay J, Wilkins A J 1985a Mechanisms of epileptogenesis in photosensitive epilepsy implied by the effects of moving patterns. Electroencephalography and Clinical Neurophysiology 61: 1–6

Binnie C D, Kasteleijn-Nolst Trenité D G A, De Korte R, Wilkins A 1985b Visual display units and risk of seizures. Lancet 1:1991

Binnie C D, van Emde Boas W, Wauquier A 1985c Geniculate spikes during epileptic seizures induced in dogs by pentylenetetrazol and bicuculline. Electroencephalography and Clinical Neurophysiology 61: 40–49

Binnie C D, Kasteleijn-Nolst Trenite D G A, De Korte R 1986a Photosensitivity as a model for acute antiepileptic drug studies. Electroencephalography and Clinical Neurophysiology 63: 35–41

Binnie C D, Van Emde Boas W, Kasteleijn-Nolst Trenité D G A et al 1986b Acute effects of lamotrigine (BW430C) in persons with epilepsy. Epilepsia 248–254

Bloom D, Jasper H, Rasmussen T 1959 Surgical therapy in patients with temporal lobe seizures and bilateral EEG abnormality. Epilepsia 1: 351–365

Bordas-Ferrer M, Talairach J, Bancaud J 1966 Incidence des accès sur l'organisation du sommeil de nuit des épileptiques. Revue Neurologique 115: 556–561

Bowden A N, Fitch P, Gilliatt R W, Willison R G 1975 The place of EEG telemetry and closed-circuit television in the diagnosis and management of epileptic patients. Proceedings of the Royal Society of Medicine 68: 246–248

Braham J 1967 An unsuccessful attempt at the extinction of photogenic epilepsy. Electroencephalography and Clinical Neurophysiology 23:558P

Brausch C C, Ferguson J H 1965 Color as factor in light-sensitive epilepsy. Neurology 15: 154–164

Brazier M A B 1973 Electrical seizure discharges within the human brain. The problem of spread. In: Brazier M A B (ed) Epilepsy, its phenomena in man. Academic Press, New York, pp 152–170

Breakell C C, Parker C S, Christopherson F 1949 Radio transmission of the human electroencephalogram and other electrophysiological data. Electroencephalography and Clinical Neurophysiology 1: 243–244

Broseta J, Barcia-Salorio J L, Lopez-Gomez L, Roldan P, Gonzalez-Darder J, Barbera J 1980 Burr-hole electrocorticography. Acta Neurochirurgica (suppl) 30: 91–96

Broughton R, Stampi C, Romano S, Cirignolta F, Barizzi A, Lugarci E 1985 Do waking ultradian rhythms exist for petit mal absences? A case report. In: Martins da Silva A, Binnie C D, Meinardi H (eds) Biorhythms and epilepsy. New York, Raven Press pp 95–105

Browne T R, Penry J K, Porter R J, Dreifuss F E 1974a A comparison of clinical estimates of absence seizure frequency with estimates based on prolonged telemetered EEGs. Neurology 24: 381–382

Browne T R, Penry J K, Porter R J, Dreifuss F E 1974b Responsiveness before, during and after spike-wave paroxysms. Neurology 24: 659–665

Bruens J H, Knijff W 1980 Ambulatory EEG monitoring with a 24 hour cassette recorder in epileptic patients. In: Epilepsy: a clinical and experimental research. Monographs in Neural Science 5: 295–297

Camfield P R, Camfield C S, Dooley J M, Tibbles J A R, Fung T, Garner B 1985 Epilepsy after a first unprovoked seizure in childhood. Neurology 35: 1657–1660

Capron E 1966 Étude de divers types de sensibilité electroencephalographique a la stimulation lumineuse intermittente et leur signification. Thesis, Foulon, Paris

Carterette E C, Symmes D 1952 Color as an experimental variant in photic stimulation. Electroencephalography and Clinical Neurophysiology 4: 289–296

Charcot J M 1887 Lecons sur les maladies du système nerveux tome III. Delahaye & Lecrosnier, Paris

Charlton M H, Hoefer P F 1964 Television and epilepsy? Archives of Neurology 2: 239–247

Chatrian G E, Lettich E, Miller L H, Green J R 1970a Pattern-sensitive epilepsy, part 1. An electrographic study of its mechanisms. Epilepsia 11: 125–149

Chatrian G E, Lettich E, Miller L H, Green J R, Kupfer C 1970b Pattern-sensitive epilepsy, part 2. Clinical changes, tests of responsiveness and motor output, alterations of evoked potentials and therapeutic measures. Epilepsia 11:151

Chatrian G E, Bergamini L, Dondey M, Klass D W, Lennox-Buchthal M, Pettersen I 1974 A glossary of terms most commonly used by clinical electroencephalographers. Electroencephalograpy and Clinical Neurophysiology 37: 538–548

Chemburkar J, Desai A D, Pabini R 1976 The sleeping pattern and incidence of seizure discharges during whole night sleep in grandmal epileptics. In: Neurology India 24: 141–147

Christodoulou G 1967 Sphenoidal electrodes. Acta Neurologica Scandinavica 43: 587–593

Connell B, Jolley D J, Lockwood P, Mercer S 1975 Activation of photosensitive epileptics whilst watching television: observations on line frequency, colour and picture content. Journal of Electrophysiological Technology 1: 281–287

Cooper R, Winter A L, Crow H J et al 1965 Comparison of subcortical, cortical and scalp activity using chronically indwelling electrodes in man. Electroencephalography and Clinical Neurophysiology 18: 217–228

Creutzfeldt O D, Watanabe S, Lux H D 1966 Relations between EEG phenomena and potentials of single cortical cells. II. Spontaneous and convulsoid activity. Electroencephalography and Clinical Neurophysiology 20: 19–37

Danesi M A 1985 Geographical and seasonal variations in the incidence of epileptic photosensitivity. Electroencephalography and Clinical Neurophysiology 61:S216

Danesi M A, Oni K 1983 Photosensitive epilepsy and photoconvulsive responses to photic stimulation in Africans. Epilepsia 24: 455–458

Darby C E, Wilkins A J, Binnie C D, De Korte R A 1980a Routine testing for pattern sensitivity. Journal of Electrophysiological Technology 6: 202–210

Darby C E, De Korte R A, Binnie C D, Wilkins A J 1980b The self-induction of epileptic seizures by eyeclosure. Epilepsia 21: 31–42

Daskalov D S 1975 Influence of the stages of nocturnal sleep on the activity of a temporal epileptogenic focus. Soviet Neurology and Psychiatry 8: 37–45

De Graaf A S, Van Wyk Kotze T J, Claassen D A 1980 Photoparoxysmal responses in the electroencephalograms of some ethnic groups of the Cape Peninsula, Electroencephalography and Clinical Neurophysiology 50: 275–281

Delange M, Castan Ph, Cadilhac J, Passouant P 1962 Study of night sleep during centrencephalic and temporal epilepsies. Electroencephalography and Clinical Neurophysiology 14:777

Delgado-Escueta A V 1979 Epileptogenic paroxysms: modern approaches and clinical correlations. Neurology 29: 1014–1022

Delgado-Escueta A V, Walsh G O 1983 The selection process for surgery of intractable complex partial seizures: surface EEG and depth electrography. In: Penry J K, Purpura D (eds) Epilepsy. Raven Press, New York pp 295–326

Delgado-Escueta A V, Mattson R H, King L et al 1981 The nature of aggression during epileptic seizures. New England Journal of Medicine 305: 711–716

Delgado-Escueta A V, Bascal F E, Treiman D M 1982 Complex partial seizures on closed-circuit television and EEG. A study of 691 attacks in 79 patients. Annals of Neurology 11: 292–300

Dement W, Kleitmann N 1957 Cyclic variations in EEG during sleep and their relation to eye movements, body mobility and dreaming. Electroencephalography and Clinical Neurophysiology 9: 673–690

Derouesne C, Golmard J L, Bilbeau H, Asselain B, Salamon 1979 Evaluation of the usual supplementary tests in neurological diagnosis. In: Alperovitch A, De Dombal F T, Gremy F (eds) Evaluation of efficacy of medical action. North Holland, Amsterdam, 179–183

De Vries J, Wisman T, Binnie C D 1981 Evaluation of a simple spike-wave recognition system. Electroencephalography and Clinical Neurophysiology 51: 328–330

Dimitrakoudi M, Harding G F A, Jeavons P M 1973 The inter-relation of the P_2 component of the V.E.R. with occipital spikes produced by patterned intermittent photic stimulation. Electroencephalography and Clinical Neurophysiology 35:416

Dondey M 1983 Transverse topographical analysis of petit mal discharges: diagnostical and pathogenic implications. Electroencephalography and Clinical Neurophysiology 55: 361–371

Doose H, Gerken H 1973 On the genetics of EEG-anomalies in childhood. IV. Photoconvulsive reaction. Neuropaediatrie 4: 162–171

Doose H, Gerken H, Hein-Völpel K F, Völzke E 1969 Genetics of photosensitive epilepsy. Neuropadiatrie 1: 56–73

Dreifuss F E (Chairman Commission on Classification and Terminology of the International League Against Epilepsy) 1981 Proposal for revised clinical and electroencephalographic classification of epileptic seizures. Epilepsia 22: 489–501

Dreifuss F E, Penry J K, Rose S W et al 1975 Serum clonazepam concentrations in children with absence seizures. Neurology 25: 255–258

Dreifuss F E, Martinez-Lage M, Roger J, Seino M, Wolf P, Dam M 1985 Proposal for classification of epilepsies and epileptic syndromes. Epilepsia 26: 268–278

Dreyer R, Wehmeyer W 1978 Laughing in complex partial seizure epilepsy: a video tape analysis of 32 patients with laughing as symptom of an attack. Fortschritte der Neurologie, Psychiatrie und ihre Grenzgebiete 46: 61–75

Driver M V, West L R, Faulk M 1974 Clinical and EEG studies of prisoners charged with murder. British Journal of Psychiatry 125: 583–587

Dumermuth G 1961 Photosensible Epilepsie und Television. Schweizerische Medizinische Wochenschrift 91: S1633–S1636

Ebersole J S 1987 Telemetered and ambulatory cassette: Review of current systems and techniques. In: Gumnit R J (ed) International conference on intensive neurodiagnostic monitoring. Raven Press, New York, 139–155

Egli M, Mothersill I, O'Kane M, O'Kane F 1985 The axial spasm – the predominant type of drop seizure in patients with secondary generalized epilepsy. Epilepsia 26: 401–415

Emerson R, D'Souza B J, Vining E P, Holden K R, Mellits E D, Freeman J M 1981 Stopping medication in children with epilepsy: predictors of outcome. New England Journal of Medicine 304: 1125–1129

Engel J 1974 Selective photoconvulsive responses to intermittent diffuse and patterned photic stimulation. Electroencephalography and Clinical Neurophysiology 37: 283–292

Engel J, Crandall P 1983 Falsely localizing ictal onsets with depth EEG telemetry during anticonvulsant withdrawal. Epilepsia 24: 344–355

Engel J, Driver M V, Falconer M A 1975 Electrophysiological correlates of pathology and surgical results in temporal lobe epilepsy. Brain 98: 129–156

Engel J, Crandall P H, Brown W J 1980 Consistent false lateralization of seizure onset with sphenoidal and scalp telemetered ictal EEG recordings in two patients with partial complex epilepsy. Electroencephalography and Clinical Neurophysiology 50:160P

Engel J, Rausch R, Lieb J P, Kuhl D E, Crandall P H 1981 Correlation of criteria used for localizing epileptic foci in patients considered for surgical therapy of epilepsy. Annals of Neurology 9: 215–224

Epstein A W, Hill W 1966 Ictal phenomena during REM

sleep of a temporal lobe epileptic. Archives of Neurology 15: 367–375

Falconer M, Kennedy W A 1961 Epilepsy due to small focal temporal lesions with bilateral spike discharging foci: a study of seven cases relieved by operation. Journal of Neurology Neurosurgery and Psychiatry 24: 205–212

Falconer M A, Serafetinides E A 1963 A follow-up study of surgery in temporal lobe epilepsy. Journal of Neurology, Neurosurgery and Psychiatry 26: 154–165

Fisher R S, Prince D A 1977 Spike-wave rhythms in cat cortex induced by parenteral penicillin. 1. Electrographic features. Electroencephalography and Clinical Neurophysiology 47: 592–596

Flor-Henry P 1969 Psychosis and temporal lobe epilepsy. Epilepsia 10: 363–395

Flor-Henry P 1972 Ictal and interictal psychiatric manifestations of epilepsy. Specific or non-specific? Epilepsia 13: 773–783

Flor-Henry P 1976 Epilepsy and psychopathology. In: Granville-Grossman (ed) Recent advances in clinical psychiatry. Churchill Livingstone, Edinburgh

Forster F M, Ptacek L J, Peterson W G, Chun R W M, Bengzon A R A, Campos G B 1964 Stroboscopic induced seizure discharges. Modification by extinction techniques. Archives of Neurology 11: 603–608

Forster F M 1977 Reflex epilepsy; behavioural therapy and conditional reflexes. Thomas, Springfield

Frantzen E, Lennox-Buchthal M, Nygaard A 1968 A longitudinal EEG and clinical study of children with febrile convulsions. Electroencephalography and Clinical Neurophysiology 24: 197–212

Frantzen E, Lennox-Buchthal M, Nygaard A, Stene J 1970 A genetic study of febrile convulsions. Neurology 20: 909–917

Gale K 1985 Mechanisms of seizure control mediated by gamma-aminobutyric acid: role of the substantia nigra. Federal Proceedings 44: 2414–2424

Garretson H, Gloor P, Rasmussen T 1966 Intracarotid amobarbital and metrazol test for the study of epileptiform discharges in man: a note on its technique. Electroencephalography and Clinical Neurophysiology 21: 607–610

Gastaut H 1948 Présentation d'une électrode pharyngée bipolaire. Revue Neurologique 80: 623–624

Gastaut H 1950 Combined photic and metrazol activation of the brain. Electroencephalography and Clinical Neurophysiology 2: 249–261

Gastaut H 1982 A new type of epilepsy: benign partial epilepsy of childhood with occipital spike-waves. In: Akimoto H, Kazamatsuri H, Seino M, Ward A (eds) Advances in epileptology (XIIIth International Symposium) Raven Press, New York, pp 19–24

Gastaut H, Tassinari C A 1966 Triggering mechanisms in epilepsy. The electroclinical point of view. Epilepsia 7: 85–138

Gastaut H, Regis H, Bostem F, Beaussart M 1960a Étude électroencéphalographique de 35 sujets ayant présenté des crises au cours d'un spectacle télévisé. Revue Neurologique 102: 533–534

Gastaut H, Poirier F, Payan H, Salamon G, Toga M, Vigouroux M H 1960b H E Syndrome: Hemiconvulsions, hemiplegia, epilepsy. Epilepsia 1: 418–447

Gastaut H, Batini C, Fressy J, Broughton R, Tassinari C A, Vitini F 1965 Étude électroencéphalographique des phénomènes épisodiques au cours du sommeil. In:

Fishgold H (ed) Sommeil de nuit normal et pathologique. Masson, Paris, pp 239–254

Geiger L R, Harner R N 1978 EEG patterns at the time of focal seizure onset. Archives of Neurology 35: 276–286

Geller M R, Geller A 1970 Brief amnestic effects of spike-wave discharges. Neurology 20: 380–381

Guerrero-Figueroa R, Darros A 1963 Experimental petit mal in kittens. Archives of Neurology 9: 297–306

Gibbs F A, Gibbs E L 1953 Atlas of Electroencephalography vol 2: Epilepsy. Addison-Wesley, Cambridge (Mass)

Gibbs F A, Gibbs E L 1960 Good prognosis of midtemporal epilepsy. Epilepsia 1: 448–453

Gibbs F A, Lennox W G, Gibbs E L 1936 The electro-encephalogram in diagnosis and in localization of epileptic seizures. Archives of Neurology and Psychiatry 36: 1225–1235

Gibbs F A, Gibbs E L, Lennox W G 1937 Epilepsy: a paroxysmal cerebral dysrhythmia. Brain 60: 377–388

Gloor P 1968 Generalized corticoreticular epilepsies. Some considerations on the pathophysiology of generalized bilaterally synchronous spike and wave discharge. Epilepsia 9: 249–263

Gloor P 1972 Generalized spike and wave discharge: a consideration of cortical and subcortical mechanisms of their genesis and synchronization. In: Petsche H, Brazier M A B (eds) Synchronization of EEG activity in epilepsies. Springer Verlag, New York, pp 382–406

Gloor P 1975 Contributions of electroencephalography and electrocorticography to the neurosurgical treatment of the epilepsies. In: Penry J K Walter R D (eds) Advances in neurology 8. Raven Press, New York, pp 59–105

Gloor P 1987 Volume conductor principles, their application to depth- and surface EEG. In: Wieser H G, Elger C E (eds) Methods of presurgical evaluation of epileptic patients. Springer, Munich, in press

Gloor P, Tsai C, Haddad F, Jasper H H 1957 The lack of necessity for sleep in the EEG or ECG diagnosis of temporal seizures. Electroencephalography and Clinical Neurophysiology 9: 379–380

Gloor P, Quesney L F, Zumstein H 1977 Pathophysiology of generalised penicillin epilepsy in the cat: The role of cortical and subcortical structures. II. Topical application of penicillin to the cerebral cortex and to subcortical structures. Electroencephalography and Clinical Neurophysiology 43: 79–94

Gloor P, Pellegrini A, Kostopoulos G K 1979 Effects of changes in cortical excitability upon the epileptic bursts in generalised penicillin epilepsy in the cat. Electroencephalography and Clinical Neurophysiology 46: 274–289

Goldensohn E S 1984 The relevance of secondary epileptogenesis to the treatment of epilepsy: kindling and mirror focus. Epilepsia 25 (suppl 2) S156–S168

Goldring S 1978 A method of surgical management of focal epilepsy, especially as it relates to children. Journal of Neurosurgery 49: 344–356

Goodridge D M G, Shorvon S D 1983 Epileptic seizures in a population of 6000: I. Demography, diagnosis and classification, and role of the hospital services. British Medical Journal 287: 641–647

Gotman J 1981 Automatic recognition of epileptic seizures in the EEG. Electroencephalography and Clinical Neurophysiology 54: 530–540

Gotman J 1982 A computer system to assist in the evaluation

of the EEGs of epileptic patients. Behavioural Research Methods 13: 525–531

Gotman J, Marciani M G 1985 Electroencephalographic spiking activity, drug levels and seizure occurrence in epileptic patients. Annals of Neurology 17: 597–603

Gotman J, Ives J R, Gloor P 1979 Automatic recognition of interictal epileptic activity in prolonged EEG recordings. Electroencephalography and Clinical Neurophysiology 46: 510–520

Gotman J, Gloor P, Quesney L F, Olivier A 1982 Correlations between EEG changes induced by diazepam and the localization of epileptic spikes and seizures. Electroencephalography and Clinical Neurophysiology 54: 614–621

Gotman J, Ives J R, Gloor P 1985 Long-term monitoring in epilepsy. Electroencephalography and Clinical Neurophysiology (suppl) 37

Gram L, Drachmann Bentsen K, Parnas J, Flachs H 1982 Controlled trials in epilepsy: a review. Epilepsia 23: 491–519

Green J B 1966 Self-induced seizures: clinical and electroencephalographic studies. Archives of Neurology 15: 579–586

Gregorie E M, Goldring S 1984 Localisation of function in the excision of lesions from the sensorimotor region. Journal of Neurosurgery 61: 1047–1055

Gross M 1983 Pseudoepilepsy. Heath, Lexington (Mass)

Gudmundsson G 1966 Epilepsy in Iceland: a clinical and epidemiological investigation. Acta Neurologica Scandinavica (suppl) 25: 4–124

Guerrero-Figueroa R, Barros A, de Balbian Verster F, Heath R G 1963 Experimental 'Petit Mal' in kittens. Archives of Neurology 9: 297–306

Guey J, Bureau M, Dravet C, Roger J 1969 A study of the rhythm of petit mal absences in children in relation to prevailing situations: the use of EEG telemetry during psychological examinations, school exercises and periods of inactivity. Epilepsia 10: 441–451

Gunn J C, Fenton G W 1971 Epilepsy, automatism and crime. Lancet 1: 1173–1176

Halász P, Dévényi E 1974 Petit mal absences in night sleep with special reference to transitional sleep and REM periods. Acta Medica Academiae Scientiarum Hungariae 31: 31–45

Harding G F A, Pearce K, Dimitrakoudi M, Jeavons P M 1975 The effect of coloured intermittent photic stimulation (IPS) on the photoconvulsive response (PCR). Electroencephalography and Clinical Neurophysiology 39:428

Harding G F A, Herrick C E, Jeavons P M 1978 A controlled study of the effect of sodium valproate on photosensitive epilepsy and its prognosis. Epilepsia 19: 555–565

Harley R D, Baird H W, Freeman R D 1967 Self-induced photogenic epilepsy. Report of four cases. Archives of Ophthalmoloty 78:730

Harris R 1972 EEG aspects of unclassified mental retardation in the brain. In: Cavanagh J B (ed) Unclassified mental retardation. Churchill Livingstone, Edinburgh

Harrison-Covello A, De Barros-Ferreira M 1975 Techniques et premiers resultats de l'enregistrement en telemetrie d'enfants presentant des elements paroxystiques (1). Revue d'Electroencephalographie et Neurophysiologie Clinique 5: 427–438

Hauser W A, Kurland L T 1975 The epidemiology of epilepsy in Rochester, Minnesota, 1935 through 1967. Epilepsia 16: 1–66

Hauser W A, Anderson E, Loewenson R B, McRoberts S M 1982 Seizure recurrence after a first unprovoked seizure. New England Journal of Medicine 307: 522–528

Heath R G 1954 Studies in schizophrenia. Harvard University Press, Cambridge (Mass)

Heath R G 1972 Pleasure and brain activity in man: deep and surface electroencephalograms during orgasm. Journal of Nervous and Mental Disease 154: 3–18

Heath R G 1975 Brain function and behaviour: emotion and sensory phenomena in psychotic patients and in experimental animals. Journal of Nervous and Mental Disease 160: 159–175

Heath R G, Mickle W A 1960 Evaluation of seven years experience with depth electrode studies in human patients. In: Ramey, O'Doherty (eds) Electrical studies on the unanesthetized brain. Hoeber, New York, pp 214–247

Hendricksen O 1986 Absence seizures: multiple and reduction of multiple drug therapy In: Schmidt D, Morselli P (eds) Intractable Epilepsy: Experimental and Clinical Aspects. Raven Press, New York, 187–193

Heppenstall M E 1944 The relation between the effects of blood-sugar levels and hyperventilation on the electroencephalogram. Journal of Neurology, Neurosurgery and Psychiatry 7: 112–118

Holmes G L 1982 Prolonged EEG and videotape monitoring in children. American Journal of Diseases of Children 136: 608–611

Holowach J, Thurston D L, O'Leary J 1972 Prognosis in childhood epilepsy: follow-up study of 148 cases in which therapy had been suspended after prolonged anticonvulsant control. New England Journal of Medicine 286: 169–174

Hopkins A, Scambler G 1977 How doctors deal with epilepsy. Lancet 1: 183–186

Huck F R, Radvany J, Avila J O et al 1980 Anterior callosotomy in epileptics with multiform seizures and bilateral synchronous spike and wave EEG pattern. Acta Neuroshirurgica (Suppl) 30: 127–135

Hughes J R 1985 Long-term clinical and EEG changes in patients with epilepsy. Archives of Neurology 42: 213–223

Hughes J R, Cayaffa J J 1973 Is the 'psychomotor variant' – 'rhythmic mid-temporal discharge' an ictal pattern? Clinical Electroencephalography 4: 42–49

Hughes J R, Grunener G 1984 Small sharp spikes revisited: further data on this controversial pattern. Clinical Electroencephalography 15: 208–213

Hunter J, Jasper H H 1949a Effects of thalamic stimulation in unanesthetized animals. Electroencephalography and Clinical Neurophysiology 1: 437–445

Hunter J, Jasper H H 1949b A method of analysis of seizure patterns. Electroencephalography and Clinical Neurophysiology 1: 113–114

Hutchinson J H, Stone F H, Davidson J R 1958 Photogenic epilepsy induced by the patient. Lancet 1: 243–245

Hutt S J, Gilbert S 1980 Effects of evoked spike-wave discharges upon short-term memory in patients with epilepsy. Cortex 16: 445–457

Hutt S J, Denner S, Newton J 1976 Auditory thresholds during evoked spike-wave activity in epileptic patients. Cortex 12: 249–257

Ishihara T and Yoshii N 1967 The interaction between paroxysmal EEG activities and continuous addition work of Uchida-Kraeplin psychodiagnostic test. Medical Journal of Osaka University 18: 75–85

Ives J R 1982a A completely ambulatory 16-channel cassette recording system. In: Stefan H, Burr W (eds) Mobile long-term EEG monitoring (Proceedings of the MLE Symposium, Bonn, 1982) Fischer, Stuttgart, pp 205–217

Ives J R 1982b Long-term EEG cassette recordings: advantages limitations and future. In: Stott F D, Raftery E B, Clement D L, Wright S L (eds) Fourth International Symposium on Ambulatory Monitoring. Academic Press, London, pp 189–194

Ives J R 1982c What time is it? Electroencephalography and Clinical Neurophysiology 54:37P

Ives J R, Woods J F 1975 4-channel 24 hour cassette recorder for long-term EEG monitoring of ambulatory patients. Electroencephalography and Clinical Neurophysiology 39: 88–92

Ives J R, Gloor P 1977 New sphenoidal electrode assembly to permit long-term monitoring of the patients' ictal or interictal EEG. Electroencephalography and Clinical Neurophysiology 42: 575–580

Ives J R, Woods J F 1980 a study of 100 patients with focal epilepsy using a four channel ambulatory cassette recorder. In: Stott F D, Raftery E B, Goulding L (eds) ISAM 1979: Proceedings of the Third International Symposium on Ambulatory Monitoring. Academic Press, London, pp 383–392

Ives J R, Thompson C J, Gloor P 1976 Seizure monitoring: a new tool in electroencephalography. Electroencephalography and Clinical Neurophysiology 41: 422–427

Jackson J H 1873 On the anatomical, physiological and pathological investigation of epilepsies. West Riding Lunatic Asylum Medical Reports, 3:315. Reprinted in: Taylor J (ed) Selected writings of John Hughlings Jackson. Hodder & Stoughton, London, pp 90–111

Janz D 1962 The grand mal epilepsies and the sleep-waking cycle. Epilepsia 3: 69–109

Jasper H H 1958 Report on the committee on methods of clinical examination in electroencephalography. Electroencephalography and Clinical Neurophysiology 10: 370–375

Jasper H H, Kershman J 1941 Electroencephalographic classification of the epilepsies. Archives of Neurology and Psychiatry 45: 903–943

Jasper H H, Droogleever-Fortuyn J 1947 Experimental studies on the functional anatomy of petit mal epilepsy. Research Publications of the Association for Research in Nervous and Mental Disorders 26: 272–298

Jasper H H, Pertuiset B, Flanigin H 1951 EEG and cortical electrograms in patients with temporal lobe seizures. Archives of Neurology and Psychiatry 65: 272–290

Jeavons P M 1969 The use of photic stimulation in clinical electroencephalography. Proceedings of the Electrophysiological Technologists Association 16: 225–240

Jeavons P M 1982 Photosensitive epilepsy. In: Laidlaw J, Richens A (eds) A Textbook of Epilepsy (2nd edition) Churchill Livingstone, Edinburgh, pp 105–211

Jeavons P M, Bower B D 1964 Infantile spasms. Clinics in developmental medicine no. 15. Heinemann, London

Jeavons P M, Harding G F A 1975 Photosensitive epilepsy. Heinemann, London.

Jeavons P M, Harding G F A, Panayiotopoulos C P, Drasdo N 1972 The effect of geometric patterns combined with intermittent photic stimulation in photosensitive epilepsy. Electroencephalography and Clinical Neurophysiology 33: 221–224

Jensen I, Larsen J K 1979 Mental aspects of temporal lobe epilepsy. Follow-up of 74 patients after resection of a temporal lobe. Journal of Neurology, Neurosurgery and Psychiatry 42: 256–265

Jones D P 1951 Recording of the basal EEG with sphenoidal electrodes. Electroencephalography and Clinical Neurophysiology 3:100

Jovaniovć U J 1967 Das Schlafverhalten der Epileptiker: I Schlafdauer, Schlaftiefe und Besonderheiten der Schṗeriodik. Deutsche Zeitschrift fü Nervenheilk. 190: 159–198

Juul-Jensen P 1964 Frequency of recurrence after discontinuance of anti-convulsant therapy in patients with epileptic seizures. Epilepsia 5: 352–363

Kaiser E 1976 Telemetry and video recording on magnetic tape cassettes in long-term EEG. In: Kellaway P, Petersen I (eds) Quantitative analytic studies in epilepsy. Raven Press, New York, pp 279–288

Kamp A 1963 Eight-channel EEG telemetering. Electroencephalography and Clinical Neurophysiology 15:164

Kamp A, Mars N J I, Wisman T 1979 Longterm monitoring of the electroencephalogram in epileptic patients. In: Amlaner C J, Macdonald D W (eds) A handbook on biotelemetry and radio tracking. Pergamon press, Oxford and New York, 499–503

Kasteleijn-Nolst-Trenité DGA, Binnie C D in preparation

Kasteleijn-Nolst-Trenité DGA, Binnie C D, Overweg J, de Korte R A 1983 Abstracts of XVth Epilepsy International Congress, Washington DC p 412

Kaufman I C, Marshall C, Walker A E 1947 Activated electroencephalography. Archives of Neurology and Psychiatry 58: 533–549

Kazamatsuri H, Kikuchi S, Jujimori M, Tokuda Y 1970 An electroencephalographic study of nocturnal sleep in the epileptic patients. Folia Psychiatrica et Neurologica Japonica 24: 1–22

Kellaway P, Frost J D 1983 Biorhythmic modulation of epileptic events. In: Pedley T A, Meldrum B S (eds) Recent advances in epilepsy. Churchill Livingstone, Edinburgh p 139–154

Kellaway P, Frost J D, Hrachovy R A 1978 Relationship between clinical state, ictal and interictal EEG discharges and serum drug levels: phenobarbital. Annals of Neurology 4:197

Kennedy W A, Hill D 1958 The surgical prognostic significance of the electroencephalographic prediction of Ammon's horn sclerosis in epileptics. Journal of Neurology, Neurosurgery and Psychiatry 21: 24–30

Kirstein L, Nilsson B Y 1977 Provokation von Spitzen im EEG mittels diffusem Licht und Lichtmustern bei epileptischen und nichtepileptischen Kranken. Zeitschrift fur Elektroenzephalographie und Verwandte Gebiete 8: 155–161

Klapetek J 1959 Photogenic epileptic seizures provoked by television. Electroencephalography and Clinical Neurophysiology 11:809

Kooi K A, Thomas M H, Mortensen F N 1960 Photoconvulsive and photomyoclinic responses in adults. Neurology 10: 1051–1058

Kostopoulos G, Gloor P 1982 A mechanism for spikewave discharge in feline penicillin epilepsy and its relationship to spindle generation. In: Sterman M B, Shouse M N, Passouant P (eds) Sleep and epilepsy. Academic Press, New York, pp 11–27

Kristensen O, Sindrup E H 1978 Psychomotor epilepsy and psychosis. Acta Neurologica Scandinavica 57: 361–377

Landolt A 1958 Serial EEG investigations during psychotic episodes in epileptic patients and during schizophrenic attacks. In: Lorenz de Haas A M (ed) Lectures on epilepsy. Amsterdam, pp 91–133

Lange L S 1961 Television epilepsy. Electroenphalography and Clinical Neurophysiology 13: 490–491

Lange H H, Lieb J P, Engel J, Crandall P 1983 Temporo-spatial patterns of pre-ictal spike activity in human temporal lobe epilepsy. Electroencephalography and Clinical Neurophysiology 56: 543–555

Laplane R, Salbreux R 1963 Les convulsions hyperpyrètiques. Revue du Praticien 13: 753–761

Lehtinen L O J, Bergstrom L 1970 Naso-ethmoidal electrode for recording the electrical activity of the inferior surface of the frontal lobe. Electroencephalography and Clinical Neurophysiology 29: 303–305

Lennox-Buchthal M A 1973 Febrile convulsions: a reappraisal. Electroencephalography and Clinical Neurophysiology (suppl) 32

Le Pestre M, Loiseau P, Larrieu E, Cohadons 1985 Stopping medication in adolescent epileptic patients (Abstracts of 16th Epilepsy International Symposium). Ciba-Geigy, Basel

Lesser R P, Dinner D S, Luders H, Morris H H 1984 Differential diagnosis and treatment of intractable seizures. Cleveland Clinic Quarterly 51: 227–240

Libo S S, Palmer C, Archibald D 1971 Family group therapy for children with self-induced seizures. American Journal of Orthopsychiatry 41: 506–508

Lieb J P, Walsh G O, Babb T L, Walter R D, Crandall P H 1976 A comparison of EEG seizure patterns recorded with surface and depth electrodes in patients with temporal lobe epilepsy. Epilepsia 17: 137–160

Lieb J P, Woods S C, Siccardi A, Crandall P H, Walter D O, Leake B (1978) Quantitative analysis of depth spiking in relation to seizure foci in patients with temporal lobe epilepsy. Electroencephalography and Clinical Neurophysiology 44: 641–663

Lieb J P, Engel J, Gevins A, Crandall P H 1981a Surface and deep EEG correlates of surgical outcome in temporal lobe epilepsy. Epilepsia 22: 515–538

Lieb J P, Engel J, Jann Brown W, Gevins A S, Crandall P H 1981b Neuropathological findings following temporal lobectomy related to surface and deep EEG patterns. Epilepsia 22: 539–549

Lieb J P, Rausch R, Engel J, Jann Brown W, Crandall P H 1982 Changes in intelligence following temporal lobectomy: relationship to EEG activity, seizure relief, and pathology. Epilepsia 23: 1–13

Lipman I J, Hughes J R 1969 Rhythmic mid-temporal discharges. An electro-clinical study. Electroencephalography and Clinical Neurophysiology 27: 43–47

Livingston S 1952 Comments on a study of light-induced epilepsy in children. American Journal of Diseases of Children 83:409

Livingston S, Torres I C 1964 Photic epilepsy: report of an unusual case and review of the literature. Clinical Pediatrics 3: 304–307

Lockard J S, Ward A A 1981 Epilepsy: a window to brain mechanisms. Raven Press, New York

Lombroso C T, Erba G 1970 Primary and secondary bilateral synchrony in epilepsy. A clinical electroencephalographic

study. Archives of Neurology 22: 321–334

Ludwig B I, Ajmone Marsan C 1975 EEG changes after withdrawal of medication in epileptic patients. Electroencephalography and Clinical Neurophysiology 39: 173–181

Lueders H, Hahn J, Lesser R L, Dinner D S, Rothner D, Erenberg G 1982 Localization of epileptogenic spike foci; comparative study of closely spaced scalp electrodes, nasopharyngeal, sphenoidal, subdural and depth electrodes. In: Akimoto H, Kazamatsuri H, Seino M, Ward A (eds) Advances in epileptology (XIIIth Epilepsy International Symposium). Raven Press, New York, pp 185–189

Maclean P D 1949 A new nasopharyngeal lead. Electroencephalography and Clinical Neurophysiology 1: 110–112

Maheshwari M C, Jeavons P M 1975 The clinical significance of occipital spikes as a sole response to intermittent photic stimulation. Electroencephalography and Clinical Neurophysiology 39: 93–95

Manson G 1974 EEG radio telemetry. Electroencephalography and Clinical Neurophysiology 37: 411–413

Marciani M G, Gotman J, Andermann F, Olivier A 1985 patterns of seizure activation after withdrawal of antiepileptic medication. Neurology 35: 1537–1543

Marcus E M, Watson C W 1966 Bilateral synchronous spike and wave electroencephalographic pattern in the cat. Interaction of bilateral cortical foci in the intact, the bilateral corticocallosal and adiencephalic preparation. Archives of Neurology 14: 601–610

Marcus E M, Watson C W, Simon S A 1968 An experimental model of some varieties of petit mal epilepsy. Electrical-behavioural correlations of acute bilateral epileptogenic foci in cerebral cortex. Epilepsia 9: 233–248

Margerison J H, Corsellis J A N 1966 Epilepsy and the temporal lobes: a clinical, electroencephalographic and neuropathological study of the brain in epilepsy, with particular reference to the temporal lobes. Brain 89: 499–530

Margerison J H, Binnie C D, McCaul I R 1970 Electroencephalographic signs employed in the location of ruptured intracranial arterial aneurysms. Electroencephalography and Clinical Neurophysiology 28: 296–306

Mars N J J, Lopes da Silva F H 1983 Propagation of seizure activity in kindled dogs. Electroencephalography and Clinical Neurophysiology 56: 194–209

Marshall C, Walker A E, Livingston S 1953 Photogenic epilepsy: parameters of activation. Archives of Neurology and Psychiatry 69: 760–765

Martins da Silva A, Aarts J H P, Binnie C D et al 1984 The circadian distribution of interictal epileptiform EEG activity. Electroencephalography and Clinical Neurophysiology 58: 1–13

Matthews W B 1964 The use and abuse of electroencephalography. Lancet 2: 577–579

Matsuo F, Knott J R 1977 Focal positive spikes in electroencephalography. Electroencephalography and Clinical Neurophysiology 42: 15–25

Mawdsley C 1961 Epilepsy and television. Lancet 1: 190–191

Maxwell R E, Gates J R, Flol M E et al 1983 Clinical evaluation of a depth electroencephalography electrode. Neurosurgery 12: 561–564

Mayersdorf A, Marshall C 1970 Pattern activation in reading

epilepsy: a case report. Epilepsia 11: 423–426

Mayersdorf A, Wilder B J 1974 Focal epileptic discharges during all night sleep studies. Clinical Electroencephalography 5: 73–87

Menini C 1976 Rôle du cortex frontal dans l'épilepsie photosensible du singe Papio papio. Journal de Physiologie 72: 5–44

Merlis J K 1970 Proposal for an international classification of epilepsies. Epilepsia 11: 114–119

Milligan N, Richens A 1981 Methods of assessment of antiepileptic drugs. British Journal of Clinical Pharmacology 11: 443–456

Milligan N, Richens A 1982 Ambulatory monitoring of the EEG in the assessment of antiepileptic drugs. In: Stott F D, Raftery E B, Clement D L, Wright S L (eds) Proceedings of the 4th International Symposium on Ambulatory Monitoring, Gent, 1981. Academic Press, London, pp 224–233

Milligan N, Dhillon S, Oxley J, Richens A 1982 Absorption of diasepam from the rectum and its effect on interictal spikes in the EEG. Epilepsia 23: 323–331

Milligan N, Oxley J, Richens A 1983 Acute effects of intravenous phenytoin on the frequency of interictal spikes in man. British Journal of Clinical Pharmacology 16: 285–289

Milstein V, Stevens J R 1961 Verbal and conditioned avoidance learning during abnormal EEG discharge. Journal of Nervous and Mental Disease 132: 50–60

Mirsky A F, Van Buren J M 1965 On the nature of the 'absence' in centrencephalic epilepsy: a study of some behavioural, electroencephalographic and autonomic factors. Electroencephalography and Clinical Neurophysiology 18: 334–348

Morrell F 1960 Secondary epileptogenic lesions. Epilepsia 1: 538–560

Morrell F, Whisler W W 1980 Secondary epileptogenic lesions in man: prediction of the results of surgical excision of the primary focus. In: Canger R, Angelieri F, Penry J K (eds) Advances in epileptology (XIth Epilepsy International Symposium). Raven Press, New York, pp 123–128

Morris H H, Lueders H 1985 Electrodes. In: Gotman J, Ives R, Gloor P (eds) Long-term monitoring in epilepsy. Electroencephalography and Clinical Neurophysiology (suppl) 37: 3–25

Morris H H, Lueders H, Lesser R L, Dinner D S 1983 Value of multiple electrodes in addition to standard 10/20 system electrodes in localizing epileptiform foci (XVth Epilepsy International Symposium, abstracts). Washington, DC.

Naquet R 1983 The clinical significance of EEG in Epilepsy. In: Nistico G, De Perri R, Meinardi H (eds) Epilepsy: An Update on Research and Therapy. Alan R Liss, New York, p 147–164

Naquet R, Louard C, Rhodes J, Vigouroux M 1961 A propos de certaines décharges paroxystiques. Leur activation par l'hypoxie. Revue Neurologique 105: 203–207

Newmark M E, Penry J K 1979 Photosensitivity and epilepsy: a review. Raven Press, New York

Niedermeyer E, Lopes da Silva F 1982 Electroencephalography. Urban & Schwarzenberg, Baltimore.

O'Kane M, O'Kane F, Mothersill I 1982 On the telemetric monitoring of ictal events. In: Stefan H, Burr W (eds) Mobile long-term EEG monitoring (Proceedings of the

MLE Symposium, Bonn, 1982). Fischer, Stuttgart, pp 137–147

Olds J 1958 Self-stimulation of the brain. Science 127: 325–323

Olivier A, Gloor P, Quesney L F, Andermann F 1983 The indications of and the role of depth electrode recording in epilepsy. Applied Neurophysiology 46: 33–36

Overweg J 1985 Antiepileptic drug withdrawal in seizure-free patients. Thesis, University of Amsterdam

Overweg J, Binnie C D 1980 Pharmacotherapy of self-induced seizures. Acta Neurologica Scandinavica (suppl) 79:98

Overweg J, Binnie C D, Oosting J, Rowan A J 1987 Clinical and EEG prediction of seizure recurrence following antiepileptic drug withdrawal. Epilepsy Research, in press

Pampiglione G 1956 Some anatomical considerations upon electrode placement in routine EEG. Proceedings of the Electrophysiological Technologists Association 7(1): 20–30

Pampiglione G, Kerridge J 1956 EEG-abnormalities from the temporal lobe studied with sphenoidal electrodes. Journal of Neurology, Neurosurgery and Psychiatry 19: 117–1292

Panayiotopoulos C P, Jeavons P M, Harding G F A 1970 Relation of occipital spikes evoked by intermittent photic stimulation to visual evoked responses in photosensitive epilepsy. Nature 228: 566–567

Panayiotopoulos C P, Jeavons P M, Harding G F A 1972 Occipital spikes and their relation to visual evoked responses in epilepsy, with particular reference to photosensitive epilepsy. Electroencephalography and Clinical Neurophysiology 32: 179–190

Pantelakis S N, Bower B D, Jones H D 1962 Convulsions and television viewing. British Medical Journal 2: 633–638

Passouant P 1967 Epilepsie temporale et sommeil. Revue Roumaine de Neurologie 4: 151–163

Passouant P, Cadillac J, Delange M 1965 Indications apportées par l'étude du sommeil de nuit sur la physiopathologie des épilepsies. International Journal of Neurology 5: 207–216

Pedley T A 1983 Differential diagnosis of episodic symptoms. Epilepsia 24: S31–S44

Penfield W, Jasper H 1954 Epilepsy and the functional anatomy of the human brain. Churchill, London

Penin H 1968 Neuartige Diagnostik und Forschungsanlagen in der Universitäts-Nervenklinik Bonn. Acta Medizinische Technologie 16: 76–78

Penry J K, Porter R J 1977 Intensive monitoring of patients with intractable seizures. In: Penry J K (ed) Epilepsy: The Eighth International Symposium. Raven Press, New York, pp 95–101

Penry J K, Porter R J, Dreifuss F E 1971 Quantification of paroxysmal abnormal discharge in the EEGs of patients with absence (petit mal) seizures for evaluation of antiepileptic drugs. Epilepsia 12: 278–279

Penry J K, Porter R J, Dreifuss R E 1975 Simultaneous recording of absence seizures with video tape and electroencephalography. A study of 374 seizures in 48 patients. Brain 3: 427–440

Perria L, Rosadini G, Rossi G F, Gentilomo A 1966 Neurosurgical aspects of epilepsy: physiological sleep as a means for focalizing EEG epileptic discharges. Acta Neurochirurgica (Wien) 14: 1–9

Polkey C E 1981 Selection of patients with chronic drug-resistant epilepsy for resective surgery: 5 years' experience. Journal of the Royal Society of Medicine 74: 574–579

Pollen D A, Perot P, Reid K H 1963 Experimental bilateral wave and spike from thalamic stimulation in relation to level of arousal. Electroencephalography and Clinical Neurophysiology 15: 1017–1028

Pond D A, Bidwell B H, Stein L 1960 A survey of epilepsy in fourteen general practices: 1. demographic and medical data. Psychiatrie, Neurologie und Neurochirurgie 63: 217–236

Porter A C 1985 Pattern sensitivity testing in routine EEG. Journal of Electrophysiological Technology 11: 153–155

Porter R J, Wolf A A, Penry J K 1971 Human electroencephalographic telemetry. American Journal of EEG Technology 11: 145–159

Porter R J, Penry J K, Lacy J R 1977 Diagnostic and therapeutic reevaluation of patients with intractable epilepsy. Neurology 27: 1006–1011

Prechtl H F R, Boeke P E and Schut T 1961 The electroencephalogram and performance in epileptic patients. Neurology 11: 296–302

Prince D A, Farrell D 1969 'Centrencephalic' spike and wave discharges following parenteral penicillin injection in the cat. Neurology 19: 309–310

Principe J C, Guedes de Oliveira P, Vaz F, Tomé A 1985 Automated event detection and characterization in EEG monitoring. Part II: Signal processing. In: Martins da Silva A, Binnie C D, Meinardi H (eds) Biorhythms and epilepsy. Raven Press, New York, pp 177–193

Prior P F, Maynard D E 1976 Recording epileptic seizures. In: Janz D (ed) Epileptology: Proceedings of the Seventh International Symposium on Epilepsy. Thieme, Stuttgart, pp 325–328

Quesney L F, Gloor P, Kratzenberg E, Zumstein H 1977 Pathophysiology of generalised penicillin epilepsy in the cat: The role of cortical and subcortical structures. I. Systemic application of penicillin. Electroencephalography and Clinical Neurophysiology 42: 640–655

Quesney L F, Gloor P, Andermann F 1981 Role of nasoethmoidal electrodes in the preoperative localization of seizure activity involving the frontotemporal convexity. Epilepsia 22: 2, 243

Quy R J, Fitch P, Willison R G 1980 High-speed automatic analysis of EEG spike and wave activity using an analogue detection and microcomputer plotting system. Electroencephalography and Clinical Neurophysiology 49: 187–189

Rabending G, Klepel H, Krell D, Rehbein D 1969 Selbstreizung bei photogener Epilepsie. Psychiatrie, Neurologie und Medizinische Psychologie 11: 427–434

Radovici A, Misirliou V, Gluckman M 1932 Epilepsie reflexe provoquée par excitations des rayons solaires. Revue Neurologique 1: 1305–1308

Rail L R 1973 The treatment of self-induced photic epilepsy. Proceedings of the Australian Association of Neurologists 9: 121–123

Ralston B L 1958 The mechanism of transition of interictal spiking foci into ictal seizure discharges. Electroencephalography and Clinical Neurophysiology 10: 217–232

Ralston B L, Papatheodorou C A 1960 The mechanism of transition of interictal spiking foci into ictal seizure discharges Part II: Observations in man. Electroencephalography and Clinical Neurophysiology 12: 297–304

Ramsay R E 1982 Clinical usefulness of ambulatory EEG monitoring of the neurological patient. In: Stott F D,

Raftery E B, Clement D L, Wright S L (eds) ISAM-GENT 1981: Proceedings of the Fourth International Symposium on Ambulatory Monitoring and Second Gent Workshop on Blood Pressure Variability. Academic Press, London, pp 234–243

Rasmussen T 1976 The place of surgery in the treatment of epilepsy. In: Morley T P (ed) Current controversies in neurosurgery. Saunders, Philadelphia, pp 463–477

Regina versus Coster 1959 The Times Law Reports 3 and 4 December

Reilly E L, Peters J F 1973 Relationship of some varieties of electroencephalographic photosensitivity to clinical convulsive disorders. Neurology 23: 1050–1057

Richter R 1960 Télévision et épilepsie. Revue Neurologique 103: 283–286

Riley T L 1983 Normal variants in EEG that are mistaken as epileptic patterns. In: Gross M (ed) Pseudoepilepsy. Heath, Lexington, pp 25–27

Riley T L, Roy A (eds) 1982 Pseudoseizures. Williams and Wilkins, Baltimore

Robin J J, Tolan G D, Arnold J W 1978 Ten-year experience with abnormal EEGs in asymptomatic adult males. Aviation, Space and Environmental Medicine 49: 732–736

Robin A, Binnie C D, Copas J B 1985 A within patients comparison of electrophysiological and hormonal responses to three types of electroconvulsive therapy. British Journal of Psychiatry 147: 707–12

Röder-Wanner U U, Wolf P, Danninger T 1985 Are sleep patterns in epileptic patients correlated with their type of epilepsy? In: Martins da Silva A, Binnie C D, Meinardi H (eds) Biorhythms and epilepsy. Raven Press, New York, pp 109–121

Rodin E A 1968 The prognosis of patients with epilepsy. Thomas, Springfield

Rodin E A, John G 1980 Withdrawal of anticonvulsant medications in successfully treated patients with epilepsy. In: Wada J A, Penry J K (eds) Advances in epileptology (The Xth Epilepsy International Symposium). Raven Press, New York, pp 183–186

Rodin E, Onuma T, Wasson J, Prozak J, Rodin M 1971 Neurophysiological mechanisms involved in grand mal seizures induced by metrazol and megimide. Electroencephalography and Clinical Neurophysiology 30: 62–72

Rodin E, Kitano H, Wasson S, Rodin M 1975 The convulsant effects of bicuculline compared with metrazol. Electroencephalography and Clinical Neurophysiology 38: 106–107

Rodin E, Kikano H, Nagao B, Rodin M 1977 The results of penicillin G administration on chronic unrestrained cats. Electrographic and behavioural observations. Electroencephalography and Clinical Neurophysiology 42: 518–527

Ross J J, Johnson L C, Walter R D 1966 Spike and wave discharges during stages of sleep. Archives of Neurology 14: 544–551

Rossi G F 1973 Problems of analysis and interpretation of electrocerebral signals in human epilepsy. A neurosurgeon's view. Brazier M A B (ed) Epilepsy, its phenomena in man. Academic Press, New York, p 259

Roubicek J, Volavka J, Matousek M 1967 Elektroencefalogram u normalni populace. Ceskoslovenska Psychiatrie 63: 14–19

Rovit R L, Gloor P, Henderson L R 1960 Temporal lobe

epilepsy – a study using multiple basal electrodes. I. Description of method. Neurochirurgia 3: 5–18

Rowan A J, Binnie C D, De Beer-Pawlikowsky N K B et al 1979 Sodium Valproate: serial monitoring of EEG and serum levels. Neurology 29: 1450–1459

Rowan A J, Overweg J, Sadikoglu S, Binnie C D, Nagelkerke N J D, Heunteler E 1980 Seizure prognosis in long-stay mentally subnormal epileptic patients: interrater EEG and clinical studies. Epilepsia 21: 219–225

Roy A 1977 Hysterical fits, previously diagnosed as epilepsy. Psychological Medicine 7: 217–273

Sato S, Dreifuss F, Penry J K 1973 The effect of sleep on spike-wave discharges in absence seizures. Neurology 23: 1335–1345

Schwab R S 1939 A method of measuring consciousness in petit mal epilepsy. Journal of Nervous and Mental Disease 89: 690–691

Schwab R S, Schwab M W, Withec D, Cock Y C 1954 Synchronized moving pictures of patients and EEG. Electroencephalography and Clinical Neurophysiology 6: 684–686

Scott D F, Furlong P F, Moffett A M, Harding G F A 1985 Is sunshine protective in photosensitive epilepsy? Electroencephalography and Clinical Neurophysiology 61: S216–S217

Seino M personal communication

Sherwin I 1981 The effect of the location of an epileptogenic lesion on the occurrence of psychosis in epilepsy. In: Koella W P, Trimble M R (eds) Temporal lobe epilepsy, mania, and schizophrenia and the limbic system. Advances in biological psychiatry 8. Karger, Basel pp 81–97

Shimazono Y, Hirai T, Okuma T, Fukuda T, Yamamasu E 1953 Disturbance of consciousness in petit mal epilepsy. Epilepsia 2: 49–55

Shinnar S, Vining E P G, Mellits E D et al 1985 Discontinuing antiepileptic medication in children with epilepsy after two years without seizures. A prospective study. New England Journal of Medicine 313: 976–980

Silverman D 1960 The anterior temporal electrode and the ten-twenty system. Electroencephalography and Clinical Neurophysiology 12: 735–737

Sindrup E 1980 Technical contributions to the differential diagnosis in epilepsy. Acta Neurologica Scandinavica (suppl) 79: 47–48

Slater F, Beard A W, Glithero E 1963 The schizophrenia-like psychoses of epilepsy. British Journal of Psychiatry 109: 95–150

Smith E B O 1982 The value of prolonged EEG monitoring to the clinician in a psychiatric liaison service. In: Stott F D, Raftery E B, Clement D L, Wright S L (eds) ISAM-GENT 1981: Proceedings of the Fourth International Symposium on Ambulatory Monitoring and Second Gent Workshop on Blood Pressure Variability. Academic Press, London, pp 162–170

So E L, Penry J K 1981 Epilepsy in adults. Annals of Neurology 9: 3–16

Soso M J, Lettich E, Belgium J H 1980 Case report: responses to stripe width changes and to complex gratings of a patient with pattern-sensitive epilepsy. Electroencephalography and Clinical Neurophysiology 48: 98–101

Spencer S S 1981 Depth electroencephalography in selection of refractory epilepsy for surgery. Annals of Neurology 9: 207–214

Spencer S S, Spencer D D, Williamson P D, Mattson R H 1981 Ictal effects of anticonvulsant medication withdrawal in epileptic patients. Epilepsia 22: 297–307

Spencer S S, Spencer D D, Williamson P D, Mattson R H 1982 The localizing value of depth electroencephalography in 32 patients with refractory epilepsy. Annals of Neurology 12: 248–253

Spencer S S, Williamson P D, Bridgers S L, Mattson R H, Ciccetti D V, Spencer D D 1985 Reliability and accuracy of localization by scalp ictal EEG. Neurology 35: 1567–1575

Sperling M R, Mendius J R, Engel J 1986 Mesial temporal spikes: a simultaneous comparison of sphenoidal, naso-pharyngeal and ear electrodes. Epilepsia 27: 81–86

Stålberg E 1976 Experiences with long-term telemetry in routine diagnostic work. In: Kellaway P, Petersén I (eds) Quantitative analytic studies in epilepsy. Raven Press, New York, pp 269–278

Stefan H, Burr W 1986 Absence signs: long term therapeutic monitoring. In: Schmidt D, Morselli P (eds) Intractable epilepsy: experimental and clinical aspects. Raven Press, New York, pp 187–193

Stefan H, Froscher W, Burr W, Hubschmann R, Penin H 1980 Diagnostik und mobile 24-Stunden-Langzeitüberwachung von Absencen unter Carbamazepinetherapie. Nervenarzt 51: 623–629

Stefan H, Burr W, Hildenbrand K, Penin H 1981 Computer-supported documentation in the video analysis of absences: preictal-ictal phenomena: polygraphic findings. In: Dam M, Gram L, Penry J K (eds) Advances in epileptology (XIIth Epilepsy International Symposium). Raven Press, New York, pp 365–373

Stefansson D B, Darby C E, Wilkins A J et al 1977 Television epilepsy and pattern sensitivity. British Medical Journal 2: 88–90

Stevens J R 1966 Psychiatric implications of psychomotor epilepsy. Archives of General Psychiatry 14: 461–472

Stevens J R 1977a The EEG spike: signal of information transmission? A hypothesis. Annals of Neurology 1: 309–314

Stevens J R 1977b All that spikes is not fits. In: Shagass, Gershon, Friedhoff (eds) Psychopathology and brain dysfunction. Raven Press, New York, pp 183–198

Stevens J R, Kodama H, Lonsbury B, Mills L 1971 Ultradian characteristics of spontaneous seizure discharges recorded by radio telemetry in man. Electroencephalography and Clinical Neurophysiology 31: 313–325

Stores G 1978 School-children with epilepsy at risk for learning and behaviour problems. Developmental Medicine and Child Neurology 20: 502–508

Storm van Leeuwen W 1982 Neuro-physio-surgery in the Netherlands since 1971. Acta Neurochirurgica 61: 249–256

Sutula T P, Sackellares J C, Miller J Q, Dreifuss F E 1981 Intensive monitoring in refractory epilepsy. Neurology 31: 243–247

Takahashi T, Tsukahara Y, Kaneda S 1980 EEG activation by use of stroboscope and visual stimulator SLS-5100. Tohoku Journal of Experimental Medicine 130: 403–409

Takahashi T, Tsukahara Y, Kaneda S 1981 Influence of pattern and red color on the photoconvulsive response and the photic driving. Tohoku Journal of Experimental Medicine 133: 129–137

Talairach J, Bancaud J 1973 Stereotactic approach to epilepsy. Progress in Neurological Surgery 5: 297–354

Talairach J, Bancaud J 1974 Stereotaxic exploration and

therapy in epilepsy. In: Vinken P J, Bruyn G W (eds) The epilepsies. Handbook of Clinical Neurology 15: 758–782

Tassinari C A, Bureau M, Dravet C, Roger J, Daniele-Natale O 1982 Electrical status epilepticus during sleep in children (ESES). In: Sterman M B, Shouse M N, Passouant P (eds) Academic Press, London, pp 465–479

Taylor D C 1972 Mental state and temporal lobe epilepsy. A correlative account of 100 patients treated surgically. Epilepsia 13: 727–765

Taylor D C 1977 Epileptic experience, schizophrenia and the temporal lobe. Mclean Hospital Journal, p 21

Tizard B, Margerison J H 1963a The relationship between generalized paroxysmal EEG discharges and various test situations in two epileptic patients. Journal of Neurology, Neurosurgery and Psychiatry 26: 308–313

Tizard B, Margerison J H 1963b Psychological functions during wave-spike discharge. British Journal of Social and Clinical Psychology 3: 6–15

Todt H 1981 Zur Spätprognose kindlicher Epilepsien: Ergbnisse einer prospektiven Längsschnittstudie. Deutsches Gesundheitswesen 30: 2012–2016

Todt H 1984 The late prognosis of epilepsy in childhood: results of a prospective follow-up study. Epilepsia 25: 137–144

Trimble M R, Perez M 1981 The phenomenology of the chronic psychoses of epilepsy. In: Koella W P, Trimble M R (eds) Temporal lobe epilepsy, mania, and schizophrenia and the limbic System: Advances in biological psychiatry 8. Karger, Basel, pp 98–105

Tükel K, Jasper H 1952 The electroencephalogram in parasagittal lesions. Electroencephalography and Clinical Neurophysiology 4: 481–494

Turski L, Cavalheiro E A, Turski W A, Meldrum B S 1986 Excitatory neurotransmission within substantia nigra pons reticulata regulates threshold for seizures produced by pilocarpine in rats. Neuroscience 18: 61–77

Van Buren J M, Ajmone Marsan C, Mutsuga N, Sadowsky D 1975 Surgery of temporal lobe epilepsy. In: Penry J K, Walter R D (eds). Advances in neurology 8. Raven Press, New York, pp 155–196

Van Egmond P, Binnie C D, Veldhuizen R 1980 The effect of background illumination on sensitivity to intermittent photic stimulation. Electroencephalography and Clinical Neurophysiology 48: 599–601

Van Heycop ten Ham M W 1980 Complete recovery from epilepsy? Discontinuation of antiepileptics after five or more seizure-free years. Huisarts en Wetenschap 23: 309–311

Van Wieringen A, Binnie C D, De Boer P T E, Van Emde Boas W, Overweg J, De Vries J (1987) Electroencephalographic findings in six antiepileptic drug trials. Epilepsy Research 3–15

Veldhuizen R, Binnie C D, Beintema D J 1983 The effect of sleep deprivation on the EEG in epilepsy. Electroencephalography and Clinical Neurophysiology 55: 505–512

Vidart L, Geier S 1967 Enregistrements teleencephalographiques chez des sujets epileptiques pendant le travail. Revue Neurologique 117: 475–480

Vignaendra V, Walsh J, Burrows S 1979 The application of prolonged EEG telemetry and videotape recording to the study of seizures and related disorders. Clinical and Experimental Neurology 16: 81–94

Wada J, Rasmussen T 1960 Intracarotid injection of sodium amytal for the lateralisation of cerebral speech dominance.

Journal of Neurosurgery 17: 266–282

Walker A E, Lichenstein R S, Marshall C 1960 A critical analysis of electroencephalography in temporal lobe epilepsy. Archives of Neurology 2: 172–182

Wallis W E 1985 Withdrawal of anticonvulsant drugs – a prospective study. Journal of Neurology (suppl) 232:260

Walter V J, Walter W G 1949 The central effects of rhythmic sensory stimulation. Electroencephalography and Clinical Neurophysiology 1: 57–86

Weir B 1964 Spikes-wave from stimulation of reticular core. Archives of Neurology 11: 209–218

Westmoreland B F, Klass D W 1981 A distinctive rhythmic EEG discharge of adults. Electroencephalography and Clinical Neurophysiology 51: 186–191

Westmoreland B F, Reiher J, Klass D W 1979 Recording small sharp spikes with depth electroencephalography. Epilepsia 20: 599–606

White J C, Langston J W, Pedley T A 1977 Benign epileptiform transients of sleep: clarification of the small sharp spike controversy. Neurology 27: 1061–1068

Wieser H G 1979 'Psychische Anfälle' und deren stereo-elektroenzephalographisches Korrelat. Zeitschrift für EEG und EMG 10: 197–206

Wieser H G 1983a Electroclinical features of the psychomotor seizure. Fischer, Stuttgart

Wieser H G 1983b Depth recorded limbic seizures and psychopathology. Neuroscience & Behavioural Reviews 7: 427–440

Wieser H G, Bancaud J, Talairach J, Bonis A, Szikla G 1979 Comparative value of spontaneous and chemically and electrically induced seizures in establishing in the lateralization of temporal lobe seizures. Epilepsia 20: 47–59

Wieser H G, Elger C E, Stodieck S R G 1985 The 'Foramen Ovale Electode': A new recording method for the preoperative evaluation of patients suffering from mesio-basal temporal lobe epilepsy. Electroencephalography and Clinical Neurophysiology 61: 314–322

Wilder B 1971 Electroencephalogram activation in medically intractable epileptic patients. Archives of Neurology 25: 415–426

Wilkins A J, Lindsay J 1985 Common forms of reflex epilepsy: physiological mechanisms and techniques for treatment. In: Pedley T A, Meldrum B (eds) Recent advances in epilepsy 2. Churchill Livingstone, Edinburgh, pp 239–271

Wilkins A J, Andermann F, Ives J 1975 Stripes, complex cells and seizures – an attempt to determine the locus and nature of the trigger mechanism in pattern-sensitive epilepsy. Brain 98: 365–380

Wilkins A J, Darby C E, Binnie C D 1977 Optical treatment of photosensitive epilepsy. Electroencephalography and Clinical Neurophysiology 43:577

Wilkins A J, Darby C E, Binnie C D 1979a Neurophysiological aspects of pattern-sensitive epilepsy. Brain 102: 1–25

Wilkins A J, Darby C E, Binnie C D, Stefansson S B, Jeavons P M, Harding G F A 1979b Television epilepsy: the role of pattern. Electroencephalography and Clinical Neurophysiology 47: 163–171

Wilkins A J, Binnie C D, Darby C E 1980 Visually-induced seizures. Progress in Neurobiology 15: 85–117

Wilkins A J, Binnie C D, Darby C E 1981 Interhemispheric differences in photosensitive epilepsy: I. pattern sensitivity thresholds. Electroencephalography and Clinical Neurophysiology 52: 461–468

Wilkus R J, Green J R 1974 Electroencephalographic investigations during evaluation of the antiepileptic agent sulthiame. Epilepsia 15: 13–25

Wilkus R J, Thompson P M 1984 Positions of sphenoidal electrodes at the beginning and end of extended EEG monitorings. Epilepsia 25:654

Williams D 1953 A study of thalamic and cortical rhythms in Petit Mal. Brain 76: 50–69

Williams D 1969 Neural factors related to habitual aggression. Brain 92: 503–520

Wolf P, Röder-Wanner U U, Brede M, Noachtar S, Sengoku A 1985 Influences of antiepileptic drugs on sleep. In: Martins a Silva A, Binnie C D, Meinardi H (eds) Biorhythms and epilepsy. Raven Press, New York, pp 137–153

Wong P K H 1985 Comparison of spike topography in typical and atypical benign rolandic epilepsy of childhood. Electroencephalography and Clinical Neurophysiology 61:S47

Wyler A R, Ojemann G A, Lettich E, Ward A 1984 Subdural strip electrodes for localizing epileptogenic foci. Journal of Neurosurgery 60: 1195–1200

Zenker C, Groh C, Roth G 1957 Probleme und Erfahrungen beim Absetzen antikonvulsiver Therapie. Neue Osterreichische Zeitschrift für Kinderheilkunde 2: 152–163

Zetterlund B 1982 Quantification of spike-and-wave episodes in 24-h tape recordings of EEG. In: Stefan H, Burr W (eds) Mobile long-term EEG monitoring (Proceeding of the MLE Symposium Bonn 1982). Fisher, Stuttgart, pp 237–244

9

Neuroradiology

B. Kendall

INTRODUCTION

The logical application of neuroradiological procedures to the study of epilepsy depends on a clear understanding of the advantages, limitations and potential morbidity of the various tests. The clinical features which influence the probability of demonstrating a causative lesion and its likely nature have been discussed in Chapter 5, and the significance of an underlying structural lesion in management and in assessment of prognosis has been stressed.

Some patients with epilepsy require no radiological study. Included in these are patients with clinically and electroencephalographically typical primary generalized seizures, in which neuropathological studies show no demonstrable underlying structural changes; and those in which clinical study resolves the nature of the lesion and decides its treatment, as, for example, most cases of uncomplicated tuberous sclerosis and disseminated known systemic neoplasm. Ideally, all other patients should have only the radiological study or selection of studies relevant to their particular treatment, preferring always the safest test if there are real alternatives. However, should it be evident that an invasive study is both necessary and likely to be sufficient, preliminary expensive and time-consuming less invasive tests should be avoided.

Neuroradiological procedures fall naturally into two groups: first, those which cause no significant discomfort to the patient, carry no risk of morbidity and do not require admission to hospital; and, secondly, those which involve injections into blood vessels or into the cerebrospinal fluid, which are unpleasant and, even in ideal

conditions, carry a small risk of permanent morbidity. In the first group, skull and chest X-ray, computer tomography (CT), magnetic resonance imaging (MRI) and isotope encephalography may be relevant to the study of epilepsy. There is no positive contraindication to the use of any or all of these procedures and the extent of their application is primarily a matter of the finance to procure the equipment and to employ a sufficient number of trained personnel to ensure an adequate service. Even with the best use of available resources, machine time tends to be limited and the study of those epileptic patients in the clinical categories which yield a relatively small number of detectable structural lesions has relatively low priority.

All neuroradiological studies need skilled radiography; the detection of slight abnormalities and the assessment of borderline normal findings is dependent on excellent technique. Good results can only be achieved when the head is completely immobile, which requires co-operating or adequately sedated patients, and the clinician should ensure that the patients whom he refers are in a suitable condition for the examination to be performed.

PLAIN RADIOGRAPHS

Plain skull radiographs are completely negative in over 85% of intracranial tumours (Hillemacher 1982) and in the presence of other significant pathology. Even abnormal appearances are frequently non-specific and rarely adequate for management. Plain skull radiographs are not a useful screening test; any patient with epilepsy requiring radiological study should first be submitted to a plain CT scan. The use of CT increased positive findings from 30% to 55% and the number of tumours detected from 5% to 10% of cases investigated when compared with all other studies, except, of course, NMR (Gastaut & Gastaut 1976) and is therefore the best widely available screening test. Where the facilities exist, this approach is both logical and economical.

Nevertheless, plain films may be made prior to referral and may reveal significant abnormalities which should be recognized. Also, skull radiographs may occasionally be useful for detailed study of bone for distinction between meningioma and other superficial intrinsic tumours shown on CT.

Raised intracranial pressure

On a good quality film there is an intact rim of cortical bone over the sella turcica in all normal cases. Raised intracranial pressure causes erosion of the inner table of the skull, which is usually first recognized by loss of part of the cortex of the sella, most frequently at the junction of the posterior wall and floor. The incidence of erosion in patients with tumours remote from the sella varies, but it is present in over 25%, reaching 44% in those studied by Mahmoud (1958); about 20% of such patients do not have papilloedema or other clinical evidence of raised intracranial pressure. Erosion of the tip of the dorsum sellae may also occur, especially when a dilated third ventricle extends down into contact; it should be noted that suprasellar tumours may cause a similar change.

Aqueduct stenosis, which may present with fits, is the commonest cause of changes in the sella characteristic of chronic hydrocephalus with enlargement of the third ventricle. Shortening of the dorsum sellae is often combined with elongation of the anterior wall of the sella and sometimes with enlargement of the anterior clinoid processes in this condition (Fig. 9.1).

When intracranial hypertension has been present since before the age of 10 years the sutures may be wider than 2 mm or have elongated interdigitations. These changes are most reliably assessed on a basal projection on which the coronal and sagittal sutures are close to the film.

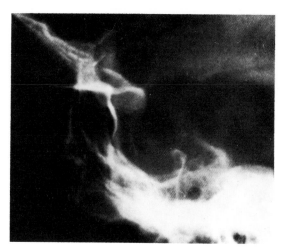

Fig. 9.1 Chronic hydrocephalus with enlargement of the third ventricle; such appearances are often due to aqueduct stenosis. Lateral radiograph of sella turcica. The dorsum sellae is short. The anterior wall of the sella is elongated.

Physiological calcification

Calcification in the pineal body and/or habenular commissure is visible on a lateral radiograph in about 60% of European adults; it is much less frequent in African and Asiatic races and in children. It is more difficult to visualize on the anteroposterior projection due to the relatively greater thickness of the frontal and occipital bones, but about 75% shown in the lateral view can be identified. Deviation of more than 2.5 mm from the midline on a straight film is usually due to displacement by a contralateral mass and rarely to ipsilateral atrophy.

Calcification in the choroid plexus of the lateral ventricles is visible in about 10% of normal adults. It is usually in the trigone region, but can be elsewhere and is not infrequently unilateral or asymmetrical. Displacement can be diagnosed definitely when the calcification is outside the range of the normal curve of the choroid plexus around the thalamus.

Plaques of ossification commonly occur in the dura lining the vault, in the falx and the tentorium. Curvilinear or circular calcified opacities are frequent in the walls of the intracavernous segments of the internal carotid artery in elderly patients. The typical shape and position of these densities facilitates recognition and distinction from significant lesions.

PATHOLOGICAL CALCIFICATION

This occurs in many conditions which may cause epilepsy. Frequently, calcification is not specific, but its appearance in a particular position may be diagnostic or it may be associated with other abnormalities making a diagnostic combination. A dense artefact may be caused by substances such as EEG paste or lacquer on the scalp and may be recognized if it is projected partly outside the line of the vault on any of the radiographs.

Tumours

Calcification is visible in 10–15% of meningiomas, sometimes outlining a considerable part of the tumour. The appearance of the calcification, and the position if close to the dura, suggests the diagnosis (Fig. 9.2), and hyperostosis at the tumour attachment or enlarged meningeal grooves leading up to it (Gold et al 1969) are confirmatory.

Calcification is visible in only 5.5% of gliomas (Kalan & Burrows 1962), being more frequent in the relatively benign tumours. Extent varies from one or two tiny or larger nodules to an irregular conglomeration of nodules or an amorphous aggregate. The most typical appearance (Fig. 9.3), which occurs in both astrocytomas and the less common oligodendrogliomas, is of one or more curvilinear streaks, suggesting gyri. Calcification in more aggressive gliomas suggests that malignant change has occurred in a more benign tumour. Hamartomas, which are most common in the temporal lobe, may show non-specific calcification indistinguishable from a glioma prior to histology.

Tuberous sclerosis

The dysplastic lesions of tuberous sclerosis often progressively calcify in older children, causing nodular and curvilinear densities. These are most frequent adjacent to the ventricular system and in the basal ganglia, though they may also occur in other sites (Fig. 9.4). Tubers may obstruct the ventricular system and cause hydrocephalus, but raised intracranial pressure is more often caused by a giant cell astrocytoma or, less commonly, other types of glioma complicating the tuberous sclerosis. CT, which is not necessary as a routine in typical tuberous sclerosis, should be performed if a tumour is suspected.

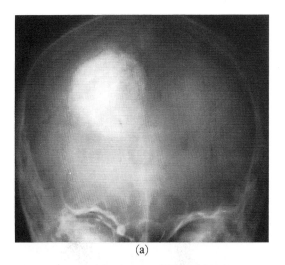

(a)

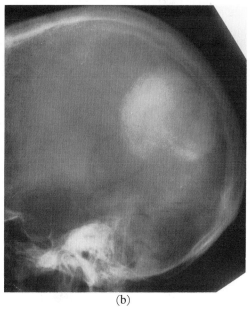

(b)

Fig. 9.2 Meningioma. Skull radiographs, **a.** antero-posterior, **b.** lateral projections. A well-defined cloud of calcification is present in the right posterior parietal parafalcine region. A prominent meningeal vascular groove ascends towards the lesion. The appearances are typical of a meningioma with calcification in psammoma bodies.

A family history, typical skin manifestations or associated mental retardation has usually suggested the diagnosis. However, these features are sometimes absent (Kingsley et al 1986) and the disease may present with predominant manifestations in other systems. Mesodermal dysplasia may occur in any of the bones, but especially in those of the

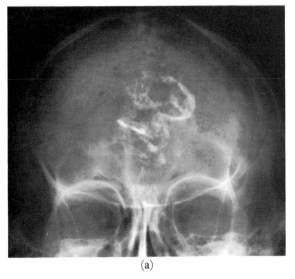

(a)

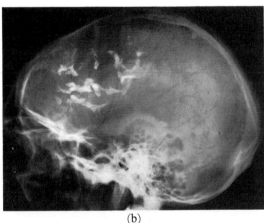

(b)

Fig. 9.3 Oligodendroglioma. Skull radiographs, **a.** antero-posterior, **b.** lateral projections. Gyriform curvilinear calcification is shown in the medial frontal region on both sides of the midline but extending further to the left. The appearances are typical of a glioma. This was an oligodendroglioma but an astrocytoma can cause similar findings.

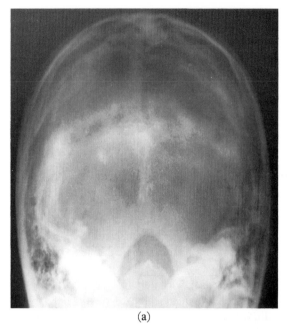

(a)

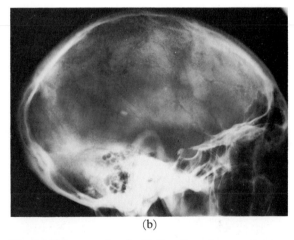

(b)

Fig. 9.4 Tuberous sclerosis. Skull radiographs, **a.** antero-posterior, **b.** lateral projections. Nodular calcification is present in the region of the basal ganglia on the right side and near the inferior surface of the right cerebellar hemisphere. Several sclerotic areas are present in the bones of the vault.

hands and feet which may show subperiosteal cysts or nodular cortical thickening (Fig. 9.5) and sclerotic areas, as well as pressure erosion from subungual fibromas. In a small number of patients the lungs are infiltrated by smooth muscle, which causes a honeycomb appearance (Fig. 9.6); spontaneous pneumothorax is a not infrequent complication of this condition. Multiple renal hamartomas, which are usually bilateral, may be shown by intravenous pyelography or computed tomography.

Intestinal polyps have also been described.

Inflammatory disease

Non-specific calcification occurs occasionally in necrotic tissues, such as old abscesses, and multiple nodules may be present in dead parasites. The history and examination will usually have

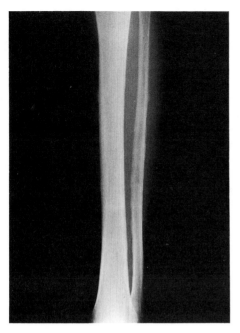

Fig. 9.5 Tuberous sclerosis. Nodular cortical thickening is shown on the tibia and fibula due to the typical periosteal nodes.

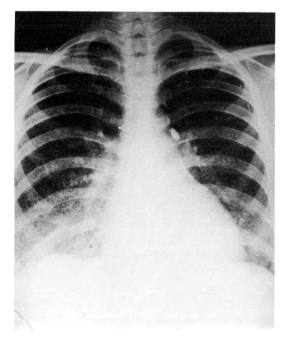

Fig. 9.6 Tuberous sclerosis. Chest radiograph. There is dense, fine, nodular and reticular shadowing, most marked towards the bases due to smooth muscle infiltration of interstitial tissues of lung.

suggested the diagnosis and the radiological findings are confirmatory.

Combined linear cortical and curvilinear basal ganglia calcifications occur in about 40% of cases of congenital toxoplasmosis and are diagnostic in the clinical context (Fig. 9.7). Hydrocephalus, due to occlusion of the aqueduct or outlets of the fourth ventricle, or microcephaly, secondary to destruction of brain substance, occur in about 50% of patients.

Cysticercosis may be confirmed by showing calcified cysts in skeletal muscles. These are typically about 3 mm in diameter and 12–15 mm in length and lie parallel to the axis of the muscle fibres. They may be recognized incidentally in the neck and shoulder girdle muscles on films of the skull and chest, but are usually searched for in soft tissue films of the thighs (Fig. 9.8). Calcification is much less frequent in cerebral cysts and is then usually confined to the scolices, which show as nodules about 3 mm in diameter. Racemose cysticerci may obstruct the fourth or third ventricle and cause raised intracranial pressure.

Tuberculomas, which are the most common intracranial masses presenting in India, may also show non-specific nodular calcification.

A very rare but typical calcification, usually in the parietal regions, occurs in the walls of cysts in the cerebral form of paragonamiasis. The disease is endemic in the Far East and may be found in visitors from Korea, China and Formosa.

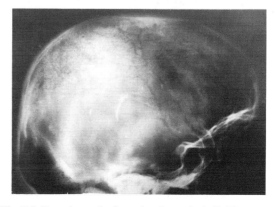

Fig. 9.7 Toxoplasmosis. Lateral radiograph skull. There are multiple nodular calcified lesions. Curvilinear calcification is present in one of the basal ganglia. The dorsum sellae is shortened due to erosion by an enlarged third ventricle, secondary to aqueduct obstruction caused by the disease.

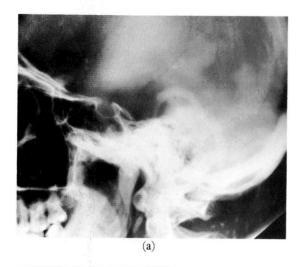

(a)

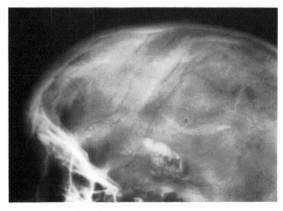

Fig. 9.9 Angiomatous malformation. Lateral radiograph skull. Aggregates of nodular calcification are shown in the inferior frontal region, confirmed by angiography to be in an angiomatous malformation.

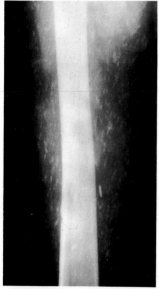

Fig. 9.8 Cysticercosis. **a.** Lateral radiograph skull. Fusiform nodular shadows of calcified cysticerci are present in the neck and facial muscles. Nodular calcification is also present in the frontal and parietal lobes in the scolices of intracerebral cysticerci. **b.** Right thigh. Large number of fusiform calcified lesions due to cysticerci in the muscles.

Vascular lesions

Fine curvilinear or nodular calcification is visible in about 15% of intracranial arteriovenous malformations (Fig. 9.9). It usually occurs in the walls of abnormal veins, forming large ring shadows, but it can also be deposited within old haemorrhages. Meningeal arteries may contribute to the blood supply of the malformation; enlargement of foramina transmitting vessels and of vascular grooves and channels in the cranial vault may support the diagnosis.

In the Sturge-Weber syndrome, characteristic sinuous double lines of calcification are laid down in superficial layers of the atrophic cortex underlying the meningeal angioma, which is usually in the occipital and posterior parietal regions (Fig. 9.10). Calcification is visible on radiographs in only 50–60% of cases; it may be seen as early as 18 months of age and tends to increase in density up to adult life. The calcification is shown more frequently and earlier in life on computed tomograms (Fig. 9.30).

New bone formation

Localized thickening of the inner table of the skull is commonly present at the site of attachment of a meningioma arising near bone. It is sometimes associated with sclerosis of the adjacent diploe and less frequently with bone formation on the outer table of the skull. Enlarged and tortuous meningeal vascular channels extending to the hyperostosis and pits in the bone where small branches from the meningeal and scalp arteries perforate the vault to supply a tumour are useful confirmatory signs (Fig. 9.11). Diploic vascular channels may also be prominent, but it is difficult to assess their significance because of considerable normal variation. Bone reaction to solitary metastases from carcinoma of the prostate or breast may simulate a meningioma; extension of sclerosis into the facial skeleton and evidence of metastases elsewhere may be helpful in differential diagnosis.

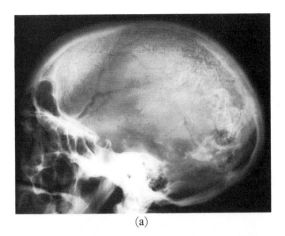

(a)

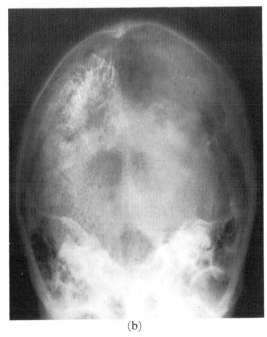

(b)

Fig. 9.10 Sturge-Weber syndrome. Skull radiographs,
a. lateral, **b.** anteroposterior. Typical gyriform calcification is
shown in the right posterior parietal and occipital regions.
The right side of the vault is considerably smaller than the
left due to associated hemiatrophy.

Meningioma-en-plaque (Fig. 9.12) typically
produces a more diffuse and extensive sclerosis of
bone, usually at the base, which could be confused
with fibrous dysplasia. The latter condition is not
a cause of epilepsy and would present an incidental finding. In its sclerotic form the bone is
thickened and has a more homogeneous chalky
density without trabecular structure.

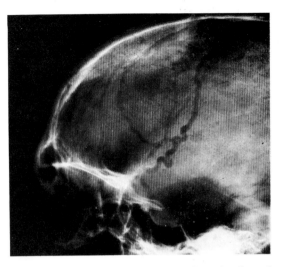

Fig. 9.11 Frontal convexity meningioma. Lateral radiograph
skull. Localized sclerosis is evident in the superior frontal
region. The groove of the middle meningeal artery is
enlarged and tortuous and branches of the vessel extend to
the abnormal bone. Large diploic vascular shadows are also
shown.

Bone erosion

Meningioma may cause isolated erosion much less
frequently than sclerosis and hyperostosis. The
erosion is usually ill defined, more extensive on
the inner aspect of the vault and is usually
accompanied by enlarged meningeal channels, a
combination which strongly suggests the diagnosis
(Fig. 9.13).

Metastases and the rare primary tumours of
bone commence within and more extensively
destroy the diploe; they are an unusual cause of
fits.

Pressure from any subadjacent mass, such as a
superficial glioma, a meningioma or a porencephalic or arachnoid cyst, may cause smooth
corticated erosion of the inner table or localized
expansion of the contiguous vault.

Cerebral hypoplasia or atrophy

Because growth of the skull is secondary to that
of the brain, which takes place mainly in the first
two years of life, radiological findings are most
marked when a lesion occurs early in this period.
Lesser changes may be seen with severe damage
occurring later but before puberty.

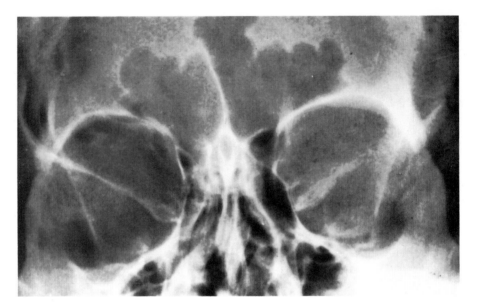

Fig. 9.12 Meningioma. Antero-posterior radiograph skull. There is sclerosis of the left lesser and greater wings of the sphenoid.

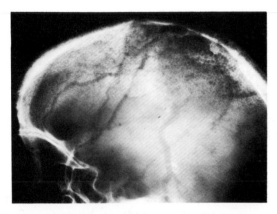

Fig. 9.13 Meningioma. Lateral radiograph skull. There is a large area of erosion high in the right parietal and fronto-parietal regions. Enlarged meningeal vascular channels extend towards the abnormal region large diploic venous channels drain away from it. The changes are diagnostic of a meningioma, but bone lysis is much less common than sclerosis in these tumours.

With predominantly unilateral involvement, the capacity of the skull over the smaller hemisphere or lobe is less than that of the corresponding normal region. This may be recognized by flattening of the curve of the vault, elevation of the base with enlargement of the air cavities in the sinuses or mastoids and deviation of the falx or superior sagittal sinus towards the affected side.

The skull overlying the atrophic lobe is usually thickened, but it may be thinned and smooth if there is a wide fluid-filled space between the atrophic lesion and the vault. CT has reduced the importance of such secondary signs by assessing atrophic lesions more directly.

Post-traumatic epilepsy

Linear fractures, especially in young patients, usually heal without trace. In depressed fractures, deformity remains and occasionally bone fragments may be shown projecting medially from the edge and are commonly associated with scarring in the adjacent brain. When the dura is torn the fracture line may widen (Fig. 9.14). In adults, this is associated with leptomeningeal cyst formation, which may cause bevelled thinning of the overlying inner table extending beyond the limits of the fracture. In children, such erosion may also be due to herniated brain, often damaged with cystic change, as well as extracerebral cyst in direct contact with the bone. The cyst sometimes herniates through the fracture line and expands under the scalp, eroding the outer table. Widening fractures, especially in children, are usually associated with underlying brain damage.

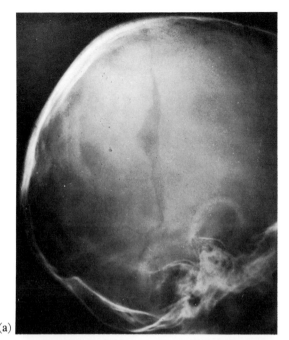

(a)

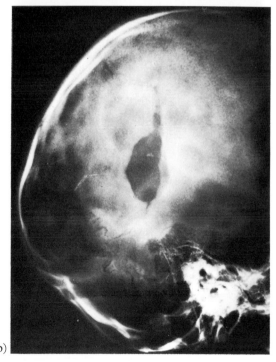

(b)

Fig. 9.14 Post-traumatic leptomeningeal cyst. Lateral radiographs skull. History of trauma three months previously. **a.** A linear cleft, wider than a fresh fracture, is shown extending vertically in one of the parietal bones. **b.** Seven months later; the fracture is considerably wider. At surgery a tear in the dura and arachnoid was associated with the leptomeningeal cyst.

A meningocerebral cicatrix may result in expansion of the ventricle or formation of an arachnoid cyst and, even in the absence of fracture, trauma may cause sufficient contusion and haemorrhage to induce formation of an intracerebral cyst. Any of these conditions may incite thinning or lateral bulging of the adjacent inner table; in all of them the pathology is well shown by CT.

CHEST RADIOGRAPHS

The importance of the lungs as a mirror of systemic disease needs no emphasis and a chest radiograph is indicated in every patient with an intracranial mass. Bronchial carcinoma is by far the most common tumour metastasizing to the brain. Cerebral metastases from other neoplasms are frequently associated with pulmonary metastases. Occasionally, unsuspected cardiac lesions or chronic lung disease is first revealed on routine chest films.

COMPUTED TOMOGRAPHY (CT)

On radiographs it is only possible to recognize four densities equivalent to bone or calcification, soft tissue or water, fat and air. CT (Hounsfield 1973) gives quantitative readings of tissue density sufficiently sensitive to discriminate between the various intracranial tissues and to distinguish white and grey matter.

The method requires that the patient lies completely still for periods of between a few seconds and a minute, varying with the type of machine, while a series of contiguous sections of the head are scanned through their edges from a large number of directions by a finely collimated beam of X-rays with a thickness of 1–13 mm. The intensity of the beam is measured before and after transmission through the head, and many readings are taken in each direction from different angles. A computer assembles the data from each section and, using a mathematical method, reconstructs it as a matrix of cells (pixels) between 0.75 mm^2 and 1.5 mm^2. A digital value approximating to within 0.5% of the average radiation absorption within the tissues contained in the volume (voxel) represented by each particular pixel is printed out in a corresponding location. This results in a format simulating the structure and shape of the original section. An image with corresponding points of variation of light intensity is displayed simultaneously on a cathode ray tube and can be recorded on film.

The most radio-opaque tissue encountered normally in the skull is compact bone and the least is air; these have been made the extremes of a scale of absorption, in which water has assigned zero value, and they have been arbitrarily designated +1000 and −1000 Hounsfield units (HU) respectively. Most of the normal intracranial soft tissues fall into the narrow range of 0 to +60 HU. The grey matter of the cortex, caudate nucleus and thalamus has a value of +36 to +56 HU and can be distinguished (Fig. 9.15) from white matter, which ranges between +20 and +38 HU with an average value of +24 HU. The pineal gland is always evident and the glomeri of the choroid plexuses are usually outlined by calcification, frequently of insufficient density to be shown on the skull radiographs. Cerebrospinal fluid, with an absorption value of between 0 and +10 HU, is shown and gives a close approximation to the configuration of the ventricles and intracranial subarachnoid spaces (Synek et al 1979); because of their small height, the normal temporal horns may be averaged out by brain tissue unless thin sections (4–5 mm) are used.

Intravenous contrast media do not cross the blood-brain barrier, so that the attenuation of the normal brain is only increased by a relatively small amount (up to 5 HU) by contrast medium retained within the bloodstream. Repeat scanning following intravenous injection of contrast medium causes an increase in the attenuation of some lesions, which is sometimes related to vascularity (see Fig. 9.21) but more commonly to interstitial extravasation of contrast medium within the lesion or to abnormalities induced in the blood-brain barrier by neoplasm, inflammation or tumour; it may also occur transiently in the cerebral cortex following prolonged status epilepticus in the absence of any other factor. Enhancement is particularly valuable for defining pathologies which are of similar attenuation to adjacent normal or oedematous brain, but it may be useful

in other cases also, to obtain the maximum information about the morphology of an abnormality. Cystic or necrotic regions, which do not increase in attenuation, are more evident when surrounding tumour tissue (see Fig. 9.23) or an abscess capsule is enhanced.

Apart from being more generally available, CT has a few advantages over magnetic resonance imaging; these include:
1. Currently shorter acquisition time, which is significant for examining restless patients
2. No limitation in the presence of magnetic materials in critical situations, such as clips on aneurysms or equipment influenced by radio waves such as cardiac pacemakers.
3. Demonstration of detail in cortical bone and calcified lesions

Pathological findings

The incidence of CT scan abnormalities is markedly influenced by clinical selection. It is increased particularly by the presence of interictal focal signs and/or focal EEG abnormalities with slowing and spikes. A coarse approximation of the incidence of CT abnormalities may be gained from analysis of the series in which the cases were either unselected (Cala et al 1977, McGahan et al 1979, Dellaportas et al 1982, Weisberg et al 1984) or only partly selected on clearly defined criteria (Bogdanoff et al 1975, Langenstein et al 1979, Yang et al 1979). Normal examinations or varying degrees of diffuse atrophy will be found in between 65% and 86%, and focal atrophy, hemiatrophy or porencephaly in between 4% and 16%. In most series, neoplasm and infarct have an incidence of just under 5%, and angiomatous malformation or aneurysm about 1.5%. In general, surgically amenable lesions are rarely detected by CT in patients without neurological symptoms or signs after more than five years' duration of seizures (Jabbari et al 1978, Gilsanz et al 1979).

Though primary generalized epilepsy was associated with CT abnormality in 10% of cases in two series (Gastaut & Gastaut 1976, Langenstein et al 1979), other series, which fit the general experience of these cases, differ from matched controls in only two respects. First, patients who had

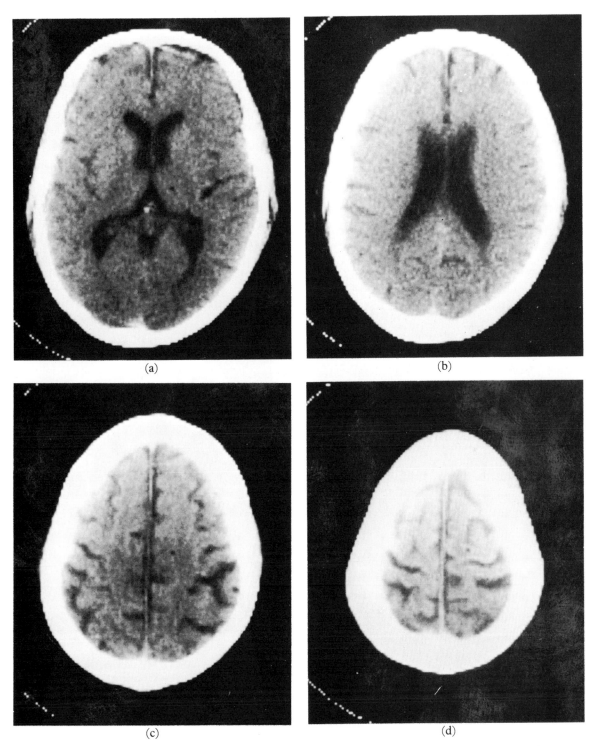

(a)

(b)

(c)

(d)

Fig. 9.15 Diffuse cerebral atrophy. Plain CT, section level **a.** third ventricle, **b.** upper parts of lateral ventricles, **c,d.** near vertex. The cerebrospinal fluid in the ventricular system and cerebral subarachnoid spaces is of lowest attenuation (0–6 H) and outlines the enlarged lateral ventricles, upper part of the third ventricle and the Sylvian and interhemispheric fissures. The hemispheric and capsular white matter (20–38 H) can be distinguished from the grey matter (36–56 H) in the basal ganglia and thalami.

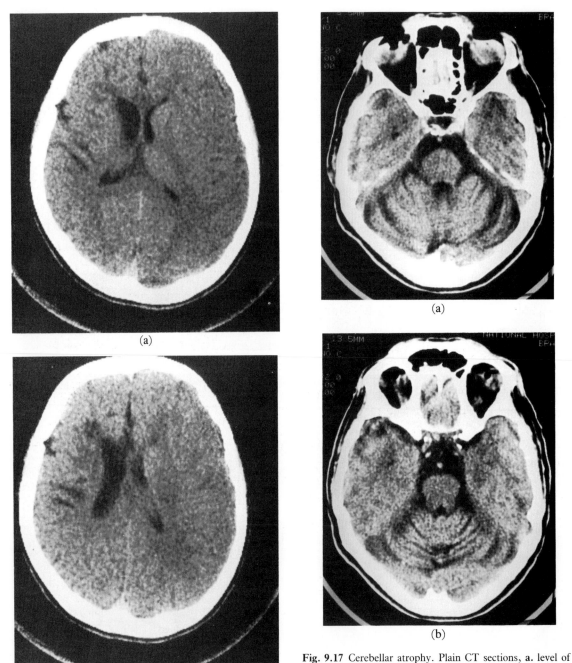

(a)

(b)

(a)

(b)

Fig. 9.16 Right hemiatrophy. **a,b.** Plain CT scan. The right hemicranium is relatively small and the vault is thickened on this side. The right lateral ventricle, the Sylvian fissure and some sulci over the frontal lobe are enlarged. There is a small region of low density in the deep frontal white matter suggesting focal accentuation of the brain damage associated with the hemiatrophy.

Fig. 9.17 Cerebellar atrophy. Plain CT sections, **a.** level of fourth ventricle, **b.** including superior surface of cerebellar hemisphere. The fourth ventricle is prominent. The basal cisterns around the brainstem are enlarged and the curvilinear dilated superior cerebellar sulci are evident.

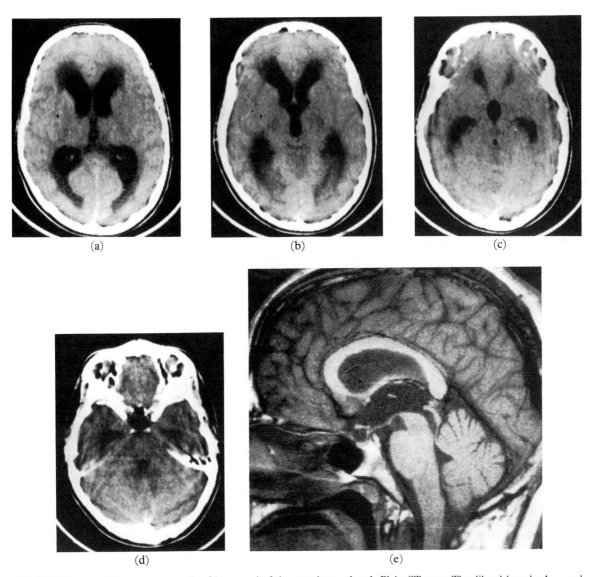

(a)　　　　　　　　　　(b)　　　　　　　　　　(c)

(d)　　　　　　　　　　(e)

Fig. 9.18 Hydrocephalus due to stenosis of lower end of the aqueduct. **a,b,c,d.** Plain CT scan. The dilated lateral **a,b,c.** and third **b,c.** ventricles and aqueduct **c** are evident. The fourth ventricle **d.**, basal cisterns and cortical sulci are not dilated. There is periventricular lucency around the frontal horns due to transependymal passage of CSF. Aqueduct stenosis (different case). **e.** MRI, sagittal section, spin echo sequence. Note the distension of the third ventricle and of the aqueduct, which tapers to stenosis at its lower end. The fourth ventricle and the basal cisterns are normal.

suffered episodes of status had a higher incidence of cerebral atrophy; and, secondly, prolonged therapy with phenytoin was occasionally associated with cerebellar cortical atrophy (Weisberg et al 1984).

In secondary generalized epilepsy atrophic changes are shown in CT in almost two-thirds of cases (Gastaut & Gastaut 1976) and an incidence

of over 90% has been recorded (Langenstein et al 1979).

The incidence of CT abnormalities is high in simple partial seizures, ranging in different series between 52% and 68%, with tumours between 4% and 38%. It is also high in complex partial seizures, ranging between 40% and 70%. Mesial temporal sclerosis is the most common abnor-

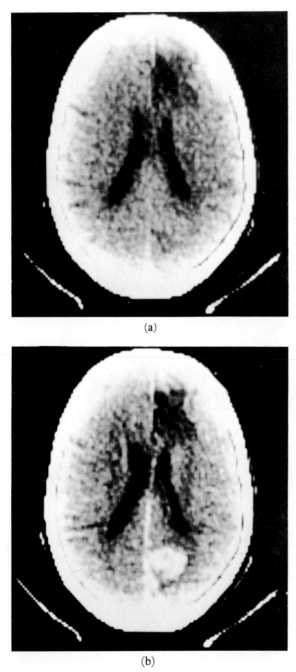

(a)

(b)

Fig. 9.19 Cerebral infarcts right frontal and parieto-occipital regions. **a.** Plain scan. Low attenuation lesions with no mass effect. **b.** After intravenous contrast medium. There is enhancement of the low attenuation parieto-occipital region and of the surrounding brain indicating injury to the blood–brain barrier and that the infarct is recent. There is no enhancement in the frontal infarct which is probably mature.

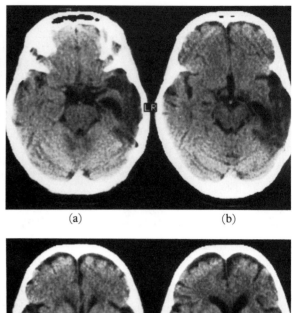

(a)   (b)

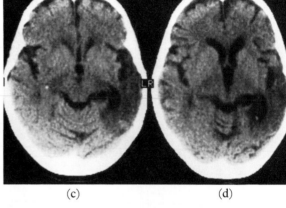

(c)   (d)

Fig. 9.20 Temporal lobe epilepsy associated with mature infarction of left temporal lobe. Plain CT scan, **a,b,c,d.** contiguous sections. There is low density involving most of the left temporal lobe. The left temporal horn is dilated. There is also more diffuse atrophy, with enlargement of cortical sulci and of the wings of the ambient cistern.

mality; it is caused by ischaemia which may be precipitated by prolonged seizures and is usually manifested as temporal lobe atrophy with dilatation of the temporal horn.

Jabbari et al (1979) reported one case with an arcuate non-enhancing region of calcification on CT. Small focal tumours, including hamartomas, have formed up to 23% of lobectomized series (Falconer & Serafetinides 1963).

The age of onset of the epilepsy considerably influences the incidence and nature of the abnormalities shown; the incidence is highest with onset during the first year of life when it may reach

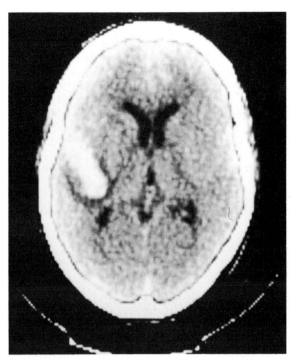

Fig. 9.21 Intracerebral haematoma. Plain CT. There is a region of homogeneously increased attenuation in the posterior part of the left temporal lobe, with well-demarcated, surrounding low attenuation blood clot from a recent haemorrhage. There is also subarachnoid blood, which accounts for the increased attenuation around the interhemispheric fissure anteriorly.

68%, with a high proportion due to congenital malformations and perinatal brain damage (Yang et al 1979). Focal seizures after the first year and under 15 years of age are uncommonly due to tumour (Holowach et al 1958); CT infrequently reveals an abnormality of therapeutic significance (Bachman et al 1976), though, occasionally, low density changes in white matter or symmetrical calcification may suggest an unsuspected metabolic disturbance. When epilepsy arises in adult life, the incidence of abnormality increases with the age of onset (Bogdanoff et al 1975, Collard et al 1976, Scollo-Lavizzari et al 1977). Under the age of 35, head injury and neoplasm predominate; between 35 and 60 cerebral ischaemia and neoplasm are dominant, with an increasing proportion of metastases; and after 55, ischaemia (Shorvon et al 1984) and degenerative disorders are most likely.

Epilepsy follows in over 12% of severe head injuries but it is rare after more minor injuries. If CT does not reveal a focal lesion soon after injury, epilepsy is unlikely; with intracerebral haemorrhage the incidence is about one in six; if both intra- and extracerebral haemorrhage are present there is about a 75% incidence of epilepsy.

Atrophy and hydrocephalus

Generalized atrophy (Fig. 9.15), hemiatrophy (Fig. 9.16), focal atrophy, cortical and cerebellar atrophy (Fig. 9.17), hydrocephalus (Fig. 9.18) and cystic expansion of the ventricles or subarachnoid space are all clearly shown. The more minor degrees of temporal atrophy associated with temporal sclerosis may be difficult to recognize, even with high resolution scanners. They are better shown with MRI, as are most midline stenosing lesions causing hydrocephalus (Figs. 9.18, 9.40).

Vascular lesions

A typical infarct (Fig. 9.19) shows as a low attenuation region involving both the white and cortical grey matter, sometimes wedge-shaped when in the distribution of a cortical artery and without displacement of adjacent structures. In a recent infarct, however, oedema may cause the lesion to appear ill defined and may produce swelling sufficient to suggest the possibility of a tumour. Repeat study may distinguish by showing a tendency of the infarct to resolve towards more typical appearances within a few days. The blood–brain barrier is damaged by infarction and enhancement may occur until recovery has taken place, which is usually less than one month after the stroke but can be up to ten weeks.

Sometimes infarction is patchy and shows as multiple regions of decreased attenuation in the distribution of the occluded vessel. An old infarct may eventually form a cyst, which causes a sharply defined region of low attenuation, or a scar, associated with focal atrophy (Fig. 9.20). Small vessel disease commonly causes patchy ill-defined low density in the deep white matter of the cerebral hemispheres, sometimes associated

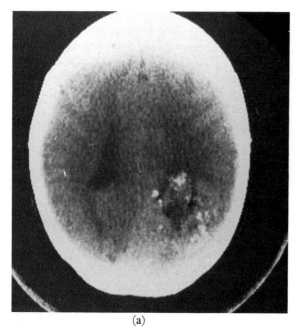

(a)

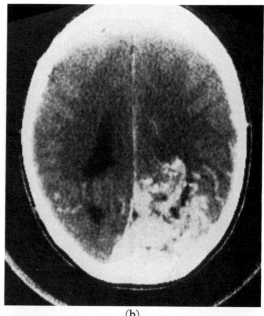

(b)

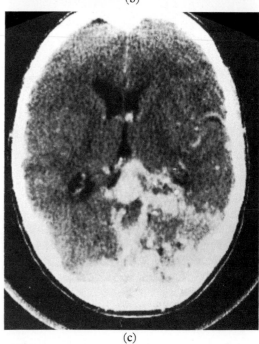

(c)

with lacunar infarcts in the white matter and/or corpus striatum.

The attenuation of clotted blood (+56 to + 80 HU), which increases as serum is expressed from the contracting clot, is sufficiently characteristic for recognition of a recent haematoma (Fig. 9.21). Angiography is necessary if details of a causative lesion need to be defined, but large aneurysms and angiomas can be identified by re-examination by CT after intravenous injection of contrast medium (Fig. 9.22). As a clot is absorbed, its density diminishes and eventually a cyst or scar, indistinguishable from an old infarct, may remain.

Tumours

Neoplasms cause mass effect of very variable degree, resulting in displacement and deformity of normal structures due to compression and/or invasion. The attenuation of tumour tissue varies markedly with the cellular structure; it may be higher, similar to or less dense than the adjacent brain. Calcified, haemorrhagic, cystic, necrotic and oedematous regions in or adjacent to tumours may cause superadded focal variations of the basic attenuation due to the tumour tissue. Grade I and II gliomas (Fig. 9.23) are mainly of diminished

Fig. 9.22 Angiomatous malformation. **a.** Plain scan. There is high density lesion containing nodular calcification in the left parieto-occipital lobes. **b.** Scan at similar level after intravenous contrast medium. There is marked enhancement throughout the high density region, with a suggestion of curvilinear structures in the anterior part of the enhancement. **c.** At a lower level after enhancement. The rounded and curvilinear structures, due to enlarged arteries supplying veins draining the angiomatous malformation, are evident.

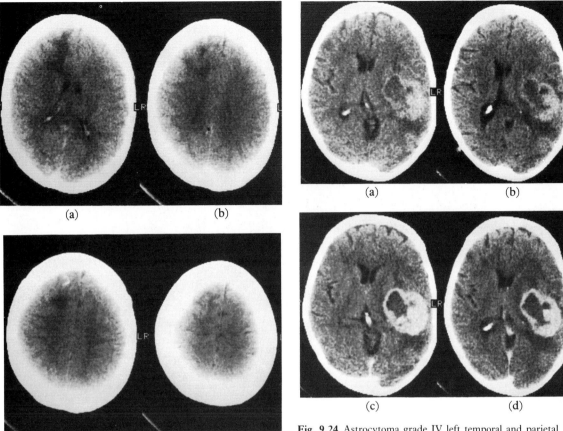

(a)　　　　　　　　(b)

(a)　　　　　　　　(b)

(c)　　　　　　　　(d)

(c)　　　　　　　　(d)

Fig. 9.23 Low grade oligodendroglioma. **a,b,c,d.** Plain scan, contiguous sections. There is extensive low density in the right frontal white matter with a little calcification peripherally near the anterior convexity. The sulci over the right hemisphere are not visible but there is no other evidence of mass effect.

Fig. 9.24 Astrocytoma grade IV left temporal and parietal lobes. Plain scan. Mass attenuation enclosing a low attenuation region which is compressing the anterior horn and trigone of the left lateral ventricle. **b,c,d.** After intravenous contrast medium, irregular ring enhancement around the low attenuation region, which was necrotic. There is also low attenuation due to oedema posterior to the mass.

attenuation, apart from calcified foci which are often evident when they are not visible on radiographs. Higher grade gliomas (Fig. 9.24) tend to be heterogeneous, usually of diminished but with areas of similar or greater attenuation than the normal white matter, and over 90% enhance with intravenous contrast medium. Fluid in cystic and necrotic parts is common in malignant tumours; it may be suspected if there are low density non-enhancing regions, but can only be definitely diagnosed when there are fluid levels. The edges of gliomas are commonly poorly demarcated although, occasionally, they may be well defined.

Metastases (Fig. 9.25) usually show as relatively well-defined masses which may vary in density from less to greater than normal brain. Not uncommonly there is irregular central necrosis and there may be extensive oedema of the adjacent white matter. If a solitary lesion is revealed, re-examination after intravenous contrast injection may show further metastases and is especially important if surgery is contemplated.

Meningiomas (Fig. 9.26) show as peripheral well-defined enhancing masses of greater attenuation in most instances, but sometimes isodense with brain. Associated cerebral oedema is not uncommon and, if the section does not pass through a small meningioma, the oedema may be mistaken for a primary intrinsic pathology.

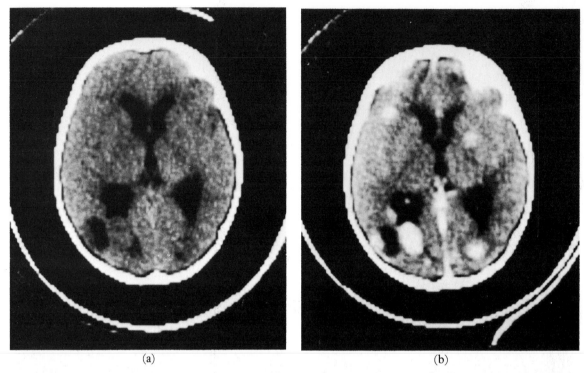

(a)   (b)

Fig. 9.25 Multiple metastases. **a.** Plain scan, **b.** same section after intravenous contrast medium. There are masses of both low and brain attenuation most of which enhance. One in the left occipital region remains of low attenuation centrally and could be cystic. There is low attenuation due to oedema around some of the lesions, but this is rather less than is usual with metastases. There is moderate hydrocephalus, which was caused by further metastases in the posterior fossa partially obstructing the fourth ventricle.

Developmental abnormalities

Dermoids, which may be recognized from the presence of fat which is less dense than water, rarely present with epilepsy; but epidermoids more frequently do so when they encroach on the surfaces of the cerebral hemispheres. They are usually low density masses, without surrounding oedema. There may be some calcification and occasionally enhancement in the capsule (Fig. 9.27).

The more gross brain malformations, in which the ventricles show characteristic anatomical deformities (Fig. 9.28), are evident on both CT and MRI imaging. Neuronal migration and proliferation abnormalities arising at a later time in development, in which the brain substance itself may be mainly affected, are more exactly depicted by MRI but may be diagnosed by CT. They include heterotopia, in which nodules of grey matter may deform the lateral ventricular outlines, expand within the white matter or

thicken the cortex causing refractory seizures, and sometimes microcephaly. Lissencephaly (Fig. 9.29), in which epilepsy is combined with retardation and microcephaly, is characterized by absence of part or all of the cerebral mantle so that the cortex appears smooth. The ventricles are large, the subarachnoid space generally wide and the Sylvian fissures shallow and wide. Recessively inherited microcephaly shows no abnormality on CT or MRI.

The dysplastic lesions of tuberous sclerosis are usually evident by the second year of life and are most commonly associated with infantile spasms. The typical subependymal, partly calcified tubers, which do not enhance, are most frequent (Fig. 9.30). Parenchymal and subcortical lesions may also be calcified, of low attenuation or less well defined. When these are solitary manifestations (Fig. 9.31) a definite CT diagnosis may not be possible, but should be recognized as consistent in the presence of clinical signs of tuberous

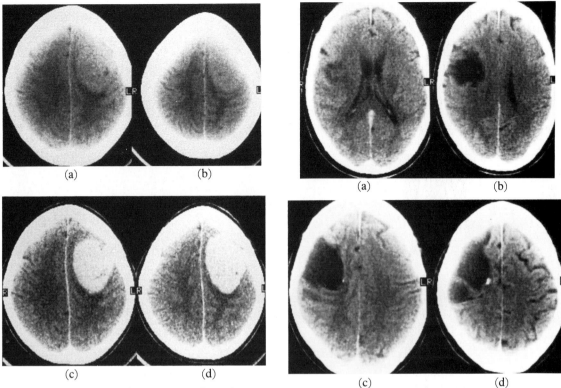

Fig. 9.26 Meningioma. **a,b.** CT above level of lateral ventricles. There is a peripheral area of increased density in the left frontal region due to a meningioma, with diminished density due to intracerebral oedema posterior to it. **c,d.** Following intravenous contrast medium, there is marked uniform enhancement of the meningioma.

Fig. 9.27 Epidermoid **a,b,c,d.** Enhanced scan. There is a low density mass adjacent to the right frontal convexity. There is a small nodule of calcification in its medial margin and there is a little enhancement along the medial margin of the mass, possibly in the adjacent cortex. There is no oedema. The sulci over the right hemisphere are occluded and the roof of the lateral ventricle is depressed.

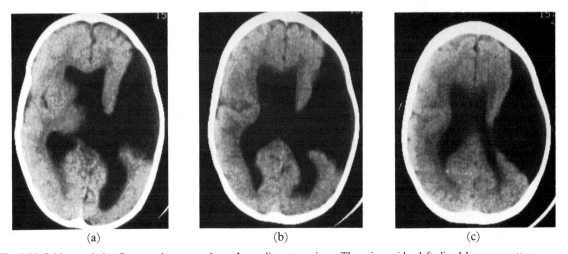

Fig. 9.28 Schizencephaly. Computed tomography, **a,b,c.** adjacent sections. There is a wide cleft, lined by grey matter, extending through the right cerebral hemisphere and linking the body of the ventricle with the subarachnoid space. The septum pellucidum is absent and parts of the margins of the dilated lateral ventricles are slightly irregular, suggesting heterotopia.

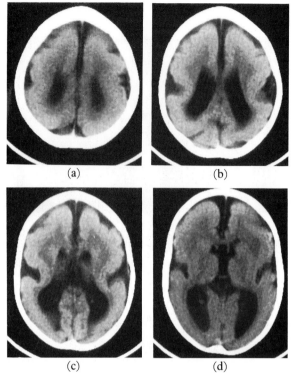

(a)   (b)

(c)   (d)

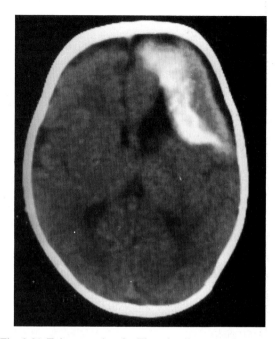

Fig. 9.31 Tuberous sclerosis. There is a large, partly calcified tuber occupying the anterior half of the left frontal lobe and associated with ventricular dilatation and dilatation of the subarachnoid space overlying it.

Fig. 9.29 Lissencephaly. Computed tomography, **a,b,c,d.** adjacent sections. The subarachnoid space is wide and outlines the abnormally smooth cortex and the shallow Sylvian fissures. The lateral and third ventricles are dilated. The septum pellucidum is absent.

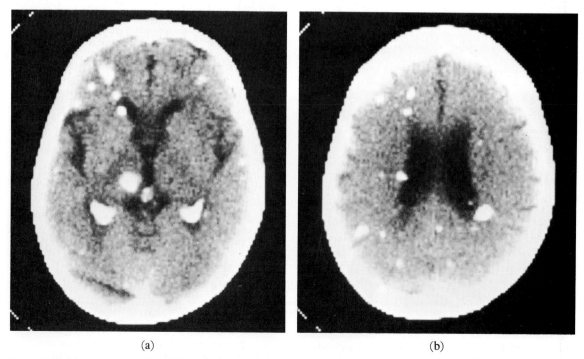

(a)   (b)

Fig. 9.30 Tuberous sclerosis. Plain CT, sections at the level of **a.** third ventricle, **b.** upper parts of bodies of lateral ventricles. There are multiple calcified paraventricular and intraparenchymal tubers. There is also physiological calcification in the pineal gland and the choroid plexuses of the lateral ventricles.

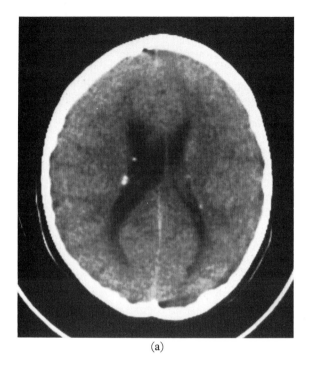

(a)

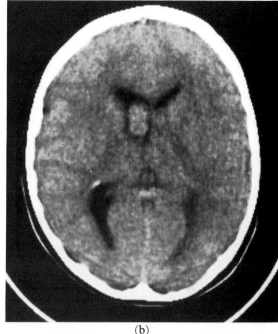

(b)

sclerosis (Kingsley et al 1986). Enhancing nodules in tuberous sclerosis are usually due to giant cell astrocytomas or occasionally to other types of glial tumours. The former are most commonly found in the region of the foramina of Monro and tend to cause obstructive hydrocephalus (Fig. 9.32).

In Sturge-Weber the subcortical calcification is shown earlier and is usually much more extensive than on skull radiographs. Abnormal enhancement occurs in affected cortex and atrophy causes enlargement of the adjacent subarachnoid space and/or ventricle (Fig. 9.33).

Inflammatory disease

Though a typical abscess is a clinical diagnosis, confirmed on CT by the presence of a relatively thin, even approximately isodense enhancing ring with a low density centre and surrounding oedema, it is an unusual cause of isolated epilepsy. However, about one-third of abscesses are atypical. These are often due to low grade organisms, sometimes in immune deficient patients. They tend to cause irregular, uneven ring or nodular enhancement on CT, with little or no central low density and relatively less oedema.

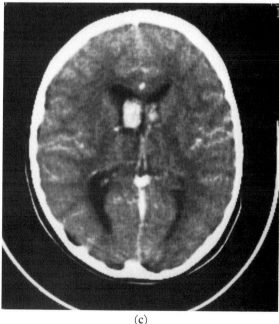

(c)

Fig. 9.32 Tuberous sclerosis, with giant cell astrocytoma. **a,b.** Plain scan. There are calcified tubers around the lateral ventricles. There are isodense masses impinging on the anterior horns of the lateral ventricles from the regions of the heads of the caudate nuclei. There is minimal dilatation of the right lateral ventricle. **c.** Similar level to **b.** after intravenous contrast medium. There is homogeneous enhancement of the tumours.

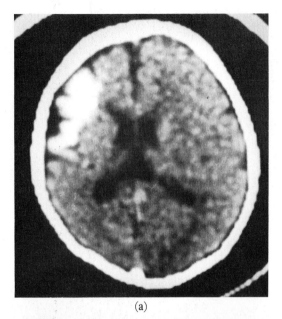

(a)

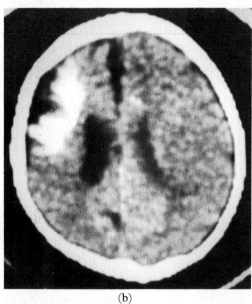

(b)

Fig. 9.33 Sturge-Weber syndrome. **a,b.** Plain scan. There is extensive calcification around the periphery of the right frontal lobe due to the Sturge-Weber syndrome but calcification was not visible on the skull radiographs. There is right sided hemiatrophy.

Tuberculomas and other granulomas are usually isodense with brain, but may be of lower density. About 40% show some calcification. There is homogeneous or irregular ring enhancement in the lesions and a variable amount of surrounding oedema, but generally less than with acute inflammatory lesions (Fig. 9.34).

Convulsions are commonly precipitated by cysticerci within the brain parenchyma at the stage when they have died and provoked granuloma formation (Fig. 9.35). Convulsions may continue at a later stage also, when the larva has undergone fibrosis and calcification (Fig. 9.8).

Hydatid cysts commonly present as slow-growing mass lesions, but convulsions occur in about 50% of cases. The CT findings are typical: a large unilocular, well-defined mass of water density, without contrast enhancement or adjacent oedema unless the cyst has burst.

Herpes encephalitis causes low density and brain swelling with predilection for the temporal lobes, which is usually evident on CT by the end of the first week of the illness and at an earlier stage on MRI. Focal haemorrhagic changes are not infrequent and patchy enhancement is usual. Early treatment may avoid the extensive brain damage which was frequently associated with considerable and rapidly progressive atrophy. In most other encephalitic illnesses, MRI is the imaging modality of choice; though CT may show brain swelling, brain density often remains normal throughout the illness (Fig. 9.36).

Antenatal infection, with toxoplasma, cytomegalic inclusion virus, rubella or herpes simplex, causes necrosis of brain tissue, which may calcify (Fig. 9.37), and atrophy leading to microcephaly, retardation and epilepsy. Cytomegalic inclusion and, less frequently, rubella cause linear calcification around the margins of the dilated ventricles. In toxoplasmosis similar changes may occur but more often there is nodular and curvilinear calcification in brain substance. Necrosis involving the aqueduct may cause hydrocephalus and surface lesions may be associated with subdural effusions resulting in macrocrania.

Carefully performed CT will detect some abnormality in about 98% of supratentorial tumours, infarcts and intracerebral haemorrhages and in most atrophic lesions. In most cases, the nature of the lesion can be suggested and in a considerable proportion its exact pathology can be predicted. In a recent analysis, 6.5% of cases diagnosed as glioma on CT were proven to be benign (Kendall et al 1979); so when CT findings

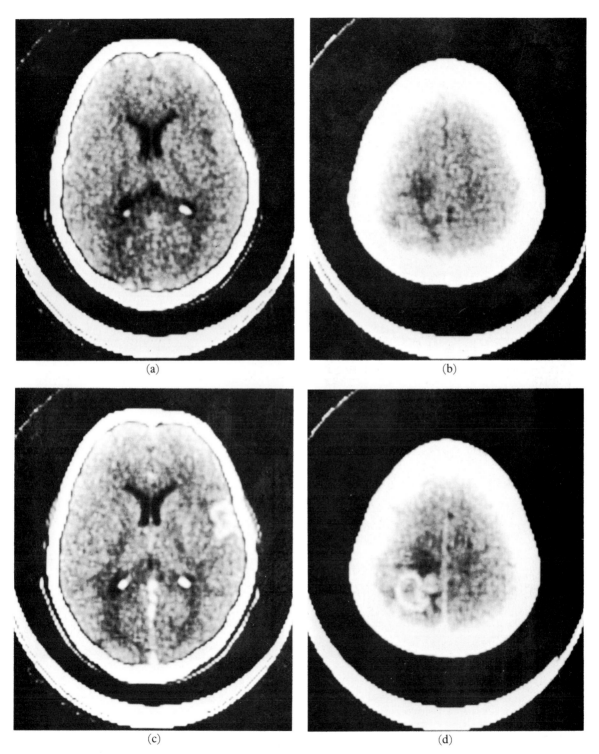

(a)

(b)

(c)

(d)

Fig. 9.34 Tuberculomas. Plain CT sections, at levels of **a.** frontal horns, **b.** at the vertex. **c,d.** Same sections after intravenous contrast medium. There are multiple lesions in the right fronto-temporal and left parietal regionis. Some are isodense with brain and others of slightly higher attenuation; all show enhancement, mostly peripheral, homogeneous in the medial right parietal region. The patient is an Asian with pulmonary tuberculosis and the lesions responded to antituberculous chemotherapy.

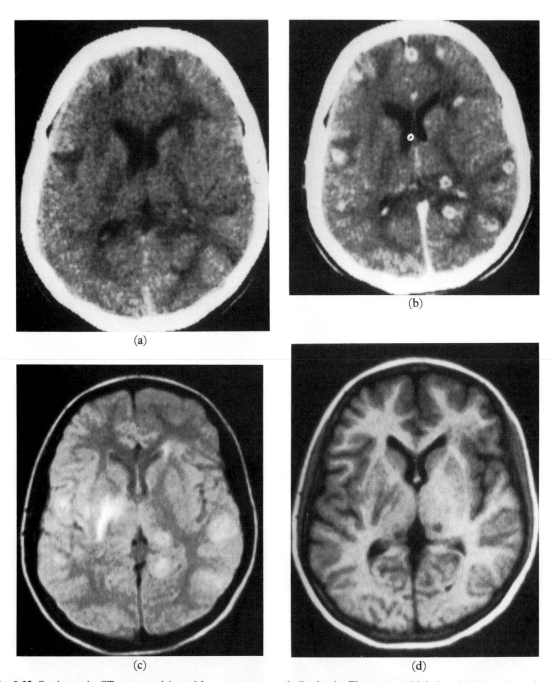

(a)

(b)

(c)

(d)

Fig. 9.35 Cysticercosis. CT scan, **a.** plain and **b.** postcontrast at similar levels. There are multiple low density regions of white matter oedema, and within or impinging on these are isodense nodules in both white and grey matter showing small ring or, occasionally, homogeneous enhancement due to granuloma formation. Some of the isodense nodules contain a high density dot representing the scolex in a cysticercus. MRI, **c.** spin echo (TR1600, TE60) and **d.** inversion recovery (TR1000, T1500) sequences. The oedematous regions give high signal in **c.** and some of the cysticerci give discrete low signal regions in **d.** Rather unusually, the abnormalities on MRI are less extensive than those shown on CT.

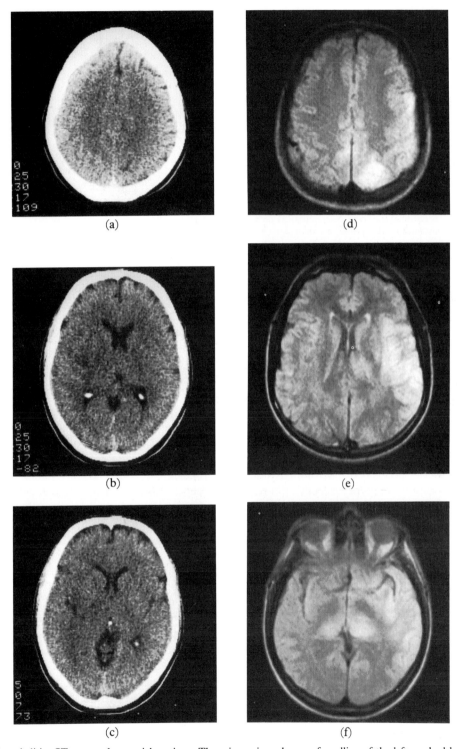

(a)

(b)

(c)

(d)

(e)

(f)

Fig. 9.36 Encephalitis. CT scan, **a,b,c.** serial sections. There is a minor degree of swelling of the left cerebral hemisphere (reader's left) with compression of the left lateral ventricle and cortical sulci. No focal abnormality. There was no abnormal enhancement. MRI, **d,e,f.** similar sections; spin echo sequence. The left hemisphere (reader's right) swelling is evident and there is increased signal from the left thalamus, occipital lobe and left temporal and parietal cortex.

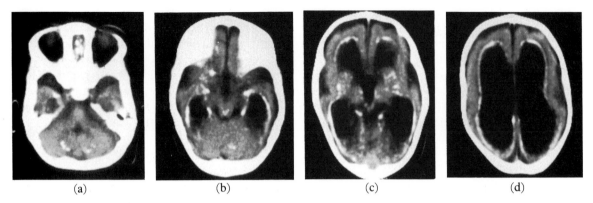

(a)   (b)   (c)   (d)

Fig. 9.37 Intra-uterine cytomegalic inclusion virus infection. Presented with retardation, epilepsy and microcrania.
a,b,c,d. Plain CT scan sections. There is irregular calcification, mainly around the dilated lateral and third ventricles but also within the brain substance. The cerebral mantle is narrow, the subarachnoid space is wide and the vault is thick due to atrophy.

favour a malignancy their compatibility with a benign lesion should always be considered.

MAGNETIC RESONANCE IMAGING

In magnetic resonance, image production is by fourier transformation of spatially coded signals produced by sensitive nucleons, which have been induced to resonate by the application of radio-frequency pulses.

Certain nucleons, by virtue of their structure, possess a magnetic moment and will therefore gyrate around the axis of a strong external magnetic field with a frequency specific for each type of nucleon. Each gyrating nucleon produces an oscillatory magnetic field and therefore induces a radio signal. If the gyrating nucleons are brought into phase, by absorption of energy induced by the application of a short external radio signal at the same frequency as the gyrating nucleons, they will produce a recordable evanescent radio signal as they lose the energy and dephase. The energy is lost by the nucleons in realigning with the magnetic field and between each other during the dephasing process. The time taken for each of these processes has considerable influence on signal strength. They are referred to as relaxation times and designated T_1 and T_2 respectively. Signal strength is also particularly influenced by the number of sensitive nucleons, movement or flow of the nucleons within or through the

magnetic field and the strength of the field. The method has some major advantages over computer tomography.

1. Ionizing radiation is not involved and, with field strengths of under 2 Tesla, the method appears to lack biological hazard. It can therefore be performed when indicated and repeated as often as necessary on clinical criteria alone. Ferro magnetic implants or foreign bodies which could move in the high magnetic field, and certain types of pacemaker which are activated in the radio-frequency field, are contraindications.

2. Each of the several parameters which influence signal intensity on magnetic resonance images can be made the dominant factor reflected in the contrasting tissues in a particular image. Variations of pulse sequence produces a series of images in which differential contrast between normal brain and different pathological processes can be accentuated. Certain lesions commonly isodense with brain on CT and, in a proportion of which CT has been completely normal, can be demonstrated by MRI; amongst these are demyelinating diseases, encephalitis (Fig. 9.36), including both direct infection, as in subacute sclerosing panencephalitis and postinfective demyelination, ischaemic lesions and low-grade gliomas (Brant Zawadski et al, 1983). In a recent study (Laster et al 1985) of 34 patients with complex partial seizures of more than 5 years duration, in which pre- and post-infusion CT

scans were negative, MRT revealed focal structural temporal lobe lesions of potential surgical therapeutic significance in four cases (11.7%); a cryptic arteriovenous malformation and a glioma were excised from two of these. The not uncommon declaration of a progressive organic lesion on a follow-up CT scan in patients with previously CT negative focal epilepsy (Young et al 1982) also supports the view that MRI will provide a worthwhile positive yield in such cases.

Magnetic resonance imaging generally shows the pathological processes revealed by CT to be more extensive (Fig. 9.37) and differences in internal structure may be more clearly defined on some of the MR sequences.

3. The image plane in MRI, being determined electronically, is unrestricted by the mechanical constraints which influence computed tomography. For practical purposes, sagittal images can only be produced on CT by computer reformatting of multiple thin sections made in an accessible plane, a process which is accompanied by loss of resolution and is also distorted by any patient movement; vertical plane images are particularly valuable in assessing the brainstem, high convexity and parasagittal regions, relationship of abnormalities to the Sylvian fissure (Fig. 9.38) and transcallosal extension of tumour. Multiple planar imaging is also useful for more exact volumetric assessment.

4. Bone-induced artefacts limit the value of CT, especially for the diagnosis of small lesions adjacent to the skull base. The mode of acquisition of MRI and the lack of signal from cortical bone has made it particularly valuable for detection of such lesions in the posterior fossa and adjacent to the floor of the middle fossa (Fig. 9.39) (Young et al 1983).

The very long T_1 of normal cerebrospinal fluid (CSF) can be used to delineate clearly the margins of the subarachnoid space and ventricles. The higher water content of the grey matter is associated with prolongation of T_1 relative to that of white matter; grey matter therefore gives a relatively lower signal when a short pulse repetition time is used and the intensity increases and eventually exceeds that from white matter as the repetition time is increased. The clear delineation of the cerebrospinal spaces (Fig. 9.40) and of the white and grey matter facilitates localization of intra-axial, extra-axial and intraventricular masses. The change in signal induced by blood flow allows flow-dependent sequences to be formulated for visualization of the major blood vessels. This is a further facility in aiding localization of intra- and extra-axial masses and defining relationships of critical structures.

In general, the most significant information from MRI has been the anatomical distribution of pathology. Tissue specific characterization is much less common, as might be expected, since increase in water content in general causes prolongation of the T_1 and T_2 relaxation time regardless of whether it is caused by oedema, infarction, encephalitis or demyelination. The paramagnetic effects of iron in methaemoglobin and of haemosiderin in subacute and chronic haematomas (Fig. 9.41), and of melanin in melanoma metastases, are manifested in short T_1 relaxation; and triglyceride fat in lipomas and teratomas, as well as in subcutaneous and intermuscular fat planes, is also characterized by a very short T_1 relaxation time. The lack of signal from rapidly flowing blood with increasing signal with turbulence and slow flow clearly delineates and specifically characterizes aneurysms and angiomatous malformations and their connecting vessels when flow-dependent sequences are used (Fig. 9.42).

The lack of clear demarcation between some tumour margins and adjacent brain or surrounding oedema has proved to be a limitation of MRI. This has been a feature of some metastases, infiltrating malignant gliomas, haemangioblastomas and meningiomas. Certain paramagnetic ions, of which gadolinium is currently the most suitable, can be administered in biocompatible compounds such as DTPA, which are, for practical considerations, retained within the normal blood–brain barrier but penetrate the disrupted barrier in damaged brain tissue and through the permeable capillaries of tumours and granulation tissue, in a very similar fashion to iodide contrast media used in CT and technetium DTPA used in radionucleide studies (Carr et al 1984). The paramagnetic agents shorten T_1 relaxation time and thus enhance contrast on T_1 weighted sequences; not

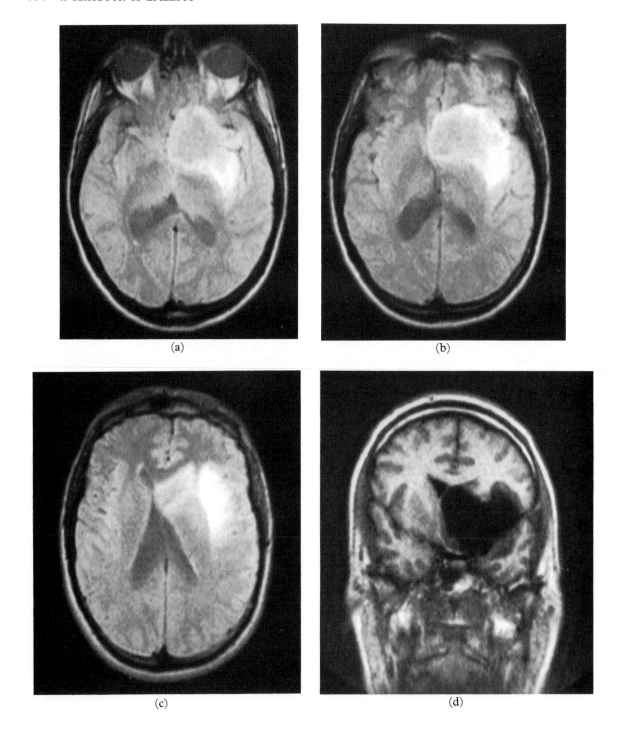

(a)

(b)

(c)

(d)

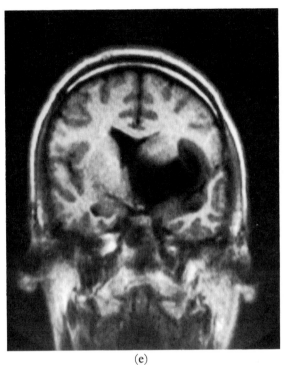

(e)

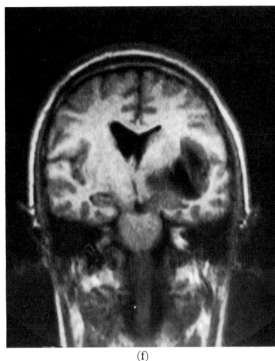

(f)

Fig. 9.38 Deep frontal-hypothalamic glioma. MRI, **a,b,c.** spin echo sequences (TR1500, TE60), contiguous sections. The tumour gives rise to a high signal. Involvement of the deep frontal region and hypothalamus is evident and the tumour extends across the midline. Precise relationship to the Sylvian fissure is difficult to assess in these sections. **d,e,f.** Inversion recovery sequence (TR2100, T1500), contiguous coronal sections. The upper border of the tumour extends up to the frontal horn and the lower margin extends across the Sylvian fissure, to involve the superior temporal white matter and hippocampal gyrus.

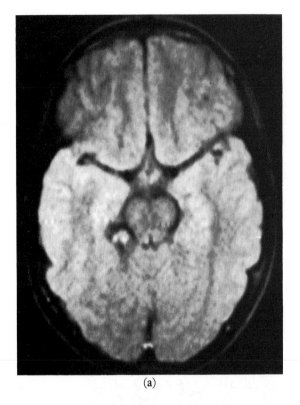

(a)

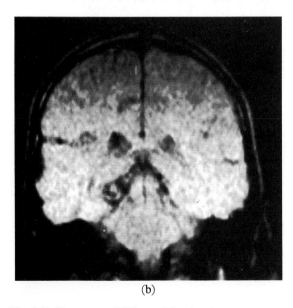

(b)

Fig. 9.39 Hamartoma. MRI, **a.** axial; spin echo sequence. High signal mass protruding from medial surface of right temporal lobe. **b.** Coronal; inversion recovery sequence. The relation of hamartoma to medial surface of temporal lobe and upper border of tentorium is shown.

only is the tumour demarcated but details of its structure tend to be better defined.

Loculated CSF, as within arachnoid cysts or porencephaly (Fig. 9.43), is distinguished by signal intensities close to those of the rest of the cerebrospinal fluid. The T_1 relaxation time shortens when protein concentration is increased (Brant Zawadski et al 1985), as within cystic or necrotic regions of tumours, though it is still generally longer than that of the solid tissues. Haemorrhagic changes are characterized by relatively short T_1 relaxation times (Fig. 9.41).

Calcification gives no signal on MRI and may be suspected for this very reason on a combination of T_1 and T_2 weighted images. However, calcification, hyperostosis and bone erosion are, in general, better revealed by CT, at least in the supratentorial compartment. Currently, the relatively long acquisition time of MRI imposes a limitation on its value for examination of restless and unco-operative patients.

If no abnormality is shown on computed tomography or magnetic resonance imaging, it is unlikely that other investigations will show a significant lesion in patients suffering from well-controlled epilepsy and no other symptoms.

ISOTOPE ENCEPHALOGRAPHY

Computed tomography or magnetic resonance imaging give more exact localization and more specific information in a much wider range of conditions than does isotope encephalography. Also, computed tomography is a simpler routine than detailed gamma encephalography performed over a period of hours. Consequently the latter has been replaced, and only when CT and MRI are not available is isotope encephalography a useful screening test for those important conditions in which isotope uptake is usually increased.

Most departments use a simple technique, employing a modern gamma camera and the isotope ^{99m}Tc, which combines the advantages of easy standardization and availability with a half-life of six hours. Both lateral, anterior and posterior views are necessary to obtain images in both planes of all regions of the brain, and for

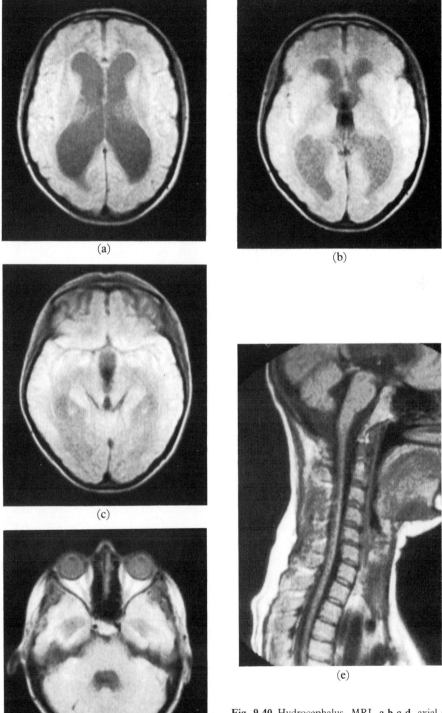

(a)

(b)

(c)

(d)

(e)

Fig. 9.40 Hydrocephalus. MRI, **a,b,c,d.** axial sections,
e. sagittal section; spin echo sequence. Communicating
hydrocephalus. There is enlargement of the whole ventricular
system and of the basal cisterns. There is slightly increased
signal around the ventricles due to transependymal passage
of fluid into the adjacent brain substance.

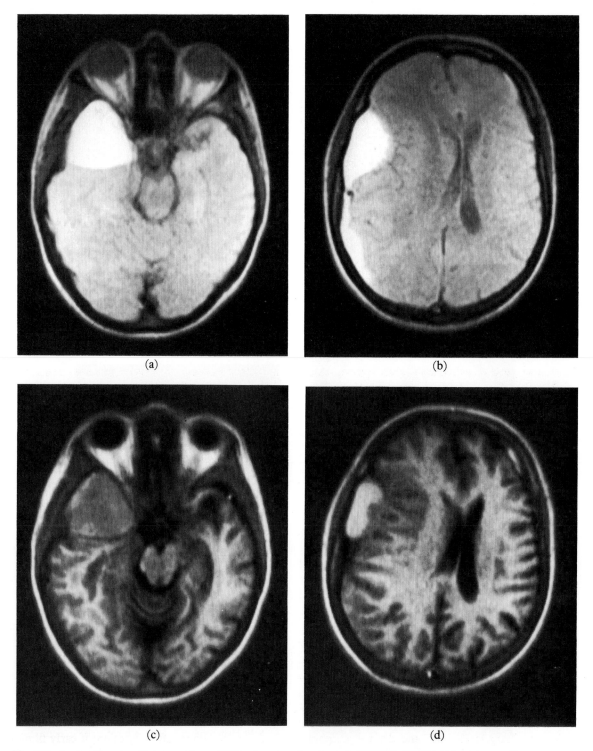

(a)

(b)

(c)

(d)

Fig. 9.41 Arachnoid cyst, with haemorrhage. MRI, **a,b.** spin echo sequence (TR1000, TE60) axial sections, and **c,d.** inversion recovery sequence (TR2000, T1500) similar sections. The high signal from the fluid over the convexity in **d.** and the slightly higher signal than cerebrospinal fluid **c.** is due to the short T_1 relaxation induced by break down products of blood in this distribution.

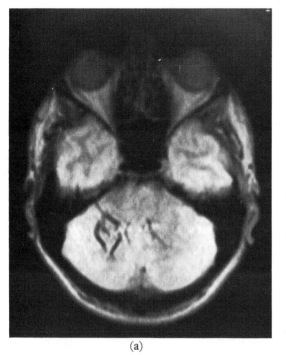
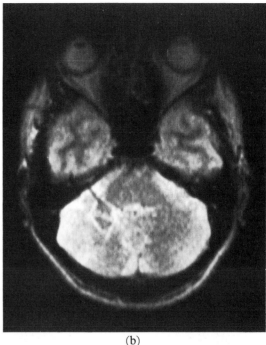

(a)   (b)

Fig. 9.42 Angiomatous malformation. MRI, spin echo sequences **a.** TR2500, TE40 and **b.** TR2500, TE80 axial sections. Note the absence of signal from flowing blood, which is particularly evident in the short echo sequence.

scanning purposes these are commonly taken at about 30 minutes after intravenous injection of the isotope. Abnormal uptake is recognized in virtually all abscesses, in over 90% of meningiomas and malignant gliomas, 85% of metastases and about 30% of benign gliomas. Abnormal uptake is not usually detected until lesions reach a critical size of about 2 cm and they may be obscured by superimposition of the normal uptake in large venous sinuses, mucous membrane and the large muscles attached to the skull base.

In most cases the appearance of the uptake is non-specific but consideration of its intensity, size, shape and position can be suggestive of a particular pathology. Multiple areas of uptake in patients with a known primary neoplasm are virtually diagnostic of metastases (Fig. 9.44), although abscesses and infarcts can also be multiple. The butterfly distribution of a corpus callosum glioma (Fig. 9.45) and diffuse peripheral uptake in a subdural haematoma are suggestive of these diagnoses. Non-specific high intensity, well-demarcated peripheral uptake is usual in

meningiomas (Fig. 9.46); the diagnosis may be confirmed by plain film changes.

Rapid serial filming immediately after injection of Technetium gives further information about the nature of the lesions. Angiomatous malformations show very early (Fig. 9.47) and fade quickly as the isotope is rapidly carried into the veins. Sometimes an irregular serpiginous shape, giving a vague outline of the vascular pattern of the malformation, is evident. Very vascular tumours, such as some meningiomas, also show early uptake, but this increases and is retained as the circulation clears. Malignant gliomas and some metastases have a slower build-up of uptake through the capillary and venous stages of transit, which then persists. Most metastases are not shown until 40–70 s after the injection and then progressively retain more of the isotope.

In gliomas and metastases the ratio of uptake between abnormal and normal tissues increases up to about four hours after injection; if early filming gives negative or equivocal findings, a later or serial study may be more reliable when such lesions are suspected.

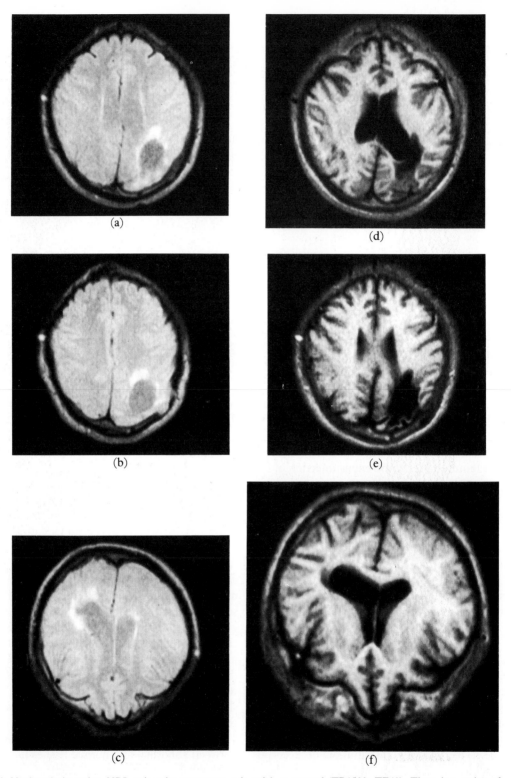

Fig. 9.43 Myelomalacic cavity. MRI, spin echo sequences, **a,b.** axial, **c.** coronal (TR1500, TE60). There is a region of diminished signal intensity, similar to that of the cerebrospinal fluid, within the left parietal lobe, with some surrounding high signal from damaged brain substance. **d,e,f.** Inversion recovery sequence (TR2100, TE500) similar sections. The myelomalacic cavity, with the dilated trigone extending towards it, is well defined on this sequence and, again, gives a similar signal to the ventricular cerebrospinal fluid.

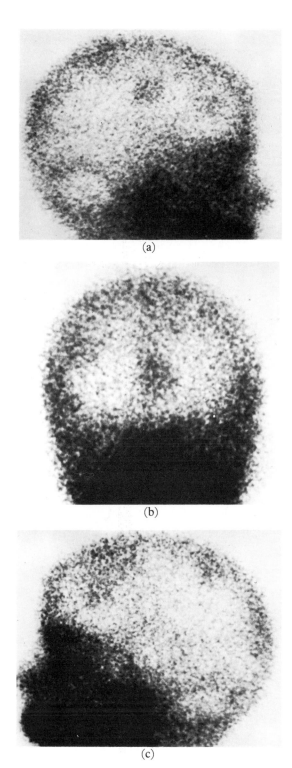

Fig. 9.44 Metastases. Gamma encephalogram, **a.** right lateral, **b.** antero-posterior, **c.** left lateral views. There are multiple areas of increased uptake in the tumours.

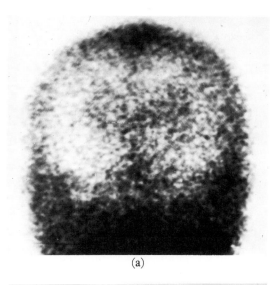

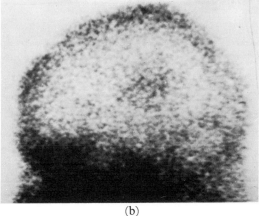

Fig. 9.45 Glioma of the corpus callosum. Gamma encephalogram, **a.** antero-posterior, **b.** lateral views. There is bilateral parietal uptake, more extensive on the left, joined across the midline.

Isotope accumulates in infarcts and haemorrhages when cellular reaction is occurring about 7–10 days from their onset and it persists for several weeks or even months, gradually diminishing; the progression on serial studies is typical.

It should be noted that occasionally abnormal uptake is found after repeated focal seizures in the absence of any demonstrable pathology. It is presumably due to alteration in the blood–brain barrier since it returns to normal on subsequent examinations.

In some instances a positive gamma encephalogram alone, or considered with plain film

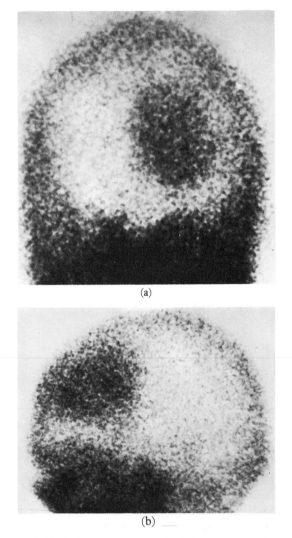

Fig. 9.46 Meningioma. Gamma encephalogram, **a.** anterior,
b. left lateral views. There is a peripheral area of dense
increased uptake in the frontal region.

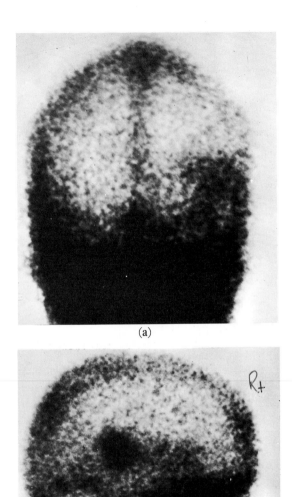

Fig. 9.47 Angiomatous malformation. Gamma
encephalogram, **a.** anterior view, **b.** right lateral view, taken
immediately after injection of isotope. There is marked
increased density in the angiomatous malformation; increased
uptake is shown extending from it in the draining veins.

studies, is diagnostic and gives sufficient information for management. More frequently, other studies are necessary to decide the diagnosis or confirm that biopsy is necessary. Many of the more benign gliomas and virtually all the atrophic processes will not be revealed by gamma encephalography so that a negative study is virtually of no value. Usually these conditions will give rise to more disturbance than well-controlled tonic-clonic seizures alone and they will be selected for further studies on clinical grounds.

POSITRON EMISSION TOMOGRAPHY (PET)

This is a high-cost research technique currently requiring a specialist operated cyclotron for the production of the so-called physiological radionucleides, including O_2^{15} (2.1 min half-life), N^{13} (10 min half-life), C^{11} (20.1 min half-life) and F^{18} (110 min half-life). The positron emission tomograph (PET) measures tomographically the uptake and distribution of these tracers in vivo and thus allows investigation of some of the biochemical processes essential to life, utilizing chemical amounts small enough not to perturb the phenomena of the study. The response within the tomograms is quantitative, reflecting absolute units of tracer concentration, enabling the method to be used for the absolute measurement of regional cerebral blood flow, oxygen and glucose utilization, amino acid synthesis, amine neurotransmitter metabolism and blood volume estimation. Such measurements have been used in the study of focal pathophysiology in epilepsy, psychosis, glioma and cerebrovascular disease amongst other pathologies.

Metabolic studies in epileptic patients have been mainly performed using fluorodeoxyglucose. These have shown diminished glucose metabolism in the region of a discrete focus, which generally includes, but tends to be more extensive than, any structural changes shown by histopathological examination of resected tissue (Engel et al 1982a). Multifocal and diffuse EEG changes are associated with a corresponding distribution of hypometabolism (Engel et al 1982b). In a few patients, diminished regional cerebral blood flow and cerebral metabolic rate for oxygen has been demonstrated on the side of the focus, mainly in the temporal lobes and basal ganglia (Kuhl et al 1980). The focus also demonstrates diminution in the stimulus-induced metabolic response to glucose metabolism. During an ictus, changes in combination with EEG abnormalities may provide useful identification of the site of the focus for surgical excision.

PET has demonstrated very variable levels of blood flow and glucose metabolic rate in middle grade and malignant gliomas, but the mean lies close to that of the corresponding contralateral brain substance: in high grade gliomas, because of the anaerobic pattern of metabolism of glucose by these tumours, there is consistent, marked reduction in oxygen extraction (Ito et al 1982, Rhodes 1983). This feature may be useful in cases in which distinction between intrinsic tumour and acute infarction is required immediately and where more simple tests have failed to elucidate. In the acute ischaemic lesion, blood flow may be reduced but oxygen extraction is increased up to 90% (normal 40–50% per passage), indicating survival, by utilization of the normal reserve in oxygen carriage, of some cerebral tissue within the infarct. After about a week, this uncoupling of flow and metabolism may be reversed as perfusion is re-established: the reduced oxygen extraction is accompanied by increased glucose utilisation related to glycolytic activity of infiltrating white cells (Wise et al 1984). After about a month, blood flow and metabolic rate of oxygen are reduced but coupling is restored (Lenzi et al 1982). In some patients with clinically transient cerebral ischaemia, cerebral vasodilatation, as shown by increase in cerebral blood volume relative to flow or focally reduced blood flow associated with increased oxygen extraction, is observed (Gibbs et al 1984) indicating chronic ischaemia.

In low grade astrocytomas glucose consumption is usually decreased, but ^{11}C-L-methionine uptake is increased in both low and high-grade gliomas and distinguishes the tumour tissue from oedema (Bergstrom et al 1983).

Radiation necrosis and recurrent high grade glioma may give markedly similar appearaces on both MRI and CT scanning. However, high grade glioma is hypermetabolic for glucose and post-irradiation necrosis is hypometabolic; PET scanning has proved useful in distinguishing between the two conditions in a number of cases.

CONTRAST STUDIES

Pneumoencephalography is no longer necessary when modern facilities are available and the use of cerebral angiography has diminished; as non-invasive studies are more accurate in the diagnosis and exclusion of structural lesions associated with epilepsy, angiography is inappropriate for this purpose, particularly if CT or MRI is negative.

Automatic serial changers and facilities for magnification and subtraction are routine requirements for conventional angiography. With modern

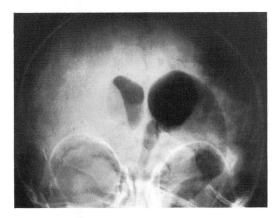

Fig. 9.48 Left hemiatrophy. Air encephalogram, brow-up antero-posterior projection. The capacity of the vault on the left side is diminished. There is dilatation of the subarachnoid space over the left cerebral hemisphere. The left lateral ventricle is dilated and the septum pellucidum and third ventricle are deviated towards it.

facilities and skilled technique, the risks of inducing a permanent neurological deficit have been reduced to about 0.2% but, even so, there should still be a definite indication and the technique adopted should ensure that the maximum amount of information is obtained.

Much of the information required from angiography can be obtained without such risk and at reduced cost by using good quality intravenous digital subtraction angiography (Takahashi et al 1983).

Pneumoencephalography

Where CT and MRI are not available and the other non-invasive studies are negative, pneumoencephalography is indicated in cases of epilepsy of recent onset, of changing or intractable nature or associated with dementia, in which there are neither lateralizing signs nor any indication of raised intracranial pressure. Generalized, hemi- or focal atrophy (Fig. 9.48) may be disclosed, as may some mass lesions, especially slightly space-occupying gliomas. The latter usually show minor displacements of the ventricles, which do not give a specific indication of the nature of the lesion unless there is also local invasion or encroachment into the wall of the ventricle or thickening of the septum pellucidum. Small infiltrating temporal gliomas (Fig. 9.49) may cause minimal distortion, narrowing or enlargement of the temporal horn;

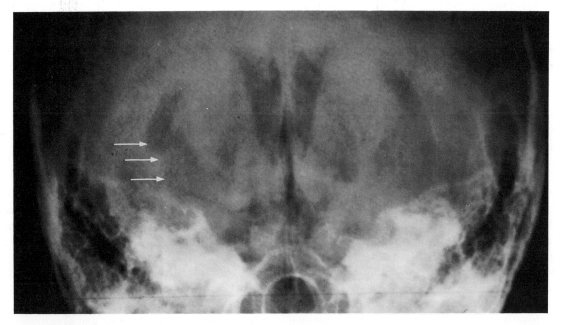

Fig. 9.49 Astrocytoma. Air encephalogram, brow-up Towne's projection. The tip of the right temporal horn is dilated and there is an irregular filling defect in its lateral part (arrows). The anterior half of the right temporal lobe was resected and contained a Grade II astrocytoma.

with hamartomas, also, there may be slight compression or displacement. Dilatation or distortion of the horn may be caused by atrophy due to mesial temporal sclerosis (Sumie et al 1978) or scarring associated with trauma, inflammation or vascular disease which has caused infarction or haemorrhage.

Tuberous sclerosis (Fig. 9.50) may be recognized from small subependymal nodules visible anywhere along the ventricular system before they develop calcification dense enough to show on

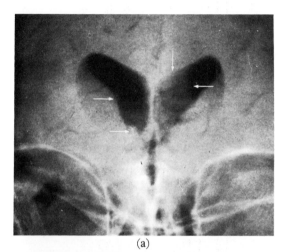

(a)

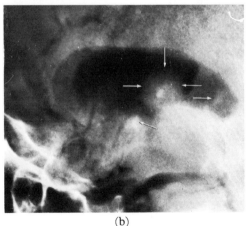

(b)

Fig. 9.50 Tuberous sclerosis. Air encephalogram, brow up **a.** anteroposterior and **b.** lateral projections. There is a large tuber, containing a calcified nodule, projecting into the medial half of the anterior part of the body of the left lateral ventricle. Two small tubers project into the right lateral ventricle; one from the floor just anterolateral to the foramen of Monro containing a little calcification, and the other from the lateral wall of the posterior part of the body (arrows).

radiographs. Heterotopic grey matter can give a similar appearance around the lateral ventricles but does not affect the third or fourth ventricles.

Epilepsy following trauma is frequently associated with meningocerebral scarring, which may be recognized by focal ventricular dilatation or porencephalic cyst formation. More diffuse atrophy may be a factor deciding against surgery.

Occasionally, cysts with a narrow connection to the main cerebrospinal fluid spaces may fill late. In post-traumatic cases a film taken several hours after injection of the air may be of value in showing such cysts.

Cerebral angiography

The localization of an intracranial mass may be evident from the stretching and splaying of cerebral vessels around the periphery of the swelling (Fig. 9.51). The gyral pattern may be distorted and the circulation locally delayed in the region of the mass. Intracerebral masses which compress the surface vessels towards the skull may be distinguished from extra-axial masses which displace the vessels away from it.

The nature of a lesion may be suspected from changes in vessel structure evident on the angiogram. The vascular bed of a tumour may show an abnormal pattern. This tends to be more florid in malignant tumours (Fig. 9.52), in which some vessels are sinusoids lined by tumour cells, through which arteriovenous shunting occurs; irregular dilatations may be formed in regions of tumour necrosis. This pattern is most usual in anaplastic primary brain tumours, occurring in about half of malignant gliomas, but is also present in some metastases. Less often, malignant tumours have fine, irregular vessels or a capillary blush which tends to be patchy in gliomas and more homogeneous in metastases; necrotic and cystic parts of tumours are avascular and residual vascularized tissue may form an irregular ring around them.

The vasculature of benign tumours tends to have a radiating or reticular basis with distal tapering, like that of normal tissues. When vascularity is increased, as is typical of most meningiomas, the capillary circulation may show

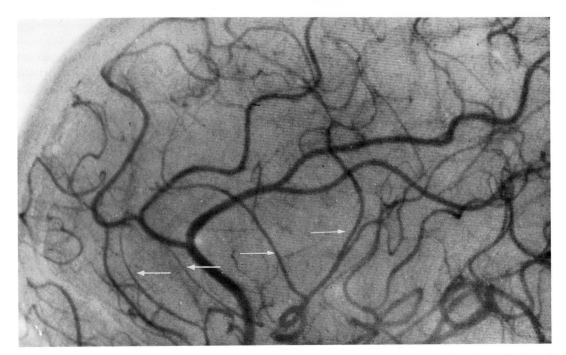

Fig. 9.51 Astrocytoma. Left internal carotid angiogram, lateral projection. Ascending frontal branches of the middle cerebral artery (arrows) are splayed apart due to a sub-adjacent swelling, without positive angiographic evidence of its nature. It proved at surgery to be a solid astrocytoma.

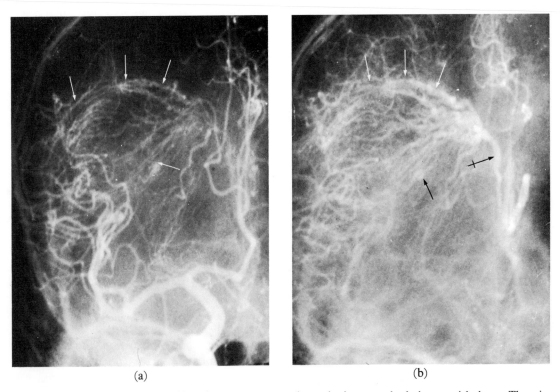

(a) (b)

Fig. 9.52 Malignant glioma. Right carotid angiogram, anteroposterior projection, **a.** early, **b.** late arterial phases. There is displacement of the anterior cerebral artery and of the internal cerebral vein to the left. Pathological vessels (arrow) are shown extending from the cortical branches of the middle cerebral artery medially through the white matter to drain into the thalamostriate vein (crossed arrow). The appearances are typical of a malignant glioma.

as a prolonged blush. In about half the malignant and a greater proportion of more benign intracerebral tumours, vascular changes are absent or minor and non-specific.

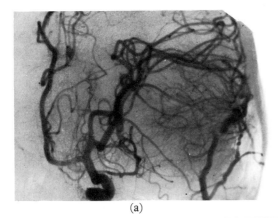

(a)

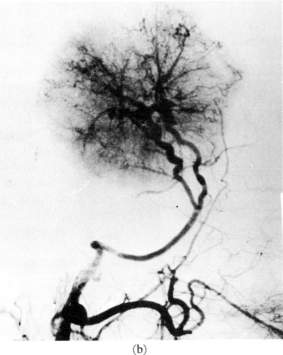

(b)

Fig. 9.53 Meningioma. **a.** Left common carotid angiogram, anteroposterior projection. The trunk of the middle cerebral artery is elevated. Its branches over the insula are displaced medially and those in the lateral ramus of the Sylvian fissure are elevated and splayed apart by an extracerebral mass which is supplied with a rich abnormal circulation from the middle meningeal artery. **b.** Left external carotid angiogram, lateral projection. The middle meningeal artery is enlarged. It gives a large number of small branches radiating from the point of attachment to supply and delineate the meningioma with a capillary blush.

Extracerebral tumours, especially meningiomas (Fig. 9.53), usually obtain a blood supply from meningeal arteries which often become enlarged and tortuous. This is not a pathognomonic feature, since intracerebral masses which invade or adhere to the dura may acquire a meningeal supply, though it is usually less pronounced than in meningiomas. Intracerebral lesions may be recognized with certainty when they receive blood from penetrating arteries or drain to subependymal veins.

The capsule of an intracerebral abscess contains small vessels which may be seen as a ring-like blush. As in any system lacking normal arteriolar resistance, arteriovenous shunting may occur in the capsule.

Arteriovenous malformations (Fig. 9.54) and occlusions of moderate-sized vessels (Fig. 9.55), which are not infrequent causes of focal epilepsy, are shown directly.

It has been emphasized that CT or MRI frequently give sufficient information for management or even suggest a specific diagnosis. Virtually all tumours, infarcts and haemorrhages, and most inflammatory lesions, are recognized; and, in some cases, where swelling is slight or absent, a lesion is obvious when angiography reveals either minimal non-specific changes or is normal. The nature of avascular masses with no

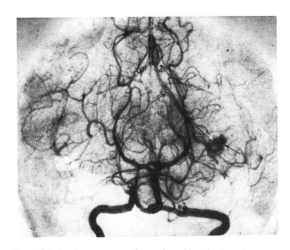

Fig. 9.54 Angiomatous malformation. Vertebral angiogram, arterial phase, anteroposterior projection. Small angiomatous malformation lying medially in the anterior part of the left temporal lobe (arrows), with early drainage to the basal vein (crossed arrow).

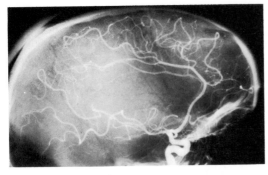

Fig. 9.55 Middle cerebral cortical arteries branch occlusion. Female, aged 55, who presented with left-sided focal fits of recent onset. Right carotid angiogram, arterial phase, lateral projection. There is marked delay of filling of the ascending frontal and anterior parietal branches of the middle cerebral artery.

evidence of the type of the pathology on angiography may also be resolved by CT. Ambiguous findings on CT are sometimes resolved by angiography but, overall, it provides positive evidence of the nature of the pathological process in only about 30% of the unusual cases in which an equivocal or inaccurate diagnosis of glioma is suggested by CT appearances.

Some information helpful for planning surgery can only be obtained by angiography. For example, the relationship of major blood vessels to the lesion, including the presence or absence of tumour cuffing, or of invasion of the venous sinuses by meningioma which may be important in this respect. When CT reveals a small infarct or focal atrophy, especially in a middle-aged or elderly patient with sudden onset of seizures, digital angiography to show the appropriate neck vessels may reveal a significant ulcerating or stenosis atheromatous plaque. Focal atrophy may be caused by an arteriovenous malformation and, if small, it may not produce a diagnostic abnormality on the non-invasive studies.

When CT and MRI are not available, the role of angiography is extended. Abnormal uptake shown on isotope encephalography is often non-specific and angiography of the appropriate vessel may be helpful in deciding the nature of the pathological process or underlying lesion. When isotope encephalography is negative and there are unexplained focal features, appropriate angiograms should be performed. Clinical or radiological evidence of unexplained raised intracranial pressure may be elucidated by non-dominant carotid angiography. This may reveal a supratentorial mass; the subependymal veins allow the size of the lateral ventricles to be assessed and, if they are dilated, deformity of the deep veins may provide a useful indicator of the cause. Venous occlusion may also be recognized, either directly or by slowing of venous flow towards the obstructed region and filling of collateral veins.

Following focal status epilepticus, capillary dilatation may temporarily occur in the affected region of the brain and rarely, show as a blush or be associated with early venous filling on angiography. Failure to consider this possibility may lead to an erroneous diagnosis of significant pathology.

REFERENCES

Bachman D S, Hodges F H, Freeman J M 1976 Computerised axial tomography in chronic seizure disorders of childhood. Pediatrics 58: 828–832

Bergstrom M, Collins V P, Ehrin E et al Discrepancies in brain tumor extent as shown by computed tomography and positron emission tomography using ^{68}Ga-EDTA, ^{11}C-glucose and ^{11}C-methionine. Case report. Journal of Computer Assisted Tomography 7: 1062–1066

Bogdanoff B M, Stafford C R, Green L, Gonzalez C F 1975 Computerized axial tomography in the evaluation of patients with epilepsy. Neurology 25: 1013–1017

Brant Zawadski M B, Davis P L, Crooks L E, Mills C M, Norman D, Newton T H, Sheldon T, Kaufmann L 1983 NMR demonstration of cerebral abnormalities: Comparison with CT. American Journal of Neuroradiology 4: 117–124

Brant Zawadski M, Kelly W, Kjos B, Newton T H, Norman D, Dillon W, Sobel D 1985 Magnetic resonance imaging and characterisation of normal and abnormal intracranial cerebrospinal fluid (CSF) spaces. Neuroradiology 27: 3–8

Cala L A, Mastaglia F L, Woodings T L 1977 Computerized tomography of the cranium in patients with epilepsy: A preliminary report. Proceedings of the Australian Association of Neurologists.

Carr D H, Brown J, Bydder G M et al 1984 Intravenous chelated gadolinium as a contrast agent in NMR imaging of cerebral tumours. Lancet i: 484–486

Collard M, Dupont H, Noel G 1976 Summary: computerized transverse axial tomography in epilepsy. Epilepsia 17: 339–340

Dellaportas G I, Dawson J M, Reynolds E H 1982

Computerised tomography in new referrals with epilepsy. British Journal of Clinical Practice Suppl 18: 201–203

Engel J Jr, Brown W J, Kuhl D E, Phelps M E, Mazziotta J C, Crandall P H 1982a Pathological findings underlying focal temporal lobe hypometabolism in partial epilepsy. Annals of Neurology 12: 518–528

Engel J Jr, Kuhl D E, Phelps M E, Mazziotta J C 1982b Interictal cerebral glucose metabolism in partial epilepsy and its relation to EEG changes. Annals of Neurology 12: 510–517

Falconer M A, Serafetinides E A 1963 A follow-up study in temporal lobe epilepsy. Journal of Neurology, Neurosurgery and Psychiatry 26:154

Gastaut H, Gastaut J L 1976 Computerised transverse axial tomography in epilepsy. Epilepsia 17: 325–336

Gibbs J M, Wise R J S, Leonders K L, Jones T 1984 Evaluation of cerebral perfusion reserve in patients with carotid artery occlusion. Lancet i: 310–314

Gilsanz V, Strand R, Barnes P, Nealis J 1979 Results of presumed cryptogenic epilepsy in childhood by CT scanning. Annals of Radiology 22: 184–187

Gold L H A, Kieffer S A, Petersonn H O 1969 Intracranial meningiomas. A retrospective analysis of the diagnostic value of plain skull films. Neurology 19: 873–878

Hillemacher A 1982 Der wert amnestischer und klinischer Daten sowie apparativer Intersuchungsbefunde bei der Diagnose von Hirntumoren. Fortschritte der Neurologie-Psychiatrie 50: 93–112

Holowach J, Thurston D L, O'Leavy J 1958 Jacksonian seizures in infancy and childhood. British Journal of Paediatrics 52: 670–686

Hounsfield G N 1973 Computerised transverse axial scanning (tomography). Part 1, description of system. British Journal of Radiology 46: 1016–1022

Ito M, Lammertsma A A, Wise R J S et al 1982 Measurement of regional cerebral blood flow and oxygen utilisation in patients with cerebral tumours using ^{15}O and positron emission tomography: analytical techniques and preliminary results. Neuroradiology 46: 1016–1022

Jabbari B, Huott A D, DiChiro G, Martins A N, Coker S B 1978 Surgically correctable lesions detected by CT in 143 patients with chronic epilepsy. Surgical Neurology 10: 319–222

Jabbari B, DiChiro G, McCarthy J P 1979 Medial temporal stenosis detected by computed tomography. Journal of Computer Assisted Tomography 3: 527–529

Kalan C, Burrows E H 1962 Calcification in intracranial gliomata. British Journal of Radiology 35: 589–602

Kendall B E, Jakubowski J, Pullicino P, Symon L 1979 Difficulties in diagnosis of supratentorial gliomas by CAT scan. Journal of Neurology, Neurosurgery and Psychiatry 42: 485–492

Kingsley D P E, Kendall B E, Fitz C R 1986 Tuberous sclerosis: A clinico-radiological evaluation of 110 cases with particular reference to atypical presentation. Neuroradiology 28: 38–46

Kuhl D E, Engel J Jr, Phelps M E, Selin C 1980 Epileptic patterns of local cerebral metabolism and perfusion in humans determined by emission computed tomography of ^{18}FDG and ^{13}NH. Annals of Neurology 8: 348–360

Langenstein D K, Sternowsky H J, Rothe M 1979 Computerized cranial transverse axial tomography (CTAT) in 145 patients with primary and secondary generalized epilepsies. I. Neuropaediatrie 10: 15–28

Laster D W, Perry J K, Moody D M, Ball M R, Witcofski R L, Riela A T 1985 Chronic seizure disorders: Contribution of MR imaging when CT is normal. American Journal of Neuroradiology 6: 177–180

Lenzi G L, Frackowiak R S J, Jones T 1982 Cerebral oxygen metabolism and blood flow in human cerebral ischaemic infarction. Journal of Cerebral Blood Flow and Metabolism 2: 321–335

Mahmoud M EI.S 1958 The sella in health and disease: Value of the radio-graphic study of the sella turcica in morbid anatomical and topographic diagnosis of intracranial tumours. British Journal of Radiology Suppl. 8

McGahan J, Dublin A B, Hill R P 1979 The evaluation of seizure disorders by computerized tomography. Journal of Neurosurgery 50: 328–332

Rhodes C G, Wise R J S, Gibbs J M et al 1983 In vivo disturbance of the oxidative metabolism of glucose in human cerebral gliomas. Annals of Neurology 14: 614–626

Scollo-Lavizzari G, Eichhorn K, Wuthrich R 1977 Computerized transverse axial tomography in the diagnosis of epilepsy. European Neurology 15: 5–8

Shorvon S D, Gilliatt R W, Cox T C S, Yu Y-L 1984 Evidence of vascular disease from CT scanning in late onset epilepsy. Journal of Neurology, Neurosurgery and Psychiatry 47: 225–230

Sumie H, Kuru Y, Kurokawa S, Kondo R 1978 Ammon's horn sclerosis on pneumoencephalotomography. Neuroradiology 16: 335–336

Synek V, Reuben J R, Gawler J, du Boulay G H 1979 Comparison of the measurement of the cerebral ventricles obtained by CT scanning and pneumoencephalography. Neuroradiology 17: 149–151

Takahashi M, Hirota Y, Bussaka W et al 1983 Evaluation of prototype equipment for digital subtraction angiography in diagnosing intracranial lesions. American Journal of Neuroradiology 4: 259–262

Weisberg L A, Nice C, Katz M 1984 Cerebral computed tomography. 2nd Edn. WB Saunders, Philadelphia

Wise R J S, Rhodes C G, Gibbs J M, Hatasawa J, Palmer T, Frackwoiak R S J, Jones T 1984 Disturbance of oxidative metabolism of glucose in recent human cerebral infarcts. Annals of Neurology 14: 627–637.

Yang P J, Berger P E, Cohen M E, Duffner P K 1979 Computed tomography and childhood seizure disorders. Neurology 29: 1084–1088

Young A C, Costanzi J B, Mohr P D, St Clair Forbes W 1982 Is routine computerised axial tomography in epilepsy worthwhile? Lancet ii: 1446–1447

Young I R, Bydder G M, Hall A S et al 1983 The role of NMR imaging in the diagnosis and management of acoustic neuroma. American Journal of Neuroradiology 4: 223–224

10

Neuropsychiatry

PART ONE
EPILEPSY AND BEHAVIOUR
T. A. Betts

INTRODUCTION

Epilepsy originates in the brain; so do our thoughts, our feelings and our behaviour. Epilepsy results from changes in chemical activity at transmitter sites and in cell membranes in the brain; so does how we comprehend the world and how we react to it. Epilepsy, therefore, can change the way we think, feel and behave; but, equally, thought, emotion and behaviour can change epilepsy.

Epilepsy is, therefore, important to the psychiatrist, and the psychiatrist is important to epilepsy. Epilepsy lies in the borderland between what is conventionally understood as a province of neurology and what is conventionally understood as a province of psychiatry. Epilepsy and its associated phenomena cannot be understood without a firm grounding in both brain and behavioural sciences.

An understanding of epilepsy requires the co-operation of several disciplines. It requires more than that, however, in that each discipline must have some understanding of the role of the others. The treatment of epilepsy is not the prerogative of any one discipline but can be a job for any doctor, whether neurologist, psychiatrist, paediatrician or general physician, providing he or she has a particular interest in epilepsy and is prepared to learn something of the skills and atti-

tudes of other branches of the profession so that total care can be offered to the patient.

This chapter is an attempt to describe the various aspects of epilepsy with which a psychiatrist is particularly concerned, and for which his or her skills have something to offer.

THE ROLE OF THE PSYCHIATRIST

There are three main ways in which the psychiatrist has a unique contribution to make to the management of people with epilepsy.

Of people with epilepsy, many are troubled, some are troublesome, and a few are mad. It is probable that psychiatric disturbance of all kinds is more common in people with epilepsy than in the general population; although this bold statement needs qualification. Most psychiatric disturbance in people with epilepsy can be seen as no more than a reaction to the stress of being epileptic. The skills of psychiatrists and their colleagues in social work and clinical psychology are very pertinent here.

Some people with epilepsy, because of concomitant brain damage or the effect that having epilepsy has had on their emotional development, grow up with persistent disturbances of behaviour or in their relationships to other people which classify them as having a personality disorder. This is one of the most contentious areas of the psychiatry of epilepsy. Again, the skills that a psychiatrist and his or her colleagues possess may have a lot to offer such people. Even more important, perhaps, if we can study these problems carefully enough, we may be in a position eventually to offer some kind of preventative treatment. A few people with epilepsy have such gross disorders of feeling, behaviour, thinking, or in the way they relate to the external world and other people, that they have to be described as actually mad; and here, of course, the psychiatrist's help is essential.

There are two other ways in which the psychiatrist has a contribution to make to the management of epilepsy. The first is in helping to diagnose attack disorder. Often the diagnosis of epilepsy is easy but sometimes it is not: particularly with complex partial seizures, it may be difficult to distinguish between a phenomenon relating to epilepsy and a phenomenon relating to psychiatric disturbance. The differential diagnosis of attacks may need psychiatric experience. Secondly, new and developing methods of treatment in psychiatry, particularly those based on learning theory, may have a great deal to offer people with epilepsy in terms of the actual treatment of their seizures. Although still largely experimental, this writer feels that behavioural treatments will eventually be a powerful adjunct to more conventional forms of therapy.

Since this is a medical textbook, a medical model has tended to be followed in describing psychological reactions to epilepsy. There are, however, other equally appropriate models that could have been used, which help to explain why people with epilepsy behave in the way they do. Although it says very little about epilepsy directly, Goffman's book (Goffman 1963) is well worth reading by those who wish to pursue this idea further. Wing (1974) presents a model of handicap, which although related to schizophrenia, is also extremely applicable to epilepsy, and, although not formally acknowledged elsewhere, it is really his structure which is being used as the emotional reactions to epilepsy are described. Wing talks of:

1. *Primary handicaps*, which are the result of chronic impairment of physiological or psychological function (e.g. loss of a limb, obsessions, or fits)
2. *Secondary handicaps* - extra handicaps which would not have been present had the primary handicap not also been present (e.g. fits leading to hospitalization which leads to institutionalisation or fits leading to fear which leads to an increased number of fits)

3. *Extrinsic handicaps*, which are pre-existing handicaps which are independent of the main one but which influence it – like poor social circumstances or a lack of social or cognitive skills which are relevant to treatment planning.

PSYCHOLOGICAL EFFECTS OF HAVING EPILEPSY

To have epilepsy is to be stressed. Stress itself can influence the frequency of fits, and it is possible sometimes for this to become a self-reinforcing phenomenon. If patients can come to terms or deal with the stress that epilepsy induces, their lives will be made much more comfortable and their seizure frequency may diminish. It is, therefore, important for any doctor who is helping people with epilepsy to know something about the effects of stress, the factors that influence the way an individual reacts to stress and the means available to help people to cope with stress. It is also important for doctors to know when reactions to stress should be classified as abnormal.

The word 'stress' itself is ill defined in the literature: sometimes it is applied to that which causes reactive and unpleasant symptoms in individuals; and sometimes it is applied to the actual symptoms themselves. In this chapter the word 'stress' implies the impact that becoming epileptic has on the patient and also the chronic effects that having epilepsy has on the individual and his or her relationships with others. In terms of its effects on the individual, help given should really be considered under two headings: first, helping him to come to terms with the diagnosis of epilepsy and secondly trying to minimize the effects that epilepsy will have on his or her life, i.e. on social life, interpersonal relationships and on his or her job.

In looking at how somebody is reacting to a particular stress, it should be remembered that stress reactions in themselves can often be considered as normal, are usually self-limiting and are part of the normal biological mechanisms of adaptation to new situations. In considering whether a particular reaction is abnormal or not, one should pay particular attention to whether the reaction is helping that person to deal with the situation, and also whether the reaction is becoming self-reinforcing (i.e. that the person is, for instance, becoming afraid of being afraid).

The term 'normal mental health' certainly does not imply an absence of stress symptoms or emotional conflicts. At any one time, the majority of the population are under some kind of stress, and so may be experiencing appropriate feelings or showing evidence of this stress in their behaviour. Indeed, if the criteria are set wide enough, almost every normal person wiil be classified as having emotional symptoms. For instance, an epidemiological study which used such broad criteria, the Manhatten Midtown Study (Srole et al 1962) found an estimated 87% of the normal population in the survey to have some emotional disturbance. In any population of supposedly ill patients, a careful distinction must, therefore, be made between normal and abnormal reactions to stress.

The way a particular individual reacts to stress depends on certain factors; some of them independent and some of them interdependent. First, there is the significance of the stress to the individual involved. It has been shown, for instance, that the psychological effects of head injury are partly dependent on the relative meaning of the injury to the individual. Dysphasia in a school-master, for instance, is of much more importance in terms of his emotional response to it than dysphasia in a farm labourer. The support which a person receives from family and friends and society will also affect his or her ability to cope with a particular stress. Someone recently bereaved, for instance, is much less able to meet the impact of physical illness.

It has also been shown (Slater & Shields 1969) that the genetic constitution of an individual and the responsiveness of his or her autonomic nervous system to stress may play an important part in shaping the particular way the stress responses are presented. Lacey et al (1953) propose the concept of response specificity: that people respond to stress in a relatively stereotyped way through their autonomic system.

Stress responses are also influenced by a person's educational and cultural background. The West Indian response to stress, for instance, is different from the British; so it is, therefore, easy to misinterpret the behaviour of immigrants. Stress is not an isolated event and a person's response is influenced by coincident problems and difficulties affecting him or her at the time. In other words, stress is easier to cope with if one is not already overburdened. Stress reactions are learned as part and parcel of growing up: children are influenced greatly in terms of the way they learn to respond to stress by the example set by their parents and by the social values of their family.

Various extra influences which fall on people with epilepsy are perhaps particularly pertinent to the way they respond to stress. There is a growing body of evidence to suggest that social learning, particularly in childhood (which will include learning about how to cope with common stresses and difficulties), is impaired by epilepsy acquired in early childhood; and it is possible that some of the chronic personality difficulties that adults with epilepsy may show are related to mal-learning in childhood.

There is no doubt as well that brain damage, particularly perhaps in the temporal lobes, impairs the ability of a person to respond in a normal way to a stressful situation: minor neurotic symptoms and hysterical reactions are probably more common in people who are brain damaged.

There is also some evidence to suggest that antiepileptic drugs needed by a person with epilepsy may also impair learning and interfere with normal responses to stress. A person with epilepsy then, not only has to suffer the normal stresses that any chronic illness would impose, but also may be handicapped in terms of responding to those stresses by the illness itself and by its necessary treatment. In some ways, then, epilepsy is a unique illness compared with other chronic handicaps.

COMING TO TERMS WITH EPILEPSY

The first problem for the patient newly diagnosed as having epilepsy is to come to terms with it. It is easy for doctors in the confines of out–patients (where patients' behaviour is usually subservient and controlled) to believe that this is easy. The patient who nods and smiles when told the diagnosis and says 'Thank you doctor, at least it's nothing more serious', is very pleasing; but one should not imagine that he or she is necessarily going to behave in the same way at home and, even if that is the case, friends, parents, spouse or children may not react similarly.

It should be remembered by all doctors that there is only a limited amount of information that patients can absorb at any one time in a medical consultation; and even that small amount is drastically reduced if the information given to the patient has emotional import.

Some doctors conceal the truth from their patients about the diagnosis of epilepsy and merely refer in a vague way to blackouts etc. This writer believes most firmly that all patients with epilepsy should know the diagnosis, but one should remember that in addition to the diagnosis the patient will require a whole range of information about lifestyle, treatment etc. If one tries to give this information at the same time as giving the patient the diagnosis it will often fall on deaf ears, and the education of the patient about all the implications of epilepsy may take several months of painstaking effort, particularly as one is often overcoming the patient's own prejudice and ignorance about the disorder.

In many chronic illnesses, including epilepsy, the use of printed handouts for the patient and his family (and even the use of videotape material) to further explain the illness is being developed. Many patients, as they come to terms with the diagnosis, will benefit from the support of fellow sufferers with the disorder. Most countries in the western world are now developing such patient support groups.

As patients come to terms with any emotionally significant or life threatening physical disability, they commonly show a range of mental mechanisms to deal with the anxieties and stress that the situation has caused. Most of these mental mechanisms are quite normal, and help to maintain emotional equilibrium under stress and preserve self-respect. The work of Bowlby (1960) and Hinton (1967) on children deprived of maternal care, and people facing unpleasant situations such as dying, shows that a very common initial reaction to such unpleasant situations is one of denial, followed by a period of struggle in which the

individual consciously tries to assimilate the new knowledge into his self-concept and image. This period of struggle and denial may be particularly painful, and may also, of course, occur in relatives. It is during this period of denial and struggle that one may see the phenomenon of the patient dragged from one useless consultation to another (often of an esoteric or fringe medicine type) because the devastating truth cannot be accepted. The consultant, flattered by being asked to provide a second opinion, should remember that the reasons for this may have much more to do with the emotional struggle that the patient is going through than with the consultant's own particular prowess.

The period of denial is often followed by a period of depression as the person begins to assimilate the unpleasant situation. This depression, providing it does not go on for too long and can be worked through, should be regarded as normal. It usually gives way eventually to a period of acceptance and resignation. These reactions need support rather than treatment, except in unusual circumstances. People passing through these emotional reactions may have transient periods of the most profound depression which, unless they become prolonged and therefore pathological, should not be treated, since there is evidence that the successful working through of grief is necessary for later emotional stability.

During this struggle to assimilate the diagnosis, both patients and their relatives may show profound feelings of guilt and anger in addition to depression. This is particularly likely to happen, of course, if there is some known reason for the epilepsy, such as a head injury or a febrile convulsion. It should be remembered that patients often invent their own mythology to explain the cause of their epilepsy, something the doctor should be aware of when discussing possible causes for a patient's epilepsy.

Although not all patients pass through a period of emotional distress on learning of the diagnosis (some may actually be relieved, having feared far worse, i.e. that they were going mad), it should be assumed that most patients will. It is important as patients go through this period of turmoil that one does not interpret it as anything else.

Case History 1

This patient was a language student at university. At the age of 19 she began to have complex partial seizures. These became frequent and, since they were rather prolonged consisting of absences in which occasionally frightened behaviour would occur, were socially disabling. Despite the concern of her friends, she initially denied there was anything wrong with her and referred to her attacks as her 'little faints'. She developed a blasé, flippant attitude to them, so much so that at one time her apparent unconcern made one doctor suspect that she had the 'belle indifférence' of hysteria (but if one talked to her for long enough, her underlying anxiety became apparent). Later, as she accepted both the diagnosis and its implications (of lifelong taking of antiepileptic drugs and restrictions on her future career) she passed through a fairly profound period of depression, but latterly has been able to accept the illness for no more or no less than it actually is, and has found comfort in being able to help others in a worse predicament. Her emotional reaction to her illness was never treated as an illness but merely supported and interpreted, and she was given the opportunity of working through it.

To have epilepsy means to be exposed to the fear of having attacks; it means being somebody who frightens and disturbs others; it means being at a disadvantage in terms of work and personal relationships; it means being open to prejudice (which exists both in the lay public and in the medical and nursing professions); and it means sometimes to suffer disturbing symptoms not always directly connected with epilepsy.

THE SOCIAL EFFECTS OF HAVING EPILEPSY

Among the many problems with which a person with epilepsy has to deal are the unpredictability of attacks, and the reactions that other people have to them. This description given by one patient is typical: 'To awaken in a street which, for a moment, I cannot recognize, lying in a filthy gutter, wet and messy because I soiled myself, my thoughts confused, surrounded by strangers who are half curious, half disgusted, this is the nightmare with which I have to live'. Many people with epilepsy will recognize those feelings. Through most of his or her life, the person with epilepsy does not appear disabled, but well. Unpredictably he or she thrusts the disability unexpectedly on unprepared and uninformed strangers.

There is widespread prejudice against epilepsy in almost all cultures. Among many primitive people, people with epilepsy are regarded with hostility and denied access to whatever medical and social care may be available. Attitudes in Africa in this regard have been particularly well studied. A person with epilepsy may become an outcast from society; exposed to social and religious taboos; sometimes denied the right to procreate; seen as different and threatening to the stability of society; and often the victim of cruel and useless medical treatment.

It is easy to be complacent, to say that such things do not happen in our own society, and that the primitive reaction to epilepsy is essentially one of rejection. However, we must remember that, until very recently, similar attitudes and practices occurred in our own societies, and to some extent still exist. In some western countries, laws forbidding people with epilepsy to marry were repealed only very recently. Officially, there is little overt prejudice against people with epilepsy. However, there is still important and significant latent prejudice even amongst those highly educated and with a tradition of liberalism and compassion – the medical, nursing and teaching professions, and the churches.

Intensive educational efforts to change public attitudes towards epilepsy have been made particularly in the United States and, as has been shown (Caveness et al 1969), these have had considerable success. As might be expected, the most favourable changes have been found amongst the better educated and younger people living in large towns in the United States. The greatest remaining prejudice against epilepsy was found in the southern states where there seems to be a relationship with racial prejudice. People with epilepsy tend to be viewed with the same hostility as the racial minorities (Bagley 1971). In western societies, both the coloured person and the person with epilepsy are feared for their supposed primitiveness and violence, and for their unpredictability (one wonders too whether guilt about how both have been treated enters into the emotional reaction to them).

In the UK 25 years ago only 57% of the population surveyed felt that people with epilepsy should be employed and 32% said that they would object to their child playing with a child with epilepsy (Office of Health Economics 1971). Can these entrenched attitudes be changed?

That attitudes may be changing in this country is illustrated by a 1979 Gallup Survey (Epilepsy News 1979) which showed that 78% of respondents then felt that people with epilepsy should be employed and 88% were happy for their children to associate with an epileptic child. Of course, what people say and what they will do are not necessarily the same. How much this poll reflects specific attitude changes to epilepsy or how much it merely reflects a general liberalization of attitudes in the British people is hard to say. A disquieting feature of the survey was that prejudice is still common in adolescents and young adults reflecting the need for better education about epilepsy in schools. Recognizing this fact, the British Epilepsy Association has recently developed a schools' pack of information about epilepsy for both teachers and pupils designed both to give unbiased information about epilepsy and to help school children to examine their attitudes towards epilepsy and those who have it. The effectiveness of this approach is currently being evaluated (Corbidge & Bullock 1986).

In purely material terms, money spent on such education in the UK would be a way in which preventative medicine might save, not only many people much unhappiness, but also an immense amount of time for psychiatrists and their colleagues in trying to relieve personality and behavioural reactions to faulty social attitudes.

It is important to emphasize that the medical and related professions themselves are not free from prejudice and may still entertain irrational attitudes about people with epilepsy. The British Medical Association Working Party on Immigration as recently as 1965 recommended that people with epilepsy should not be allowed to enter this country 'for social and economic reasons'. It is difficult for people even with well-controlled epilepsy to enter the medical, nursing or teaching professions (Betts 1986).

Doctors, nurses and school teachers (and their own teachers in universities and training colleges) are an important source of unbiased education for the public, and removal of prejudice in these groups is therefore very important. The teacher, whether medical, nursing or lay, has a vital role

in educating others about epilepsy. In the classroom the teacher, by his or her acceptance of the child with epilepsy and calmness and unconcern if a child has a fit, by example helps to dispel fear and prejudice in the rest of the class. It is easy for busy doctors immersed in their clinical work to forget the importance that such preventative work may have, and the effect that it may have even on their own practice.

A large number of problems with family relationships can be averted by the understanding, sympathy and common sense of the family doctor. Those problems which are more severe or which have been allowed to develop unnoticed need the special experience of the psychiatrist, and his or her psychologist and social work colleagues to put them right. Reactions of rejection or hostility against the child with epilepsy by parents are common and as previously mentioned, are often associated with feelings of guilt. Some parents, aware of their hostile feeling, will compensate for them with over concern and overprotection; others will be overtly hostile with equally damaging results, although it is a moot point whether overt hostility or kindly over protection lead to more damage in the long run.

Case History 2

At the age of 8, this girl sustained a cerebrovascular accident of unknown aetiology in the territory of the right middle cerebral artery. After investigation in a neurosurgical unit, she recovered quite well although she was left with residual hemiplegia. This, however, did not interfere with her school performance and she eventually obtained a job in the Civil Service and married. She was the youngest of her family and, particularly after her stroke, was babied by the rest of the family, so that she grew up with a rather histrionic and attention-seeking personality. About a year after her marriage she began to develop brief absences accompanied by bilateral twitching in the arms. The attacks worsened rapidly. There had always been a defnite startle component to them, but now, instead of lasting a few seconds and being followed by instant recovery, they started to last up to half an hour. She would respond to unexpected sounds in her environment by a brief akinetic absence plus a few bilateral jerks of the arms. This was followed by weeping, kicking, screaming and rolling about. She would frequently cry out 'get off' and appeared to be struggling with an imaginary, evil and presumably lecherous assailant. (This change in her attack pattern had followed her visit to hospital for a brain scan which involved an intravenous injection – which she hated – and also a visit to a film called 'The Exorcist'.)

The family's reaction to these very noisy attacks was interesting in that, when she had them, they would rush to her and start rubbing her legs, patting her on the face, and mopping her brow with a damp cloth. At the same time, the mother and the husband would have a bitter quarrel over the struggling body of the young woman, the mother accusing the husband of being the cause of the attacks, saying, 'she wasn't like this until she married you', whilst the husband would be hurling similar accusations back at the mother. Eventually the mother took the girl back into her own home to live with her. The frequency of the attacks increased until she was admitted to hospital, having up to half-a-dozen in a single day, exhausting both herself and her family. She was rapidly transferred from a general medical ward to a psychiatric unit where the attacks were treated simply by ignoring them and they disappeared fairly rapidly. The startle seizures were controlled with clonazepam. When she went home on weekend leave, the post-ictal elaboration returned and it became apparent that they were the woman's reaction to pre-existing family stresses which had been intensified by the development of her genuine attacks. A family conference was held in which a common policy for dealing with the attacks was thrashed out, and they declined in frequency at home. Over the next few years the elaborated attacks reappeared at times of family stress, and occasionally at such times she also had other brief hysterical symptoms like total aphonia.

She developed a good therapeutic relationship with her social worker who encouraged her to develop independence and self-reliance, which was particulary needed after the birth of her child. As she became more mature in her relationships and more self-assertive, family attitudes to her changed and, eventually, her husband left home taking the child with him; she was then rejected by her mother, so that she is now having to make her own way in the world. It seems that neither the family nor the husband were able to accept the girl when she was no longer in a relationship emotionally dependent on them. It is interesting that, as she has developed a more mature personality, she has ceased having even her genuine attacks and she has recently been withdrawn from medication.

Overprotection during childhood may well lead to the kind of battle which I have just described, with mother and husband competing to give unnecessary succour to the daughter or wife. It is often as difficult and painful for the victims of such family battles to break away as it is for the family.

Case 3
This 24-year-old woman, born of a prolonged and difficult labour and who later had several febrile convulsions, developed complex partial seizures originating in the left temporal lobe at the age of 11. The seizures consisted of an absence lasting a couple of minutes, during which the girl felt intense jamais vu and had micropsia; occasionally, seizures would continue for a great deal longer. They were frequent and showed little response to medication and were most likely to occur in the early morning.

The family's reaction to them was pathological. Mother and father denied themselves the opportunity of having other children and devoted themselves to the care of their child. The mother gave up work, the child was kept in a school near home; due to frequent seizures, school attendance was poor. She was never allowed to play with other children or to go out on her own, but had to be accompanied everywhere by her mother. She eventually left school and tried to obtain employment. Her mother was so anxious that the young woman might possibly have an attack whilst on her own, that her anxieties were communicated to the daughter. She, in turn, became so tense and anxious at the prospect of new employment, that she had many seizures, and she could not keep the job. Consequently, she spent a very restricted life at home merely helping her mother with domestic tasks. Occasionally, she would go to a youth club but, again, was always accompanied by her mother. At the club she met and fell in love with a young man with whom she had a prolonged courtship, marrying six years after they first met. They moved into a house only a few doors away from her parents' house. The woman now finds herself in a very difficult situation. A combination of intensive behavioural treatment and new chemotherapy has made her far more independent and has taught her to deal with her anxieties better, and has significantly reduced the number of her attacks, but she is still trapped in a dependency situation with her mother, who interprets independence as ingratitude and her husband, who is the kind of man who wanted a dependent domesticated woman to look after him.

Several studies (Pond & Bidwell 1959, Bagley 1971) have shown that the earlier the age of the onset of epilepsy, the more likely it is that the child will have behavioural problems during childhood and also in later life. Pathophysiological factors are obviously important, but psychological ones even more so.

STRESS DISORDERS

Many stress responses are normal. They become abnormal either when they are very severe, so that they interfere significantly with the person's life or with the life of others; when they become prolonged and continue to exist long after the stress itself has resolved; when they are maladaptive (in other words they inhibit a person's correct response to a particular stress so that it cannot be solved); or when they become self-reinforcing so that the stress symptoms themselves become the stress.

Reinforcement can also occur because of the effect that the patient's symptoms have on other people, or because the patient's symptoms do, in an unhealthy way, solve the problem. Psychiatrists talk about 'primary gain' which the patient may obtain from his or her symptoms; and 'secondary gain', which is the reinforcement or encouragement that other people may unwittingly give to the patient's symptoms. As we have seen, some parents have a need for a child to be totally dependent on them, and may, as the child comes to adolescence, encourage such dependency needs. The patient whose symptoms are cutting him or her off from a stressful situation (like the development of paraplegia in a teenager who is in conflict about whether or not to leave home) may find that there is a kind of collusion between him or herself and other people so that the symptoms are unintentionally reinforced by other people who cheerfully push the paralysed teenager around in a wheelchair and help the person to adapt to the life of somebody who is paralysed.

Just as we cannot consider epilepsy in isolation (epilepsy is certainly not just about having fits), so we cannot consider psychiatric symptoms in isolation – we have to take into account not only the patient's reaction to them but also the reaction of other people, and the situation in which they are occurring.

The particular stress disorder which occurs in an individual is the sum of many forces and influences acting on him or her and is partly determined by constitution and by previous experience. Stress disorders tend to be fairly consistent, although modified by the factors we have already considered, and they can also be modified by treatment.

The most common stress disorder is probably an anxiety state, which may be seen as a 'flight or fight' reaction which has become distorted by the requirements of civilization. Some people under stress develop disabling depressive symptoms; some may show maladaptive ritualistic or obsessional behaviour, others (although this is now rare), 'cut off' from their stress and develop hysterical conditions. Occasionally, people under stress may break down into acute psychotic states. Stress is, of course, also a most important causative factor in some physical illnesses and a significant adjunct to many others. The role of stress in the precipitation of epilepsy itself will be considered later on in this chapter. The types of maladaptive responses to stress which have been described are not necessarily exclusive: many people who are anxious, for instance, can also feel depressed and vice versa.

By and large, stress disorders should not be seen as illnesses. There is no doubt that psychiatric illnesses in the true sense do occur in people with epilepsy and these will be considered later in this chapter. Except perhaps in rare situations, however, it is unhelpful to see anxiety, mild depression or hysteria as an illness, particularly as this tends to imply that there is a 'medical' treatment.

Do stress disorders occur more commonly in people with epilepsy than in the general population? The answer is that they probably do, and that epilepsy, in some ways, is unique in causing stress disorders (it should be remembered, however, that life experiences may be pathogenic in a disorder; in other words they may actually cause the disturbance or they may be pathoplastic, in that they alter the form that the disturbance takes in the particular individual.)

Studies of the epidemiology of stress disorders and psychiatric illness in people with epilepsy have been made, but there are many difficulties in carrying out an accurate epidemiological survey of the psychological difficulties of people with a chronic relapsing disorder like epilepsy. It is known, for instance, that in the UK only about half the people with epilepsy in the community treated by their general practitioners will be seen at a hospital clinic. Those that are seen are often referred, not because of the severity of their epilepsy as such, but because of other handicaps, both physical and mental, or because of co-existent personality and stress disorders. Any studies that concentrate on a hospital population of people will, therefore, be biased by the selected population being studied.

Although general practitioners frequently know a great deal about their patients' social problems, emotional disorders and psychological difficulties, such information may not be recorded or assessed accurately. It is also true that there are, in the general population, some people with epilepsy (and certainly many people with mental disorders) who do not seek help from their general practitioners. The sickest people often may be those least likely to seek help. Again, therefore, it is likely that those who do seek help from their general practitioner will be a biased sample. Some people with epilepsy may not themselves realize that they have it, or their families may accept it without asking for help. In one study (Betts 1974) of people with epilepsy admitted to psychiatric hospitals, it was found that 28% of the sample (who had proven epilepsy) had never consulted their general practitioners about their attack disorder, and were not receiving medication.

Therefore, to accurately determine the relationship between epilepsy, stress disorders and mental illness, field studies should be carried out in which a total population of a particular town or district is sampled by specially trained personnel who can carry out a formal examination of all people with a particular disorder. Even such a study as this will miss those people in the population who have been removed to institutions.

The results, therefore, of the studies carried out in the past few years should be interpreted cautiously. There does seem to be general agreement, however, that stress disorders (neurotic disorders) are more common in people with epilepsy than in the general population (Gudmundsson 1966).

A survey of all handicapped children on the Isle of Wight (Graham & Rutter 1968) suggested that about one-third of children with epilepsy had significant psychiatric disturbance. This proportion rose in those cases that had associated neurological symptoms; and was particularly high in those who were also mentally handicapped. The survey showed that the prevalence of psychiatric disorder was twice as frequent in children with epilepsy compared with children who had other chronic disabilities, e.g. asthma, and was about four times the expected rate in the general child population.

It may be that one other unique factor in the burden that epilepsy imposes on people (apart from the fear of the attacks themselves and the limitations on day-to-day living) is the fear of loss of control which epilepsy engenders. In this regard a comparison can be made between people with epilepsy and sufferers from Ménière's syndrome, some of whom may also be toppled to the ground by their vertigo. Patients with this disease may also feel very keenly the ignominy of their disability, which they are also helpless to control, and it has been shown that they too are

particularly liable to develop anxiety and depression (Pratt & Mackenzie 1958).

ANXIETY

As has already been said, anxiety is part of normal experience; it becomes pathological when it becomes overwhelming or self-reinforcing, or when it prevents the individual from dealing with the problem which is causing the anxiety. Anxiety has a psychological – a feeling of morbid dread or fear, which is subjectively most unpleasant – and a somatic component, which consists of symptoms referrable to stimulation of the sympathetic and the parasympathetic autonomic nervous systems (palpitation, nausea, diarrhoea, muscle aching, shaking etc). In some patients, the psychological component is prominent and in some the somatic component. Since anxiety often presents with somatic symptoms, it can easily be mistaken for physical illness, and the corollary is also true. In epilepsy, it is particularly important to distinguish between querulousness, irritability and agitation found in organic brain disease and anxiety itself. Likewise, anxiety is often a component of depression and, in somebody who is agitated, it is important to look for a possible underlying depressive illness.

Anxiety may be generalized and, therefore, be with the person all the time (so-called 'free-floating anxiety') or it may be situational, occurring in response to certain definite identifiable stimuli to which the patient is exposed (so-called 'phobic anxiety', occurring only when the patient is travelling, going into shops or encountering, say, cats or moths). In somebody who has anxiety symptoms, it is important to distinguish any phobic element, as this may alter the management. As will be seen later, patients who become acutely anxious often have so-called 'panic attacks' and these can be sometimes difficult to distinguish from epilepsy itself. A variety of severe phobic anxiety is 'agoraphobia'; the patient is crippled by intense anxiety when stepping over the threshold of home, and may, in fact, become totally housebound.

In this writer's experience, phobic anxiety and

agoraphobia seem particularly common in people with epilepsy and relate clearly to the patient's fear of having a seizure in a crowded place or in the street. Often, as we shall see later, the patient's anxiety increases the likelihood of having seizures so that, as the seizure anxiety increases so does the frequency of seizures, with each reinforcing the other. Indeed, the relationship between anxiety and epilepsy is extremely complex: an understanding of the nature of anxiety; its role in exacerbating and complicating epilepsy; and its management is necessary for anyone who cares for people with epilepsy. It is particularly important to distinguish between 'state' and 'trait' anxiety – between anxiety as a response to a situation or anxiety as a permanent part of a person's personality.

Betts (1981a), suggested a classification of the relationship between anxiety and epilepsy, which is slightly modified as follows:

1. Anxiety reaction to acquiring the label of epilepsy
2. Anxiety reaction to the social and family stigmatization of epilepsy
3. Prodromal anxiety
4. Anxiety as an aura
5. Ictal anxiety
6. Anxiety (agitation) occurring in an epileptic psychosis
7. 'Organic anxiety'
8. True phobic anxiety related to seizures
9. Anxiety which precipitates a seizure

Anxiety as already indicated is a common reaction to the stress of the discovery that one has epilepsy or of family, friends or society's bad reaction. But anxiety can also occur as a prodromal symptom of epilepsy – in other words, often for several days before an attack a definite increase in a person's anxiety levels is apparent, culminating in a fit (usually tonic-clonic) and usually with relief of the anxiety afterwards.

Case History 4
This simple man of 40, despite taking phenobarbitone in adequate dosage, has had tonic-clonic seizures about once a month ever since a closed head injury 20 years before. Both he and his family notice that about one week before his seizure he becomes irritable, restless and agitated, sweats more, his pulse rate rises and he becomes hypo-chondrial and preoccupied with bodily sensations. About two days before his attack he develops an urticarial rash on his trunk and arms, his sleep becomes disturbed and he develops a feeling of anxious expectation. At this time his sensorium is intact, physical examination normal and an EEG normal. Within two days of the rash developing he will have a tonic-clonic seizure, usually in his sleep. When he wakes, he is his usual calm, sunny self.

On one occasion full control of his seizures was obtained with phenytoin and for nearly a year he had no attacks; but his distraught relatives approached his doctor requesting that he be allowed to have the occasional seizure as without them he had become anxious and irritable all the time, and the phenytoin was withdrawn. Later it was found that if he took clobazam 30 mg for 10 days from the onset of his anxiety he had neither the anxiety nor the rash nor the fit; and he has now been successfully maintained on this regimen (plus his usual phenobarbitone) for two years.

What the mechanism of prodromal anxiety is, is anybody's guess, although it is unlikely to be directly related to the epilepsy. What is clear is that occasionally anxiety is experienced as part of the ictal experience, either as an aura or as the ictus itself.

Case History 5
This 15-year-old girl was referred when she grew too old for the paediatric service with a diagnosis of probable pseudo-seizures. Her attacks consisted of shouting, screaming, and rolling on the floor with kicking and jerking. She was a very reserved girl, difficult to get to know and the despair of a harrassed and divorced mother who was finding her daughter's behaviour more and more difficult to cope with.

Ambulatory EEG monitoring showed that there was no discernible paroxysmal activity during the convulsive struggling, but that these episodes were always preceded by a 30 s spike discharge from the right temporal lobe. Observation of the girl's attack in hospital showed that the attacks started with the girl looking frightened: her eyes would glaze and she would rub her lower abdomen with her left hand; she would then give a sudden start, throw herself on the floor and begin to scream and kick.

She eventually revealed that her attacks started with an intense feeling of fear 'as though the end of the world was coming'. This fear was felt in the pit of her stomach which tightened and tightened and the feeling would then rise up into her throat; she felt that when it reached her throat she would die. It was to escape from these feelings that she would scream and struggle. She found it difficult to tell others of these terrifying experiences lest she be judged mad.

Subsequently, these attacks lessened in frequency and she no longer reacts to them with her previous dramatic behaviour.

Case History 6
This 20-year-old girl was referred with a diagnosis of panic attacks. From the age 3 she had suffered from brief episodes of anxiety. From 3 until 12 she had had sudden feelings of anticipatory anxiety ('like going to the circus').

These would come on suddenly, last a few seconds and go as quickly as they came. She found them mildly pleasant: 'like something nice was going to happen', could not relate them to any particular event or circumstance and held them of no consequence.

When she was about 12 the attacks continued but the nature of the feeling changed. Now the anxiety was unpleasant, 'like going to the dentist', and tended to last longer and she became visibly upset by them. She became afraid that others might notice them and laugh and stopped going out or mixing with people. At the time of change in the emotional tone of the attacks there was a great deal of family turmoil.

By the time she was seen she had had a year of psychiatric treatment to no avail (including interpretive psychology and behaviour therapy) and was housebound, as she was having several attacks a day. Observation in hospital showed that she would suddenly go quiet; consciousness would be clouded; and there would be some swallowing followed after about 10–20 s by brief tachypnoea; sometimes she would rub her nose. Ambulatory EEG monitoring showed at these times that there was a clear-cut spike discharge in the right posterior temporal region.

Treatment with carbamazepine has reduced both the frequency and duration of these attacks, but they still occur, and tend to increase during times of stress. The girl needed a great deal of counselling to enable her to accept her epilepsy and admit its existence to others.

Case History 7
This woman believed herself to be a witch, as did many of the inhabitants of the small Herefordshire village where she lived. She had been able to predict many natural disasters and had become an object of fear and veneration in her village. She eventually became greatly distressed by her prophecies and by the effect they were having on others; she had several episodes of depression and was referred for further investigation. A careful history showed that she was not predicting natural disasters in a direct way, but would develop sudden brief intense feelings of apprehension of impending disaster. These would repeat themselves at intervals until a natural disaster would occur, and her reputation would then be further enhanced. These forebodings did not occur every time there was a natural disaster, and it was clear that selective forgetting of occasions when she did not predict correctly and retrospective falsification of memory were responsible for her reputation. Careful nursing observation on the ward revealed that she was having a brief attack disorder in which she would suddenly slump forward for a few seconds, breathing stertorously with a vacant glazed expression. During the attacks she could not be roused, and would wake up suddenly, although she was dazed for a few seconds afterwards; she was quite unaware of having had an attack although she remembered a premonitory feeling before it. The relationship between her attacks and the premonitory experiences became clear when it was found that there was EEG evidence of a right temporal lobe epileptic focus.

Case History 8
This woman had had an undiagnosed attack disorder thought to be psychogenic for eight years before she was referred for a second opinion. Her turns started the day after the delivery of her third child. Although she had had

them for eight years, only her husband had ever witnessed one. She could only describe them vaguely, although she knew that in them she was very badly frightened. She described feeling hot and very anxious for no apparent reason and thought they lasted for about 15 min. At first they might come on at any time, but for some time they had occurred invariably on a particular day of her menstrual cycle. In addition to these symptoms, she was undoubtedly prone to depression and anxiety and had a marked obsessional personality. She had had a very unhappy childhood, with a complete disruption of normal family relationships. Over the eight years she had had frequent EEG examinations, all of which revealed no abnormality, and had taken a large amount of psychotropic medication, including tranquillisers and antidepressants, all of which had failed completely to relieve her symptoms. Most doctors who had seen her over this eight-year period thought she was suffering from anxiety attacks. For some reason it was eight years before anyone got a description from her husband, the only witness of the attacks. What he had observed was very different from his wife's account. He said the attacks were very brief, seldom lasting more than 30 s; he appreciated when she was having one since she became vacant and clouded and he was not able to reassure her. After the attacks, she was intensely anxious and frightened. She was admitted to a specialized unit for observation at the phase of her menstrual cycle when an attack might be expected. The attacks began, as anticipated, and were as her husband had described. They began quite suddenly; for 20–30 s she was dazed and unrousable and was observed to flush violently over the face and upper arms and she chewed and smacked her lips. She came to suddenly, although she appeared somewhat dazed and confused for some seconds afterwards, and was also intensely frightened (it was this part of the attack she remembered).

During the day of the attacks themselves, but at no other time, her EEG showed evidence of strong epileptic activity in her left temporal lobe. She is an example of how, during a temporal lobe attack, time sense may become distorted so that the patient gives an inaccurate estimate of how long the attack lasts.

Williams (1956) in his classic paper on ictal emotion felt ictal anxiety to be the most common of the ictal feelings and to be confined to the anterior part of the temporal lobes, either the left side or bilateral. This writer's experience, as shown above, is different. Ictal anxiety can be accompanied by automatic manifestation of anxiety like sweating, belching, vomiting, piloerection, tachycardia or, as in one patient, even micturition. Automatism related to the anxiety may occur, and visual hallucinations of a frightening nature may be observed. Williams felt that the fear often has an unnatural quality like fear of the supernatural, rather than being reality based. It is clear from the above case histories that ictal anxiety may not be recognized and carry a psychiatric label. Occasionally, the converse is true and anxiety attacks may be mistaken for an ictus.

Case History 9

This woman, aged 38, had a long history of psychiatric illness. For some years before admission to a psychiatric hospital she had become agoraphobic, being unable to pass over the threshold of her front door without experiencing symptoms of anxiety. She became particularly anxious when entering shops and, shortly before her admission to hospital, began to experience peculiar attacks of depersonalization in this situation, eventually falling to the floor if she entered a supermarket. She was aware of a rising tide of anxiety before these phenomena happened; suddenly, the anxiety would seem to leave her, and was replaced by intense depersonalization. She became aware of a feeling of lightheadedness, tingling in her hands and feet, followed by tetany of the hands and feet, and she would then pass into a brief period of apparent unconsciousness. When one of these attacks was witnessed, she was put into an ambulance and initially taken to a nearby general hospital, but from there transferred to the local psychiatric hospital. During the course of her investigations there, an EEG was performed which showed some dysrhythmia in the right temporal lobe (a not uncommon finding in people with phobic anxiety). On the basis of this abnormal EEG she was diagnosed as having temporal lobe epilepsy and was referred for neurosurgical advice. She was seen at the request of the neurosurgeon before surgery was contemplated; admitted to a general hospital psychiatric unit; treated with intensive behaviour therapy; and, eventually, made a full recovery from the attacks which were clearly not epilepsy but panic attacks. The phenomena of lightheadedness, tingling, tetany, and then apparent unconsciousness, which were considered as epileptic, are of course symptoms and signs of hyperventilation which, rarely, may even cause a major convulsion.

Case History 10

This man of 36 was referred from another consultant with a diagnosis of intractable temporal lobe epilepsy which large doses of several antiepileptic drugs had failed to control. Two years previously, following a road accident, he had begun to develop attacks which were described as starting with 'an aura of fear' and which were accompanied by stereotyped behaviour described as an automatism. This was sometimes followed by a tonic-clonic seizure. The attacks were occurring many times a week and had totally disrupted his life and the life of his family – he had also been dismissed from a couple of jobs because of his epilepsy.

On admission to hospital, he was noted to be intoxicated with the various antiepileptic drugs he was taking and the usual policy of gradually withdrawing them was pursued. He became very apprehensive as they were withdrawn, and warned that he would have many fits as a result. It was interesting that, as so often happens both with people with epilepsy and also those with pseudoseizures, he did not have an attack for about ten days after his admission to hospital. He had several attacks on his first weekend visit home, however, being returned to hospital in an ambulance accompanied by various worried relatives. He then began to have many attacks whilst in hospital and most of them followed the same curious stereotyped form. Nurses would notice that he had become somewhat distant and vague; he would then suddenly jump to his feet, run to the nearest water tap which he would turn on (it was always the cold tap), and then allow a stream of cold water to flow over his head whilst holding his nose and groaning incoherently. His attacks would usually terminate after this, and he would lie on his bed for about half an hour recovering, declaring himself to have a headache and to feel sleepy. On two or three occasions, however, whilst kneeling with the cold water pouring over his head, he would have an undoubted tonic-clonic seizure.

If he was arrested in his dramatic flight down the ward to find the nearest cold tap, however, it was possible to hold a rational if somewhat fraught conversation with him, and there was no evidence of a diminution in or clouding of conciousness and he would express himself at that time as feeling intensely anxious and frightened and said that the sensation of cold water, plus the act of holding his nose, seemed to prevent the anxiety from becoming more intense. It was also noted that at these times he was hyperventilating and it seemed that his nose holding was a way of slowing his breathing.

EEGs before and after a seizure failed to reveal any significant abnormality, and, during one of his EEGs, hyperventilation precipitated one of his seizures up to nose holding with no concomitant EEG change. There was no doubt, however, that occasionally, what came to be regarded as acute panic attacks were followed by genuine tonic-clonic seizures. As he came to be better known (when detoxified he became a somewhat amiable rogue) the connection between his anxiety attacks and his road accident became more clear: the car he was driving when he had the accident was stolen, he was uninsured, he did not have a driving licence and he was also drunk. He had been terrified ever since that the police might investigate the accident and charge him with the various offences that he had committed. However, in the accident itself he had suffered a head injury with slight concussion afterwards and it was interesting that air encephalography of the brain revealed a discrete area of cortical atrophy in the right parietal area consistent with the previous head injury.

He was treated by an intensive regime of behaviour therapy aimed at anxiety reduction and whilst on the ward he completely stopped having his anxiety attacks and after this no spontaneous tonic-clonic seizures were seen. It was concluded that he was suffering primarily from anxiety attacks, which occasionally were severe enough to precipitate a tonic-clonic seizure from hyperventilation, due perhaps to a low convulsive threshold induced by his head injury. He was eventually discharged and attended an employment rehabilitation unit.

Unfortunately, with the stresses of work and family life, he began to have panic attacks again and eventually had another tonic-clonic seizure and persuaded his general practitioner to put him back on antiepileptic drugs. The reason that he was keen to go back on drugs was to gain respectability in the eyes of his family who, when told that his attacks were primarily anxiety attacks, rejected him and told him to 'pull himself together'. When he had a futher tonic-clonic seizure at home following rehabilitation they became very angry with the hospital, insisted he change consultants and complained to their Member of Parliament who instituted enquiries into the 'gross incompetence' of the hospital. It was difficult to convince the MP that one could have an epileptic attack without necessarily being 'an epileptic'.

In this writer's experience anxiety attacks (or panic attacks) can be a trap for the unwary and can be confused with epilepsy. In a personal series of patients with pseudoseizures, panic attacks account for about 30% of the total. Their recognition and management will be dealt with further in Part Two of this chapter.

Sometimes anxiety or agitation may accompany a psychosis associated with epilepsy or be part of complex partial status. A peculiar form of agitation can also be seen in the brain-damaged, often accompanied by obsessionality (or 'organic orderliness'). Sometimes, in all the above, the agitation can be so prominent that the underlying cause is unrecognized. The management of phobic anxiety about epilepsy and anxiety that precipitates a seizure will be described later.

The management of anxiety involves careful investigation of the patient and his or her symptoms, with a physical history and examination followed by detailed analysis of emotional symptoms and life situation. Some patients with anxiety need counselling to help them to discover the best way of dealing with the situation that is making them anxious. Some, whose anxiety relates to interpersonal conflict, may need formal psychotherapy (in other words, a therapeutic relationship with a professional therapist who uses interpersonal skills and the emotional relationship that develops between therapist and patient to lead to an understanding of the emotional or interpersonal conflict causing the anxiety). Formal psychotherapy is a skilled undertaking with a large investment in terms of time and resources and, although sometimes extremely useful, need not be applied routinely in every patient who is anxious.

Behavioural methods of treatment, i.e. treatment aimed at helping the patient to overcome symptoms or to control them without worrying too much about the antecedents of the anxiety, are gaining popularity. They were originally used successfully in patients with phobic anxiety, but are now being used in those with free-floating anxiety. There are various available methods of teaching a patient to control his or her anxiety, involving types of relaxation training or biofeedback which will be described in the section on the self-control of seizures. The advantages of behavioural methods is that they teach the patient self-reliance and self-control.

In this writer's view, the use of psychotropic medication in those who are anxious should be kept to an absolute minimum. Far too many people in this country are given minor tranquillizers or hypnotic drugs to deal with neurotic symptoms which can be much better dealt with by other methods. Once started, tranquillizers are difficult to stop: they lead to dependence, they are a potent source of overdoses, and they teach the patient nothing about self-reliance. These views against the use of psychotropic medication in anxiety may seem severe, but they do apply particularly to patients with epilepsy, as most minor tranquillizers of the benzodiazepine group have antiepileptic properties and it may be even more difficult to take a patient with epilepsy off diazepam or chlordiazepoxide than somebody who is not epileptic. Occasionally, other medication may be temporarily useful in treating anxiety, particularly beta-blocking drugs if the anxiety has a large somatic component (Tyrer 1974). If tranquillizers are used, they should be given in short courses of two or three weeks during which time the patient must be encouraged to deal with the situation which is causing the anxiety.

DEPRESSION

'Depression' is a term much used but often little defined. As a symptom of a reaction to stress it is probably less common than anxiety, but can be much more disabling.

Depression, like anxiety, has both psychological and somatic components. It is a feeling of pathological sadness or lowness of spirits (which may pass beyond ordinary human understanding), often accompanied by feelings of guilt, unworthiness and self-blame.

In severe depression, delusions and hallucinations of a gloomy nature may occur. These psychological symptoms are accompanied by biological symptoms of a change in sleep pattern, loss of weight, loss of appetite and loss of libido. In milder forms of depression, the appetite and sleep changes sometimes go in the reverse direction and there is oversleeping and overeating, with a consequent weight gain.

Classically, two forms of depression are described, reactive and endogenous (or neurotic and psychotic), implying that in some people depressive symptoms are a clear result of life stress or interpersonal difficulty; in other patients no such relationship can be seen, and it is assumed that depression is an illness sui generis. This is sometimes a useful concept, although it is probable that in the majority of patients with a depressive illness no clear separation can be made. Endogenous depressive illnesses do seem to be more common in people with epilepsy, as will be described later.

The relationship between depression and epilepsy is basically similar to that between anxiety and epilepsy (reviewed by Betts 1981a). As already indicated, depression is a natural component of the grief reaction, although it can be suppressed or denied (Williams 1981). Likewise, it can be the product of a person's reaction to family or social stress caused by the epilepsy.

Prodromal depressive symptoms have been described (this writer has one current case), although, like ictal depression, they are much rarer than prodromal anxiety. Depression as part of an aura is likewise less common. In a personally observed series of 2000 patients with epilepsy Williams (1956) knew of 100 who felt emotion as part of the attack: the majority felt frightened (61), 21 depressed and the rest had some other feeling.

Since both anxiety and sadness is so much part of our life it might be difficult to distinguish normal sadness from ictal sadness, but the sadness often has a bizarre quality and is so out of context that it is easy to recognize. Almost invariably, if looked for, something else recognizably part of a complex partial seizure will be present.

Case History 11

This 63-year-old man tumbled off a ladder in a fit whilst painting his house. One of his lumbar vertebrae was shattered. Whilst lying in an orthopaedic ward, alone in the early hours of the morning, he cut his throat with a razor blade, and his life was barely saved. On admission to the psychiatric ward he was in a profound depressive stupor; he had had lifelong poorly controlled epilepsy and was still having several major seizures a week, despite heroic

attempts to control them with antiepileptic drugs. He had had several previous psychiatric admissions for depressive illnesses. Because of his precarious physical condition, his depression was not treated for a few days. In that time it was noted that he was passing very rapidly from the depth of profound despair and depression to near normality and back again. In the middle of a sentence he might slump forward into an intense stupor, the picture of unhappiness, responding painfully and slowly to all questions, and full of suicidal ideas, only suddenly, some minutes or an hour or so later, to lift in mood back to an almost normal state. His EEG showed generalized spike-and-wave discharge. He was treated with clonazepam. A relatively small dose of this drug rendered him attack-free and within a few days of starting it his depressive mood changes disappeared and have not returned.

Peri-ictal depression will sometimes persist after the ictus is over for a variable length of time. Although persistent depression more usually comes on as attack frequency is declining (Flor-Henry 1969, Betts 1974), occasionally it is found as part of an increase in attack frequency and this writer has rarely seen it as a kind of 'depressive delerium' (Betts 1981a). William (1956) likewise describes depression as being associated with 'a bad phase in the epilepsy'.

Case History 12

At the age of 14, this girl developed brief complex partial seizures supposedly from a closed head injury at the age of 7. At 16, tonic-clonic seizures developed and tended to run in clusters a few months apart. They continued despite treatment with phenytoin and phenobarbitone and, when she was 22, she began to develop severe but short-lived depressive illnesses that came on when there was an exacerbation of her epilepsy, and in which several determined attempts at suicide occurred. Antidepressant medication had little effect but both the fits and the depression would paradoxically disappear quickly if electroconvulsive therapy was used. In these depressive episodes she was not confused or disorientated, but developed profound guilt feelings, woke early, was retarded, lost weight and heard hallucinatory voices in the second person telling her she was unworthy and should kill herself. Eventually, episodes of frequent seizures and depression occurred several times a year. Depot flupenthixol was tried and since then, despite having occasional clusters of major fits there has been no recurrence of the depression.

Depression can be part of what otherwise would be seen as a schizophrenic illness occurring in relation to epilepsy. Indeed, careful studies of the phenomenology of epileptic psychosis (Perez & Trimble 1980) suggest that an affective component to these states is common.

The management of depression involves a detailed history and examination of the patient, both physically and mentally, and an enquiry into life circumstances. Some depressions can be supported and worked through using techniques of counselling or psychotherapy. In contrast to anxiety, however, some patients will need chemical support as well; the indications for using drugs even in reactive depression are much stronger than in anxiety. The tricyclic antidepressants should be considered first, although their convulsant action needs to be remembered.

The drug treatment of the depression of epilepsy has recently been reviewed (Robertson 1985). Theoretically a non-convulsant antidepressant like nomifensine might be more appropriate because of the risk of induced seizures but, in practice, Robertson found that neither amitriptyline nor nomifensine (which has subsequently been withdrawn because of untoward side-effects) were particularly effective in the depressive states of epilepsy, the depressions often spontaneously remitting. Neither drug had any effect on fit frequency. This writer has found that occasionally electroconvulsive therapy (ECT) is needed.

Case History 13
This 23-year-old girl developed complex partial seizures at the age of 16. There was a previous history of febrile convulsions as a child. The attacks were initially frequent and responded poorly to antiepileptic drugs. Physical examination showed no abnormality although an EEG showed some right posterior spike-and-wave activity. A year before her admission to hospital, her seizures spontaneously declined in frequency and she had not had one for three months. Shortly after her attacks stopped, she quite suddenly became profoundly depressed with early morning waking, loss of weight and appetite, loss of sexual interest and marked diurnal variation in mood. She developed profound ideas of guilt related to childhood masturbatory episodes, and was admitted to hospital following a determined attempt at suicide with her antiepileptic drugs. Treatment with amitriptyline in hospital failed to resolve the depression (although there was a concominant return of her seizures and, in addition, she had two tonic-clonic attacks which she had never had before). Amitriptyline was, therefore, stopped. Because of the severity of her depression and her continuing suicidal feelings, she was treated with a course of electroconvulsive therapy. After six applications of ECT, her depression had largely resolved and she was able to go home. It is interesting that the electrically induced seizures produced a remission in her depression which the spontaneous tonic-clonic seizure had not (this is not always the case). Over the subsequent year she had two further short-lived episodes of depression which did not require hospitalization or treatment as they

resolved fairly rapidly, and since then she has been both depression- and seizure-free.

Apart from the drug treatment, patients with depression need the support of somebody who understands how disabling depression can be. As a person's depression starts to improve, so he or she will need careful rehabilitation, because, like anxiety, there is no doubt that depression can be self-reinforcing. The loss of confidence in one's abilities which depression can engender may eventually be more disabling than the depression itself, and can persist long after the depression is over.

In the management of depression the risk of suicide must always be kept in mind. Those with epilepsy have a readily available source of dangerous antiepileptic drugs with which to overdose. It is probable that suicide attempts, as well as completed suicide, (Barraclough 1981) are more common in people with epilepsy than in the general population (Mackay 1979). A patient with epilepsy is also more likely to repeat previous overdoses. Part of the explanation for the increased incidence of repeated overdoses in people with epilepsy may, of course, lie in the chronic nature of the epileptic patient's problems which are not resolved by the overdose attempt.

In a busy general hospital, this writer sees many people with epilepsy who have taken overdoses of their antiepileptic drugs. One particular phenomenon which is not well described in the textbooks is worth reporting: following recovery of consciousness in patients who have taken large overdoses of such drugs as phenytoin, phenobarbitone, primidone or the benzodiazepines, there may be an interval of several days of unruly acting-out behaviour which may be mistaken for the patient's normal state.

Case History 14
A 17-year-old girl with poorly controlled epilepsy (probably because of her reluctance to take antiepileptic drugs because of their side-effects) discovered herself to be pregnant and immediately swallowed a large quantity of the phenobarbitone and phenytoin she was supposed to take. She was admitted to hospital unconscious, and recovered consciousness 24 h later. Shortly after regaining consciousness she was found on a window ledge of the general hospital to which she had been admitted, threatening to jump. When taken back to bed and restrained, she bit, fought and scratched the nursing staff, broke two thermometers on her bedside locker and attempted to swallow them, and later broke a cup and attempted to cut her

wrists. Unless constantly watched, she would get out of bed and dash round the wards, screaming and shouting and attempting to leave the hospital. She was, therefore, transferred to a psychiatric unit (where this kind of behaviour after antiepileptic drug overdosage was well known), and her behaviour was contained rather than treated, as it has been found that sedating such disturbed patients merely makes them worse.

An EEG at this time showed changes compatible with drug intoxication, but there was no evidence of subictal epileptic activity (which might have been the cause of her mental state). Three days after her admission to the psychiatric unit her behaviour rapidly settled and a pleasant and co-operative, if somewhat troubled, teenager emerged from underneath it. Her antiepileptic medication was changed to carbamazepine; her compliance with treatment improved, and she was counselled about her pregnancy, which she decided to keep.

In patients with epilepsy, threats of suicide should always be taken seriously and carefully assessed. Any patient who is depressed should be asked specifically about whether or not he or she has had any thoughts or plans of self-harming. (Many patients are relieved to be asked this question). It has been shown that most people who succeed in killing themselves have given clear warning to somebody of their intention beforehand. Patients who are considered likely to make active attempts at suicide (whether their depression is reactive or endogenous) should be admitted to hospital for treatment of their depression and, if necessary, they should be compelled to come into hospital.

Even if initial assessment suggests that the patient is not potentially suicidal, it is important to keep in close touch with him or her until the depression has clearly resolved. It should also be remembered that somebody with intractable epilepsy, which has not responded to treatment, may attempt to take his or her life, not because of depression but because it is felt to be a rational solution to an intolerable situation.

A high-seizure frequency may make effective treatment of the depression more difficult and concomittant with the treatment of depression every effort should be made to bring the patients' seizures under as good control as possible, short of intoxication. (It should be remembered that the symptoms of depression can resemble those of drug intoxication and vice versa). It cannot be emphasized too strongly that, if a family doctor or neurologist has any doubts about the suicidal intentions of a depressed patient whom he or she is treating, it is important that the patient be referred urgently for a psychiatric opinion.

Symptomatic alcoholism is common in depression and may also occur in people with epilepsy; although one survey has suggested that drinking problems are less common in people with epilepsy than in the general population (Mackay 1979). If alcoholism does occur in somebody with epilepsy, it complicates considerably the management of the epilepsy. Excessive alcohol intake may cause fits in the predisposed (as may alcohol withdrawal), although it can be debated whether such 'Rum Fits' constitute established epilepsy. However, alcohol affects the metabolism of antiepileptic drugs, and it is difficult to control serum levels if they are liable to be influenced by excessive and erratic alcohol intake. Patients who drink excessively are usually unreliable in the taking of prescribed drugs.

There is no evidence that moderate drinking needs to be forbidden in people with epilepsy (who are already subject to many restrictions); although in view of the potential epileptogenic effects of over-hydration, an excessive fluid intake should be avoided. A very few people with epilepsy are very sensitive to the effect of alcohol and regularly have attacks induced by even a very small amount: the writer knows of two patients who *only* have attacks if they drink alcohol, and have been able to abolish their attacks (and need not take antiepileptic drugs) by avoiding it. It should also be remembered that those who are brain damaged are probably more sensitive to the effects of alcohol: occasionally, a small amount of alcohol in some people may produce 'mania à potu', an excited, aggressive state, induced by what would otherwise have been a non-intoxicating amount of alcohol, and resembling to some extent epileptic furore.

Those patients with anxiety and depression who are faced with a loss of employment or severe social disadvantage (like the break-up of a marriage), will need further measures to help them. Antidepressants or a therapeutic relationship will not be enough, and skilled help from a social worker can be of tremendous importance to such patients. Despair which has evoked a call for psychiatric help will often be associated with an increased frequency of fits, and this in its turn exacerbates the psychiatric problems which then exacerbate the difficulties in controlling the epilepsy. Inpatient care, which provides a constant refuge with careful observation of fits, good medical management, adjustment of antiepileptic drugs, and a controlled programme of work rehabilitation is essential. Even specialized neurological units with good psychiatric support may not be able to look after patients long enough or provide adequate work programmes, and specialized psychiatric units, which in some ways are more suitable, may not have all the necessary medical facilities. For the patients just described with multiple handicaps the Special Centres for Epilepsy, where there are complementary hospital and residential units, may be particularly useful but may not be able to take the very disturbed.

Effective treatment and management of the patient depends not on the skills of one particular discipline but rather on the understanding by each specialist discipline of the skills of the others and on their constructive co-operation. A member of any discipline who treats people with epilepsy must have a good working knowledge of the skills of the other disciplines which are necessary for the total care of a patient with epilepsy, and must know when to call in other specialized help. Any psychiatrist who sets out to treat the psychological complications of epilepsy must also have a very sound knowledge of epilepsy itself.

The psychological opposite to depression is mania or hypomania in which there is elevated mood, sleeplessness, overactivity, often grandiose delusions, flights of ideas, irritability and weight loss. The condition is much rarer than depression and there is no evidence that it is more common in people with epilepsy than could be expected by chance. It can be difficult to distinguish between an excited schizophrenic state and hypomania: affective symptoms are certainly common in the psychoses of epilepsy which may explain the apparent lack of connection.

Certainly, this writer cares currently for two patients who have in the past carried the label of schizophrenia in addition to having epilepsy. Both, in his opinion, however, have recurrent attacks of hypomania with grandiose religious delusions; both have right temporal lobe epileptic foci; both get an increase in focal EEG paroxysmal activity during their episodes of excitement. Neither has ever exhibited a first-rank symptom of schizophrenia. Episodes are short-lived and the patients have normal personalities in between.

OTHER STRESS DISORDERS

Some people under stress develop compulsive ritualized behaviours (such as compulsive hand washing, checking or thinking) which can be seen as an attempt to ward off the anxiety induced by the particular stress. Compulsive disorders are particularly likely to become self-reinforcing and are subjectively most unpleasant. There is no evidence that they are more common in people with epilepsy than in the general population. They seem to respond best to behavioural methods of treatment. (They should be distinguished from the 'obsessional personality' which is a rigid pedantic personality structure not uncommon in those who are brain damaged.)

Some people under stress, in order to escape an intolerable situation, develop hysterical symptoms. There is no word in psychiatry which has been more abused and misunderstood than hysteria. To a psychiatrist, hysteria means the unconscious adoption of conversion symptoms of an organic nature (often of a pseudoneurological character) which resolve the conflict or stress for the patient often in a symbolic way (e.g. the paralysis of the writing hand which prevents a student from writing his or her final examination papers). Most psychiatrists would agree that the symptoms or signs presented are adopted unconsciously in hysteria, although the borderline between conscious simulation of a disorder and conscious malingering is difficult to define. Hysteria nowadays in Britain is rare, and usually easy to recognize, particularly as it usually results from an acute traumatic situation for the patient.

Problems in recognition arise with chronic symptoms which may be hysterical. It is certainly true that acute hysterical symptoms, unless rapidly treated, may become chronic; particularly as they are easily reinforced by the reaction of other people to them. However, it cannot be emphasized enough that, in a patient with chronic neurological symptoms for which no adequate cause can be found, the diagnosis of hysteria must only be made on positive diagnostic criteria for hysteria and not just be a diagnosis of exclusion. Many patients with a definite organic lesion may over-elaborate their symptoms in order to draw the attention of an often doubting medical profession to them. Cases of firmly diagnosed hysteria often turn out later to have either organic or other psychiatric pathology to account for them (Slater 1965).

Hysteria has usually been treated by some form of psychotherapy but there is a growing interest in treating hysteria along behavioural lines (Bird 1979). A full account of the management of hysteria will be found in Mersky (1979). The condition will be considered further in Part Two of this chapter on simulated seizures. Simulated seizures which are those of true hysteria (the distinction between malingering – deliberate simulation – hysteria – unconscious simulation – and what might be called temper tantrums is not always easy to make) are sometimes accompanied by other neurological signs.

Occasionally, people under stress break down into what appears to be an acute psychotic illness of either an undifferentiated or schizophrenic type. In some patients who break down like this under acute stress, there is no doubt that it is an unconsciously simulated psychotic disorder (like the Ganser syndrome), which can be seen as a variant of hysteria, often with a clear message from the patient to the outside world, 'Look how mad you have made me'; but occasionally an acute schizophrenic illness can be precipitated by stress. Such illnesses have a good prognosis if the stress can be removed and in people with epilepsy need to be distinguished from those psychotic illnesses of a schizophrenic type which are found in association with epilepsy itself, or from complex partial status.

PERSONALITY DISORDERS IN PEOPLE WITH EPILEPSY

There is a long-held belief that people with epilepsy are more prone to disorders of personality than people without epilepsy. This question needs to be considered critically, without the prejudices of those who have preconceived ideas or those who are over-anxious to alleviate the problems that their patients have by refusing to accept that some people with epilepsy may have problems in interpersonal relationships.

A personality disorder is not easy to define. It is true, however, that some people seem to have chronic problems of adjustment to society, with living, or with relating to other people, which appear to be persistent and longstanding (often dating from childhood) producing stress symptoms either in the person concerned or in those who have to live with him or her. Problems arise in the definition and measurement of such apparent personality disorders, as the definition of a personality disorder is very much bound up with the values of the particular society which is defining it. A particular trait may be seen by one society as pathological; in another it may even be the norm. In societies such as ours, which are changing rapidly, definitions become even more difficult.

The diagnosis of a personality disorder must rest on definitive reliable criteria and not on the personal prejudices either of the psychiatrist making the diagnosis or of society. Attempts have been made recently to try to clarify and refine the concept of personality disorder, and even to develop rating scales which can be used to define it accurately (Walton & Presly 1973, Tyrer & Alexander 1979, Tyrer et al 1979).

Most of the published observations on the relationship between personality disorder and epilepsy, however, are not based on reliable criteria which have been scientifically evaluated but merely on descriptions of the patient's behaviour. Such descriptions (which classify people as, for example, 'obsessional' or 'hypochondriacal' or 'overdependent') miss 90% of the patient's other behaviours; and it may be better to see patients on a continuum from normality in terms of a particular personality trait and also to see their personalities as multidimensional. As Walton & Presly (1973) point out, any classification of personality disorder should be based on clinical observation of behaviour rather than intuitive hunches. No symptom of neurotic or psychotic illness is required to make the diagnosis, the abnormality is in the personality itself and is based on the clinical history and examination and the observation of behaviour, and as Tyrer et al (1979) point out, on a history from a relative who has known the patient for some time. Deviation from normal behaviour shows itself primarily in the patient's relationship with other people and is a continuing, not an episodic, phenomenon.

Various personality traits have been attributed to people with epilepsy from time to time. The most famous (or infamous) personality type historically related to epilepsy is, of course, the 'epileptic personality' itself.

The balance of evidence suggests that a small number of patients with chronic epilepsy living under conditions of institutionalization or environmental handicap may develop a characteristic pattern of personality change which has attracted many descriptive adjectives in its time; many of them pejorative. Such patients are commonly described as pedantic, circumstantial, meticulous, religiose, egocentric, hypercritical, hypochondriacal, suspicious and quarrelsome and possessing a slowness and stickiness of thought which may suggest subnormality or early dementia. Such patients in an institution, even if few in number, are bound to colour opinion and must also represent a continuing problem in management. It is surprising how widely this view is still held. Indeed, not so very long ago (Henderson & Gillespie 1950) it was held that this epileptic personality was an accentuation of a pre-existing epileptic constitution which was responsible for the fits and any medical deterioration that occurred.

The problem in an institution is that if one has ideas about the personality of patients it is extremely easy to find evidence which supports one's hypothesis and, indeed, the hypothesis may even become self-filling. If one is expecting a certain form of behaviour from a patient one may well behave towards him or her in such a way as actually to induce the behaviour. The other problem about having a fixed belief that certain patients have an abnormal personality characteristic, is that one is then not motivated to change them, (although there is some evidence that even organic personality traits can be treated and changed).

However, there is little doubt that the constellation of personality traits described above does occur and is found in people with epilepsy. This apparent association is due to factors of selection in that those with unfavourable personality traits will tend to enter institutions more often than those whose personalities enable them to manage much better in the outside world, and, once admitted, they tend to stick there. Referral of patients with epilepsy to general hospital outpatients unconnected with psychiatry is still more likely to occur if the patient has psychological problems (Pond et al 1960).

The epileptic temperament, if it exists, or when it occurs, is the result of multiple handicap: childhood environmental and physical deprivation; brain damage; and, perhaps, the chronic effects of antiepileptic drugs. A temperament in many ways similar can be found in patients with other non-epileptic prolonged disabilities, e.g., rheumatoid arthritis and chronic pain cause personality change (Merskey & Tonge 1974).

Some authors suggest that the 'epileptic personality' may be a brain damage syndrome (Guerrant et al 1962) and there is some evidence that a similar clinical picture may occur in those with bitemporal lobe damage but without epilepsy (Slater et al 1963). It is certainly true that the epileptic personality has lost its importance in the thinking of those psychiatrists with an interest in epilepsy as, indeed, has the interest in trying to substantiate the relationship between epilepsy and other types of personality disorder. The methodological drawbacks and difficulties are well described by Tizard (1962). Another widely believed 'fact' has been that people with epilepsy are overly religious. However, when put to proper enquiry the opposite appears to be the case (Sensky 1983).

There remains, however, a generally held view in the literature and elsewhere that people with epilepsy are aggressive. Whether aggressiveness is more common in people with epilepsy than in the general population has never been tested formally, except in children where the evidence is conflicting. One study (Mellor et al 1974) suggested that epileptic children are somewhat more miserable than their peers but, if anything, are less aggressive. Bagley (1971) found an increase in aggressiveness in certain types of epilepsy in children. (It should be remembered that aggression in someone with epilepsy may be the result of severe subnormality or a symptom of associated mental illness) The evidence has recently been reviewed by Rodin (1982) and Fenton (1983), particularly the 1980 International Workshop on Aggression and Epilepsy.

Whether or not aggressiveness is more common in adults with epilepsy than in the general population is open to question, but there is no doubt that people with epilepsy are feared for their aggressiveness. In this writer's experience this is an irrational fear which stems from a small group of hospitalized epileptic patients who may show aggressiveness, and from the general fear of epilepsy itself; and, as shown elsewhere (Betts 1981b) from experiences in the asylums at the turn of the century.

Some people may, following their epileptic seizure, have outbursts of self-limiting, extreme, undirected violence – so-called 'epileptic furore'. Whether this is itself an ictal phenomenon is uncertain. What is true is that it is becoming very rare nowadays. Violence may also occur after temporal lobe attacks, which in themselves may pass almost unnoticed or may be part of the ictus itself. A few patients with epilepsy may have clear-cut episodes of rage in between their epileptic attacks which may be difficult to control.

The management of those few patients with epilepsy who do show extreme rage, whether it is ictal, peri-ictal or apparently unassociated with ictal events, may be difficult and require the resources of a secure unit until the aggression can be controlled or contained. In many cases, the rages can be intentionally or unintentionally reinforced.

Case History 15

This man was first seen by the writer in 1967 when he had been in hospital for 11 years having been admitted at the age of 35. He had a history of meningitis as a child and also of a forceps delivery. His epilepsy began at the age of 11, and was described as 'grand mal' in type. From the age of 20 he almost invariably suffered epileptic furore after each fit, and was eventually admitted to a mental hospital because of these furores. Following his admission to hospital he continued to have many epileptic fits (up to about 20 a month) and for a long time was the terror of the hospital being confined to a locked room on a locked ward; and there was a record of several homicidal attacks on staff

and patients. Most of the homicidal episodes occurred after a major tonic-clonic seizure but occasionally, in between his major seizures, he would have sudden short-lived outbursts of homicidal violence. They would start without warning or obvious precipitant and last for 5 to 30 min (during which time he was entirely unapproachable). He seemed to have no memory of them afterwards. At the time of his admission he appeared to be suffering also from a paranoid psychosis, in which he was described as having ideas of reference, grandiose delusions and auditory hallucinations. This psychotic state cleared within a few months after his admission without specific treatment.

He had been taking large doses of phenytoin and phenobarbitone since his admission. His epilepsy had not been investigated until 1967 when an EEG showed phase reversal of spike and wave activity in the right anterior midtemporal region. In addition to his regular antiepileptic drugs, chlordiazapoxide, 25 mg three times a day was added in 1967. Subsequently, he had no further fits and there were no further aggressive outbursts. His whole personality seemed to change in that he become pleasant and sociable, and within six months of starting chlordiazapoxide he was allowed out into the grounds for the first time ever. He eventually started work in the occupational therapy unit. He was seen again in 1979 (Betts & Skarrott 1979). He was still in hospital, although clearly he would have been quite suitable for hostel accommodation if any had been available. He was a pleasant, cheerful man with a wry sense of humour, and a good grasp of current affairs. There was no evidence of a dementing process. The chlordiazapoxide had been withdrawn in 1974; he had occasional short-lived aggressive episodes since that time (but none for two years) and he had had no seizures since originally taking chlordiazapoxide, although he remained on heavy doses of phenobarbitone and phenytoin.

Case History 16

This man had already been in hospital for 29 years when first seen by the writer in 1967. He was 19 years old on admission. His epilepsy was known to have begun at the age of 13 and was simply described in his notes as 'grand mal' in type. In 1967 he was still having a couple of fits a month. He was admitted originally 'confused and demented, and elated with auditory hallucinations. This seems to have been an acute organic psychosis of paranoid type, which disappeared quite rapidly after his admission to hospital without any specific treatment. Subsequently, he suffered from many attacks of epileptic furore following his tonic-clonic seizures and occasionally would suffer from acute aggressive outbursts in between his major seizures. These rages occurred without provocation, although it was noted that a specific phrase 'who's got wooden legs' would always precipitate an aggressive outburst.

This, at one time, unfortunately became a source of amusement for some of the nursing staff. In 1967 he was taking 240 mg of phenobarbitone a day in divided doses; this dosage has continued until the present day. His medical notes had continued to describe him as suffering from 'epileptic insanity', although no psychotic features had been observed in his mental state for many years and he was also described as suffering from 'epileptic dementia', although in fact he was correctly orientated in space and time and had a reasonable knowledge of current events. On review in 1979 he was found to be pleasant and equable in temperament. He was a somewhat simple man of 60 who showed no evidence of a dementing process and no psychotic features. His last seizure occurred in 1974, and since then there had been no further episodes either of furore or of aggressive outbursts.

Case History 17

This 30-year-old publican had been in good health and there was no evidence of previous seizure activity. One evening, whilst working with his wife in their public house, he went down into the cellar to change a beer cask and failed to return after a few minutes. His wife, who suspected that he was having an affair with one of the barmaids, crept down to the cellar to see what was going on. When she got into the cellar she saw her husband in the throes of a tonic-clonic seizure. Shortly after the attack ended, her husband rose in a dazed fashion from the floor and kicked in several of the barrels in the cellar. His wife remonstrated with him and was irritably pushed out of the way by her husband, who then ran upstairs into the bar and began to assault his customers. Although he hurt several of them, his violence did not seem to be directed against any one in particular. If people kept out of the way he failed to pursue them, but if they tried to restrain him, he would respond with violence. The police were summoned and he was eventually taken away with some difficulty to a local hospital where, in the casualty department, further attempts were made to restrain him. During the struggle, two members of the staff were injured but attempts to inject him with a sedative were fruitless. He was eventually locked in a side room where, left to himself, he quietened down very rapidly and fell asleep. Subsequent, investigations revealed a temporal glioma which was ultimately fatal. Similar behaviour occurred following further seizures but without the violence as no further attempts were made to restrain him and he was just confused and irritable. Attempts at conversation with him during such states were fruitless as, although he was clearly awake, he rarely made any reply.

These patients are representative of the epileptic patients with aggressive outbursts that can be found in mental hospitals. In them there seems to be a relationship, even if not a direct one, between seizures and the aggressive outbursts as both seem to wane at about the same time. They do not resemble at all closely the patients decribed by Maletzky (1973) with the 'episodic dyscontrol syndrome'. These were men without epilepsy (but many of them had temporal lobe EEG abnormality) who were subject to episodes of senseless, unprovoked violence in the setting of severe personality disorder; some improved with phenytoin.

The treatment of such violent aggressive outbursts is difficult and somewhat controversial. Occasionally, patients may respond well to the exhibition of benzodiazepine drugs, whether intravenously or by chronic oral medication; but not all will do so, and it should be remembered that these drugs, like alcohol and the barbiturates, may have a disinhibiting action, making the violence worse. Some patients will be better controlled with parenteral butyrophenone drugs or chlormethiazole. A particularly useful drug for calming the acutely disturbed is droperidol which can be given safely intravenously. Patients with acute aggressive outbursts are often better left alone and unrestrained, as the outburst is usually self-limiting.

Some patients, then, do have episodes of severe aggression. It is widely reported in the literature, although no controlled studies have been done, that many patients with epilepsy are chronically irritable and aggressive. It is not certain that this is necessarily more than one would find in an equivalent population of either institutionalized patients or normal people; but if it is accepted for a moment that perhaps some people with epilepsy do show undue aggressiveness, is it possible to find any correlation between the aggression and their social and epileptic history? There have been several reviews (Taylor 1969b, Serafetinides 1965, and an unpublished Birmingham study). All three studies suggested that men with epilepsy are more likely to be aggressive than women and also showed that the earlier the onset of the epilepsy, the more likely it was that aggression would develop later, which would suggest strongly the importance in the pathogenesis of aggression of early social disadvantage and failures of social learning. Taylor and Serafetinides suggested that there is a connection between aggression and temporal lobe epilepsy, but no such relationship was found in the Birmingham study. Serafetinides suggested that patients with left temporal lobe lesions are more likely to be aggressive but his figures, though persuasive, were not statistically significant.

The populations studied, however, are not comparable. The first two studies were considering patients with intractable epilepsy selected for surgery because of unilateral temporal lobe lesions, whereas the Birmingham study covered a much wider and probably more representative population of patients with epilepsy admitted to mental hospitals (Betts 1974). Many questions about the relationship between aggression and epilepsy remain unanswered and further work using control populations is clearly necessary.

The evidence to date suggests that, although brain mechanisms may be important, the influence of social and learning factors may be paramount in causing aggression in people with epilepsy. This is important because prevention may be possible with better management of children with epilepsy.

One important factor that has come out of studies of aggressiveness in epilepsy (Taylor 1969a) is that, in those patients going forward for temporal lobe surgery, aggressiveness is a good prognostic sign in terms of successful rehabilitation after the operation and cessation of fits. It is interesting that the other psychiatric disorders that may occur in association with temporal lobe epilepsy are seldom improved by temporal lobectomy, and may even be made worse. It has been suggested that some of the depressive illnesses which occur after otherwise successful temporal lobe surgery, (Hill et al 1957) are the result of the 'turning in' of this aggression onto the patient himself. Postoperative depression is certainly common after temporal lobectomy but may have other causes.

Gunn (1969) in his study of people with epilepsy in prisons, found little evidence of an increased degree of aggressiveness and violence in epileptic prisoners, although he recognised that some more difficult patients might have been sent to the special hospitals. He also found that in those people with epilepsy in prisons who were aggressive there was no particular correlation with any type of epilepsy. Others also have found no evidence that aggressiveness is especially common in temporal lobe epilepsy (Guerrant et al, 1962, Small et al 1966). Lishman (1968) in his study of the psychiatric sequelae of brain injury found that aggressiveness was more common after frontal rather than temporal lobe injuries.

EPILEPSY AND CRIME

If there is uncertainty about a relationship between epilepsy and aggressiveness, what is the relationship between epilepsy and crime itself? It has long been held that there is such a relationship (Lombroso 1889). In a survey of prison and borstal receptions in England and Wales, followed by a study of a representative sample of male epileptic prisoners (Gunn 1969), it was shown that the prevalence of epilepsy in the prison population is well above that to be expected. Many of these epileptic prisoners were also psychiatrically abnormal, but they were no more aggressive than the general population of prisoners. They did, however, have significantly more depressive symptoms than their fellow prisoners and had attempted suicide more often. There was no relationship between the kind of crime the prisoners had committed and whether or not they had epilepsy, and no relationship between type of crime and type of epilepsy.

No explanation could be found for the apparent increase in criminal acts in people with epilepsy, although it is likely to be a social one rather than a physiological one.

A further study (Gunn & Fenton 1971) of epileptic patients in a special hospital to assess the possible connection between criminal acts and epileptic automatism showed automatism to be an extremely rare explanation for crime in people with epilepsy, and crime related to an attack tends to be post-ictal rather than ictal. Those people in England and Wales whose crimes are directly related to the ictus or automatism are particularly disadvantaged as English case law (Regina v. Sullivan) defines such a state as insanity, with the likelihood that an offender will be committed to a special hospital. For a full discussion see Fenwick (1985).

Many people with epilepsy are socially disadvantaged and deprived, and tend to drift into crime and possibly are caught more easily. Most people with epilepsy in prison are there for thieving, as is the general prison population, and the increased prevalence of people with epilepsy in prison is almost certainly related to social rather than medical factors.

EPILEPSY AND SEXUALITY

The general public again tends to equate epilepsy with hypersexuality, in the same way as they tend to associate it with criminality and violence. How much of this prejudice can be blamed on Lombroso (1889) is uncertain, but the actual facts about sexuality in epilepsy are very different.

There is a relationship between sexuality and temporal lobe epilepsy (Shukla et al 1979). Temporal lobe lesions may produce disturbances of sexual function, usually hyposexuality with lowered sex drive, occasionally total impotence, and, in women, loss of sexual response (Hierons & Saunders 1966). Social and psychological factors may play at least as important a part as biological ones, although accumulating evidence does suggest that there is a neurophysiological factor present.

There is some evidence that successful treatment of the epilepsy, particularly by surgery, may improve sexual performance (Taylor 1969a). It may be that treatment of epilepsy by enzyme-inducing drugs may affect sexual performance, as such drugs lead to the rapid metabolism of testosterone with lowering of free testosterone blood levels. Testosterone has a relationship with sexual arousal and activity although it is a complex one. It has been suggested that this effect on testosterone metabolism causes the hyposexuality of epilepsy (Toone et al 1981). Testosterone depot injections have been suggested as a remedy but a formal trial has not been undertaken. Regular testosterone injections are not without their dangers and tend to induce non-specific feelings of well-being and increased appetite that may be mistaken for therapeutic improvement.

Free testosterone blood levels are difficult to measure (usually bound and free levels are measured together). Interpretation of the significance of low levels is also difficult (unless they are pathologically low), particularly as infrequent intercourse leads to a low level of testosterone: a high frequency of intercourse tends to increase testosterone levels. Except for patients with hypogonadism, however, there is little evidence that increasing testosterone levels artificially leads to increased intercourse.

Most of the work on the relationship between sexuality and epilepsy (as might be expected in a male-dominated medical profession!) has been on male sexuality. However, testosterone does have a relationship with female sexual arousal and so

changes in its metabolism may affect sexual response in women.

The writer's own experience (Betts 1984) suggests that social and psychological factors are important in the causation of sexual difficulty and lack of responsiveness in both men and women with epilepsy. In a review of people with epilepsy attending a psychosexual clinic (Betts 1984) they were shown to have the same kind of problems as the non-epileptic in roughly the same proportion (the over-representation of people with epilepsy within the clinic was probably due to the writer's interest both in epilepsy and in sexual disorder). The recovery rate of the sexual problems of people with epilepsy was also the same as those without epilepsy, using standard behavioural methods of treatment (and without testosterone supplements).

However, two aetiological factors did seem prominent in those with epilepsy who had a sexual problem: lack of practice due to social isolation and, more important, the inhibitory effect of fear of an attack during sexual activity. This fear usually inhibited the person with epilepsy, but occasionally would inhibit the partner. Because of the bonding effect of a happy sex life and its effect on morale and feelings of well-being, help to achieve a satisfactory sexual union, where appropriate, seems to me to be an important part of the rehabilitation of someone with epilepsy. The fear of a fit during intercourse is common, but may well not be volunteered and must be directly enquired for.

Case History 18
This man of 50 had had tonic-clonic seizures since the age of two. They had not responded well to medication (he was taking a mixture of phenytoin and phenobarbitone). He had grown up friendless and isolated and had shunned the company of women believing that they would not want 'an epileptic like me'. He suppressed his sexual feelings because a doctor had told him when he was young that masturbation led to attacks and he obeyed this injunction rigorously.

In his late forties his attacks began to abate and he was befriended at work by a woman 10 years younger. As the romance developed she indicated that she wanted it to sexualize and he was confronted with his lack of experience and low levels of sexual arousal. He became miserable and, as his feelings for the woman deepened, suicidal. He was referred for professional help. He was treated with a behavioural programme (a modified sexual growth programme of Lopiccolo) which included the development and shaping of masturbatory fantasies and developed a strong sexual response which he was able to develop into a fully satisfying sexual relationship with his partner, with the aid of some joint counselling. His self-esteem grew as he was able to allow the warm and tender part of his nature to show itself for the first time. When last seen he was contemplating marriage and he had been attack-free for nearly a year.

Case History 19

This girl of 24 was referred from a family planning clinic for advice as a 'case of oral contraceptive induced epilepsy'. When younger she had had tonic-clonic seizures (probably secondarily generalized) and, although these had stopped when she was 12, she continued to have occasional brief complex partial attacks which passed almost unnoticed (she stopped antiepileptic medication at 16). At the age of 18 she became engaged and started taking an oral contraceptive and a month later had a tonic-clonic fit whilst in bed at night. Her fiancé, who had known nothing of the epilepsy, fled and the relationship ended. Six years later she was engaged again, took the pill, and again a week or two later had a nocturnal tonic-clonic attack. Her present fiancé was made of sterner stuff than the last and stayed with her.

It became clear that the problem had nothing to do with the pill. Both attacks had occurred when she was attempting intercourse for the first time. She had hated and feared her major attacks and was terrified that during the abandonment and loss of control of sexual activity they would return. This fear was reinforced by the experience of her first attempt, so that she approached a sexual encounter rigid with fear and overbreathing as soon as a direct sexual approach was made. She was treated with a sexual growth programme, which allowed her to develop a sexual relationship with her fiancé with her fear confronted and controlled by anxiety reduction techniques. She has now developed a satisfactory sexual relationship and has had no further tonic-clonic attacks.

There is possibly a slight increase of perverse sexuality in temporal lobe epilepsy, although the evidence for this is slight. It has recently been reviewed by Hoenig & Kenna (1979), and, again, neurophysiological factors as well as social ones may be playing a part. The temporal lobes, after all, are probably the seat of sexual awareness in humans and it is, therefore, not surprising that aberrations in functions in these areas in the brain may give rise to aberrations in sexual behaviour. There is very little evidence that hypersexuality – except of a primitive kind such as excessive masturbation – occurs in epilepsy, although it may do so in very rare cases. Often, of course, hypersexuality is bound up with mental illness or severe brain damage.

Occasionally, sexual functioning may get bound up in the epileptic event itself, as in those patients whose attacks sometimes have a sexual component (Mitchell et al 1954), or in those patients whose major seizures are triggered off by a sexual experience as a form of reflex epilepsy (Hoenig & Hamilton 1960).

Case History 20

This girl of 16 had brief complex partial seizures, often premenstrual. After they occurred she would become disturbed, tearful and angry, and would sometimes show acting-out behaviour, running round the room and screaming. Even when the attacks came under much better control with carbamazepine the acting-out continued. Ambulatory EEG monitoring showed that her complex partial seizures were brief and the acting-out was not an ictal event.

She eventually made a confiding relationship with her clinic doctor (particularly when her mother was encouraged not to accompany her daughter during every interview) and the cause of her acting-out behaviour was revealed. Her partial complex seizure was a brief abrogation of consciousness followed by lip-smacking, of which she was dimly aware. In addition, she revealed this was accompanied by an intense, pleasurable, erotic feeling arising in her vagina and apparently rising upwards towards her throat. She was sexually inexperienced and her mother had given her such strong warnings about sexuality that she was frightened and confused by her feelings and her acting-out behaviour was an attempt to escape from their overwhelming presence. She was counselled and educated about sexual feelings and lost her fear of them and the acting-out behaviour disappeared.

Case History 21

This 26-year-old woman had a history of abruptly broken relationships (including two engagements). She had had a ten-year history of secondary generalized epilepsy partly controlled by phenytoin. Her partial attacks, which were not always followed by a tonic-clonic seizure, were a feeling of warmth in her vagina which rose in intensity until she had an orgasmic feeling (but only on one side of her vagina and pelvis). A tonic-clonic fit might then follow. Unfortunately, when having intercourse she discovered that a sexually induced orgasm would be followed by a tonic-clonic fit. Although one of her partners claimed not to notice, she found the event embarrassing and distressing and several of her partners (she enjoyed her sexuality) abruptly broke off the relationship. It had been planned to try some form of behavioural management of her reflex epilepsy (perhaps by habituation therapy) and she was the subject of one of the clinic's more unusual requests to the ambulatory monitoring service, but a change of medication to carbamazepine lead to complete control of her attacks, both reflex and otherwise, and further investigation and treatment was not needed.

There is a recognized relationship between previous incest and the later development of pseudoseizures (Goodwin et al 1982). Occasionally, sexual assaults or an incestuous sexual relationship may be followed by true epilepsy and this writer has had three patients with undoubted epilepsy whose attacks followed closely upon such a traumatic event. In two of them the behaviour they show during a complex partial seizure has sexual connotations. Both have found psychotherapy helpful. In both, it initially lead to an increase in attacks as painful memories were uncovered.

EMOTIONAL AND PSYCHOLOGICAL CONTROL OF FITS

It has been known for a long time that certain physical and emotional stimuli and certain somatic and mental states can influence, either directly or indirectly, the number of attacks which a patient is having. Occasionally, patients may have a measure of control over their fits. This writer feels that a great deal more attention should be paid to these phenomena, partly because they may help to explain one of the fundamental problems of epilepsy – why do fits occur when they do? – and partly because they may hold out therapeutic possibilities.

Such states should be of increasing interest to the psychiatrist. Physical stimuli adequate to precipitate attacks may, on occasion, be replaced by the psychological equivalent of such stimuli, and many of the methods of psychological treatment whose aim is a reduction of anxiety or a lowering of arousal, may have some therapeutic benefit in these forms of epilepsy and, indeed, in epilepsy in general.

Photic epilepsy induced by flickering light, sudden changes in light intensity or complex patterns, is the commonest form of reflex epilepsy. A variation of this is television epilepsy, which is particularly common in young adolescents. Rarely, reading may provoke attacks in which initial twitching of the jaw progresses to a generalized convulsion if the subject does not stop reading at once. There is an excellent recent review by Wilkins & Lindsay (1985).

Case History 22
This 20-year-old student was referred with a study phobia to a psychiatrist. He gave a history that, in the previous year at university, whenever he attempted to study hard at night, he had a blackout and was either found by his friends wandering in a dazed state outside his room or slumped before his open books. He said that when reading he suddenly became aware of a throbbing in his throat, followed by a twitching in his jaw, and then remembered no more for up to an hour. This was clearly reading

epilepsy which disappeared when he was given antiepileptic drugs.

Photic stimulation is the commonest way in which subjects, usually children, physically induce their own seizures; although in this writer's experience this type of directly self-induced epilepsy is rare. Visual self-inducers are characterized by exceptionally high light sensitivity, frequent seizures and subnormal intelligence. Most of these visually induced attacks are of the generalized absence or myoclonic type, and the frequency of attacks depends to a certain extent on the available light intensity. For example, they are more common in Australia than in the UK.

Most children that do this cannot give an adequate explanation of their behaviour, although it would seem from observation that pleasure and escape from stress or boredom are important aetiological factors. Some seem almost compelled to do it, in the same way that some children with television epilepsy seem irresistibly drawn towards a television set. Whether this urge is an epileptic phenomenon or related to some other phenomena, like counter-phobic behaviour, is not known. Self-induced visual epilepsy is very difficult to treat and, in many cases, it is necessary to help the family rather than the child, and advise them on how the child and his or her symptoms should be handled.

Hyperventilation is a common form of induced epilepsy in children and adolescents: some people with self-induced epilepsy seem able to produce an attack at will, or on request, but without any realization of how they do it; some unconsciously hyperventilate; others do it by an effort of concentration.

Seizures may be precipitated by other sensory stimuli, such as loud unexpected sounds; an element of startle is essential since a loud sound that the patient is expecting will not induce an attack (Doube 1965).

Musicogenic epilepsy, another rare condition, has aroused considerable interest. In most patients with musicogenic epilepsy, an affective associative response to the music is required to bring on a fit. In a few cases, however, there is evidence that the musical sound itself is the epileptogenic stimulus, possibly at a subcortical level.

A number of other stimuli effective in inducing fits have been described, including voice and language; movement; skin touching or tapping; vibration; eating food or the sight of it; immersion in hot or cold water; taste; and sexual stimulation (Gastaut & Tassinari 1966)

The important emotional and psychological component to most cases of reflex epilepsy is perhaps best illustrated by Goldie & Green's (1959) classic study. They described a man who could produce a reflex fit by rubbing his face. The psychological stimuli of preparing to rub his face, or thinking about rubbing it, were as effective as actually rubbing it in provoking epileptic EEG activity or the actual attack itself.

The reflex epilepsies are difficult to treat: it may be impossible to shield the patient from the provoking stimulus without great difficulty, or it may be that the patient does not want to be shielded, either because he or she likes the stimulus or because it gives some kind of emotional pleasure. Antiepileptic drugs are often unsatisfactory. Recently attempts have been made, mainly by Forster (1972) to use conditioning or extinction techniques which may have great possibilities in treating the reflex epilepsies, although they are at present too time consuming for widespread use. They may also work by a therapeutic shift of the patient's attention away from the triggering stimulus (Mostofsky & Balaschak 1977).

Forster (1972) presents the particular triggering stimulus to the patient continually, until the convulsive and EEG responses to the stimulus have extinguished. He may also train the patient to give himself a different stimulus if he encounters the actual triggering stimulus (as say when reading) which prevents the usual convulsive response. Forster appears to have had a great deal of success with these techniques and is also engaged in developing portable devices which can continue the patient's treatment at home, as much of the treatment at the moment is laboratory based.

SELF-CONTROL

The phenomenon of the self-control of seizures has been well known since the days of Hughlings Jackson and Gowers but seems to have been studied curiously little and, in many cases, little effort seems to have been made to discover exactly what it is that some patients actually do to stop their attacks. Symonds (1959), Fenton (1983) and Lubar & Deering (1981) reviewed the evidence that voluntary mental and physical activity could inhibit seizures. It is well known that patients with sensory or motor epilepsy can sometimes inhibit their attacks, once they have started, either by vigorous sensory stimulation of the involved area or by brisk muscular activity.

In the writer's experience, patients who can stop their seizures in this way do not always feel comfortable afterwards and they may feel better if they allow themselves to have an attack at a time and place of their own choosing. Symonds was more concerned with those patients who could inhibit seizures by an effort of concentration or an effort of will. This may involve thinking very hard about not having an attack or the repetition of some phrase which has the property of stopping the attacks, or occasionally the induction of an emotional state in which the attack will not occur. Of Symonds' patients, 5.3% could stop their attacks in this way, although how they did it was not usually obvious. Patients may not volunteer to their doctors that they have these control mechanisms and they may only be discovered by accident.

Although little is known about how these patients actually stop their seizures, it is known that desynchronizing and other control mechanisms do exist in the brain and quite possibly they could be better utilized. That certain psychological methods of treatment might be used in potentiating such control mechanisms is illustrated by the example of the woman that Efron (1956) described, where a controlling mechanism which the patient herself had noticed and brought to the attention of her doctor was shaped and refined, so that it became easier to use. It would be interesting to see whether patients with other sensory auras could be treated in the same way.

It has been held for a long time that emotional states can lead to an increase in the number of patients' attacks and, therefore, one could suppose that altering such states could reduce seizure frequency. Direct induction of seizures by emotional stimuli is probably rare and certainly Gastaut & Tassinari (1966) in their extensive review could find very little evidence that direct induction occurs. However, most doctors experienced in epilepsy are aware that changes in a patient's emotional state often towards higher arousal may lead to an increased number of attacks (Servit et al 1963). In recent years, a fair amount of laboratory evidence has emerged to support these beliefs.

Mattson et al (1970) carried out a detailed and important neurophysiological study of the effects of psychic stress on the frequency of seizures, although not as a direct stimulus. In other words, in a patient under stress more seizures than usual are likely to occur but not as a direct result of the stress itself. A search was made for any measure of an increase in arousal or stress that could be related to the increase in seizure frequency. There was little relationship between any of the usual parameters of arousal (e.g. plasma cortisol levels) and seizure frequency, but it was noted that increase in seizure frequency under stress was related to involuntary hyperventilation, with a resulting fall in carbon dioxide concentration. The aetiological importance of this finding was supported by the observation that such an increased seizure frequency under stress could be prevented if the patient was made to breathe an increased concentration of carbon dioxide. It is suggested that involuntary overbreathing may be an important psychophysiological precipitant of seizures, as it is in those patients who induce their attacks deliberately by hyperventilation.

Gotze et al (1967) using telemetered EEG recordings, showed that physical exercise tended to normalize the EEGs of patients with epilepsy. After exercise, in patients who were made to hyperventilate, less EEG abnormality was produced than if they had hyperventilated without previous physical exercise. It would seem, therefore, that physical exercise raises the seizure threshold and reduces the likelihood of seizures occurring.

It may be that involuntary hyperventilation was also responsible for the effect that Stevens (1959) noticed in her experiment which showed that emotionally stressful interviews had an adverse effect on EEG stability in a large proportion of people with epilepsy. Hyperventilation is often seen in those who are anxious and, of course, is amenable to behavioural manipulation.

The telemetered EEG is a powerful tool in the study of the effects of various kinds of stress and emotional states on both EEG and seizure activity. Two studies in this field (Vidart & Geier 1968, Bureau et al 1968) are of interest. Vidart was concerned with adults, and measured the occurrence of diffuse episodes of spike-and-wave activity in the EEGs of patients with known epilepsy as they went about a normal life. Intellectual work which did not overtax the capacity of the patient to deal with it, such as mental arithmetic, caused a reduction in EEG abnormalities, and presumably, therefore, a reduction in seizure frequency. If the intellectual effort required to solve the problem exceeded a level critical for the patient, the number of abnormalities increased again (Bureau et al 1968). As might be expected, fatigue and tiredness increased the amount of spike and wave activity in the EEG. The relationship between a patient's mental state and abnormalities in the EEG was shown to be complex. Changes in mood might either increase or decrease the amount of abnormal epileptic activity.

Stressful events always seemed to increase the amount of abnormal activity occurring; whereas, if interest was shown in the patient, the number of abnormalities would decrease. In adults or children, boredom or inactivity led to the most abnormalities per unit time in the EEG, whereas if their attention were engaged and they were interested in their work, the amount of EEG activity decreased dramatically.

Such states as emotional stress, sleep deprivation, fatigue, boredom and prolonged overtaxing intellectual effort and hyperventilation seem, therefore, to be important factors in precipitating seizures. Physical exercise and interesting intellectual work seem to decrease seizures. In this field, it is clear that psychological methods may have an important part to play in the management of seizures and that further research is necessary. There is no doubt that psychological methods of treatment along behavioural lines are probably the treatments of choice for people who self-induce their seizures; and it is also a reasonable assumption to make that those seizures which are associated with an increase in anxiety will also be amenable to psychological methods of treatment aimed at reducing anxiety levels.

Scattered reports occur in the literature (Mostofsky & Balaschak 1977) which suggest that anxiety-reducing treatment using relaxation or desensitization are effective in treating patients whose anxiety levels are increasing their seizure frequency, and the behavioural treatment results in the frequency of seizures or even their disappearance. These are reviewed by Betts (1983). The problem of assessing the results of behavioural treatment is that like all treatments there may be non-specific factors present in the therapy which may be responsible for the patient's improvement, rather than the specific therapeutic technique itself. Thus, relaxation therapy is common to many behavioural treatments; it may just be this that is producing the improvement. Likewise, many behavioural techniques have an indirect cognitive effect (i.e. change the way an individual thinks about him or herself). Again, cognitive restructuring may actually provide the benefit.

Case History 23

This 28-year-old woman had had occasional tonic-clonic fits between the ages of 5 and 11, and had then remained seizure-free until the age of 26 when she suddenly had an attack in a supermarket. At the time this happened, she was under a great deal of marital and personal stress and had been feeling anxious for some weeks. She was still taking antiepileptic drugs. She was extremely embarrassed about the spectacle she had made of herself and, although the marital and personal stress later resolved itself, she continued to feel anxious whenever she approached the particular supermarket in which the fit had occurred. On several occasions, her anxiety levels were so high that further seizures occurred there. As a result, she became more generally anxious and attacks began to occur in other places, at home or in the street, and she eventually became so frightened of going out that she become totally housebound. Her antiepileptic drugs were increased but had no apparent effect on her seizure frequency.

She was admitted to hospital for behavioural treatment of her agoraphobia. This consisted of intensive relaxation training so that she would have some control over her anxiety feelings, followed by gradual exposure to the outside world, with encouragement and verbal reward as she was able to progress outside the hospital. As a result, her anxiety symptoms diminished markedly but she was still afraid of having a seizure in a supermarket or public place. Accordingly, Standage's (1972) method of getting the patient, whilst relaxed, to imagine themselves having a seizure (desensitization in imagination) was used. As a

result, she lost her fear of attacks and from that time she has not had another one despite being able now to go anywhere. Her drugs were subsequently withdrawn.

Case History 24

This 24-year-old man had developed secondary generalized complex partial seizures from a right anterior lobe focus six years before. Despite medication with carbamazepine and sodium valproate, his attacks occurred on a daily basis. Ambulatory EEG monitoring confirmed their epileptic nature and he was referred for a second opinion as to his suitability for surgery. Observation during his hospital stay showed that he had no attacks in hospital but invariably had half a dozen on his return home for the weekend. This was initially thought to be due to family stresses but he eventually revealed that he almost invariably had a fit when walking past a particular lamppost at the end of his street. Since he lived at the bottom of a cul-de-sac there was little he could do to avoid it. The cause of this lamppost-induced reflex epilepsy was initially obscure, but eventually he recalled that it was the spot where he had had his first attack and he now approached this lamppost feeling that he was bound to have another one. He was taught a relaxation method that involved breathing control which he could apply when he approached the lamppost; he also had some desensitization in imagination before attempting this and was also taught to think positive thoughts about not having an attack as he passed the lamppost. This combination of relaxation, desensitization and cognitive therapy certainly worked, in that he lost his lamppost attacks (and had so few spontaneous attacks afterwards that he declined surgery), but which of these techniques was the effective one?

Sometimes, too, a technique may be effective but for reasons other than those the therapist thinks are the effective ones. For instance, an interesting variant of desensitization was described by Feldman & Paul (1976), in which video-tape recordings of their seizures were played back to five patients. The authors believed that the video tapes provided a means by which the patients could acquire otherwise unrecognized or forgotten information and thereby identify specific emotional triggers which precipitated their seizures. The video tapes were therefore used as a specific adjunct to classical psychotherapy. Another way of seeing the procedure, however, would be as a desensitization to the patients fear of their own seizures and this is the more likely explanation. It is clearly a useful method and should be tried further. Certainly in the patients this writer sees, where the epilepsy is made worse by anxiety, behavioural methods of treatment have now an established place in management. The question arises as to whether behavioural methods of treatment, or indeed psychotherapy itself, has a part to play in the management of epileptic fits when neither self-inducement, anxiety or high arousal appear to be playing a precipitating part. This matter is still controversial and has not been subjected to vigorous experimental proof, but there are indications (Mostofsky & Balaschak 1977, Betts 1983) that, even in patients where there does not appear to be an emotional precipitant, behavioural methods aimed at extinguishing seizure behaviour may be beneficial.

These behavioural methods include relaxation; operant conditioning (rewarding non-seizure behaviour and 'punishing' seizure activity); desensitization; psychotherapy; extinction and habituation techniques; and biofeedback (which has not lived up to its early promise). In individual cases, the techniques work well, though few studies have controlled for placebo effects (placebo effects are, of course, also psychological in nature) or for non-specific effects of treatment.

Because behavioural treatment is time consuming it tends only to be applied when obvious seizure-related anxiety is present, or when the patients attacks are unusual or have a marked behavioural component. This means that some of the case reports in the literature are probably accounts of the treatment of pseudo-seizures (whose treatment is obviously psychological). What is needed is a formal trial of these techniques in epilepsy uncomplicated by anxiety or other special features. The brain has its own mechanisms for preventing or aborting seizure activity; behavioural treatment should be directed at enhancing or reinforcing these mechanisms and thus become a truly holistic technique.

ORGANIC MENTAL ILLNESS AND EPILEPSY

Brain damage and impairment of brain function is often found in epilepsy. It may be responsible for, or a factor in, mental illness occurring in people with epilepsy.

In a person with epilepsy who is of limited or subnormal intelligence, almost invariably both the epilepsy and the subnormality are related to a single aetiological cause. In general terms,

epilepsy itself does not cause reduction in intelligence, and studies which have suggested that it does have usually looked at highly selected populations. However, there is now good evidence that both ictal activity (Jus & Jus 1962) and subictal activity (Goode et al 1970) may interfere with registration of information and also occasionally cause a brief retrograde amnesia. Epileptic activity occurring in specific brain areas, particularly the left temporal lobe, may also interfere with intellectual functioning and learning in children, and therefore cause behaviour problems (Stores 1978). There is also growing evidence that antiepileptic drugs may play a part in learning difficulty in children with epilepsy (Stores 1978) and these effects, occurring at an early age, may partly account for the observation that patients with temporal lobe epilepsy have a lower intelligence the earlier the onset of their epilepsy (Taylor & Falconer 1968). It has been shown that actual mental retardation in children with epilepsy is restricted to those who have suffered acute cerebral insults in the form of perinatal damage, head injury or infection, or who have had status epilepticus at an early age (Ounsted et al 1966).

Up until recently, discussion about the effects of brain damage and epileptic .activity, whether ictal or subictal, and medication on intelligence and learning, was difficult to quantify due to the relative crudity of tests of intelligence, intellect and cortical functioning. However, recent advances in the neuropsychology of epilepsy (Dodrill 1978), have led to more discriminatory tests of intellectual and cognitive function. Also being developed are reliable tests of vigilance, attention, performance and learning in a laboratory setting (Hutt & Fairweather 1971, Hutt 1979). There is little doubt from these studies that specific cognitive, learning and performance deficits do occur in people with epilepsy and, that, for some children with epilepsy, special teaching methods and skills are necessary to obtain optimum learning performance (Ch. 16).

EPILEPSY AND DEMENTIA

It used to be accepted without much question that people with epilepsy were liable to dement, and the concept of epileptic dementia was a part of older psychiatric teaching. This concept requires critical examination.

Dementia may be described as a syndrome of chronic, irreversible and usually progressive intellectual and memory loss in which both recall and retention of information are affected. Usually, recent memory is more affected than distant memory. An important early sign of dementia is an emotional lability with which may go a 'catastrophic reaction' in which the patient over-reacts emotionally to quite trivial changes in his or her environment.

As the disorder progresses, so there is a deterioration of judgement and critical faculties which may lead to inappropriate behaviour. There may also be a release of previously controlled elements in the patient's personality, revealing themselves for the first time, so that, for instance, antisocial behaviour may be expressed in a previously well-behaved middle-aged man.

Poverty of thought and ideation occurs. Patients show difficulty in shifting from one topic to the next and eventually develop severe perseveration. They lose the ability to think logically or handle symbols and develop 'concrete thinking'. Later they may become disorientated in time and place, but very rarely in person, and they suffer from episodes of confusion; infection and sedatives may make confusion worse. Very often chronic emotional changes occur, usually those of depression and may appear when the patient is aware of his or her failing powers.

The diagnosis of dementia is largely a clinical diagnosis, although assisted by psychological tests and radiological investigation. It should not be a diagnosis that is made lightly and only after the fullest possible investigation. The value of careful investigation of people suspected of having dementia has been shown by Marsden & Harrison (1972), who found that a proportion of patients referred with a diagnosis of dementia did not have the condition at all and that some who were demented had treatable causes of the dementia.

Follow-up studies of patients with dementia (Mann 1973) show that, even in patients diagnosed radiologically as having dementia, some turn out on follow-up not to have the disorder at all. Both clinical, radiological, and also psycho-logical investigations in patients with suspected dementia may therefore give rise to misleading results, particularly in the case of psychological testing which is relatively crude and inaccurate except in advanced cases. However, the recent introduction of more specific and sensitive psychological tests is to be welcomed, particularly the Halstead Reitan Neuropsychological Battery, a version of which has been prepared for patients with epilepsy (Dodrill 1978). It should lead to improved accuracy of psychological investigation as it becomes more widely used in this country.

The inaccuracies in the diagnosis of dementia should be particularly borne in mind in considering the relationship between epilepsy and dementia. Whether epilepsy itself is associated with progressive dementia is uncertain. The term 'epileptic dementia' occurs quite commonly in the psychiatric literature but is often mistaken, either for the chronic changes of psychotic illnesses, for the personality changes that occur in epilepsy, for institutionalization, for depression, which so often occurs in epilepsy, or for chronic drug intoxication. In this writer's experience chronic depression and unrecognized intoxication with phenytoin are easily labelled as dementia in people with epilepsy.

Apart from those children who suffer devastating brain insults as a result of febrile status epilepticus, it is unlikely that even repeated epileptic fits lead to any degree of dementia. In those people who do have epilepsy and have presenile dementia, almost certainly the two syndromes are the result of a single brain disease of a progressive nature (for an example see Betts et al 1968). Some dementing illnesses are associated with symptomatic epilepsy, especially in the later stages (e.g. Alzheimer's disease and multi-infarct dementia). Occasionally, therefore, epilepsy may be the presenting sign of such a condition or even, occasionally, of something more exotic like porphyria (Scane et al 1986). It is occasionally speculated that some people with epilepsy are suffering from chronic viral infections or from the punch-drunk syndrome (traumatic encephalopathy). These hypotheses are unproven, apart from occasional case reports, and are still speculative.

It should be expected, however, that people with epilepsy who are brain damaged, even if the brain damage is static, will tend to dement earlier than the general population, as they have already lost some of their cortical reserves. It is still generally accepted that considerable neuronal damage may occur without any apparent loss of intellectual function but that, after a critical level of brain tissue has been lost, there will be a rapid and obvious loss of function.

In assessing a patient with suspected dementia associated with epilepsy, full investigation should be undertaken, both neurological and psychiatric. Psychological testing should be employed by using relevant tests (Dodrill 1978). Psychiatric illness, drug intoxication, and apathy and inertia due to chronic illness should be rigorously excluded. Computer assisted tomography (CT) of the brain should also be carried out, although it should be noted that the procedure is not as helpful in the diagnosis of dementia as was thought originally (reviewed by Ashworth 1986) and, when fully evaluated, investigative procedures such as magnetic resonance imaging (MRI) may well be more valuable. Occasionally, cerebral biopsy may be necessary to elucidate the cause of a particular dementing syndrome (Sim et al 1966), although use of this particular form of investigation is becoming rare.

THE CONFUSIONAL STATES OF EPILEPSY

Various organic mental states occur in people with epilepsy either with a time relationship to a clinical seizure or occurring at the same time as subictal seizure activity in the EEG. They are becoming increasingly recognized and have both psychiatric and forensic importance. Their classification has been confused and arbitrary and they have gone under a bewildering variety of names. A division of these states into three groups has been made by continental authors (Bruens 1974).

Post-ictal twilight states

These may occur after any type of fit; any attempt to restrain the confused patient may lead to outbursts of aggression. The EEG shows profuse irregular slow activity. Hughlings Jackson thought that such states might be due to the exhaustion of cerebral neurones, but it is possible that they may represent a continuing ictal event. It is also possible that the now very rare epileptic furore is related to these states. Some patients, however, after their seizures are not aggressive but remain in a prolonged confused dreamlike state which seems to occur regularly after their attacks (twilight state).

Generalized absence status

This is a mental state directly related to generalized epileptic discharges. Since its first description by Lennox in 1945, in which it was termed petit mal status, it has been described by several authors under different names. This writer would use a term coined by Roger et al (1974), that of generalized status epilepticus expressed as a confusional state. This describes a clinical picture and avoids using terms like absence and petit mal because not all patients who develop absence status have either a previous history of convulsions or of absences (Roger 1974, Ellis & Lee 1978). Indeed, these states do sometimes seem to start de novo in middle age without a previous epileptic history. They are characterized by a confusional state which varies in intensity and presentation from patient to patient and also varies within the same patient from time to time. There may be only a slight degree of confusion, often then accompanied by apparent histrionic or neurotic behaviour, but with clear-cut evidence of an organic deficit on formal psychological testing. There may be episodes of severe confusion, often with a patchy loss of intellectual function (i.e. the patient may remember one thing but forget others during the attack, or may have transient signs of parietal lobe disturbance). There may be the most profound stupor. Those confusional states, which are related to previous epilepsy of a generalized nature, seem to respond well to intravenous diazepam or clonazepam, but often respond poorly to other antiepileptic drugs; whereas the ictal confusional states of middle age seem to respond to conventional drugs, once the underlying epileptic diathesis is identified.

Occasionally, during the ictal period, in addition to the confusion previously described, frank psychotic symptoms may appear. These can often be seen as the patient's attempt to explain puzzling internal feelings which cannot be understood. This phenomenon is more common in the acute prolonged confusional states of later life (Ellis & Lee 1978).

Case History 25

This 13-year-old girl, who had had recurrent generalized absences and tonic-clonic seizures since the age of 3, poorly controlled with conventional medication, was admitted from a neurological ward to a psychiatric unit with the diagnosis of schizophrenia made by the neurologists. On admission she was fatuous and giggling, appeared to have visual hallucinations, and described herself as married to a well-known pop singer. In addition to this, however, she was vague and distant, appeared to be disorientated and had little memory of recent events. She had been admitted to the neurological unit in this state some days previously. EEG examination on her admission to the psychiatric unit showed generalized 3 per second spike-and-wave activity. Oral nitrazepam was given and, within a day, the EEG abnormality had stopped and a somewhat bewildered but now normal 13-year-old girl emerged from underneath the apparent psychotic behaviour. On reviewing her history it would seem that, in the preceding few years, she had had many attacks like this lasting up to a day which had greatly interfered with her school work. Under a small dose of nitrazepam these attacks no longer occurred although she continued to have the occasional tonic-clonic seizure. Her school work improved markedly.

Complex partial status

This involves a prolonged alteration in mental state resulting from epileptic discharge in the cortex, usually in the temporal lobes. This has not been described extensively in the British literature and is said to be rare (Fenton 1983) but in this writer's experience it is more common than is generally thought. The condition is better described in the continental literature and the patients this writer has seen follow quite closely the descriptions given there: five case histories have been appended to illustrate the clinical features. Some twilight states which resemble complex partial status but which are chronologically related to seizures, appear to occur in other types of epilepsy. These are the ones particularly described by Landolt (1985) who maintained that such twilight states can result from overdosage of antiepileptic drugs – a statement with which one would agree.

Case History 26

This 40-year-old man had never sought help for the brief seizures which he had had for 20 years, and which were of a brief muddled feeling accompanied by a déjà vu experience. He had had one of his usual attacks on the bus on his way to work; after the attack he walked away from his regular bus stop in a dazed state, removing his clothing as he did so. Completely naked, he wandered up and down a shopping precinct muttering incoherently. He was arrested, struggling violently, and covered in the regulation blanket, removed to a police station. When questioned he did not make coherent replies except occasionally to mutter 'protest'. He remained in this state for 12 hours and then suddenly recovered his senses, and demanded to know where he was and who had removed his clothing. He has not shown similar behaviour since, but passed through a transient period of depression on knowing what he had done. Subsequent investigation showed a right temporal epileptic focus on EEG examination.

Case History 27

A man of 23 was found wandering in a dazed fashion in the middle of a large city. He had given no coherent reply to questions by the police, and search of his clothing revealed no identifying mark or documents. He was accordingly admitted to a psychiatric hospital where he was observed to spend most of his time in a catatonic-like stupor, crouched in a chair. Occasionally he was thought to be visually hallucinating as he seemed to be watching some insect or bird flying round his room. Rarely he would become violently aggressive, when he would dash up out of his chair and fly around the ward overturning tables and chairs and smashing windows for a few minute before returning to his previous still posture. He was thought to have catatonic schizophrenia and was treated with psychotropic drugs but with little effect. A week after admission whilst asleep in bed he was observed to have a tonic-clonic fit. On awakening the next morning he was lucid and rational, knew his name and where he came from, and was surprised to find himself in hospital. Over the next few hours, the previous psychotic state returned; an EEG at this time showed continuous spike and wave discharge from the left temporal lobe. He was given intravenous diazepam and his mental state returned to normal, at the same time as the abnormal EEG discharges stopped. He made a complete recovery with regular antiepileptic drugs.

Case History 28

A woman with left temporal lobe epilepsy stopped her antiepileptic drugs suddenly. A day later she passed into a peculiar clouded mental state in which she was irritable and tearful and had obvious memory difficulty. Definite organic impairment was confirmed on formal mental state testing. She would not eat, lost weight rapidly and complained of bone pain. She would wander distracted round the house in a confused state and was incapable of looking after her children. An EEG showed continual epileptic activity in the left temporal area, which previously had only been present during her actual attacks. Ten days after this episode started she awoke one morning in a normal frame of mind; on that day the EEG abnormality had disappeared and has not returned.

Case History 29

A girl of 18 had had complex partial seizures originating in the right temporal lobe since the age of 7: their aetiology was obscure. She had occasional tonic-clonic attacks as well. Her attacks became more frequent, despite increasing dosages of carbamazepine. It had been intended to try sodium valproate but publicity about the side-effects of this drug in the national press made the patient request the use of another drug. Clobazam was tried and the girl rapidly passed into a peculiar mental state of perplexity and irritability, and left to herself would sit listlessly all day avoiding her usual pursuits. If questioned, she would appear orientated in time and place but was very slow to respond and would not co-operate in psychological testing. An EEG (and ambulatory EEG monitoring) showed dense spike and wave activity originating in the posterior part of the right temporal lobe. Clobazam was withdrawn and within a few days the original bright vivacious teenager returned. Subsequently she has been taking sodium valproate and her attack frequency has declined markedly and she has returned to college.

Case History 30
This 15-year-old girl is an identical twin, both of whom have generalized epilepsy although their attacks are infrequent. They had been treated by their general practitioner with phenobarbitone. This girl suddenly developed an acute mental illness where she became mute and immobile; except to occasionally ejaculate the words 'British Constitution' and wander about. She was sleepless and incontinent. An EEG showed a continual spike focus in the left temporal area. Intravenous clonazepam temporarily altered her mental state, but it would return a few hours later. Oral carbamazepine was ineffectual, as was oral clonazepam. After a week she was given one treatment with electroconvulsive therapy under brietal anaesthesia (brietal anaesthesia on its own was ineffective) and the mental state cleared and has not returned: the left temporal focus on EEG has also not returned and she has had no further attacks whilst taking carbamazepine. A year after this her twin sister developed a rather similar mental state but this was not accompanied by EEG changes and was found to be a deliberate imitation of her sister's attack for purposes of gaining more attention. Firm persuasion abolished it.

These cases illustrate the wide variety of phenomena which may be seen in association with continual epileptic activity occurring in one temporal lobe though, if looked for, confusion and evidence of organic impairment can always be found. Pseudoneurotic behaviour may also be prominent. Sometimes, automatisms are the main feature to be seen in the patient's mental state and, occasionally, the patient may wander away in the twilight state in a kind of fugue. Twilight states may be prolonged and last for several days.

More profound confusional states can also occur in epilepsy and some people with epilepsy develop a frank delirium although not apparently as an ictal experience. Epileptic delirium was frequently described in the older literature on epilepsy and is in fact still encountered (Betts 1981b). The usual characteristics of delirium are present:

psychomotor overactivity; perceptual distortions; hallucinatory experiences, usually of a visual nature; confusion; disorientation in time and place; and a degree of clouding of consciousness. Delusional ideas may also be present, usually persecutory, although this writer has seen the occasional patient with a depressive element to his delirium.

Landolt (1958) associates these delirious states with suppression of fits and forced normalization of the EEG. However, the writer would agree with other continental authors (Bruens 1974) that forced normalization does not occur in states in which there is also clouding of consciousness. It has been his experience that these delirious conditions are relatively common, often associated with the patient's admission to hospital, and usually seem to be associated with a sudden increase in attack frequency and carry a relatively good prognosis (Betts 1974). It has usually not been possible to do an EEG at the time of the patient's admission but it has been his clinical impression that one is seeing a confusional state related to frequent seizures rather than to ictal activity itself.

Case History 31
This man of 60 had had about four tonic-clonic fits a year from the age of 30 which had never been investigated, although he had been taking phenobarbitone for years. Just before his sixtieth birthday he had eight attacks within a week, possibly connected with a reduction in his antiepileptic drugs. During this period he became suspicious, truculent and hostile, and later became physically aggressive and overactive and developed florid paranoid ideas; imagining that he was being spied upon, that his neighbours were pumping gas under his doors; he appeared to have auditory hallucinations and began to see visions of the devil. Finally he attacked his son-in-law with an axe, mistaking him for the devil himself. On removal to hospital he was noted to have the classical symptoms of delirium, and was markedly confused with severe disorientation and a poor retentive memory. His antiepileptic drugs were increased and within a few days the exited delirious state disappeared pari passu with cessation of his seizures, and the mental state has not returned.

This patient seems to have been left with no residual organic deficit although in the writer's mental hospital experience some patients who develop a delirious state related to epilepsy seem afterwards to have a permanent organic defect state, although it can be difficult to say whether or not they had had it before.

REFERENCES

Ashworth B 1986 Who needs a CT brain scan? British Medical Journal 292: 845–846

Bagley C 1971 The social psychology of the child with epilepsy. Routledge & Kegan Paul, London

Barraclough B 1981 Suicide and epilepsy. In: Reynolds E, Trimble M (eds) Epilepsy and psychiatry. Churchill Livingstone, Edinburgh, pp 72–76

Betts T A 1974 A follow-up study of a cohort of patients with epilepsy admitted to psychiatric care in an English city. In: Harris P, Mawdsley C (eds) Epilepsy: Proceedings of the Hans Berger Centenary Symposium Churchill Livingstone, Edinburgh, pp 326–336

Betts T 1981a Depression, anxiety and epilepsy. In: Reynolds E, Trimble M (eds) Epilepsy and psychiatry. Churchill Livingstone, Edinburgh, pp 60–71

Betts T 1981b Epilepsy and the mental hospital. In: Reynolds E, Trimble M (eds) Epilepsy and psychiatry. Churchill Livingstone, Edinburgh, pp 175–184

Betts T 1983 The psychological management of epilepsy. In: Rose F (ed.) Research progress in epilepsy. Pitman, London, pp 315–325

Betts T 1984 Sexual problems in people with epilepsy. Paper presented at British Danish Dutch Epilepsy Symposium, Elsinore, October 1984

Betts T 1987 The employment of people with epilepsy within the National Health Service. In: Espir M, Edwards F, Oxley J (eds) Epilepsy and employment. Royal Society of Medicine London, to be published

Betts T A, Skarott P H 1979 Epilepsy and the mental hospital. Paper presented at International League Against Epilepsy Scientific Meeting, Oxford. November 1979

Betts T A, Smith W T, Kelly R E 1968 Adult metachromatic leucodystrophy (sulphatide lipidosis) simulating acute schizophrenia. Neurology 18: 1140–1142

Bird J 1979 The behavioural treatment of hysteria. British Journal of Psychiatry 134: 129–137

Bowlby J 1960 Grief and mourning in infancy and early childhood. Psychoanalytic Study of the Child 15:9

Bruens J H 1974 Psychoses in epilepsy. In: Vinken P L, Bruyn L W (eds) Handbook of clinical neurology 15. North Holland, Amsterdam, pp 593–610

Bureau M, Guey J, Dravet C, Roger J 1968 A study of distribution of petit mal absences in the child in relation to his activities. Electroencephalography and Clinical Neurophysiology 25:513

Caveness W, Merritt H, Gallup G 1969 A survey of public attitudes towards epilepsy in 1969. US Dept. of Health Education and Welfare, Public Health Service, Washington DC

Corbidge P, Bullock K 1968 Production of a teaching package about epilepsy – an analysis. Paper presented at Northern European Epilepsy Meeting, York, September 1986

Dodrill C 1978 A neuropsychological battery for epilepsy. Epilepsia 19: 611–623

Doube J R 1965 Sensory precipitated seizures – a review. Journal of Nervous and Mental Disease 141: 524–539

Efron R 1956 The effect of olfactory stimuli in arresting uncinate fits. Brain 79: 267–281

Ellis J M, Lee S I 1978 Acute prolonged confusion in late life as an ictal state. Epilepsia 19: 119–128

Epilepsy News 1979 12

Feldman R G, Paul N L 1976 Identity of emotional triggers in epilepsy. Journal of Nervous and Mental Disease 162: 345–353

Fenton G 1983 Epilepsy, personality and behaviour. In: Rose F (ed.) Research progress in epilepsy. Pitman, London, pp 188–209

Fenwick P 1981 Precipitation and inhibition of seizures. In: Reynolds E, Trimble M (eds) Epilepsy and psychiatry. Churchill Livingstone, Edinburgh, pp 306–321

Fenwick P 1985 Regina v. Sullivan; the trial and judgement. In: Fenwick P, Fenwick E (eds) Epilepsy and the law. Royal Society of Medicine, London, pp 3–8

Flor-Henry P 1969 Psychosis and temporal lobe epilepsy. Epilepsia 10: 363–395

Forster F M 1972 The Classification and conditioning treatment of the reflex epilepsies. International Journal of Neurology 9: 73–86

Gastaut H, Tassinari C A 1966 Triggering mechanisms in epilepsy. Epilepsia 7: 85–138

Goffman E 1963 Stigma. Notes on the management of spoiled identity. Prentice Hall, New Jersey

Goldie L, Green J M 1959 A study of the psychological factors in a case of sensory reflex epilepsy. Brain 82: 505–524

Goode D J, Penry J K, Dreifuss F E 1970 Effects of paroxysmal spike wave on continuous visual motor performance. Epilepsia 11: 241–254

Goodwin J, Zouhar M, Bergman R 1982 Hysterical seizures in adolescent incest victims. In: Goodwin J Sexual abuse. Incest victims and their families. John Wright, Boston, pp 101–108

Gotze W, Kupicki S T, Munter F, Teichman J 1967 Effect of exercise on seizure threshold. Diseases of the Nervous System 28: 664–667

Graham P, Rutter M 1968 Organic brain dysfunction and child psychiatric disorder. British Medical Journal 3: 695–700

Gudmundsson D 1967 Epilepsy in Iceland. Acta Neurologica Scandinavica 43 (suppl 25): 1–124

Guerrant J, Anderson W W, Fisher A, Weinstein M R, Jaros R M, Deskins A 1962 Personality in epilepsy. Thomas, Springfield

Gunn J C 1969 Epileptics in prison. MD Thesis, University of Birmingham, England

Gunn J C, Fenton G 1971 Epilepsy, automatism and crime. Lancet 1: 1173–1176

Henderson D, Gillespie R D 1950 A textbook of psychiatry. 7th edn. Oxford University Press, London

Hierons R, Saunders M 1966 Impotence in patients with temporal lobe lesions. Lancet 2: 761–763

Hill D, Pond D A, Mitchell W, Falconer M A 1957 Personality changes following temporal lobectomy for epilepsy. Journal of Mental Science 103: 18–27

Hinton J 1967 Dying. Penguin, Harmondsworth

Hoenig J, Hamilton C M 1960 Epilepsy and sexual orgasm. Acta Psychiatrica Scandinavica 35: 448–456

Hoenig J, Kenna J C 1979 EEG abnormalities and transexualism. British Journal of Psychiatry 134: 293–300

Hutt S J 1979 Cognitive processes and EEG activity in patients with epilepsy. Paper presented at the International Conference on Psychology and Medicine. University College of Swansea, Wales.

Hutt S J, Fairweather H 1971 Some effects of performance

variables upon generalized spike wave activity. Brain 94: 321–326

Jus A, Jus K 1962 Retrograde amnesia in petit mal. Archives of General Psychiatry 6: 163–167

Lacey J T, Bateman D E, Van Lehn R 1953 Autonomic response specificity. Psychomatic Medicine 15: 8–21

Landolt H 1958 Serial electroencephalographic investigations during psychotic episodes in epileptic patients & during schizophrenic attacks. In: Lorentz de Haas A M (ed.) Lectures in epilepsy. Elsevier, Amsterdam, pp 91–133

Lishman W A 1968 Brain damage in relation to psychiatric disability and head injury. British Journal of Psychiatry 114: 373–410

Lombroso C 1889 L'uomo delinquente. Bocca, Turin

Lubar J, Deering W 1981 Behavioural approaches to neurology. Academic Press, New York

Mackay A 1979 Self- poisoning – a complication of epilepsy. British Journal of Psychiatry 134: 277–282

Maletzky B M 1973 The episodic dyscontrol syndrome. Diseases of the Nervous System 34: 178–185

Mann A H 1973 Cortical atrophy and air encephalography: a clinical and radiogical study. Psychological Medicine 3: 374–378

Marsden C D, Harrison M J 1972 Outcome of investigation of patients with presenile dementia. British Medical Journal 2: 249–252

Mattson R H, Heninger G R, Gallagher B B, Glaser G H 1970 Psychophysiologic precipitants of seizures in epileptics. Neurology 20:407

Mellor D H, Lowitt I, Hall D J 1974 Are epileptic children behaviourally different from other children? In: Harris P, Mawdsley C (eds) Epilepsy: Proceedings of the Hans Berger Centenary Symposium. Churchill Livingstone, Edinburgh, pp 313–316

Merskey H 1979 The analysis of hysteria. Baillière Tindall, London

Merskey H, Tonge W L 1974 Psychiatric illness. 7th edn. Baillière Tindall, London

Mitchell W, Falconer M A, Hill D 1954 Epilepsy with fetishism relieved by temporal lobectomy. Lancet ii: 626–630

Mostofsky D I, Balaschak B A 1977 Psychobiological control of seizures. Psychological Bulletin 84 (No. 4): 723–759

Office of Health Economics 1971 Epilepsy in society. London

Ounsted C, Lindsay J, Norman R 1966 Biological factors in temporal lobe epilepsy. Heinemann, London

Perez M, Trimble M 1980 Epileptic psychosis – diagnostic comparison with process schizophrenia. British Journal of Psychiatry 137: 245–249

Pond D A, Bidwell B H 1959 A survey of epilepsy in 14 general practices. II. Social and psychological aspects. Epilepsia 1: 285–299

Pond D A, Bidwell B H, Stein L 1960 A survey of epilepsy in 14 general practices. I. Demographic and medical data. Psychiatrica, Neurologica, Neurochirugia 63: 217–236

Pratt R T C, Mackenzie W 1958 Anxiety states following vestibular disorders. Lancet 2: 347–349

Robertson M 1985 Depression in patients with epilepsy: an overview and clinical study. In: Trimble M (ed.) The psychopharmacology of epilepsy. John Wiley, Chichester, pp 65–82

Rodin E 1982 Aggression and epilepsy. In: Riley T L, Roy A (eds) Pseudoseizures. Williams and Wilkins, Baltimore/London, pp 185–212

Roger J, Lob H, Tassinari C A 1974 Generalized status epilepticus expressed as a confusional state (petit mal status or absence status epilepticus). In: Vinken P L, Bruyn G W (eds) Handbook of clinical neurology 15. North Holland Publishing, Amsterdam, pp 145–188

Scane A, Wight J, Godwin-Austin R 1986 Acute intermittent porphyria presenting as epilepsy. British Medical Journal 292: 946–947

Sensky T 1983 Religiosity, mystical experience and epilepsy. In: Rose F (ed.) Research progress in epilepsy. Pitman, London, pp 214–220

Serafetinides E 1965 Aggressiveness in temporal lobe epileptics and its relation to cerebral dysfunction and environmental factors. Epilepsia 6: 33–42

Servit Z, Machek J, Stercova A, Kristof M, Servenkova V A, Dudas B 1963 Reflex influences in the pathogenesis of Epilepsy in the Light of Clinical Statistics. In Servit Z (ed.), Reflex Mechanisms in the Genesis of Epilepsy. Amsterdam: Elsevier

Shukla G D, Srivastava O N, Katiyar B C 1979 Sexual disturbances in temporal lobe epilepsy – a controlled study. British Journal of Psychiatry 134: 288–292

Sim M, Turner E, Smith W T 1966 Cerebral biopsy in the investigation of presenile dementia. British Journal of Psychiatry 112: 119–133

Slater E, Beard A W, Glithero E 1963 The schizophrenia-like psychoses of epilepsy. British Journal of Psychiatry 109: 95–150

Slater E 1965 The diagnosis of hysteria. British Medical Journal 1: 1395–1399

Slater E, Shields J 1969 Genetical aspects of anxiety. In: Lader M H (ed.) Studies in anxiety. Headley Brothers, Ashford

Small J, Hayden M, Small I 1966 Further psychiatric investigations of patients with temporal and non-temporal lobe epilepsy. American Journal of Psychiatry 123: 303–310

Srole L, Langner T S, Michael S T, Opler M K, Rennie T A C 1962 Mental Health in the Metropolis, the Mid-town Manhattan study. McGraw Hill, New York

Standage K F 1972 Treatment of epilepsy by reciprocal inhibition of anxiety. Guys Hospital Reports 121: 217–219

Stevens J R 1959 Emotional activation of the electroencephalogram in patients with convulsive disorders. Journal of Nervous and Mental Disease 128: 339–351

Stores G 1978 School children with epilepsy at risk for learning and behaviour problems. Developmental Medicine and Child Neurology. 20: 502–508

Symonds C 1959 Excitation and inhibition in epilepsy. Brain 82: 133–146

Taylor D C 1969a Aggression and epilepsy. Journal of Psychosomatic Research 13: 229–236

Taylor D C 1969b Sexual behaviour and temporal lobe epilepsy. Archives of Neurology 21: 510–516

Taylor D C, Falconer M A 1968 Clinical socio-economic and psychological changes after temporal lobectomy. British Journal of Psychiatry 114: 1247–1261

Tizard B 1962 The personality of epileptics. Psychological Bulletin 59: 196–210

Toone B, Wheeler M, Fenwick P 1980 Sex hormone changes in male epileptics. Clinical Endocrinology 12: 391–395

Tyrer P 1974 The role of bodily feelings in anxiety. Oxford University Press, London

Tyrer P, Alexander J 1979 Classification of personality

disorder. British Journal of Psychiatry 135: 163–167

Tyrer P, Alexander J, Cicchetti D, Cohen M, Remington M 1979 Reliability of a schedule for rating personality disorder. British Journal of Psychiatry 135: 168–174

Vidart L, Geier S 1968 Work, fatigue and the psychic state in epileptic patients: a telemetric EEG study. Electroencephalography and Clinical Neurophysiology 25:511

Walton H J, Presly A S 1973 Use of category system in the diagnosis of abnormal personality. British Journal of Psychiatry 122: 259–268

Wilkins A, Lindsay J 1985 Common forms of reflex

epilepsy: physiological mechanisms and techniques for treatment. In: Pedley A, Meldrum B (eds) Recent advances in epilepsy 2. Churchill Livingstone, Edinburgh pp 239–271

Williams D 1956 The structure of emotions reflected in epileptic experiences. Brain 79: 29–67

Williams D 1981 The emotions and epilepsy. In: Reynolds E, Trimble M (eds) Epilepsy and psychiatry. Churchill Livingstone, Edinburgh pp 49–59

Wing J 1974 Paper 5. In: People with handicaps need better trained counsellors. Central Council for Education and Training of Social Workers

PART TWO
DIFFERENTIAL DIAGNOSIS OF NON-EPILEPTIC ATTACKS
M. R. Trimble

INTRODUCTION

Although textbooks since the contribution of Gowers (1881) have given advice as to how to distinguish between epileptic and non-epileptic seizures, few authors have actually studied this problem. It is reasonable to say that, with the exception of the addition of electroencephalography and neurohormonal data, the stated criteria have altered little in the last 100 years. However, while they may help in the differential diagnosis of perhaps 90% of patients presenting at the clinic, it is the remaining 10% who present the problem as the diagnosis still remains in doubt, even after careful analysis of the description of the seizure pattern.

In these patients, a purely symptom-orientated approach, concentrating solely on the seizures, may lead to the wrong conclusions. As is the general rule in medicine, the essential part of the investigation is the history, together with an understanding of the patient in whom the symptoms are presenting. In addition, information regarding such obvious factors as seizure-precipitating events should be sought, paying particular attention to the setting and timing of the very first attack. It is a truism that seizures occurring many times a day in the presence of a normal interictal electroencephalogram are most likely to be non-

epileptic, and that talking, screaming or displays of emotional behaviour during or immediately after the attack are likely to lead to a similar conclusion. However, the presence of paroxysmal abnormalities on the EEG do not necessarily prove a diagnosis of epilepsy, and it should be recalled that paroxysmal discharges such as generalized spike-wave complexes are found in approximately 3% of healthy people (Fenton 1982). In particular, paroxysmal theta activity or sharp waves, especially in the posterior temporal location should not be misinterpreted as confirming a clinical impression that the patient has epilepsy.

RECENT STUDIES

EEG assessment

Several groups have reported their experience with additional electroencephalographic methods such as ambulatory monitoring or video telemetry in adults (Ramani et al 1980, Desai et al 1982, Luther et al 1982, King et al 1982) and in children (Holmes et al 1980). Unfortunately, even with the more advanced monitors, the pattern of the electroencephalogram is often obscured during the seizure itself by muscle artifact which may be misinterpreted as spike-wave activity. Nevertheless, helpful data can be obtained from ictal traces, particularly if flattening of the EEG or an increase in spike-wave activity is detected prior to the episode or asymmetry is noted post-ictally with the appearance of slow waves. While it would be a rare event to have a generalized tonic-clonic convulsion that was not associated with ictal electroencephalographic discharges, the same is not true of partial seizures. Ambulatory monitoring, particularly with a restricted number of electrodes may fail to detect electrical activity from an epileptic focus and give rise to the suggestion that the seizure is non-epileptic.

Clinical features

From a different viewpoint, Roy (1977, 1979) studied 22 patients with a final diagnosis of hysterical seizures and compared them to a control group of patients with well-defined epilepsy using a number of variables.

A clinical history was obtained, and both groups were given rating scales of psychopathology, including the General Health Questionnaire, the Wakefield self-assessment depression inventory, and an anxiety inventory. Significant differences included, for the experimental group, a family history of psychiatric disorder; personal history of psychiatric disorder; attempted suicide; sexual maladjustment; and increased scores on the anxiety and depression inventories. A clinical diagnosis of current affective disorder was made in 19 of the 22 subjects at the time of the investigation and the author's conclusion was that five factors – namely, family history and past history of psychiatric disorder, attempted suicide, sexual maladjustment and current affective syndrome – helped differentiate hysterical from epileptic seizures. This important study emphasizes the value of seeking information beyond the phenomenology of the seizures in making a diagnosis, in particular the past history and present affective state. Similar data, notably with regard to present and past psychiatric disorder and suicide attempts were reported by Stewart et al (1982).

Henry & Woodruff (1978) described a physical sign which provides a positive basis for the diagnosis of some non-epileptic seizures during an attack, based on variation of ocular deviation with the patient's posture. In non-neurological states resembling coma or seizures the following signs were observed when the patient is lying on the ground and is turned from one side to another. The eyes are always deviated to the ground, thus changing their position with posture. In the case of epileptic seizures, any deviation of the eyes tends to be constant and not related to body position. In the study, this variation of ocular position was absent in 20 cases of coma where there was a clear 'organic' diagnosis.

Fenton (1982) lists the following features as useful for the diagnosis of non-epileptic seizures:

> variability in seizure pattern with bizarre features not consistent with a seizure discharge spreading within the brain; vague, inconsistent, and changing descriptions of subjective sensations as auras or initial seizure phenomena; evidence of responsiveness to environmental stimuli (retention of corneal reflexes, resistance to eye opening, head retraction on supra-orbital notch pressure, retrospective recall of some or all of the events of the seizure, change of position to avoid discomfort, etc) in spite of apparent unconsciousness during the attacks; verbal expression of obscenities, combative behaviour, histrionic behaviour, and emotional display during and after the attacks; the occurrence of other hysterical conversion phenomena, either of transient appearance as post-seizure events or persistently present between attacks.

He does not include, as several other authors have done, the absence of such phenomena as incontinence of urine or tongue biting during the attacks which, while they may be rare, certainly do occur in non-epileptic seizures. Also, positive Babinski responses and diminished corneal reflexes have been reported (see Lesser 1985). Furthermore, self-injury is not uncommon, this often occurring at body sites different from those in epilepsy, which in the latter very often involve head injury and inconsistent cuts and bruises which are seen according to where the patient falls.

In non-epileptic seizures, the site of the lesion is often inconsistent with damage during a fall, reflecting self-injury during the attack, and may involve the same part of the body, thus reopening old wounds.

The main difficulty with drawing up the clinical characteristics of epileptic and non-epileptic seizures is that, in difficult cases, the pattern of attacks is, as noted, remarkably similar in both, the history may initially be unhelpful, and even such techniques as ambulatory monitoring and video telemetry do not clarify the diagnosis. Furthermore, all of those with experience in this field have seen the most unusual manifestations of some epileptic seizures, which, without the benefit of much detailed investigation, would otherwise clearly have been hallmarked as 'hysterical'.

Neuroendocrine findings

Recently, neurohormonal markers have been used to help identify epileptic seizures. Since stimulation of the medial basal hypothalamus increases prolactin levels, it was hypothesized that abnormal electrical activity in epilepsy, which passed through the midbrain, should raise serum prolactin concentrations. Thus, investigations were begun at the National Hospitals and The Chalfont Centre for Epilepsy into post-ictal changes of various anterior and posterior pituitary neurohormones.

In one of the first reports, Trimble (1978) studied three groups of patients. These were: a group with generalized epilepsy and tonic-clonic seizures; a control group undergoing unilateral ECT and full neuromuscular relaxation; and a smaller group of seven patients with 'hysteria' which resembled tonic-clonic seizures. Significant elevations in prolactin occurred, maximal between 15 and 20 minutes, in the generalized epilepsy and the ECT groups, and in the majority of cases the levels rose to greater than 1000 IU/ml, in the presence of normal baseline values before the ictus. In contrast, the patients diagnosed with hysteria showed little change in their serum prolactin levels after the attack, and none rose above 500 IU/ml. It was thus suggested that the use of post-ictal prolactin could be helpful in distinguishing epileptic and non-epileptic seizures if the following considerations were taken into account. First, it was essential to ensure that the patient had a normal baseline prolactin. Secondly, the seizure needed to be bilateral and last for at least 30 s and, finally, the post-ictal change needed to be in excess of 1000 IU/ml. Thus, in a patient showing such elevations, it was hypothesized that hypothalamic stimulation had occurred consequent on the spread of seizure discharge.

Since that early investigation, several replications have been carried out (Oxley et al 1981, Dana-Haeri et al 1983, Trimble et al 1985). In the first of these, three groups of patients were evaluated using a four channel tape EEG monitor in association with clinical evaluation and post-ictal prolactin levels. The first group consisted of patients with epileptic seizures only; the second group had patients with epileptic and non-epileptic seizures; and the third group consisted of those with non-epileptic seizures only. The psychiatric diagnosis was based upon past history of psychiatric symptoms, evidence of personality disorder; or evidence of previous conversion phenonena. The clinical assessments were made blind to the electroencephalographic and prolactin data. In this study, all patients in the first group showed electoencephalographic abnormalities, in seven out of nine this being demonstrated during the seizure. A serum prolactin elevation over 1000 IU/ml was seen in all four subjects with tonic-clonic seizures from the first two groups; less significant elevations were seen with some of the other seizure types. In the third group (non-epileptic seizures), no patient showed seizure-related epileptic activity and there were no changes in serum prolactin levels. Generally, psychiatric diagnosis based on history, taped EEG and prolactin estimations provided similar diagnostic groupings, emphasizing the importance of a positive contribution of the psychiatric history to the analysis of a patient.

Recent data (Dana-Haeri et al 1983, Trimble et al 1985) has extended the observations further to look at other pituitary hormones and seizure types. Thus, the occurrence of significant prolactin elevations in association with generalized seizures has been confirmed, with nearly 60% of patients showing a rise to greater than 1000 IU/ml and 96% showing levels greater than 500 IU/ml in the presence of a normal baseline. Follicle stimulating hormone (FSH) levels change little in male patients, but significantly increase in female patients at a 20-min sample. Luteinizing hormone (LH) levels are significantly elevated following generalized seizures in males and females. In these investigations, samples were taken at 1 min, 20 min and 60 min after the ictus and compared to baseline, and it was interesting that prolactin levels returned to baseline values at 60 min, whereas elevated LH levels were still raised at this time. Further, prolactin levels were found to be significantly elevated at the 1 min sample, suggesting possible release of prolactin from the anterior pituitary even prior to the clinical manifestations of the seizure.

Following complex partial seizures with alteration of consciousness, a rise in prolactin was noted for male patients immediately, and 20 min after the attack for both sexes. LH levels were elevated at 20 min only in females, and no alteration in FSH was seen. The elevations in prolactin were less than for generalized seizures, only 63% having a rise to greater than 500 IU/ml at 20 min. Changes after simple partial seizures were minimal and non-significant. Arginine vasopressin levels have also been examined in an attempt to see if this was a valuable marker of epileptic activity within the first minute of a seizure. While some patients markedly increased their levels of vasopressin, the rise was not constant, even in patients with generalized tonic-clonic seizures.

Other authors have confirmed and extended most of these findings. Abbott et al (1980), Hoppener et al (1982), Collins et al (1983), Wyllie et al (1984) and Laxer et al (1985) reported that plasma prolactin is elevated following generalized tonic-clonic seizures, and the peak rise occurs around 15–20 min after the seizure. Collins et al noted that patients with partial seizures (90% of whom had elementary (simple) partial seizures) did not show a change of prolactin levels and Pritchard et al (1983), in a study of six patients with complex partial seizures, noted elevations of prolactin from 2.5 to 10 times the baseline values. Wyllie et al (1984) noted a rise three times that of the baseline in 43% of complex partial seizures, and Laxer et al (1985) commented specifically on a rise seen in patients with automatisms and posturing. These results bear out the data mentioned above (Dana-Haeri et al 1983) in which prolactin thus distinguished complex from simple partial seizures with regard to the neuroendocrine response. Hoppener et al (1982), Collins et al (1983) and Laxer et al (1985) confirmed that the plasma prolactin levels were unchanged following pseudoseizures, and that estimations of plasma prolactin are useful in the differentiation of generalized attacks with regard to their epileptic or non-epileptic etiology.

In an extension of the methodology for this type of investigation, Gallagher et al (1984) reported adrenocorticotrophic hormones (ACTH) and prolactin levels during electrical stimulation of medial temporal lobe structures. Electrodes were placed in the amygdalae and hippocampi of 18 patients, and plasma samples collected after stimu-lation. Those which led to a complex partial or generalized tonic-clonic seizure always resulted in a rise of both hormones (and cortisol), but stimulation without the elicitation of an after-discharge did not change hormone levels.

Berkovic (1984) also carried out an extensive study in a variety of patients, some of whom had electrodes implanted intracerebrally. He confirmed a post-ictal rise in prolactin in all patients with tonic-clonic seizures 5–30 fold above baseline levels, with a peak at 19 min. However, in six patients with multiple tonic-clonic seizures and status epilepticus the rise was less, suggesting that exhaustion of central prolactin supplies may occur and raising doubts as to the value of the test in status epilepticus if the result is negative. Following tonic seizures, the pattern was similar to tonic-clonic attacks, but during absence status and after myoclonic and simple partial seizures there was no rise. After complex partial seizures, abnormal elevations were seen in 80% of patients, less than that seen for generalized tonic-clonic seizures.

The depth electrode recordings allowed more accurate estimates of seizure length and spread. No relationship was seen between the peak post-ictal prolactin levels and seizure length, but in those with bilateral temporal lobe activity, peak levels were significantly greater than in those with only unilateral activity.

In keeping with the other reported data, non-epileptic seizures (14 attacks studied in 10 patients) did not influence prolactin, but in two patients with syncope, one did show a large rise suggesting that 'convulsive syncope' may also change hormonal output.

The conclusion from these data with regard to the use of prolactin in the assessment of patients with seizures of as yet undetermined etiology would be as follows. First, it is essential to ensure that the baseline prolactin is within the normal range. Secondly, following a tonic-clonic seizure with bilateral neuromuscular activity lasting longer than 30 s, a several fold rise in prolactin from baseline levels (we have adopted a level of 1000 IU/ml for diagnostic purposes) is seen in patients where the seizures are epileptic, changes being present within a few minutes of the ictus and being maximal some 15–20 min later. If there is uncertainty, a further prolactin level at one hour should reveal a decline in the prolactin level towards normal limits. Patients with non-epileptic seizures, excepting perhaps those of cardiac or vascular origin, do not show these elevations, and neither do patients with simple partial seizures or possibly status epilepticus. In patients with complex partial seizures and alteration of consciousness, the changes that occur post-ictally are of lesser magnitude and the test is less reliable in those cases. Nonetheless, a clearly significant elevation from baseline values at 20 min with return to normal at one hour may provide important information which can be added to other information about the patient which has been collected in the assessment of their seizures.

PSYCHOPATHOLOGY AND NON-EPILEPTIC SEIZURES

The only systematic study of the classification of psychopathology in patients with pseudoseizures is that of Stewart et al (1982). They compared patients with epileptic to those with non-epileptic seizures, and a group with a combination of attacks. The psychopathology was evaluated with standardized rating scales and Research Diagnostic Criteria and Diagnostic and Statistical Manual III (DSM III) (American Psychiatric Association 1980) criteria. The most frequent diagnoses in the epileptic sample (n=11) were alcoholism, anxiety and minor affective disorder. In the mixed group (n=13), five had major depressive disorder, four had antisocial personalities, four had Briquet's hysteria, and one schizophrenia. In the pseudoseizure only group (n=13), eight had 'major character pathology', two Briquet's hysteria, and one the histrionic personality. It is germane to consider the following psychiatric diagnoses in relationship to non-epileptic seizures: depressive illness, anxiety, hysteria, schizophrenia and malingering.

Affective disorders

The study of Roy (1977) emphasizes the importance of seeking possible affective disturbances, in particular a major affective disorder as a cause of non-epileptic seizures. In some cases this is most obvious when the seizures are presenting as a new problem, and at first sight the affective disturbance may not be readily apparent. However, once initiated as a clinical pattern, the non-epileptic seizures may continue for a considerable amount of time and, once the patient is on the epileptic 'roundabout' and receiving polytherapy with antiepileptic drugs, the situation may be compounded. The association between depressive symptoms and conversion phenomena in this group, is similar to patients with other conversion symptoms (Wilson-Barnett & Trimble 1985) and is in line with reports of several authors, including Gadd & Merskey (1975). This has important therapeutic and theoretical implications. From the therapeutic point of view it again underlines the need for careful psychiatric assesment of these cases and, theoretically, it raises the possibility that, in some of them, the pathophysiology of the conversion is interlinked with the underlying affective disorder. Treatment in these cases should obviously be orientated tcwards management of the underlying depressive illness and, in this writer's experience, should rely heavily on both psychotherapeutic and pharmacotherapeutic methods. Antiepileptic medication, particularly polytherapy, tends to exacerbate affective disturbance (Thompson & Trimble 1982) and clearly is inappropriate for the management of these patients. A caveat here is to emphasize that epilepsy itself may provoke psychiatric morbidity, including depression (Robertson & Trimble 1985); thus, unravelling the problem requires a great deal of clinical expertise in understanding not only the presentation and natural history of epilepsy, but also that of psychiatric illnesses, such as depression.

Hysteria

Hysteria, as already noted, has a long historical association with non-epileptic seizures. The position with regard to the theoretical understanding of hysteria has changed within the last 30 years, following the writings of such authors as Chodoff & Lyons (1958), Guze & Purley (1963), and Slater (1965). The first authors clearly made the distinction between the hysterical personality, a specific style emphasizing an individual's trait, and hysteria, a particular kind of psychosomatic symptomatology, often referred to as conversion hysteria or conversion reaction. In psychiatric practice, there are few who would not doubt the existence of the hysterical personality. However, the point was made by Chodoff & Lyons (1958) and re-emphasized by others (Merskey & Trimble 1979) that it is possible to have conversion symptoms without conforming to the classical hysterical personality style. Indeed, only approximately 21% of patients with conversion phenomena have the hysterical personality. Clinically, therefore, while detection of the hysterical personality may hint that the patient's symptoms are more a reflection of psychopathology than epilepsy, this feature alone is not sufficient to make a diagnosis of 'hysterical' seizures.

The essential features of the hysterical personality include: histrionic display; emotional lability and fragility; flamboyance; a history of impulsive actions with 'short circuiting' of decision making; verbal imprecision; and a tendency to overt seductiveness in the presence of a history of sexual problems including frigidity. It is generally more common amongst females, although it occurs in males and should always be sought for when attempting to piece together the clinical details of these patients.

Guze & Purley (1963) have suggested the existence of a certain specific pattern of hysteria referred to as Briquet's hysteria. These patients are almost all females and are always polysymptomatic. They characteristically have a history of an excessive number of surgical operations and hospitalizations, with the presentation of numerous somatic complaints. Frigidity and dyspareunia are often reported and sociopathic personality traits are noted in the families. Although some have implied that this group is really a form of hypochondriacal neurosis, or one end of the spectrum of hysterical personality disorder, Guze & Purley (1963) claim that it is a recognizable entity with a well-defined natural history. Of more importance to the theme of this chapter, however, is the fact that some 1% to 2% of consecutive female patients attending hospital for investigations, and up to 10% of psychiatric in-patients have the condition. Furthermore, non-epileptic

seizures are common in this group. Since the definition of the condition contains the fact that it is an intractable disorder and difficult to treat, recognition of such patients is of paramount importance clinically in order to avoid unnecessary surgical and medical intervention, including the prescription of antiepileptic drugs.

Schizophrenia and malingering

Of the disorders mentioned above, schizophrenia is rarely associated with non-epileptic convulsions, and the most common cause of seizures in this disease is probably the spontaneous occurrence of convulsions or the prescription of neuroleptic or other psychotrophic drugs which lower the seizure threshold. Malingering is likewise rare, although non-epileptic seizures occurring in the setting of compensation are not infrequently seen, but then the arguments concern whether or not the patient is malingering, has hysteria, or has some other condition driven by the compensation, disguised by such eponyms as 'compensation neurosis' (Trimble 1981).

PSYCHIATRIC SYNDROMES RESEMBLING EPILEPSY

A number of psychiatric syndromes may be confused with epileptic seizures. These include panic attacks, anxiety, rage attacks and fugues.

Panic attacks

Panic attacks are noted in patients who give a prior history of anxiety neurosis, and often occur in a setting of stress. The recognized clinical criteria for panic disorders are given in Table 10.1 (American Psychiatric Association 1980). It should be emphasized that, in some patients with temporal lobe epilepsy and complex partial seizures, the aura of panic may resemble in entirety the panic attacks of patients with this psychiatric condition. The clue to the diagnosis of epilepsy may be given in the somewhat more stereotyped nature of the auras of panic; their more fleeting nature; their greater paroxysmalness with the absence of a build-up of anxiety sometimes hours before the attack; the lack of the continuing

Table 10.1 Diagnostic criteria for panic disorder (American Psychiatric Association 1980)

A. At least three panic attacks within a three-week period in circumstances other than during marked physical exertion or in a life-threatening situation. The attacks are not precipitated only by exposure to a circumscribed phobic stimulus

B. Panic attacks are manifested by discrete periods of apprehension or fear, and at least four of the following symptoms appear during each attack:
   1. dyspnoea
   2. palpitations
   3. chest pain or discomfort
   4. choking or smothering sensations
   5. dizziness, vertigo, or unsteady feelings
   6. feelings of unreality
   7. paresthesiae (tingling in hands or feet)
   8. hot and cold flushes
   9. sweating
   10. faintness
   11. trembling or shaking
   12. fear of dying, going crazy or doing something uncontrolled during an attack

C. Not due to a physical disorder or another mental disorder, such as major depression, somatization disorder, or schizophrenia

D. The disorder is not associated with agoraphobia

presence of anxiety after the attack; and, no past history of psychopathology. The unpleasant fear-like aura of temporal lobe epilepsy is often initially an epigastric feeling and has a clear quality, rising up the midline of the body into the throat before the patient loses consciousness. In panic disorder, although again the feeling is often epigastric in origin, the pattern of radiation is more diffuse often spreading to involve the whole body. Further, hyperventilation, tachycardia, sweating, shortness of breath and other manifestations of anxiety will often be reported by the patient. Loss of consciousness may occur in non-epileptic seizures, and there are a small group of patients who hyperventilate and then, on account of this, have an epileptic seizure. Thus, careful attention to the time of onset, length and accompanying clinical features of the phenomena, taken together with the clinical history, will often enable the patients with panic disorder to be distinguished from those with epilepsy.

Phobic anxiety-depersonalization syndrome

A related condition is the phobic anxiety-depersonalization syndrome discussed by Harper & Roth (1962). In this disorder, a combination of phobias occurs in association with depersonalization. Often there is a clear precipitating event or the onset may be protracted. In particular, a sudden onset and the features of the depersonalization may suggest a diagnosis of temporal lobe epilepsy and other clinical features, such as déjà vu experiences and perceptual disorders, may further lead to difficulties with diagnosis. In Harper & Roth's study, 30 cases of phobic anxiety-depersonalization syndrome were compared with 30 patients with clearly defined epilepsy, which was probably temporal lobe epilepsy. A number of features were found to clearly distinguish these two group of patients. Thus, the phobic group had an older age of onset than the epileptic sample, and in 28 of the former, the disorder could be related to traumatic experiences immediately preceding the onset. The first epileptic attacks usually began out of the blue, while bereavement was a particularly common precursor of the depersonalization syndrome. The depersonalization itself was often associated with a sensation of fear and some reported being drowsy. In no case, however, was it accompanied by aphasia or clinical evidence of clouding of consciousness. Interestingly, déjà vu and jamais vu were equally common in both the epileptic and psychiatric patients, although in the epileptic group the experience was often extremely vivid, while in the phobic anxiety-depersonalization syndrome it often continued for long periods. The attacks occurred more frequently in the neurotic patients but, in both groups, were preceded by a feeling of tension or anxiety and tended to begin abruptly. However, the speed at which the attacks terminated was markedly different in the two groups, except where post-ictal confusion was noted. The EEG helped to discriminate between the groups, although over one third of the patients would fail to be classified by this index alone. Often, mild non-specific abnormalities, or even sharp waves over the temporal regions, were described in the neurotic patients and were not of value in the differential diagnosis.

Harper & Roth (1962) had 15 patients in whom the diagnosis was extremely difficult, presenting with features of both the neurosis and epilepsy. The mean age of the group was higher than for the two groups alone, as was the mean age of onset of the illness. In nearly all of these patients, the attack began after stress and a history of phobic anxiety, depression or suicidal attempts was common, as were neurotic personality traits in the past history. On a follow-up three to nine years later it was concluded that 12 did not have epilepsy.

Rage attacks

Rage attacks as ictal events are described as rare, although it is acknowledged that aggression may occur ictally and post-ictally, especially in a confused patient who is badly managed (Fenwick 1986). In such situations the aggression is often poorly directed and there is more danger of the patient harming himself than others. Recurrent outbursts of aggressive behaviour are not usually epileptic, often being related to a personality disorder, or to a lowered threshold for the release of aggression following brain damage. The episodic dyscontrol syndrome (Mark & Ervin 1970) is a condition of repeated paroxysmal episodes of violence, often associated with abnormal electroencephalographic activity, especially temporal lobe disturbance, which may respond to antiepileptic therapy. The relationship of this condition to temporal lobe epilepsy remains an area of controversy.

Fugue states

Fugue states are prolonged episodes of amnesia associated with wandering that are interlinked with a variety of psychopathologies. The amnesia lasts hours, weeks or occasionally years and, if related to psychiatric disablity such as depression, is usually seen in the setting of escape from difficult or intolerable circumstances. Unlike epileptic automatisms, which are briefer, the patient remains in contact with the environment, manipulates it successfully and appropriately, and often fails to draw much attention to him or herself. This is unlike episodes of transient global amnesia, which tend to be shorter lived and during which the patient often behaves inappropriately, asking repeatedly the same questions and appearing in a state of confusion.

Finally, attention should be brought to a small group of seizure patients who, following attempts to dissect out underlying neurological and psychiatric morbidity, Briquet's hysteria and other entities, still have an unclear diagnosis. These patients, with negative neurological evidence of epilepsy, are often assumed to be a psychiatric problem, although psychopathology is difficult to uncover and depressive illness or psychosis does not appear to be part of the current mental state. Some of these patients, well described in the last century by, for example Charcot, have associated stigmatas, such as hemianaesthesia or tunnel vision, or a clear history of other conversion phenomena suggestive of hysteria. Whether or not the existence of this group of patients justifies the retention of the term 'hysteria' as an independent entity is not clear; nevertheless, recognition that such a group exists is important, since a diagnosis of epilepsy is probably inappropriate.

REFERENCES

Abbott R J, Browning M C K, Davidson D L W 1980 Serum prolactin and cortisol concentrations after grand mal seizures. Journal of Neurology Neurosurgery and Psychiatry 43: 163–167

American Psychiatric Association 1980 DSM III Washington DC

Berkovic S 1984 Clinical and experimental aspects of complex partial seizures. Doctor of Medicine Thesis, University of Melbourne

Chodoff T, Lyons H 1958 Hysteria, hysterical personality and hysterical conversion. American Journal of Psychiatry 114: 734–740

Collins W C J, Lanigan O, Callaghan N 1983 Plasma concentrations following epileptic and pseudoseizures. Journal of Neurology, Neurosurgery and Psychiatry 46: 506–508

Dana-Haeri J, Trimble M R, Oxley J 1983 Prolactin and gonadotrophin changes following generalized and partial seizures. Journal of Neurology Neurosurgery and Psychiatry 46: 331–335

Desai B T, Porter R J, Penry J K 1982 Psychogenic seizures. Archives of Neurology 39: 202–209

Fenton G W 1982 Hysterical Alterations of conciousness. In: Roy A (ed.) Hysteria. John Wiley, Chichester, pp 229–246

Fenwick P 1986 Aggression and epilepsy. In: Trimble M R,

Bolwig T (eds) Some psychiatric aspects of epilepsy. John Wiley, New York, p 31–60

Gadd R A, Merskey H 1975 Middlesex hospital questionnaire scores in patients with hysterical conversion symptoms. British Journal of Medical Psychology 48: 367–370

Gallagher B B, Murvin A J, King D W, Flanigin H F 1984 ACTH and prolactin secretion in man during electrical stimulation of medial temporal lobe structures. Neurology 34 (S):125

Gowers W R 1881 Epilepsy. Churchill, London

Guze S D, Perley M J 1963 Observations on the natural history of hysteria. American Journal of Psychiatry 119: 960–965

Harper M, Roth M 1962 Temporal lobe epilepsy and the Phobic anxiety–depersonalisation syndrome. Comprehensive Psychiatry 3: 129–151, 215–226

Henry J, Woodruff G A J 1978 A diagnosis sign in states of apparent unconsciousness. Lancet 2: 920–921

Hoppener R J E A, Rentmeester T H, Arnoldkssen W, Hulsman J A, Gumnit R J, Meijers C A M 1982 Changes in serum prolactin levels following partial and generalized seizures. British Journal of Clinical Practice. (suppl. 18): 193–195

Holmes G L, Sackellares J C, McKiernan J, Ragland M, Dreifus F E 1980 Evaluation of childhood pseudoseizures using EEG telemetry and video tape monitoring. Journal of Paediatrics 97: 554–558

King D W, Gallagher D B, Murvin A J et al 1982 Pseudoseizures: diagnostic evaluation. Neurology 32: 18–23

Laxer K D, Mulloly J P, Howell B 1985 Prolactin changes after seizures classified by EEG monitoring. Neurology 35: 31–35

Lesser R P 1985 Psychogenic seizures. In: Pedley T, Meldrum B S (eds) Recent advances in epilepsy vol. 2. Churchill Livingstone, Edinbugh, pp 273–296

Luther J S, McNamara J O, Carwile S, Miller P, Hope R 1982 Pseudoepileptic seizures: methods of video-analysis to aid diagnosis. Annals of Neurology 12: 458–462

Mark V H, Ervin E R 1970 Violence and the brain. Harper & Row, London

Merskey H, Trimble M R 1979 Personality, sexual adjustment and brain lesions in patients with conversion

symptoms. American Journal of Psychiatry 136: 179–182

Oxley J, Roberts M, Dana-Haeri J, Trimble M R 1981 Evaluation of prolonged 4-channel EEG tape recordings and serum prolactin levels in the diagnosis of epileptic and non-epileptic seizures. In: Dam M, Gram L, Penry J K (eds) Advances in epileptology. Raven Press, New York, pp 343–357

Pritchard P B, Wannamaker J, Sagel J, Nair R, De Villier C 1983 Endocrine function following complex partial seizures. Annals of Neurology 14: 27–32

Ramani S V, Quesney L F, Olson D, Gumnit R J 1980 Diagnosis of hysterical seizures in epileptic patients. American Journal of Psychiatry 137: 705–709

Robertson M M, Trimble M R Depression and epilepsy: a review. British Journal of Clinical Practice (suppl. 18): 48–51

Roy A 1977 Hysterical fits previously diagnosed as epilepsy. Psychological medicine 7: 271–273

Roy A 1979 Hysterical seizures. Archives of Neurology 36:447

Slater E 1965 Diagnosis of hysteria. British Medical Journal 1: 1395–1399

Stewart R S, Lovitt R, Stewart R M 1982 Are hysterical seizures more than hysteria? American Journal of Psychiatry 139: 926–928

Thompson P, Trimble M R 1982 Anticonvulsant drugs, cognitive function and behaviour. Epilepsia 24 (suppl. 18): 21–22

Trimble M R 1978 Serum prolactin in epilepsy and hysteria. British Medical Journal 2:1682

Trimble M R 1981 Post traumatic neurosis. John Wiley, Chichester

Trimble M R, Dana-Haeri J, Oxley J, Baylis P H 1985 Some neuroendocrine consequences of seizures. In: Porter R et al (eds) Advances in Epileptology. 15th Epilepsy International Symposium. Raven Press, New York, pp 201–208

Wilson-Barnett J, Trimble M R 1985 An investigation of hysteria using the illness behaviour questionnaire. British Journal of Psychiatry 146: 601–608

Wyllie E, Luders H, MacMillan J P, Gupta M 1984 Serum prolactin levels after epileptic seizures. Neurology 34: 1601–1604

PART THREE
THE PSYCHOSES OF EPILEPSY
M. R. Trimble

HISTORICAL BACKGROUND

Although it has recently become a subject of great interest, the relationship between psychosis and epilepsy goes back many years and one of the earlier British contributions came from Willis (Dewhurst 1980). It was, however, the continental authors of the nineteenth century who made the first substantial contributions (Berrios 1979). For example, Griesinger (1857) stated that 'a very great number of epileptics are in a state of chronic mental disease even during the intervals between their attacks'; and Morel (1860) introduced the term 'larval epilepsy' for those cases in which automatic activity and acute behavioural disturbances, such as outbursts of anger or violence, were seen without necessarily including loss of consciousness. He drew attention to the paroxysmal nature of the clinical features of these associated states and noted certain personality characteristics of chronic epileptic patients which later crystallized into the concept of the epileptic character.

One of the earlier French contributions was from Esquirol (1838) who reported that some four-fifths of chronic female in-patients had some form of mental disorder. The early reports of Bouchet & Cazauvielh (1825) contained associations between temporal lobe pathology and insanity, and they commented that many patients did not become psychotic until a number of years had passed since starting epilepsy.

Falret (1860) drew attention to the association between the timing of seizures and the subsequent mental state. He thus classified the psychiatric disorders of epilepsy into those which were peri-ictal, those which were interictal, and the long-term insanities, the latter being 'those phenomena of longer duration constituting true madness'.

British views at this time were found to vary. Authors such as Reynolds (1861) were unable to accept that there was any special mental state related to epilepsy, while Hughlings Jackson (1875) recognized epilepsy as a cause of insanity in 6% of cases, identifying mainly the ictal variety. In seeking explanations for a link, Clouston (1887) suggested that the area of brain which, when disturbed, leads to epilepsy might also be responsible for the abnormal mental state. Maudsley (1879) accepted the notion of masked epilepsy and interestingly referred to the 'exaggerated development of the religious sentiment' in epileptic patients which could be associated with visions and revelations from on high. Turner (1907) reported on paroxysmal psychoses which either preceded, succeeded, or replaced convulsive episodes and which could include hallucinatory, delusional, maniacal, melancholic or psychasthenic states. He also noted that a number of epileptic patients passed eventually into a state of continued delusional insanity requiring asylum treatment.

Thus, by the turn of the nineteenth century, many authors had commented on associations between epilepsy and psychosis; although the explanations for this varied. Some authors felt that the seizure discharges were related to this, while others suggested that the seizures and the insanity were both reflections of an underlying, similar, but not necessarily the same, pathology. A third

link was also noted. Thus Savage, in his contribution to Daniel Tuke's *Dictionary of psychological medicine* (Tuke 1892), suggested that some patients who were relieved of their seizures could then deteriorate mentally, but further that in other cases epileptic seizures were followed by an improvement in the mental state.

One consequence of these various contributions was that 'epileptic insanity' held a separate place in the majority of classifications of insanity that were put forward at that time, as distinctive, for example, as 'general paralysis of the insane'. Although in part this was linked with ideas of hereditary degeneration, which were prevalent in neurological and psychiatric circles towards the end of the nineteenth century, it also reflected the bias of referral populations that these various authors examined. The psychiatrists, especially the asylum doctors, saw institutionalized patients, and thus were more inclined to comment on the longer term alterations of the mental state in patients with intractable seizures, while others, such as Hughlings Jackson, dealt more with the acute paroxysms as were seen on a neurological in-patient ward.

In the early part of the twentieth century, the relationship between epilepsy and psychosis attracted little attention and, indeed, the pendulum swung to suggest that, if anything, epilepsy and psychosis were less often found together than would occur by chance (Glaus 1931), and so an antagonism between the two conditions was suggested.

Increasing use of the electroencephalogram and the identification of temporal lobe epilepsy, led to a recrudescence of the idea that psychiatric disorders were more common in patients with epilepsy, but this time the association was more with focal temporal lobe epilepsy (Gibbs 1951). Other authors commented on a chronic paranoid hallucinatory state in epilepsy, referring to it as a definitive entity and suggesting that patients with this condition usually had temporal lobe epilepsy with typical complex auras (Pond 1957). The fact that the psychotic episodes began several years after the onset of the seizures and often occurred in the setting of a diminishing seizure frequency was reiterated; similar findings being reported by Hill (1953) and Slater & Beard (1963). The latter authors were most influential with their report on 69 cases of epileptic psychosis which they referred to as being 'schizophrenia-like'. They also commented that the psychoses tended to develop a number of years after the seizure disorder had started, and that the majority of patients had temporal lobe abnormalities and were diagnosed as having temporal lobe epilepsy. They were referred to as schizophrenia-like because many of them had classical first-rank symptoms of Schneider, but differences between this epileptic psychosis and a process schizophrenia were acknowledged. These included the maintenence of a warm affect; the presentation often with intense affective symptoms; and the absence of any clearly defined pre-morbid personality style, such as the schizoid personality.

CLASSIFICATION

A simple classification of the relationship between seizures and psychosis is shown in Table 10.2. It acknowledges the earlier division into ictal and interictal states, and distinguishes between episodic and chronic forms of the condition. Thus, peri-ictal disturbances are clearly related to abnormal electrical activity in the brain, which can be seen on the electroencephalogram if it is recorded at the time of the behaviour disturbance; in contrast to the interictal disturbances which are seen between seizures and not clearly interlinked with the acute neurophysiological disturbance. It

is now clear, however, that this does not mean that abnormal electrical activity is not present somewhere in the central nervous system which may be directly linked to the psychotic picture.

Peri-ictal

The most frequent peri-ictal disturbance is an acute organic brain syndrome which occurs shortly after partial or generalized seizures. In these cases, patients in a state of confusion may appear psychotic and sometimes complain of hallucinations or delusions. A patient may wander in a confused fashion, but is rarely aggressive unless inappropriately handled. In some cases, particularly following several bouts of seizures, a prolonged organic psychosyndrome can ensue which goes on for hours or occasionally days. Certainly, if during a seizure, anoxic brain damage or severe head injury has occurred, then a prolonged psychosis may emerge which again reflects the organic brain syndrome and for which further investigation is mandatory.

Complex partial and absence seizures may present as a form of status epilepticus. While rare, these probably occur more frequently than suspected, and appropriate electroencephalographic monitoring at the time of the disturbance is mandatory to make the diagnosis. In both, consciousness is clouded and the patient shows overt confusion and difficulty in manipulating cognitive tasks which may, however, particularly with complex partial seizure status, be subtle.

Table 10.2 A suggested outline of the psychoses associated with epilepsy

	Disturbance of consciousness	EEG: most common disturbances
Episodic:		
Post-ictal automatism	+	Slow waves
Absence status	+	3/s spike and wave
Complex partial seizure status	+	Continuous temporal lobe abnormality
Psycho-organic episodes	+	Very abnormal EEG with slow dysrhythmia
Forced normalization states	−	Normal
Chronic:		
Paranoid states	−	Temporal lobe abnormalities
Schizophrenic-like states	−	Temporal lobe abnormalities (left side)
Manic depressive states	−	Temporal lobe abnormalities (?)

Such episodes can continue for many days and the patient may present with a variety of psychopathological phenomena including hallucinations, delusions and affective symptoms. The absence status is less likely to be associated with clearly defined psychotic manifestations than temporal lobe status, the patient often appearing in a prolonged twilight state with fluctuating levels of arousal and periodic bursts of rapid eyeblinks or myoclonic jerks.

Interictal

In contrast, interictal psychoses occur between seizures and cannot directly be linked to the ictus. However, clinically there are some patients who develop a psychosis following an increase in seizure frequency and, when their seizures resolve, continue to display psychotic symptoms for a prolonged period. In one variety, patients usually, after a bout of seizures, have a lucid interval of some 24 to 48 hours and then switch into a psychotic state with over-activity, elation and dysphoria, delusions, illusions and hallucinations, often with a marked aggressive or religious content. Clouding of consciousness may be seen if the appropriate clinical testing is carried out, and the EEG is found to be abnormal. The condition may last days or even weeks, slowly resolving into a chronic often well-encapsulated psychotic state or gradually dissipating. This clinical picture emphasizes the close relationship between the peri-ictal disturbances and interictal states as commented on by Ferguson & Rayport (1984). Thus, in these patients it is difficult in the later stages of the psychosis to be certain that the psychotic phenomena, which may not be accompanied by surface electroencephalographic abnormalities, are not related to continuing electrophysiological disturbances in deep structures. Certainly, there is strong evidence that many patients with psychosis and *no* epilepsy may show spike-wave disturbances in various regions of the limbic system when they have electrodes implanted in those areas (Heath 1977). In addition, psychotic symptoms can be provoked by stimulation of limbic system structures in experimental circumstances.

Clinically, the interictal disturbances are seen as chronic psychotic states with a fairly typical psychiatric picture. Manic-depressive psychoses, presenting with fluctuating states of overactivity, flight of ideas and pressure of speech in which the patient is euphoric, irritable and aggressive, are seen; but sudden mood swings are not uncommon, and often, on close questioning, patients describe a dysphoria rather than a euphoria. True cyclical manic-depressive illness seems rare, although depressive illness with a psychotic, especially paranoid flavouring, is more common. These patients demonstrate a classical paranoid state with vigilance, overt hostility and suspiciousness with over-sensitiveness towards their environment. Delusions may occur which have a persecutory content and, in chronic states, patients may accumulate vast amounts of documentary information supporting their contentions and grievances. The schizophreniform psychoses have the form of a schizophrenic illness, although some differences have already been noted and were reported on by Slater & Beard (1963). Delusions of persecution and religious delusions are often reported, although hebephrenic deterioration and catatonic phenomena are rare. The long history of religiosity in association with epilepsy was reviewed by Dewhurst & Beard (1970), who presented a number of cases of their own, all of which were diagnosed as having temporal lobe epilepsy.

One study has recently used intensive monitoring in a group of epileptic patients with psychotic episodes. Ramani & Gumnit (1982) monitored 10 patients with video telemetry: 65% of their group had complex partial seizures, or complex partial seizures with secondary generalization, while 26% had generalized seizures. The patients all had longstanding epilepsy (average duration 17.9 years) and their psychosis had been present for a mean of 12.3 years. Nine patients were diagnosed as having a schizophrenia-like presentation and in no patient did the episode of psychosis last longer than about three weeks. One patient showed a striking reduction of the spikes on EEG during the psychotic phase; two others showed a tendency towards aggravation of psychosis with a reduction of seizure frequency brought about by prescription of antiepileptic drugs. In all patients, interictal paroxymal abnormalities were reported, in eight of a bilateral or generalized nature. This comprehensive study of psychosis confirms that schizophrenia-like states can occur in association with various form of epilepsy, and that a reciprocal link between the seizures and psychotic symptoms occurs in some cases.

ON THE ANTAGONISM BETWEEN EPILEPSY AND PSYCHOSIS

Closely allied to the ictally related psychoses, but interictal in nature and often of brief duration and paroxysmal in presentation, are short-lived psychotic bouts in which there is some form of antagonism, either between seizure frequency or between abnormal EEG discharges and the psychotic symptoms. Landolt (1958) recorded changes in the EEG during pre-seizure dysphoric episodes and limited periods of overt psychosis lasting days or weeks. During these he noted improvement in previously abnormal EEGs and referred to this phenomenon as 'forced normalization'. At the end of the psychotic episodes, the EEGs were again abnormal. In the extensive collection reported by Dongier (1959), EEG data on 536 psychotic episodes that occurred in 516 patients were reported. EEG abnormalities disappeared during the psychosis in 78 cases and in 53% of these there was no obvious clouding of consciousness. Delusions were particularly frequent in patients in whom a pre-existing focal discharge disappeared, and in these patients the episode lasted a particularly long time, sometimes several weeks. Both Landolt and Dongier suggested that paranoid and schizophreniform states were more likely to be seen following the suppression of focal, particularly temporal focal, as opposed to generalized, discharges.

The theme has been taken up more recently by Wolf (Wolf 1984, Wolf & Trimble 1985). It has been pointed out that the term 'forced normalization' was poorly translated into English, implying in that language some form of active force which in German was not the intention; for Landolt it was purely descriptive. Although Landolt initially concentrated on partial seizures, in his later writing he also recognized forced normalization to occur with generalized attacks, particularly following the introduction of the succinimide drugs. These observations are supported by the studies of Wolf (1984). In addition, the latter points out that forced normalization may result in a number of differing clinical patterns, not necessarily psychotic ones. He includes such phenomena as pre-psychotic dysphoria which may herald a psychotic state, but also hypochondriacal states, episodes of hysterical symptomatology, depressive states, manic states and twilight states.

The term 'alternative psychosis' was introduced by Tellenbach (1965) to provide a shortened term which paid more attention to the presence or absence of seizures, rather than EEG phenomena. It implied that, in some cases, the control of seizures did not mean cure of the clinical problem or even inactivity of any underlying disease process, and that psychoses may flower as a result.

ON THE AFFINITY BETWEEN EPILEPSY AND PSYCHOSIS

Prevalence

There are few careful epidemiological studies of psychopathology in patients with epilepsy, and therefore estimating the incidence of psychosis is difficult. In Pond & Bidwell's study (1959) nearly 30% of their patients had 'psychological difficulties', 7% having been in a psychiatric hospital before or during the survey year. A temporal lobe group had a higher rate of hospitalization to psychiatric hospitals and a higher rate of severe personality change and psychosis. Gudmundsson (1966), in a survey of the population of Iceland, was able to compare the prevalence rates for psychiatric illness in epilepsy to those without epilepsy. In the epilepsy population, some 8% were psychotic, again being greater in his temporal lobe sample. In a similar extensive survey, Zielinksi (1974) provided further data on non-selected epileptic patients from a population in Poland: 58% showed some 'mental abnormality' and approximately 3% had psychotic symptoms. In that survey, psychopathology was over-represented in those with temporal lobe epilepsy and secondary generalization.

Despite these data, a number of authors still question whether psychosis is more likely to occur in epilepsy than, for example, in other chronic disorders and, further, whether there is a link to temporal lobe epilepsy. An important investigation was carried out by Hermann & Whitman (1984). As part of a review of the literature on epilepsy and behaviour they examined psychopathology as rated by the Minnesota Multiphasic Personality Inventory (MMPI) in a large number of patients with epilepsy using chronic non-neurological or neurological disorders as controls, taken from published findings in the literature. When they examined those patients with psychopathology, the epilepsy group showed a significantly higher rating of psychosis than the neurological controls; who in turn showed a higher rate than the chronically medically ill controls. They thus suggested that, if a special type of psychopathology was manifest in patients with epilepsy, there was a higher probability that it was a psychotic disorder.

In summary then, there does appear to be evidence, stemming from several different investigations, that patients with epilepsy may be more prone to the development of psychosis. Some authors suggest an over-representation of temporal lobe epilepsy, or temporal lobe epilepsy where the seizures secondarily generalize.

Risk factors

It is obvious that most patients with temporal lobe epilepsy do not develop psychosis, and therefore attempts to clarify those who may be more at risk have been carried out. Hermann & Whitman (1984) have listed some of these as determined from the literature. They include a past history and present findings suggestive of organicity; being left handed or ambidextrous; having automatisms or secondarily generalized seizures; having a lower frequency of complex partial seizures; showing focal spike activity in medial as opposed to lateral temporal cortical recording leads; showing more independent spike foci and a higher frequency of maximal spike foci at such leads and bilateral medio-basely located spike abnormalities.

Hermann et al (1982), again using the MMPI, made a significant contribution when comparing patients with temporal lobe epilepsy to generalized epilepsy by separating out a temporal lobe group that had an aura of fear, in contrast to those who had different auras. The fear group displayed pathological elevations on several MMPI scales, especially for schizophrenia. Since ictal fear results from activity of the medial temporal lobes, especially the amygdala and hippocampus (Gloor 1972), these data reinforce suggestions that medial temporal lesions, in other words those more clearly identified with the limbic system, may be more associated with the likelihood of development of psychosis.

Another important factor which seems to be emerging is the relationship, not between temporal lobe epilepsy per se and psychosis, but between complex partial seizures that secondarily generalize and psychopathology; suggesting either a more widespread epileptic disturbance or a greater propensity for seizures to generalize through limbic system structures. This has emerged from several studies, including that of Rodin et al (1976) who noted that most mental disturbances in patients with temporal lobe epilepsy occurred in those that had more than one seizure type; and the data of Bruens (1980), who noted that the highest incidence of psychosis was in patients with a temporal lobe EEG focus and bilateral spike-wave activity suffering from both psychomotor and generalized seizures.

The studies of Taylor (1975) identified the possible importance of 'alien tissue lesions' in temporal lobe structures and, in addition, age of onset of seizures after the age of 10. This latter factor has been investigated in more detail by Hermann et al (1980) who examined MMPI scales in relation to age of onset and type of seizures. An adolescent onset, with temporal lobe epilepsy, was associated with the highest scores on the schizophrenia scale. In general, a group with generalized epilepsy of adolescent onset scored lower on most of the scales than did the group with temporal lobe epilepsy, suggesting an age/seizure type interaction.

Phenomenology

A criticism of much of the work in this field is that the term 'psychosis' has been used without definition by some authors and little attempt has been made to specify the precise phenomenology of the patients who are examined. It is noteworthy that the Anglo-Saxon authors who have written on this subject tend to use the concepts of Kurt Schneider for the diagnosis of schizophreniform illness, in particular relying on the presence of first-rank symptomatology. The importance of being precise is emphasized by more recent techniques that have used standardized and validated methods for quantifying psychopathology in the psychoses of epilepsy (Perez & Trimble 1980.)

Using such methodology it has been possible to compare as objectively as possible the presentation of psychosis in epilepsy with process schizophrenia, in the absence of epilepsy. In the first report of this kind, Perez & Trimble (1980), using the Present State Examination (PSE) of Wing, presented data on 24 patients with epilepsy and psychosis referred prospectively. The psychosis occurred in the setting of clear consciousness and was present for at least a month. This technique, which allowed for diagnosis to be made by the CATEGO computer programme, gave a PSE syndrome profile for the epileptic group which was compared with non-epileptic schizophrenic controls. In this study, 50% of the patients with epilepsy and psychosis were categorized as having schizophrenic psychosis; 92% having a profile of nuclear schizophrenia based on the first-rank symptoms of Schneider. The syndrome profile of the patients with schizophrenia and epilepsy compared with those with schizophrenia showed few significant differences, emphasizing the similarity of the clinical presentation of these two disorders. Recently, Toone et al (1982b), in a retrospective study, also using the PSE, have reported similar findings. These data thus suggest that, in a group of patients with psychosis and epilepsy, a significant number will have a schizophrenia-like presentation virtually identical with regard to presenting symptoms to nuclear schizophrenia in the absence of epilepsy. One important aspect of this is to stress at least some common pathophysiological link for the two disorders.

Perez & Trimble (1980) further examined in their sample the differences in presentation between psychotic patients with temporal lobe epilepsy and those with generalized epilepsy. All patients who were diagnosed by the CATEGO as having nuclear schizophrenia had temporal lobe abnormalities on their electroencephalogram and received a clinical diagnosis of complex partial seizures. Patients with psychosis and generalized epilepsy had a variety of psychopathological presentations, which included schizophrenia without first-rank symptoms and manic and depressive psychoses. This study was thus a confirmation of the direct link between certain types of epilepsy and certain patterns of clinical presentation, suggested by others extending back to the early reports of Hill (1953) and Pond (1957).

These recent studies clarify some of the rather obscure issues which have perplexed some non-medical authors on the subject of psychosis and epilepsy. Thus, the link between temporal lobe epilepsy and psychosis has provoked considerable argument, almost as vociferous as that which relates to the link between temporal lobe changes and personality disorder. In general, most authors who have looked at this area do find an over-representation of temporal lobe abnormalities. It is pointed out that patients with temporal lobe epilepsy tend to be over-represented in populations presenting to hospitals and, further, that non-clinical studies (using for example, rating scales such as the MMPI) or even some clinical studies, often fail to note differences between those with temporal lobe and other seizure types (Hermann & Whitman 1984). However, it would appear that a link emerges between a certain nuclear form of schizophrenia-like illness and temporal lobe epilepsy. This does not mean that patients with other forms of epilepsy may not also develop psychosis; although the clinical presentation of it may well be different. It is unfortunate that in much of the literature authors make accurate attempts to note epileptic variables, but in contrast show considerable laxity in precision with regards to psychiatric variables.

LATERALITY

A further important consideration was introduced by Flor-Henry in 1969. He suggested that left-sided temporal lobe lesions in particular were associated with a schizophreniform presentation, contrasting with a right-sided abnormality linking with a manic-depressive picture. The hint of this laterality difference is noted further in the work of Taylor (1975), Pritchard et al (1980) and Sherwin (1981). In the follow-up study of Ounsted & Lindsay (1981), in which patients earlier diagnosed as having temporal lobe epilepsy were reassessed 13 years later, 9 patients developed a schizophreniform psychosis with first-rank symptoms of Schneider, 7 had a left-sided focus, and 2 had bilateral discharges. Trimble & Perez (1982), using electroencephalographic criteria for lateralization of focus, compared the PSE syndrome profiles of patients with left-sided to those with right-sided lesions. In their group, 8 patients had consistent left-sided EEG abnormalities, 2 had bilaterally independent foci, 4 had right-sided abnormalities, and 2 had a unilateral focus (one left and one right) in all EEG recordings except their most recent. Comparison of the profiles of those with left-sided versus those with right-sided abnormalities noted two significant differences: namely, the left-sided patients had significantly more nuclear schizophrenia and ideas of reference, than the right-sided patients.

Although in these studies the clinical documentation of patients was as precise and objective as possible, it is clear that evaluation of laterality from surface electroencephalographic recordings is open to criticism. In order to circumvent this difficulty, Sherwin (1982) carried out several studies of patients who, while awaiting temporal lobe surgery, had the laterality of their focus established by depth recording of ictal episodes and ensuing cessation of seizures following temporal lobectomy. Again he was able to conclude that patients with left-sided temporal lobe epileptogenic lesions were at special risk for the development of the schizophrenia-like psychoses, and that psychosis was a rare complication in patients with other focal (non-temporal) epileptic lesions. Toone et al (1982a) in a retrospective study, using the syndrome check-list (SCL) derived from the PSE, have also examined the question of laterality using computerized axial tomography (CT): 57 patients with psychosis and epilepsy were examined and a tendency towards an excess of left-sided abnormalities in schizophreniform cases was reported. Unlike the studies using electroencephalographic techniques, however, this difference was not significant, although hallucinations were seen exclusively in the patients with left-sided lesions.

These data taken together would suggest that a pattern of psychosis, resembling nuclear schizophrenia, does occur in patients with temporal lobe epilepsy more commonly than in other forms of epilepsy, and that, when present, it is much more likely to be associated with a left-sided or predominantly left-sided lesion. Moreover, since the studies using the electroencephalogram have been more convincing in demonstrating this relationship than those using CT scan data, the evolution of the clinical pattern would seem more likely to be dependent on functional as opposed to strictly structural abnormalities. Further evidence for this suggestion derives from a second recent study of CT scan data in patients with schizophreniform psychoses of epilepsy. Trimble and colleagues (Perez et al 1985) quantitatively evaluated the CT scans of 10 patients with epileptic psychosis and nuclear first-rank symptoms; 10 patients with non-nuclear psychoses of epilepsy; and 8 with schizophrenia who were not epileptic. All these psychotic groups had high values for the bilateral septum caudate distance, and the size of the third and fourth ventricles compared to expected normal data, but no laterality differences were noted on such indices, nor on measures of cortical abnormality.

Three further points should be made. The first is that several authors have failed to detect a relationship between the laterality of focus and presentation of the psychosis (e.g. Kristensen & Sindrup 1978, Jensen & Larsen 1979), although such authors have also failed to use precise diagnostic criteria as outlined above. The second is that there is a growing, and now extensive, literature on laterality in non-epileptic psychiatric patients which points in a similar direction; namely, to abnormalities of left hemisphere function in schizophrenia (Gruzelier 1981). Finally, the literature on the link between manic-depressive illness and right-sided lesions is less substantial and, to date, this second hypothesis emerging from Flor-Henry's (1969) data has yet to be confirmed.

MECHANISMS

Further questions may be asked with regard to the mechanism of the development of psychosis. A number of different explanations have been put forward, and the majority take as their starting point the now established relationship between the temporal lobe-limbic system and affective experiences.

There are two main contrasting hypotheses. The first is that the schizophrenia-like illnesses are epileptic in origin and should be referred to as 'epileptic psychoses'. The second is that they are a manifestation of organic neurological damage and thus not specific for epilepsy. The former view has been most strongly expressed by Flor-Henry (1969). He criticized the absence of a control population in some of the earlier studies, and noted that in his series, as well as in others (e.g. Hill 1953, Pond 1957), an inverse relationship between the frequency of psychomotor seizures and the onset of the psychosis had been recorded in some patients. He suggested that it was not structural damage but the characteristics of the seizures that lead to the clinical picture. Support for this suggestion comes from other studies in which depth electrodes have been implanted in psychotic patients who do not have epilepsy. Abnormal electrical activity in the deep temporal structures is shown to be associated with suppression of surface cortical activity and, when patients display psychotic behaviour, abnormal spike-wave activity may be detected in deep areas, notably the septal region, which is not seen on conventional surface electrodes (Heath 1977).

The alternative position was taken by Slater & Beard (1963). They noted that a significant proportion of the psychotic patients had a defined organic basis for their epilepsy, and that the onset of the psychosis seemed linked to the duration of the epilepsy. Their conclusion stressed the importance of an underlying structural lesion in the temporal lobe. A similar view was taken by Kristensen & Sindrup (1978). Kiloh (1971) made the point that almost any diffuse brain disease may on occasion be associated with a similar clinical picture, and epilepsy is often not present. He suggested that psychoses were a reflection of a certain stage of what, in the long run, was a dementing process. Follow-up studies of such patients do not, however, lend support to this view (Slater & Beard 1963).

Bruens (1980) put forward the idea that both organic and psychodynamic events potentiate each other. The patient is unable to protect him or herself against the vicissitudes of life except by using pathological defence mechanisms, which result in psychosis. Pond (1962) suggested it was the abnormal experiences associated with temporal lobe epilepsy which gradually became integrated into a person's psychic life that led to the development of psychosis. However, these explanations do not account for the laterality findings, and as Slater & Beard (1963) point out, do not take into account the volitional disturbances, thought disorder and hebephrenic symptoms noted in some of these patients.

Symonds (1962) pointed to the 'epileptic disorder of function'. It was, he suggested, not the loss of neurones in the temporal lobe that was responsible for the psychosis, but the disorderly activity of those that remain. A similar view was stressed by Taylor (1975) who stated 'perhaps it is better, from the point of view of avoiding psychosis, for the (temporal) lobe to be nonfunctional rather than dysfunctional'. However, the well-documented cases of psychoses in epilepsy that develop after temporal lobectomy (e.g. Jensen & Larsen 1979, Sherwin 1982), and the similarity of certain neuropathological abnormalities recently described in patients with schizophrenia and schizophreniform psychosis of epilepsy, which include not only focal pathology in the temporal lobes, but gliosis in periventricular, peri-aqueductal, midbrain tegmentum and basal forebrain areas (Stevens 1982), suggest that we must look beyond the temporal lobes for our fuller understanding of this condition.

One theory recently advanced is that chronic temporal lobe ictal lesions may lead to kindling of activity in other regions of the brain, especially forebrain limbic areas, and these changes lead to the development of psychosis. It is extremely difficult to kindle epileptic seizures in certain parts of the limbic system, particularly those that are catecholaminergic. Kindling of the mesolimbic dopamine system leads, not to seizures, but to marked behaviour changes which persist after the kindling has ceased (Stevens & Livermore 1978). The possibility arises that in humans similar mechanisms exist, such that chronic subictal activity leads to a kindling process within dopaminergic pathways, overactivity of which leads to the development of abnormal behaviour patterns and psychosis. It is difficult here to ignore the growing literature on the pathology of schizophrenia, in which the same dopamine-rich areas of the limbic forebrain are suggested as sites for abnormalities that are, at least in part, responsible for the development of the psychosis (Crow 1980). Since behaviour changes associated with kindling of the mesolimbic dopamine system are enhanced by the administration of dopamine agonists, it is possible that the kindling itself is associated with altered postsynaptic function of dopamine receptors. Since dopamine agonism is probably anticonvulsant in action, and raises the seizure threshold (Trimble 1977), these neurophysiological observations may be invoked to explain the clinical findings of an association between persistent abnormal temporal lobe activity and psychosis, and the tendency of its development to be associated with a declining seizure frequency.

Further information on mechanism derives from recent studies of positron emission tomography (PET) with radioactive labelled oxygen to measure cerebral blood flow (rCBF) and metabolism (rCMRO$_2$) in a group of epileptic patients whose psychosis was assessed using the PSE (Gallhofer et al 1985). In the PET investigations, patients with epilepsy and psychosis were compared with patients with epilepsy and no psychosis; the groups being matched for age, type of epilepsy, IQ and seizure frequency. The rCMRO$_2$ was lower in most regions examined in the psychotic group, especially in frontal and temporal cortices, and the basal ganglia. Again laterality differences were recorded with the psychotic sample (most of which had nuclear symptoms) showing lower rCMRO$_2$ on the left side, especially in the temporal regions. Since none of these patients had severe epilepsy, and mainly infrequent partial seizures, these findings imply that any explanation for the development of psychosis in epilepsy must take into consideration

'down regulation' of activity in certain brain structures, especially those linked to the basal ganglia and the limbic system.

Finally, the possible role of antiepileptic drugs should be considered. Considerable evidence has now accumulated that polytherapy, and perhaps certain of the older antiepileptic compounds such as phenobarbitone and phenytoin, can provoke cognitive changes and alteration of mood and personality (for review see Trimble & Reynolds 1984). However, apart from some idiosyncratic reactions, the phenomenon of forced normalization, and the production of an organic brain syndrome with gross toxicity, the link between chronic antiepileptic drug therapy and the provocation of psychosis has never been substantiated, even by those authors who have looked at this question (Slater & Beard 1963).

In summary, therefore, at the present time the evidence for a functional as opposed to a structural change in limbic system structures, both within the temporal lobes and downstream in forebrain limbic structures, may be the most useful hypothesis to follow with regard to understanding the development of at least some of the psychoses of epilepsy. Alternative mechanisms, including recurrent brain damage with anoxia or head injury, may, along with polytherapy, be responsible for cognitive dulling and the development of a dementia-like picture. While in the older texts this was confused with psychosis, thinking and methodologies have progressed considerably. Animal models, particularly the kindling model; behaviour disturbances observed following other temporal lobe lesions in animals and humans; and the EEG abnormalities recorded in association with psychosis in limbic system structures, also point in this direction.

TREATMENT

Ictal psychoses

The management of the interictal and ictal psychoses clearly differ. The ictal psychoses occur because of acute electrical disturbances in the central nervous system that are associated with the epileptic seizures and the correct management involves better control of seizures and, in particular, the prevention of clusters of seizures which may so disrupt cerebral activity that the psychosis becomes inevitable. Sadly, for many patients with epilepsy, treatment is still with unbridled polypharmacy and they have not had access to either intensive monitoring of their seizures for better diagnosis, or of their treatment for better management. In patients with psychosis and epilepsy, particularly those on polypharmacy, it is always worthwhile reconsidering the antiepileptic drug load and attempting to achieve monotherapy where possible. In view of the now substantial literature that patients without epilepsy, but who have manic depressive psychosis, seem to respond to carbamazepine (Post et al 1985), it might be expected that carbamazepine monotherapy would be the drug of choice. Certainly replacing more sedative antiepileptic drugs by carbamazepine can bring with it improvement of cognitive performance and mood and, indeed, an improvement in seizure frequency (Thompson & Trimble 1982), which is clearly important in terms of preventing these ictal psychoses. Although there have been no controlled trials, generally for patients with temporal lobe epilepsy and associated psychiatric impairments, carbamazepine is to be seen as the drug of choice. It is also indicated in the longer term management of patients prone to complex partial seizure status, while those developing absence status require either sodium valproate or ethosuximide for continued therapy.

Psychosis should not be seen as a bar to temporal lobe surgery, particularly if the psychotic state is peri-ictal, and if a unilateral site of origin of the seizure is demonstrated.

Sometimes during psychotic episodes antipsychotic drugs are required, and haloperidol or pimozide are preferable in these ictally related episodes. They may need to be given intravenously or intramuscularly, but oral administration should be used if possible. It is important that patients with only ictally related psychoses are not kept on these medications chronically and, when the psychosis is resolved, they should be slowly withdrawn.

Wolf (1984) has suggested the use of benzodiazepines in prepsychotic dysphorias of forced normalization, and has pointed out that, with generalized absence seizures, forced normalization is less likely to occur if the patient is treated with sodium valproate as opposed to ethosuximide.

Interictal psychoses

In contrast to these ictally related states, interictal psychoses should be treated as psychiatric disorders in the absence of epilepsy. It is probable that, in these situations, temporal lobectomy has little impact on the psychosis, although that should not be seen as a reason to bar patients from consideration, and some improve. Manic-depressive psychoses can be treated with lithium, although rationalization of therapy with the introduction of carbamazepine monotherapy would appear to be the most appropriate management initially. Individual episodes of manic psychosis may require the prescription of a major tranquillizer such as a phenothiazine or a butyrophenone, although the treatment should be selected carefully (see below). In depressive psychosis, antidepressants should be considered, and ECT is not contraindicated if required.

Paranoid states and schizophrenia-like psychoses need to be evaluated, not only from the point of view of their psychiatric phenomonology but also in relationship to the seizure frequency. Thus, patients who stop having seizures or have a diminished seizure frequency prior to the onset of their psychosis require a neuroleptic which lowers the seizure threshold, such as a phenothiazine. Indeed, such patients may require the application of ECT to bring about a therapeutic seizure if their psychosis is life threatening. Alternatively, where patients are seen to have an increase in or no alteration of their seizure frequency in association with the interictal psychosis, a neuroleptic drug less likely to precipitate seizures is probably more appropriate. Generally, these are the butyrophenones, such as haloperidol and pimozide. Longer term intramuscular preparations such as flupenthixol can be used and there is no evidence that they interfere with the control of seizures. At the present time there are few data on the interaction between antipsychotic and antiepileptic drugs, although idiosyncratic interactions between phenytoin and chlorpromazine have been reported and deterioration of either the mental state or seizure frequency following the initiation of these drugs should lead to further assessment of anti-epileptic drug levels.

PROGNOSIS

The only follow-up series reported is that of Slater & Beard (1963). Generally, the prognosis was better than for process schizophrenia, with many patients staying in employment and many living permanently at home. Their epilepsy tended to be less troublesome over time, and one-third were in remission with regards to their psychotic symptoms; 11 patients had received a temporal lobectomy, and in 8 the psychotic symptoms had receded.

REFERENCES

Berrios G E 1979 Insanity and epilepsy in the 19th century. In: Roth M, Cowie V (eds) Elliot Slater: a tribute. Gaskel Press, pp 161–171

Blumer D, Walker A E 1975 The neural basis of sexual behaviour. In: Benson D F, Blumer D (eds) Psychiatric aspects of neurologic disease. Grune and Stratton, New York, pp 199–217

Bouchet D, Cazauveilh M 1825 De l'épilepsie considéré dans ces rapports avec l'alienation mentale. Archives Général de Médicine 9: 512–542

Bruens J H 1980 Psychoses in epilepsy. Historic concepts and new developments. In: Canger R, Aangeleri F, Penry J K (eds) Advances in epileptology: XIth Epilepsy International Symposium. Raven Press, New York, pp 161–166

Clouston T S 1887 Clinical lectures on mental diseases. Churchill, London

Crow T 1980 Molecular pathology of schizophrenia: more than one disease process. British Medical Journal 280: 66–68

Dewhurst K 1980 Thomas Willis' Oxford lectures. Sandford, Oxford

Dewhurst K, Beard A W 1970 Sudden religious conversions in temporal lobe epilepsy. British Journal of Psychiatry 117: 497–507

Dongier S 1959 Statistical study of clinical and electroencephalographic manifestations of 536 psychotic episodes occurring in 516 epileptics between clinical seizures. Epilepsia 1: 117–142

Esquirol J E D 1838 Des maladies mentales considérées sous les rapports médicale, hygienique et médico-legal. Ballière, Paris

Falret J 1860 De l'état mental des epileptiques. Archives Générales de Médicine 16: 661–679

Ferguson S M, Rayport M 1982 Psychosis and epilepsy. In: Blumer D (ed.) Psychiatric aspects of epilepsy. APA Press, Washington DC, p 229–270

Flor-Henry P 1969. Psychosis and temporal lobe epilepsy. Epilepsia 10: 363–395

Gallhofer B, Trimble M R, Frackwiak R, Gibbs J, Jones T 1985 A study of cerebral blood flow and metabolism in epileptic psychosis using positron emission tomography and oxygen-15. Journal of Neurology, Neurosurgery and Psychiatry 48: 201–206

Gibbs F A 1951 Ictal and non-ictal psychiatric disorders in temporal lobe epilepsy. Journal of Nervous and Mental Diseases 113: 522–528

Glaus A 1931 Über Combinationen von Schizophrenie und Epilepsie. Zeitschrift für Diegesante Neurologies und Psychiatrie 135:450

Gloor P 1972 Temporal lobe epilepsy: its possible contribution to the understanding of the functional significance of the amygdala and its interaction with neocortical-temporal mechanisms. In: Eleftheric N B (ed.) The neurobiology of the amygdala. vol. 1. Plenum, New York, pp 423–457

Griesinger W 1857 Mental pathology and therapeutics. (transl. Lockhart Robertson C, Rutherford J) New Syndenham Society, London

Gruzelier J H 1981 Cerebral laterality and psychopathology. Fact or fiction. Psychological Medicine 11: 219–227

Gudmundsson D 1966 Epilepsy in Iceland. Acta Neurologica Scandinavica 43 (suppl. 25): 1–124

Heath R G 1977 Subcortical brain function correlates of psychopathology and epilepsy. In: Shagass C, Gershon S, Friedhoff A J (eds) Psychopathology and brain dysfunction. Raven Press, New York, p 51–63

Hermann B P, Whitman S 1984 Behavioural and personality correlates of epilepsy. Psychological Bulletin 95: 451–493

Hermann B P, Schwartz M S, Karnes W E et al 1980 Psychopathology in epilepsy: relationship of seizure type to age at onset. Epilepsia 21: 15–23

Hermann B P, Dickem S, Schwartz M S, Karnes W E 1982 Interictal psychopathology in patients with ictal fear: a quantitive investigation. Neurology 32: 7–11

Hill D 1953 Psychiatric disorders of epilepsy. The Medical Press 229: 473–475

Hughlings Jackson J 1875 On temporary mental disorders after epileptic paroxysms. In: Taylor J (ed.) Selected writings of John Hughlings Jackson vol. 1. Staples Press, London, p 119–134

Jensen I, Larsen J K 1979 Psychoses in drug-resistant temporal lobe epilepsy. Journal of Neurology, Neurosurgery and Psychiatry 42: 948–954

Kiloh L G 1971 Psychiatric aspects of epilepsy. In: Winton R R (ed.) Geigy symposium on epilepsy. Geigy, Australia, p 46–50

Kristensen O, Sindrup E H 1978 Psychomotor epilepsy and psychosis. Acta Neurologica Scandinavica 57: 361–370

Landolt H 1958 Serial encephalographic investigations during psychotic episodes in epileptic patients and during schizophrenic attacks. In: de Hass, L (ed.) Lectures on epilepsy. Elsevier, London p 91–133

Maudsley H 1879 The pathology of the mind. MacMillan, London

Morel B A 1860 D'une forme de délire suite d'une

surexcitation nerveuse se rattachant à une variété non encore décrite d'épilipsie. Gazette Hebdomadaire de Médicine et de Chirugie 7: 773–775

Ounsted C, Lindsay J 1981 The long-term outcome of temporal lobe epilepsy in childhood. In: Reynolds E H, Trimble M R (eds) Epilepsy and psychiatry. Churchill Livingstone, Edinburgh, pp 185–215

Perez M M, Trimble M R 1980 Epileptic psychosis – a diagnostic comparison with process schizophrenia. British Journal of Psychiatry 137: 245–249

Perez M M, Trimble M R, Reider I, Murray N M 1985 Epileptic psychosis, a further evaluation of PSE profiles. British Journal of Psychiatry 146: 155–163

Pond D A 1957 Psychiatric aspects of epilepsy. Journal of the Indian Medical Profession 3: 1441–1451

Pond D A 1962 The schizophrenia-like psychosis of epilepsy – discussion. Proceedings of the Royal Society of Medicine 55:311

Pond D A, Bidwell B H 1959 A survey of epilepsy in 14 general practices. Epilepsia 1: 285–299

Post R M, Uhde T W, Joffe R T, Roy-Byrne P P, Kellner C 1985 Anticonvulsant drugs in psychiatric illness. In: Trimble M R (ed.) The psychopharmacology of epilepsy. John Wiley, Chichester, pp 141–172

Pritchard P B, Lombroso C T, McIntyre M 1980 Psychological complications of temporal lobe epilepsy. Neurology 30: 227–232

Rodin E A, Katz M, Lennox K 1976 Differences between patients with temporal lobe seizures and those with other forms of epileptic attacks. Epilepsia 17: 313–320

Ramani V, Gumnit R J 1982 Intensive monitoring of interictal psychosis of epilepsy. Annals of Neurology 11: 613–622

Reynolds E H, Trimble M R 1984 Adverse Neuropsychiatric effects of anticonvulsant drugs. Drugs 29: 570–581

Reynolds J R 1861 Epilepsy. Livingstone, London

Sherwin I 1981 Psychosis associated with epilepsy: significance of laterality of the epileptogenic lesion. Journal of Neurology, Neurosurgery and Psychiatry 44: 83–85

Sherwin I 1982 The effect of location of an epileptogenic lesion on the occurrence of psychosis in epilepsy. In: Koella W P, Trimble M R (eds) Temporal lobe epilepsy, mania, schizophrenia and the limbic system. Karger, Basel, pp 81–97

Slater E, Beard A W 1963 The schizophrenia-like psychoses of epilepsy. British Journal of Psychiatry 109: 95–150

Stevens J R 1982 Risk factors for psychopathology in individuals with epilepsy. In: Koella W P, Trimble M R (eds) Temporal lobe epilepsy, mania, schizophrenia and the limbic system. Karger, Basel, pp 56–80

Stevens J R, Livermore A 1978 Kindling in the mesolimbic dopamine system: animal model of psychosis. Neurology 28: 36–46

Symonds C 1962 The schizophenia-like psychoses of epilepsy – discussion. Proceedings of the Royal Society of Medicine 55:311

Taylor D C 1969 Sexual behaviour and temporal lobe epilepsy. Archives of Neurology 21: 510–516

Taylor D C 1975 Factors influencing the occurrence of schizophrenia-like psychosis in patients with temporal lobe epilepsy. Psychological Medicine 5: 249–254

Tellenbach C H 1965 Epilepsie als Anfallsleiden und als Psychose. Der Nervenartzt 36: 190–202

Thompson P J, Trimble M R 1982 Anticonvulsant drugs and cognitive functions. Epilepsia 23: 531–544

Toone B K, Dawson J, Driver M V 1982a Psychoses of epilepsy. A radiological evaluation. British Journal of Psychiatry 140: 244–248

Toone B K, Garralda M E, Ron M A 1982b The psychosis of epilepsy and the functional psychoses: a clinical and phenomenological comparison. British Journal of Psychiatry 141: 256–261

Trimble M R 1977 The relationship between epilepsy and schizophrenia: a biochemical hypothesis. Biological Psychiatry, 12: 299–304

Trimble M R, Perez, M M 1980 Psychosocial functioning in adults. In: Kulig B M, Meeinardi H, Stores G (eds) Epilepsy and behaviour. Swets and Zeitlinger BV, Lisse, p 118–127

Trimble M R, Perez M M 1982 The phenomenology of the chronic psychoses of epilepsy. In: Koella W P, Trimble M R (eds) Temporal lobe, epilepsy, mania, schizophrenia and the limbic system. Karger, Basel, pp 98–105

Trimble M R, Reynolds E H 1984 Neurospychiatric toxicity of anticonvulsant drugs. In: Mathews B (ed.) Recent advances in neurology. Churchill Livingstone, Edinburgh, pp 261–280

Tuke D H 1892 Dictionary of psychological medicine. Churchill, London

Turner W A 1907 Epilepsy – a study of the idiopathic disease. Churchill, London

Wolf P 1984 The clinical syndromes of forced normalisation. Folia Psychiatrica et Neurologica Japonica 38: 187–192

Wolf P, Trimble M R 1984 Biological antagonism and epileptic psychosis. British Journal of Psychiatry 146: 272–276

Zielinsk J J 1974 Epidemiology and medical-social problems of epilepsy in Warsaw. Warsaw Psychoneurological Institute, Warsaw

11

Neuropsychology

C. B. Dodrill

INTRODUCTION

As applied to the study of human beings, *neuropsychology* is the discipline which deals with the ability, personality and behavioural correlates of brain lesions and other pathological conditions of the nervous system. It is of great importance in a complete evaluation of a person with epilepsy.

By definition, a person with a seizure disorder has a dysfunctional brain, at least during the attacks. However, EEG studies accomplished between episodes are frequently abnormal and suggest that there are irregularities in brain functioning even between attacks. Since the brain constitutes the biological basis of abilities and adjustive skills, one might expect to find indications of decreased abilities also between attacks. Indeed, this has already been demonstrated when a reasonably comprehensive battery of neuropsychological tests has been used (Dodrill 1978). Furthermore, numerous problems in adjustment have been documented by many investigators, as detailed in other chapters in this volume. Thus, a study of the underlying deficiencies in brain functions is essential to a thorough understanding of patients with this common disorder.

In this chapter, comments will initially be offered concerning the nature of neuropsychological testing. The remaining sections will then be directed towards topics in epilepsy of specific relevance to neuropsychology, including antiepileptic drugs and performance, neuropsychological aspects of surgical intervention, mental deterioration in epilepsy, and the prediction of later performance in life through neuropsychological tests.

THE NATURE OF NEUROPSYCHOLOGICAL EVALUATION

Since the brain is a complex organ with many functions, it is evident that the extent to which these functions are intact cannot be determined without assessing a number of them. Furthermore, it is entirely reasonable to assume that epilepsy is likely to present various conditions of neuropsychological relevance including EEG epileptiform discharges, immediate and long-term effects of attacks upon the brain, and the presence of antiepileptic drugs on a continuing basis. In addition, it is clear that the brain provides the basis for all higher level adaptive abilities of the organism and that, if brain functioning is compromised, adaptive abilities are likely to be compromised as well. All of these facts and others argue for a systematic and comprehensive neuropsychological assessment of patients with epilepsy. Such an assessment should be undertaken with tests having both a demonstrated sensitivity to brain functions generally and to types of impairment which are likely to be encountered in this particular disorder.

Despite the apparent reasonableness of the basic strategy for neuropsychological assessment presented in the previous paragraph, this is rarely followed. Usually, no more than one or two hours are allowed for the psychological/neuropsychological evaluation of a person with epilepsy and, typically, half of this time is devoted to interviewing rather than objective testing. The tests selected tend to be those which are given to patients generally, regardless of the nature of their medical problems, and thus are not directed towards deficits which may be related to antiepileptic medication, effects of seizures etc. Moreover, the testing is often fragmentary, with only portions of tests being administered such as the Wechsler scales plus a few other brief measures.

This general approach to neuropsychological evaluation is the rule rather than the exception both in the UK and elsewhere, for reasons pertaining to limited funding and time available. After working in this area for more than a decade, it has been the author's experience that only in the United States have more exacting evaluations been conducted on a regular basis and then only with a minority of people with epilepsy. Furthermore, in only one case has a battery of neuropsychological tests been assembled specifically directed towards the deficiencies found in people with epilepsy and also standardized upon that group. This is the Neuropsychological Battery for Epilepsy (Dodrill 1978). It is briefly described below, not because it represents the best possible approach, but because it recognizes the complexity of brain functions through comprehensive and systematic objective assessment, because it was developed with the needs of people with epilepsy in mind, and because it was standardized on this patient group.

The Neuropsychological Battery for Epilepsy

Before development of this battery was undertaken, research work for several years was accomplished on people with epilepsy which focused upon the effects of antiepileptic drugs, upon the effects of both epileptiform and non-epileptiform changes, upon the effects of attacks, and upon the effects of underlying brain damage on performance. From these studies, it became apparent that two categories of tests would be needed. First, tests were needed which would give three general types of information and thus provide the foundation for the assessment of each patient. Secondly, specific neuropsychological tests were required.

General tests

Wechsler Adult Intelligence Scale-Revised. Although tests of general intelligence have well known limitations, they provide an index of overall functioning which is helpful in the interpretation of the more specialized neuropsychological tests. As is true throughout the battery, no effort is made to abbreviate tests and all 11 subtests are given on every testing.

Lateral Dominance Examination (Reitan & Davidson 1974). Preference in handedness, footedness, and eyedness is important information which is obtained by actual testing rather than by patient self-report. This information is then used in the interpretation of the neuropsychological tests.

Minnesota Multiphasic Personality Inventory. This test provides an indication of the types and magnitudes of emotional factors for each case. It is curious that objective evaluation of this area is often omitted, especially since emotional problems are frequently documented in this patient group and since such factors may affect the results on the neuropsychological tests.

As can be seen from the above, there is a significant commitment to establishing a basis for the interpretation of the specialized neuropsychological test measures. While other tests could have been selected to establish this foundation, the primary point is that such a foundation is important before proceeding with the neuropsychological measures.

Special neuropsychological tests

In selecting the neuropsychological tests, a series of steps was systematically followed. Initially, a broad range of approximately 100 test variables were considered, which arose from a variety of tests. The only restriction at this point was that the test had to have some prospect of sensitivity to the types of deficits often seen in epilepsy. In a pilot study, obviously overlapping and deficient variables were eliminated and 35 remained. Three studies were then initiated to select the final test measures. First, the requirement of Reitan (Reitan & Davidson 1974) was adopted that each test measure must be shown to be sensitive to the neurological problems in the patient group. In particular, it was required that each test statistically differentiate epileptic from normal control subjects. Second, the extent of test overlap was minimized by eliminating test variables selectively, using specific guidelines. Finally, entirely new groups of subjects were examined to be certain that these test characteristics held. All of the above procedures are described in detail elsewhere (Dodrill 1978) and the result was a series of 16 test variables which are obtained from the administration of 11 different tests. These tests are briefly described below:

Stroop Test. A single colour plate is used in which colour names are printed in incongruous colours ('red' is printed in green print, 'orange' is printed in blue print etc.). In the first part of this procedure, the person simply reads the words as quickly as possible and ignores the colours of the print. The neuropsychological indicator is the number of seconds required to complete the test. In the second part of the test, the person must read the colours of the print while ignoring what the words say. This second part is very difficult and it requires a great deal of concentration. Furthermore, when the time for the first part is subtracted from the longer time for the second part, a measure of interference is provided, and this is the second neuropsychological score obtained from this test. The test appears to be a good index of distractability.

Wechsler memory scale (Form I). The two parts of this test, which were ultimately adopted as neuropsychological measures, include the total score from the Logical Memory subtest and the usual score from the Visual Reproduction portion. These measures provide indicators of verbal and non-verbal memory, respectively. In the former, stories are used; in the latter, drawings.

Reitan- Klove Perceptual Examination. This test, and most of those which follow, are described by Reitan & Davidson (1974). Tactile, auditory and visual perception are systematically evaluated under conditions of unilateral and bilateral simultaneous stimulation. In addition, there are a series of tests evaluating agraphagnosia, finger agnosia and astereognosis. A fixed number of trials is undertaken for each task with respect to each body side and the total number of errors made is the neuropsychological indicator.

Name writing procedure. The full name is written by the patient first with the preferred hand and then with the non-preferred hand. The number of letters written per second is the neuropsychological

cal measure from this test. Interestingly, this simple measure appears to be an indicator of phenytoin toxicity.

Category Test. This is the 208 item adult version of this test which employs an apparatus including a slide projector and a bell/buzzer system of feedback concerning correctness/incorrectness of responses. The test appears to evaluate abstractive capabilities and concept formation, as well as a person's ability to adapt to a novel situation and to utilize effectively feedback which is given about performance. The neuropsychological score is the total number of errors.

Tactual Performance Test. The patient is blindfolded and is required to put blocks of various sizes and shapes in their holes on a board. The Time Component consists of the total time required to place the blocks in with the preferred hand, the non-preferred hand, and both hands taken together. After the board is taken away, the person is asked to draw a picture of the board. The number of blocks remembered out of ten is the Memory Component. The number correctly localized in the drawing is the Localization Component. Thus, this test provides three critical test scores.

Seashore Rhythm Test. Using a tape recorder, 30 series of rhythmic beats are presented in pairs and the patient indicates if the rhythms are the same in each pair or if they are different. The score is the number correct.

Seashore Tonal Memory Test. This is another test given with the tape recorder. In this test, a series of notes is played twice. In the second playing, one note is changed in tone and this note is to be indicated by number. The score is the number of correct items. Both this test and the Rhythm Test appear to evaluate attention to the task and short term memory.

Finger Tapping Test. This test employs a small apparatus which measures oscillation speed of the index finger over ten second periods. The average scores of the two hands are added together to obtain a single critical score on this simple test of motor speed.

Trail Making Test. In Part A, the patient connects in order circles numbered 1 to 25 on a piece of paper as quickly as possible. In Part B,

25 circles are also connected as quickly as possible but with orderly alternation between numbers and letters (1–A–2–B–3–C etc.). As with the Stroop Test, errors must be corrected before the test can proceed. The time for Part B is the critical score on this test.

Aphasia Screening Test. This is a test of various aspects of language function. Items requiring naming, spelling, reading, pronunciation, calculation etc are scored for errors made. As a secondary part of this test, drawings are required which provide a basis for judging the extent to which there is constructional dyspraxia or distortion in visual–spatial relationships. One neuropsychological indicator summarizes the language area and one the visual–spatial area.

Evaluation of test results

The results from the above tests are evaluated in four ways which complement one another. First, the general level of performance can be compared with a normal control group and for each of the 16 test measures, ranges of normal and abnormal performance have been identified (Dodrill 1978). Secondly, the relative efficiencies of the right and left body sides are compared on a variety of perceptual and motor tests. Thirdly, the tests facilitate a search for specific signs of neurological deficit such as various aspects of dysphasia. Finally, patterns of deficits can be sought out. These are all methods by which brain related deficits can be documented. The methods are used in such a way that the limitations of one can be offset by the strengths of another. For example, while the level of performance method is very helpful in identifying performance relative to the general population, many factors other than neurological problems may affect performance. This problem does not affect the approach by which the performance of the sides of the body are compared. Thus, these methods are used in a complementary manner and the result is much more satisfactory than a procedure (such as an intellectual assessment) which relies primarily or solely upon level of performance indicators.

The application of the Neuropsychological Battery for Epilepsy to individual cases will be illustrated later in this chapter. The battery is also effective when applied to groups of patients for various purposes (see references by Dodrill at end of chapter).

ANTIEPILEPTIC DRUGS AND PERFORMANCE

Undoubtedly this is the most commonly researched area in the neuropsychology of epilepsy today. The number of investigations in recent years has increased markedly, and the focus of the research in the UK is especially strong. Indeed, there have been so many papers published that there have been at least 15 *reviews* of the area within the last decade. These have included summaries by Reynolds (1983), Schmidt (1982), Thompson (1983), Trimble (1981, 1983), and Wittels & Stonier (1981). Except possibly for a very recent paper (Dodrill 1986b), these reviews are routinely negative and credit antiepileptic drugs with greater or lesser degrees of adverse mental effects. The conclusions typically reached for the drugs are very briefly summarized below.

Reported adverse effects

Phenytoin

Perhaps in part because of its availability for many years and its wide use, this drug has been attributed with a number of negative effects. The most prominent of these appear to relate to decreased motor speed which is noted in a number of studies. However, there are also reports of diminished memory, attentional skills and similar functions (e.g. Matthews & Harley 1975, Thompson & Trimble 1982, Thompson 1983).

Phenobarbitone

Adverse effects of this drug upon attention, memory and behaviour have most frequently been reported and the studies cited have frequently emphasized work with children (Hutt et al 1968, Trimble 1983, Trimble & Corbett 1980). Of the negative effects, adverse behavioural changes are perhaps the most clearly documented, but subtle changes in attention and concentration are likely which may not be noticed by the patients until this drug is discontinued.

Carbamazepine

This is the only agent for which serious questions have been raised about a positive or psychotropic effect. This is now generally disbelieved (Parnas et al 1979) but it is nevertheless widely thought that this medication is less intoxicating than others. The positive findings with this medication may therefore be at least in part due to the removal of more intoxicating agents. The fact that it appears to be equally effective in controlling seizures as other drugs which have better demonstrated adverse effects (Troupin et al 1977) has contributed to its popularity in recent years.

Sodium valproate

As with carbamazepine, few adverse cognitive or behavioural effects have been associated with this drug (Sommerbeck et al 1977, Trimble 1983). Furthermore, it has been demonstrated to be efficacious in controlling several types of seizures approximately as well as more sedating agents, (Covanis et al 1982, Shakir et al 1981), and this fact has contributed to its increased use in recent years.

Methodological problems

The above constitutes a brief summary of the major findings from a large number of studies of the principal antiepileptic drugs. Other agents have not been studied with sufficient frequency to permit definitive statements. In general, the studies in the area tend to have a negative tone by reporting adverse effects of antiepileptic agents or, at best, neutral reports such as in the case of carbamazepine and sodium valproate. These conclusions, however, may ultimately prove to be excessively pessimistic. In his recent review of the area, Dodrill (1986b) came to a number of conclusions which are summarized below. If these conclusions are ultimately found to be correct, they may modify currently accepted notions

concerning drug effects since at least some of these may be attributed to other factors.

1. Approximately 50% of all studies use normal subjects and single active agent versus placebo experimental designs. It is doubted that this is an appropriate design for psychological studies since the results routinely show adverse effects regardless of which drug is considered (if the dose is sufficient and the tests are sensitive) or no effect (if the dose is small and the tests are insensitive). Even ignoring the obvious differences between epileptic and normal subjects and the short time course of these studies, they do not appear to simulate the situation with which the physician is confronted; namely, what drug to give rather than whether or not a drug should be given. Very good drugs can appear toxic when studied using this design since they are usually more toxic than placebo. Yet, many conclusions reached by reviews in the area are significantly based upon studies of this type.

2. Approximately 50% of all studies of patients with epilepsy are based upon single or multiple testings of patients who are placed on their drug regimens solely for clinical reasons. Two groups of patients on different drug regimens may be matched for age, sex, education etc and the conclusion drawn that any differences in performance between the groups must be due to the drugs. However, drugs are not prescribed randomly, and it is likely that the groups are intrinsically different and thus cannot be compared in this manner. For example, if one group of patients is given a certain drug (e.g. phenytoin) for clinical reasons and a second group is given another drug (e.g. carbamazepine), differences in performance cannot be attributed to the drugs even if the groups do not differ for age, sex etc. This is true since there are subject-related reasons why one drug is given in one case and the other in another case. This experimental error has been made repeatedly.

In a second common design, patients are tested at two points in time and two or more groups are formed who for clinical reasons had their drug regimens changed in similar ways (or not changed). It is concluded that changes in test scores on the second occasion represent generalizable characteristics of the basic type of drug alteration accomplished. Using actual data, Dodrill (1986b) shows that these study designs lead to the evaluation of only selected patients with findings that may be different than if all patients are studied. In a similar manner, it appears that patients who are reduced from polytherapy to monotherapy are different from those who could not so be reduced, and it is not clear that results obtained with the former group can be generalized to the latter. This is true since there is neither a random assignment of subjects nor a general application of a particular drug change to all persons in a specified population in these studies. Thus, this type of study design tends to attribute inappropriately differences between subject groups to the drugs with which they are treated.

3. Statistical problems are found in many studies. The most frequent of these is to report a small number of findings as drugs effects when numerous statistical tests have been run. Such findings may not exceed chance expectations, especially when the obvious intercorrelations of statistically significant variables are taken into account. Another error is to use a control group which is much smaller than the experimental group with the result that practice effects or other changes are less likely to be found. Finally, variability in test scores, seizure counts, or related measures may be so high that actual differences may be obscured. Unfortunately this variability is rarely reported, such as in the form of standard deviations.

4. The effects of seizures are often not adequately considered. In one cross-sectional study (Dodrill 1986a), for example, it was shown that substantial differences in performance normally attributable to drugs were more likely the products of lifelong histories of tonic-clonic seizures. This variable is rarely reported by investigators. Indeed, actual data including means and standard deviations on even intercurrent seizures are rarely reported and, if the variability is high, important adverse effects may be obscured since statistical significance is artificially lost.

5. The choice of test has a major bearing on the outcome of studies. In general, highly timed tests are most likely to result in the discovery of statistically significant findings. Batteries of tests which have a timed component in all or nearly all measures may really be measuring only one factor (speed of response) and not memory, decision making etc which happen to represent the content of the test where speed is evaluated. The fact that the inventor of a test claims that it measures 'reasoning' cannot be taken as proof that it measures this construct.

The effects of the criticisms stated above upon research in this area will not be known for some time but, if they prove to be accurate, part of the adverse effects currently ascribed to drugs will eventually be attributed to other factors. Obviously, this will be an area of great interest in the future.

SURGERY FOR EPILEPSY

The administration of standardized neuropsychological tests in connection with surgery for seizure relief has had three basic purposes:

1. Identification of areas of brain-related deficit for correlation with EEG and other data and thus to assist in the prediction of likelihood of relief from seizures
2. Description of surgical candidates with establishment of baseline presurgical ability levels
3. Postsurgical evaluation to identify effects of surgery. Work in each of these areas will be briefly discussed.

Presurgical identification of brain-related deficits

The first work showing that the results from neuropsychological tests could be used to help locate seizure foci was done at the Montreal Neurological Institute. In a major paper by Bengzon et al (1968), it was demonstrated that relief from seizures was more likely when the neuropsychological tests identified dysfunction which lateralized to the cerebral hemisphere where surgery was ultimately performed. It was also shown that there was increased likelihood of a favourable outcome when these tests specifically localized to the temporal lobes. No relationship was found between surgical outcome and general neuropsychological abnormalities or intelligence.

Several other studies have also produced positive findings, although they have not always been in exact agreement as to which variables are the best predictors.

Perhaps the most comprehensive paper on the prediction of surgical outcome is that of Dodrill et al (1986) who utilized 71 variables from a broad range of medical specialities including neuropsychology, EEG, neurology (seizure-related variables) and neuroradiology. Of special note were 48 neuropsychological variables arising from the Wechsler Adult Intelligence Scale (WAIS), the Minnesota Multiphasic Personality Inventory (MMPI) and the Neuropsychological Battery for Epilepsy (Dodrill 1978) and related measures. The subjects were 100 patients with refractory seizure disorders who were randomly assigned to predictive (n = 75) and cross-validation (n = 25) samples. These patients had undergone cortical resection in a variety of areas. The evaluation of seizure relief was based upon seizures appearing in the second postoperative year with classification as follows:

1. Seizure-free – no attacks during the second postoperative year
2. Significantly improved – a minimum of 75% reduction in seizure frequency with no more than 10 seizures in the second postoperative year regardless of the number in the year just prior to surgery
3. Not significantly improved – less than a 75% reduction in seizures or more than ten attacks in the second postoperative year.

The outcome of this study failed to identify any seizure history or radiological variable as a consistent predictor of surgical success. Four neuropsychological variables were identified which, with their ranges of favourable prediction, are as follows:

1. WAIS Digit Symbol (scaled score of nine or greater or raw score of 47 or greater on the WAIS-R)
2. Marching Test (time of 20 s or quicker with the preferred hand)
3. MMPI Hysteria Scale (score of 75 or less)
4. MMPI Paranoia Scale (score of 80 or less).

Four reliable EEG predictors were also found:

1. Single focus
2. Discharges from the anterior midtemporal area
3. Discharges only from side of surgery
4. Discharges from surgical area no more frequent than one per minute on average.

From these eight predictors, it was possible to forecast whether or not individual patients would be significantly helped by the surgery and to do so with an 80% accuracy rate. It was also possible to construct a probability table of the various surgical outcomes (Table 11.1). This table provides estimates of the likelihood of being seizure-free, significantly improved or not significantly improved in the second year following surgery. It is clear that this table could not have been constructed without the neuropsychological variables and it appeared that the neuropsychological variables and the EEG variables contributed about equally to prediction. Thus, it appears that neuropsychological tests have a role in the prediction of seizure relief from cortical resection surgery which is not duplicated by variables arising from other specialities.

Table 11.1 Surgical outcomes with patients grouped by number of favourable preoperative prognostic indicators (n = 100)

Number of favourable prognostic indicators	Outcome		
	Seizure-free	Significantly improved	Not significantly improved
0–3	0%	0%	100%
4	9%	9%	82%
5	37%	20%	43%
6	27%	53%	20%
7	64%	32%	4%
8	75%	25%	0%

Establishment of baseline presurgical functioning

The decision to undertake surgery for epilepsy is a major one and is not made lightly. As such, it is well to have as much basic information about the surgical candidate as possible. In particular, it is well to have at hand a basic estimate of intelligence, an indication of the nature and extent of neuropsychological deficits and an evaluation of emotional adjustment. With such information the potentials of each surgical candidate which might be salvaged by stopping the seizures can be judged. Warning may also be given about neuropsychological difficulties or emotional problems which might complicate the postoperative course and even, upon occasion, argue against performing the surgery altogether.

The tests used in preoperative assessment vary markedly from one surgical centre to the next and depend upon the training and orientation of the psychologist, the time and equipment available and so on. It is highly desirable that the areas of intelligence, neuropsychological functioning and emotional adjustment are included, as suggested above. Although a comprehensive battery of tests obviously cannot be administered in every instance due to various constraining factors, an example of the administration of such is offered below to show how it can contribute to the overall evaluation of surgical candidates and also provide a baseline against which the effects of surgery may be evaluated.

Case History

K. B. was an 18-year-old girl who had just completed high school when she was hospitalized for her presurgical work-up. She had experienced generalized tonic-clonic seizures beginning at the age of 18 months during an episode of high fever. Although she had been taking antiepileptic medication constantly since her first attack, she soon began to experience other types of seizures. Complex partial seizures began at 6 and by the age of 18 were the only type of attack reported. They occurred on average ten times per month and were poorly controlled by a wide variety of drug regimens. EEG studies including closed circuit television/long-term monitoring investigations captured eight seizures, all of which arose from the left sphenoidal area. The interictal tracings also demonstrated occasional diffuse atypical spike-wave patterns as well as moderate to marked generalized abnormalities. Her cerebral angiogram was normal, but a CT scan revealed herniation of the left mesial temporal structures. The intracarotid sodium amytal procedure

(Wada test) showed speech and language to be associated with the left hemisphere and left hemisphere only in this strongly right-handed person. The study also demonstrated a substantial loss in short-term memory when the left hemisphere was perfused and thereby suggested that structures on the right were unable to support memory by themselves. A complete battery of neuropsychological tests was administered and the results are presented in Table 11.2 (scores *not* in parentheses). At the top of this table, basic descriptive information is given. At the bottom, the results of general test measures are reported. As can be seen, this young lady was above average in intelligence with the somewhat unusual finding in epilepsy that visual-spatial skills on the WAIS were slightly better developed than those in the verbal or language-related area. Her good level of mental abilities was encouraging in terms of ultimate potential and the MMPI failed to identify any emotional or psychosocial problem. Likewise, only three of the 16 specialized or discriminative measures of the Neuropsychological Battery for Epilepsy fell outside normal limits and a good general level of performance was thereby indicated. This means that her performances across a broad range of perceptual, motor and cognitive tasks were normal. However, it was noted that verbal memory as evaluated by the Wechsler Memory Scale was deficient and fell outside normal limits, whereas non-verbal memory as evaluated by the same test was entirely normal. Also, the right hand was relatively deficient on the Finger Tapping Test since the preferred hand is expected to perform about 10% better than the non-preferred hand. These findings implicate the posterior inferior frontal and anterior temporal areas of the left hemisphere and closely correspond with the focus. (Of secondary interest is the relatively poor performance with the left hand on the Tactual Performance Test and the mild constructional dyspraxia noted in her pencil and paper drawings; these findings may reflect the bilateral disturbance noted on the EEG tracings).

A review of the predictors of surgical outcome revealed that because of the generalized EEG discharges and because discharges in the area of surgical interest were very frequent, only one of the four EEG indicators was positive. All four neuropsychological indicators were positive, however, so that the overall score was five and the overall outlook was moderately favourable (Table 11.1). She was taken to surgery where a markedly gliotic left temporal lobe was noted along with 4–5 mm of uncal herniation over the incisura. A left temporal lobectomy was performed which was guided by corticography and language testing. At the conclusion of surgery, the resection was noted to extend 7 cm posteriorly at the level of the inferior temporal gyrus and about 3.5 cm posteriorly at the level of the superior temporal gyrus. The resection included the uncus, the amygdala and the anterior hippocampus. Follow-up two years later revealed that she had been entirely seizure-free since surgery.

Postsurgical neuropsychological evaluation

A number of investigations have now been completed concerning changes in abilities following cortical resection surgery for epilepsy. Initially,

Table 11.2 Preoperative and one year postoperative neuropsychological test results on a woman who underwent a left temporal lobectomy. (postoperative scores are given in parentheses).

Name .... Hospital No. .... Date (6 Aug 82) No. 4048

9 Jun 81

18	12	R	C	Unemployed
Age (19)	Education (12+)	Handedness (R)	Race (C)	Occupation (Waitress)

NEUROPSYCHOLOGICAL BATTERY FOR EPILEPSY

Discriminative Measures

Stroop Test

Category Test 7 (4)

Part I　68 (72)
Part II　165 (165)
II — I　97
84

Wechsler Memory Scale (Form I)

Tactual Performance Test 3.9 11.0
　Preferred (2.9) Total Time (6.8)
　　4.5 8
Verbal (Stories)　14* (21)
　Non-preferred (2.5) Memory (8)
　　12 2.7 5
Visual-Spatial (Drawings)　12 (12)
　Both Hands (1.4) Localization (3*)

Perceptual Examination

Seashore Rhythm Test 30 (28)

Seashore Tonal Memory Test 29 (27)

	R	L
	0	0
Misperceptions	(8)	(0)
	0	0
Suppressions	(8)	(0)
	0	0
Finger Agnosia	(0)	(0)
	0	0
Agraphagnosia	(0)	(0)
	0	0
Astereognosis	(0)	(0)
	2	1	3
Total Errors	(16)	(0)	(16*)
	8	8
Astero. Time	(8)	(8)

Finger Tapping
　51　49　100
Preferred (52) Nonpreferred (47)　(99)

Trail Making Test
　13　32
Part A (17)　Part B (33)

Aphasia Screening Test
　(0)　(2)　(2)
Expressive (0) Receptive (0)　(0)

Name Writing (Let/S)
　1.86　0.52　0.81*
Pref. (1.62) Nonpref. (0.81)　(1.08)

Constructional Dyspraxia Mild* (Ques.)

* Performance falls outside normal limits.　Total tests outside normal limits: 3/16 (2/16)

General Measures

Wechsler Adult Intelligence Scale					Minnesota Multiphasic Personality Inventory					Lateral Dominance Examination		
	109		9	11		50		41	41		R	L
VIQ	(111)	Info	(7)	Dig Sym (10)	?	(50)	Pd	(41)	Es (40)		7	0
	111		9	9		46		59	23	Hand	(7)	(0)
PIQ	(113)	Comp	(10)	Pic Com (11)	L	(46)	Mf	(55)	Ep (21)		2	0
	110		13	12		53		47	10	Eye	(2)	(0)
FSIQ	(112)	Arith	(15)	Bl Des (16)	F	(58)	Pa	(41)	A (11)		2	0
	66		11	11		57		48	24	Foot	(2)	(0)
VSS	(68)	Simil	(11)	Pic Arr (11)	K	(59)	Pt	(58)	R (21)		26.5	24.5
	58		15	15		52		55	Man 13	Dyna.	(27.5)	(26)
PSS	(59)	Dig Sp	(15)	Obj Ass (11)	Hs	(48)	Sc	(60)	Anx (13)		10	0
	124		9			40		50	Cr. 3	ABC	(10)	(0)
TSS	(127)	Vocab	(10)		D	(40)	Ma	(60)	In. (2)		7	7
						49		49		March	(9)	(11)
					Hy	(49)	Si	(53)				

there was a concern about a possible general intellectual loss, but there is now only occasionally such a report (Polkey 1983). Instead, the primary attention has turned to memory and to adverse changes in various aspects of speech and language when surgery is on the speech-related hemisphere.

Undoubtedly, the most detailed work on changes in memory following surgery has been accomplished by Milner and her associates at the Montreal Neurological Institute. Although presented in many papers, a brief summary is to be found in Milner (1975). Various procedures are presented which are sensitive to changes in verbal memory when the operation is on the speech-related side and others are used when surgery is contralateral to speech. Losses in the expected areas are often reported, but the losses are selective and they are (typically) not incapacitating in everyday life. The losses appear most frequently when the mesial resection is extensive (including much of the hippocampus) and may be devastating when the contralateral hippocampus is already dysfunctional. Fortunately, the latter condition is routinely detectable preoperatively by the intracarotid sodium amytal procedure.

There have now been several reports that memory functions contralateral to the surgery side may show improvement following surgery, especially when the surgery is successful. This is occasionally reported as a general finding (Cavazzuti et al 1980) but more typically when surgery is on the speech-related side (Novelly et al 1984, Rausch & Crandall 1982). Efforts to minimize language-related deficits, including memory, have also been reported and these have typically included corticography, intra-operative mapping of speech and memory through stimulation and the individualization of resections. The results of these procedures appear promising (Ojemann & Dodrill 1985) and show that a substantial reduction in seizure frequency can often be obtained without significant losses in verbal abilities. Such procedures were used in the planning of the resection for K. B., the case already described, and the postoperative neuropsychological findings are described below.

Case History
One month and one year after surgery, K. B. received a repeat neuropsychological assessment, and the findings obtained at one year are presented in Table 11.2. Scores on the measures of intelligence increased very slightly and were probably the products of practice effects. On the neuropsychological battery there was a mild but very clear improvement. The greatest positive change was on the verbal or Logical Memory portion of the Wechsler Memory Scale where there were 21 correct recollections immediately after the material was presented instead of 14. Likewise, after a 30 min. delay there were 18 correct recollections whereas preoperatively there had been 12 (these scores are not reported in Table 11.2). This is a greater improvement than is typically seen, but it illustrates the point that with appropriate intra-operative procedures, an extensive (7 cm) resection can be carefully undertaken on the speech-related side with no discernable losses in verbal memory as evaluated by these tests. Other indications of mild improvement were noted on several of the neuropsychological tests. For example, the relationship between the performances of the right and left hands became normal on both the Tactual Performance Test and the Finger Tapping Test. The mild constructional dyspraxia seen previously decreased to the point that it was no longer clearly discernable. Only the Perceptual Examination demonstrated more deficits than preoperatively, but it was noted that these deficits were entirely attributable to a right superior homonymous quadranopic visual field defect. The MMPI demonstrated no adverse change in emotional adjustment. At the end of the second postoperative year, the patient reported that she was seizure-free, off medication and was making an excellent psychosocial adjustment.

MENTAL DETERIORATION IN EPILEPSY

Role of seizures

In their recent comprehensive review of this topic, Lesser et al (1986) document that mental deterioration in epilepsy has been described for millenia and at least as far back as the early Greek physicians. Indeed, in 1885, William Gowers wrote, 'The mental state of epileptics. . . as is well known, frequently presents deterioration. . . Every grade of intellectual defect may be met with down to actual imbecility' (Gowers 1885). While the defect in mental abilities exists before the first seizure in some cases, Gowers clearly attributed the deterioration to the seizures themselves in the majority of cases. In 1907, Turner in his book, *Epilepsy – A Study of the Idiopathic Disease*, makes a very similar statement:

> The *frequency of the attacks* materially affects prognosis; the more frequent the seizures the greater the percentage of confirmed cases, and the greater the degree of mental impairment, and *vice versa*. Fits recurring in series are accompanied by a high grade of dementia. (Turner 1907, p. 223).

A number of modern papers have provided empirical evidence to support the observations of these earlier physicians. Lennox & Lennox (1960), for example, provided data to suggest a direct relationship between the estimated lifetime number of tonic-clonic seizures and 'mental impairment'. Rodin (1968) attributed losses in intelligence to the effects of seizures themselves in a longitudinal study, and noted that deterioration occurred regardless of etiology or presence of brain damage. In identical twins, single convulsive attacks have also been related to substantial losses in abilities (Dodrill & Troupin 1976) and this was subsequently reaffirmed by a larger study from the same laboratory (Dodrill 1986a).

In the latter investigation, it was shown that persons having 100 or more individual and uncomplicated convulsive attacks were significantly demented, and the dementia could not be attributed to early brain damage, age at onset of seizures, antiepileptic drugs or a host of other factors. In agreement with this study was an earlier paper by Markiewicz & Dymecki (1969) who found diffuse cortical damage at post-mortem examination of patients who had experienced numerous tonic-clonic seizures, even when there was no record of status epilepticus.

Studies of status epilepticus have shown perhaps even more clearly the adverse effects of serial seizures upon mental abilities. These studies have been comprehensively reviewed by Delgado-Escueta et al (1983) and Hauser (1983). Investigations in the area have focused upon changes in intelligence and have demonstrated significant intellectual decreases in both children and adults. Physical neurological changes have also been reported. Convulsive status epilepticus is particularly deleterious to mental abilities.

Studies of induced convulsions in animals also point to adverse effects of seizures upon the brain. This area has been reviewed in a detailed manner by Wasterlain & Dwyer (1983). Seizures inhibit brain protein synthesis, brain growth and behavioural development. Ischaemic cellular changes have been associated with prolonged seizures under conditions of hyperpyrexia, arterial hypotension, hypoxia and acidosis (Meldrum & Brierly 1973). Although the exact effects of each of these factors in producing cellular change may be under

discussion for some time, the important point is that, at least with repeated seizures, careful experimental studies have indeed documented pathological cellular changes in animals.

Age of onset of epilepsy

The extent of deterioration has often been related to age at onset of epilepsy. Bourgeois et al (1983), for example, found that children whose intelligence decreased with time had an earlier onset of seizures. Their study included multiple testings of children and was therefore somewhat easier to interpret than investigations which attempt to relate age at onset to intelligence after an assessment at only one point in time. Pre-existing brain damage significantly complicates the interpretation of the latter studies, although the fact remains of decreased achievement in later life with a history of early onset of epilepsy (Harrison & Taylor 1976). With respect to the long-term effects of seizures themselves, at least one author (Dodrill 1986a) has now provided evidence to suggest that it may not be early age at onset *per se* which is of importance but rather that an early age at onset permits a larger number of seizures to accumulate by any given point in time. At any rate, early age at onset is certainly not an asset, and a number of cases have been observed in which early age at onset combined with frequent convulsive attacks has resulted in substantial losses in mental abilities over time. The following is an example of such a case.

Case History
At age 11 months, a Caucasian male experienced a febrile illness and from that time on began to have single convulsive attacks. At first, the tonic-clonic seizures occurred only with illness and high fever, but soon spontaneous attacks began to appear. The EEG demonstrated a generalized dysrhythmia by the age of $2\frac{1}{2}$ years. Although he sat alone at 7 months, other developmental landmarks began to be delayed and he did not walk independently until 17 months nor put words together until 30 months. Negativistic behaviour was observed as early as 18 months and he began to bite and hit others. Convulsive attacks occurred at the rate of one per week or more, and sometimes as frequently as one per day. Despite extensive efforts to control his seizures at a specialized medical facility, this goal was never achieved. A wide variety of drug regimens was attempted over the years but by the early school years he was having generalized non-convulsive attacks and later he manifested complex partial seizures. As the school years began, the behavioural problems intensified, and special school place-

ment was undertaken with an individualized behaviour modification program. This met with limited success.

The boy's intellectual abilities were evaluated on six occasions known to the medical staff. At the age of 4 he had been administered the Stanford-Binet Intelligence Scale. At ages 5, 6, 7 and 9 the Wechsler Intelligence Scale for Children had been given. Finally, the Wechsler Adult Intelligence Scale was administered at age 17. The changes in overall intelligence are presented in Figure 11.1. The general shape of the curve is of interest. With a fairly constant seizure frequency of one convulsive attack per week to one per day, the loss in mental abilities is more rapid earlier in life. It was of interest to note that both parents had college degrees and were professionals. Thus, it is entirely possible if not likely, that initially this boy's intellectual level was higher than the 97 found with the Stanford-Binet at the age of 4. Another point of interest is that the intellectual losses continued indefinitely. Indeed, in counselling with the parents and in making plans for the future, it was possible to estimate how low his intellectual level might be at age 30, age 40 etc. However, a few months following the last testing, he had a nocturnal convulsion and suffocated in his pillow.

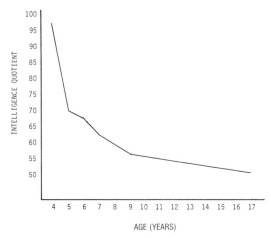

Fig. 11.1 Deterioration in intellectual performance of one male with frequent seizures beginning at the age of 11 months.

Role of antiepileptic drugs

One source of possible mental deterioration which has not yet been considered is that of antiepileptic drugs. In the case example just given, for instance, it is simply not possible to be certain that some of the losses in intelligence might not have been attributable to the variety of medication taken over the years. This is true even though it is known in this particular case that the parents kept the boy at subtoxic levels whenever possible. Indeed, it was felt by the medical staff that fewer seizures would have occurred had the parents

administered more medication as was occasionally suggested to them. However, it is also recognized that, since blood levels were routinely in the normal range, toxicity would have resulted more frequently.

The possible adverse effects of antiepileptic drug use over long periods of time has been a particular focus of research in the UK. Studies in the area have been well reviewed by Reynolds (1983) and by Trimble (1983) and are discussed earlier in this chapter. In general, these investigators have tended to relate deterioration to the drugs themselves. However, as Trimble & Corbett (1980) have pointed out, while children who are deteriorating are administered larger drug doses, seizure frequency is related to psychomotor slowing in the same patients. Furthermore, it is obvious that larger doses tend to be given to patients whose seizure disorders are more difficult to manage. Simply matching subject groups for variables such as age, sex, and even seizure frequency, does not necessarily assure control of the severity factor.

Conclusions

In summary, it is apparent that the complexities in this area will require a great deal of careful evaluation in the future. A few conclusions can be drawn however:

1. While substantial deterioration definitely does occur in some cases, it is not the typical result of epilepsy. Data here are tentative, but it may occur in 10–20% of cases (Bourgeois et al 1983, Trimble & Corbett 1980) or even less if all persons with epilepsy are considered
2. Significant deterioration is not usually seen unless a large number of seizures has occurred (especially generalized con-vulsive seizures) or unless status epilepticus has been experienced
3. Intellectual deterioration was clearly described centuries before antiepileptic drugs were used.
4. Seizures themselves may result in pathological cellular changes but it is not clear that all seizures result in such changes. Much research will be necessary before the reliable prediction of losses or absence thereof can be made in individual patients.

5. Underlying brain disease apart from epilepsy may be of great importance in mental deterioration
6. Antiepileptic drugs undoubtedly contribute to deterioration in some cases, but much remains to be known about their contribution and their interaction with other relevant factors

PERFORMANCE IN LIFE

In this section, an area will be discussed which is of importance but in which there has yet been limited formal work. This is the area in which scores on neuropsychological tests are related to demonstrated ability to perform in everyday life. It is very easy to devise tests, but it is more difficult to document that they are truly related to performance in life. That is, if statistically significant differences are found between two groups of patients on any particular test, is there an empirical basis for presuming that the poorer of the groups will perform discriminately worse on one task or another which reasonably might be encountered in everyday life? That is not a trivial point, and the problem will be illustrated below.

In a highly controlled experiment (MacLeod et al 1978), access to short- and long-term memory were evaluated in patients with epilepsy before and after their phenobarbitone doses were increased by 60% to 100%. The experiment was set up so that accuracy was perfect and the outcome measure was response time as measured in milliseconds. Although this was a very well designed experiment in most respects, it is noted that the outcome measure is not really memory at all but rather time. With the increase in phenobarbitone dose, time to access short-term memory was increased reliably until under the most complex experimental condition the delay was just over 100 ms. The difference easily reached statistical significance and the paper was published in a very prestigious journal.

The above experiment may well be of significance to cognitive psychologists on a theoretical basis, but it is reasonable to ask (as we ultimately must) about its practical significance. It basically suggests that after about one week following a major increase in phenobarbitone dose, there will be no decrease in accuracy of either long or short-term memory and no increase in access time to long-term memory. However, there will be a reliable increase of approximately 0.1 s in access to recently acquired materials provided they are complex. Any application of the study to performance in life would therefore require a situation in which complex new materials were repeatedly presented and where split-second response time was at a premium. Although there are very few situations where this might be applicable, occasionally one might be found, such as with an air traffic controller. Here, images of multiple airplanes are constantly changing across a screen and, if a person with epilepsy was at the controls and had just had a major increase in phenobarbitone dose and an emergency arose, the delay might in fact be 0.1 s in response to the situation. Whereas none of us would wish the controller to respond in a delayed manner (especially if we were on one of the airplanes!), it is not really clear that a delay of this magnitude would be of significance, even in this extreme situation. Under normal conditions, delays of 0.1 s would be completely undetectable.

The very difficult problem of relating test performance to life was reviewed by Heaton & Pendleton (1981). They identified areas of great practical significance to everyday living and in particular focused upon adults with ability to maintain employment and to live independently. Fortunately, a number of studies which they reviewed utilized persons with epilepsy as subjects. In both investigations of persons with epilepsy and studies of other subject groups, tests of intelligence (such as the Wechsler Adult Intelligence Scale) and tests from the Halstead-Reitan Neuropsychological Battery were best correlated with either vocational adjustment or skills in independent living. These reviewers did not report response time as relevant to adjustment in these major areas. It is also noted that the Halstead-Reitan Battery contains no measures of true reaction time (in milliseconds).

The majority of the studies reviewed by Heaton & Pendleton (1981) related neuropsychological tests to performance in life at the point in time when the tests were taken. In an additional paper since the 1981 review, Dodrill & Clemmons (1984) attempted to predict vocational adjustment and ability to live independently in adult life from the Halstead-Reitan Battery which was administered in adolesence. They found that it was possible to predict whether or not there would be problems in one area or another with an 85% accuracy rate. They were less able to predict which area would represent a problem for a given patient in adulthood, however.

The above findings are of significance in the identification of tests to be used in evaluating persons with epilepsy. Their significance, however, may not be fully apparent until it is pointed out that tests of reaction time are quite possibly the most sensitive measures to antiepileptic drugs. In a recent major review, Dodrill (1986b) found that the type of test was related to the likelihood of demonstrating a drug effect as follows: reaction time (measured in milliseconds), 85%; other tests timed in whole seconds, 79%; tests of intelligence (usually partially timed), 59%; all other (untimed) tests, 43%. Thus, while at present it has by no means been demonstrated conclusively, the possibility has been raised that tests of reaction time may be more sensitive to antiepileptic drug effects but less sensitive to performance in life, whereas other tests may have converse strengths and weaknesses. Should this ultimately be proved accurate, it will certainly have a bearing on test selection in clinical and investigative work. This may be the case especially in clinical settings where there are not the resources to administer a large battery of neuropsychological tests in many instances.

There is one additional point which arises from the study of MacLeod et al (1978), and which was mentioned briefly above. This is the point that although the test was identified as a test of 'memory' and the study one of 'memory impairment', in reality the study was one of speed of response. Thus, the wary reader will wish to examine the tests closely to be sure that the differences in mental abilities reported really represent those abilities and not some common factor such as speed of response.

CONCLUSIONS

Neuropsychological evaluation of the patient with epilepsy is of great importance. This chapter has dealt with major areas of current interest, including the effects of antiepileptic drugs, surgery for epilepsy, mental deterioration and the relevance of neuropsychological tests to adjustment in everyday life. In each of these areas, neuropsychological assessment contributes to a more complete understanding of the person with epilepsy. However, it is also apparent that much remains to be known about each of these areas and that there are many important investigations yet to be conducted. Work in each of these areas should prove to be as rewarding as it is challenging.

ACKNOWLEDGMENTS

The preparation of this chapter and a portion of the research reported herein was supported by grants NS 17277, NS 17111, and NS 21706 awarded by the National Institute of Neurological and Communicative Disorders and Stroke, PHS/DHHS, USA. Appreciation is extended to Drs Allan S. Troupin and Arthur A. Ward for assistance with the case material.

REFERENCES

Bengzon A R A, Rasmussen T, Gloor P, Dussault J, Stephens M 1968 Prognostic factors in the surgical treatment of temporal lobe epileptics. Neurology 18: 717–731

Bourgeois B F D, Prensky A L, Palkes H S, Talent B K, Busch S G 1983 Intelligence in epilepsy: A prospective study in children. Annals of Neurology 14: 438–444

Cavazzuti V, Winston K, Baker R, Welch K 1980 Psychological changes following surgery for tumors in the temporal lobe. Journal of Neurosurgery 53: 618–626

Covanis A, Gupta A K, Jeavons P M 1982 Sodium valproate: monotherapy and polytherapy. Epilepsia 23: 693–720

Delgado-Escueta A V, Wasterlain C G, Treiman D M, Porter R J (eds) 1983 Status epilepticus: mechanisms of brain damage and treatment. Advances in neurology vol 34. Raven Press, New York

Dodrill C B, Troupin A S 1976 Seizures and adaptive

abilities: a case of identical twins. Archives of Neurology 33: 604–607

Dodrill C B 1978 A neuropsychological battery for epilepsy. Epilepsia 19: 611–623

Dodrill C B 1986a Correlates of generalized tonic-clonic seizures with intellectual, neuropsychological, emotional, and social function in patients with epilepsy. Epilepsia 27: 399–411

Dodrill C B 1986b Effects of antiepileptic drugs on psychological abilities. In:Penry J K (ed) Epilepsy: diagnosis, management, and quality of life. Raven Press, New York, in press

Dodrill C B , Clemmons D 1984 Use of neuropsychological tests to identify high school students with epilepsy who later demonstrate inadequate performances in life. Journal of Consulting and Clinical Psychology 52: 520–527

Dodrill C B, Wilkus R J, Ojemann G A, et al 1986 Multidisciplinary prediction of seizure relief from cortical resection surgery. Annals of Neurology 20: 2–12

Gowers W R 1885 Epilepsy. Churchill, London

Harrison R M, Taylor D C 1976 Childhood seizures: a 25-year follow-up: social and medical prognosis. Lancet 1: 948–951

Hauser W A 1983 Status epilepticus: frequency, etiology, and neurological sequelae. In: Delgado-Escueta A V, Wasterlain C G, Treiman D M, Porter R J (eds) Status epilepticus: mechanisms of brain damage and treatment. Advances in neurology, vol 34. Raven Press, New York, pp 3–14

Heaton R K, Pendleton M G 1981 Use of neuropsychological tests to predict adult patients' everyday functioning. Journal of Consulting and Clinical Psychology 49: 807–821

Hutt S J, Jackson P M, Belsham A, Higgins G 1968 Perceptual-motor behaviour in relation to blood phenobarbitone level: a preliminary report. Developmental Medicine and Childhood Neurology 10: 626–632

Lennox W G, Lennox M A 1960 Epilepsy and related disorders. Little, Brown, Boston

Lesser R P, Luders H, Wyllie E, Dinner D S, Morris III, H H 1986 Mental deterioration in epilepsy. Epilepsia, in press

MacLeod C M, Dekaban A S, Hunt E 1978 Memory impairment in epileptic patients: selective effects of phenobarbital concentration. Science 202: 1102–1104

Markiewicz D, Dymecki J 1969 Neuropathological changes in epilepsy with behavioral and intellectual disorders. Polish Medical Journal 8: 181–192

Matthews C G, Harley J P 1975 Cognitive and motor-sensory performances in toxic and nontoxic epileptic subjects. Neurology 25: 184–188

Meldrum B S, Brierly J B 1973 Prolonged epileptic seizures in primates: ischemic cell change and its relationship to ictal physiological events. Archives of Neurology 28: 10–17

Milner B 1975 Psychological aspects of focal epilepsy and its neurosurgical management. In: Purpura D P, Penry J K, Walter R D (eds) Advances in neurology vol 8. Raven Press, New York, pp 299–321

Novelly R A, Augustine E A, Mattson R H et al 1984 Selective memory improvement and impairment in temporal lobectomy for epilepsy. Annals of Neurology 15: 64–67

Ojemann G A, Dodrill C B 1985 Verbal memory deficits

after left temporal lobectomy for epilepsy. Journal of Neurosurgery 62: 101–107

Parnas J, Flachs H, Gram L 1979 Psychotropic effects of anti-epileptic drugs. Acta Neurologica Scandinavica 60: 329–343

Polkey C E 1983 Effects of anterior temporal lobectomy apart from relief of seizures: a study of 40 patients. Journal of the Royal Society of Medicine 76: 354–358

Rausch R, Crandall P H 1982 Psychological status related to surgical control of temporal lobe seizures. Epilepsia 23: 191–202

Reitan R M, Davison L A (eds) 1974 Clinical neuropsychology: current status and applications. Winston, New York

Reynolds E H 1983 Mental effects of antiepileptic medication: a review. Epilepsia 24: S85–S95

Rodin E A 1968 The prognosis of patients with epilepsy. Thomas, Springfield

Schmidt D 1982 Adverse effects of antiepileptic drugs. Raven Press, New York

Shakir R A, Johnson R H, Lambie D G, Melville I D, Nanda R N 1981 Comparison of sodium valproate and phenytoin as single drug treatment in epilepsy. Epilepsia 22: 27–33

Sommerbeck K W, Theilgaard A, Rasmussen K E, Lohren V, Gram L, Wulff K 1977 Valproate sodium: evaluation of so-called psychotropic effect. A controlled study. Epilepsia 18: 159–167

Thompson P J 1983 Phenytoin and psychosocial development. In:Morselli P L, Pippenger C E, Penry J K (eds) Antiepileptic drug therapy in pediatrics. Raven Press, New York, pp 193–200

Thompson P J, Trimble M R 1982 Comparative effects of anticonvulsant drugs on cognitive functioning. British Journal of Clinical Practice Symposium (suppl.) 18: 154–156

Trimble M 1981 Anticonvulsant drugs, behaviour, and cognitive abilities. Current Developments in Psychopharmacology 6: 65–91

Trimble M R 1983 Dementia in epilepsy. In: Melin K-A (ed) Third workshop on memory functions. Acta Neurologica Scandinavica (suppl. No. 99) 69: 99–104

Trimble M, Corbett J 1980 Anticonvulsant drugs and cognitive function. In: Wada J A, Penry J K (eds) Advances in epileptology: the Xth Epilepsy International Symposium. Raven Press, New York, pp 113–120

Troupin A S, Ojemann L M, Halpern L et al 1977 Carbamazepine – a double-blind comparison with phenytoin. Neurology 27: 511–519

Turner W A 1907 Epilepsy: a study of the idiopathic disease. Macmillan, London

Wasterlain C G, Dwyer B E 1983 Brain metabolism during prolonged seizures in neonates. In: Delgado-Escueta A V, Wasterlain C G, Treiman D M, Porter R J (eds) Status epilepticus: mechanisms of brain damage and treatment. Advances in neurology vol 34. Raven Press, New York, pp 241–260

Wittels P Y, Stonier P D 1981 The effects of benzodiazepines on psychomotor performance in patients. In: Hindmarch I, Stonier P D (eds) Clobazam (Royal Society of Medicine International Congress and Symposium Series, No 43). Royal Society of Medicine, London

12

Clinical pharmacology and medical treatment

E. M. Rimmer
A. Richens

INTRODUCTION

With the currently available drugs, approximately 80% of patients presenting with epilepsy will have their fits controlled. This leaves a significant number of patients, particularly those with complex partial seizures or symptomatic epilepsy, who will continue to have seizures which will prove refractory to optimal drug therapy. Others will develop unacceptable acute or chronic adverse effects from their antiepileptic medication. Thus there is an urgent need for new antiepileptic drugs with greater efficacy and less toxicity.

Although we are still far from understanding completely the underlying neurochemical mechanisms of epilepsy or the mode of action of most of the antiepileptic drugs in use today, advances have been made in our understanding of central nervous system neurotransmitters and the pathophysiological changes underlying seizures. Consequently, a more rational approach to the development of new antiepileptic drugs is evolving and we look forward to a time when new drugs will be identified which will specifically modify the abnormal mechanisms that cause seizures.

Advances have been made in the management of epilepsy over recent years although a study in 1977 showed that patient care was still far from optimal (Hopkins & Scambler 1977). With the exception of sodium valproate, there have been no major innovations in the treatment of epilepsy over the last 20 years. However, we have learnt a great deal more about the presently available drugs and how to use them to better effect. Increased knowledge of antiepileptic drug pharmacokinetics has been invaluable and the use of serum drug concentration monitoring can be very useful for selected antiepileptic drugs. Because of our greater awareness of the hazards of polytherapy, in particular the risks of chronic drug toxicity and the dangers of drug interactions, monotherapy has become the general policy. No longer should a newly diagnosed patient presenting for the first time with seizures be immediately assigned to combination therapy.

However, there are still many unanswered questions about the natural history and optimal drug management of epilepsy, many of which are being currently investigated. When should drug treatment be started? How long should drugs be continued after a patient has been rendered seizure free? Does drug treatment really influence the natural history of epilepsy? Can we predict which patients will respond well to drug therapy? Which drugs are best for which seizure types? In time it is hoped that clear and definite guidelines will emerge so that a concensus on the best management of epilepsy will be achieved.

In this chapter we describe the principal drugs currently available to treat epilepsy and outline some general principles of management. In the last section we will describe recent advances in the neuropharmacology of epilepsy and the prospects for new drug development.

PART ONE
PRINCIPAL DRUGS USED IN THE TREATMENT OF EPILEPSY

PHENYTOIN

Phenytoin (5,5-diphenylhydantoin) was first ident-ified as an antiepileptic drug in 1938, and since then has been extensively used. Of the various antiepileptic drugs in common use, phenytoin has been studied in greatest depth because it is the most widely used, is relatively easy to measure in serum and has some interesting pharmacokinetic properties which are responsible for the wide variation in response to the drug.

Structure

The structure of phenytoin is given in Figure 12.1. Phenytoin is usually administered as the acid or as the sodium salt.

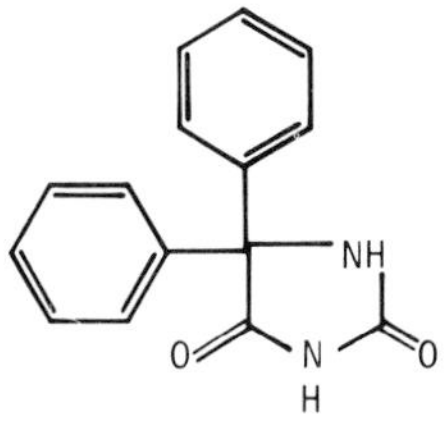

Fig. 12.1 Structure of phenytoin

Mode of action

Despite widespread clinical use and intensive investigation, the principal mechanism of action of phenytoin remains elusive. Many actions of the drug have been identified experimentally but the relevance of these to its antiepileptic action in humans is still not clear. Non-synaptic actions include reduction of sodium ion conductance, blockade of repetitive firing and reduction in post-tetanic potentiation (MacDonald 1983). Post-synaptic effects include enhancement of GABA-mediated inhibition and reduction of excitatory synaptic transmission. It also has presynaptic effects on calcium entry into neurones and may

block neurotransmitter release. However, many of these actions on neuronal excitability and synaptic transmission do not occur at therapeutically relevant free drug concentrations. The reduction of repetitive firing of neurones due to slowing of the recovery of sodium channels from inactivation does occur at low concentrations of phenytoin and may turn out to be an important factor in pheny-toin's anticonvulsant action.

Pharmacokinetics

These are summarized in Table 12.1. The reader is referred to Richens (1979) for a detailed review of the pharmacokinetics of phenytoin.

Table 12.1 Summary of pharmacokinetic data for phenytoin

Range of daily maintenance dose	Adult: 150–600 mg/day Child: 5–15 mg/kg/day
Minimum dose frequency	Adult: once daily Child: twice daily
Time to peak serum level	4–12 h (oral) Many hours (intramuscular)
Percentage bound to plasma proteins	85–90%
Apparent volume of distribution	0.45 l/kg
Elimination half-life in adults	9–140 h (saturation kinetics)
Time to steady state after starting therapy	7–21
Major metabolite	5-(p-hydroxyphenyl)-5-phenylhydantoin (inactive)

Absorption

The acid form of phenytoin is poorly soluble in water but the sodium salt is much more soluble. The acid, unless in the microcrystalline form, is poorly and erratically absorbed, whereas the sodium salt which is macrocrystalline in form is reliably absorbed. The excipient in a formulation may influence bioavailability by altering the rate of deaggregation of the particles. In Australasia in 1968, an outbreak of phenytoin intoxication occurred when the manufacturers of Dilantin capsules changed the excipient from hydrated calcium sulphate to lactose, which resulted in an unexpected increase in bioavailability (Tyrer et al 1970). Elsewhere, similar problems have arisen with inequivalence between the various marketed preparations. In the UK and USA a chewable microcrystalline tablet formulation for paediatric use (Epanutin Infatabs) appears to be better absorbed than standard tablets (Stewart et al 1975), although only marginally better than capsules (Smith & Kinkel 1976). However, Infatabs contain 50 mg of phenytoin acid, which is equivalent to 54 mg of the sodium salt contained in standard tablets and capsules.

Parenteral preparations of phenytoin exist and, although they are recommended for intramuscular administration, crystals of drug precipitate and phenytoin is very poorly and unreliably absorbed by this route (Wilensky & Lowden 1973). Also considerable muscle damage may (Serrano & Wilder 1974) occur. The serum concentrations produced by intramuscular administration may be inadequate and a change from oral to intramuscular administration to cover, for instance, an abdominal operation, may cause seizures. On the other hand, rebound intoxication may occur on resumption of the oral therapy because considerable quantities of drug remain in the tissues to be absorbed (Wilder & Ramsay 1976). Thus it is more satisfactory to give phenytoin by intravenous infusion (into a saline drip) in a single daily dose when oral administration is not possible for a short period.

Distribution and plasma protein binding

Phenytoin is approximately 90% bound to plasma proteins in adults (Porter & Layzer 1975). The binding is mainly to albumin (Odar-Cedarlöf & Borga 1976), but there are also secondary low affinity sites on other proteins. Although there is controversy over the degree of intersubject variation in protein binding, it would appear that in most epileptic patients, who do not have a medical condition known to alter drug protein binding and are not taking concurrent drugs which interfere with phenytoin binding, the amount of variability in protein binding is very small. However, hypoalbuminaemia reduces protein binding as do liver and renal disease (see below). Only the free (unbound) drug is available to produce a phar-

macological effect at the site of action and, therefore, ideally it would be more relevant to measure free drug concentrations in serum as a therapeutic guide. However, the currently available methods for doing this are too time consuming and costly and are not yet reliable enough. Thus routine measurement of free serum phenytoin concentrations is not indicated at present. An alternative approach is to measure saliva phenytoin concentration, which is closely related to free drug concentration in serum. The salivary glands act as a simple dialysis membrane across which free drug molecules are able to diffuse and equilibrate (Reynolds et al 1976, Paxton et al 1977). There are methodological difficulties to this technique and it is necessary to take precautions to avoid direct contamination of the saliva by the oral formulation.

Phenytoin diffuses rapidly into the tissues including the brain. Following intravenous administration the distribution phase lasts about two hours. Brain binding is of the same order of magnitude as protein binding in serum and thus brain concentrations are very similar to serum concentrations (Houghton et al 1975b). Penetration into brain tissue is rapid and this explains the efficacy of phenytoin in the treatment of status epilepticus (Wilder et al 1977). Cerebrospinal fluid concentrations mirror serum free drug concentrations (Houghton et al 1975b).

Metabolism and excretion

Phenytoin is extensively metabolised by hydroxylase enzymes in the liver and less than 5% appears unchanged in the urine. The rate of hepatic metabolism is under genetic (polygenic) control and varies between individuals (Richens 1979). There is a continuous unimodal distribution of rates of metabolism, with very slow and very fast metabolizers at the extreme ends of the distribution. Race may also be an important determinant of the rate of metabolism as Negroes metabolize phenytoin more slowly than Caucasians. The major metabolite of phenytoin is 5-p-hydroxyphenyl-5-phenylhydantoin (p-HPPH) which is pharmacologically inactive. This is conjugated to glucuronide and excreted in the urine. The conversion of phenytoin to this metabolite by liver microsomal enzymes is saturable within the therapeutic range of serum concentrations, i.e. the liver is unable to increase its rate of metabolism proportionately as the drug serum concentration rises (Richens 1979). Instead, it moves towards a situation in which a fixed amount of drug is removed regardless of increases in the serum level (zero order kinetics). The ratio of metabolite to parent drug is influenced both by genetic differences in drug metabolism and by steady state serum concentrations of parent drug. As the latter rises, the hydroxylation mechanism becomes saturated and p-HPPH production fails to rise in proportion, and relatively more parent drug appears in the urine (Houghton & Richens 1974). p-HPPH appears to be actively excreted by the renal tubules as its renal clearance exceeds the glomerular filtration rate.

Plasma half-life and dose interval

The plasma half-life of the parent compound determines the time taken to reach a plateau serum level, and the time taken for complete elimination of the drug following its withdrawal. A knowledge of half-life is essential in estimating the frequency of drug administration of doses and the time interval which should elapse between changes in dose. The effective plasma half-life gradually lengthens as the steady-state concentration rises as a result of the saturable nature of phenytoin metabolism (Richens 1979). On average, the effective half-life at very low serum concentrations is about 13 hours, but this lengthens to 46 hours when the steady-state concentration reaches the top of the therapeutic range. The time to steady state (approximately equal to five half-lives)

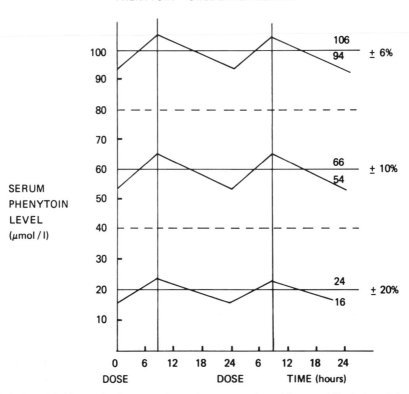

Fig. 12.2 Theoretical plot of the fluctuation in serum phenytoin concentration with once–daily dosing. Calculations have been made at three steady-state concentrations: subtherapeutic, therapeutic and toxic. The therapeutic range of serum concentrations 40–80 μmol/l (10–20 μg/ml) is indicated with dotted lines. Half-life data provided by Houghton & Richens (1974) have been used. Peak and trough concentrations, together with the percentage fluctuations, have been calculated. The fluctuation decreases as the serum concentration rises because saturation kinetics effectively lengthen the elimination half-life. (Reproduced with permission from Richens 1979).

depends upon the dose and the final concentration reached, and may be as long as two weeks or more in a patient given a dose yielding a high therapeutic or toxic concentration. Similarly, the rate of elimination of phenytoin on discontinuing therapy may be much slower than expected, particularly in a patient who started with toxic serum concentrations.

Also, the fluctuations in serum concentrations may be less than expected (Richens 1980). The higher the steady-state serum concentration, the smaller (in percentage terms) is the fluctuation in

serum concentration. Figure 12.2 represents a theoretical plot of the fluctuations in serum concentration with once-daily dosing at a subtherapeutic, therapeutic and toxic steady-state concentration. The degree of fluctuation in serum levels throughout 24 hours is quite acceptable for clinical purposes and this accords with the finding (Strandjord & Johannessen 1974) that once-daily dosage in adults is compatible with effective control of seizures. However, in children twice-daily dosing is preferable because the serum half-life of phenytoin is shorter. If a more immediate

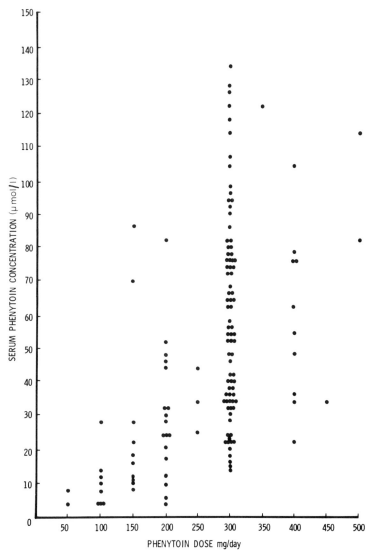

Fig. 12.3 Relationship between phenytoin dose and serum level in 137 patients treated chronically with phenytoin and usually at least one other antiepileptic drug (N.B. 4 μmol/l = 1 μg/ml)

therapeutic effect is required a loading dose may be administered (Wilder et al 1973), but such dosing schedules may be associated with a higher incidence of adverse effects. When intravenous administration for the treatment of status epilepticus is needed a dose of 10–15 mg/kg body weight given over 5–10 min will lead to plasma levels of 40–80 μmol/l (10–20 μg/ml).

Dose–serum concentration relationship

As a consequence of the great variability in rate of phenytoin metabolism between individuals, the steady state serum concentrations achieved with a given dose of phenytoin will vary greatly (Fig. 12.3). A dose of 200 mg/day of phenytoin may be enough to produce a therapeutic concentration in one adult patient, while another may require in excess of 500 mg/day. Although age, sex and body weight influence the dose–serum concentration relationship, in adults the relative contribution of each is fairly small (Houghton et al 1975a). If the data in Figure 12.3 is replotted to take into account body weight there is only a marginal improvement in the dose–level relation-

ship. Body surface area correlates most strongly with dose requirements in adult patients.

In children, body size becomes a major determinant of dose. The dose/kg of body weight required to produce a given serum concentration increases as body weight falls. Although dosing related to body surface area is the most reliable guide in practice, it is usually satisfactory to dose according to body weight (Table 12.2). However, because there is such a wide interindividual variation in serum levels produced by a given dose of

Table 12.2 Starting doses of phenytoin in children and infants. the doses have been chosen to produce an average serum concentration of 40 μmol/l (10 μg/ml)

Body weight kg	Phenytoin dose mg/kg/day	mg/day*
6–10	10.0	100
11–15	9.0	125
16–20	8.0	150
21–25	7.0	175
26–30	6.5	200
31–35	5.5	200
36–40	5.5	225
41–45	5.5	250
46–50	5.0	250
51–60	5.0	300

* Doses rounded off to suit 25 mg dose units

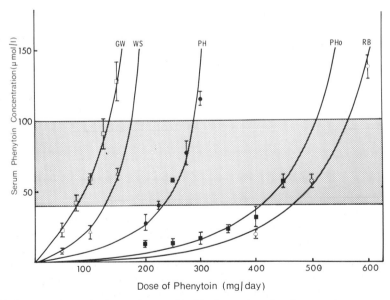

Fig. 12.4 Relationship between phenytoin dose and serum level in five patients in whom steady-state concentrations were measured at several different doses. Each point represents the mean ± S.D. of 3–8 separate estimations of the serum level. The curves were fitted by computer using the Michaelis-Menten equation. The stippled area indicates the 'therapeutic range' of serum levels but is more generous than the usually quoted 40–80 μmol/l (N.B. 4 μmol/l = 1 μg/ml). (Reproduced from Richens & Dunlop 1975, by kind permission of the editor)

phenytoin, the doses suggested will give levels that are too low in some and toxic in a few.

The saturable nature of phenytoin metabolism is of considerable practical importance because it leads to a non-linear relationship between dose and serum level in each patient (Richens & Dunlop 1975). Figure 12.4 illustrates the relationship between phenytoin dose and serum level in five patients in whom steady-state concentrations were measured at several different doses. In patient PH, an increment of only 55 mg would carry the serum level from the lower limit to the upper limit of the therapeutic range. Thus, on a dose of 200 mg daily, the serum level is below the therapeutic range, yet on a daily dose of 300 mg the level is above the range and could be causing symptoms of toxicity. The same pattern is seen in each patient although the dose range yielding a therapeutic level varies considerably, presumably because of genetic differences in the rate of hydroxylation in the liver. The steepness of the dose–serum level relationship within the therapeutic range is important in a number of ways:

1. If phenytoin therapy is regulated by monitoring serum levels, increments in dose should be limited to 50 mg or less once the level comes close to the lower end of the therapeutic range
2. Monitoring serum phenytoin levels is essential if the dose is to be correctly tailored
3. A small increase in the bioavailability of the drug will readily increase a therapeutic level to a toxic one
4. The effects of drug interactions will be exaggerated. Addition of a second drug which either inhibits or induces phenytoin metabolism will produce a disproportionate change in phenytoin level

These practical problems make phenytoin therapy difficult to manage. In order to assist the prescriber in achieving levels within the therapeutic range, various schemes have been designed to assist dosage adjustment (Flint et al 1985). Each demands at least one measurement of phenytoin serum concentration, from which a prediction can be made of the increment in dose necessary to increase the level into the therapeutic range. Of the methods requiring one dose-concentration pair, the nomogram illustrated in Figure 12.5 is

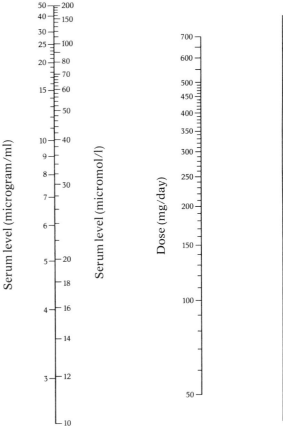

Fig. 12.5 Nomogram for adjusting phenytoin dose. Given a single reliable serum concentration on a known dose of phenytoin, the dose required to achieve a desired level can be predicted. A line is drawn connecting the observed serum concentration (left-hand scale) with the dose administered (centre scale) and extended to intersect the right hand vertical line. From the point of intersection, another line is drawn back to the desired serum level (left-hand scale). The dose required to produce this level can be read off the centre scale. N.B.: This nomogram will give misleading predictions if the serum concentration measurement is inaccurate, if the patient's compliance is in doubt or if a change in concurrent treatment has been made since measurement of the serum level. (Reproduced with permission from Rambeck et al 1979.)

probably the best predictor of phenytoin concentrations. The methods requiring two known doses and plasma concentrations are more accurate, but no method is sufficiently precise to substitute for confirmatory serum phenytoin concentrations (Flint et al 1985).

Concentration–effect relationship

In view of the great variability between individuals

in phenytoin kinetics and the narrow therapeutic ratio of the drug, the case for monitoring serum levels of phenytoin is well established. Buchthal et al (1960) were the first to attempt to define a therapeutic range of serum concentrations of phenytoin. In a prospective study in 12 hospitalized patients with frequent fits, they found no clinical response until the serum concentration exceeded 40 μmol/l (10 μg/ml). As clinical signs of toxicity were frequently encountered with levels above 80 μmol/l (20 μg/ml) they considered that a therapeutic range of 40–80 μmol/l (10–20 μg/ml) would give optimal control of fits without toxicity. This view was reiterated by Kutt & McDowell (1968) and this range has been widely used in the management of phenytoin therapy. However, Buchthal and his colleagues studied only a small number of patients with severe epilepsy and their conclusions may not be valid for ambulatory

patients with mild or moderate epilepsy. A number of retrospective studies were performed subsequently but the results were conflicting (Haerer & Grace 1969, Travers et al 1972, Lund 1973). Because retrospective studies are unsatisfactory with too many factors uncontrolled, Lund (1974) set up a three-year prospective study in 32 patients with grand mal seizures. The patients were selected because they had at least one seizure during a two-month control period. During the first year, plasma phenytoin levels averaged 24.4 μmol/l (6.1 μg/ml) but during the second and third years the levels were increased to 46.8 μmol/l (11.7 μg/ml) and 60 μmol/l (15.0 μg/ml) respectively by a change in the brand of phenytoin or a change in dose. The total number of fits occurring during the three years were 186, 132 and 52 respectively. Although the improvement in control was independent of the

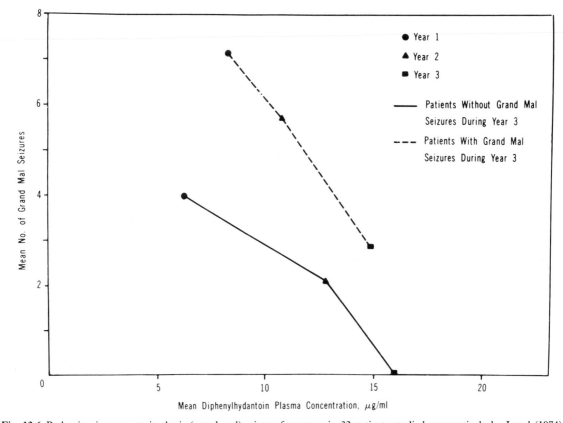

Fig. 12.6 Reduction in mean tonic clonic (grand mal) seizure frequency in 32 patients studied prospectively by Lund (1974). Phenytoin (diphenylhydantoin) dose was increased over a 3-year period in order to achieve plasma concentrations within the therapeutic range of 10–20 μg/ml (40–80 μmol/l). A dose-related reduction in seizure frequency was seen regardless of whether the patients were seizure free at the end of the study. (Reproduced with permission from Lund 1974.)

type of seizures, the optimal phenytoin level for each patient was dependent on the severity of the epilepsy (Fig. 12.6). This last observation is important because it suggests that many patients with mild epilepsy may be controlled with serum levels below the therapeutic range suggested by Buchthal et al (1960).

Recent studies of therapeutic ranges of phenytoin serum concentrations (Gannaway & Mawer 1981, Schmidt & Haenel 1984, Turnbull et al 1984) have emphasized that the efficacy of serum phenytoin concentrations varies not only between patients, but also with the type of seizure within an individual patient. The variation in therapeutic plasma concentration appears to be primarily related to the type and severity of the individual patient's epilepsy. Thus the concept of the lower limit of the therapeutic range of phenytoin concentrations of 40 μmol/l (10 μg/ml) should probably be abandoned. There is general agreement that clinical signs of phenytoin intoxication become more frequent when the serum level rises to between 80 and 120 μmol/l (20–30 μg/ml) but the absolute incidence of toxic effects at a particular concentration varies considerably from one report to another, partly depending on the clinician's criteria for intoxication. However, the rigid use of an upper limit to the therapeutic range is unnecessary and may deny some patients the benefit of extra therapeutic effect without the occurrence of toxicity. The quoted therapeutic range for phenytoin should be used as a guide to dosage adjustment but should not be a substitute for clinical judgement.

Pharmacokinetics in special situations

In neonates who have not been exposed to enzyme-inducing drugs in utero, the metabolism of most drugs will be very slow at birth (Morselli 1977). During the first few months of life, the enzyme systems mature and are capable of metabolizing antiepileptic drugs much faster than in the adult (Blain et al 1981). During childhood the rate of metabolism gradually slows until it reaches adult levels. In neonates who have been exposed to enzyme-inducing drugs such as phenytoin in utero, the half-life of transplacentally transferred phenytoin has been shown to be 6.6 to 34 hours.

The plasma protein binding of phenytoin is also lower in neonates. Serum antiepileptic drug levels tend to fall progressively throughout pregnancy due to an increased metabolic capacity of the maternal liver, the development of drug metabolizing activity in the fetal liver and a reduction in plasma protein binding of drugs (see Ch. 15 Pt 2). Only small quantities of phenytoin are excreted in breast milk. Disease states can alter phenytoin kinetics. Hypoalbuminaemia causes a decrease in the plasma protein binding of phenytoin which can result in drug toxicity appearing at apparently therapeutic serum levels. The plasma protein binding of phenytoin is also reduced in cirrhosis, and hepatocellular diseases can reduce the systemic metabolism (Blaschke 1977). In renal disease the binding of phenytoin to serum albumin is reduced, partly because of hypoalbuminaemia but also more importantly because of the presence of endogenous inhibitors of phenytoin binding (Reidenberg & Drayer 1978).

Drug interactions

Pharmacokinetic

Numerous interactions between phenytoin and other drugs have been described (Perucca & Richens 1980, 1985). Most of these are pharmacokinetic and many occur because of the enzyme-inducing effects of phenytoin.

Effect of phenytoin on other drugs Phenytoin itself is a potent inducer of hepatic microsomal drug metabolizing enzyme activity and this is probably the mechanism responsible for reducing the plasma concentrations or the therapeutic effect of oral anticoagulants, oral contraceptive steroids, carbamazepine, benzodiazepines and other drugs (Perucca 1978).

The effect of other drugs on phenytoin The steep dose–serum concentration relationship and narrow therapeutic ratio of phenytoin makes drug interactions which alter phenytoin serum concentration very important; in particular, those in which phenytoin metabolism is inhibited resulting in elevation of the serum level. Phenytoin is a poor substrate for drug metabolizing enzymes and inhibition of metabolism is relatively common when phenytoin-treated patients are exposed to other drugs, including sulthiame, pheneturide, chloramphenicol, propoxyphene and isoniazid. Reduction of serum phenytoin concentrations by enzyme induction have been reported with carbamazepine co-medication and chronic ethanol intake. There are, however, conflicting reports on the effect of phenobarbitone on phenytoin metabolism. As phenytoin is highly protein bound, it is also susceptible to displacement from protein binding sites by drugs such as sodium valproate and salicylic acid (Perucca et al 1980). This will result in a fall in protein binding and in a higher free fraction of phenytoin. In the case of valproic acid, which also inhibits the metabolism of phenytoin, the interaction is very complex and results in a higher free phenytoin concentration but a lower total phenytoin concentration than prior to addition of valproate to therapy.

Pharmacodynamic

Interactions between drugs at their site of action in the tissues are termed 'pharmacodynamic interactions'. Combination drug therapy for epilepsy increases the incidence of central nervous system adverse effects, such as drowsiness and incoordination.

Adverse drug reactions

The acute dose-dependent adverse effects of phenytoin consist of vertigo, tremor, ataxia, dysarthria, diplopia, nystagmus and headache (Kutt et al 1964). Severe side effects are rare at serum phenytoin levels below 120 μmol/l (30 μg/ml) but great individual variation occurs and some patients experience adverse effects with levels within the therapeutic range while others do not develop toxic reactions with serum levels well above this range.

Peripheral and central nervous system

Evaluation of subtle effects of long-term antiepileptic drug therapy on cognitive function and behaviour can be difficult, but there have been several studies in both volunteers and epileptic patients which have shown a negative effect of phenytoin on cognitive function although this effect is potentially reversible. In a study by Thompson et al (1981) phenytoin was shown to impair performance of volunteer subjects significantly, compared with placebo, in tests of memory, concentration, mental and motor speed. These neuropsychological impairments seem to be associated with high serum drug levels (Thompson & Trimble 1983). More severe toxic effects of phenytoin on mental function can result in a reversible confused state which has been referred to as encephalopathy, delirium or psychosis. Intellectual deterioration, depression, impairment of drive, initiative and psychomotor slowing are common findings. These changes may develop subacutely or chronically, usually in association with high serum phenytoin concentrations and may be unaccompanied by other signs of phenytoin toxicity, such as nystagmus or ataxia. Occasionally, unusual neurological signs such as dyskinesias have been noted. Such encephalopathy seems more common in children.

Although it is well known that acute toxicity with phenytoin can lead to a reversible cerebellar syndrome, there has been some controversy as to whether permanent pathological or clinical changes can occur (Alcala et al 1978). Seizures themselves can cause loss of Purkinje cells but it appears that the drugs may be responsible in many cases for permanent cerebellar syndromes. Such long-term damage may occur more often in brain-damaged and mentally retarded patients.

There have been several reports of reversible involuntary movement disorders with phenytoin, in particular dyskinesias, similar to those produced by neuroleptics (Chadwick et al 1976). In many cases, the abnormal movements coincided with a period of high serum phenytoin concentrations and again the patients most at risk appeared to be those with pre-existing brain damage.

In recent years there have been many studies of peripheral neuropathy, often asymptomatic, associated with chronic antiepileptic therapy, and the drug most often incriminated is phenytoin. However, there are several difficulties in their interpretation: in many of the studies the patients were taking polytherapy; acute reversible electrophysiological changes were not always distinguished from chronic irreversible abnormalities; and variables, such as length of drug therapy, periods of drug toxicity and folate levels, were not always considered. A study of 51 previously untreated epileptic patients followed prospectively on carefully monitored monotherapy with either CBZ or DPH for 1–5 years revealed no clinical evidence of neuropathy, although slight abnormalities of sensory conduction were found in 18% of patients on phenytoin, but in none of those on carbamazepine (Shorvon & Reynolds 1982).

Hepatic toxicity

Hepatic toxicity induced by phenytoin is a rare occurrence. It usually develops within six weeks of the first phenytoin exposure and appears unrelated to phenytoin dosage or serum levels (Parker & Shearer 1979). The hepatotoxicity is usually accompanied by a rash, fever and lymphadenopathy, and eosinophilia is a common occurrence. These features suggest that the mechanism may be a hypersensitivity reaction. Liver histology shows mixed hepatocellular damage with cholestasis and necrosis.

Long-term therapy with phenytoin may cause asympatomatic biochemical changes such as increased serum alkaline phosphatase and alanine aminotransferase, and enlargement of the liver may also occur (Andreasen et al 1973). These changes are thought to be due to the enzyme-inducing properties of phenytoin and will result in altered metabolism of both endogenous and exogenous substances.

Endocrine and metabolic disorders

A number of different endocrine and metabolic effects have been associated with phenytoin treatment (Bennet 1977). Phenytoin has been shown to accelerate cortisol metabolism due to its effect on hepatic microsomal enzymes. This is compensated for by an increased cortisol secretion rate, presumably due to increased ACTH secretion from the anterior pituitary gland (Werk et al 1964). The increased rate of steroid hormone metabolism may be of clinical importance in epileptic patients who require steroid replacement therapy or steroids for disease suppression, e.g. renal allograft recipients.

Phenytoin also has been shown to have an effect on the secretion of thyroid hormones with reduction in free thyroid hormones and enhanced peripheral conversion of T_4 to T_3 (Finucane & Griffiths 1976). Phenytoin may also have an effect on the pituitary to suppress release of TSH but this is rarely accompanied by clinical features of thyroid dysfunction.

The role of antiepileptic drug therapy in the problems of infertility and impotence in epileptic patients is as yet unclear. Phenytoin causes an increase in sex hormone binding globulin and increases the breakdown of oestrogens and androgens (Richens 1984). However, other factors such as an effect on the pituitary or direct toxicity to the germinal tissue are possibly also important.

High serum concentrations of phenytoin have been shown to inhibit insulin release from the pancreas in response to hyperglycaemia.

Long-term antiepileptic drug therapy is associated with a significant incidence of hypocalcaemia and osteomalacia although rarely is the bone disease symptomatic (Richens & Rowe 1970, Editorial 1976, Bell et al 1978, Hahn 1976). The biochemical mechanisms involved have not yet been fully elucidated, although phenytoin has been shown to reduce plasma levels of the biologically active vitamin D metabolites.

Haematological toxicity

Phenytoin therapy has been implicated in the development of megaloblastic anaemia, aplastic anaemia, leucopenia and lymphadenopathy. In many patients there is a mild macrocytosis which does not require treatment. Other patients with more severe changes usually respond well to folate therapy without discontinuation of the drug. A transient leucopenia sometimes occurs on starting phenytoin therapy; rarely, phenytoin can cause a pure red cell aplasia or agranulocytosis. Long-term phenytoin treatment can lead to a reversible lymphadenopathy with histology resembling lymphoma and this is thought to be the result of a hypersensitivity reaction (Editorial 1971). Phenytoin has also been shown to cause IgA immunoglobulin deficiency (Shakir et al 1978, Meissner et al 1984).

Skin and soft tissue reactions

Skin rashes are a fairly rare adverse reaction to phenytoin therapy, although the incidence appears to be higher if high loading doses of phenytoin are used (Wilson et al 1976). The rash is usually morbilliform. Rarely, more severe skin disorders such as erythema multiforme may occur. Facial coarsening and thickening of subcutaneous tissue have also been reported as complications of long-term phenytoin treatment. Gum hyperplasia is an adverse effect peculiar to phenytoin. It occurs quite frequently in minor degree and its severity increases with larger drug doses and longer duration of therapy.

Teratogenicity (See also Ch. 15 Pt 2)

There is substantial evidence of an increased incidence of developmental abnormalities in the children of mothers with epilepsy: estimated to be two to three times the usual rate (Janz 1982). The common major abnormalities include cleft lip and palate, congenital heart lesions and malformations of the skeleton, central nervous system and gastrointestinal tract. The increased frequency of malformations has been attributed to the teratogenic effects of the antiepileptic drugs themselves (most are teratogenic in animals), but it is very difficult to differentiate drug effects from the other complicating factors including the seizures and the genetic risk from the maternal epileptic disorder. The occurrence of the so-called 'fetal hydantoin syndrome', including various craniofacial and distal limb anomalies, retarded growth and mental handicap has been disputed. Strickler et al (1985) postulated that a genetic defect in arene oxide detoxification may contribute to susceptibility to phenytoin-induced birth defects.

Indications for the use of phenytoin

Phenytoin has been used extensively over the years although it has been superseded to some extent by the newer drugs such as carbamazepine and valproate, primarily because of its high incidence of adverse effects and difficult pharmacokinetic profile. It is an effective drug in the treatment of tonic-clonic and partial seizures but is ineffective in absence seizures. It also has a role in the emergency treatment of status epilepticus.

Methoin (mephenytoin) and ethotoin

Methoin and ethotoin are hydantoin compounds related to phenytoin (Sjö et al 1975, Troupin et al 1976). Although methoin has been shown to have marked antiepileptic activity and has been used clinically for more than 30 years its use has declined due to excessive risk of serious toxicity, particularly rashes and blood dyscrasias. Ethotoin is rarely used because of its low efficacy, despite its minimal incidence of adverse effects.

CARBAMAZEPINE

Carbamazepine was developed in the late 1950s and its anticonvulsant properties were demonstrated in animals in 1963. Over the last 20 years it has been used extensively as an antiepileptic drug. It is an iminostilbene derivative and is closely related structurally to the tricyclic antidepressant drug imipramine.

Structure

The structure of carbamazepine is shown in Figure 12.7. Carbamazepine behaves as a neutral lipophilic substance and is virtually insoluble in water.

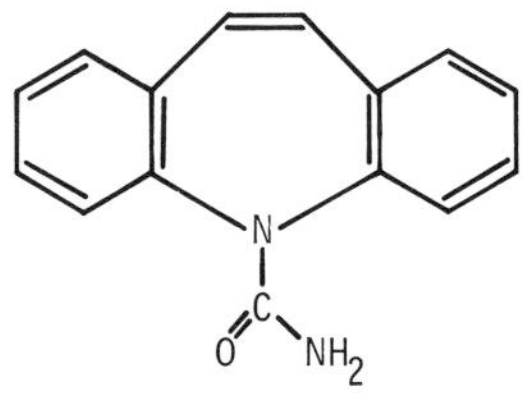

Fig. 12.7 Structure of carbamazepine

Mode of action

The mechanism of carbamazepine's antiepileptic effect remains uncertain, but it seems to share many of the actions of phenytoin. Many studies have used doses far in excess of the clinically relevant drug concentration and its insolubility in water has presented problems to investigators. Its most likely mode of action is to limit high frequency sustained repetitive firing, an action similar to that of phenytoin (MacDonald et al 1985). The 10,11-epoxide metabolite has a similar effect at clinically relevant drug concentrations.

Pharmacokinetics

These are summarized in Table 12.3. The reader is referred to Pynnönen (1979) for a general review of the pharmacokinetics of carbamazepine.

Table 12.3 Summary of pharmacokinetic data

Range of daily maintance dosage	Adult: 400–1800 mg/day Child: 10–30 mg/kg/day
Time to peak serum level	4–8 h (but may be delayed up to 24 h)
Percentage bound to plasma proteins	75%
Apparent volume of distribution	1.2 l/kg
Elimination half-life	Single doses: 20–55 h After chronic therapy: 10–30 h (adults) 8–20 h (children)
Time to steady state after starting therapy	Up to 10 days (but subsequent fall may occur due to autoinduction)
Major metabolite (active)	10, 11-epoxide
Others:	Dihydrodiol Hydroxy-metabolites Iminostilbene
Minimum dose frequency	Adult: twice daily Child: twice daily

Absorption

Carbamazepine is absorbed slowly and erratically after oral administration. Absorption is inversely dependent on dose and may be enhanced by giving the drug with food (Levy et al 1975). Because of the lack of an intravenous formulation, the absolute bioavailability of carbamazepine in humans is not known precisely, but is probably of the order of 75–85%.

Distribution and plasma protein binding

Carbamazepine is highly lipid soluble and it distributes rapidly to tissues. The apparent volume of distribution has been calculated as 0.8–2.0 l/kg by various workers. The plasma protein binding of carbamazepine is 70–80% and of the epoxide metabolite is 48–53%. The interindividual variation in carbamazepine plasma protein binding is small and is unlikely to be of clinical importance due to the fairly high free fraction under normal conditions. Other antiepileptic drugs do not appear to influence carbamazepine binding. Concentrations of carbamazepine in the brain are similar to those in plasma, as are those of carbamazepine epoxide. Cerebrospinal fluid carbamazepine concentrations are between 17% and 31% of those in plasma. Saliva concentrations of carbamazepine and the epoxide also reflect the free fraction of the drug in plasma and measurement of saliva drug concentrations has been used for monitoring of free plasma concentrations (Chambers et al 1977).

Metabolism and excretion

Carbamazepine is largely metabolized into a stable epoxide metabolite, carbamazepine 10,11-epoxide, which is pharmacologically active (Faigle et al 1977, Bertilsson & Tomson 1986). It is further metabolized to hydroxy-derivatives which are excreted in the urine. Only about 2% of the drug is excreted unchanged in the urine.

Carbamazepine exhibits dose-independent kinetics. The plasma half-life may be up to 55 hours after a single dose of carbamazepine but following repeated treatment the half-life decreases to between 5 and 24 hours. This is due to 'autoinduction' of the hepatic microsomal enzyme systems and leads to what is known as 'time-dependent kinetics'. As the clearance of carbamazepine increases during chronic therapy, increases in dose of the drug are required to maintain the same plasma carbamazepine level. It takes three to four weeks for maximal autoinduction to occur. Autoinduction of carbamazepine metabolism seems to accelerate preferentially the elimination reaction of the epoxide by increasing the production of the dihydroxide. The metabolism of carbamazepine is also induced by other antiepileptic drugs, such as phenytoin. Thus the dose of carbamazepine required by epileptic patients who are already taking enzyme-inducing antiepileptic drugs is higher than in drug naive patients (Cereghino et al 1975). Heteroinduction by other drugs preferentially induces the formation of the epoxide rather than its subsequent oxidative product. Reported plasma half-lives for the carbamazepine 10,11-epoxide range from 3 to 23 hours.

Dose–serum concentration relationship

There is little correlation between dose of carbamazepine and serum concentration when blood samples from different patients are analysed. In addition to the usual variation in the rate of metabolism between individuals, there are two other probable reasons for this: the variable bioavailability of the drug; and autoinduction of metabolism. When carbamazepine is given with other drugs, such as phenytoin, phenobarbitone and primidone, heteroinduction of carbamazepine metabolism complicates the picture further. Levels of the 10,11-epoxide also vary widely between individuals. The serum concentration of the epoxide in adults is reported as between 15 and 55% of the concentration of unchanged drug and may be higher in children (Morselli et al 1975). The ratio of epoxide to carbamazepine also varies according to the co-medication, being higher in patients on other enzyme-inducing antiepileptic drugs (Rane et al 1976). There is a cross reaction on enzyme immunoassay testing between carbamazepine itself and the epoxide. This interference is probably not a problem for routine plasma determinations, but immunoassay methods may overestimate carbamazepine concentrations in cerebrospinal fluid or saliva due to a relatively higher proportion of epoxide in these fluids.

Concentration–effect relationship

A relationship between serum concentration and antiepileptic efficacy has been demonstrated for carbamazepine (Cereghino et al 1974, Sillanpää et al 1979). The commonly quoted therapeutic range is 20–40 μmol/l (approximately 5–10 μg/ml)

although patients with mild epilepsy may be controlled with much lower levels. Adverse effects do not usually occur until serum levels reach 40–50 μmol/l (9.5–12 μg/ml). Although the 10,11-epoxide possesses antiepileptic activity in animals equivalent to that of the parent drug itself, its antiepileptic potency in humans is uncertain. However, it probably contributes to the overall pharmacological effect of carbamazepine, particularly when allowance is made for its lower degree of plasma protein binding. In children, its relative concentration in plasma can be much higher and its contribution may therefore be greater. There is, however, insufficient data as yet to justify routine measurement of the epoxide metabolite during therapeutic drug monitoring. In children, measurement of saliva concentrations of carbamazepine may be preferable to serum level monitoring. These correlate closely (Chambers et al 1977).

Dose interval

With half-life values of 10–30 hours after chronic dosing in the adult, twice-daily dosing is appropriate. Johannessen et al (1977) showed that the variation in serum level with twice-daily dosing is about 50% of the mean value. However, with large total daily doses in some patients, adverse effects may occur 2–4 hours after drug administration and it may then be necessary to divide the total daily dose into three or more divided doses to avoid high peak serum concentrations.

Pharmacokinetics in special situations

In neonates whose mothers take carbamazepine during pregnancy, placental transfer of carbamazepine occurs, resulting in fetal enzyme induction in utero. Thus, clearance of the drug in such neonates may be similar to adults. In children, carbamazepine metabolism is greater than in adults and the epoxide:carbamazepine ratio is significantly higher (Rane et al 1976). The plasma protein binding of carbamazepine in children may be lower than in adults. In pregnancy, there is evidence of increased metabolism of carbamazepine resulting in lower carbamazepine levels but higher epoxide levels (Battino et al 1985).

Although carbamazepine binding may be reduced by liver or renal disease, an increased toxicity of the drug due to this mechanism is unlikely. Severe liver disease may also be associated with reduced metabolism of carbamazepine.

Drug interactions

Most of the documented interactions are pharmacokinetic (Perucca & Richens 1980, 1985).

Effect of carbamazepine on other drugs

Carbamazepine can induce the metabolism of other drugs given concomitantly, including other antiepileptic drugs such as sodium valproate, ethosuximide, phenytoin and clonazepam and other medications, such as warfarin and the oral contraceptive steroids.

Effect of other drugs on carbamazepine

Levels of carbamazepine are significantly lowered when phenytoin, phenobarbitone or primidone are added to carbamazepine therapy, but the ratio of the 10,11-epoxide to parent drug may be increased. Enzyme-inhibiting drugs, such as cimetidine, propoxyphene and verapamil, can elevate carbamazepine levels. Protein binding interactions do not appear to be important for carbamazepine.

Adverse drug reactions with carbamazepine

Adverse effects occur in approximately one-third of patients treated and are more frequent in patients on polytherapy. In 5%, withdrawal of carbamazepine is necessary. Carbamazepine causes various dose-related neuropsychiatric adverse drug reactions including alteration in mental function and impaired co-ordination. The more serious idiosyncratic side-effects, including toxic hepatitis and blood dyscrasias, are exceedingly rare. Experience with carbamazepine over recent years has confirmed its relatively low toxicity.

Neuropsychiatric

The most common dose-related adverse effects of carbamazepine are those that affect co-ordination

and they usually consist of a disturbance of eye movements resulting in dizziness, blurred vision and diplopia, or a disturbance of balance causing ataxia. Other more complex eye movement disturbances are seen more rarely. Such dose-related side-effects often occur early on in the course of treatment and are transient. If the starting dose of carbamazepine is small and the dose is increased gradually there are usually fewer problems. It is not unusual for patients to complain of intermittent side effects, often occurring between two and four hours after a dose and coinciding with peak serum carbamazepine concentrations. This is due to the fluctuations in plasma levels which occur during the dosing intervals, and these fluctuations are greater when other antiepileptic drugs are taken concomitantly. It can be managed by administering the drug in three or four divided doses. If very high serum carbamazepine levels occur, for example after acute overdose, enhancement of seizures may occur.

Carbamazepine appears to have relatively less adverse effect on mental functioning than some of the other antiepileptic drugs. The reported incidence of neurotoxicity varies considerably, but there are no published reports of irreversible neurological toxicity. In volunteers, deficits in association with carbamazepine occurred in relation to motor rather than mental speed and in one task measuring processing speed and perceptual registration the administration of carbamazepine was associated with a significant improvement in performance (Thompson et al 1981). In studies of epileptic patients where medication was altered by reducing the number of different antiepileptic drugs prescribed, and in some cases substituting carbamazepine for the original medication, improvement in the performance of psychological tests was recorded (Thompson & Trimble 1982). Those patients who changed to carbamazepine, either alone or in combination with existing treatment, displayed more widespread improvements in test performance particularly on measures of memory. It was not clear whether these improvements were due to withdrawal of polytherapy, better seizure control or an independent beneficial effect of carbamazepine on psychomotor performance.

Dyskinesias and asterixis have been reported to

occur rarely with carbamazepine. Psychoses provoked by carbamazepine have been rarely reported. There is no evidence to incriminate carbamazepine in the development of peripheral neuropathy (Shorvon & Reynolds 1982).

Haematological disorders

Adverse haematological reactions to carbamazepine are very rare but are potentially serious (Pisciotta 1982). They include bone marrow depression in the form of leucopenia, anaemia and thrombocytopenia, and more rarely proliferative effects such as eosinophilia and leucocytosis. The incidence of aplastic anaemia has been estimated at 0.5/100 000/yr. It has been observed more often in patients being treated with carbamazepine for trigeminal neuralgia than for epilepsy. Haematological disturbances other than agranulocytosis and aplastic anaemia are almost always reversible. Transient leucopenia occurs in about 10% of patients, usually in the first month of therapy. More substantial persistent leucopenia is rare and responds to discontinuation of carbamazepine (Hart & Easton 1981).

Gastrointestinal disturbances

Gastrointestinal disturbances during carbamazepine therapy are mostly found in the first few weeks of treatment. They include anorexia, nausea and vomiting.

Hepatic disturbances

Hepatic toxicity has been reported in association with carbamazepine therapy but is a very rare occurrence: 21 cases reported in the literature during the first 20 years of use. Mostly, symptoms occurred within the first month of therapy, which suggests a hypersensitivity reaction. On withdrawal of the drug most patients recovered.

Skin reactions

The incidence of skin reactions with carbamazepine is at least 3%, although some studies have found a higher rate of skin reactions which may have been related to higher initial dose of the drug (Chadwick et al 1984). Most occur early in the course of treatment. Many of the skin rashes are mild maculopapular, morbilliform, urticarial or vesicular eruptions which do not necessitate cessation of the drug. Less frequently, exfoliative dermatitis may occur and this type of reaction necessitates discontinuation of carbamazepine. Reversible alopecia has also been reported.

Endocrine disturbances

Hyponatraemia and low plasma osmolality may occur in patients receiving carbamazepine (Perucca et al 1978). The mechanism of this effect is not clear. There is some evidence of increased release of antidiuretic hormone from the posterior pituitary gland, but other investigators have suggested that there is increased renal sensitivity to normal plasma concentrations of antidiuretic hormone. Hyponatraemia may result in weight gain, oedema, irritability and loss of seizure control. Carbamazepine can also alter circulating thyroid hormone concentrations, possibly by inducing their metabolism, but clinical hypothyroidism is rare. Carbamazepine therapy has been associated with changes in circulating androgens and exaggerated luteinizing hormone (LH) responses to gonadotrophin-releasing hormone consistent with enhanced sex hormone metabolism due to hepatic enzyme induction (Richens 1984). Induction of hepatic metabolism by carbamazepine leads to reduced levels of exogenous contraceptive hormones and may result in oral contraceptive pill failure (see Ch 15 Pt 2).

Biochemical features of osteomalacia have been found in patients on carbamazepine but without clinical evidence of bone disease (Hahn 1976).

Teratogenicity

There is little evidence from animal studies to implicate carbamazepine as a teratogen. Clinical studies also support minimal teratogenic effects of carbamazepine. However, the possibility of the epoxide metabolite possessing teratogenic potential has been raised, based on the observation of a high rate of congenital abnormalities after prenatal exposure to certain combinations of antiepileptic drugs which result in accumulation of the epoxide (Lindhout et al 1984).

Indications for the use of carbamazepine

Carbamazepine is an effective drug in the control of partial and tonic-clonic seizures but has no therapeutic effect in absence seizures. Its low incidence of adverse effects and possible beneficial psychotropic effect makes it the preferred therapy in many patients, particularly in women of child-bearing age.

Oxcarbazepine

Oxcarbazepine is a new antiepileptic drug chemically closely related to carbamazepine. Preliminary clinical studies indicate that oxcarbazepine has an antiepileptic efficacy similar to carbamazepine while adverse effects, especially sedation, may be fewer. Preliminary studies have shown that only 25% of patients allergic to carbamazepine will show a cross-reaction to oxcarbazepine, so its main therapeutic potential would appear to be in patients who have derived therapeutic benefit from carbamazepine but have developed allergic reactions necessitating withdrawal of the drug. The reduced incidence of adverse effects with oxcarbazepine has been suggested to be due to the absence of an epoxide metabolite of the drug.

SODIUM VALPROATE

Sodium valproate is the sodium salt of valproic acid (dipropylacetic acid, 2-propylpentanoic acid or 2-propylvaleric acid). The acid itself, the magnesium salt and the amide are also marketed as antiepileptic drugs in some countries. It was first used to treat epileptic patients in 1964 and has been licensed for clinical use in the UK since 1973 and the USA since 1978 (limited indications only).

Structure

The structure of valproic acid is shown in Figure 12.8. It differs from that of the traditional anti-

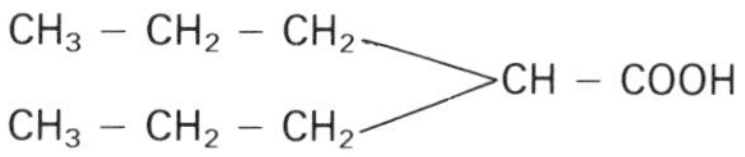

$$CH_3 - CH_2 - CH_2 \diagdown$$
$$ CH - COOH$$
$$CH_3 - CH_2 - CH_2 \diagup$$

Fig. 12.8 Structure of valproic acid

epileptic drugs in that its structure is that of a simple two-chain fatty acid.

Mode of action

Sodium valproate has been shown to have anticonvulsant properties in a variety of experimental animal models of epilepsy. Although a number of hypotheses have been advanced to account for the anticonvulsant activity of the drug, the mechanism of action is far from clear (Chapman et al 1982). Suggested mechanisms include:

1. Increasing the brain concentrations of the inhibitory neurotransmitter, gamma-amino-butyric acid (GABA); it has been shown to interact with several enzymes involved in the synthesis and degradation of GABA but these enzymatic effects only occur at relatively high drug concentrations
2. Selective enhancement of post-synaptic responses to GABA
3. A direct effect on neuronal membranes, e.g. by altering potassium conductance
4. Reduction of brain concentrations of the excitatory amino acid neurotransmitter, aspartic acid

Pharmacokinetics

These are summarized in Table 12.4. The reader is referred to Pinder et al (1977) and Gugler & von Unruh (1980) for a detailed account of the pharmacokinetics of sodium valproate.

Absorption

Sodium valproate has been shown to be completely absorbed following oral administration, with peak plasma concentrations of valproic acid occurring at one to four hours after ingestion of the plain tablets or syrup and at four to eight hours after enteric-coated tablets. Absorp-

Table 12.4 Summary of pharmacokinetic data on sodium valproate

Range of daily maintenance dosage	Adult: 600–3000 mg/day Child: 20–30 mg/kg/day
Time to peak serum level	1–4 h (plain tabs) 2–8 h (enteric- coated)
Oral absorption	>95%
Percentage bound to plasma proteins	Approx. 90% (see text)
Apparent volume of distribution	0.1–0.4 l/kg
Elimination half-life (adults)	9–21 h
Time to steady state after starting therapy	4 days
Major metabolites	β, ω and ω-1 oxidation products.
Minimum dose frequency	? Once daily

tion may be delayed if the drug is taken after a meal.

Distribution and plasma protein binding

The distribution of valproic acid is largely restricted to the extracellular water. Values for the apparent volume of distribution have been reported as 0.1–0.4 l/kg. Concentrations in brain and cerebrospinal fluid are much lower than plasma levels and appear to be related to the free drug concentration in plasma. In humans, the brain concentration has been shown to be 6.8–27.9% of plasma concentrations. At plasma levels within the accepted therapeutic range, valproic acid is highly bound (approx. 90%) to the plasma proteins, mainly albumin, but the binding is concentration dependent and the free fraction increases as total plasma valproate concentrations rise (Gugler et al 1980). This gives rise to a non-linear relationship between dose and serum level and affects the interpretation of total serum valproic acid concentrations during therapeutic drug monitoring (Gram et al 1980). Valproic acid binding is reduced by free fatty acids as well as in patients with hypoalbuminaemia, liver and renal disease (Gugler & Mueller 1978). Because of the drug's low pka (4.95) it is secreted into saliva in small amounts which do not reflect the free plasma concentration.

Metabolism and excretion

Valproic acid is almost completely metabolized prior to excretion, only 1–3% of the ingested dose being excreted unchanged in the urine. Its metabolism is complex and the identification and quantification of the many metabolites has proved difficult (Jakobs & Löscher 1978). The major elimination pathway is via conjugation with glucuronic acid (20–70%). The remainder is largely metabolized via oxidative pathways (β, ω and ω-1) particularly ω-oxidation. Some of the metabolites of valproic acid possess antiepileptic activity, although mostly less than that of the parent compound. The clinical significance of this is uncertain but it has been calculated that the parent drug itself is responsible for more than 90% of the therapeutic effect.

Plasma half-life

The plasma half-life varies between 9 and 21 hours, with a mean of 12–13 hours. In patients, who are taking other antiepileptic drugs, shorter values can be measured and this is the result of the induction of the oxidation of valproic acid. Because of the relatively short half-life, it is generally administered two to three times daily. However, there is evidence from animal and patient studies (Lockard & Levy 1976, Rowan et al 1979) that the antiepileptic effect may come on more slowly than would be predicted from the time to peak plasma concentration following a single dose, and that it may long outlast the presence of drug in the plasma. Thus, once-daily administration appears feasible and patient studies have shown that seizure control was at least as good with once-daily dose as with divided dosage (Covanis & Jeavons 1980).

Concentration–effect relationship

Because sodium valproate appears to have a prolonged pharmacological effect in epilepsy, with delayed onset of action and carry-over of effect, it would not be expected that measurements of plasma drug concentration would correlate closely with antiepileptic effect. A therapeutic range for seizure control of 350–700 μmol/l (approximately 50–100 μg/ml) was first suggested by Schobben et al (1975) but many subsequent studies have failed to show such a relationship. Some of the toxic effects of valproic acid, such as tremor, appear to be related to plasma concentrations of the drug and are more common with levels greater than 700 μmol/l. Besides interindividual variations in serum valproic acid concentrations when patients are given the same dose there are large intra-individual fluctuations in the concentrations throughout the day depending on the frequency and time of drug administration. Thus, standardization of sampling times is necessary. Furthermore, the extent of protein binding is very variable due to concentration-dependent binding and disease states which alter binding. As it is the free drug concentration that is responsible for the therapeutic action, it would perhaps be more relevant to attempt to relate free valproate concentration to clinical effect.

Consequently, the value of therapeutic drug monitoring for valproate is uncertain.

Pharmacokinetics in special situations

The half-life of valproic acid is prolonged in neonates (20–67 hours) but falls rapidly in the first few months of life so that in older infants it reaches adult values. Placental transfer of valproate and its metabolites has been demonstrated with reports of higher concentrations in cord than in maternal blood. Small amounts of the drug are secreted into breast milk with levels reported as 0.17–5.4% of maternal plasma concentrations and therefore unlikely to affect the baby adversely (see Ch. 15 Part 2). Doses of valproate in patients with renal disease should be reduced and valproate should be avoided in patients with liver disease.

Drug interactions

Unlike most of the other antiepileptic drugs in common use, sodium valproate does not induce hepatic metabolism but rather appears to act as a non-specific inhibitor of drug metabolism (Perucca et al 1979, 1980). Below are most of the significant interactions which have been documented so far.

Pharmacokinetic interactions

Effect of valproate on other drugs Serum phenobarbitone concentrations may increase when sodium valproate is introduced concurrently and result in excessive sedation. This interaction is thought to arise because of the inhibition of the metabolism of phenobarbitone by valproic acid resulting in a prolonged elimination half-life. The interaction between phenytoin and valproic acid is more complex. The latter drug displaces phenytoin from its binding site on albumin and also inhibits the metabolism of phenytoin, thus reducing its intrinsic clearance. This results in increased free levels of phenytoin and either decreased or unchanged total levels (Perucca et al 1980). Because of these conflicting effects on phenytoin kinetics, in some circumstances it may be necessary to measure free rather than total phenytoin concentrations in patients on phenytoin–valproate combination therapy. Valproic acid can also inhibit the metabolism of primidone but its effects on carbamazepine and ethosuximide kinetics are less consistent.

Effect of other drugs on valproate Several antiepileptic drugs can reduce serum concentrations of valproic acid by increasing the intrinsic clearance by enzyme induction. Such an interaction is seen with phenytoin, carbamazepine and phenobarbitone. Salicylates have been reported to displace valproic acid from plasma protein binding sites.

Pharmacodynamic interactions

Sodium valproate may enhance the effects of central nervous system depressants including ethanol.

Adverse drug reactions (Turnbull 1983)

The incidence of adverse effects with sodium valproate is difficult to gauge exactly because many patients are on polytherapy and the method of determining side effects varies between studies.

Schmidt (1984b) estimated the incidence of adverse reactions based on analysis of 16 trials on a total of 1140 patients as 26%, but in only 2% were problems so severe that discontinuation of valproate therapy was necessary.

Gastrointestinal disorders

Recognized problems include anorexia, nausea, vomiting, dyspepsia, diarrhoea and constipation. The incidence of gastrointestinal adverse reactions is reduced by use of the enteric-coated preparation. They may also be minimized by starting valproate in a low dose and gradually increasing it, and by taking the drug with food and in divided doses. Pancreatitis has occasionally been reported in association with valproate therapy and rare deaths have occurred.

Weight gain

An increase in weight is a recognized problem with sodium valproate; the reason is uncertain.

Skin and hair

Rashes are a rare occurrence with valproate but reversible hair loss occurs quite frequently with a reported incidence between 2.6 and 12%. Occasionally the hair regrows curly.

Haematological disorders

Thrombocytopenia and bruising may occur during therapy with valproate. There have also been reports of abnormal platelet function.

Neurological

Tremor is a well-recognized adverse effect of sodium valproate. It is usually of the benign essential type and is probably dose related and reversible. Reports on the effects of sodium valproate on cognitive function conflict, probably due to difficulty in interpretation when patients are on multiple drug therapy and have variable seizure frequency. In normal volunteers, impairment in decision making was found but the adverse effects were much less than with phenytoin.

Hepatotoxicity

Severe hepatotoxicity, occasionally with a fatal outcome is a rare adverse effect of valproate. It appears to be due to an idiosyncratic reaction and usually occurs during the first six months of treatment. Most of the reported cases have occurred in children and many had already been noted to have developmental delay or associated neurological disease. Most were taking other enzyme-inducing drugs and in some cases the causative role of sodium valproate was not clear cut. It has been suggested that the drug is not normally hepatotoxic but in the presence of a metabolic abnormality it may become so. The incidence of liver toxicity is low, approximately one in 50 000, but the risk increases when treating children with severe epilepsy, progressive neurological disease and taking multiple drug therapy. Asymptomatic elevations of hepatic transaminases are not uncommonly found and usually respond to dose reduction.

Hyperammonaemia

Valproate may cause various metabolic disturbances because it inhibits several enzymes involved in intermediary cell metabolism (Kay et al 1986). Moderate asymptomatic elevations in blood ammonia levels are common during valproate therapy, but in a few cases encephalopathy has resulted, occasionally with fatal outcome.

Teratogenicity

Sodium valproate has been shown to be teratogenic in animals and reports of abnormalities in the offspring of epileptic mothers taking sodium valproate have been published (see Ch. 15 Pt 2). One from the Rhône-Alps Region of France first drew attention to a possible causal relationship between sodium valproate and spina bifida.

Indications for the use of sodium valproate

Sodium valproate has been used in a wide range of seizure disorders but its major use has been in the treatment of the primary generalized epilepsies. It is very effective therapy for absence seizures, with success rates approaching 100% in uncomplicated previously untreated absence seizures. Valproate is comparable with phenytoin and carbamazepine in the control of tonic-clonic seizures and is the drug of choice in patients with photosensitive epilepsy. It may also be beneficial in the treatment of myoclonic seizures. Although sodium valproate is less effective for the treatment of partial seizures than it is in primarily generalized seizures, it appears to be as effective as phenytoin or carbamazepine. Valproate has also been shown to be effective for the prophylaxis of febrile convulsions. It is unsuitable for use in status epilepticus because its onset of action occurs several hours after administration.

PHENOBARBITONE

Phenobarbitone was introduced into the drug treatment of epilepsy in 1912. Phenobarbitone is a substituted barbituric acid and it was the first effective organic epileptic agent. It is much more potent as an anticonvulsant than as a sedative.

Structure

The structure of phenobarbitone is shown in Figure 12.9. The free acid is only sparingly water soluble, but the sodium salt is freely soluble. The pKa is 7.3 and it is a stronger acid than other barbiturates.

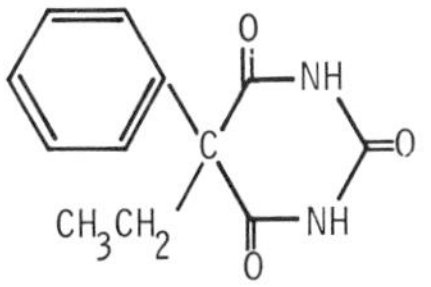

Fig. 12.9 Structure of phenobarbitone

Mechanisms of action

In humans, phenobarbitone is effective against generalized tonic-clonic and partial seizures but has very little effect on absence seizures. All the different barbiturates are not equally effective as antiepileptic drugs in ambulatory patients with epilepsy. The sedative-anaesthetic barbiturates, such as pentobarbitone produce marked sedation at anticonvulsant doses, whereas phenobarbitone is clinically useful because it has antiepileptic activity without causing excessive sedation.

Barbiturate drugs have been shown to have numerous different actions on central nervous system neurones including:

1. Modification of postsynaptic neurotransmitter responses, to enhance GABA-mediated inhibition and to diminish glutaminergic and cholinergic excitation; they also directly increase membrane chloride ion conductance
2. Presynaptic action to reduce calcium entry into the neurones and block neurotransmitter release.
3. Non-synaptically to reduce voltage dependent sodium and potassium conductances and block repetitive firing.

Augmentation of GABA responses and antagonism of glutamate excitation occur at clinically relevant phenobarbitone concentrations and thus may be the underlying mechanism of anticonvulsant activity (Schultz & MacDonald 1981). Other actions, e.g. direct increase in chloride conductance, may be more important for the sedative and anaesthetic properties of barbiturates. Enhancement of GABAergic responses appears to be effected by facilitating GABA binding to GABA receptors, as phenobarbitone does not directly alter chloride channel conductance at low drug concentrations.

Pharmacokinetics

These are summarized in Table 12.5. The reader is referred to Butler (1978) and Wilensky et al (1982) for a detailed review of the pharmacokinetics of phenobarbitone.

Absorption

Absorption of phenobarbitone after oral administration is virtually complete but the rate of absorption is variable. Jalling (1974) found peak serum concentrations 1–6 hours after oral dosing but slower absorption has been described in earlier reports (Sjögren et al 1965). This may be due to differences in pharmaceutical formulation, and the

Table 12.5 Summary of pharmacokinetic data on phenobarbitone

Range of daily maintenance dose	Adult: 30–240 mg/day Child: 2–6 mg/kg/day
Minimum dose frequency	Once daily
Time to peak serum levels	1–6 h
Percentage bound to plasma proteins	45%
Apparent volume of distribution	0.5 l/kg
Elimination half-life	Adult: 50–160 h Child: 30–70 h
Time to steady state after starting therapy	Up to 30 days
Major metabolite (inactive)	Para-hydroxyphenobarbitone

effect of food on absorption may be important. Intramuscular injections of phenobarbitone reach peak serum concentrations in 0.5–6 hours (Graham 1978, Wilensky et al 1982) but this is too slow for the emergency treatment of status epilepticus.

Distribution and plasma protein binding

Although the distribution of phenobarbitone to vascular tissues occurs fairly rapidly after absorption, the penetration of the drug into the brain is slow and this is another reason why phenobarbitone is not an ideal drug for the treatment of status epilepticus. The later phases of drug distribution result in almost equal phenobarbitone concentrations in all tissues of the body. The distribution of phenobarbitone is sensitive to variations in the pH of plasma because it has a pKa close to physiological plasma pH. Acidosis causes a shift of the drug from plasma to tissues, and alkalosis results in an increased phenobarbitone concentration in the plasma (Waddell & Butler, 1957).

Phenobarbitone is about 45% bound to plasma proteins. This relatively low degree of protein binding means that the drug is less susceptible to alterations in plasma protein concentrations and is unlikely to be significantly involved in drug interactions in which there is competition for binding sites. Cerebrospinal fluid concentrations of phenobarbitone reflect the free drug concentrations in plasma (Houghton et al 1975b) but the saliva concentrations do not because they are sensitive to pH changes (Schmidt & Kupferberg 1975). It is therefore unwise to use saliva for serum drug level monitoring in the case of phenobarbitone.

Metabolism and excretion

Phenobarbitone is partly metabolized and partly excreted unchanged in the urine (Butler 1978). Studies in patients have reported between 11 and 55% of the dose is excreted unchanged by the kidneys. The remainder is hydroxylated in the para position to p-hydroxyphenobarbitone, which is then excreted both unchanged and as the glucuronide by the kidneys.

Para-hydroxyphenobarbitone lacks antiepileptic activity. Both the biotransformation and renal clearance of phenobarbitone proceed slowly. The plasma half-life in adults ranges from 50–160 hours (mean 96 h). Thus, once-daily dosing with phenobarbitone is possible. Because of phenobarbitone's pKa of 7.3, the rate of excretion of the parent compound by the kidneys can be altered significantly by changes in urine pH. Alkalinization of the urine increases the renal excretion of unchanged phenobarbitone by reducing the non-ionic back diffusion from the distal renal tubule to the plasma. This property has been exploited in the treatment of phenobarbitone overdose. The renal clearance can be increased from 4–6 ml/min to 30 ml/min by bicarbonate administration.

Dose–serum concentration relationship

Over the therapeutic range of serum concentrations there is a nearly linear relationship between dose and serum level within subjects. Thus phenobarbitone is an easier drug to manage clinically than phenytoin. However, there is considerable variation between subjects in the serum level produced by a given dose. Children metabolize the drug more quickly than adults and therefore require proportionally larger mg/kg doses.

Concentration–effect relationship

Although studies examining the relationship between plasma level of phenobarbitone and seizure control have produced some conflicting results, it would appear that plasma pheno-barbitone levels greater than 42 μmol/l (10 μg/ml) are associated with improved clinical efficacy (Buchthal et al 1968). With plasma levels over 172 μmol/l (40 μ/ml) the additional therapeutic benefits decline and there is a higher incidence of adverse effects (Plaa & Hine 1960). However, it is well recognized that tolerance occurs to the sedative effects of the drug so that a serum level of 20 μmol/l (4.8 μg/ml) produced acutely may have a greater sedative effect than a level of 200 μmol/l (48 μg/ml) which has been maintained chronically. However, it is less certain whether tolerance to the antiepileptic effect occurs in humans. A therapeutic range of 42–170 μmol/l (10–40 μg/ml) has been suggested as a guide to therapy but, because of the phenomenon of tolerance, it could be argued that the value of therapeutic drug monitoring for this drug may be less than previously thought.

Pharmacokinetics in special situations

Phenobarbitone can cross the placental barrier and enter the fetus. The amount in breast milk is fairly small and the dose reaching the breast-fed infant is unlikely to result in side-effects (Kaneko et al 1979). Phenobarbitone's half-life is prolonged in neonates but in children is less than in adults. Because phenobarbitone is cleared partly by renal excretion patients with poor renal function (creatinine clearance <30 ml/min) may be at risk of phenobarbitone toxicity.

Drug interactions

Most of the reported drug interactions involving phenobarbitone occur in situations where pheno-barbitone has altered the kinetics of other drugs (Perucca & Richens 1980, 1985). Alteration in protein binding has not been implicated as an important factor in any reported interactions. However, phenobarbitone is a potent inducer of hepatic mixed function oxidase enzymes and thus can alter the metabolism of numerous drugs, e.g. warfarin and oral contraceptive steroids and various endogenous substances. However, the effect of enzyme induction by phenobarbitone on other drugs in individual patients is largely unpredictable and seems to depend on genetic factors and previous contact with environmental inducing agents. There is no evidence of autoinduction of phenobarbitone metabolism in humans. Inhibition of phenobarbitone's own metabolism by other drugs may also occur, e.g. the valproate–phenobarbitone interaction which can result in phenobarbitone toxicity.

Adverse reactions to phenobarbitone

Phenobarbitone has been widely used for over 70 years and thus experience with the drug has led to the accumulation of considerable information about its toxicity. Serious systemic adverse reactions appear to be very uncommon. The most frequent problems encountered are neuro-psychiatric toxicity.

Neuropsychiatric toxicity

Even with serum concentrations of pheno-barbitone within the therapeutic range of 42–170 μmol/l (10–40 μg/ml) adverse changes in affect, behaviour and cognitive function are often encountered. High serum concentrations can result in nystagmus, dysarthria and ataxia (Plaa & Hine 1960). The most common adverse reaction in adults is sedation, although marked tolerance to it can develop. In children and the elderly a paradoxical effect may occur resulting in insomnia and hyperkinetic activity. The incidence of behaviour disturbances in children has been reported as over 50% in some studies (Wolf & Forsythe 1978). Those children most at risk are the ones with organic brain disease. Phenobarbitone therapy can cause alteration in mood, particularly depression. Cognitive function may also be disturbed, and the resulting deficits in attention and memory may be subtle and difficult to measure.

Dependence, habituation and withdrawal

Physical dependence on phenobarbitone occurs and abrupt discontinuation after high dosage produces abstinence symptoms, including anxiety, insomnia, tremors, confusion and seizures. If a decision is made to stop phenobarbitone therapy, it must be tapered off very slowly to avoid withdrawal seizures. A neonatal withdrawal syndrome has been described in infants born to epileptic mothers taking phenobarbitone.

Haematological toxicity

Megaloblastic anaemia and macrocytosis have been described during therapy with phenobarbitone alone or more commonly when in combination with other antiepileptic drugs, especially phenytoin. As with phenytoin, folate deficiency occurs, but does not require treatment unless anaemia results.

Coagulation defects can occur in neonates whose epileptic mothers take phenobarbitone during pregnancy (Mountain et al 1970). They are due to a deficiency of vitamin K dependent clotting factors, and vitamin K administration to the baby post partum will prevent this coagulation deficiency.

Bone disorders

Biochemical osteomalacia can occur in epileptic patients treated with phenobarbitone but clinical demineralization of bone is rare (see p. 431).

Hepatic toxicity

There is a low incidence of liver damage resulting from treatment with phenobarbitone.

Endocrine changes

Phenobarbitone stimulates the peripheral metabolism of T_4 which is countered by an increased secretion of T_4 from the thyroid gland so that most patients remain euthyroid.

Skin reactions

Various types of skin rashes have been reported with phenobarbitone. They are usually mild maculopapular or morbilliform eruptions. The incidence of such reactions is low and more serious skin problems, such as exfoliative dermatitis are extremely rare.

Teratogenicity

As previously discussed (see p. 432) there is an increased risk of fetal malformations in the offspring of epileptic mothers, but the role played by the various antiepileptic drugs in their etiology is far from clear. Evidence for the teratogenic potential of phenobarbitone is much less than for phenytoin.

Other barbiturates

Over the past 30 years other barbiturate derivatives have been developed but none has been shown to be clinically superior to phenobarbitone itself. One such compound, methylphenobarbitone, is less reliably absorbed than phenobarbitone and following absorption it is demethylated to phenobarbitone with a half-life of about 20 hours (Eadie et al 1978). Most of its pharmacological effect resides in its phenobarbitone metabolite. Thus, there is no advantage in giving methylphenobarbitone rather than phenobarbitone itself and the drug has not achieved any widespread popularity.

PRIMIDONE

Primidone is a desoxybarbiturate which was first marketed as an antiepileptic drug in 1952.

Structure

The structure of primidone and its two major metabolites, phenobarbitone and phenylethylmalonamide (PEMA) are shown in Figure 12.10

Mechanism of action

Primidone is metabolized to phenobarbitone and PEMA in the liver (Baumel et al 1972). In experimental models of epilepsy both primidone itself and PEMA have antiepileptic activity. However, it is far from clear how much they contribute to the clinical effect in epileptic

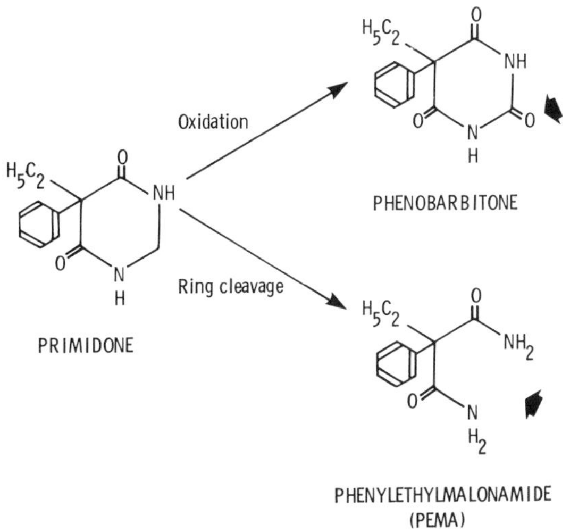

Fig. 12.10 Structure of primidone and its two major metabolites

Table 12.6 Summary of pharmacokinetic data on primidone

Range of daily maintenance dosage	Adult: 250–1500 mg/day Child: 15–30 mg/kg/day
Minimum dose frequency	Twice daily
Time to peak serum level	2–5 h
Percentage bound to plasma proteins	Less than 20%
Apparent volume of distribution	0.6 l/kg
Major active metabolites	Phenobarbitone Phenylethylmalonamide (PEMA)
Elimination half-life (adults)	Primidone 4–12 h Derived phenobarbitone 50–160 h Derived PEMA 29–36 h
Time to steady state after starting therapy	Up to 30 days for derived Phenobarbitone

patients. There is little information about possible modes of action of these two substances and certainly a large part of the anticonvulsant effect of primidone must be due to its conversion to phenobarbitone. (For postulated mechanisms of action of phenobarbitone see p. 441).

Pharmacokinetics

A summary of the pharmacokinetics of primidone is given in Table 12.6. The reader is referred to Baumel et al (1972) for a detailed review.

Absorption

Peak serum concentrations are achieved within 2–5 hours after administration of a single dose but after chronic administration peak levels appear to occur later (Booker et al 1970, Schottelius 1982).

Distribution and plasma protein binding

Studies of the distribution of primidone in humans are not extensive. Reported CSF:serum ratios range from 0.53–1.13 and brain concentrations have been shown to correlate well with plasma concentrations with a brain:plasma ratio 0.87 (Houghton et al 1975b). Saliva:serum ratios are 73–100%. The degree of protein binding of primidone is low, unbound primidone levels being about 80% of the total serum level.

Metabolism and excretion

Primidone is metabolized in the liver to phenobarbitone and phenylethylmalonamide (PEMA) although a relatively high percentage of primidone may be excreted unchanged via the kidneys (Kaufmann et al 1977). On average 20–25% is converted to phenobarbitone but there is extensive interindividual variation in the degree of conversion and this leads to a wide scatter of serum phenobarbitone:primidone concentration ratios (Booker et al 1970). The metabolism to phenobarbitone is very slow after single dose administration but after chronic dosing the conversion occurs more rapidly. Metabolism to PEMA is rapid following a single dose of primidone. Primidone has a half-life of 4–12 hours and therefore considerable fluctuation in serum concentrations occur throughout the day. The derived phenobarbitone has a much longer half-life and therefore the serum concentration of this metabolite exceeds the serum concentration of the parent drug despite the fact that only a relatively small proportion of primidone is metabolized to phenobarbitone. PEMA also accumulates because it is eliminated more slowly than primidone. The ideal dose interval for primidone administration is uncertain because the role played by unchanged primidone and PEMA in the anticonvulsant effect of the drug is uncertain. In animals both primidone and PEMA have antiepileptic activity against experimental seizures (Bourgeois et al 1983) but whether they contribute significantly in the treatment of epileptic patients is not certain. However, Oxley et al (1980) have shown that, in some patients, primidone is a superior antiepileptic drug to phenobarbitone when given in doses which produce similar serum phenobarbitone concentrations. Whether the parent drug itself or the derived PEMA accounts for this additional activity is not known. In view of all the uncertainty it is probably wise to administer primidone in twice-daily divided dosage.

Dose–serum concentration relationship

An approximately linear relationship exists between primidone dose and derived serum phenobarbitone concentrations. The ratio of the primidone:phenobarbitone concentrations at steady state is an average 1:2.5 but there is wide variation between subjects. The co-administration of other enzyme-inducing antiepileptic drugs, e.g. phenytoin, increase the ratio by increasing the rate of metabolism of primidone to phenobarbitone and leading to accumulation of phenobarbitone, and possibly a potentiation of pharmacological effect. Changes in the primidone:phenobarbitone ratio during pregnancy have been reported with a fall during later pregnancy, although the mechanism of this change is not clear and the possibility of non-compliance with medication has not been excluded (Battino et al 1984).

Serum concentration–effect relationship

Correlation of plasma concentrations of primidone with clinical control of seizures is complicated because of its conversion into two active metabolites as well as possibly being active in its own right. Thus for a full assessment it may be necessary to monitor plasma levels of all three compounds. The most practical approach is to monitor derived phenobarbitone. The potential benefit of also measuring unchanged primidone is in detection of non-compliance because those patients who have only started to take the primidone a few days prior to clinic attendance will have a low serum phenobarbitone:primidone ratio. Plasma primidone concentrations in excess of 70 μmol/l (15 μg/ml) are likely to be accompanied by side-effects.

Adverse effects of primidone

Many patients experience side-effects of drowsiness, weakness and dizziness at the initiation of primidone therapy. These symptoms may be severe and last several days. They may occur even when the starting dose is low, and appear to be related to serum concentrations of the parent drug rather than the metabolites. When primidone is added to other enzyme-inducing antiepileptic drug therapy, this initial intolerance is usually less, due to the more rapid conversion of the parent drug to its metabolites. These adverse effects usually subside with time due to functional tolerance to side-effects of primidone (Leppik et al 1984) so that the dose of primidone may be gradually increased. Primidone shares much of the adverse reaction spectrum of phenobarbitone. Only rarely has primidone been implicated in severe haematological or idiosyncratic reactions. There is some evidence that primidone intake during pregnancy may be important in the pathogenesis of minor abnormalities and poor somatic development in the children of epileptic women (Rating et al 1982).

ETHOSUXIMIDE

The clinical effectiveness of ethosuximide against pure absence seizures was first reported in 1958, and it remains an important drug for this indication.

Structure

The structure of ethosuximide is shown in Figure 12.11.

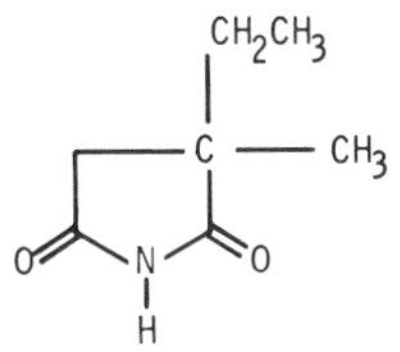

Fig. 12.11 Structure of ethosuximide

Mechanism of action

The high degree of therapeutic specificity of ethosuximide in human seizure disorders is reflected by its selective antiepileptic action against experimental seizures. It will prevent pentylenetetrazole seizures in animals but has no effect on maximal electroshock seizures. Despite its widespread use in the treatment of absence seizures, ethosuximide's mode of action is unknown. It has been reported to inhibit cortical Na^+K^+-ATPase activity; to reduce slightly the activities of succinate dehydrogenase and aldehyde reductase; to alter cerebral neurotransmitter levels; and has several actions on synaptic transmission. It is ineffective against repetitive neurone firing and there is no evidence for enhancement of GABA inhibition. Because of the limited data available it is not possible to advance a definite hypothesis on the antiepileptic mechanism of action of ethosuximide.

Pharmacokinetics

These are summarized in Table 12.7. The reader is referred to Sherwin (1978) for a detailed account.

Absorption

Ethosuximide is rapidly and completely absorbed from the gastrointestinal tract, peak plasma levels occurring after 1–4 hours (Buchanan et al 1973). Absorption is quicker with syrup preparations.

Drug distribution and plasma protein binding

Plasma protein binding of ethosuximide is negligible and therefore the drug is present in saliva and CSF in concentrations which approximate

Table 12.7 Summary of pharmacokinetic data on ethosuximide

Range of daily maintenance dosage	Adult: 500–1500 mg/day Child: 10–15 mg/kg/day
Minimum dose frequency	Once daily
Time to peak serum level	1–4 h
Percentage bound to plasma proteins	Negligible
Apparent volume of distribution	0.7 l/kg
Major metabolites (inactive)	2 (1-hydroxyethyl)-2-methylsuccinimide 2-(2-hydroxyethyl)-2-methylsuccinimide 2-acetyl-2-methylsuccinimide
Elimination half-life	Adult: 40–70 h Child: 20–40 h
Time to steady state after starting therapy	Up to 14 days (adult) Up to 7 days (child)

to that of plasma (McAuliffe et al 1977). Ethosuximide appears to be distributed throughout body water, without much selective regional concentration. It crosses the placenta to the fetus rapidly and ethosuximide concentrations in breast milk are about 94% of the plasma levels (Kaneko et al 1979).

Metabolism and urinary excretion

Ethosuximide is extensively metabolized to two hydroxylated metabolites and a ketone derivative. These are largely excreted as glucuronides. Only 10–20% of the drug is excreted unchanged in the urine.

Elimination half-life and dose interval

The elimination half-life is longer in adults than children, but at all ages is long enough for once daily administration to be feasible (Buchanan et al 1976). However, with larger doses, gastrointestinal adverse effects may make divided dosing preferable.

Dose–serum concentration relationship

Although there is some evidence that the dose–serum concentration relationship may not be linear over the therapeutic range it is not sufficient to have important practical implications for prescribing of ethosuximide. A daily dose of 20 mg/kg yields a serum level of about 450 μmol/l (65 μg/ml) on average (Browne et al 1975).

Concentration–effect relationship

There is good evidence from clinical studies that control of absence seizures is related to the plasma level of the drug and that most patients require a level in the range 200–700 μmol/l (40–100 μg/ml) to achieve optimal control, although some patients may benefit from increased doses to produce levels of 850 μmol/l (120 μg/ml) or more (Sherwin et al 1973, Sherwin 1982). There does not appear to be a clear relationship between serum levels and adverse effects. Saliva levels of ethosuximide are an alternative way of monitoring ethosuximide therapy in children.

Drug interactions

Because ethosuximide does not bind to plasma proteins and does not induce hepatic microsomal enzymes the number of documented interactions with other drugs is relatively small, and most are of little clinical importance (Perucca & Richens 1980, 1985). Occasionally, addition of valproate to a patient's ethosuximide therapy has caused elevation of plasma ethosuximide levels resulting in toxicity. Also, when enzyme inducing drugs such as carbamazepine are given concurrently, higher doses of ethosuximide may be required to achieve the same plasma ethosuximide levels.

Toxicity

Ethosuximide has a relatively good record regarding incidence of adverse effects. Most problems relate to the acute dose-related side-effects, such as nausea, abdominal discomfort, drowsiness, anorexia and headache. Nausea is the most common adverse effect and usually occurs within the first few days of ethosuximide administration. It frequently responds to dose reduction. Ethosuximide has also been reported to cause exacerbation of various types of seizures, particularly tonic-clonic convulsions. However, because tonic-clonic seizures occur at some time during the course of absence seizures in about 25% of patients it is difficult to be sure whether the tonic-clonic seizures were coincidental or causally related to the ethosuximide therapy. Behavioural and cognitive adverse effects have been ascribed to ethosuximide including psychotic episodes, but it is difficult to be sure about how frequently this occurs from the reported studies. They may be a manifestation of drug intoxication.

Skin reactions

Skin rashes have been frequently described with ethosuximide and include erythema multiforme and the Stevens-Johnson syndrome. They usually remit on discontinuation of the drug. Systemic lupus erythematosus-like syndromes have been reported in association with ethosuximide administration.

Haematological toxicity

Blood dyscrasias have been reported with ethosuximide but are very rare.

Teratogenicity

There is little information available regarding the risk to the fetus exposed to ethosuximide.

Phensuximide and methsuximide (Porter et al 1977)

Phensuximide is less potent than ethosuximide and its clinical use is declining. Methsuximide's antiepileptic activity rests almost entirely with its metabolite, N-desmethyl-methsuximide. It is used relatively little compared with ethosuximide.

BENZODIAZEPINES

The 1,4-benzodiazepines were first synthesized in 1933. They have antiepileptic activity in addition to tranquillizing and hypnotic effects. They are the most potent agents for the emergency treatment of status epilepticus but their value in the long-term treatment of epilepsy is severely limited by their adverse effects of sedation and psycho-motor retardation; the development of tolerance to their antiepileptic effects; and by the problem of withdrawal reactions. There is some evidence that clobazam, a 1,5-benzodiazepine, impairs psychomotor performance less than the 1,4-benzo-diazepines, but it suffers from the other draw-backs of this class of drug.

The individual benzodiazepine drugs which are most frequently used in the clinical management of epilepsy will be selected for discussion.

Structure

The structures of two important benzodiazepine drugs used in the treatment of epilepsy, diazepam and clonazepam, are shown in Figure 12.12.

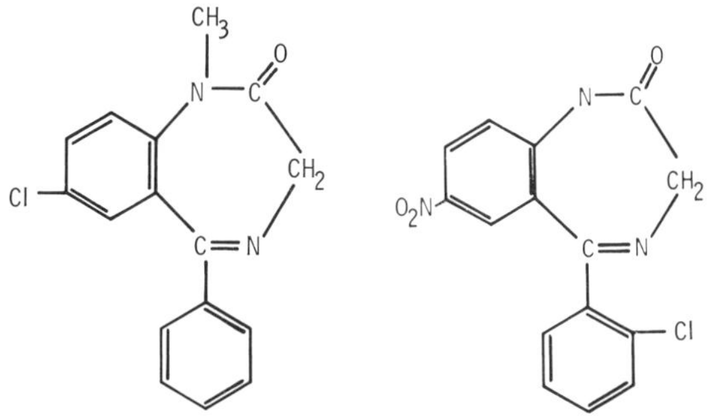

Fig. 12.12 Structure of diazepam and clonazepam

Mechanism of action

The major inhibitory neurotransmitter in the mammalian brain, gamma-aminobutyric acid (GABA) exerts its effects through increased permeability of the post-synaptic membrane to chloride ions, resulting in hyperpolarization of the neurone. The GABA receptor and associated chloride ion channel appear to be part of a protein complex which contains receptor sites for GABA, benzodiazepines and picrotoxin/barbiturates as well as the chloride ionophore. It is thought that many of the actions of benzodiazepines, particu-larly the antiepileptic effects, occur by modu-lation of the postsynaptic responses to GABA. Benzodiazepines bind to highly specific receptor sites at the GABA receptor complex and thereby augment the inhibitory effects of GABA itself. (For reviews see Squires & Braestrup 1977, Haefely 1980, Olsen 1981).

Pharmacokinetics

Tables 12.8, 12.9 and 12.10 summarize the main pharmacokinetic properties of diazepam, clona-zepam and clobazam (Mandelli et al 1978, Richens 1983).

Diazepam

When given orally, diazepam is rapidly absorbed with peak plasma concentrations occurring within

Table 12.8 Summary of pharmacokinetic data on diazepam and its N-desmethyl metabolite

	Diazepam	*N-Desmethyldiazepam*
Range of daily adult maintenance dosage	5–60 mg/day	
Minimum dose frequency	twice daily	
Time to peak serum level (oral)	0.5–2 h	
Percentage bound to plasma proteins	97%	97%
Apparent volume of distribution	1–2 l/kg	
Major active metabolite	N-desmethyyl-diazepam Temazepam Oxazepam	Oxazepam
Inactive metabolites	Conjugated derivatives	Conjugated derivatives
Elimination half-life	20–60 h	30–90 h
Time to steady state after starting therapy		Up to 20 days

Table 12.9 Summary of pharmacokinetic data on clonazepam

Range of daily adult maintenance dosage	1–10 mg/day
Minimum dose frequency	Once daily
Time to peak serum level (oral)	1–3 h
Percentage bound to plasma proteins	85%
Apparent volume of distribution	2–5 l/kg
Inactive metabolites	7-aminoclonazepam 7-acetaminoclonazepam
Elimination half-life	20–60 h
Time to steady state after starting therapy	Up to 14 days

Table 12.10 Summary of pharmacokinetic data on clobazam

Range of daily adult maintenance dosage	20–60 mg/daily
Minimum dose frequency	Once daily
Time to peak serum level (oral)	1–4 h
Percentage bound to plasma proteins	Approx. 90%
Apparent volume of distribution	?
Elimination half-life	18 h (42 h N-desmethylclobazam)
Active metabolite	N-desmethylclobazam
Time to steady state after starting therapy	Up to 4 weeks for N-desmethyclobazam 1 week for clobazam

30–90 minutes (Hillestad et al 1974, Gamble et al 1975). Although the presence of food in the stomach delays oral absorption, the extent of absorption may actually increase (Greenblatt et al 1978). Diazepam is very insoluble in water and is prepared for parenteral use in a vehicle which is irritant and often causes local thrombophlebitis on intravenous administration. There is a preparation in an emulsion form which is less irritant. The drug will come out of solution if it is diluted with small amounts of saline but it may be diluted with large amounts for intravenous infusion. However, administration of diazepam by intravenous in-

fusion is not altogether satisfactory because diazepam and its active metabolite, N-desmethyldiazepam accumulate and prolonged coma can result. It also adsorbs on to the intravenous tubing. When given intramuscularly, its absorption is slow and unreliable (Hillestad et al 1974, Gamble et al 1975, Kanto 1975) and it is therefore inadvisable to administer diazepam by this route for the emergency treatment of status epilepticus where a rapid effect is required. The absorption of diazepam solution from the rectum is rapid and peak serum levels occur within 6–10 minutes in most patients (Knudsen 1977, Dulac et al 1978, Meberg et al 1978, Milligan et al 1981). Rectal diazepam can be used prophylactically for febrile convulsions but is less satisfactory than in travenous diazepam for the treatment of acute convulsions (Knudsen 1979). Suppositories of diazepam are much more slowly and erratically absorbed and produce lower serum levels.

Following intravenous diazepam, drug distribution to body tissues is rapid. Peak brain concentrations are seen within 1–5 minutes. The apparent volume of distribution is 1–2 l/kg. It is highly bound to plasma proteins (approx. 97%) and CSF and salivary concentrations correspond to the free serum diazepam concentrations.

Diazepam is extensively metabolized by demethylation and hydroxylation. Its major metabolite, N-desmethyldiazepam, is pharmacologically active and accumulates because it has a longer half-life than the parent drug. The hydroxylated derivatives of diazepam and N-desmethyldiazepam are temazepam and oxazepam, which are both pharmacologically active but have short half-lives. All three metabolites are conjugated with glucuronic acid and excreted in the urine. Only traces of the parent drug are eliminated unchanged. The long half-life of diazepam (20–60 h) and N-desmethyldiazepam (30–90 h) allows the drug to be administered once daily. However, when larger doses are given, the sudden rise in serum concentration may cause adverse effects and divided dosage may then be preferable. The half-life is reduced in patients on enzyme-inducing antiepileptic drugs and may be prolonged in the elderly and in patients with liver disease. Diazepam itself does not significantly induce hepatic enzymes.

Clonazepam (Pinder et al 1976)

Clonazepam is fairly rapidly absorbed with peak serum levels at 1–3 hours. It distributes to body tissues equally rapidly and is approximately 85% bound to plasma proteins. It is extensively metabolised to 7-aminoclonazepam and 7-acetaminoclonazepam, both of which are inactive. The elimination half-life of clonazepam is 20–60 hours in adults so that once daily dosing is possible. Clearance of the drug is more rapid in children. Enzyme-inducing antiepileptic drugs, e.g. phenytoin can lower serum clonazepam concentrations.

Clobazam (Schmidt, 1984a)

In humans, clobazam is virtually completely absorbed after oral administration with peak plasma levels within 1–4 hours. It is 90% protein bound. The terminal half-life of elimination of the parent compound is approximately 18 hours. The major metabolite is N-desmethylclobazam which is active but has considerably less potency than the parent drug. The elimination half-life of the N-desmethyl metabolite is much longer than that of the parent compound (approximately 42 h). The metabolism of clobazam is induced by concomitant antiepileptic medication (Jawad et al 1984).

Serum concentration–effect relationship

Tolerance occurs to the therapeutic effects of the benzodiazepines. Diazepam has been used principally in the emergency treatment of status epilepticus and should not normally be used for the long-term treatment of chronic epilepsy. Thus there is little data on therapeutic serum concentrations in chronic use of diazepam. Clonazepam has been used more extensively in the chronic treatment of epilepsy as well as in the acute therapy of status epilepticus. The correlation between plasma concentrations and therapeutic effect has been found to be somewhat variable although levels greater than >100 nmol/l (0.03 μg/ml) are recommended. In view of the development of receptor tolerance, the value of serum level monitoring is unlikely to be great.

There may also be technical difficulties in the actual measurement of the low plasma concentrations of the drug giving rise to misleading values. Intermittent therapy with benzodiazepines in chronic epilepsy may be valuable and avoid the development of tolerance, e.g. in catamenial epilepsy (Feely et al, 1982).

Adverse reactions to benzodiazepines

Adverse reactions such as drowsiness, ataxia, dizziness and behavioural changes occur commonly at the beginning of treatment. Irritability, inattention, sedation and hypotonia are more common in children. These dose-related adverse effects tend to lessen with the duration of treatment because of the development of tolerance. Older patients do appear to be more sensitive to the effects of benzodiazepines. There may be additive effects on the central nervous system when benzodiazepines are administered with other sedating drugs or alcohol. Clobazam may cause less psychomotor impairment than the 1,4-benzodiazepines but otherwise it seems to share all the other adverse features. There is little evidence for haematological, hepatic or renal toxicity of the benzodiazepines. Occasionally, skin rashes occur.

Teratogenicity has been reported with diazepam in particular an increased risk of cleft palate, but the evidence is far from conclusive.

Dependence develops with benzodiazepines and in adults, agitation, anxiety, insomnia, tremor, hallucinosis and tonic-clonic seizures have been seen in relation to diazepam withdrawal. A neonatal withdrawal syndrome has also been reported in newborn babies who have been exposed to long-term benzodiazepine treatment in utero.

When benzodiazepines are given intravenously for the emergency treatment of seizures the most serious adverse effects are respiratory depression, hypotension and cardiac arrest. The incidence of such problems is low, but equipment and personnel prepared for cardiopulmonary resuscitation should be available. Newborns of mothers who have been given a dose of diazepam in the 24 hours preceding delivery may have transient respiratory depression, hypotension and poor feeding.

TROXIDONE

Troxidone (trimethadione) is an oxazolidinedione drug used primarily in the treatment of absence seizures. Over recent years its use has declined because of the greater clinical efficacy of ethosuximide and sodium valproate in absence seizures.

Mechanism of action

The mechanism of action of troxidone and its active metabolite, dimethadione remains unknown.

Pharmacokinetics (Withrow 1982)

Troxidone is rapidly and almost completely converted in vivo to dimethadione which because of its very slow excretion rate accumulates in large quantities during chronic troxidone therapy. Dimethadione concentrations in plasma are about 20 times higher than the parent compound.

Although troxidone itself can protect against seizures, it is thought that the dimethadione active metabolite accounts for most of the antiseizure effects of troxidone treatment. Because of the long half-life of dimethadione it could probably be given once daily, although traditionally it is prescribed in divided doses. It may take several weeks for plasma concentrations of dimethadione to reach steady state.

Plasma concentration-seizure control relationship

Retrospective studies indicate that most patients whose absence seizures are controlled by the drug have concentrations of dimethadione, the active metabolite, greater than 5400 μmol/l (700 μg/ml) (Jensen 1962, Booker 1982). There is often delay in response of two weeks or more because it takes such a long time for dimethadione levels to reach steady state.

Toxicity

The known complications of troxidone therapy were summarized by Wells (1957) and little has been added since. Most of the adverse effects on the central nervous system are dose dependent and reversible. Day blindness and photophobia are the most common side-effects. Sedation, lack of concentration, dizziness and ataxia are recognized problems; and insomnia, confusion and psychotic reactions have also been reported. The milder reactions can usually be controlled by dose reduction. Skin reactions are common and include serious eruptions such as erythema multiforme and exfoliative dermatitis. The most serious adverse drug reactions include bone marrow depression, and fatal pancytopenia has been reported. Maternal ingestion of troxidone has been closely linked with an increased incidence of fetal anomalies, sometimes so characteristic that the term 'fetal trimethadione syndrome' has been applied (Feldman et al 1977). The evidence for teratogenicity of trimethadione is stronger than for any other antiepileptic drug and thus its use in pregnancy is absolutely contraindicated.

Indications for use

It would appear from clinical trials that troxidone is a less effective drug for the treatment of absence seizures than ethosuximide and sodium valproate. In view of the serious adverse effects of troxidone its use should seldom be necessary.

PART TWO
GENERAL PRINCIPLES IN THE DRUG TREATMENT OF EPILEPSY

WHEN TO START ANTIEPILEPTIC DRUGS?

It is essential that before antiepileptic drug therapy is started a correct diagnosis is made. A clear distinction between epileptic and non-epileptic attacks is of major importance because the attachment of the label of 'epilepsy' to a person has grave medical, therapeutic and social implications that will greatly influence his future life. When diagnostic difficulty persists despite appropriate investigations, it is often the best course to let time make matters clear. Therapeutic trials of antiepileptic drugs in cases of doubt are rarely justified and often only make the management of the patient more difficult. An erroneous diagnosis of epilepsy is a frequent cause of treatment failure.

The variable prognosis of epilepsy makes it difficult to decide when to start drug treatment in the individual patient or indeed when to stop it. The clinical management of epilepsy is based as much on empirical practice as on scientific evidence. It is not certain to what extent antiepileptic drug therapy alters the outcome of seizure states – do the drugs control fits or do they cure the underlying disorder (Chadwick & Reynolds, 1985)?

The decision to start treatment in an individual patient should take into account not only the number of attacks experienced but also, the circumstances in which they occurred, the presence or absence of precipitating factors; the type and severity of the attacks; whether or not there are any accompanying neurological, psychiatric or social problems; and whether the patient wants treatment.

There are no hard and fast rules but most neurologists in the UK would not recommend treatment after a single tonic-clonic seizure. In the United States, there is a greater tendency to start drug therapy after single seizures, although this may be primarily for medicolegal reasons. The reports on the prognosis of a single untreated seizure are conflicting, and this is probably due to variation in the delay between the occurrence of the first seizure and the time of medical review. In their retrospective general practice study, Goodridge & Shorvon (1983) found that a single seizure was followed by others in 80% of patients; whereas some hospital studies have reported lower recurrence rates of 27% and 38% (Hauser et al 1982, Cleland et al 1981). A study of prognosis after a first untreated tonic-clonic seizure (Elwes et al 1985) showed that the cumulative probability of recurrence was 20% by one month, 28% by two months, 32% by three months, 46% by six months, 62% by one year and 71% by three and four years. Thus further seizures appeared to be likely to occur in the majority of patients after a single seizure. The risk of recurrence is greatest in the first month and declines from then on.

Although most doctors would not treat an isolated seizure, if two or more seizures occur within a short time interval, e.g. one year, antiepileptic drug treatment is generally considered advisable. Nevertheless, there is considerable variation in practice, because no studies exist on the clinical course of untreated epilepsy. The risk of recurrence is greater after two seizures than after one (Hauser et al 1982). Generally, the longer seizures continue during treatment, the less likely are patients to go into remission (Elwes et al 1984). This supports the view of Gowers (1881) that epilepsy tends to escalate and would lend support to the idea that seizures should be suppressed by treatment as soon as possible (Reynolds et al 1983). However, it is by no means certain that drug therapy can alter the predetermined course of a patient's epilepsy. It may be that there are some patients who have only a mild tendency to fits and others who have inherently more severe epilepsy. There is no definite evidence yet that the prognosis of the latter group of patients can be modified by drugs. Shorvon et al (1985) call for placebo-controlled trials of antiepileptic drugs to be performed in newly diagnosed patients with epilepsy in order to resolve this issue. If antiepileptic drug treatment does prevent subsequent evolution to chronic epilepsy, then the use of such drugs is imperative. If, however, it is shown that treatment merely suppresses the fits without any fundamental effect on the disease process itself, then in selected patients with less severe epilepsy, the self-limiting nature of the disease would make routine drug treatment unnecessary.

DRUG TREATMENT OF THE EPILEPSIES

There is a lack of agreement as to choice of drugs for the different seizure disorders. This is because there is a paucity of scientific evidence on which to base rational choice. In a review of 250 antiepileptic drug trials, Coatsworth (1971) first documented and emphasized the inadequacies of almost all studies up until then. Although the general quality of clinical trials has improved

Table 12.11 Drug treatment of seizures based on an abbreviated version of the International Classification of Epileptic Seizures (Gastaut 1970)

Types of seizure	Drugs of choice

1. Partial Seizures
  i. With elementary symptomatology (focal motor, sensory & autonomic)
  ii. With complex symptomatology (impaired consciousness & cognitive, affective, psychosensory & psychomotor symptomatology)
  iii. Becoming secondarily generalised (focal seizure leading to tonic-clonic seizure)
	Carbamazepine
	Phenytoin
	Sodium valproate
	Primidone
	Phenobarbitone

2. Generalized Seizures (seizures which do not produce clinical manifestations referable to part of one hemisphere) i. absences	Sodium valproate Ethosuximide
ii. bilateral massive epileptic myoclonus (myoclonic jerks)	Sodium valproate Clonazepam
iii. infantile spasms	ACTH Clonazepam
iv. clonic seizures	Phenytoin Carbamazepine
v. tonic seizures	Primidone Phnenobarbitone Sodium valproate
vi. tonic-clonic seizures	
vii. atonic seizures viii. akinetic seizure	Sodium valproate Clonazepam
3. Unilateral Seizures (tonic, clonic or tonic-clonic seizures which are unilateral)	As for 2.iv–vi above

greatly since then, it is hardly surprising that in clinical practice the choice of drugs has often been based on opinion, fashion and marketing pressures. Even with the established drugs, there is insufficient information to make a completely rational choice of initial drug therapy in a newly diagnosed epileptic patient (Table 12.11).

Drugs effective in tonic-clonic and partial seizures

Tonic-clonic seizures can be primary in origin or can result from secondary generalization of a focal discharge. Drugs effective against tonic-clonic seizures are in general also active against partial seizures. However, partial seizures and generalized tonic-clonic seizures which start focally tend to show a poorer response to medical treatment.

Recent trials comparing the drugs most commonly used to treat tonic-clonic seizures allow some conclusions about relative efficacy to be made (Mattson et al 1985, Shorvon et al 1978, Callaghan et al 1985, Turnbull et al 1982, 1985). In a comparative trial by Mattson et al (1985)

carbamazepine and phenytoin gave the highest overall treatment success, with intermediate success for phenobarbitone and lowest for primidone. Primidone's poor performance was mainly due to a high incidence of intolerable acute adverse effects. Control of tonic-clonic seizures did not differ significantly between the four drugs but carbamazepine provided complete control of partial seizures more frequently than primidone or phenobarbitone. The authors recommended carbamazepine or phenytoin as drugs of first choice for single-drug therapy of adults with partial and/or generalized tonic-clonic seizures. Unfortunately, sodium valproate was not one of the test drugs included in this study.

However, Turnbull et al (1982, 1985) found no significant difference in efficacy between phenytoin and sodium valproate in a group of newly diagnosed patients with epilepsy. Similar results were obtained by Callaghan et al (1985) in their prospective study between carbamazepine, phenytoin and sodium valproate. The success rate for medical treatment of patients with partial seizures seems consistently lower than for those with primary generalized tonic-clonic seizures. However,

Chadwick & Turnbull (1985) conclude that, on current evidence, it is not possible to suggest that any individual drug is preferable against the two types of seizure in adult patients.

Dose scheme for tonic-clonic and partial seizures

Once a decision has been made to treat a patient with epilepsy, one of the drugs of choice (Table 12.11) should be selected and started in a low to average dose (Table 12.12). Sufficient time should then be allowed for the serum drug level to reach steady state and for the patients response to therapy to be assessed. If the response is inadequate, the dose should be increased gradually until seizure control is achieved or until signs of drug toxicity occur. If monitoring of serum drug levels is available, the dose of drug can be adjusted more skilfully, particularly for phenytoin but, ultimately, the decision that the correct dose has been reached is largely a clinical one. If intoxication occurs before an acceptable degree of control is achieved, the best option is to change to an alternative drug, the first drug being tailed off slowly whilst gradually introducing the second. If the second drug fails, a third drug may be tried. Alternatively, a combination of two drugs can be prescribed, although it needs to be borne in mind that the addition of a second drug often fails to achieve improved control of seizures. Indeed the patient may sometimes have more fits and is at greater risk of experiencing adverse drug effects (Shorvon & Reynolds 1979, Schmidt 1982). Recent studies of monotherapy in previously untreated adolescent or adult epileptic patients

with tonic-clonic and/or partial seizures have shown a success rate of about 75% (Shorvon et al 1978).

One of the most common reasons for seizure recurrence is poor compliance with therapy (Elwes et al 1984). Sudden withdrawal of antiepileptic drug treatment may predispose to seizures, particularly with phenobarbitone or benzodiazepine therapy. The management of epilepsy in patients whose fits do not respond well to the initial drug therapy can be difficult. If the response to full doses of two drugs is inadequate, addition of a third is probably seldom justified. It may be that the drugs are actually making the patient's seizures worse or are causing unacceptable adverse effects in exchange for little therapeutic benefit. Good records of fit frequency during the period of drug therapy are invaluable and checks on compliance are also necessary. It may be difficult to assess how much benefit the patient is deriving from drug treatment when several years have elapsed since its initiation, especially if many drugs have been tried in a variety of permutations.

Recent studies have shown that reductions in drug therapy are often justified and will occasionally produce a dramatic improvement in the patient's mental state whilst at the same time not affecting, and sometimes even reducing fit frequency (Shorvon & Reynolds 1979, Fischbacher 1982, Callaghan et al 1984, Lesser et al 1984). However, such drug reductions are not without hazards and need to be done slowly and carefully to prevent withdrawal seizures during the period of drug reduction. Occasionally, a

Table 12.12 Satisfactory starting dose of the commonly used antiepileptic drugs in adults

Drug	Dose units available in UK (mg)	Starting dose	Range of maintenance doses (mg/day)
Phenytoin	25, 50, 100	100 mg twice daily	150–600
Carbamazepine	100, 200	100 mg twice daily	400–1800
Phenobarbitone	15, 30, 60, 100	30 mg at night	30–240
Primidone	250	125 mg at night	250–1500
Sodium valproate	200, 500	200 mg twice daily	600–3000
Ethosuximide	250	250 mg twice daily	500–1500
Troxidone	300	300 mg twice daily	900–2100
Diazepam	2, 5, 10	5 mg twice daily	5–60
Nitrazepam	5	2.5 mg twice daily	5–20
Clonazepam	0.5, 2	0.5 mg twice daily	1–10

patient who has been well controlled on combination therapy may relapse when converted to monotherapy and control may not be regained despite return to polytherapy. A message from such experience is that it is more difficult to reduce polytherapy than to avoid it in the first place.

Drugs effective in absence seizures

The two major drugs for the treatment of absence seizures are ethosuximide and sodium valproate. Clinical trials have shown them to be equally effective, with success rates approaching 100% in patients with simple classical absence seizures (Suzuki et al 1972, Callaghan et al 1982, Sato et al 1982). The response is less impressive in patients with atypical absence seizures and the Lennox-Gastaut syndrome. An advantage of sodium valproate over ethosuximide is that it is also effective against tonic-clonic seizures so that in patients with coexisting absences and tonic-clonic fits sodium valproate would be the initial treatment of choice. Troxidone appears less effective than either sodium valproate or ethosuximide and is seldom used. In patients who fail to respond to sodium valproate and ethosuximide given alone, the combination of the two may prove effective. Long-term benzodiazepine therapy has been used to treat absence seizures but usually in patients whose seizures have not been controlled by other antiepileptic drugs and have had a benzodiazepine added to their other medication. A number of studies report a beneficial effect of benzodiazepines, but there are major deficiencies in most of the trials, e.g. lack of uniformity of seizure type in the patients described, small numbers of patients, lack of blind techniques. The major disadvantages of benzodiazepines in the treatment of absence seizures are the marked sedative effects and the development of tolerance to the antiepileptic effect. Thus benzodiazepines should not normally be used to treat absence seizures.

Dose scheme for the management of absence seizures

Sodium valproate should be started in a dose of 10 mg/kg/day and this can be increased according to clinical response to approximately 30 mg/kg/day in children. Occasionally, higher doses of 40–60 mg/kg/day are required in refractory absence seizures provided there is no evidence of drug toxicity. Because of its short half-life, sodium valproate is usually administered as two or three divided doses to minimize fluctuations in serum levels. However, this practice has been questioned in the light of evidence that the pharmacodynamic effect of the drug is prolonged. Indeed, studies have shown the equivalence, or even superiority of, a single daily dose over divided dosing schedules. There is no greater incidence of toxicity and administration as a single daily dose aids compliance.

The value of the measurement of serum levels of valproic acid to assist in adjustment of dose is controversial (see p. 439). If sodium valproate fails to control the absence attacks, ethosuximide should be substituted. It should be started in a dose of 10 mg/kg and increased until seizure control is achieved. Serum level monitoring of ethosuximide can be helpful in selection of the correct dose. If ethosuximide in full dose is not effective then the combination of ethosuximide and sodium valproate should be tried, as this has been shown to be effective in some refractory patients (Rowan et al 1983). If the seizures are still not controlled either troxidone or a benzodiazepine such as clonazepam can be used. The EEG can be very useful in the assessment of response to treatment in patients with absence seizures. Clinical response correlates well with the reduction in number of spike-wave paroxysms on the EEG.

Treatment of myoclonic epilepsies

The myoclonic epilepsies of early childhood represent a heterogeneous group of disorders. In infantile spasms, ACTH or corticosteroid therapy has become a conventional form of treatment and there is good evidence that an immediate improvement in the clinical and electroencephalographic abnormalities occurs (Jeavons & Bower 1974, Hrachovy et al 1979). There seems to be little difference in the efficacy of the two treatments but there is general agreement that the long-term prognosis is not influenced by this treatment and is usually poor (Jeavons & Bower 1974, Pollack et al 1979).

Of the other myoclonic epilepsies, there are those which are notoriously drug resistant, such as the Lennox-Gastaut syndrome; while others are more amenable to therapy, such as true myoclonic epilepsy or myoclonic epilepsy of childhood. The coexistence of atonic-akinetic seizures in general signifies a more resistant epilepsy. Head-nodding attacks, atypical absences or tonic-clonic fits may occur in addition.

In general, myoclonic phenomena respond best to treatment with a benzodiazepine drug, sodium valproate or ethosuximide. Six large studies reviewed by Browne & Penry (1973) reported a 50% or greater reduction in myoclonic seizure frequency in 36–100% of patients treated with chlordiazepoxide, diazepam or nitrazepam. Studies in which the latter two drugs have been compared indicate that nitrazepam is equal in efficacy or perhaps slightly superior to diazepam.

A number of uncontrolled reports has been published describing the use of clonazepam in myoclonic epilepsies and the results have been uniformly favourable (Pinder et al 1976, Browne 1976). Atonic-akinetic seizures also appear to benefit (Pinder et al 1976).

A satisfactory comparative study of the response of myoclonic epilepsies to clonazepam and to sodium valproate has not been performed. Sodium valproate, however, appears to be of a similar efficacy to benzodiazepine drugs (Jeavons et al 1977). Patients with myoclonic epilepsy of childhood or adolescence seem to do best; those with Lennox-Gastaut syndrome did less well, although half derived considerable benefit which is worthwhile in such a notoriously drug-resistant condition.

Other drugs such as phenytoin, phenobarbitone and primidone are used in myoclonic and akinetic epilepsies, particularly when other types of fit co-exist, but no controlled trials of these drugs have been performed. On the whole, the response of myclonic seizures to these drugs is poor.

Treatment of photosensitive epilepsy

Drug treatment is only one aspect of management of photosensitive epilepsy (see p. 275). Sodium valproate would appear to be the drug of first choice in patients with photically induced seizures and the majority of such patients achieve complete seizure control (Harding et al 1978). Clonazepam is also effective but is more sedative (Nanda et al 1977).

Value of the EEG in regulating therapy

The EEG is invaluable as an aid to identify the type of seizures from which a patient is suffering and therefore in enabling a logical choice of drug to be made. As a guide to the regulation of therapy, however, it is less useful. It should be remembered that the routine clinical EEG records cerebral activity for a period of only 30 minutes or so during a patient's waking day, and on one occasion the recording may coincide with a period of normal electrical activity and on the next day with an episode of disturbed function. Single records may therefore be unhelpful or even misleading. This has been noted in a number of therapeutic trials, but particularly when carbamazepine has been the drug under study (Cereghino et al 1974). Even prolonged EEG telemetry has failed to show a correlation between the clinical and EEG response to carbamazepine (Rodin et al 1974). When assessing the efficacy of a new drug in an individual patient it is the improvement in seizure control which is important, not changes in EEG activity, which may or may not parallel the changes in the patient's clinical condition.

On the other hand, the improvement in the incidence of absences produced by ethosuximide therapy is accompanied closely by a reduction in the number of spike-waves paroxysms in the EEG (Penry et al 1972). Thus, when treating patients with absence seizures, the EEG can be a very useful monitor of drug therapy.

Hazards of polytherapy

A survey of four European countries by Guelen et al (1975) found that among 11 700 patients from 15 centres, the mean number of drugs per patient was 3.2 of which 84% were antiepileptic. It would seem likely that such figures are representative of the situation in most developed countries. Many factors contribute to the evolution of polytherapy. By its nature, epilepsy is often a chronic disorder and in those patients with chronic drug-resistant epilepsy, the natural response to this is to add more drugs. Traditional approaches to drug treatment often included commencement of a patient on two drugs at presentation and the addition of more drugs when the initial drugs failed.

However, awareness of the hazards of poly-pharmacy in epilepsy has increased in recent years (Shorvon & Reynolds 1979). The points against this type of management are that drug toxicity and interactions become increasingly common as the number of drugs administered increases; the difficulty in identifying the cause of an adverse reaction becomes greater; and errors in drug dosing and deliberate non-compliance become frequent. Although the therapeutic effects of several drugs may be additive, so are the toxic effects.

Thus it is desirable that polypharmacy is avoided and that, wherever possible, one antiepileptic drug should be used alone (Reynolds & Shorvon 1981). However, 20–25% of patients developing epilepsy will not have their seizures adequately controlled by one drug and combinations of two drugs may therefore be necessary, but only rarely should three drugs be used together.

Factors carrying a poor prognosis for successful therapy

There appear to be some patients with epilepsy who prove to be highly resistant to drug treatment (Rodin 1968, Shorvon & Reynolds 1982). However, these patients probably only account for about 20% of all patients presenting with seizures and they are over-represented in specialist epilepsy clinics. Features associated with a poor prognosis include: additional neurological or psychosocial handicap; partial seizure types; mixed seizures; and symptomatic epilepsy. Initial response to treatment may also be determined by the number of seizures prior to the onset of therapy. It is not clear whether this is due to these patients having more severe epilepsy to start with or whether the occurrence of seizures renders more seizures likely as suggested by Gowers in 1881.

Compliance with antiepileptic therapy

It is well recognized that poor compliance is a major reason for drug failure. It may also precipitate status epilepticus and the phenomenon of sudden unexpected death in epilepsy. Peterson et al (1982) identified the following key determinants of patient compliance with antiepileptic drug therapy: concern about health; generalized tonic-clonic seizures; and the absence of barriers to compliance. They have also shown that strategies to improve compliance, such as counselling, special medication containers, self-recording of medication intake and seizures etc, could be effective and lead to a reduction in seizure frequency (Peterson et al 1984). The recent trend towards monotherapy is obviously an aid towards patient compliance. Whenever possible, drugs should be prescribed to be taken once or twice daily rather than three or four times a day. Regular review of patients' treatment is helpful and rationalization of the treatment regime can greatly improve compliance. Serum drug level monitoring can be helpful when poor compliance is suspected.

WHEN TO STOP ANTIEPILEPTIC DRUGS

The fact that antiepileptic drugs are not without toxic effects is a strong argument for considering drug withdrawal in epileptic patients who have achieved remissions from their seizures for several years. The benefits of drug withdrawal have to be balanced against the consequences of seizure recurrence, particularly for driving and employment. The clinical practice between specialists varies greatly on the subject of drug withdrawal. Most paediatricians are keen to try and withdraw drugs early, whereas adult neurologists tend to be more cautious because of the potential problems of loss of driving licence and dismissal from employment.

Several studies have been performed to determine the factors influencing the success of drug withdrawal in epileptic patients and they have been reviewed by Chadwick (1985). Overall it appears that approximately one-third of patients who have 2–3 years remission from seizures will have recurrence of seizures on drug withdrawal and most seizures will occur during drug reduction or within the first year after stopping drugs. The patients most at risk of relapse appear to be those with the most severe fits and the longest duration of epilepsy. Relapse of primary generalized seizures including absences is rare. Patients with secondary generalized seizures, partial seizures and mixed seizure types appear to be at greatest risk. The presence of a neuropsychiatric abnormality or structural cerebral disorder are adverse prognostic factors (Juul-Jensen 1964, Holowach et al 1972). The value of electroencephalographic abnormalities in predicting the likelihood of relapse is controversial (Emerson et al 1981, Thurston et al 1982, Juul-Jensen 1968, Janz & Sommer-Burkhardt 1975, Holowach et al 1972).

There are many unanswered questions about the correct policy for drug withdrawal. The best advice at present is that drug withdrawal should be considered in all patients who have been completely fit-free for at least two years. Favourable prognostic factors include primary generalized seizures of relatively short duration without any evidence of neuropsychiatric disorder and a normal EEG. In all patients, informed consent must be obtained after thorough discussion. Weight must be given to the patient's occupation and whether they currently hold a driving licence. If a decision is taken to withdraw antiepileptic medication then this should be done very slowly, probably over six months or longer to prevent seizures arising in close association with drug withdrawal.

ANTIEPILEPTIC DRUG PROPHYLAXIS FOLLOWING HEAD INJURY AND NEUROSURGERY

Only a small percentage of patients who sustain a significant head injury will suffer from fits once they have recovered from the acute stage of the illness. But, because head injuries occur so frequently, there are a considerable number of patients with late post-traumatic epilepsy in the community and fits are a serious cause of long-term morbidity after head injury. The incidence of epilepsy varies according to the nature of the injury. More than 50% of the patients have their first fit within a year of the head injury but the onset of epilepsy may be delayed by several years. Risk factors for the development of late onset epilepsy (i.e. fits occurring after the first week following head injury) have been evaluated (Jennett 1975). Important predictive factors are: the presence of a depressed skull fracture, the development of early epilepsy (within the first week); and the need to evacuate an intracranial haematoma within two weeks of the injury. However, the place of prophylactic antiepileptic drug therapy in the management of such patients, especially those at high risk of developing post-traumatic epilepsy, is far from clear. Will the use of drugs early after the cerebral insult prevent the development of an epileptic focus? Which drugs should be used and in what dose? When should they be started and for how long should they be administered?

A study by Young et al (1983a) in which 244 patients were randomly assigned to either phenytoin or placebo within 24 hours after head injury failed to show any significant beneficial effect of phenytoin on the incidence of early post-traumatic seizures. A further paper by these authors, looking at the incidence of late epilepsy in this same group of patients failed to show any effect on late seizures either. However, patient compliance was not good in this second study and the serum phenytoin concentrations were often low (Young et al, 1983b). If those patients who develop early fits are excluded from analysis, the incidence of late seizures is relatively low and therefore clinical trials with large numbers of patients (2000) would be necessary in order to prove the efficacy of antiepileptic drug therapy in the prevention of late post-traumatic epilepsy (McQueen et al 1983). Thus the benefit of routine prescription of antiepileptic drugs in severely head-injured patients remains uncertain and any treatment policy for long-term prophylaxis has to consider the likely high level of non-compliance with the drug regime, the risks of adverse drug effects and the uncertain benefit conferred on a group of patients with relatively low risk of developing seizures.

Similar questions arise about the efficacy of prophylactic antiepileptic drug therapy to prevent seizures following neurosurgery. The risk of developing fits following supratentorial procedures for non-traumatic pathology is well recognized and has led to many neurosurgeons giving routine antiepileptic prophylaxis. A retrospective study defined the overall risk of seizures as 17% but it varies according to the condition for which the patient had surgery (Foy et al 1981). Studies of antiepileptic prophylaxis have given mixed results (North et al 1983, Shaw et al 1983) and there is need for larger placebo-controlled studies to determine whether such policies really are of benefit.

PROPHYLAXIS OF FEBRILE CONVULSIONS

Febrile convulsions are discussed in detail in Chapter 4. About 4% of children have a febrile convulsion and in most of them simple febrile convulsions do not lead to epilepsy or produce neurological or learning deficits. There is a small risk that if further febrile convulsions occur, they may be severe or prolonged with the risk of causing structural damage in the temporal lobe leading to chronic epilepsy. Febrile convulsions are, however, a distressing experience for the child and his family. The fits recur in 30–40% of patients. Measures to reduce pyrexia during febrile episodes are essential – increasing fluid intake, removal of clothes and administration of aspirin or paracetamol – but the place of prophylactic treatment with antiepileptic drugs is still under debate (Editorial 1980, 1981). It is clear that certain anticonvulsants, if taken properly, will prevent recurrent febrile convulsions. Well-controlled trials comparing daily phenobarbitone therapy with no treatment or intermittent treatment have established its efficacy in the prevention of recurrent febrile convulsions (Wolf et al 1977) and several studies with continuous sodium valproate medication have shown that it is equally effective (Ngwane & Bower 1980, Wallace & Aldridge-Smith 1980, Lee & Melchior 1981, Herranz et al 1984). However, phenytoin and carbamazepine have been shown to be ineffective (Melchior et al 1971, Bacon et al 1981, Antony & Hawke 1983). Unfortunately prophylaxis with both phenobarbitone and sodium valproate has

drawbacks. There is high incidence of behaviour disorders in children treated with phenobarbitone and it is likely to impair learning ability (Wolf & Forsythe 1978). Consequently, compliance with therapy may be low. Sodium valproate is less frequently associated with adverse effects but there is the rare but very serious problem of hepatotoxicity. Thus neither drug is ideal for treating large numbers of apparently normal children.

An alternative approach is to give intermittent treatment whenever a child who has had a previous febrile convulsion becomes febrile. Phenobarbitone is not a suitable drug for this kind of therapy as effective serum levels are not achieved rapidly enough. Similarly, sodium valproate may have a delayed onset of action. Rectal administration of diazepam solution is satisfactory for such intermittant prophylaxis of febrile convulsions because it is rapidly absorbed and can be administered at home by a parent. Knudsen & Vestermark (1978) showed that prophylactic rectal diazepam at a temperature above 38.5°C is as effective as long-term treatment with phenobarbital. In both groups, 6% of all febrile episodes lead to new convulsions. There were no significant side-effects of such therapy. However, although such treatment strategies can reduce the frequency of subsequent febrile convulsions the risk of subsequent epilepsy does not appear to be altered.

TREATMENT OF EPILEPSY IN DISEASE STATES

Most of the reported pharmacokinetic studies of antiepileptic drugs have been performed in normal volunteers or in patients who were healthy apart from having epilepsy. Sometimes it is necessary to administer these drugs to patients with diseases of other systems and these diseases may alter the way in which they are handled.

Gastrointestinal disease

It is likely that the absorption of drugs can be modified in patients who have undergone gastric or small bowel surgery, or who have small bowel conditions such as coeliac disease. This possibility has been little investigated although one study showed good absorption of phenytoin and ethosuximide in a patient with a jejuno-ileal bypass (Peterson & Zweig 1974).

Hypoalbuminaemia

Changes in plasma albumin concentration can have important effects on the protein binding of some antiepileptic drugs, principally phenytoin and sodium valproate. For a given serum drug concentration, the amount of a highly bound drug which remains unbound increases as the plasma albumin falls and, because it is the latter fraction which produces the concentration gradient for drugs to enter the brain, a reduced albumin level may cause drug toxicity at apparently therapeutic serum levels. This possibility should be borne in mind if a patient shows unexpected toxicity at normal serum levels.

Liver disease (Blashke 1977, Asconape & Penry 1982)

Antiepileptic drug disposition may be altered in several ways by liver disease: (a) bioavailability may be increased because of the development of portal-systemic anastomoses in cirrhosis which may allow drugs to bypass the liver on absorption; (b) systemic metabolism may be reduced by hepatocellular disease; (c) plasma protein binding of drugs may be reduced by hypoalbuminaemia, particularly affecting highly protein- bound drugs such as phenytoin, sodium valproate and diazepam.

Renal disease (Reidenberg & Drayer 1978, Asconape & Penry 1982)

Although renal excretion plays a small part in the elimination of most antiepileptic drugs, renal failure can indirectly alter the distribution of drugs by reducing their binding to plasma proteins. The free fraction may be increased at least two-fold for phenytoin and valproate. The impaired binding may be partly due to a lowered serum albumin concentration but a more important factor is probably a change in the molecular configuration of albumin or the presence of circulating endogenous inhibitors of binding (Reiden-berg & Drayer 1978). Thus, when serum levels of phenytoin and sodium valproate are interpreted, allowance must be made for the reduced protein binding of these drugs. Phenobarbitone is cleared partly by urinary excretion, and creatinine clearance values below 30 ml/min may be associated with phenobarbitone toxicity.

Other diseases

It is likely that other diseases such as cardiac failure will alter the disposition of antiepileptic drugs but this has not been systematically studied. Acute viral infections may inhibit the metabolism of drugs, and symptoms of drug toxicity may be mistaken for symptoms of intercurrent infection. Drugs given for concomitant diseases may also influence the pharmacokinetics of antiepileptic drugs. The treatment of epilepsy in pregnancy is dealt with in Chapter 15 Part 2.

TREATMENT OF ACCOMPANYING PSYCHIATRIC DISORDERS

The various types of psychiatric disturbance which can accompany chronic epilepsy are discussed in Chapter 10. Several therapeutic problems can be encountered in treating disorders of this nature in the epileptic patient. Phenytoin, carbamazepine, phenobarbitone and primidone induce the activity of liver enzymes and this effect can result in a much more rapid turnover and excretion of drugs such as the tricyclic antidepressants and phenothiazines. The epileptic patient is likely, therefore to have therapeutically ineffective levels of these psychotropic drugs if standard doses of the latter are used. If failure occurs when treating these patients, there should be no hesitation in increasing the dose beyond the usual limits.

The convulsant activity of tricyclic antidepressants and phenothiazines is now well documented and should be borne in mind when prescribing for an epileptic patient (Betts et al 1968, Legg & Swash 1974, Edwards et al 1986). Some tricyclics appear more likely than others to precipitate fits. Of the newer drugs, maprotiline seems to be especially prone to produce convulsions.

Compliance with antiepileptic drug therapy may also be a problem in those epileptic patients with accompanying psychiatric disorders, and seizures may be precipitated by sudden withdrawal of their antiepileptic medication. Such patients are also at risk of drug overdose which may include their antiepileptic drugs. Drug coma has to be distinguished from the post-ictal state. Although these are additional problems when treating patients who also have psychiatric disorders, on no account should severe depression or psychosis go untreated.

Antiepileptic drug intoxication can present as a psychotic behaviour disorder and should be borne in mind in the differential diagnosis of this condition in the epileptic patient.

DRUG LEVELS IN THE MANAGEMENT OF EPILEPSY (Richens 1976, Reynolds 1980).

Since the development of spectrophotometric techniques for measuring phenobarbitone and phenytoin in the late 1940s and early 1950s a variety of methods have been described for estimating concentrations of these compounds. The most widely used are gas chromatography, high performance liquid chromatography and immunoassay techniques. Each method has its advantages and drawbacks (Pippenger et al 1978). Careful attention to quality control within the laboratory is necessary if the clinician is to have confidence in the results and incorrect decisions based on the results are to be avoided (Ayers et al 1980). Several inter-laboratory quality control schemes have been set up to assist the analyst to achieve accuracy (Pippenger et al 1978, Griffiths et al 1980). Whether the report is helpful to the clinican, however, depends upon the drug being measured, and the reasons for requesting a drug level.

Not all drugs are suitable for therapeutic drug monitoring. The original criteria were as follows:

1. The action of the drug in question should be reversible
2. No tolerance should occur at receptor sites
3. The drug should have no active metabolites

4. The unbound concentration of the drug in plasma should equate with the unbound drug at the receptor site
5. The therapeutic response should be clearly related to the plasma concentrations of that drug
6. The therapeutic effects of the drug should be measurable with accuracy

It was expected that most benefit would be obtained with drugs having a narrow therapeutic index. Phenytoin fulfils the above criteria and a therapeutic range of drug in plasma was suggested by Lund (1974) and confirmed clinically (Gannaway & Mawer 1981, Reynolds et al 1981). There is little doubt that the availability of plasma phenytoin assays has greatly improved the clinical use of phenytoin, which can be a difficult drug with which to deal. The same cannot be said for all the other antiepileptic drugs for which plasma concentration assays are available.

There are a number of sound reasons in clinical practice for measuring the serum level of a drug, whether an antiepileptic drug or any other compound. These should be borne in mind whenever a decision to monitor a drug is made:

1. When there is wide interindividual variation in the rate of metabolism of a drug, producing marked differences in steady state levels between patients
2. When saturation kinetics occur, causing a steep relationship between dose and serum level within the therapeutic range
3. When the therapeutic ratio of a drug is low, i.e when the therapeutic doses are close to toxic doses, most of the available antiepileptic drugs have a low ratio
4. When signs of toxicity are difficult to recognize clinically or where signs of overdosage or underdosage are indistinguishable
5. During pregnancy, or when gastrointestinal, hepatic or renal disease is present, which is likely to disturb drug absorption, metabolism or excretion
6. When patients are receiving multiple drug therapy with the attendant risk of drug interaction. If a drug is being added which is known to alter the metabolism of an existing drug, it is wise to monitor the level of the latter

7. Where there is doubt about the patient's compliance. Up to 50% of epileptic outpatients do not take what is prescribed (Mucklow & Dollery, 1978); serial samples, particularly on admission to hospital may identify these patients

8. During research studies such as controlled therapeutic trials, a correlation between the serum level of a drug and its therapeutic or toxic effect is sound evidence that the effect really is due to the drug

Obviously for research studies the decision to measure serum levels will be based on different criteria from routine estimations performed to improve the clinical management of the individual patient. Sufficient evidence from prospective studies relating serum levels and effect must be available in order that the results can be interpreted in a way that will lead to improved management. For some drugs there is little to be gained by measuring levels – indeed the clinician may be deluding himself by using an apparently scientific approach to the control of epilepsy and succeed only in treating the serum level and not the patient. Thus it is important to examine each antiepileptic drug in turn and consider the evidence for and against monitoring levels.

Phenytoin

The soundest case can be made out for measuring phenytoin levels. It is a difficult drug to use clinically and therefore most of the reasons given above for monitoring drug levels apply to phenytoin. The rate of metabolism of the drug varies widely from person to person and this is exaggerated by saturation of the enzyme system involved. There is a narrow therapeutic index, so that the therapeutic range of serum levels is close to the toxic range. Sometimes phenytoin intoxication is difficult to recognize when it presents in an unusual way such as with odd psychiatric symptoms, encephalopathy or even as increased fit frequency, and these signs may be misinterpreted as an indication for more intensive antiepileptic drug therapy. These are all compelling reasons why measurement of phenytoin serum levels is worthwhile and aids the clinical management of

epilepsy. Perhaps it would be helpful to spell out typical situations in which measuring serum phenytoin levels may be of value:

1. When fits are not controlled by greater than average doses of the drug – the important question here is whether an optimum level of drug has not been yet achieved because the patient is a rapid metaboliser or is failing to take his tablets, or whether his epilepsy is resistant to phenytoin

2. If a patient shows clinical signs of phenytoin intoxication, namely coarse nystagmus, ataxia and slurred speech, it is useful to confirm that they are drug-induced by estimating the serum level; sometimes a low or normal level may be found in a patient whose cerebellar signs are caused by cerebellar pathology rather than intoxication

3. If a patient presents with odd neuropsychiatric symptoms or dyskinetic movements; these can result from phenytoin intoxication even in the absence of nystagmus

4. If a previously well-controlled patient has a sudden increase in fit frequency; this can result from a fall in serum level (e.g. because he is failing to take his tablets) or from a rise to toxic levels (e.g. from a change in bio-availability of a formulation)

5. If another drug which might interfere with phenytoin metabolism is added to the patient's treatment

6. In the management of status epilepticus in a patient who has been receiving maintenance doses of phenytoin

7. In the management of childhood epilepsy in which dose adjustment can be more difficult

8. If the epilepsy is complicated by other diseases which might affect phenytoin handling

9. During pregnancy

The serum concentration–effect relationship is discussed on page 427. The accepted therapeutic range is 40–80 μmol/l (10–20 μ/ml). However, a number of patients with mild epilepsy will be controlled with serum levels which are below this range, and in some patients therapeutic benefit without evidence of toxicity may be achieved with levels above the therapeutic range. Thus it is essential not to stick rigidly to this range but rather to use it as a guide only when evaluating individual patients.

More recently the question of whether we should be monitoring free phenytoin serum concentrations (i.e. unbound drug concentrations) rather than total drug values has been raised. Monitoring of total plasma concentrations assumes lack of variability in plasma protein binding of a drug so that there is a constant relationship between total and free drug concentration. For phenytoin, the degree of variability of protein binding in epileptic patients without evidence of other medical disorders or co-administration of interacting drugs which alter protein binding (e.g. valproate) is probably small (Rimmer et al 1984). The currently available methods for measuring free concentrations are time consuming, expensive and insufficiently robust for routine use; the results therefore may be less reliable than measurement of total levels. In conditions such as hypoalbuminaemia, renal and liver disease and pregnancy, the free fraction of phenytoin may be considerably increased and, under these circumstances, monitoring of free serum phenytoin concentrations may be preferable. Saliva drug concentrations are an alternative, provided precautions are taken during collection to avoid contamination from orally administered drug.

In conclusion, therefore, the object in the management of phenytoin therapy should be to increase the serum concentration until fit control is achieved, whether this is at 20 μmol/l for a patient with mild epilepsy or 100 μmol/l in severe disease. A knowledge of the serum level makes it possible to achieve this optimal treatment without risk of overdosage. The therapeutic range of 40–80 μmol/l should not be used inflexibly. Serum level monitoring used sensibly and possibly in conjunction with the use of one of the various dosage nomograms available can greatly assist dosage adjustment in many patients.

Phenobarbitone

Despite the widespread availability and use of phenobarbitone assays, one of the essential criteria for the validity of monitoring is absent in the case of this drug. It is well recognized that tolerance occurs to the sedative effects (Butler 1978), such

that a low serum level produced acutely may have a much greater sedative effect than a much higher level which has been maintained chronically. It is less certain whether tolerance occurs to the antiepileptic activity. It is seen in mice (Schmidt et al 1980) but has not been formally studied in humans. Thus the relationship between serum concentration of phenobarbitone and its actions on the central nervous system may not be a constant one and probably depends on the degree of tolerance which has developed. The therapeutic range which was suggested by Buchthal et al (1968) of 40–105 μmol/l is probably too low, and the upper level depends on the degree of tolerance that the patient and the physician have for the sedative effects of the drug. In conclusion, the value of measuring phenobarbitone levels may be much less than previously thought.

Primidone

With primidone, the situation is more complicated because it is converted to two active metabolites, phenobarbitone and PEMA as well as probably being active in its own right. Thus for a full assessment it may be necessary to measure levels of all three compounds. However, for this to be justified, the relative potencies of the three compounds would need to be known so that the overall antiepileptic drug effect could be assessed. This is not possible on present evidence. The most practical approach is to monitor derived phenobarbitone.

One potential value of measuring unchanged primidone is in detecting non-compliance; for the patient who arrives at the clinic having taken the drug for only a few days beforehand will have a low ratio of phenobarbitone to primidone in his or her serum. Apart from this, primidone estimations for routine purposes are not helpful.

Carbamazepine

Serum levels of this drug show considerable variation from patient to patient and are markedly influenced by the presence of other enzyme-inducing drugs. However, carbamazepine has an active metabolite, carbamazepine 10,11-epoxide, although its contribution to the overall therapeutic effect of carbamazepine is not certain in humans. Levels of the 10,11-epoxide vary widely between individuals, being relatively high especially in children in whom it may have a substantial therapeutic effect. The ratio of epoxide to parent drug is increased by co-administration of enzyme inducing drugs.

Despite these reservations, a therapeutic range of 20–40 μmol/l (5–10 μg/ml) has been suggested for carbamazepine (Cereghino et al 1974). Adverse effects do not usually occur until serum levels of around 40–50 μmol/l (10–12 μg/ml) are achieved and usually consist of blurring of vision and diplopia. However, there is considerable variability between patients. Although these symptoms are often a good indication of pending toxicity some patients may become hyponatraemic and show impaired water balance before other signs of toxicity develop (Perucca et al 1978). This may be why carbamazepine toxicity can be associated with an increase in fit frequency. As carbamazepine has a relatively short half-life on chronic dosing, standardization of time of blood sampling is preferable.

Sodium valproate

The position regarding monitoring of valproic acid is not clear at present. It has a greater therapeutic ratio than some of the other drugs. The therapeutic range of serum concentrations of valproic acid is poorly defined. A range of 350–700 μmol/l (50–100 μg/ml) was first suggested by Schobben et al (1975), and Gram et al (1980) found that serum concentrations greater than 350 μmol/l (50 μg/ml) had a superior clinical effect compared with lower serum concentrations. Other groups have found similar ranges (Adams et al 1978, Henriksen & Johannessen 1980, Klotz & Schweizer 1980) but others have disputed the existence of a therapeutic range (Schobben et al 1980, McQueen et al 1982). Some of the toxic effects of valproate, such as tremor, appear to be related to plasma concentrations of the drug and are more common with levels greater than 700 μmol/l (Turnbull 1983).

Besides interindividual variation in valproic acid levels, there are large intraindividual fluctuations during the day depending on the times of drug administration so that standardization of sampling times is necessary. Also, the extent of protein binding is variable and thus monitoring of total serum concentrations may be less relevant to clinical effect. More importantly, it appears that sodium valproate may have a non-reversible effect (Lockard & Levy 1976, Rowan et al 1979) which, if confirmed, lessens the value of monitoring because fluctuations in the level will not correlate closely with the antiepileptic effect.

In conclusion, because of these reservations, serum concentrations of valproic acid would not be expected to correlate with clinical effect and thus the position at present regarding the value of monitoring this drug is far from established. There is little evidence that measuring serum levels of valproic acid improves the clinical use of the drug.

Clonazepam

As with phenobarbitone, tolerance occurs to the effect of clonazepam (and other benzodiazepines) therefore the same limitations apply to the monitoring of the drug. Furthermore, serum levels of clonazepam are much lower than for most of the other antiepileptic drugs and technical difficulties in measurement loom large. In fact, the poor quality of results returned in quality control checks indicate that they may be more misleading than helpful (Griffiths et al 1980). There are no satisfactory studies of the relationship between serum levels and clinical effect, although Morselli (1978) reported that plasma levels over 580–640 nmol/l (180–200 ng/ml) were associated with an increase in seizure frequency, improvement occurring on reduction to 130–180 nmol/l (40–50 ng/ml). Thus, routine monitoring of clonazepam levels are not justified on present evidence.

Ethosuximide

As it is used mainly in children, routine monitoring may have a place, although the serum level appears to be fairly predictable for a given dose in mg/kg provided the age of the patient is taken into account (Sherwin 1982). Regular monitoring was found to reduce non-compliance and allowed drug requirements to be individualized, resulting in an improvement of control (Sherwin et al 1973). Two prospective studies have been carried out to study the relationship between control of absence seizures and plasma levels of ethosuximide. One showed that plasma levels in the completely controlled patients were in the range 290–500 μmol/l (41–70 μg/ml). However, as only four of the 18 patients achieved 100% control, it is difficult to draw firm conclusions about the therapeutic range (Penry et al 1972). In a second study involving 117 patients (Sherwin et al 1982), 45% · were completely controlled with ethosuximide and most of these patients had plasma levels above 280 μmol/l (40 μg/ml). A number of patients had levels in excess of 700 μmol/l (100 μg/ml) and the authors suggest that the therapeutic level for some may be as high as 850 μmol/l (120 μg/ml). There is thus good evidence that control of absence seizures is related to the plasma level of the drug and that most patients require a level of up to 700–850 μmol/l (100–120 μg/ml) to achieve optimum control. There does not appear to be a clear correlation between serum levels and adverse effects (Sherwin 1978). The active metabolite of methsuximide (N-desmethylmethsuximide) is responsible for the therapeutic activity of this drug. A therapeutic range of up to 200 μmol/l (40 μ/ml) for the metabolite has been suggested.

Timing of blood sampling

The shorter a drug's elimination half-life the greater the fluctuation in serum levels throughout a 24-hour period. Although the frequency of dosing is adjusted to compensate for this, it is seldom practical to administer a dose during the night, and therefore an early morning trough occurs which, for a drug like sodium valproate may be only about one half of the peak level. With phenobarbitone and phenytoin this fluctuation can usually be ignored and a random sample will give a reasonable estimate of the steady-state level. With carbamazepine, the fluctuation is greater and, therefore, standardization is preferable. Probably a sample taken six hours after dosing, using a twice-daily regime, is reasonable. For sodium valproate, a shorter interval of about four to five hours would be better.

In practice, blood samples will usually coincide with the time of a patient's clinic visit. The advantage to be gained from attempting to achieve the pharmacokinetic ideal is usually too small to be justified.

Abuse of drug monitoring

Table 12.13 summarizes the evidence discussed above and attempts to rank the value of therapeutic drug monitoring for each of the commonly used antiepileptic drugs. Knowledge of plasma concentrations of some of these drugs can be invaluable for the clinical management of the patient, particularly for phenytoin, and less so for ethosuximide and carbamazepine. However, rigidity of interpretation of serum concentrations should be avoided and alterations of drug dosage only made after clinical evaluation.

Monitoring of free drug concentrations

The usefulness of plasma monitoring of drugs rests on the assumption that plasma total drug concentrations reflect free, therapeutically active concentrations and, therefore, depend on protein binding remaining constant. This is especially important for highly bound drugs such as phenytoin and sodium valproate. Situations in which protein binding may be disturbed include pregnancy, old age, liver and renal diseases and when other drugs are prescribed which alter protein binding. However, for most routine measurements it is probably unnecessary to measure free drug concentrations. So far, the methods available for measuring free drug are not completely reliable and are time consuming and expensive and are therefore not applicable for everyday use. Some clinicians routinely use saliva drug concentrations instead. Measurement of antiepileptic drugs in saliva samples reflects free serum drug concentrations for phenytoin, primidone and carbamazepine, but is less reliable for phenobarbitone and is unhelpful in the case of sodium valproate. Saliva sampling is less traumatic for the patient than venepuncture, but there are risks of contamination

Table 12.13 Which drugs should be monitored?

Drug	Therapeutic levels[†] μmol/l (μg/ml)	Value rating[‡]	Comments
Phenytoin	40–80 (10–20)	*****	Monitoring essential for good therapy. Accurate dosing difficult without serum levels, because of saturable metabolism. Low therapeutic ratio, disguised toxicity and frequency of drug interactions add weight to the case for routine monitoring.
Carbamazepine	20–40 (5–10)	***	Monitoring useful. Clinical symptoms (especially eye symptoms) are often helpful in determining dose limit, but water intoxication and increase in fit frequency may be caused by high serum level. Standardization of sampling time advisable.
Ethosuximide	350–700 (50–100)	***	Monitoring in children is less acceptable, but can be helpful as a guide to correct dose.
Phenobarbitone	70–180 (15–40)	**	Tolerance develops and therefore therapeutic range difficult to define.
Primidone (unchanged)		*	Phenobarbitone is major metabolite therefore this should be monitored if indicated. Occasional measurement of primidone useful in slow metabolizers.
Valproic acid	350–700 (50–100)	*	Timed specimens essential. Little evidence that management is improved by monitoring. Possibility of 'hit and run' effect.
Clonazepam		*	Sedation is usually dose limiting; serum levels unhelpful because of development of receptor tolerance.

† Evidence for these ranges is, in some cases, inadequate. ‡ The more asterisks, the greater the value of routine monitoring.

of samples when patients are taking elixirs and uncoated tablets. It is probably of most value in monitoring drug therapy in children (Knott 1983).

TREATMENT OF STATUS EPILEPTICUS

Major status epilepticus is a grave medical emergency in which mortality can be as high as 21% (Rowan & Scott 1970, Oxbury & Whitty 1971). Prolonged seizure activity by itself damages the brain and the severity of the neuronal injury is proportional to the duration of seizure activity. The associated physiological alterations, in particular hypoxia and hyperthermia, hasten this damage (Meldrum et al 1973). Thus, apart from the immediate mortality, the incidence of neurological and mental sequelae is high and it seems likely that damage to the vulnerable temporal lobes during status epilepticus in childhood may cause Ammon's Horn sclerosis leading to chronic temporal lobe epilepsy. Status epilepticus therefore requires prompt and effective treatment if

uneventful recovery is to occur. The prognosis is related to the time interval between the onset of status and the start of effective treatment (Rowan & Scott 1970, Whitty & Taylor 1949, Meldrum et al 1973). There are many unresolved questions about the best treatment of status epilepticus and many aspects of the pharmacological therapy remain empirical. However, the following points are useful guidelines:

1. Initial doses of drugs should be given intravenously not intramuscularly. Some drugs, such as diazepam and phenytoin are slowly and unpredictably absorbed from intramuscular injection sites and it is therefore inappropriate to use them this way in status. Rectal administration of drugs is not appropriate, except when medical help is not immediately available.

2. Adequate doses of the drugs should be administered from the start (Janz & Kautz 1964).

3. There should be no hesitation about repeating the dose if status returns.

4. If status returns despite two or three single-dose administrations a continuous infusion may be

tried, e.g. chlormethiazole. Diazepam is not ideal for intravenous infusion because an active metabolite, N-desmethyldiazepam, has a long half-life and therefore accumulates.

5. Other measures may need to be taken, such as tepid sponging for febrile convulsions in children. Administration of aspirin, however, is no longer recommended because of the risk of precipitating Reye's syndrome. Rehydration and correction of acidosis may be necessary. Care should be taken to maintain an unobstructed airway and if impaired oxygenation is present intubation and ventilation should be instituted.

6. Any possible metabolic or drug toxic causes should be considered as the underlying precipitant of the episode of status. Metabolic abnormalities should be corrected as the status often responds poorly to the use of antiepileptic drugs. Hypoglycaemia, hyponatraemia, hepatic encephalopathy, hypocalcaemia and hyperosmolar states may all cause status epilepticus. Drugs such as aminophylline, lignocaine, isoniazid, tricyclic antidepressants and cocaine can also precipitate seizures (Chadwick 1983).

7. The drug treatment of status epilepticus, particularly in refractory cases, may require polytherapy. As the different classes of antiepileptic drugs have different mechanisms of action (Spero 1982) there is probably some reasonable rationale behind this approach.

8. Once seizure activity is controlled, careful consideration should be given to the patient's maintenance therapy. Measurement of drug levels on a specimen taken immediately on admission will be invaluable but, in the heat of the moment, will often be forgotten. If facilities are available it is reasonable to request an urgent result, for it may influence the early management. Rowan & Scott (1970) found that omission or reduction of antiepileptic therapy was a common precipitating factor. If the serum level is low, administration of parenteral supplements of phenytoin or phenobarbitone may prevent a recurrence of the status epilepticus and serial measurements of the levels while the patients remain in hospital will allow an optimum therapeutic level to be achieved.

9. A switch from parenteral to oral therapy should not be made too early.

Although there are many reports testifying to the effectiveness of various drugs in treating status epilepticus, very few studies have been performed where two drugs have been compared. Of the drugs available, the consensus of opinion is that an intravenous injection of diazepam or clonazepam is the most effective initial treatment for status. Although intravenous short-acting barbiturates, e.g. thiopentone, are also very effective, the incidence of respiratory depression is much greater. Intravenous injection of phenytoin may also be effective, particularly if the patient has not been receiving this drug chronically or if the episode of status has been precipitated by failure to take it as prescribed; but intoxication can occur if the patient already has a therapeutic level in his or her serum. Chlormethiazole given by intravenous infusion is very effective. Although paraldehyde has unpleasant physical properties it remains an effective drug. If fits continue despite administration of full doses of the above drugs, general anaesthesia and full curarization can be used with intermittent positive pressure ventilation. This will suppress the peripheral motor manifestations of the convulsions but the abnormal electrical activity on the EEG may continue. Thus administration of antiepileptic drugs must be continued, guided by continuous EEG monitoring.

Benzodiazepines

Benzodiazepines are probably the most potent agents available for the emergency treatment of status epilepticus. Intravenous administration of either diazepam or clonazepam is currently the initial treatment of choice for status epilepticus in infants, children and adults. They appear to suppress most types of status, although absence seizures in patients with Lennox-Gastaut Syndrome appear to respond poorly (Browne & Penry 1973, Tassinari et al 1983, Schmidt 1984a). They have also been used successfully in the acute treatment of febrile convulsions. Diazepam and clonazepam seem to be similarly effective (Schmidt 1984a) although experience with clonazepam is less extensive. Both drugs may fail in patients with acute brain damage underlying the episode of status epilepticus, with severe metabolic derangement or in status epilepticus of long duration. Either drug may be effective in patients where the other drug has failed.

The rapid effect of diazepam is due to its speed of brain penetration. After an initial rapid rise, the brain and serum levels of diazepam fall quickly after intravenous administration because the drug redistributes to other tissues and therapeutic levels are maintained for only one to two hours at most. Thus recurrence of seizures after an interval is a well recognized problem. Clonazepam has a longer duration of action so that recurrence of seizures may be less of a problem (Congdon & Forsythe 1980). In a study of recurrent seizures in the same child, the mean duration of action was 24.5 hours for clonazepam and 8.8 hours for diazepam. However, because doses of clonazepam are lower, 1 mg or less, it may be harder to titrate the dose than for diazepam.

In adults, intravenous administration of one ampoule (10 mg in 2 ml) of diazepam is usually adequate to terminate major status. Larger doses, however, are sometimes necessary. In children 0.2–0.3 mg/kg is usually sufficient, although neonates may require up to 0.5 mg/kg. On a weight-for-weight basis clonazepam is about ten times more potent than diazepam. Adults require 0.01–0.05 mg/kg but children may need 0.01–0.1 mg/kg. During the emergency drug treatment of status, the intravenous dose may be titrated directly in relation to the efficacy of the drug. There is little information on the therapeutic plasma concentrations of diazepam during acute treatment of status. Schmidt (1984a) reported preliminary data suggesting that levels of 500 ng/ml are necessary for acute seizure control and that 150 ng/ml are sufficient to maintain control. However, the rate of rise of plasma concentration may influence the therapeutic effect.

Intravenous diazepam and clonazepam are relatively safe drugs but they can cause cardiorespiratory depression, especially in the elderly and if they are administered after other sedative drugs (Prensky et al 1967, Bell 1969). The underlying cause of the status may also be an important determinant of toxicity (Tassinari et al 1983). Schmidt & Seldon (1982) describe mild to severe hypotension or respiratory depression in 5.2% of 246 status epilepticus patients treated with intravenous diazepam.

The recent introduction of rectal solutions has greatly improved the clinical use of diazepam for acute treatment. Absorption from the rectum is more rapid than with oral or intramuscular administration and is the closest approximation to intravenous injection (Moolenaar et al 1980). However, rectal diazepam should be reserved for use when medical attention is not immediately available, as the peak serum levels obtained are much lower than after intravenous diazepam.

Diazepam may be given by intravenous infusion but this is not altogether satisfactory. There are solubility problems, the drug adsorbs into the tubing, the dose must be very carefully titrated and, lastly, accumulation of the drug and its active desmethyl metabolite occur so that coma may last for several days after status has been controlled.

Phenytoin

Phenytoin given intravenously is effective in the acute management of status epilepticus, either alone as initial therapy or following the administration of diazepam. It crosses the blood–brain barrier rapidly, although the onset of action is slower than that of diazepam. For initial therapy, doses of up to 1000 mg in adults (15 mg/kg) infused at a rate of 50 mg/min are recommended. Wilder (1983) summarized his experience in over 200 patients, and status was controlled in 30% within 10 min, 50% in 15 min and 80% at 20 min. It must not be infused too rapidly because large doses of the solvent given too quickly can produce hypotension, apnoea and cardiac arrest. The drug should not be given intramuscularly because of the tissue damage produced and the erratic and slow absorption. The dose administered should be sufficient to produce therapeutic concentrations for the next 24 hours (40–80 μmol/l, 10–20 μg/ml) when maintenance treatment may be started. Cranford et al (1978) produced plasma levels at 24 hours of 7.1 ± 1.5, 13.5 ± 3.6 and 15 ± 2.9 μg/ml following 12, 15 and 18 mg/kg of intravenous phenytoin. The dose of phenytoin infused during treatment of status may have to be modified if the patient has previously been receiving phenytoin therapy. Monitoring serum phenytoin concentrations will enable the optimal level to be achieved and minimise the risk of intoxication.

Chlormethiazole

Intravenous infusion of 0.8% solution of chlormethiazole has been shown to be effective in terminating status epilepticus (Laxenaire et al 1966, Harvey et al 1975). Too rapid an infusion may result in hypotension and apnoea, and it is always necessary that the patient is kept under close and constant observation during the infusion. In adults 40–100 ml of chlormethiazole 0.8% solution administered over a period of five to ten minutes will usually stop convulsions. Thereafter, the rate of infusion is slowed down and titrated against the patient's response. Chlormethiazole has the great advantage of a short duration of action and therefore control over the patient's state is good; the degree of sedation can be rapidly altered by a change in infusion rate. Its chief disadvantage is its propensity to cause thrombophlebitis. It is probably underused in the acute treatment of status epilepticus: it is a good second line treatment if bolus doses of benzodiazepines are ineffective.

Phenobarbitone

Although often given by intramuscular injection in major status, phenobarbitone is not rapidly absorbed, taking up to six hours to reach a peak serum level (Jalling 1974). Even when given intravenously, phenobarbitone has a rather delayed onset of action because equilibration between serum and brain occurs slowly. Up to 800 mg may have to be given by slow or intermittent intravenous injection before adequate brain levels are achieved. Thus, phenobarbitone is no longer the drug of choice for immediate treatment of status although it still has a part to play in the maintenance therapy once the acute episode is controlled.

Paraldehyde

Before the introduction of the benzodiazepine drugs, paraldehyde was considered to be the treatment of choice for major status epilepticus. It has been used extensively with success in the past.

Whitty & Taylor (1949) recommended giving 8–10 ml intramuscularly as soon as possible, massaging the injection site to promote absorption, although it takes up to 30 minutes to act. If status continues, they suggested that further injections of 5 ml every 30 minutes be given until it ceases. The drug may also be given intravenously in normal saline, but there is limited solubility so a 4% solution should be used. Rectal administration of 4–8 ml may be used. The unpleasant smell of the drug, its irritant nature, occasionally resulting in a cold abscess at the site of injection or, if badly placed, sciatic nerve palsy, and its ability to dissolve some of the earlier plastic syringes has led to a decline in its use. However, it may still have a useful place in the emergency treatment of status epilepticus when only the intramuscular route is available (peak levels are reached more rapidly with paraldehyde than with diazepam, phenytoin and phenobarbitone following intramuscular injection) or where patients are allergic to the drugs of first choice. Modern plastic syringes are unaffected by paraldehyde.

Sodium valproate

Although sodium valproate therapy in status epilepticus has been described by oral (Manhire & Espir 1974), nasogastric (Barnes et al 1976) and rectal routes (Vajda et al 1977) the long delay from the time of drug administration to control of seizures is a major drawback.

General anaesthesia

If fits continue despite administration of the above drugs it may be necessary to anaesthetize and paralyse the patient to suppress the clinical manifestations of the seizure, which would, if they continued, prove ultimately fatal. A short-acting barbiturate, e.g. thiopentone, may be used together with a neuro-muscular blocking drug. Continuous EEG monitoring is necessary in order to follow the progress of seizure activity.

Treatment of absence status

Both diazepam and clonazepam are highly effective in terminating absence status due to primary epilepsy. However, in patients with Lennox-Gastaut syndrome, the response may be less satisfactory and, on occasion, tonic status may be precipitated by the administration of benzodiazepines (Tassinari et al 1983).

Treatment of cluster seizures

Some patients with severe epilepsy frequently have a cluster of seizures occurring at close intervals during the course of a day. Although these episodes may not fall within the definition of status epilepticus, there is nevertheless reason for concern lest the fits evolve into status. Intravenous diazepam may not be necessary in these patients and oral or rectal diazepam may be preferable (Milligan et al 1984). Intramuscular diazepam is very painful in conscious patients and it is very slowly absorbed. Midazolam, a water-soluble benzodiazepine, is absorbed rapidly from intramuscular injection sites, but its duration of action is shorter than that of diazepam (Jawad et al 1986).

PART THREE
NEW DRUGS FOR EPILEPSY

FUTURE PERSPECTIVES IN THE DRUG TREATMENT OF EPILEPSY

Although drug therapy is not the only approach to the management of epilepsy, it is likely to retain a central role for the foreseeable future. Presently available drugs are far from ideal. They fail to render all patients fit-free – approximately 20% of patients are drug resistant – and there is also the problem of acute and chronic antiepileptic drug toxicity. Thus there is an urgent need for new drugs which are more potent but less toxic. The ideal antiepileptic drug would have the following features.

1. It should be at least as effective as the currently available drugs with an improved therapeutic ratio

2. It should possess no serious toxicity
3. Tolerance should not develop to it
4. It should be easy to use:
   active orally
   long half-life (24 hours or so)
   simple pharmacokinetic characteristics (i.e. no saturable metabolism or binding)
   no effect on hepatic enzymes

The traditional approach to the development of new antiepileptic drugs has involved the screening of all newly synthesized compounds to identify antiseizure activity by testing them in rodent models of epilepsy. It was by this approach that phenytoin was discovered in 1938. The most widely used initial screening test involves the use of two complementary test models which together will identify the anticonvulsant activity of all the major antiepileptic drugs in clinical use (Krall et al 1978). The maximal electroshock test in mice involves the detection of a modification of the seizure pattern by the test drug and correlates fairly well with the potency of the drug against partial and generalized tonic-clonic seizures in patients. The second test uses a chemical convulsant, pentylenetetrazole, in mice; activity in this test predicts drugs likely to be effective in the suppression of absence seizures. Recently, various genetic models of epilepsy have been described where seizures occur either spontaneously or in response to specific sensory stimulation (e.g. auditory seizures in certain mice) and these models may be more analogous to human epilepsy than the experimental seizures caused by unnatural chemicals and electrical methods (Löscher & Meldrum 1984). Primate models of epilepsy have been developed such as the alumina gel model of focal epilepsy in monkeys (Lockard 1980) and the spontaneously photosensitive Senegalese baboon, *Papio papio* (Naquet & Meldrum 1972). Although the results of drug testing in such primate models are more likely to be predictive of probable efficacy in human epilepsy, they are impractical for initial screening of large numbers of chemicals.

A second approach to the development of new antiepileptic drugs is to modify the chemical structures of existing drugs in order to increase the potency but with fewer undesirable features. After the anticonvulsant potency of phenobarbitone was recognized in 1912, many other barbiturates were synthesized but none had antiepileptic activity superior to phenobarbitone. Similarly, none of the many analogues of phenytoin proved clinically superior to the original drug. More recently, following the discovery of the anticonvulsant activity of the 1,4-benzodiazepines, the possible advantages of the 1,5-benzodiazepines are being explored in an attempt to reduce sedative and psychomotor adverse effects. Oxcarbazepine, an analogue of carbamazepine, also has been developed with the aim of finding a compound with a lower incidence of adverse effects.

Thus many of the antiepileptic drugs currently in use have been discovered largely by chance and these haphazard methods are still used in the search for new drugs for epilepsy. However, recently a more rational approach to the development of new anticonvulsants has evolved based on increased understanding of neurotransmission in the mammalian central nervous system. The pathophysiological changes which occur in nervous tissue during seizure discharges have been studied and chemicals have been specifically designed to alter the threshold for the initiation of seizure activity or to limit the development and spread of the abnormal electrical activity. Much research has also been directed towards identification of the cellular mechanisms of action of existing drugs in an attempt to elucidate which effects are fundamental to their antiseizure activity; so far, multiple biochemical and physiological actions have been demonstrated for most of the currently available drugs and uncertainty remains as to which are most important.

The neurochemistry of the mammalian central nervous system is exceedingly complex. There are more than 40 putative transmitters which have been identified in brain tissue (Iversen 1982). In addition to the established neurotransmitters, such as acetylcholine and the monoamines, amino acids and many small peptides are believed to act as neurotransmitters; some being primarily excitatory and others inhibitory. It is thought that the transmitters used by the great majority of fast point-to-point neural pathways in the CNS are amino acids. Gamma-aminobutyric acid (GABA) and glycine are the major inhibitory transmitters. Glycine plays a major role in the spinal cord and

brain stem, while GABA is the principle inhibitory transmitter in the rest of the brain, the cortex, hypothalamus, thalamus, cerebellum and basal ganglia. GABA may be the transmitter used at up to a third of all neural synapses.

The powerful excitatory amino acids, aspartate and glutamate, cause depolarization of neurones and they appear to be the most commonly used excitatory transmitters for CNS interneurones.

In contrast, the monoamines (acetylcholine, adrenaline, noradrenaline and serotonin) are mainly associated with more diffuse neural pathways, which appear to perform modulatory functions of various types including arousal responses, control of movement and emotions and the regulation of the sleep–wake cycle. More than 30 neuropeptides have been identified as possible neurotransmitters. As yet, relatively little is known of their roles in the central nervous system functioning. Evidence so far suggests that they too have a neuromodulatory role with effects on various behavioural responses, including analgesia, locomotor activity and learning.

Normal functioning of the brain depends on the interplay between inhibitory and excitatory activity. Seizures occur as a result of recurrent paroxysmal excessive discharges of neuronal tissue and the characteristic pathophysiological event is thought to be the paroxysmal depolarization shift of neuronal membrane potentials and associated burst discharge (Prince & Wong 1981). These abnormal discharges could occur because of an imbalance in the brain between excitatory and inhibitory systems – either an excess of excitatory activity or a deficiency in the inhibitory network. In the past, researchers have investigated the possibility that abnormalities in the monoamine neurotransmitter systems may underlie the development of seizure activity (Meldrum 1978). Although these chemicals do modify seizure thresholds, it is now believed that their importance in the genesis of seizures is relatively minor compared with the amino acid transmitters. So far, there is no significant evidence for a role for the neuropeptides in epilepsy.

It is thought that the excitatory amino acid transmitters, glutamate and aspartate may be involved in the initiation and spread of the seizure discharge and that the inhibitory system using the transmitter GABA is responsible for the termination of seizure activity. Thus seizures could result from excessive release of the excitatory amino acids or from impairment of the inhibitory mechanisms mediated by GABA. Although it is unlikely that a single common abnormality will underlie the whole spectrum of the different types of epilepsy, this simplistic model has greatly assisted the development of new drugs for epilepsy. Most attention to date has been focused on the hypothesis that the underlying neurochemical defect in epilepsy may be a functional impairment in the inhibitory GABAergic neuronal network. There is some insubstantial evidence to support this view. In animals, manoeuvres which reduce cerebral GABA concentrations provoke seizures (Meldrum 1975). In some experimental models of focal epilepsy, neurotransmitter analysis reveals evidence for reduced GABA function in the epileptic foci (Ribak et al 1979, Bakay & Harris 1981). Similarly, in human epileptic foci removed at temporal lobectomy for intractable epilepsy, some but not all workers have found similar changes (Lloyd et al 1981). Also, some of the existing antiepileptic drugs, including benzodiazepines, sodium valproate, barbiturates and possibly phenytoin, are now believed to work at least in part by enhancing GABA-mediated inhibition (Spero 1982) and this would provide indirect support for this theory. Lastly, the understanding of GABA as a neurotransmitter is more advanced than the knowledge of the excitatory amino acid transmitters and pharmacological techniques for investigation and manipulation of GABA pathways are now available.

The idea that excessive excitation is the fundamental abnormality in seizure etiology has also been explored. Again, there is some experimental evidence to support this hypothesis. Aspartate and glutamate are excitatory when applied iontophoretically in the mammalian CNS (Curtis & Johnston 1974). They also initiate seizure activity when given systemically or by focal intracerebral injection in animals (Johnston 1972, Bradford & Dodd 1975). Release of glutamate into superfusates is observed during seizures (Dodd et al 1980). A role for synaptically released excitatory amino acids in epilepsy is most clearly established by the finding that antagonists acting selectively at excitatory

amino acid receptors possess antiepileptic properties in animal models of epilepsy (Meldrum 1984).

Because of the complex inter-relationships between the excitatory and inhibitory neurones in the brain, it is likely that any pharmacological intervention is likely to have multiple effects, both desirable and undesirable, and it would be necessary for any chemical to be effective in clinical epilepsy that it should have an overall stabilizing effect. Thus, pharmacological intervention to enhance inhibition in the CNS by raising GABAergic activity and/or to reduce excitation by modification of excitatory amino acid transmission is currently being explored.

Enhancement of inhibition

GABAergic neurones are widely distributed in the brain and spinal cord and mainly function as local inhibitory interneurones in the neocortex, hippocampus, cerebellum and other brain regions. These intrinsic inhibitory interneurones act to hyperpolarize the soma of pyramidal neurones and suppress the excessive synchronous or sustained discharges of pyramidal neurones which constitute the epileptic discharge.

GABA is synthesized from glutamate by the enzyme, glutamic acid decarboxylase (GAD) (Fig. 12.13). It is broken down to succinic semialdehyde by GABA-transaminase (GABA-T) and glutamate is regenerated. Succinic semialdehyde

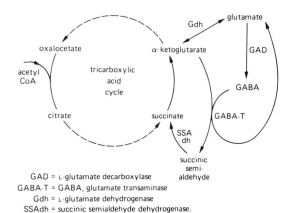

GAD = L-glutamate decarboxylase
GABA-T = GABA, glutamate transaminase
Gdh = L-glutamate dehydrogenase
SSAdh = succinic semialdehyde dehydrogenase.

Fig. 12.13 Synthesis and breakdown of GABA in nervous tissue. Vigabatrin (γ-vinyl-GABA) inhibits GABA-transaminase, the enzyme which destroys GABA, and causes an increase in GABA in the central nervous system

is further metabolized to succinic acid which re-enters the Krebs tricarboxylic acid cycle. This diversion pathway from carbohydrate metabolism is known as the 'GABA shunt'.

When an action potential is generated in a neurone which uses GABA as its transmitter, the depolarization of the nerve terminal results in the calcium dependent release of GABA from synaptic vesicles into the synaptic cleft. The GABA molecules then attach to the GABA_A receptors on the postsynaptic membrane. Occupation of the GABA_A receptor by GABA results in the opening of chloride channels. The influx of chloride ions causes hyperpolarization of the neurone, making the neurone less susceptible to excitatory influences. The action of GABA is terminated by active reuptake of GABA into neurones and glia, where some of the GABA is metabolized by GABA-T and some is recycled in the transmitter pool. The GABA_A receptor complex embedded in the postsynaptic membrane has become better characterized over recent years. It consists of several interrelated subunits.

1. *The chloride ion channel*, which opens to allow the influx of chloride ions resulting in hyperpolarization of the neurone.

2. *The GABA receptor* itself which when occupied by GABA or another agonist molecule causes opening of the chloride channel. Bicuculline is an antagonist at this site.

3. *The benzodiazepine receptor* which is adjacent to the GABA receptor and when occupied by agonist molecules, e.g. diazepam enhances the effect of GABA by favouring the opening of the chloride channel. Antagonists and inverse agonist molecules also act at the same receptor site. The benzodiazepine receptor and the GABA receptor are thus coupled with the benzodiazepine acting as a 'gain control' on the GABA receptor function. Thus the action of antiepileptic benzodiazepines would appear to be intimately linked with the action of GABA.

4. *Barbiturates* have also been shown to bind to the GABA receptor complex but at a site associated with the chloride channel. They increase the length of time the chloride channel is open in response to GABA receptor agonists.

5. *Other receptor sites* have been proposed for phenytoin and sodium valproate.

There is also evidence for a second type of GABA receptor which responds to a different range of GABA agonists such as baclofen and which is not bicuculline sensitive. This second receptor type, the GABA_B receptor is not linked to chloride channels and is found on monoamine terminals and possibly on excitatory amino acid terminals. GABA_B receptor agonists cause reduced entry of calcium and diminished transmitter release. Less is known about the GABA_B receptor.

There are various possible pharmacological manoeuvres which could enhance GABAergic inhibition.

GABA agonists and prodrugs

Because GABA itself does not cross the blood–brain barrier it is not possible to give GABA systemically to patients with epilepsy. Thus various compounds have been synthesized as GABA prodrugs. They contain a lipid-soluble moiety that facilitates brain penetration and subsequently they undergo enzymic conversion within the brain to release GABA itself or a related analogue, e.g. progabide, cetyl GABA. Progabide was found to be effective against seizures in animals (Worms et al 1982, Cepeda et al 1982), but appears less impressive in human epilepsy (Dam et al 1983, Loiseau et al 1983, Van der Linden et al 1981). Another approach has been the design of lipid-soluble agonist molecules which act at the postsynaptic GABA_A recognition site to reproduce the hyperpolarising action of GABA itself, e.g. 4,5,6,7-tetrahydroisoxazolo (5.4-c) pyridin-3-01 (THIP), muscimol. THIP is an effective anticonvulsant in some animal seizure models, but was ineffective when tried in baboons with photosensitive epilepsy and in patients with epilepsy (Meldrum & Horton 1980, Petersen et al 1983). Why these agonists are ineffective in clinical epilepsy is not clear – possibly they have a too diffuse an inhibitory action or perhaps they are not specific for the GABA_A receptor.

GABA-transaminase inhibitors (e.g. ethanolamine-o-sulphate, γ-vinyl GABA (vigabatrin), γ-acetylenic GABA)

These compounds are specific enzyme-activated, irreversible (suicide) inhibitors of the enzyme

GABA-transaminase and they thus prevent the breakdown of GABA in neurones and glia. The brain concentration of GABA is raised after administration of these compounds to animals and it is thought that the pool of GABA available for synaptic release from nerve terminals is also increased. Most research so far has been done with vigabatrin, which has been shown to be anticonvulsant in animal models of epilepsy, both rodents (Schechter et al 1979) and primates (Meldrum & Horton 1978). Studies using the drug in patients with epilepsy have confirmed its antiepileptic activity and have shown it to be well tolerated (Gram et al 1983, Rimmer & Richens 1984). However, preclinical animal toxicity tests have demonstrated vacuolation in the white matter of the CNS of rats, mice and dogs, and this aspect of potential toxicity in humans will require careful monitoring during further clinical trials.

GABA uptake inhibitors (e.g. nipecotic acid, 4,5,6,7-tetrahydroisoxazolo (4,5-c) pyridin-3-ol (THPO))

Synaptically released GABA is taken up into neurones and glia by specific sodium-dependent uptake mechanisms. Compounds which inhibit this re-uptake will enhance the inhibitory effect of the GABA. Those chemicals which are selective inhibitors of glial reuptake are likely to have the most consistent anticonvulsant action. Many of the available uptake inhibitors do not cross the blood–brain barrier but, when evaluated by intracerebral injection in mice, they have been shown to be anticonvulsant (Schousboe et al 1983). None of the GABA-reuptake inhibitors so far developed are sufficiently promising to be tested in patients.

Enhancement of GABA action at the GABA receptors (e.g. benzodiazepines)

Another possible way to augment GABA inhibition is by using drugs which bind to the various sites on the GABA receptor complex and enhance the effect of synaptically released GABA. Theoretically, this type of pharmacological action should preserve the necessary spatial and temporal linkage to suppress abnormal neuronal output but have little effect on normal neuronal function.

This is how benzodiazepines and anticonvulsant barbiturates are thought to exert their antiepileptic effect. Thus the development of other compounds which act at the GABA receptor complex is a possible source of new drugs which might lack the limitations of those currently available, i.e. habituation/dependence, development of tolerance, undue sedation.

Diminishing excitatory transmission

Knowledge about the excitatory amino acid transmitters is much less extensive than knowledge about GABA. Glutamate and aspartate are widely distributed in the CNS and seem to be the most commonly used excitatory transmitters for interneurones in the brain and spinal cord. Some neurones use aspartate and others glutamate, but it is difficult to identify specific pathways with certainty because of lack of suitable biochemical markers. Glutamate is present in large amounts in nervous tissue as one of the predominant intracellular organic cations found in all excitable cells and its important role in intermediary metabolism makes study of its putative role as a neurotransmitter difficult. Glutamate and aspartate depolarize neurones by activating membrane sodium channels. It appears that there are multiple receptor subtypes distinguishable by using selective agonist and antagonist drugs. The classes of receptors identified so far include kainate, quisqualate, N-methyl-D-aspartate (NMDA) and glutamate. The endogenous transmitters acting at each receptor type is not definitely known. The different receptor subtypes seem to be linked to different ionic conductances. Quisqualate and glutamate receptors produce a steady depolarization with an increased firing rate, whilst NMDA produces a pattern of paroxysmal shifts in membrane potential and burst discharges similar to those seen in epilepsy. This suggests the NMDA receptor class may be important in epilepsy (Meldrum 1984).

When glutamate or aspartate are applied iontophoretically to mammalian neurones they are excitatory, and when they are injected focally in large doses into animal brains epileptic discharges are provoked. Thus synaptic release of excitatory transmitters may initiate the paroxysmal burst discharges of epilepsy and cause spread of the epileptic activity throughout the brain. Manoeuvres to decrease excitatory transmission could therefore be effective in epilepsy. There are several different approaches to this outlined below.

Impaired maximal rate of synthesis of excitatory transmitters

This could theoretically have a selective action on the pool of glutamate and/or aspartate available for neurotransmission. However, the routes of synthesis of the excitatory amino acids are not known with certainty. Sodium valproate has been shown to decrease brain aspartate concentrations but how this is done and the significance of this effect is unknown.

Decreased synaptic release of excitatory transmitters

Release of excitatory amino acid transmitters might be achieved by an effect on autoreceptors on presynaptic terminals or via GABA$_B$ receptors.

Lamotrigine, a new drug under clinical trial, is thought to act in this way (Leach et al 1986).

Decreased postsynaptic action

Analogues of the excitatory amino acids that act as antagonists at the postsynaptic receptors have been synthesized. Such compounds have been evaluated in test animals and are anticonvulsant against audiogenic and various chemically induced seizures in mice. The most potent specific antagonists are 2-amino-5-phosphonovalerate (2APV) and 2-amino-7-phosphonoheptanoic acid (2APH) which are selective for the NMDA receptor site. 2APH is also effective against photically induced seizures in baboons. Unfortunately, when these compounds are administered systemically, there is only limited entry into the brain because of poor lipid solubility. Thus none of the excitatory amino acid antagonists so far synthesized are yet at the stage of testing in patients. However, this approach to the production of new antiepileptic drugs appears to be a very promising one.

REFERENCES

Adams D J, Luders H, Pippenger C 1978 Sodium valproate in the treatment of intractable seizure disorders: a clinical and electroencephalographic study. Neurology 28:152

Alcala H, Lertratanangkoon K, Stenbach W, Kellaway P, Horning M G 1978 The purkinje cell in phenytoin intoxication; ultrastructural and Golgi studies. Pharmacologist 20:240

Andreason P B, Lyngbye J, Trolle E 1973 Abnormalities in liver function tests during long-term diphenylhydantoin in epileptic out-patients. Acta Medica Scandinavica 194:261

Anthony J H, Hawke S M B 1983 Phenobarbital compared with carbamazepine in prevention of recurrent febrile convulsions. American Journal of Diseases of Childhood 137:892

Asconape J J, Penry J K 1982 Use of antiepileptic drugs in the presence of liver and kidney diseases: a review. Epilepsia 23 (Suppl.1):565

Ayers G, Burnett D, Griffiths A, Richens A 1980 Quality control of drug assays. Clinical Pharmacokinetics 6:106

Bacon C J, Mucklow J C, Rawlin M D et al 1981 Placebo-controlled study of phenobarbitone and phenytoin in the prophylaxis of febrile convulsions. Lancet ii:600

Bakay R A E, Harris A B, 1981 Neurotransmitter, receptor and biochemical changes in monkey cortical epileptic foci. Brain Research 206:387

Barnes S E, Bland D, Cole A P, Evans A R 1976 Use of sodium valproate in a case of status epilepticus. Development Medicine and Child Neurology 18:236

Battino D, Binelli S, Bossi L et al 1984 Changes in

primidone/phenobarbitone ratio during pregnancy and the puerperium. Clinical Pharmacokinetics 9:252

Battino D, Binelli S, Bossi L et al 1985 Plasma concentrations of carbamazepine and carbamazepine 10, 11-epoxide during pregnancy and after delivery. Clinical Pharmacokinetics 10:27

Baumel I P, Gallagher B B, Mattson R H 1972 Phenylethylmalonamide (PEMA). An important metabolite of primidone. Archives of Neurology 27:34

Bell D S 1969 Dangers of treatment of status epilepticus with diazepam. British Medical Journal 1:159

Bell R D, Pak C Y C, Zerwekh J, Barilla D E, Vasko M 1978 Effect of phenytoin on bone and vitamin D metabolism. Annals of Neurology 5:374

Bennet E P 1977 Influence of phenytoin and carbamazepine on endocrine function. Epilepsia 18:294

Bertilsson L, Thomson T 1986 Clinical pharmacokinetics and pharmacological effects of carbamazepine and carbamazepine 10, 11-epoxide: an update. Clinical Pharmacokinetics 11:177

Betts T A, Kalra P L, Cooper R, Jeavons P M 1968 Epileptic fits as a probable side effect of amitriptyline. Lancet 1:390

Blain P G, Mucklow J C, Bacon C J, Rawlins M D 1981 Pharmacokinetics of phenytoin in children. British Journal of Clinical Pharmacology 12: 659–661

Blaschke T F 1977 Protein binding and kinetics of drugs in liver disease. Clinical Pharmacokinetics 2:32

Booker H E 1982 Trimethadione. Relation of plasma concentration to seizure control. In: Woodbury D M, Penry

J K, Pippenger C E (eds) Antiepileptic Drugs, p 697 New York, Raven Press

Booker H E, Hosokowa K, Burdette R D, Darcey B 1970 A clinical study of serum primidone levels. Epilepsia 11:395

Bourgeois B F D, Dodson W E, Ferendelli J A 1983 Primidone, phenobarbital and PEMA: seizure protection, neurotoxicity, and therapeutic index of individual compounds in mice. Neurology 33:283

Bradford H F, Dodd P R 1985 Convulsions and activation of epileptic foci induced by monosodium glutamate and related compounds. Biochemical Pharmacology 26:253

Browne T R 1976 Clonazepam. A review of a new anticonvulsant drug. Archives of Neurology 33:326

Browne T R, Penry J K 1973 Benzodiazepines in the treatment of epilepsy. A review. Epilepsia 14:277

Browne T R, Dreifuss F E, Dyken P R et al 1975 Ethosuximide in the treatment of absence (petit mal) seizures. Neurology 25:515

Buchthal F, Svensmark O, Schiller P J 1960 Clinical and electroencephalographic correlations with serum levels of diphenylhydantoin. Archives of Neurology 2:624

Buchthal F. Svensmark O, Simonsen H 1968 Relation of EEG and seizures to phenobarbital in serum. Archives of Neurology 19:567

Buchanan R A, Kinkel A W, Smith T C 1973 The absorption and excretion of ethosuximide. International Journal of Clinical Pharmacology and New Drugs 7:213

Buchanan R A, Kinkel A W, Turner J L, Heffelfinger J C 1976 Ethosuximide dosage regimens. Clinical Pharmacology and Therapeutics 19:143

Butler T C 1978 Some quantitative aspects of the pharmacology of phenobarbital. In:Pippenger C E, Penry J K, Kutt H (eds) Antiepileptic drugs: quantitative analysis and interpretation. Raven Press, New York, p 261

Callaghan N, Kenny R A, O'Neil B, Crowley M, Goggin T 1985 A prospective study between carbamazepine, phenytoin and sodium valproate as monotherapy in previously untreated and recently diagnosed patients with epilepsy. Journal of Neurology, Neurosurgery and Psychiatry 48:639

Callaghan N, O'Dwyer R, Keating J 1984 Unnecessary polypharmacy in patients with frequent seizures. Acta Neurologica Scandinavica 69:15

Callaghan N, O'Hare J, O'Driscoll D, O'Neill B, Daly M 1982 Comparative study of ethosuximide and sodium valproate in the treatment of typical absence seizures (petit mal). Developmental Medicine and Child Neurology 24:830

Cepeda C, Worms P, Lloyd K G, Naqvet R 1982 Action of progabide in the photosensitive baboon, Papio papio. Epilepsia 23:463

Cereghino J J, Brock J T, Van Meter J C, Penry J K, Smith L D, White B G 1974 Carbamazepine for epilepsy. A controlled prospective evaluation. Neurology 24:401

Cereghino J J, Brock J T, van Meter J C, Penry J K, Smith L D, White B G 1975 The efficacy of carbamazepine combinations in epilepsy. Clinical Pharmacology and Therapeutics 18:733

Chadwick D (1983) Drug induced convulsions. In:Rose F C (ed) Research progress in epilepsy. Pitman, London, p 151

Chadwick D 1985 The discontinuation of antiepileptic therapy. In: Meldrum B M, Pedley T A (eds) Recent advances in Epilepsy Vol. 2 Churchill Livingstone, Edinburgh, 2, p 111

Chadwick D, Reynolds E H 1985 When do epileptic patients need treatment? Starting and stopping medication. British Medical Journal 290:1885

Chadwick D, Turnbull D M 1985 The comparative efficacy of antiepileptic drugs for partial and tonic-clonic seizures. Journal of Neurology, Neurosurgery and Psychiatry 48:1073

Chadwick D, Shaw M D M, Foy P, Rawlins M D, Turnbull D M 1984 Serum anticonvulsant concentrations and the risk of drug induced skin eruptions. Journal of Neurology, Neurosurgery and Psychiatry 47:642

Chadwick D, Reynolds E H, Marsden C D 1976 Anticonvulsant-induced dyskinesias: a comparison with dyskinesias induced by neuroleptics. Journal of Neurology, Neurosurgery and Psychiatry 39:1210

Chambers R E, Homeida M, Hunter K R, Teague R H 1977 Salivary carbamazepine concentrations. Lancet i:656

Chapman A, Keane, P E, Meldrum B S, Simiand J, Vernieres J C 1982 Mechanism of anticonvulsant action of valproate. Progress in Neurobiology 19:315

Cleland P G, Mosqvera I, Steward W P, Foster J B 1981 Prognosis of isolated seizures in adult life. British Medical Journal, 283:1364

Coatsworth J J 1971 Studies on the clinical effipacy of marketed antiepileptic drugs. NINDS Monograph No. 12.US Government Printing Office Washington DC

Congdon P J, Forsythe W I 1980 Intravenous clonazepam in the treatment of status epilepticus in children. Epilepsia, 21:97

Covanis A, Jeavons P M 1980 Once-daily sodium valproate in the treatment of epilepsy. Developmental Medicine and Child Neurology 22:202

Cranford R E, Patrick B, Anderson C B, Kostick B 1978 Intravenous phenytoin: clinical and pharmacokinetic aspects. Neurology 28:874

Curtis D R, Johnston G A R 1974 Amino acid transmitters in the mammalian central nervous system. Physiology 69:97

Dam M, Gram L, Philbert A et al 1983 Progabide: a controlled trial in partial epilepsy. Epilepsia 24:127

Dodd P R, Bradford H F, Abdul-Ghani, A S, Cox D W G, Coutinhonetto J 1980 Release of amino acids from chronic epileptic and subepileptic foci in vivo. Brain Research 193:505

Dulac O, Aicardi J, Rey E, Olive G 1978 Blood levels of diazepam after single rectal administration in infants and children. Journal of Pediatrics 93:1039

Eadie M J, Bochner F, Hooper W D, Tyrer J H 1978 Preliminary observations on the pharmacokinetics of methylphenobarbitone. Clinical and Experimental Neurology 15:131

Editorial 1971 Is phenytoin carcinogenic? Lancet ii:1071

Editorial 1976 Anticonvulsant ostemalacia. British Medical Journal 2:1340

Editorial 1980 Febrile convulsions: a suitable case for treatment. Lancet ii:680

Editorial 1981 Febrile convulsions: long-term treatment. British Medical Journal 282:673

Edwards J G, Long S K, Sedgwick E M, Wheal H V 1986 Antidepressants and convulsive seizures: clinical, electroencephalographic, and pharmacological aspects. Clinical Neuropharmacology 9:329

Elwes R D C. Chesterman P, Reynolds E H 1985 Prognosis after a first untreated tonic-clonic seizure. Lancet ii:752

Elwes R D C, Johnson A L, Shorvon S D, Reynolds, E H 1984 The prognosis for seizure control in newly diagnosed epilepsy. New England Journal of Medicine 311:944

Emerson R, D'Souza B J, Vining E P et al 1981 Stopping medication in children with epilepsy. New England Journal of Medicine 304:1125

Faigle J W, Feldmann K F, Baltzer V 1977 Anticonvulsant effect of carbamazepine. An attempt to distinguish between the potency of the parent drug and its epoxide metabolite. In:Gardner-Thorpe C, Janz D, Meinardi, H, Pippenger C E (eds) Antiepileptic drug monitoring, Pitman Press, Avon p 104

Feely M, Calvert R, Gibson J 1982 Clobazam in catamenial epilepsy: a model for evaluating anticonvulsants. Lancet ii:71

Feldman G, Weaver D, Lovrien E, 1977 The fetal trimethadione syndrome: report of an additional family and further delineation of their syndrome. American Journal of Diseases of Childhood 131:1389

Finucane J F, Griffiths R S 1976 Effect of phenytoin therapy on thyroid function. British Journal of Clinical Pharmacology 3:1041

Fischbacher E, 1982 Effect of reduction of anticonvulsants on well being. British Medical Journal 285:423

Flint N, Lopez L M, Robinson J D, Williams C, Salem R B 1985 Comparison of eight phenytoin dosing methods in institutionalized patients. Therapeutic Drug Monitoring. 7:74

Foy P M, Copeland G P, Shaw M D M 1981 The incidence of postoperative seizures. Acta Neurochirugica 55:253

Gamble J A S, Dundee J W, Assaf R A E 1975 Plasma diazepam levels after single oral and intramuscular administration. Anaesthesia 30:164

Gannaway D J, Mawer G E 1981 Serum phenytoin concentration and clinical response to patients with epilepsy. British Journal of Clinical Pharmacology 12:833

Gastaut H 1970 Clinical and electroencephalographical classification of the epileptic seizures. Epilepsia 11:102

Goodridge D M G, Shorvon S D 1983 Epileptic seizures in a population of 6000. II.Treatment and prognosis. British Medical Journal 287: 645.

Gowers W R 1881 Epilepsy and other chronic convulsive diseases. Churchill, London

Graham J 1978 A comparison of the absorption of phenobarbitone given via the oral and the intramuscular route. Clinical and Experimental Neurology. 15:154

Gram L, Flachs H, Wurtz-Jorgensen, A, Parnas J, Andersen B 1980 Sodium valproate, relationship between serum levels and therapeutic effect: a controlled study. In: Johannessen S I et al. (eds) Antiepileptic therapy: advances in drug monitoring. Raven Press, New York, p 217.

Gram L, Lyon B B, Dam M, 1983 Gamma-vinyl GABA: a single-blind trial in patients with epilepsy. Acta Neurological Scandinavica 68:34

Greenblatt D J, Allen M D, McLaughlin D S, Harmatz J S, Shader R I 1978 Diazepam absorption: effects of antacids and food. Clinical Pharmacology and Therapeutics 24:600

Griffiths A, Hebdige S, Perucca E, Richens A 1980 Quality control in drug measurement. Therapeutic Drug Monitoring 2:51

Guelen P J M, Van der Kleijn E, Woudstra U 1975 Statistical analysis of pharmacokinetic parameters in epileptic patients chronically treated with antiepileptic drugs. In:Schneider H, Janz D, Gardner-Thorpe C, Meinardi H, Sherwin A C (eds) Clinical pharmacology of Antiepileptic Drugs. p 2 Springer-Verlag, Berlin

Gugler R, Mueller G 1978 Plasma protein binding of

valproic acid in healthy subjects and in patients with renal disease. British Journal of Clinical Pharmacology 5.441.

Gugler R, von Unruh G E 1980 Clinical pharmacokinetics of valproic acid. Clinical Pharmacokinetics 5:67

Gugler R, Eichelbaum M, Schell et al 1980 The disposition of valproic acid. In: Johannessen S I et al (eds) Antiepileptic therapy: advances in drug monitoring. Raven Press, New York, p 125

Haefely W E 1980 GABA and the anticonvulsant action of benzodiazepines and barbiturates. Brain Research Bulletin 5(suppl.2):873

Haerer A F, Grace J B 1969 Studies of anticonvulsant levels in epileptics. 1. Serum diphenylhydantoin concentrations in a group of medically indigent outpatients. Acta Neurologica Scandinavica 45:18

Hahn T J 1976 Bone complications of anticonvulsants. Drugs 12:201

Harding G F A, Herrick C E, Jeavons, P M 1978 A controlled study of the effect of sodium valproate on photosensitive epilepsy and its prognosis. Epilepsia 19:555

Hart R G, Easton J D 1981 Carbamazepine and hematological monitoring. Annals of Neurology 11:309

Harvey P K P, Higenbottam T W, Loh L 1975 Chlormethiazole in treatment of status epilepticus. British Medical Journal 2:603

Hauser W A, Andersen V E, Loewenson R B, McRoberts S M 1982 Seizure recurrence after a first unprovoked seizure. New England Journal of Medicine 307:522

Henriksen O, Johannessen 1980 Clinical observations of sodium valproate in children: an evaluation of therapeutic serum levels. In: Johannessen, S I et al (eds) Antiepileptic therapy: advanced in drug monitoring. Raven Press, New York, p 253

Herranz J L, Armijo J A, Artega R 1984 Effectiveness and toxicity of phenobarbital, primidone and sodium valproate in the prevention of febrile convulsions controlled by plasma levels. Epilepsia 25:89

Hillestad L, Hansen T, Melsom H, Driveness A 1974 Diazepam metabolism in normal man. 1. Serum concentrations and clinical effects after intravenous intramuscular, and oral administration. Clinical Pharmacology and Therapeutics 16:479

Holowach J, Thurston D L, O'Leary J 1972 Prognosis in childhood epilepsy. New England Journal of Medicine. 286:169

Hopkins A, Scambler G 1977 How doctors deal with epilepsy. Lancet 1:183

Houghton G W, Richens A 1974 Rate of elimination of tracer doses of phenytoin at different steady-state serum phenytoin concentrations in epileptic patients. British Journal of Clinical Pharmacology. 1:155

Houghton G W, Richens A, Leighton M, 1975a Effect of age, height, weight and sex on serum phenytoin concentration in epileptic patients. British Journal of Clinical Pharmacology 2:251

Houghton G W, Richens A, Toseland P A, Davidson S, Falconer M A 1975b Brain concentrations of phenytoin, phenobarbitone and primidone in epileptic patients. European Journal of Clinical Pharmacology 9:73

Hrachovy R A, Frost J D, Kellaway P, Zion T 1979 A controlled study of prednisone therapy in infantile spasms. Epilepsia 20 403

Iversen L C 1982 Neurotransmitters and CNS disease. Introduction. Lancet ii:914

Jakobs C, Loscher W 1978 Identification of metabolites of

valproic acid in serum of humans, dog, rat and mouse. Epilepsia 19 591

Jalling B 1974 Plasma and CSF concentrations of phenobarbital in infants given single doses. Developmental Medicine and Child Neurology 16:781

Janz D 1982 On major malformations and minor abnormalities in the offspring of parents with epilepsy. In: Janz D, Dam M, Richens A, Bossi L, Helge H, Schmidt D (eds) Epilepsy, Pregnancy and the Child. Raven Press, New York, p 211

Janz D, Kautz G 1964 The aetiology and treatment of status epilepticus. German Medical Monthly 9:451

Janz D, Sommer-Burkhardt E M 1975 Discontinuation of antiepileptic drugs in patients with epilepsy who have been seizure free for more than two years. In: Janz D (ed.) Epileptology. Thieme-Verlag, Stuttgart, p 228

Jawad S, Oxley J, Wilson J, Richens A 1986 Pharmacodynamic evaluation of midazolam as an antiepileptic compound. Journal of Neurology, Neurosurgery and Psychiatry 49:1050

Jawad S, Richens A, Oxley J, 1984 Single dose pharmacokinetic study of clobazam in normal volunteers and epileptic patients. British Journal of Clinical Pharmacology 18:873

Jeavons P M, Bower B D 1974 Infantile spasms. In: Vinken, P J, Bruyn G W (eds) Handbook of clinical neurology vol 15: the epilepsies. American Elsevier, New York, p 219

Jeavons P M, Clark J E, Maheshwari M C 1977 Treatment of generalised epilepsies of childhood and adolescence with sodium valproate (Epilim). Developmental Medicine and Child Neurology. 19:9

Jennett W B 1975 Epilepsy after non-missile head injuries. Heinemann, London 2nd Ed.

Jensen B 1962 Trimethadione in the serum of patients with petit mal. Danish Medical Bulletin 9:74

Johannessen S I, Barruzzi A, Gomeni R, Strandjord R E, Morselli, P L 1977 Further observations on carbamazepine and carbamazepine-10,11-epoxide kinetics in epileptic patients. In:Gardner-Thorpe C, Janz D, Meinardi H, Pippenger C E (eds) Antiepileptic drug monitoring. Pitman Press, Avon, p 110

Johnston G A R 1972 Convulsions induced in 10-day-old rats by intraperitoneal injection of monosodium glutamate and related excitant amino acids. Biochemical Pharmacology 22:137

Juul-Jensen P 1964 Frequency of recurrence after discontinuance of anticonvulsant therapy in patients with epileptic seizures. Epilepsia 5:352

Juul-Jensen P 1968 Frequency of recurrence after discontinuation of anticonvulsant therapy in patients with epileptic seizures. A new follow up study after 5 years. Epilepsia 9:11

Kaneko S, Sato T, Suzuki K 1979 The levels of anticonvulsants in breast milk. British Journal of Clinical Pharmacology 7:624

Kanto J 1975 Plasma concentrations of diazepam and its metabolites after per oral, intramuscular and rectal administration. International Journal of Clinical Pharmacy and Biopharmaceutics 12:427

Kaufmann R F, Habersang R, Lansky, L 1977 Kinetics of primidone metabolism and excretion in children. Clinical Pharmacology and Therapeutics 22:200

Kay J D S, Hilton-Jones D, Hyman N 1986 Valproate toxicity and ornithine carbamoyltransferase deficiency. Lancet ii:1283

Klotz U, Schweizer C 1980 Valproic acid in childhood epilepsy: anticonvulsive efficacy in relation to its plasma levels. International Journal of Clinical Pharmacology, Therapy and Toxicology 18:461

Knott C 1983 Measurement of saliva drug concentrations in the control of antiepileptic medication. In:Pedley T A, Meldrum B S (eds) Recent Advances in epilepsy vol 1. Churchill Livingstone, Edinburgh, p 57

Knudsen F E 1977 Plasma-diazepam in infants after rectal administration in solution and by suppository. Acta Paediatrica Scandinavica. 66:563

Knudsen F U 1979 Rectal administration of diazepam in solution in the acute treatment of convulsions in infants and children. Archives of Diseases in Childhood 54:855

Knudsen F U, Vestermark S 1978 Prophylactic diazepam or phenobarbital in febrile convulsions: a prospective controlled study. Archives of Diseases of Childhood 53:600

Krall R L Penry, J K White B G, Kupferberg H J, Swinyard E A 1978 Antiepileptic drug development. II. Anticonvulsant drug screening. Epilepsia, 19:409

Kutt H, McDowell F 1968 Management of epilepsy with diphenylhydantoin sodium. Journal of the American Medical Association 203:969

Kutt H, Winters W, Kokenge R, McDowell F 1964 Diphenylhydantoin metabolism, blood levels, and toxicity. Archives of Neurology 11 642

Laxenaire M, Tridon P, Poire P 1966 Effect of chlormethiazole in treatment of delirium tremens and status epilepticus. Acta Psychiatrica Scandinavica 42 (suppl.) 192:87

Leach M J, Marden C M, Miller A A 1986 Pharmacological studies on lamotrigine, a novel potential antiepileptic drug. II. Neurochemical studies and mechanism of action. Epilepsia 27:490

Lee K, Melchior J C 1981 Sodium valproate versus phenobarbital in the prophylactic treatment of febrile convulsions in childhood. European Journal of Paediatrics 137:151

Legg N J, Swash M 1974 Clinical note: Seizures and EEG activation after trimipramine. Epilepsia 15:131

Leppik I E, Cloyd J C, Miller K 1984 Development of tolerance to the side effects of primidone. Therapeutic Drug Monitoring 6:189

Lesser R P, Pippenger C E, Luders H, Dinner D S 1984 High dose monotherapy in the treatment of intractable seizures. Neurology, 34:707

Levy R H, Pitlick W H, Troupin A S, Green J R, Neal J M 1975 Pharmacokinetics of carbamazepine in normal man. Clinical Pharmacology Therapeutics, 17:657

Lindhout D, Hoppener R J E A, Meinardi H 1984 Teratogenicity of antiepileptic drug combinations with special emphasis on epoxidation (of carbamazepine). Epilepsia 25:77

Lloyd K G, Munari C, Bossi L, Stoeffels C, Talairach J, Morselli P L 1981 Biochemical evidence for the alterations of GABA-mediated synaptic transmission in pathological brain tissue (stereo-EEG or morphological definition) from epileptic patients. In: Morselli P C, Lloyd K G, Löscher W, Meldrum B, Reynolds, E H (eds) Neurotransmitters, seizures and epilepsy. Raven Press, NewYork, p 325

Lockard J S 1980 A primate model of clinical epilepsy: mechanisms of action through quantification of therapeutic effects. In: Lockard J S, Ward A A (eds) Epilepsy. A window to brain mechanisms. Raven Press, New York, p 11

Lockard J S, Levy R H 1976 Valproic acid: reversibly acting drug? Epilepsia 17:477

Loiseau P, Bossi L, Guyot M, Orofiamma B, Morselli P L 1983 Double-blind cross-over trial of progabide versus placebo in severe epilepsies. Epilepsia 24:703

Löscher W, Meldrum B S 1984 Evaluation of anticonvulsant drugs in genetic animal models of epilepsy. Federation Proceedings 43:276

Lund L 1973 Effects of phenytoin in patients with epilepsy in relation to its concentration in plasma. In:Davies D S, Prichard B N C (eds) Biological effects of drugs in relation to their plasma concentration, Macmillan, London, p 227

Lund L, 1974 Anticonvulsant effect of diphenylhydantoin relative to plasma levels. A prospective three-year study in ambulant patients with generalised epileptic seizures. Archives of Neurology 31:289

McAuliffe J J, Sherwin A L, Leppik I E, Fayle S E, Pippenger C E 1977 Salivary levels of anticonvulsants: a practical approach to drug monitoring. Neurology 27:409

MacDonald R L 1983 Mechanisms of anticonvulsant drug action. In: Pedley T A, Meldrum B S (eds) Recent Advances in epilepsy Vol 1. Churchill Livingstone, Edinburgh, p 1

MacDonald R L, McLean M J, Skerritt J H 1985 Anticonvulsant drug mechanism of action. Federation Proceedings 44:2634

McQueen J K, Blackwood D H R, Harris P, Kalbag R M, Johnson A L 1983 Low risk of late post-traumatic seizures following severe head injury: implications for clinical trials of prophylaxis. Journal of Neurology, Neurosurgery and Psychiatry 46:899

McQueen J K, Blackwood D H R, Minns R A Brown J K 1982 Plasma levels of sodium valproate in childhood epilepsy. Scottish Medical Journal 27;312

Mandelli M, Tognoni G, Garatini S 1978 Clinical pharmacokinetics of diazepam. Clinical Pharmacokinetics. 3:72

Manhire A R, Espir M 1974 Treatment of status epilepticus with sodium valproate. British Medical Journal 3:808

Mattson R H, Cramer J A, Collins J F et al 1985 Comparison of carbamazepine, phenobarbital, phenytoin and primidone in partial and secondarily generalized tonic clonic seizures. New England Journal of Medicine 313:145

Meberg A, Langslet A, Bredesen J E, Lunde P K M 1978 Plasma concentration of diazepam and n-desmethyldiazepam in children after a single rectal or intramuscular dose of diazepam. European Journal of Clinical Pharmacology 14:273.

Meissner O, Joubert P H, Joubert H F, Van der Merwe C A 1984 The IgA immune system in epileptics on anticonvulsant therapy. European Journal of Clinical Pharmacology. 27:81

Melchior J C, Buchthal R, Lennox-Buchthal M 1971 The ineffectiveness of diphenylhydantoin in preventing febrile convulsions in the age of greater risk, under 3 years. Epilepsia 12:55

Meldrum B S 1975 Epilepsy and GABA-mediated inhibition. International Reviews of Neurology 17:1

Meldrum B 1978 Neurotransmitters and epilepsy. In:Legg N J (ed.) Neurotransmitter systems and their clinical disorders, Academic Press, London, p 167

Meldrum B, 1984 Amino-acid neurotransmitters and new approaches to anticonvulsant drug action. Epilepsia 25: (suppl. 2):S140

Meldrum B, Horton R 1978 Blockade of epileptic responses in the photosensitive baboon, Papio papio by the two irreversible inhibitors of GABA-transaminase, Y-acetylenic GABA (4-amino-hex-5-ynoic acid) and γ-vinyl GABA (4-amino-hex-5-enoic acid). Psychopharmacology 59:47

Meldrum B S, Horton R W 1980 Effects of bicyclic GABA agonist, THIP, on myoclonic and seizure responses in mice and baboons with reflex epilepsy. European Journal of Pharmacology 61:231

Meldrum B S, Vigouroux R A, Brierley J B 1973 Systemic factors and epileptic brain damage. Archives of Neurology 29:82

Milligan N M, Dhillon S, Griffiths A, Oxley J, Richens A 1984 A clinical trial of single dose rectal and oral administration of diazepam for the prevention of serial seizures in adult epileptic patients. Journal of Neurology, Neurosurgery and Psychiatry 47:235

Milligan N, Dhillon S, Richens A, Oxley J, 1981 Rectal diazepam in the treatment of absence status: a pharmacodynamic study. Journal of Neurology, Neurosurgery and Psychiatry

Moolenaar F, Bakker S, Visser J, Huizinga J 1980 Biopharmaceutics of rectal administration of drugs in man. IX. Comparative biopharmaceutics of diazepam after single rectal, oral, intramuscular and intravenous administration in man. International Journal of Pharmaceutics 5:127

Morselli P L 1977 Antiepileptic drugs. In:Morselli P L (ed.) Drug disposition during development. Spectrum, New York, p 311

Morselli P L 1978 Clinical significance of monitoring plasma levels of benzodiazepine tranquillisers and antiepileptic drugs. In: Deniker P, Radouco-Thomas C, Villeneuve A (eds) Neuropsychopharmacology. Pergamon Press, Oxford, p 877

Morselli P L, Gerna M, de Maio D, Zanda G, Viani F, Garattini S 1975 Pharmacokinetic studies on carbamazepine in volunteers and in epileptic patents. In: Schneider H, Janz D, Gardner-Thorpe C, Meinardi H, Sherwin A (eds) Clinical pharmacology and antiepileptic Drugs. Springer-Verlag, Berlin, p 166

Mountain K R, Hirsch J, Gallus A S 1970 Neonatal coagulation defect due to anticonvulsant drug treatment in pregnancy Lancet 1:265

Mucklow J C, Dollery C T 1978 Compliance with anticonvulsant therapy in a hospital clinic and in the community. British Journal of Clinical Pharmacology 6:75

Nanda R N, Johnson R H, Keogh H J, Lambie D G, Melville I D 1977 Treatment of epilepsy with clonazepam and its effects on other anticonvulsants. Journal of Neurology, Neurosurgery and Psychiatry 40:538

Naquet R, Meldrum B S 1972 In: Purpura D, Penry J K, Tower D B, Woodbury D M Walter R Q, (eds) Experimental models of epilepsy. Raven Press, New York, p 373

Ngwane E, Bower B 1980 Continuous sodium valproate or phenobarbitone in the prevention of 'simple' febrile convulsions. Archives of Diseases of Childhood 55:171

North J B, Penhall R K, Hanieh A, Frenwin D B, Taylor W B, 1983 Phenytoin and post-operative epilepsy, a double blind study. Journal of Neurosurgery 58:672

Odar-Caderlöf I, Borga 0 1976 Impaired protein binding of phenytoin in uremia and displacement effects of salicylic acid. Clinical Pharmacology and Therapeutics, 20:36

Olsen R W 1981 GABA-benzodiazepine-barbiturate receptor interactions. Journal of Neurochemistry 37:1

Oxbury J M, Whitty C W M 1971 Causes and consequences of status epilepticus in adults. A study of 86 cases. Brain 94:733

Oxley J, Hebdige S, Laidlaw J, Wadsworth J, Richens A 1980 A comparative study of phenobarbitone and primidone in the treatment of epilepsy. In: Johannessen S I et al (eds) Antiepileptic therapy: advances in drug monitoring. Raven Press, New York, p 237

Parker W A, Shearer C A 1979 Phenytoin hepatotoxicity: a case report and review. Neurology 29:175

Paxton J W, Whiting B, Stephen K W 1977 Phenytoin concentrations in mixed parotid and submandibular saliva and serum measured by radioimmunoassay. British Journal of Clinical Pharmacology, 4:185 Penry J K, Porter R J, Dreifuss F E 1972 Ethosuximide. Relation of plasma levels to clinical control. In: Woodbury D M

Penry J K, Schmidt R P (eds) Antiepileptic drugs. Raven Press, New York, p 431

Perucca E, 1978 Clinical consequences of microsomal enzyme induction by antiepileptic drugs. Pharmacology and Therapeutics 2:285

Perucca E, Garratt S, Hebdige S, Richens A, 1978 Water intoxication in epileptic patients receiving carbamazepine. Journal of Neurology, Neurosurgery and Psychiatry 41:713

Perucca E, Hebdige S, Gatti G, Lecchini S, Frigo G M, Crema A 1980 Interaction between phenytoin and valproic acid: plasma protein binding and metabolic effects. Clinical Pharmacology and Therapeutics 28:779

Perucca E, Hedges A, Makki K, Hebdige S, Wadsworth J, Richens A 1979 The comparative enzyme-inducing properties of antiepileptic drugs. British Journal of Clinical Pharmacology 7:414

Perucca E, Richens A 1980 Antiepileptic drug interactions. In: Tyrer J (ed) The treatment of epilepsy. MTP Press, Lancaster

Perucca E, Richens A, 1985 Antiepileptic drug interactions. In: Frey H-H, Janz D (eds) Handbook of experimental pharmacology vol 74: Antiepileptic drugs. Springer-Verlag, Berlin, p 831

Peterson D I, Zweig R W 1974 Absorption of anticonvulsants after jejuno-ileal bypass. Bulletin Los Angeles Neurological Society 39:51

Peterson G M, McLean S, Millingen K S 1982 Determinants of patient compliance with anticonvulsant therapy. Epilepsia 23:607

Petersen H R, Jensen I, Dam M 1983 THIP: a single blind controlled trial in patients with epilepsy. Acta Neurologica Scandinavica 67:114

Peterson G M, McLean S, Millingen K S 1984 randomized trial of strategies to improve patient compliance with anticonvulsant therapy. Epilepsia, 25:412

Pinder R M, Brogden R N, Speight T M, Avery G S 1976 Clonazepam: a review of its pharmacological properties and therapeutic efficacy in epilepsy. Drugs 12:321

Pinder R M, Brogden R N, Speight T M, Avery G S 1977 Sodium valproate: a review of its pharmacological properties and therapeutic efficacy in epilepsy. Drugs 13:81

Pippenger C E, Penry J K, Kutt H (eds) 1978 Antiepileptic drugs: quantitative analysis and interpretation. Raven Press, New York

Pisciotta A V 1982 Carbamazepine. Haematological toxicity. In: Woodbury D M, Penry J K, Pippenger C E (eds) Antiepileptic drugs. Raven Press, New York, p 533

Plaa G L, Hine C H 1960 Hydantoin and barbiturate blood levels observed in epileptics. Archives internationales de pharmacodynamie (et de therapie) 128:375

Pollack M A, Zion T E Kellaway P 1979 Long-term prognosis of patients with infantile spasms following ACTH therapy. Epilepsia 20:255

Porter R J, Layzer R B 1975 Plasma albumin concentration and diphenylhydantoin binding in man. Archives of Neurology 32:298

Porter R J, Penry J K, Lacy J R, Newmark M E, Kupferberg H J 1977 The clinical efficacy and pharmacokinetics of phensuximide and methsuximide. Neurology 27:375

Prensky A I, Raff M C, Moore M J, Schwab R S 1967 Intravenous diazepam in the treatment of prolonged seizure activity. New England Journal of Medicine 276:779

Prince D A, Wong R K S 1981 Human epileptic neurons studied in vitro. Brain Research 210:323

Pynnönen S 1979 Pharmacokinetics of carbamazepine in man: a review. Therapeutic Drug Monitoring 1:409

Rambeck B, Boenigk H E, Dunlop A, Mullen P W, Wadsworth J, Richens A 1979 Predicting phenytoin dose: a revised nomogram. Therapeutic Drug Monitoring 1:325

Rane A, Höjer B, Wilson J T 1976 Kinetics of carbamazepine and its 10, 11-epoxide metabolite in children. Clinical Pharmacology and Therapeutics. 19:276

Rating D, Nau H, Joauager-Roman E, et al 1982 Teratogenic and pharmacokinetic studies of primidone during pregnancy and in the offspring of epileptic women. Acta Paediatrica Scandinavica 71:301

Reidenberg M M, Drayer D E 1978 Effects of renal disease upon drug disposition. Drug Metabolism Reviews 8:293

Reynolds E H 1980 Serum levels of anticonvulsant drugs. Interpretation and clinical value. Pharmacology and Therapeutics 8:217

Reynolds E H, Shorvon S D 1981 Monotherapy or polytherapy for epilepsy. Epilepsia 22:1

Reynolds E H, Elwes R D C, Shorvon S D 1983 Why does epilepsy become intractable? Prevention of chronic epilepsy. Lancet ii:952

Reynolds F, Ziroyanis P, Jones N, Smith S E 1976 Salivary phenytoin concentrations in epilepsy and in chronic renal failure. Lancet 2:384

Reynolds E H, Shorvon S D, Galbraith A W, Chadwick D, Dellaportas C I, Vydelingom L 1981 Phenytoin monotherapy for epilepsy: a long-term prospective study, assisted by serum level monitoring, in previously untreated patients. Epilepsia 22:475

Ribak C E, Harris A B, Vaughn J E, Roberts E, 1979 Inhibitory GABAergic nerve terminals decrease at sites of focal epilepsy. Science 205:211

Richens A, 1976 Drug treatment of epilepsy. Henry Kimpton, London

Richens A 1979 Clinical pharmacokinetics of phenytoin. Clinical Pharmacokinetics 4:153

Richens A 1983 Clinical pharmacokinetics of benzodiazepines. In: Trimble M R (ed.) Benzodiazepines divided. John Wiley, Chichester, p 187

Richens A 1984 Enzyme induction and sex hormones. In: Porter et al (eds) Advances in epileptology: XVth Epilepsy International Symposium. Raven Press, New York

Richens A, Rowe D J F 1970 Calcium metabolism in patients with epilepsy. British Medical Journal 4:803

Richens A, Dunlop A 1975 Serum phenytoin levels in the management of epilepsy. Lancet ii:247

Rimmer E M, Buss D C, Routledge P A, Richens A 1984 Should we routinely measure free plasma phenytoin concentration? British Journal of Clinical Pharmacology 17:99

Rimmer E M, Richens A 1984 Double-blind study of γ-vinyl GABA in patients with refractory epilepsy. Lancet i:189

Rodin E A 1968 The prognosis of patients with epilepsy Thomas, Springfield

Rodin E A, Rim C S, Rennick P M 1974 The effects of carbamazepine on patients with psychomotor epilepsy: results of a double-blind study. Epilepsia 15:547

Rowan A J, Scott D F 1970 Major status epilepticus. A series of 42 patients. Acta Neurologica Scandinavica 46:573

Rowan A J Binnie C D, Warfield L A, Meijer J W A 1979 Epilepsia 20:61

Rowan A J, Meijer J W A, de Beer-Pawlikowski N, Van der Geest P, Meinardi H 1983 Valproate-ethosuximide combination therapy for refractory absence seizures. Archives of Neurology 40:797

Sato S, White B G, Penry J K et al (1982) Valproic acid versus ethosuximide in the treatment of absence seizures. Neurology 32:157

Schechter P J, Tranier Y, Grove J 1979 Attempts to correlate alterations in brain GABA metabolism by GABA-T inhibitors with their anticonvulsant effects. In: Mandel P, De Feudis F V (eds) GABA-Biochemistry and CNS functions. Plenum, New York p 43

Schmidt D 1982 Two antiepileptic drugs for intractable epilepsy with complex partial seizures. Journal of Neurology, Neurosurgery and Psychiatry 45:1119

Schmidt D 1984a Benzodiazepines – an update. In: Pedley J A, Meldrum B S (eds) Recent advances in epilepsy Vol 1. Churchill Livingstone, Edinburgh, p 125

Schmidt D 1984b Adverse effects of valproate. Epilepsia 25 (Suppl. 1):S44

Schmidt D, Kupferberg H J 1975 Diphenylhydantoin, phenobarbital and primidone in saliva, plasma and cerobrospinal fluid. Epilepsia 16:735

Schmidt D, Haenel F 1984 Therapeutic plasma levels of phenytoin, phenobarbital, and carbamazepine: individual variation in relation to seizure frequency and type. Neurology 34:1252

Schmidt D, Kupferberg H J, Yonekawa W, Penry J K 1980 The development of tolerance to the anticonvulsant effect of phenobarbital in mice. Epilepsia 21:141

Schmidt D, Seldon L (eds) 1982 Adverse effects of antiepileptic drugs. Raven Press, New York

Schobben F, Van der Kleijn E, Gabreels F J M 1975 Pharmacokinetics of di-n-propylacetate in epileptic patients. European Journal of Clinical Pharmacology 8:97

Schobben F, Van der Kleijn E, Vree T B 1980 Therapeutic drug monitoring of valproic acid. Therapeutic Drug Monitoring 2:61

Schottelius D D 1982 Primidone. Biotransformation. In: Woodbury D M, Penry J K, Pippenger C E (eds) Antiepileptic drugs. Raven Press, New York, p 415

Schousboe A, Larsson O M, Wood J D, Krogsgaard-Larson P 1983 Transport and metabolism of γ-amino-butyric acid in neurons and glia: implications for epilepsy. Epilepsia. 24:531

Schultz D W, MacDonald R L 1981 Barbiturate enhancement of GABA-mediated inhibition and activation of chloride ion conductance: correlation with anticonvulsant and anaesthetic actions. Brain Research 209:177

Serrano E E, Wilder B J 1974 Intramuscular administration of diphenylhydantoin. Histologic follow-up. Archives of Neurology 31:276

Shakir R A, Behan P O, Dick H, Lambie D G 1978 Metabolism of immunoglobin A, lymphocyte function, and histocompatibility antigens in patients on anticonvulsants. Journal of Neurology, Neurosurgery and Psychiatry 41:307

Shaw M D M, Foy P, Chadwick D 1983 Effectiveness of prophylactic anticonvulsants following neurosurgery. Acta Neurochirurgica. 69:253

Sherwin A L 1978 Clinical pharmacology of ethosuximide. In: Pippenger, C E, Penry J K, Kutt H P (eds) Antiepileptic drugs: quantitative analysis and interpretation. Raven Press, New York, p 283

Sherwin A L 1982 Ethosuximide. Relation to plasma concentration of seizure control. In: Woodbury D M, Penry J K, Pippenger C E Antiepileptic drugs. Raven Press, New York, p 637

Sherwin A L, Robb J P, Lechter M 1973 Improved control of epilepsy by monitoring plasma ethosuximide. Archives of Neurology 28:178

Shorvon S D, Reynolds E 1979 Reduction of polypharmacy for epilepsy. British Medical Journal ii:1023

Shorvon S D, Reynolds E H 1982 Early prognosis of epilepsy. British Medical Journal 285:1699

Shorvon S D, Chadwick D, Galbraith A W, Reynolds E H 1978 One drug for epilepsy. British Medical Journal 1:474

Shorvon S D, Espir M L E, Stever T J, Dellaportas C I, Clifford Rose F 1985 For debate: is there a place for placebo controlled trials of antiepileptic drugs? British Medical Journal 291:132

Sillanpää M, Pynnönen S, Laippala P, Säklauo E 1979 Carbamazepine in the treatment of partial epileptic seizures in infants and young children: a preliminary study. Epilepsia 20:563

Sjö O, Hvidberg E F, Larsen N E, Lund M, Naestoft J, 1975 Dose dependent kinetics of ethotoin in man. Clinical and Experimental Pharmacology and Physiology 2:185

Sjögren J, Solvell L, Karlsson I 1965 Studies on the absorption rate of barbiturates in man. Acta Medica Scandinavica 178:553

Smith T C, Kinkel A 1976 Absorption and metabolism of phenytoin from tablets and capsules. Clinical Pharmacology and Therapeutics 20:738

Spero L 1982 Neurotransmitter and CNS disease: epilepsy. Lancet ii:1319

Squires R F, Braestrup C 1977 Benzodiazepine receptors in rat brain. Nature 266:732

Stewart M J, Ballinger B R, Devlin E, Miller A, Ramsay A C 1975 Bioavailability of phenytoin – a comparison of two preparations. European Journal of Clinical Pharmacology 9:209

Strandjord R E, Johannessen S I 1974 One daily dose of diphenylhydantoin for patients with epilepsy. Epilepsia 15:317

Strickler S M, Dansky L, Miller M A, Seni M-H, Andermann E, Spielberg S P 1985 Genetics predisposition to phenytoin-induced birth defects. Lancet. ii:746

Suzuki M, Maruyama H, Ishibashi Y et al 1972 A double-blind comparative trial of sodium dipropylacetate and ethosuximide in epilepsy in children, with special emphasis on pure petit mal seizures. Medical Progress 82:470

Tassinari C A, Daniele O, Michelucci R, Bureau M, Dravet C, Roger J 1983 Benzodiazepines: efficacy in status epilepticus. In: Delgado-Escueta A V, Wasterlain C G,

Trieman D M, Porter R J (eds) Advances in epileptology vol 34: Status epilepticus. Raven Press, New York

Thompson P, Huppert F A, Trimble M R 1981 Phenytoin and cognitive function: effects on normal volunteers and implications for epilepsy. British Journal of Clinical Psychology 20:155

Thompson P J, Trimble M R 1982 Anticonvulsant drugs and cognitive functions. Epilepsia 23:531

Thompson P J, Trimble M R 1983 The effect of anticonvulsant drugs on cognitive function: relation to serum levels. Journal of Neurology, Neurosurgery and Psychiatry 46:227

Thurston J H, Thurston D L, Hixon B B, Keller A J 1982 Prognosis in childhood epilepsy. New England Journal of Medicine 306:831

Troupin A S, Ojemann L M, Dodrill C B 1976 Mephenytoin: a reappraisal. Epilepsia 17:403

Turnbull D M 1983 Adverse effects of valproate. Adverse Drug Reactions and Acute Poisonings Review 2:191

Turnbull D M, Rawlins M D, Weightman D, Chadwick D W 1982 A comparison of phenytoin and valproate in previously untreated adult epileptic patients. Journal of Neurology, Neurosurgery and Psychiatry 45:55

Turnbull D M, Rawlins M D, Weightman D, Chadwick D W 1983 Long-term comparative study of phenytoin and valproate in adult onset epilepsy. British Journal of Clinical Practice 27:3

Turnbull D M, Rawlins M D, Weightman D, Chadwick D W 1984 'Therapeutic' serum concentrations of phenytoin: the influence of seizure type. Journal of Neurology, Neurosurgery and Psychiatry 47:231

Turnbull D M, Howel D, Rawlins M D, Chadwick D W 1985 Which drug for this adult epileptic patient: phenytoin or valproate? British Medical Journal 290:815

Tyrer J H, Eadie M J, Sutherland J M, Hooper W D 1970 Outbreak of anticonvulsant intoxication in an Australian city. British Medical Journal 3:271

Vajda F J E, Symington G R, Bladin P F 1977 Rectal valproate in intractable status epilepticus. Lancet i:359

Van der Linden G J, Meinardi H, Meijer J W A, Bossi L, and Gomeni C 1981 A double blind crossover trial with progabide (SL 76002) against placebo in patients with secondary generalized epilepsy. In: Dam M, Gram L, Penry J K (eds) Advances in epileptology: 12th Epilepsy International Raven Press, New York, p 141

Waddell W J, Butler T C 1957 The distribution and excretion of phenobarbital. Journal of Clinical Investigation 36:1217–1226

Wallace S J, Aldridge-Smith J 1980 Successful prophylaxis against febrile convulsions with valproic acid or phenobarbitone. British Medical Journal 280:353

Wells C 1957 Trimethadione: its dosage and toxicity.

Archives Neurology and Psychiatry 77:140

Werk E E, McGee J, Scholiton L J, 1964 Effect of diphenylhydantion on cortisol metabolism in man. Journal of Clinical Investigation 43:1284

Whitty C W M, Taylor M 1949 Treatment of status epilepticus. Lancet 2:591

Wilder B J 1983 Efficacy of phenytoin in treatment of status epilepticus. In:Delgado-Escueta, A V, Wasterlain, C G, Treiman D M Porter R J (eds) Advances in neurology vol 34: Status Epilepticus. Raven Press, New York, p 441

Wilder B J, Ramsey R E 1976 Oral and intramuscular phenytoin. Clinical Pharmacology and Therapeutics 19:30

Wilder B J, Serrano E E, Ramsay E 1973 Plasma diphenylhydantoin levels after loading and maintenance doses. Clinical Pharmacology and Therapeutics 14:797

Wilder B J, Ramsay E, Willmore L J et al 1977 Efficacy of intravenous phenytoin in the treatment of status epilepticus; kinetics of central nervous system penetration. Annals of Neurology 1:511

Wilensky A J, Lowden J A 1973 Inadequate serum levels after intramuscular administration of diphenylhydantoin. Neurology 23:318

Wilensky H J, Priel P N, Levy R H, Comfort C P, Kaluzny S P 1982 Kinetics of phenobarbital in normal subjects and epileptic patients. European Journal of Clinical Pharmacology 23:87

Wilson J T, Hojer B, Rane A 1976 Loading and conventional dose therapy with phenytoin in children; kinetic profile of parent drug and main metabolite in plasma. Clinical Pharmacology and Therapeutics 20:48

Withrow C D 1982 Trimethadione: biotransformation. In: Woodbury D M, Penry J K, Pippenger C E (eds) Antiepileptic drugs. Raven Press, New York, p 689

Wolf S M, Forsythe A 1978 Behaviour disturbance, phenobarbitone and febrile seizures. Paediatrics 61:728

Wolf S M, Carra A, Davis D C et al 1977 The value of phenobarbital in the child who has had a single febrile seizure: a controlled prospective study. Paediatrics 59: 378

Worms P, Depoortere H, Durand A, Morselli P L, Lloyd K G, Bartholini G 1982 γAminobutyric acid (GABA) receptor stimulation. I. Neuropharmacological profiles of progabide (SL 76002) and SL 75102 with emphasis on their anticonvulsant spectra. Journal of Pharmacology and Experimental Therapeutics 220:660

Young B, Rapp R P, Norton J A, Hack D, Tibbs P A, Bean J R 1983a Failure of prophylactically administered phenytoin to prevent early post-traumatic seizures. Journal of Neurosurgery 58:231

Young B, Rapp R P, Norton J A, Hack D, Tibbs, P A, Bean J R 1983b Failure of prophylactically administered phenytoin to prevent late post-traumatic seizures. Journal of Neurosurgery, 58:236

13

Neurosurgery

C. E. Polkey

INTRODUCTION

Although epileptic seizures are common in general neurosurgical practice as a symptom of underlying disease or, occasionally, as a consequence of neurosurgical interference, when they are the main symptom, and the underlying pathology is initially obscure; they constitute a separate problem; it is with the neurosurgical solution to this problem that this chapter is concerned.

There is a large volume of animal experimental work on the neurophysiological basis of epilepsy, but little of this can be shown to be relevant to the natural history of the disease in humans. It is thought that secondary epileptogenesis in humans is imperfect and that, if it occurs at all, proceeds only to an intermediate stage (Morrell & Whistler 1980). It is difficult to relate this to the surgical treatment of the disease and so this aspect will not be covered in detail, but touched on as and where it seems appropriate. Details of the neurophysiology relating to electrocorticography are provided by Dr Binnie in Chapter 8. It should also be remembered that epilepsy results from the interaction between some cerebral disease process, whether identifiable or not, and the individual brain; the identical disease process in the same location in different patients will not necessarily give rise to the same severity of epilepsy or even the same manifestations. For this reason, therefore, the realistic achievement of surgical treatment must be to control the disease rather than eradicate it and, although the long follow-up periods for the early and now classical procedures indicate that in many cases this control is almost perfect, it is possible for patients, even many years after a successful operation, to experience further epileptic attacks.

The physician who wishes to decide whether a patient with chronic epilepsy would benefit from surgery is faced with the multitude of techniques used to assess such patients, together with a number of different operative procedures apparently available to treat the same condition. The purpose of this chapter is to resolve some of this confusion and to give a rational account of the scope of surgery in this situation. With modern practice, the mortality and morbidity of the neurosurgical techniques used in the treatment of epilepsy is acceptably low. By contrast, it is agreed by all authorities that chronic epilepsy leads to a decreased life expectancy especially when poorly controlled or as part of an underlying cerebral pathology. Thus, Penning et al (1969) noted that the average life expectancy of 202 patients was about 50 years and that the life expectancy was diminished by 43.6% in men and 51.4% in women; they quote similar figures from other authors.

Operations have been used in the treatment of epilepsy since neurosurgery first became practicable and the work of the early pioneers is very impressive, as recounted in the review by Talairach et al (1974). However, the first rational approach came from the Montreal Neurological Institute where Wilder Penfield, expanding the ideas he had worked upon with Foerster, began to try to show that possible epileptogenic areas of cerebral cortex, identified by stimulation at surgery, could be resected with benefit to the patient. The addition of electrical recording from the surface of the brain at operation and then from the deep structures, together with careful observational and surgical techniques, enabled this group to build up an unrivalled experience of resective surgery, described in their numerous publications and continuing to the present time.

However, as the Montreal group was becoming established, it became clear that this technique of local cortical resection was not suitable for all types of chronic epilepsy and so in other centres different philosophies and means of treatment were developed. The identification of the limbic system and the Papez circuit outlined a system of widespread connections which, in experimental animals, seemed to be especially vulnerable to epileptic-type discharges. Also, with his description of 'kindling', Goddard (1967) demonstrated experimentally that repeated electrical stimulation of the same neural pathway would cause a permanent change in its neurophysiological properties. These observations suggested that chronic epilepsy might alter the electrical activity of the brain so as to increase, or even perpetuate, the problem. It was then reasoned that, if these mechanisms could be modified in circumstances where the basic cause of the epilepsy was either unidentifiable or untreatable by surgery, then some relief from chronic seizures might follow. With the advent of human stereotactic surgery, the principles of which are described later, a number of workers began to explore this approach. The operations consisted of making, by various means, destructive lesions in one or more sites in the brain. Finally, there are a number of other procedures of a functional nature, including cerebellar stimulation introduced by Cooper (1973) which will also be discussed.

Because the number of centres carrying out surgical treatment for epilepsy is small, and the number of patients treated at each is also small, there is a tendency for each centre to rely on a few techniques, each well known to them; so patients with the same problem might be offered functional surgery in one centre and resective surgery in another. Further confusion is introduced by the fact that the personality problems which frequently accompany chronic epilepsy, and temporal lobe epilepsy in particular, may be alleviated by stereotactic procedures which have then been applied to patients who present with the same personality problems and no epilepsy. This has tended to make the assessment of some reports of these procedures difficult. In many of the earlier reports of the results of this kind of surgery, the period of follow-up was rather brief. For these reasons, this review tends to refer to reports in which the period of follow-up is five years or more and the surgical techniques are clearly defined. Especially valuable are reports from workers such as Talairach and his group or Vaernet where both types of techniques have been used.

PRINCIPLES OF ASSESSMENT OF PATIENTS FOR SURGERY

In all cases it must be established that the patient's epilepsy is both chronic and drug resistant. This, of course, includes the patient's record of drug compliance. The frequency of fits which is regarded as disabling will naturally vary from centre to centre, and even from patient to patient: most patients do not have attacks at regular intervals but an average of one attack per week seems reasonable. It must also be established that relieving the epilepsy will be of measurable benefit to the patient, or those who care for the patient, and that there is only the minimal possibility of producing an adverse effect from the operation which would be more disabling than the original epilepsy. A careful and complete psychiatric history is also of importance and an attempt should be made to distinguish clearly between those psychiatric complaints which are known to be associated with chronic epilepsy, and those of independent conditions. Finally, what the surgeon hopes to accomplish in terms of seizure relief, together with the possible hazard, should be conveyed realistically to the patient, the relatives and the referring physician. In order to produce the best results and also avoid false optimism or pessimism, it is better that such surgery should be carried out in a few centres with a reasonable turnover rather than occasionally in a general neurosurgical practice. In the case of resective surgery, it is now generally agreed that the success of the surgery depends upon demonstrating that the fits originate in one part of the brain and that frequently one can link them with some structural change in that part of the brain. Secondary to these considerations is the need to show that the remainder of the cerebral hemisphere is healthy and that resecting the affected part, large or small, will have a minimal effect. In the case of stereo-tactic or other functional procedures, similar information will be needed to justify lesions inter-rupting or modifying abnormal neurophysiological pathways.

Clinical

History

This is taken with perseverance and care for detail, and independent corroboration should be obtained both from relatives and previous hospital case notes. Two themes should be pursued in such history taking: the first is an attempt to establish that all the patient's attacks have a common source; the second is to seek evidence of, or a reason for, structural abnormality in the appro-priate part of the patient's brain.

In the first case, a careful history of the type of attack which the patient suffers must be obtained. In trying to locate the origin of a fit clinically attention should be paid to the aura, to any focal or lateralizing features in the attack, as well as its nature, and to any post-ictal phenomena such as a Todd's palsy. Any inconsistencies must be accounted for, or taken as evidence of multiple origins of the attacks. Particular difficulty may be experienced with speech phenomena for two reasons. First, it may be difficult to establish precise hemisphere dominance and, secondly, certain phenomena may arise in the non-dominant hemisphere as described by Falconer (1967a). Good descriptions of the localizing value of various epileptic phenomena are to be found in Penfield & Jasper (1954). It is essential to get a good description of the fit in layperson's terms, not accepting the use of expressions such as 'petit mal' or 'minor seizure' at face value. Witnesses, especially relatives, may display a kind of mirror description in which they attribute the patient's lateralizing features to the opposite side of their own body, but this can usually be clarified by careful questioning (Falconer, unpublished obser-vation). For purposes of careful follow-up the frequency of fits should be carefully established. Because such attacks are rarely regular it seems

reasonable to note, for the year prior to referral, the average frequency of attacks, together with the greatest number in one day and the longest fit-free interval, and to make a note of any obvious clustering.

The second point to be established from the history is whether there is any possible cause for the structural change. In an elegant monograph Ounsted et al (1966) showed that in 66 out of 100 children with psychomotor epilepsy a definite history could be obtained of birth injury or infan-tile febrile convulsions; and that, in the remainder, where the age of onset was later, miscellaneous lesions such as small tumours were found. In a similar vein, Falconer (1974) clearly demonstrated that in patients whose temporal lobectomy specimens showed the changes of mesial temporal sclerosis, there was a high inci-dence of previous febrile convulsions, whereas patients with other lesions did not show this.

Such history taking may require several hours, perhaps even several sessions, and considerable background research, but will amply repay the time spent.

Physical signs

Except in the case of previous brain damage or in patients with expanding lesions, physical signs during the interictal period are rare and when present tend to be soft and solitary. Examination in the immediate post-ictal period should always be carried out whenever possible, and special weight placed on lateralizing or localizing signs found during this period.

Observation

It is well known that when these patients are admitted to hospital for observation they often enter a fit-free period. Since it is necessary, for a number of reasons, to see the patient's attacks it would seem reasonable to reduce their antiepi-leptic medication. It is unwise to remove it al-together but a reduction, usually to one or two drugs, may be safely made without provoking status epilepticus. Direct observation of the attacks by suitably instructed medical and nursing staff is also of considerable value. A period of at least two weeks observation is necessary preoperatively and, occasionally, this period may have to be extended to several weeks.

Investigations

Neurophysiological studies

There are chapters elsewhere in this book on neurophysiology and this account is written from a neurosurgeon's point of view, but it is important to emphasize that close co-operation with an experienced clinical neurophysiologist is essential in the management of these patients. From the surgeon's point of view, the aim of the neurophysiological studies in these patients is to demonstrate the presence or absence of focal abnormality. The EEG itself is a dynamic phenomenon which changes with age and circumstances, and it is therefore important to obtain a sight of any previous records. In patients being considered for stereotactic lesions, complex studies using stereotactically placed electrodes will be necessary to demonstrate the presence of deep foci or irritable pathways. Furthermore, neurophysiological studies in the postoperative period are valuable, especially as a prognostic indicator (Van Buren et al 1975, Brazier et al 1975).

Although routine EEG studies may be helpful, they are frequently without focal features and so further studies become necessary; preferably after a reduction of antiepileptic medication, as we have already discussed. This manouevre allows the basic abnormalities to emerge and also removes drug effects which may be confusing. It is known that sleep will produce or heighten abnormalities in these records and so advantage is taken for natural sleep or drowsiness during long records. However, sleep may be induced either by prior sleep deprivation or the use of drugs, and we have used quinalbarbitone (Seconal) in a dose of 200 mg in adults; other workers describe the use of diazepam (Brazier et al 1976) and short-acting barbiturates (Wilder 1971). In examining records made under these circumstances, one is looking for the appearance of, or an increase in, the sharp waves and spikes; and, when drugs are used to induce sleep, the absence of the drug-induced fast activity that is usually seen from normal cortex.

The use of stimulants such as megimide (Bemegride) to provoke attacks is one that we have not used now for some years. The test itself is unpleasant and cannot be repeated more than once or twice, so that the relevant answer may not be forthcoming. In addition, attacks produced in this way may not be like the patient's habitual fits and it then becomes difficult to use the results of the test as a basis for surgery. Wieser et al (1979) showed that chemically induced seizures have the least correlation with spontaneously occurring seizures seen in depth recordings. It is of course of great value to obtain neurophysiological recordings during one of the patient's habitual seizures, especially if a visual record of the seizure can be made at the same time.

Certain parts of the cerebral cortex are poorly served by scalp electrodes and, in the case of the inferior part of the temporal lobes, extracranial access to the base of the skull can be used. There are a number of ways of doing this or obtaining equivalent recordings, including electrodes placed on the zygoma or in the nasopharynx and, as used at the Maudsley for many years, a technique of using small wires inserted under the zygoma so as to come to rest on the underside of the sphenoid bone. This technique, often combined with thiopentone sodium (Pentothal) narcosis, will be referred to as Pentothal-sphenoidal recording. The use of electrodes inserted through the foramen ovale has been described by Wiesser et al (1985) and abnormalities recorded by this route are said to correspond well with those seen in stereotactic recordings from the mesio-basal limbic structures.

An even more detailed assessment of intracerebral electrical activity may be needed, as in certain cases of frontal epilepsy, when it may be necessary to use more invasive techniques. One consists of passing electrodes into the cranium under stereotactic control, so as to be reasonably sure of the area from which the recordings are being obtained. Sometimes quite large areas of cortex are investigated by this means, but some teams restrict themselves to areas of particular interest. The general methods and advantages of this technique of stereo-electroencephalography (SEEG) are to be found in a review of their use by the Paris group (Talairach et al 1974). They state that, using SEEG techniques, they can outline a 'zone épileptogénie' in 85% of cases and that surgery in these cases has a very good result. They do, however, note in the same review that, although 428 patients have been investigated using this technique, they have carried out 236 operations, 160 of which were resective operations. There is no doubt that the use of these techniques, especially in regard to temporal lobe foci, can increase the number of patients who can be offered operations with a good chance of success. Thus Rasmussen (1983) notes that in 10–15% of patients, extensive investigation without depth electrodes failed to identify a temporal lobe focus. Subsequent investigation of this group of patients using depth electrodes reveal such a focus and allowed successful operation in two-thirds of them. In addition, the use of depth recording has also thrown some light on the mechanism of epileptic discharge in these patients. Data presented by Lieb et al (1982a), from a retrospective study of 52 patients investigated and treated at UCLA, showed that it was the ictal rather than the interictal neurophysiological data which were relevant in predicting the outcome of operation. A companion paper (Lieb et al 1982b) details the neurophysiological characteristics associated with the type of pathology found in the resected temporal lobe. Crandall et al (1981) and Delgado-Escueta & Walsh (1983) describe schemes of assessment of patients for temporal lobectomy in which stereotactic recordings are only performed on patients in whom there is not a clear lateralization on surface or sphenoidal electrodes. Delgando-Escueta & Walsh (1983) describe findings similar to those of Crandall et al (1983) but claim, in addition, that the findings correlate well with the patient's seizure type and the results of operation; a view not confirmed by other workers. They suggest that stereotactic exploration is justified when surface and sphenoidal recordings show bilateral ictal paroxysms; when they show diffuse ictal patterns; when discrepancies exist between ictal and interictal EEG patterns and the clinical seizure pattern; or when there is a suggestion from the clinical or neurophysiological data of an extratemporal origin for the fits.

Modern technology now provides arrays of electrodes which can be implanted at open operation and used for short periods of chronic recording from the extradural space in the central and parietal regions (Goldring 1979, Gregorie & Goldring 1984) This technique is particularly valuable in children, yielding information which would be obtained in adults by acute cortical stimulation and recording at craniotomy. Similar strip electrodes have been used in the subdural space to record from the inferior cortex (Wyler et al 1984) and the mesial surface of the frontal lobes and provide an alternative, and sometimes better, technique to that of stereotactic recording. Acute electrocorticography is used chiefly at operation and will be discussed later in relation to that topic.

The intracarotid amylobarbitone (Amytal) injection technique first described by Wada (1949) can be used for three purposes, the first two of which have to be conducted under local anaesthetic:

1. to determine hemispheric dominance for speech
2. to carry out tests of memory function to determine whether one temporal lobe may be safely removed (often conbined with (1); we have found this test useful and for a detailed description Milner (1975) should be consulted
3. to discover whether bilateral discharges originate from independent foci, or are due to secondary synchrony.

These tests are uncomfortable and carry some risk and should therefore only be used with good reason.

Neuroradiological studies

Neuroradiology, as applied to epilepsy in general, is dealt with in Chapter 9, but this section deals with neuroradiology in relation to surgery. The object of these neuroradiological studies is to seek evidence of a focal lesion. Although less fashionable, plain skull radiographs and tomography may reveal asymmetries relating to underlying brain atrophy or calcification denoting a structural brain lesion. During the last ten years CT (computer tomography) scanning of the intracranial structures has become generally available and improved the quality. The early use of the technique in virtually doubling the number of known structural abnormalities in epileptic populations is well known (Gastaut & Gastaut 1976). Furthermore, lesions which produce a definite change in the tissue density on CT scan, even if unaffected by contrast, are now detected by fourth generation scanners, even when quite small. Thus Rasmussen (1983) states that 90% of indolent gliomas and similar lesions are now detectable on CT scan. However, small atrophic lesions, in which a cerebral structure is reduced slightly in size but unaltered in density over a significant area, such as in mesial temporal sclerosis, are more difficult to detect. Placing a contrast medium in the basal cisterns may help, but even then this may need a complex computer programme to detect the condition. Using such a method Wyler & Bolender (1983) successfully diagnosed mesial temporal sclerosis in 16 out of 17 cases. The place of MRI (magnetic resonance imaging) scanning in investigating these patients is not yet clear since it has only recently become available. However, anecdotal evidence suggests that it will be good at revealing anatomical details, including the size and shape of the temporal horns, and occasionally it will show indolent tumours invisible to CT scanning. Because of the limitations of CT scanning and the cost and rarity of MRI facilities, there is still a place for air studies in demonstrating the size and shape of the temporal horns in hippocampal sclerosis. Cerebral angiography has diminished considerably in usefulness, but it should be noted that a normal angiogram on the side of an electrical focus is not evidence of the absence of a surgically treatable lesion.

Finally, mention should be made of the use of positron emission tomography (PET). It is becoming clear from various publications by the group in UCLA that this technique, using a radioactive fluorine sugar analogue, can show increased uptake in the temporal lobe during ictal activity and the reverse during the post-ictal and interictal state (Engel et al 1982, Engel 1984). These findings correlated well with the neurophysiological findings and are regarded by this group as a good supplementary test to help decide lateralization. A further refinement of this technique, single photon emission computerized tomography (SPECT) which does not need a cyclotron, shows a good correlation between abnormal uptake in epileptogenic areas and focal abnormalities on SEEG.

Psychometric studies

These are devoted to seeking a specific deficit which may be related to an organic brain lesion, and also to assessing the extent of any more widespread brain damage which might be a limiting factor to the size of any planned resection. The chief areas of interest relate to speech and memory function. This latter is especially intriguing when trying to determine whether temporal lobe disease is unilateral or bilateral. Such studies are also useful in gauging the extent and duration of any postoperative deficit. The data on these matters chiefly concern temporal lobe operations and, to a lesser degree, hemispherectomy, and will be dealt with in more detail in discussing those procedures.

The first requisite in assessing the results of surgery is to have the solid base of a good preoperative assessment. There should be a follow-up period of at least five years, since the number of patients remaining fit-free diminishes with time (Van Buren et al 1975). Where possible, the pathology in the resected specimen should be known. Finally, although for reasons already given it is desirable that such surgery should be carried out in a few centres, nevertheless, the technical details of this surgery should be such that it can be repeated by an adequately trained neurosurgeon, otherwise the procedure dies with its originator. In general, however, it is reasonable to assert that much of the success of such surgery tends to rest upon the selection techniques rather than the technical details of the surgery.

The purpose of this introduction is to set out the kind of considerations which must be taken before surgery is contemplated. Clearly, the final decision with regard to surgery in any particular case will depend upon the result of the foregoing investigations in a way which will emerge later. Because temporal lobe attacks are still the most common type of epilepsy for which surgical assistance is asked, it will be convenient to discuss the details of the surgical management of this condition first.

RESECTIVE SURGERY

Temporal lobectomy

We have already noted that temporal lobe epilepsy is the most common seizure for which surgery is sought; and a survey of the literature shows that temporal lobectomy is the most common and most widely reported surgical operation. Rasmussen (1979), reviewing the Montreal experience with resective surgery, notes that out of a total of 1407 operations between 1928 and 1974, 722 were temporal lobe resections. Jensen (1975a) was able to assemble data on 2282 published temporal lobe resections. She points out, quite correctly, that the results of these operations vary, but that those surgeons who have included the deep structures of the temporal lobe in their resection have obtained better relief of seizures. This is confirmed by Van Buren et al (1975), who noted that there were only 20% failures with complete operations compared with 50% with gyrectomies, topectomies and other techniques.

Assessment and investigation

The clinical features in the selection of these patients have already been outlined. They should have chronic complex partial seizures of at least five years duration in the case of an adult. The history should be such as to establish the complex partial nature of the attacks and also where possible to lateralize their origin.

It should be recalled that the 'auras' or complex partial seizures (i.e. the early sensory components) can be very bizarre and, to some extent, they have a predictive value. Their origin is still uncertain. Although they accompany electrical discharges in electrodes implanted in the deep structures of the temporal lobe (Babb & Crandall 1976) it is difficult to reproduce them by stimulation of these structures (Halgren et al 1978). Falconer & Taylor (1968) found that an aura was more likely to be present in patients with mesial temporal sclerosis in the resected temporal lobe and that, in those cases, the aura was more likely to have a somatosensory content, such as a rushing cephalic aura or a rising epigastric aura, rather than the taste or smell auras more usually associated with other lesions such as hamartomas. The way in which the

attack begins is held by some to be of importance. Thus, Delgado-Escueta & Walsh (1983) claim that those attacks which begin with a motionless stare, especially if consistent when the attacks are videotaped, have their origin in the mesial temporal structures and respond well to surgery. The seizures themselves, in addition to the recognized features of mumbling, lip smacking, swallowing, fumbling etc may have more bizarre components such as rushing about, trying to hide and so on; and, finally, frequently terminate in automatisms for which the patient is usually amnesic and which are associated with the seizure discharge becoming bilateral. Serafetidines & Falconer (1963) made a careful study of the speech disturbances in 100 patients and divided them into (a) paroxysmal dysphasia, consisting of an inability of the patient to express himself during a period of awareness and usually found in patients subsequently offered left temporal lobectomy; and (b) speech automatisms, consisting of identifiable words and phrases for which the patient is subsequently amnesic; this situation was more common in patients undergoing right temporal lobectomy.

The occurrence of other kinds of attacks as well as complex partial seizures has not been considered a bar to operation by most authors. Falconer & Serafetidines (1963) noted that the results of operation in patients who suffered tonic-clonic seizures were the same as those obtained in patients who suffered solely with complex partial seizures. Van Buren et al (1975) also noted that 50% of their patients suffered tonic-clonic attacks. However, Jensen (1976a) analysing 74 cases operated upon by Vaernet, sees tonic-clonic seizures as a bad prognostic indicator.

The interictal history is also of importance in these patients. Many of them have personality, social and behavioural difficulties. The proportion varies between one series and another, presumably because of variation in the referral sources and Jensen (1975a), surveying the world literature, states that the proportion varies between 15% and 56%. In the majority of cases the disorder corresponds to that described by Pond (1974), consisting of irritability, unpredictable mood variation, quarrelsome behaviour and so forth. There is no ready explanation for the aggressive, difficult behaviour displayed by these patients. It has been linked by some to a loss of control associated with amygdalar disease (Mark & Ervin 1970); a more sophisticated explanation is put forward in a series of papers by Bear and his co-workers. They suggest that these behavioural changes are related to a 'hyperconnection' syndrome caused by fortuitous connections between various limbic functions fuelled by the epileptic focus (Bear & Fedio 1977, Bear 1979, Bear et al 1982). Such 'aggressive' behaviour is not a bar to operation and may be relieved by it.

By contrast, only a small number of these patients exhibit a frank psychosis. The level of about 12% quoted by Falconer (1973) seems general for the epileptic population seen in psychiatric hospitals and clinics (Fenton 1978). However, in a large population of unselected temporal lobe patients (Currie et al 1971), the proportion was much lower, being of the order of 2%. The majority of these psychoses are of a paranoid type but lacking the cardinal features of schizophrenia. There is a tendency for this type of psychosis to be associated with left, i.e. dominant, hemisphere lesions (Flor-Henry 1969) and with the presence of alien tissue within the temporal lobe (Taylor 1975). Even when the surgery is successful in relieving the fits, the psychosis is usually unaffected, although it tends to mellow or burn out with time.

Finally, the previous medical history is important in looking for possible causes of structural brain damage to account for the epilepsy. In this respect the association between mesial temporal sclerosis and a previous history of a severe febrile convulsion is now well accepted, and the evidence for this, and some possible mechanisms of its pathogenesis, are well summarized by Falconer (1974). As suggested by the work of Ounsted (1967), the absence of a history of birth trauma or a febrile convulsion, together with a later onset for the epilepsy and the preservation of normal intelligence, suggests the presence of a small 'tumour like' lesion in the temporal lobe. These guidelines are fairly loose but valuable in the overall prediction of aetiology.

The results of temporal lobectomy in children will be dealt with later, but it is our experience that if drug-resistant epilepsy is established prior to puberty, especially when associated with a structural abnormality, it seldom remits with age; this is a constant feature in taking the histories of patients in their late teens and early twenties. In general, as shown by Falconer & Davidson (1974), criteria similar to those used in assessing adults can be successfully applied to children.

The investigation of these patients as already mentioned consists of psychometric, neuroradiological and neurophysiological tests. The importance of psychometric testing has already been outlined. A full-scale IQ of 70 points or more is thought to be necessary before a patient can benefit from temporal lobectomy. Using appropriate tests, a disparity between verbal and performance IQ may be found, although it is admitted by Milner (1975) that such differences do not have a high reliability. A recent study of 59 Maudsley patients (Powell et al 1985) showed that there were small non-significant trends, with patients who subsequently underwent a left lobectomy having a better performance on non-verbal tasks and the converse for right lobectomy candidates, as had been suggested earlier by Blakemore & Falconer (1967). However, it was also noted that the age of onset of the seizures influenced both the preoperative findings and the effects of operation. Of equal importance is the assessment of memory function and here poor performance in either the Wechsler Logical Memory (dominant temporal lobe) or the Rey-Osterreith Tests (non-dominant temporal lobe) is well accepted as evidence of appropriate damage.

When the psychometric findings conflict with other evidence there may be several explanations. One is that the patient is of mixed hemispheric dominance; another is that the patient may have sustained major unilateral temporal lobe damage at an early age and performs poorly because all the remaining memory function is subserved by one temporal lobe. A third explanation is that the patient has true bitemporal damage. The Wada test is useful in distinguishing between these possibilities and, in particular, it will give a good assessment of the memory function of the temporal lobe that will remain after a proposed lobectomy.

The variety of neuroradiological tests available has already been described. If the results of these tests are normal, then the decision for operation must be made on other grounds. As Newcombe & Shah (1975) pointed out, contralateral dilatation of the temporal horn was found in 13% of cases and operation was then carried out on the basis of the EEG findings. However, if there is a psychometric deficit corresponding to such a dilatation, but contralateral to the predominant EEG abnormalities, then care should be taken that one is not dealing with a situation in which the more damaged temporal lobe is electrically quieter. The use of the CT scanner has revealed discrete lesions in patients with widespread unilateral or bilateral EEG abnormalities. Our experience has confirmed the earlier observations of Falconer & Kennedy (1961) and the more recent ones of Wieser & Yasargil (1982) that the removal of such lesions results in an improvement in the epilepsy and the resolution, over a year or so, of the EEG abnormalities.

Neurophysiological studies are clearly of paramount importance. As already mentioned, many centres use a staged method of neurophysiological investigation, so that only in a proportion of cases is it necessary to use prolonged, invasive, expensive methods of investigation. To some extent, the more exhaustive the investigation the more successful is the surgery. Recent figures, such as those provided by Delgado-Escueta & Walsh (1983) or Wieser (1986), suggest that if a definite antero-mesial onset for the seizures can be demonstrated then the proportion of fit-free patients increases significantly; but this is only so when the location of the onset of the seizures has been confirmed by depth electrode recordings. This improvement is likely to be related to the ability to remove these structures completely, compared with other epileptogenic areas such as lateral temporal or extratemporal cortex, as much as to the improved localization of the epileptogenic discharge. We have already noted that in many centres where all these techniques are available a staged method of investigation is used. The simplest assessment consists of interictal sleep and Pentothal-sphenoidal recordings as already mentioned. The interpretation of the results of these tests and their use in recommending temporal lobe surgery is dealt with in detail by Engel et al (1975). However, some 40% of patients

may show bilateral independent discharges on scalp interictal recordings (Van Buren et al 1975) and, occasionally, the seizure onset may be contralateral to the predominant interictal discharge (Engel et al 1981). The use of sphenoidal electrodes with ictal recording may improve the localization but, even so, there remains a residual group of patients in whom no convincing lateralization or localization is obtained. Crandall (1975) noted that, whereas scalp recordings would give adequate information in 30% of patients when depth electrode recording was used, a focus was revealed in 73% of patients. Delgado-Escueta & Walsh (1983) point out that, in many patients, the ictal onset can be adequately demonstrated in nasopharyngeal or sphenoidal electrodes as an initial low-voltage fast rhythm which corresponds to unifocal or regional paroxysms in the amygdalo-hippocampal regions. Only if certain lateralization is unavailable by these means should depth electrode implantation be used. The use of subdural strip electrodes in this region, as described by Wyler et al (1984) is thought to be an adequate substitute for SEEG by some, although others dispute this. Although SEEG is relatively free of complications it is a technique which is expensive in staff and time. The advantages of SEEG exploration in the investigation of temporal lobe epilepsy are best seen in attempting to define hemisphere lateralization in patients with bitemporal discharges, or localization in patients where it is uncertain whether discharges are frontal or temporal in origin. There is much detailed information published about the use of these SEEG techniques, and good reviews by Delgado-Escueta & Walsh (1983) and Flanigin et al (1985). It can be argued either that the use of such implanted chronic recording systems improves the success rate of surgery by improving localization, or that it brings a constant success rate to a wider population. The precise application of these techniques will depend upon each centre's expertise and experience, nevertheless it has been accepted that they are both necessary and justified.

Summary

Although each case must be decided upon the detailed results of these investigations, and in particular the neurophysiology, it is possible to obtain some idea of the likelihood of a successful result from a temporal lobectomy by looking at the various factors involved in a simple way. It can be shown, using a crude point-scoring system, that patients in whom a good result is obtained have certain features in common, whereas the reverse is true of those who do badly. Thus if a complex partial seizure with an aura, lateralized temporal EEG abnormalities in the interictal records, appropriate psychometric deficits and a positive lesion on a CT scan each score 2 points, then a score of 5 or more invariably puts a patient in the improved group (Polkey 1983). If this is combined with the idea that the presence of a definite pathology in the specimen is also correlated with a good result (Falconer 1969, Lieb et al 1982b) and that most pathology can be predicted preoperatively on consideration of the history and radiological findings, then clearly the surgeon can form a shrewd idea as to which patients will do well.

Operative methods and technique

It is not appropriate, in this text, to give a detailed technical account of the surgery involved, merely to indicate its nature and extent. The view could be taken that having demonstrated a probable antero-mesial abnormality by the preoperative assessment, the object of the surgery should be to remove this abnormality. The standard Falconer 5–6 cm 'en bloc' resection, appropriately modified in the dominant hemisphere would suffice to deal with this situation, except in special circumstances which will be described later. The empirical evidence is that a resection is more effective in terms of seizure relief than any form of disconnection or stereotactic ablation (Ojemann & Ward, 1975, Talairach et al 1974, Turner 1982, Vaernet 1972). A complete lobectomy may be more effective than the other procedures for each of three cogent reasons: first, it accomplishes a clear and extensive disconnection; secondly, it removes a large mass of neural tissue, thus reducing the possibility of achieving the theoreticians 'critical mass'; and lastly, it is more likely to remove the pathology.

This is a suitable point to discuss the place of electrocorticography and the use of local anaesthesia in these procedures. The anatomical boundaries of temporal lobectomy are set to minimize the neurological complications of the procedure. These limits are a posterior distance of 6.5 cm from the pole to avoid a hemianopia, sparing part of the superior temporal gyrus in the dominant hemisphere and no 'spike chasing' in the insula to avoid a hemiplegia. If within these limits there does not seem to be any advantage in sparing tissue, then it is not essential to carry out cortical recording. However, it does have a prognostic value in that patients with persistent abnormalities in the post-resection ECoG tend to have a poor result from the operation (Van Buren et al 1975). The use of local anaesthesia is equally contentious. The assertion made in the past that the corticogram was more useful in planning the resection and more 'natural' under these conditions is not so important now, for the reasons already given. When operating on the dominant, usually left, temporal lobe, local anaesthesia may be useful in allowing cortical stimulation to delineate the speech areas. However, there is no reliable comparison of the results of operations carried out under such conditions (that minimize speech problems whilst maximizing the size of the resection) with patients operated upon under general anaesthesia using anatomical landmarks. These landmarks are either a limit of the first 1–1.5 cm of the superior temporal gyrus, as suggested by Falconer (1971a), or to where the first sulcus crosses the superior temporal gyrus as suggested by Rasmussen (personal communication). Recently Ojemann & Dodrill (1985) have described a method of dominant hemisphere memory mapping which enables them to tailor the resection so as to minimize any verbal memory deficit. However, this does result in a smaller resection, which they admit may be less effective in controlling the epilepsy. It should be emphasized that in most extratemporal resections the use of electrocorticography and local anaesthesia is essential.

The methods of anaesthesia used by most centres are similar, the choice of basal sedation may vary. If general anaesthesia is used, non-barbiturate agents are usually employed together with controlled respiration and the patient is run as light as possible during corticography. It is not usually necessary to use diuretics or Mannitol during these operations. If local anaesthesia is used, infiltration is carried out with 0.5% lignocaine with adrenaline at a dilution of 1:200 000; details of this technique are to be found in Van Buren et al (1975). After the corticogram, which is activated with 100–150 mg of thiopentone given intravenously, the anaesthesia is supplemented with additional thiopentone during the resection and closure. If necessary the skin may be reinfiltrated at the end of the procedure. We have not found blind endotracheal intubation necessary during this part of the procedure.

The technique of the resection by the 'en bloc' method, in which the pathology is preserved, is well described by Falconer (1971a). His account can be followed by any well-trained neurosurgeon. The operation is technically easier when some atrophic process is present. In performing the craniotomy, it is important to get right down on to the floor of the middle fossa and to within 1–2 cm of the temporal pole, otherwise subsequent manoeuvres become more difficult. In carrying out the resection several points are important. First, the appropriate part of the superior temporal gyrus must be preserved on the dominant side. Secondly, care is necessary in dissecting the temporal cortex off the insula so as to avoid damage to the main trunk and branches of the middle cerebral artery; in this respect the subpial technique described by Falconer is excellent. Thirdly, it is necessary to remove the anterior 1–2 cm of the hippocampus without encroaching on the structures in the tentorial hiatus. The closure is performed in the usual way, as after any craniotomy; we do not routinely use antibiotics or steroids. The patient is usually maintained on two antiepileptic drugs after operation, phenytoin and carbamazepine or primidone are useful. If the patient remains free of attacks for two or three years after operation then consideration is given to the removal of the drugs. The usual postoperative complications of craniotomy occur rarely, but can be effectively treated and have no influence on the eventual outcome of the surgery (Falconer & Serafetidines 1963)

Recently, Wieser (Wieser & Yasargil 1982) has described a group of patients in whom there are unilateral discharges which are shown by depth recordings to emanate from the medial temporal structures, often in association with radiological evidence of a structural abnormality such as a hamartoma. In these patients, resection of the amygdala and hippocampus, using a microsurgical technique is effective and spares the lateral temporal cortex and avoids psychometric deficits. This operation of 'amygdalo-hippocampectomy' however is not suitable for many patients who currently benefit from an 'en bloc' resection.

Neuropathology

It is impossible to discuss resective surgery for epilepsy without reference to the pathology found in the specimens, and in this respect the data is most abundant for temporal lobectomy. Because the results of operation are also related to the pathology this discussion is appropriate at this point. Murray Falconer, collaborating with Professor J. A. N. Corsellis and Dr C. Bruton produced the largest and most comprehensively examined series of temporal lobectomy specimens in which the resection included the anterior 1–2 cm of the hippocampus. As described by Falconer (1971b), the pathological material divided itself into four groups. Gross lesions, which would have been treated on their own account, such as meningiomas, have of course been excluded. The results of surgery in relation to pathology are shown in Table 13.1. for a group of 90 patients followed up for between two and seven years. The pathological groups are described below.

Mesial temporal sclerosis

Classically, this lesion consists of a loss of neurones from the H_2 or Sommer sector of the hippocampus, together with a lesser degree of neuronal loss from the endfolium (H_3 and H_4) but with sparing of the resistant or H_2 sector. This pathology, originally described by Bouchet & Cazauvieihl in 1825, was also described by Sano & Malamud (1953) and Margerison & Corsellis (1966) in the brains of patients with chronic epilepsy dying in psychiatric institutions. Both

Table 13.1 Outcome of temporal lobectomy in relation to the pathology in the specimen

Pathology	No. of patients	Worthwhile improvement		Remainder	
		Group I	Group II	Group III	Group IV
M.T.S.	46	61%	19%	9%	11%
Tumour or hamartoma	25	80%	16%	0%	4%
Other lesions	5	20%	40%	20%	20%
Cortical dysplasia	4	75%	0%	0%	25%
All pathology	80	65%	19%	6%	10%
Non-specific findings	10	10%	30%	10%	50%

papers note that the lesion was frequently either unilateral or more pronounced on one side. Margerison & Corsellis (1966) found a good correlation between the clinical and neurophysiological features and the pathological findings. This lesion was found in 50% of Falconer's material and similar findings are reported by other authors, though in different proportions (Jann Brown 1973, Talairach et al 1974, Mathieson 1975, Van Buren et al 1975). The extent of the sclerosis may be important. The UCLA group have subdivided this pathology into those where the sclerosis is restricted to the Ammon's horn and those where it involves other structures, such as the amygdala, parahippocampal and fusiform gyri. They claim that those with the more extensive lesion get a better result from the lobectomy (Lieb et al 1982b).

Hamartomas and small cryptic tumours

This kind of lesion was found in 20–25% of the surgical material. It was absent from the autopsy studies of Margerison & Corsellis (1966) and it had been suggested that these lesions, with the passage of time, become frank glial tumours (Falconer 1967b). Although it is well known that glial tumours can become more active after a long period, we are now seeing with the CT scanner similar small calcified lesions in older people and so its seems that these lesions can remain static throughout life. Occasionally, mixed lesions known as gangliogliomas are seen. In addition, there are a small number of other lesions such as

angiomas and cortical dysplasia (see Taylor et al 1971).

Scars and infarcts

These were less common, accounting for 10% or less of the total.

Non-specific lesions

These formed about 25% of Murray Falconer's material and that from other centres. This term is deliberate since there were some changes in the form of astrocyte proliferation and subpial gliosis in these specimens. The use of the CT scanner and a better interpretation of the other data has reduced the proportion of patients with non-specific findings; and in 86 consecutive lobectomies at the Maudsley between 1976 and 1984 there were non-specific findings in only 9 cases (9%) and none in the last 19 specimens.

Results of temporal lobectomy

These have been well summarized by Jensen (1975a), and her bald statement remains true that 'two-thirds of the patients were either free or almost free of seizures and over half of these patients who were mentally abnormal before operation were normalized or had obtained a marked improvement'. If we make use of her figures for each of the three centres with over 100 resections, namely, the Montreal Neurological Institute, Murray Falconer's figures from the

Table 13.2 Results of unilateral temporal lobectomy for chronic epilepsy (data taken from Jensen 1975a)

Centre	No. of patients	Worthwhile improvement		Remainder		Operative deaths
		Group I	Group II	Group III	Group IV	
Guy's Maudsley London	152	61 (39.8%)	25 (16.7%)	39 (25.5%)	24 (16.2%)	2 (1.3%)
Salpetriere, Paris	110	32 (29.1%)	40 (36.4%)	20 (18.2%)	17 (15.5%)	1 (0.9%)
Montreal Neurological Institute	569	249 (43.8%)	120 (21.0%)	200 (35.1%)		1 (0.2%)
Total	831	342 (41.1%)	185 (22.3%)	300 (36.0%)		4 (0.5%)

Maudsley Hospital, London and those from the Salpetriere in Paris, then we obtain the results shown in Table 13.2. The result of operation with regard to seizure control are grouped according to the scheme proposed by Jensen (1975a), in which the divisions are: Group I, free from seizures; Group II, marked improvement in frequency, meaning at least 75% better; Group III, some improvement; and Group IV, no improvement. These series combine a total of 831 patients and it will be seen that 42% were completely free of seizures and a further 22% fell into Group II giving a worthwhile result from operation in 64% of cases. The mortality rate is extremely low at 0.5% and ever declining. More recent studies confirm these figures. Rasmussen (1983), summarizing the Montreal experience with 1034 patients, finds 50% of patients having only occasional seizures with a further 13% showing a marked reduction in seizure frequency; and Crandall et al (1983), reviewing the UCLA experience, find 54% of patients had either rare seizures or no seizures and a further 22% were improved. We have recently reviewed 90 patients operated upon at the Maudsley and found 58% having less than one fit per year of follow-up, with 25% free of seizures, and a further 21% with their seizure frequency reduced at least 75%; giving an overall improvement in 79% of patients operated upon. The results in terms of seizure or relief in children are similar to those seen in adults (Falconer & Davidson 1974).

We are also interested in the durability of the result of operation. It has been noted by others that the longer the patients are followed then the smaller is the proportion remaining fit-free (Van Buren et al 1975). We found that this was true of our patients, but also noted that patients who achieved a reduction in fit frequency better than 75% by the end of the first year after operation never reverted to a seizure frequency greater than this in periods of follow-up extending to 15 years. We also noted a small group of patients who had recurrent infrequent fits after fit-free intervals of two years or more. In half these patients the recurrent seizure was a generalized seizure occurring during or after the withdrawal of antiepileptic medication and responded to its reintroduction.

Neurological sequelae do occur and their documentation varies from series to series. The 'neighbourhood' fits described by Falconer & Serafetidines (1963) consisted of twitching of the contralateral face and arm. They occurred in the first postoperative week and had no effect upon the ultimate outcome. In our hands, the chief neurological complications from the most minor to the most serious have been: visual field defects, usually an upper quadrantanopia; homolateral third nerve palsy; speech disturbance when operating in the dominant hemisphere; hemipareses. It is difficult to know the extent of these problems in the published series because the assessment of them is clearly dependent upon how long they persist and the accuracy of observations. Jensen (1975a) pointed out that there is a great disparity in the recording of visual field defects between the different centres. If the resections are greater than 6–6.5 cm from the temporal pole in an adult then a complete homonymous hemianopia is more likely to result, becoming almost certain beyond 7 cm. When the resection lies between 5 cm and 6 cm from the pole then the chance of a complete hemianopia is 5% or less, depending upon the vagaries of Meyer's loop (Falconer & Wilson, 1958). The upper quadrantanopia appears in about 60% of patients, normally recedes over the next year and does not seriously inconvenience those in whom it persists. Similarly, although Falconer reported homolateral third nerve palsies in about 15% of his patients, they were usually of short duration disappearing in fewer than six months. Likewise, if patients are carefully observed during the first week after a dominant temporal lobe resection, they invariably show some degree of expressive dysphasia; but even in patients where the speech difficulty is more evident social speech is quickly regained. The level of 5% given by Jensen (1975a) seems reasonable. Any hemiparesis is usually transient and again the level of 2% quoted by Jensen (1975a) is realistic.

In summary, the neurological sequelae of temporal lobectomy, although occurring, are not so frequent or permanent as to be a serious deterrent to operation.

The intellectual sequelae of temporal lobectomy have already been hinted at; in general, psychometric scores one month after operation show a slight decline but thereafter tend to improve. The danger of producing a disabling amnesic syndrome when both temporal lobes are damaged is well known, and the autopsy findings under such circumstances have been described by Penfield (1974). The auditory learning deficit described by Blakemore & Falconer (1967), which may follow left temporal lobectomy, is said to recede in the majority of cases over two to three years. Jones (1974) found that patients who had undergone a left temporal lobectomy needed mnemonic aids to overcome their learning difficulties, whereas those patients who had a right temporal lobectomy did not need these aids. The subject is well reviewed by Milner (1975). In the study already mentioned (Powell et al 1985), it was shown that when the pathology was acquired early in life there was little change in the intellectual function measured

one month after temporal lobectomy; but when it occurred in a previously healthy temporal lobe, the results of a lobectomy, especially on the dominant side, could be disabling and this point is echoed by Delgado-Escueta & Walsh (1983). In some patients this may be an acceptable price to pay for seizure relief, but not in others.

A relatively high proportion of the patients investigated and selected for surgery have psychiatric abnormalities. In the Copenhagen series of 74 patients, only 8.5% were considered psychiatrically normal (Jensen 1976b); and in the series of 100 patients described by Taylor & Falconer (1968) only 13% could be considered psychiatrically normal. As we have already mentioned, the chief abnormalities observed were social maladjustment and aggression. Although a recent review suggests that personal aggression is a rare accompaniment of temporal lobe epilepsy (Delgado-Escueta et al 1981), nevertheless, occasionally a murderous impulse may form part of the attack, and Falconer certainly had one case in which such attacks ceased after lobectomy; a similar case is described by Hamlin & Delgado (1977). It is the experience of all those who have been concerned with these matters that social adjustment is improved by operation (Taylor & Falconer 1968, Jensen 1976b) so that more than half of these patients can live independently and be employed afterwards. Those patients who did best in this way also had a good relief from seizures. Jensen (1976b) states that an improvement in personality problems was associated with good seizure relief, normal intelligence and operation undertaken before the age of fifteen years. It was hoped and expected that treating children during their formative years, if successful, would not only lead to control of their seizures but also to a neutralization of all the adverse social and educational effects of chronic uncontrolled epilepsy. A study of the fate of a group of 50 children from the Park Hospital at Oxford, whose epilepsy was treated surgically with a variety of operations including temporal lobectomy, emphasizes the successful results which can be obtained in terms of education, employment and social adjustment; however, they also note that such patients may need extensive postoperative rehabilitation in the widest sense (Lindsay et al 1984) As far as frank aggression is concerned, Falconer (1973) surveying 100 patients noted that 27 were aggressive prior to surgery, that 10 of these were improved by temporal lobectomy, and in 7 of these 10 cases the pathology in the resected temporal lobe was mesial temporal sclerosis.

With regard to psychoses, it has already been stated that these usually failed to improve if they were schizophreniform; indeed, they were made worse by operation. Serafetidines & Falconer (1962), describing twelve cases, noted that when there was a confusional psychosis related to the epilepsy (Fenton 1978) this usually disappeared; that paranoid delusional psychosis accompanied by depression might improve; and that schizophrenic like states usually persisted.

The operation itself may produce psychiatric disorders; thus Falconer & Taylor (1968) reported 3 patients so affected; Jensen and Larsen (1979) described 9 patients, 6 of whom were free of seizures; and Sherwin (1981) described a patient worse after surgery. We have observed psychosis in two out of 86 patients and in one of these it was transient. Both of these patients had a non-dominant lobectomy on neurophysiological grounds but had adverse psychometric scores. Taylor (1975), studying Falconer's series, noted a greater occurrence of schizophreniform psychosis in patients with 'alien tissue' lesions in the resected temporal lobe and also that there seemed to be a higher proportion of left-handers amongst these patients. He discusses the possible explanations for these findings. Depressive episodes after right temporal lobectomy are well known and may culminate in suicide.

The overall effect of the operation upon the psychiatric state, summarized by Jensen (1975a) is that 23.5% of patients were mentally normal at the time of follow-up compared with 6.2% prior to operation; and that a further 40.9% had improved, leaving only 35.6% who had remained unchanged or had deteriorated.

The long-term fate of these patients has also been studied. Jensen (1975b), surveying the long-term mortality in 820 patients surviving the operation, found a late mortality of 4.76%, one-third of these patients dying of epilepsy, one-third committing suicide and the remaining third dying of natural causes. Taylor & Marsh (1977) made a

detailed study of the cause of death in 37 patients out of 193 operated upon by Murray Falconer: 8 of these deaths were due to persisting epilepsy, 9 were due to suicide, 3 of these patients having been free of fits since operation; 11 of the deaths were clearly due to natural causes, including recurrent tumours; and the remaining 9 deaths occurred in unclear circumstances. Although, as Jensen (1975b) notes, the death rate observed in these patients (47.6/1000) is in excess of that for an equivalent Danish population aged 10–59 years (2.9/1000), it is still better than the rate of 59.4/1000 quoted for a representative group of Danish epileptic patients by Brink-Henriksen et al (1970).

OTHER CORTICAL RESECTIONS INCLUDING MAJOR RESECTIONS

The remaining resections fall into two groups: First, are resections of other parts of the cortical mantle involving parts of one or two lobes, the commonest being the frontal lobe and then the central or parietal areas and rarely the occipital lobe. Second, are really major resections involving removal of the whole cerebral cortex or all except one part of one lobe, amounting to total or subtotal hemispherectomies. With the exception of the Montreal Neurological Institute, the experience of most centres with these operations is quite small. Thus in the Maudsley Neurosurgical Unit, where over 300 operations for epilepsy were carried out between 1950 and 1974, only 21 were focal resections with about 20 hemispherectomies. The material described in this section therefore derives chiefly from the experience of the Montreal group as published by Rasmussen with the lesser experience of ourselves, the Paris group (Talairach et al 1974), and a small group from Scandinavia (Bhatia & Kollevold 1976).

The principles of assessment for frontal lobectomy are similar to those used in temporal lobectomy, but the decision may be more difficult for a number of reasons. Typical adversive seizures are common enough, but when associated with other kinds of seizure these latter do not have the same benign prognostic significance as other types of epilepsy associated with temporal lobe attacks.

According to Rasmussen (1975a), frontal lobe seizures may begin in one of six ways each of which may have a specific localizing value. Although it is probable that adversion is a reasonable lateralizing feature in frontal lobe epilepsy, it may not be absolutely reliable. Robillard et al (1983) have shown with depth electrode studies that the onset of frontal lobe adversive seizures may be equally contralateral and ipsilateral.

A further difficulty arises when trying to localize neurophysiological abnormalities within the frontal lobe by scalp EEG, especially when these abnormalities are near the midline. The prevalence of apparent bifrontal abnormalities in these patients makes selection difficult even when special tests are used to try to differentiate bilateral secondary synchrony (Rasmussen, 1975a). The impressive results described with SEEG by Talairach et al (1974) and a similar philosophy adopted by Rossi et al (1978) in suggesting that the current failure rate of this kind of surgery of 30–40% may be improved by a better definition of the 'zone epileptogenie' using depth electrodes, indicate that these techniques may be especially useful in improving the results of surgery in this area. Access to the medial and inferior parts of the frontal lobes by use of the strip and grid electrodes described earlier may also improve localization in this region.

In their series of 91 patients, Bhatia & Kollevold (1976) carried out 22 frontal lobectomies as against 36 temporal lobectomies; in the Paris series (Talairach, Bancaud et al 1974) there were 24 frontal lobectomies compared with 68 temporal lobectomies, and, in the Montreal material (Rasmussen 1975a), 760 temporal lobectomies were performed and 244 frontal lobectomies. The pathology found in these frontal lobe resections is more heterogeneous than in the temporal lobe material. Rasmussen (1975a) describes the pathology in their 244 non-tumourous frontal lobe resections as follows: cicatricial or anoxic, 68%; miscellaneous, 10%; unknown, 21%. The other groups do not give a separate analysis.

The technique of operation in the frontal lobe is similar to that used elsewhere, and, provided that a reasonable posterior limit is set to the resection, the neurological sequelae are fewer than with temporal lobectomy. If the procedure is performed under local anaesthesia, then electrocorticography and cortical stimulation may be used to plan the resection, especially in the dominant hemisphere where speech may be at risk. If the craniotomy is large, or has to come near to the midline, then it is often convenient to stage the procedure making the craniotomy under general anaesthesia and then, within a few days, carrying out the recording, stimulation and definitive resection under local anaesthesia with antibiotic cover in between. The results of operation are reasonable, though not as good as for temporal lobectomy. In the Montreal series of 236 patients (Rasmussen, 1975a) the operative mortality was 1.7% and, of the remainder, 23% were in Group I and 32% in Group II, giving a worthwhile improvement in 55% but with a greater proportion in Group II. In the Paris series (Talairach et al 1974) a success rate of 54.2% (equivalent to Groups I and II) was obtained in 24 frontal lobe resections.

The surgery of other parts of the cortex is equally rare and here reliance must be placed almost totally on the results from Montreal, of whose material this group forms 30% (Rasmussen 1975b). In lesions involving the central area, the attacks are more stereotyped and virtually always have a somato-motor or somato-sensory component. These patients also present with either focal status or epilepsia partialis continuans more frequently than other groups. Because many of the causative lesions are gross and acquired early in life, a higher proportion of these patients have a pre-existing neurological deficit than other patients and they tend to come to operation at an earlier age. In these cases also, whenever possible, local anaesthesia, ECoG and cortical stimulation are employed and these techniques become more useful.

The technical arrangements for electrocorticography should be such as to allow a good recording to be obtained free of artefacts, including pulse and movement artefacts, with the minimum of disturbance. Some of the electrodes will be placed on the exposed surface of the brain whilst others of a more flexible design will be slipped onto the inferior and medial surfaces of the cortex. Although there is sometimes a visible abnormality on the surface, at other times there is not; but in either event the cortical recording must serve as a means of delineating the extent of the resection. In this respect, attention should be paid, as with the scalp recordings, to those features which denote structural damage as distinct from epileptic activity. There is no reliable way of distinguishing spikes which are likely to persist from those that may disappear some while after a resection. Rasmussen (1979) concludes, on the basis of his long experience, that whenever possible the maximum spiking area should be removed. He claims that 45% of patients achieved almost complete seizure control in a group where re-operation was deemed advisable because of poor control following a small resection. It should be noted that extensive preoperative investigations should be undertaken because the view of cortical activity obtained at acute corticography is limited both in space and in time; although the latter objection can be overcome, to some extent, by the use of Goldring's grid technique (Goldring 1979). The use of cortical stimulation in eloquent areas is also important and can easily be undertaken using a small battery-powered constant current stimulator. Cortical stimulation as a means of identifying areas of low epileptic threshold is no longer thought to be very useful. If a fit is provoked by cortical stimulation it can easily be controlled by intravenous anaesthesia, such as thiopentone, and after 20 or 30 minutes the cortical exploration can be continued. The surgical technique in carrying out the actual resection should be meticulous, the excision being taken to the gyral margins and down to the white matter wherever possible.

Although the question of postoperative neurological deficit is a thorny one in these areas Rasmussen's experience in this respect is fairly encouraging (Rasmussen 1975b). He states that removal of the motor face area leaves a persisting deficit in only half the patients; that the post-central leg area can be removed with only a slight decrease in the proprioception in the foot; and that the precentral leg area should only be removed if it is already damaged; but that on those occasions when it has been thought necessary a flaccid paralysis of the leg resulted which may show some recovery after three to four months. Although portions of the arm area may be removed there will always be some deficit, even if it is very slight. The results of surgery in these areas are quite good with 31% of patients in Group I and 26% in Group II,' giving a worthwhile improvement in 57%. In the French series (Talairach et al 1974), a success rate of 60% was obtained with resections of the central cortex. Details of the results of occipital and parietal resections can be found in the same review of the Montreal material (Rasmussen 1975b). We have carried out cortical resections on 27 patients in the decade 1975 to 1985. These comprised 13 frontal resections, 10 central or parietal and 4 occipital. Where the pathology has been discrete, small and non-progressive, the results have been good. A few patients, who in retrospect are suffering from the syndrome described by Rasmussen (1978) as encephalitis with epilepsy, did badly with such limited resections, as one might expect. Among the others the results were in line with those already discussed. The pathology found in these specimens covered a wide spectrum including traumatic and perinatal scarring, cortical dysplasia and a variety of other pathologies which were represented by single cases.

In summary, resective surgery in these other parts of the cortex can also be rewarding. The investigation of such patients, especially the neurophysiological investigation, is more time consuming than with temporal lobe epilepsy. However, the side-effects of these operations, except where taking a calculated risk, are relatively minor and infrequent. The overall effects in terms of seizure relief are reasonable: Rasmussen (1975b) has 64% in Groups I and II; Talairach et al (1974) obtained 67% in these groups; and in our small series there were 26% fit-free and 55% improved.

Major resections

Major resective procedures in the form of total or subtotal hemispherectomy have in recent years lacked popularity because of the late complications of such procedures and because of a natural aversion to such major surgery, which is unfortunate because these operations were in many ways very successful. The indications for operation are as follows.

The subject should suffer from intractable

epilepsy and, in addition, should have a complete infantile hemiplegia usually accompanied by a complete homonymous hemianopia, although the conversion of a partial field defect to a complete hemianopia would be justified in exchange for the benefits of the operation. It is debatable as to whether a progressive hemiparesis rendered complete by the Todd's palsy of an epilepsia partialis continuans, as we have seen especially in Rasmussen's encephalitis, is effectively the same thing as a complete hemiplegia, but we have certainly considered it so upon occasion. In spite of their severe hemiplegia, virtually all of these patients are able to walk preoperatively, and many will have undergone orthopaedic procedures to try to help their walking. In addition, there should be evidence that only one hemisphere is involved in the disease process: the degree of mental retardation should be acceptable; and there should be good parental collaboration. The onset of progressive dementia, preferably supported by psychometric data, should be regarded as an indication for urgent action especially if all the other parameters are right (Griffith 1967), otherwise the situation may become irretrievable. These patients often have a behaviour disorder and this is not a bar to operation and may indeed be improved by surgery. These patients may also experience a number of different types of fit, although Wilson (1970) reviewing 50 hemispherectomies carried out by McKissock, notes that major seizures occurred in 56% of patients but predominated in only 40%. Minor seizures occurred as the sole form of epilepsy in only 12%, but occurred in all of the group which were subject to a variety of fits, and these comprised 38% of the total. Exclusively focal or unilateral fits were uncommon, comprising 10% of the series. In the same series of patients, 72% were subject to a behaviour disorder, sometimes episodic, which was severe enough to disrupt home, insitutional or working life. Generally, there was a clear-cut cerebral insult early in life to account for the gross hemispheric damage and Wilson (1970) describes two main causes. The first was an episode of perinatal trauma or hypoxia, which occurred in 54% of cases; the other was an acute febrile illness between 1 and 4 years of age. This illness was accompanied or followed by convulsions which

were frequently focal or unilateral, and during the convalescent phase of the illness the hemiplegia was first noticed. These cases constituted 30% of the series, but, in a small number of cases, the aetiology is different and with improvements in perinatal and infant care the grosser causes of unilateral hemispherical damage are disappearing. However, as discussed previously, a group of patients is emerging with the syndrome described by Rasmussen (1978) as encephalitis with epilepsy, and a similar syndrome has been described in five children by Gupta et al (1984). This is a progressive disease, usually manifest by intractable focal motor seizures and a progressive hemiparesis. This illness progresses over a variable length of time, tends to begin before 15 years of age in a previously healthy child and has pathological appearances suggestive of a chronic encephalitis. Although the disease may become stationary, it often progresses to the point where a major resection is feasible and beneficial.

Psychometric studies usually show a low level of function. In the patients described by Wilson (1970), 66% of the patients had IQ scores of less than 65 points. With the gross early insults the fate of speech after hemispherectomy is not a problem since it is usually present before operation and preserved. Thus, in the patients described by Wilson (1970), there was no alteration in speech in 84% of the patients as a result of the operation. However, postoperative dysphasia or aphasia occurred in six of the patients (12%), in five of these the left hemisphere had been removed and in the sixth where the right hemisphere was removed the patient was reputed to be right-handed. In half of these patients it was thought that the deficit had persisted, although accurate assessment was difficult because of the degree of mental retardation. The available literature on this point is unhelpful. There are certainly reports in the literature of adult patients surviving dominant hemispherectomy for glioma and regaining some speech function (Smith, 1966). The fate of speech when there is early damage to the left hemisphere is not as clear as it once seemed and it is now thought that speech transference may be either incomplete or inefficient; details are to be found in a review by Rasmussen & Milner (1977). From the standpoint of a patient undergoing a major resection, if the damage occurs before speech acquisition then it will be unaffected by the operation. However, our experience suggests that in patients where the disease process has started after the age of 6 or 7 then pre-existing verbal problems may persist after operation.

A CT scan will demonstrate the changes of hemiatrophy very elegantly. Preoperative angiography may be advisable to show how the anterior cerebral arteries are fed: they may both fill from the internal carotid on the affected side, but even in cases where an acute vascular episode was thought to be the basis of the original insult, angiography at this stage often fails to demonstrate an appropriate lesion (Till & Hoare 1962). The EEG changes in these patients at first sight seem contradictory in that there are frequently more abnormalities to be seen over the 'good' hemisphere, whereas the activity over the affected hemisphere may be relatively flat. However, it is known that these neurophysiological abnormalities in the 'good' hemisphere respond well to surgery; indeed, it was in part this neurophysiological deterioration in the better hemisphere which lead Krynauw (1950) to propose the operation and he was gratified to find that these changes were reversible.

The operative technique of the classical operation is well known. The practice is to carry out a hemicorticectomy in which all the neocortex and hippocampus is removed, leaving only the basal ganglia and thalamus. With experience this is a relatively safe procedure to perform and details can be found in the appropriate references (Rasmussen 1975b, Kempe 1968). Because of the problem of delayed haemorrhage described below, the Montreal group have suggested that a buttress of frontal or occipital cortex should be left on the affected side. This mechanical buttress prevents small movements of the falx which they believe are responsible for this complication and, using this method of subtotal hemispherectomy, Rasmussen (1975b) states that they have carried out 48 such operations without any cases of delayed haemorrhage. Latterly, they have achieved a functional total hemispherectomy by dividing the remainder of the corpus callosum.

In modern times, the operative mortality of these operations is low: both Rasmussen (1975b) and Wilson (1970) report only one death, although two more of the Montreal patients died within a year as a result of progression of 'encephalitis'. In the early postoperative period it is common to see a form of aseptic meningitis characterized by irritability, drowsiness, headache, fever and meningism. It occurred in 28% of the cases described by Wilson (1970). It usually resolves within one to two weeks and may be ameliorated by daily lumbar puncture or, if severe, by washing out of the cavity; it may also respond to steroids. The possible neurological sequelae have already been discussed. After the period of aseptic meningitis has passed, the patient is mobilized but may need a period of three to four weeks intensive physiotherapy to relearn his walking. The late morbidity of the classical operation has already been described. As well as the late delayed haemorrhage which presents as headache and vomiting accompanied by neurological and intellectual deterioration, as described by Oppenheimer & Griffith (1966), there can sometimes be progressive hydrocephalus of the remaining lateral ventricle, presumably from the same cause. Although with early and energetic treatment the condition can be ameliorated (Falconer & Wilson 1969), the use of either the subtotal technique of Rasmussen or the modification described below should abolish this problem in the future. Adams (1983) has described a form of total hemispherectomy in which the various cavities created in the classical removal are separated by means of a plug of muscle in the foramen of Monro and a flap of dura sewn over the falx and tentorium. He gives good reasons to believe that this will reduce the occurrence of late delayed haemorrhage.

The results of both total and subtotal hemispherectomy are good, although those patients undergoing subtotal hemispherectomy without a total corpus callosum split tend to fare slightly worse than those who had the classical total hemispherectomy. In the cases of total hemispherectomy described by Wilson (1970) and Rasmussen (1975b), the results are very similar, with 68% of paients in Group I and 80–85% of patients showing a marked improvement. The corresponding figures for subtotal hemispherectomy were 45% in Group I and 70%, showing a marked improvement. A similar improvement was seen in patients with a behaviour disturbance, 53% became normal and a further 40% were improved.

In view of the major surgery involved and the problems with late delayed haemorrhage, alternatives to hemispherectomy have been sought. Callosal section, which we will discuss later, is thought by some to be an appropriate lesser procedure. Balasubramanian and Kanaka (1975) reported 10 patients of the kind normally considered for hemispherectomy, in whom a stereotactic amygdalotomy was performed in the affected hemisphere with improvement in fit frequency and behaviour in seven of them followed for between 2 and 9 years. If similar experience was obtained by others then this, or callosal section, could be a way round the disadvantages of hemispherectomy. If however this approach seems disappointing, then the use of the subtotal hemispherectomy with complete callosal section, or the modified total hemispherectomy of Adams (1983), would seem to be justified in properly selected patients.

STEREOTACTIC PROCEDURES

Introduction

The application of the techniques of stereotactic neurosurgery to chronic epilepsy is a superficially attractive idea. The basis of such surgery is well known, from its application to the treatment of movement disorders and to a lesser extent in the treatment of psychiatric illness. The original method, developed by Horsley and Clarke for experimental use, was subsequently adapted by others for use in the human brain. In essence, if an accurate map in three dimensions can be made of the brain with reference to fixed points, then a needle inserted through a small drill hole in the skull can be guided under X-ray control, using co-ordinates from the fixed points in three planes, to any particular structure known as the target. This target can then be made the subject of neurophysiological recording and stimulation as has already

been described under the topic of SEEG. In addition, it is possible to destroy such targets using a variety of means. Provided that they are reasonably accurate, these small intracerebral lesions are likely to have less mortality and morbidity than major open surgery.

The idea that the persistence of chronic epilepsy may be equally attributable to the electrical properties of the neural paths over which the seizure discharge travels and to whatever basic pathology is responsible, gathers some support from experimental work. If we accept this, then the bulk of the clinical and experimental evidence would be in favour of a subcortical midbrain origin for such pathways, occurring in reverberating circuits between the reticular formation, thalamus and cerebral cortex, as in the concept of 'centrencephalic epilepsy'. It was therefore suggested that interruption of these 'circuits' by judiciously placed stereotactic lesions would help to control generalized epilepsies which were not otherwise amenable to surgical treatment. Earlier methods used to achieve the interruption of such pathways involved open surgery but, if stereotactic techniques were available, then targets in various subcortical structures such as the internal capsule, thalamus, basal ganglia and hypothalamus would be accessible.

By contrast, the use of targets in the deep structures of the temporal lobe emerged as a consequence of placing stereotactic lesions in these areas to try to control aggressive behaviour, as pioneered by Narabayashi et al (1963). It was noted that if such patients had poorly controlled epilepsy, which a significant proportion did, then if the amygdala lesion was successful in controlling their behaviour it would also frequently ameliorate their epilepsy. Since it was also known that poorly controlled complex seizures were often associated with structural lesions in one or both temporal lobes, this seemed an added reason why targets in these areas would be rewarding. Finally, there was the theoretical justification from the properties of the 'Papez' circuit and the basolateral limbic system (Livingston & Escobar 1972), for supposing that such lesions would be effective. Likewise, McLardy (1969) believes that the interruption of the pathways between the amygdala and the CA_2

part of the hippocampus is the effective part of all temporal lobe surgery.

Technique

The nature of the lesion-making process does not seem to be important and various methods have been tried, including warm wax and lipiodol, radio-frequency currents and radioactive seeds. Also, the particular stereotactic technique used in setting up the target does not seem to be important.

There are three factors which must be considered in assessing the usefulness of stereotactic lesioning in the treatment of epilepsy. The first is that, since these procedures are free of mortality, direct verification of the position of the lesions is difficult, if not impossible, although modern CT and MRI scanning techniques may produce some kind of verification. Therefore, an error in the placing of these lesions may result in a good target being misreported or vice versa. Secondly, when experimental results from animal work are looked at, they are not sufficiently consistent to serve as valid models for human lesions. Thirdly, the numbers of patients reported in the literature, with their considerable diversity of clinical disease, number and placement of lesions and reporting of the results, makes any attempt to utilize a specific target for a particular patient almost impossible. In review articles both Talairach et al (1974), and Ojemann & Ward (1975) state that this method of surgery, even in the best reported series, is much less effective than resective surgery and largely empirical. A very recent review by Flanigin et al (1985) merely reports the results of these operations in a relatively brief section.

Stereotactic lesions in subcortical structures

The targets in this group have included the internal capsule, pallidium, thalamic nuclei, fields of Forel and the hypothalamus. There is little to be gained from a catalogue of the papers in this field, most of which relate to a diversity of lesions in a small number of patients. Good reviews are to be found in the references cited above and it will suffice to mention a few examples. Thus,

Spiegel et al (1958) report the effect of pallidal lesions and in their later papers they note that the combination of these with amygdala lesions is particularly effective. Typically, however, of their nine patients, three only were free of seizures and three others improved. Likewise, Pertuiset et al (1969) describe the effect of stereotactic thalamotomy on ten patients with tonic-clonic seizures but note that their results are inconclusive. Jelsma and his co-workers (Jelsma et al 1973) describe how various capsular lesions will improve partial seizures, but not primary or secondary generalized seizures. Finally, lesions made in the fields of Forel are also disappointing in their results (Jinnai et al 1976), although this may depend in part upon the accuracy of the placing of the lesion (Jinnai & Mukawa 1970). Because of the considerable variation in the case and target selection when subcortical lesions are used, these must still be regarded as largely speculative without clear indications which can be perceived by those not directly concerned with this work.

Stereotactic lesions in temporal structures

Here the prospect seems more hopeful. A greater number of cases are described and the effect of the lesions seems more evident. In most series, lesions were made in the amygdala but these were often combined with other targets including the anterior commissure and fornix.

Narabayashi has summarized the results of stereotactic amygdalotomy upon 47 children, and notes that 44 of them had poorly controlled epilepsy (Narabayashi & Shima 1973). As a result of this procedure 22 of the children were improved both in respect of their seizures and their behaviour, and in a subsequent paper he reports similar results in adults (Narabayashi 1979). Likewise, Umbach (1966) describes 25 cases where unilateral or bilateral fornicectomy was combined in some patients with lesions of the amygdala, lamella medialis or hypothalamus, and in 18 of these patients where the follow-up was adequate five of the patients were free of epilepsy. They suggested that it might be possible in some cases with bitemporal abnormalities to combine an open resection on one side with a stereotactic lesion on the other. Adams & Rutkin (1969) found only one patient free of epilepsy out of 16 treated by amygdalectomy. By contrast 15 of 36 patients treated by Bouchard et al (1975) were improved. It is significant that the best results were found in patients with complex partial seizures requiring only unilateral lesions, precisely the group which might be expected to benefit from resective surgery. Mundinger et al (1976) noted the same kind of results in 33 cases; treatment of unilateral foci being twice as successful as that of bilateral foci. They found that the best combination of lesions was fornicotomy and anterior commissurotomy. The results of other groups are equally scattered. Balasubramanian & Kanaka (1976) obtained complete relief in 36 out of 76 cases using limbic lesions: Flanigin & Nashold (1976) had 4 out of 16 patients who would have been in Groups I and II; Barcia-Solario & Broretta (1976) followed 42 patients who had undergone fornicotomy over 8 years and 43% had an improvement in their epilepsy and 58% in their behaviour.

Particular attention should be paid to the results reported by Vaernet (1972), who carried out amygdalectomies on 45 patients. When unilateral lesions were necessary, 5 out of 27 patients were fit-free, or virtually so, and with bilateral lesions 3 out of 18. Significantly, 8 out of 12 patients with unilateral foci who did not do well with amygdalectomy were subsequently treated with temporal lobectomy, with a good result in all cases. Also Talairach et al (1974) describing their results in 44 patients, note that only 23% of patients obtained complete relief of their seizures. They felt that this method of treatment was less successful than open resection and were also anxious about possible memory difficulties in patients with bilateral disease, having encountered some problems in three of their patients. A final warning is also given by Narabayashi & Mitzutani (1970) who note that complex partial seizures are especially prone to return after 6 to 12 months.

How can one summarize this work? It is clear that both the selection procedures used and the multiplicity of lesions produced, makes a comparison between the results of the various groups difficult. The kind of patients treated by Narabayashi are clearly different from those treated by Vaernet but, in spite of these differences, a number of common themes may be discerned. As the selection procedures approach those for open surgery, the results of stereotactic intervention improve. However, it is clear that some patients who do not fulfil the strict criteria for open surgery may be helped by stereotactic lesions. Other workers do not mention the memory problems encountered by the Paris group and, indeed, many of them positively record the absence of such problems.

Other procedures

Brief mention should be made of three other procedures. The first, described by Turner (1963) and unique to him, consists of cutting either unilaterally or bilaterally the deep temporal fibre connections. He has recently summarized the results of several decades using this procedure Turner (1982). In respect of fit frequency, unilateral and bilateral lesions seem equally effective making 20–30% of the patients fit-free with complete failure in 11% for both procedures, but his results are difficult to interpret because many patients needed additional lesions elsewhere in the brain and he describes the psychiatric results of the operation as disappointing.

The second procedure, section of the corpus callosum, is currently undergoing a minor revival. Originally proposed by Van Wagenen & Herren (1940) as a means of preventing the spread of epileptic discharges from one hemisphere to the other, it was also taken up by Bogen and his colleagues, who noted an improvement in the epilepsy, but also found that when the section was complete there could be undesirable neuropsychological sequelae which were ameliorated if the splenium was spared (Gordon et al 1971). The operation was subsequently applied to a different group of patients, namely children who would otherwise merit a hemispherectomy; and Luessenhop et al (1970) reported some modification of seizure frequency in these patients. About the same time Wilson began to use the procedure for patients similar to those originally treated with it (Wilson et al 1975) and then evolved a microsurgical technique which improved the results and reduced complications (Wilson et al 1982). Rayport found that 10% of the patients assessed in their epilepsy surgery programme were suitable for this procedure (Rayport et al 1983). They found the procedure useful in reducing seizure frequency but noted that there could be serious neuropsychological sequelae. A recent discussion of this topic at an international symposium on the surgical treatment of epilepsy suggested that this procedure was of benefit in trying to confine the seizure discharge to one hemisphere, preserve consciousness and to reduce the frequency and severity of fits. Various groups in describing their experiences found that akinetic or drop attacks were reduced by it, that the EEG would be desynchronized but would not become normal. The patients could be subject to a number of complications including transient hemiparesis, temporary mutism and the neuropsychological problems already mentioned. At present this procedure must still be regarded as potentially useful but under trial.

The third procedure is anterior cerebellar stimulaion. This was based on physiological studies and in particular those of Cooke & Snider (1955) and Dow & Moruzzi (1958). The treatment was pioneered by Irving Cooper (Cooper 1973, Cooper et al 1976) and he apparently demonstrated a beneficial effect. However, double-blind controlled stimulation trials such as those reported by Van Buren et al (1978) have shown that the procedure has no objective effect and it has been largely abandoned.

Summary

The history of stereotactic and functional surgery in the treatment of epilepsy is much briefer than that of resective surgery, and the case material is of necessity more heterogeneous. The indications for these procedures are therefore less clear and, because they lack easily identifiable success, they have been used more sparsely. However, they are not without some success and the possibilities they represent should continue to be explored so that eventually we might arrive at some more definite indications for their use.

CONCLUSION

This review, after a brief historical introduction, summarizes the factors used to select patients for the classical resection procedures used to treat chronic drug-resistant epilepsy. Since the beginning of Penfield's work in 1930, over a period of more than 50 years, it has become possible to predict the value of these procedures to individual patients; achieving freedom from seizures in 30% or more, with a further worthwhile improvement in at least the same proportion, leaving only about 20% unaffected. Over the same period the mortality of these procedures has become negligible, the incidence of serious side-effects has fallen to less than 10%, and many of the patients are better adjusted to their social environment. Although the results of stereotactic and functional surgery are less impressive they can still bring about a cessation of seizures in 20% of patients with a lower risk of side effects or fatality.

REFERENCES

Adams C B T 1983 Hemispherectomy – a modification. Journal of Neurology, Neurosurgery and Psychiatry 46: 617–619

Adams J E, Rutkin B B 1969 Treatment of temporal lobe epilepsy by stereotactic surgery. Confinia Neurologica 31: 80–85

Babb T L, Crandall P H 1976 Epileptogenesis of human limbic neurones in psychomotor epileptics. Electroencephalography and Clinical Neurophysiology 40: 225–243

Balasubramanian V, Kanaka T S 1975 Why hemispherectomy? Applied Neurophysiology 38: 197–205

Balasubramanian V, Kanaka T S 1976 Stereotactic surgery of the limbic system in epilepsy. Acta Neurochirugica suppl. 23: 225–234

Barcia-Solario J L, Broretta J 1976 Stereotactic fornicotomy in temporal lobe epilepsy: indications and long term results. Acta Neurochirugica suppl. 23: 167–175

Bear D M 1979 Temporal lobe epilepsy – a syndrome of sensory-limbic hyperconnection. Cortex 15: 357–384

Bear D M and Fedio P 1977 Quantitative analysis of interictal behaviour in temporal lobe epilepsy. Archives of Neurology 34: 454–467

Bear D M, Levin K, Blumer D, Chetham D, Ryder J 1982 Interictal behaviour in hospitalised temporal lobe epileptics; relationship to idiopathic psychiatric syndromes. Journal of Neurology, Neurosurgery and Psychiatry 45: 481–488

Bhatia R, Kollevold T 1976 A follow-up study of 91 patients operated on for focal epilepsy. Epilepsia 17: 61–66

Blakemore C B, Falconer M A 1967 Long-term effects of anterior temporal lobectomy on certain cognitive functions. Journal of Neurology, Neurosurgery and Psychiatry 30: 364–367

Bouchard G, Kim Y K, Umbach W 1975 Stereotactic methods in different forms of epilepsy. Confinia Neurologica 37: 232–238

Bouchet & Cazauvieihl 1925 De l'épilepsie considereé dans ses rapports avec l'alienation normale. Archives Générales d Médecine 9:510

Brazier M A B, Crandall P H, Jann-Brown W 1975 Long term follow-up of EEG changes following therapeutic surgery in epilepsy. Electroencephalography and Clinical Neurophysiology 38: 495–506

Brazier M A, Crandall P H, Walsh G O 1976 Enhancement of EEG lateralizing signs in temporal lobe epilepsy: a trial of diazepam. Experimental Neurology 51: 241–258

Brink-Henriksen P, Jurel-Jensen P, Lund M 1970 The mortality of epileptics. In: Brackenridge R D C (ed.) Life assurance medicine. Proceedings 10th International Congress Life Assurance Medicine, Pitman, London, pp 139–148

Cooke P, Snider R S 1955 Some cerebellar influences on electrically induced cerebral seizures. Epilepsia 4: 19–28

Cooper I S 1973 Chronic stimulation of the paleocerebellar cortex in man. Lancet i:206

Cooper I S, Amin I, Riklan M, Waltz J, Poon T P 1976 Chronic cerebellar stimulation in epilepsy. Archives of Neurology 33: 559–570

Crandall P H 1975 Post-operative management and criteria for evaluation. In: Purpura D P, Penry J K, Walter R D (eds) Advances in Neurology vol 8. Raven Press, New York, pp 265–279

Crandall P H, Engel J, Rausch R 1983 Indications for depth electrode recordings in complex partial epilepsy and subsequent surgical results. In: Rose F C (ed.) Research progress in epilepsy. Pitman, London, pp 507–526

Currie S, Heathfield K W G, Henson R A 1971 Clinical course and prognosis of temporal lobe epilepsy. A surgery of 666 patients. Brain 94: 173–190

Delgado-Escueta A V, Walsh G O 1983 The selection process for surgery of intractable complex partial seizures: surface EEG and depth electrography. In: Ward A A, Penry J K, Purpura D P (eds) Epilepsy. Raven Press, New York, pp 295–326

Delgado-Escueta A V, Mattson R H, King L et al 1981 Special report: the nature of aggression during epileptic seizures. New England Journal of Medicine 305: 711–716

Dow R S, Moruzzi G 1958 The physiology and pathology of the cerebellum. University of Minnesota Press, Minneapolis

Engel J 1984 The use of positron emission tomographic scanning in epilepsy. Annals of Neurology 15: S180–S194

Engel J, Driver M V, Falconer M A 1975 Electrophysiological correlates of pathology and surgical results in temporal lobe epilepsy. Brain 98: 129–156

Engel J, Lieb J P, Rausch R, Kuhl D E, Crandall P H 1981 Correlation of criteria used for localising epileptic foci in patients considered for surgical therapy of epilepsy. Annals of Neurology 9: 215–224

Engel J, Jann-Brown W, Kuhl D E, Phelps M E, Maziotta J C, Crandall P H 1982 Pathological findings underlying focal temporal lobe hypometabolism in partial epilepsy. Annals of Neurology 12: 518–528

Falconer M A 1967a Brain mechanisms suggested by neurophysiologic studies. In: Brain mechanisms underlying speech and language. Grune and Stratton, New York, pp 185–203

Falconer M A 1967b Surgical treatment of temporal lobe epilepsy. New Zealand Medical Journal 66: 539–542

Falconer M A 1969 The surgical treatment of temporal lobe epilepsy. In: Herrington R N (ed.) Current problems in neuropsychiatry. Headley Bros, Ashford, pp 95–101

Falconer M A 1971a Anterior temporal lobectomy for epilepsy. In: Logue V (ed.) Operative surgery vol 14. Neurosurgery. Butterworths, London, pp 142–149

Falconer M A 1971b Genetic and related aetiological factors in temporal lobe epilepsy. Epilepsia 12: 13–31

Falconer M A Reversibility by temporal lobe resection of the behavioural abnormalities of temporal lobe epilepsy. New England Journal of Medicine 289: 451–455

Falconer M A 1974 Mesial temporal (Ammon's Horn) sclerosis as a common cause of epilepsy. Aetiology, treatment and prevention. Lancet ii: 767–770

Falconer M A, Wilson J L 1958 Visual field changes following anterior temporal lobectomy: their significance in relation to 'Meyer's loop' of the optic radiation. Brain 81: 1–14

Falconer M A, Kennedy W A 1961 Epilepsy due to small focal temporal lesions with bilateral independent spike-discharging foci. A study of seven cases relieved by operation. Journal of Neurology, Neurosurgery and Psychiatry 24: 205–212

Falconer M A, Serafetidines E A 1963 A follow-up study of surgery in temporal lobe epilepsy. Journal of Neurology, Neurosurgery and Psychiatry 26: 154–165

Falconer M A, Taylor D C 1968 Surgical treatment of drug-resistant epilepsy due to mesial temporal sclerosis. Etiology and significance. Archives of Neurology 19: 353–363

Falconer M A, Wilson P J E 1969 Complications related to delayed haemorrhage after hemispherectomy. Journal of Neurosurgery 30: 413–426

Falconer M A, Davidson S 1974 The rationale of surgical treatment of temporal lobe epilepsy with particular reference to childhood and adolescence. In: Harris P, Mawdsley C (eds) Epilepsy. Proceedings of the Hans Berger Centenary Symposium. Churchill Livingstone, Edinburgh, pp 209–214

Fenton G W 1978 Epilepsy and psychosis. Journal of the Irish Medical Association 71: 315–324

Flanigin H F, Nashold B S 1976 Stereotactic lesions of the amygdala and hippocampus in epilepsy. Acta Neurochirugia suppl 27: 235–239

Flanigin H, King B, Gallagher B 1985 Surgical treatment of epilepsy. In: Pedley T A, Meldrum B S (eds) Recent advances in epilepsy no 2. Churchill Livingstone, Edinburgh, pp 517–559

Flor-Henry P 1969 Psychosis and temporal lobe epilepsy: a controlled investigation. Epilepsia 10: 363–395

Gastaut H, Gastaut J L 1976 Computerised transverse axial tomography in epilepsy. Epilepsia 17: 325–336

Goddard G V 1967 Development of epileptic seizures through brain stimulation at low intensity. Nature 214: 1020–1021

Goldring S 1979 A method for the surgical management of focal epilepsy, especially as it relates to children. Journal of Neurosurgery 49: 344–356

Gordon H W, Bogen J E, Sperry R W 1971 Absence of deconnexion syndrome in two patients with partial section of the neocommissure. Brain 94: 327–336

Gregorie E M, Goldring S 1984 Localisation of function in the excision of lesions from the sensorimotor region. Journal of Neurosurgery 61: 1047–1055

Griffith H B 1967 Cerebral hemispherectomy for infantile hemiplegia in the light of the late results. Annals of the Royal College of Surgeons 41: 183–201

Gupta P C, Rapin I, Houroupian D S, Roy S, Llena J, Tandon P N 1984 Smouldering encephalitis in children. Neuropediatrics 15: 191–197

Halgren E, Walter R D, Cherlow D G, Crandall P H 1978 Mental phenomena evoked by electrical stimulation of the human hippocampal formation and amygdala. Brain 101: 83–117

Hamlin H, Delgado J R 1977 Case report: juvenile psychomotor epilepsy and associated behavior disorder – 20 year follow-up of temporal lobectomy. In: Sweet W H, Obrador S, Martin-Rodriguez J G (eds) Neurosurgical treatment in psychiatry, pain and epilepsy. University Park Press, Baltimore, pp 569–571

Jann-Brown W 1973 Structural substrates of seizure foci in the human temporal lobe. In: Brazier M A (ed.) Epilepsy; its phenomena in man. UCLA Forum in medical sciences no 17. Academic Press, Mew York, pp 339–374

Jelsma R K, Bertrand C M, Martinez S N, Molina-Negro P 1973 Stereotactic treatment of frontal lobe and centrencephalic epilepsy. Journal of Neurosurgery 39: 42–51

Jensen I 1975a Temporal lobe surgery around the world. Acta Neurologica Scandinavica 52: 354–373

Jensen I 1975b Temporal lobe epilepsy. Late mortality in patients treated with unilateral temporal lobe resections. Acta Neurologica Scandinavica 52: 374–380

Jensen I 1976a Temporal lobe epilepsy. Type of seizures, age, and surgical results. Acta Neurologica Scandinavica 53: 335–357

Jensen I 1976b Temporal lobe epilepsy: social conditions and rehabilitation after surgery. Acta Neurologica Scandinavica 54: 22–44

Jensen I, Larsen J K 1979 Mental effects of temporal lobe epilepsy. Follow-up of 74 patients after resection of a temporal lobe. Journal of Neurology, Neurosurgery and Psychiatry 42: 256–265

Jinnai D, Mukawa J 1970 Forel-H-tomy for the treatment of epilepsy. Confinia Neurologia 32: 307–315

Jinnai D, Mukawa J, Kobayashi K 1976 Forel-H-tomy for the treatment of intractable epilepsy. Acta Neurochirurgica suppl. 23: 159–165

Jones M K 1974 Imagery as a mnemonic aid after left temporal lobectomy: Contrast between material-specific and generalised memory disorders. Neuropsychologica 12: 21–30

Kempe L G 1968 Hemispherectomy. In: Operative neurosurgery vol 1. Springer-Verlag, New York, pp 180–189

Krynauw R A 1950 Infantile hemiplegia treated by removing one cerebral hemisphere. Journal of Neurology, Neurosurgery and Psychiatry 13: 243–267

Lieb J P, Engel J, Gevins A, Crandall P H 1982a Surface and deep EEG correlates of surgical outcome in temporal lobe epilepsy. Epilepsia 22: 515–538

Lieb J P, Engel J, Jann-Brown W, Gevins A S, Crandall P H 1982b Neuropathological findings following temporal lobectomy related to surface and deep EEG patterns. Epilepsia 22: 539–550

Lindsay J, Glaser G, Richards P, Ounsted C 1984 Developmental aspects of focal epilepsies of childhood treated by neurosurgery. Developmental Medicine and Child Neurology 26: 574–587

Livingston K E, Escobar A 1972 The continuing evolution of the limbic system concept. In: Hitchcock E, Laitinen L, Vaernet K Psychosurgery. Thomas, Springfield, pp 25–33

Luessenhop A J, Dela-Cruz T C, Fairchild D M 1970 Surgical disconnection of the cerebral hemispheres for intractable seizures. Results in infancy and childhood. Journal of the American Medical Association 213: 1630–1636

Margerison J H, Corsellis J A N 1966 Epilepsy and the temporal lobes: a clinical electroencephalographic and neuropathological study of the brain in epilepsy, with particular reference to the temporal lobes. Brain 89: 499–536

Mark V H, Ervin F R 1970 Violence and the brain. Harper & Row, New York

Mathieson G 1975 Pathological aspects of epilepsy with special reference to surgical pathology. In: Purpura D P, Penry J K, Walter R D (eds) Advances in neurology vol 8. Raven Press, New York, pp 107–138

McLardy T 1969 Ammon's norn pathology and epileptic dyscontrol. Nature 221: 877–878

Milner B 1975 Psychological aspects of focal epilepsy and its neurosurgical management. In: Purpura D P, Penry J K, Walter R D (eds) Advances in Neurology vol 8. Raven Press, New York, pp 299–314

Morrell F, Whistler W W 1980 Secondary epileptogenic lesions in man: prediction of the results of surgical excision of the primary focus. In: Canger R, Angeleri F, Penry J K (eds) Advances in epileptology. The XIth International Symposium. Raven Press, New York, pp 123–128

Mundinger F, Becker P, Grolkner E, Bachschmid G 1976 Late results of stereotactic surgery of epilepsy predominantly temporal lobe type. Acta Neurochirugica suppl 23: 177–182

Narabayashi H, Mitzutani T 1970 Epileptic seizures and the stereotaxic amygdalotomy. Confinia Neurologica 32: 289–297

Narabayashi H, Shima F 1973 Which is the better amygdala target, the medial or lateral nuclei? (For behaviour problems and paroxysm in epileptics). In: Laitinen L V, Livingstone K E (eds) Surgical Approaches in Psychiatry. U.K.:MTP Lancaster, pp 129–134

Narabayashi H, Nagao T, Sato Y, Yoshida M, Nagahata M 1963 Stereotactic amygdalotomy for behaviour disorder. Archives of Neurology 9: 1–16

Narabayashi H 1979 Long range results of medial amygdalotomy on epileptic traits in adult patients. In: Rasmussen T, Marino R (eds) Functional neurosurgery. Raven Press, New York, pp 243–252

Newcombe R L, Shah S H 1975 Radiological abnormalities in temporal lobe epilepsy with clinico-pathological correlates. Journal of Neurology, Neurosurgery and Psychiatry 38: 279–287

Ojemann G A, Ward A A 1975 Stereotactic and other procedures for epilepsy. In: Purpura D P, Penry J K, Walter R D (ed) Advances in neurology vol 8. Raven Press, New York, pp 241–263

Ojemann G A, Dodrill C B 1985 Verbal memory deficits after left temporal lobectomy for epilepsy: mechanism and intraoperative prediction. Journal of Neurosurgery 62: 101–107

Oppenheimer D R, Griffith H B 1966 Persistent intracranial bleeding as a complication of hemispherectomy. Journal of Neurology, Neurosurgery and Psychiatry 29: 229–240

Ounsted C 1967 Temporal lobe epilepsy: the problem of aetiology and prophylaxis. Journal of the Royal College of Physicians of London 1: 273–284

Ounsted C, Lindsay J, Norman R 1966 Biological factors in temporal lobe epilepsy. Heinemann, London

Penfield W D 1974 Autopsy findings and comments on the role of hippocampus in experiential recall. Archives of Neurology 31: 145–154

Penfield W D, Jasper H 1954 Epilepsy and the functional anatomy of the Human Brain. Little, Brown, Boston

Penning R, Müller C, Ciompi L 1969 Mortalité et cause de décès des épileptiques. Psychiatrica Clinica 2: 85–94

Pertuiset B, Hirsch J F, Sachs M, Landau-Ferey J 1969 Selective stereotactic thalamotomy in 'Grand Mal' epilepsy. Excerpta. Med. Amst. ICS No 193, item 190, p 72

Polkey C E 1983 Prognostic factors in selecting patients with drug-resistant epilepsy for temporal lobectomy. In: Rose F C (ed.) Research progress in epilepsy. Pitman, London, pp 500–506

Pond D A 1974 Epilepsy and personality disorders. In: Vinken P J, Bruyn G W (eds) Handbook of clinical neurology vol 15. The epilepsies. North Holland Publishing Amsterdam, pp 576–592

Powell G E, Polkey C E, McMillan T 1985 The new Maudsley series of temporal lobectomy. I. Short term cognitive effects. British Journal of Clinical Psychology 24: 109–124

Rasmussen T 1975a Surgery of frontal lobe epilepsy. In: Purpura D P, Penry J K, Walter R D (eds) Advances in neurology vol 8. Raven Press, New York, pp 197–205

Rasmussen T 1975b Surgery for epilepsy arising in regions other than the frontal and temporal lobes. In: Purpura D P, Penry J K, Walter R D (eds) Advances in neurology vol 8. Raven Press, New York, pp 207–226

Rasmussen T 1978 Further observations on the syndrome of chronic encephalitis and epilepsy. Applied Neurophysiology 41: 1–12

Rasmussen T 1979 Cortical resection for medically refractory focal epilepsy: results, lessons, questions. In: Rasmussen T, Marino R (eds) Functional Neurosurgery, Raven Press, New York, pp 253–269

Rasmussen T 1983 Surgical treatment of complex partial seizures: results, lessons and problems. Epilepsia 24: S65–S76

Rasmussen T, Milner B 1977 The role of early left brain damage in determining the lateralisation of cerebral speech functions. Annals of the New York Academy of Science 299: 355–369

Rayport M, Ferguson S M, Corrie W S 1983 Outcomes and indications of corpus callosum section for intractable seizure control. Applied Neurophysiology 46: 47–50

Robillard A, Saint-Hilaire J M, Mercier M, Bouvier G 1983 The lateralising and localising value of adversion in epileptic seizures. Neurology 33: 1241–1242

Rossi G F, Colicchio G, Gentilomo A, Scerrati M 1978 Discussion on the causes of failure of surgical treatment of partial epilepsies. Applied Neurophysiology 41: 29–37

Sano K, Malamud N 1953 Clinical significance of sclerosis of the cornu ammonis. Archives of Neurology and Psychiatry 70: 40–53

Serafetinides E A, Falconer M A 1962 The effects of temporal lobectomy in patients with psychosis. Journal of Mental Science 108: 584–593

Serafetinides E A, Falconer M A 1963 Speech disturbances in temporal lobe seizures: a study in 100 epileptic patients submitted to anterior temporal lobectomy. Brain 86: 333–346

Sherwin I 1981 Psychosis associated with epilepsy: significance of the laterality of the epileptogenic lesion. Journal of Neurology, Neurosurgery and Psychiatry 44: 83–85

Smith A 1966 Speech and other functions after left (dominant) hemispherectomy. Journal of Neurology, Neurosurgery and Psychiatry 29: 467–471

Spiegel E A, Wycis H T, Baird H W 1958 Long-range effects of electropallido-ansotomy in extra-pyramidal and convulsive disorders. Neurology 8: 734–740

Talairach J, Bancaud J et al 1974 Approche nouvelle de la neurochirugie de l'épilepsie. Neurochirurgie 20:suppl. 1

Taylor D C 1975 Factors influencing the occurrence of schizophrenia like psychosis in patients with temporal lobe epilepsy. Psychological Medicine 5: 249–254

Taylor D C, Falconer M A 1968 Clinical, socio-economic and psychological changes after temporal lobectomy for epilepsy. British Journal of Psychiatry 114: 1247–1261

Taylor D C, Falconer M A, Bruton C J, Corsellis J A N 1971 Focal dysplasia of the cerebral cortex in epilepsy. Journal of Neurology, Neurosurgery and Psychiatry 34: 369–387

Taylor D C, Marsh S M 1977 Implications of long-term follow-up studies in epilepsy: with a note on the cause of death. In: Penry J K (ed.) Epilepsy, the eighth international symposium. Raven Press, New York, pp 27–34

Till K, Hoare R D 1962 Cerebral angiography in investigation of acute hemiplegia in childhood. Little Club. Clinics in Developmental Medicine 6: 69–73

Turner E A 1963 A new approach to unilateral and bilateral lobotomies for psychomotor epilepsy. Journal of Neurology, Neurosurgery and Psychiatry 26: 285–299

Turner E A 1982 Temporal lobe operations. In: Surgery of the mind. Carver Press, Birmingham, pp 126–169

Umbach W 1966 Long term result of fornicotomy for temporal epilepsy. Confinia Neurologica 27: 121–123

Vaernet K 1972 Stereotaxic amygdalotomy in temporal lobe epilepsy. Confinia Neurological 34: 176–180

Van Buren J M, Ajmone-Marsan C, Mutsuga N, Sudowsky D 1975 Surgery of temporal lobe epilepsy. In: Purpura D P, Penry J K, Walter R D (eds) Advances in neurology vol 8. Raven Press, New York, pp 155–196

Van Buren J, Wood J H, Oakley J, Hambricht F 1978 Preliminary evaluation of cerebellar stimulation by double-blind stimulation and biological criteria in the treatment of epilepsy. Journal of Neurosurgery 48: 407–416

Van Wagenen W P, Herren R Y 1940 Surgical division of commissural pathways in the corpus callosum. Archives of Neurology and Psychiatry 44: 740–759

Wada J 1949 A new method for the determination of the side of cerebral speech dominance. A preliminary report on the intra-carotid injection of sodium amytal in man. Medicine and Biology 14: 221–222

Wieser H G 1986 Proceedings of an international conference on the surgical treatment of epilepsy. Raven Press, New York (in press)

Wieser H G, Bancaud J, Talairach J, Bonis A, Szikla G 1979

Comparative value of spontaneous and chemically and electrically induced seizures in establishing the lateralisation of temporal lobe seizures. Epilepsia 20: 47–59

Wieser H G, Yasargil M G 1982 Die "Selektive Amygdala-Hippokampektomie" als chirugische Behandlung du mediobasal-Limbischen Epilepsie. Neurochirugia 25: 39–50

Wieser H G, Elger C E, Stodieck S R G 1985 The 'Foramen Ovale Electrode': a new recording method for pre-operative evaluation of patients suffering from medio-basal temporal lobe epilepsy. Electroencephalography and Clinical Neurophysiology 61: 314–322

Wilder B 1971 Electroencephalogram activation in medically intractable epileptic patients: activation techniques including surgical follow-up. Archives of Neurology 25: 415–426

Wilson D H, Culver C, Waddington M, Gazzaniga M 1975 Disconnection of the cerebral hemispheres. An alternative to hemispherectomy for the control of intractable seizures. Neurology 25: 1149–1153

Wilson D H, Reeves A G, Gazzaniga M 1982 "Central" commissurotomy for intractable generalised epilepsy: series two. Neurology 32: 687–697

Wilson P J E 1970 Cerebral hemispherectomy for infantile hemiplegia. A report of 50 cases. Brain 93: 147–180

Wyler A R, Bolender N F 1983 Preoperative CT diagnosis of mesial temporal sclerosis for surgical treatment of epilepsy. Annals of Neurology 13: 59–64

Wyler A R, Ojemann G A, Lettich E, Ward A A 1984 Subdural strip electrodes for localising epileptogenic foci. Journal of Neurosurgery 60: 1195–1200

14

Epilepsy in developing countries

PART ONE
EPILEPSY IN INDONESIA
B. Chandra

One of the most important health problems facing developing countries has been epilepsy. First of all because of its incidence and prevelance, which in Indonesia for instance is of the same magnitude as tuberculosis (both have an incidence of 7 per 1000). A second reason is that leading causes of epilepsy like birth injury, childhood infections, febrile seizures and head injuries because of traffic accidents are all very frequent in developing countries. The third reason is that because of lack of paramedical personnel, physicians and funds it is often difficult to diagnose and treat the patient with epilepsy. Many developing countries face the same problem as Indonesia: how to reach with few doctors and nurses epileptic patients in a population of 135 million people spread over a distance equal to that from London to Turkey. Finally, in the future these problems will grow as most of the world population increase will occur in developing countries, especially in Asia (Tower 1978).

In this chapter epilepsy in developing countries will be discussed under five headings:

1. Identifying patients
2. Etiological factors
3. Clinical management
4. Prevention
5. Rehabilitation

IDENTIFYING PATIENTS

Every doctor working in a village in a developing country knows that one of the main problems is how to identify the epileptic patient. Some factors which need to be considered are as follows.

The belief that epilepsy is always hereditary and cannot be cured

Several foreign physicians, whom this writer invited to visit some rural areas, were astonished to hear the negative answer given by the people in the village to a simple question like: 'Do you suffer from convulsions?' Nearly everyone answered this question with a firm 'no'. If, however, the question was phrased: 'Did you ever suffer an attack of *twitchings* and *cramps* of your arms and legs followed by unconsciousness and sometimes urinary incontinence?' To this question many people responded with an affirmative 'yes'.

The reason for this behaviour was, that for most people in the village, convulsions (*ayan* in Indonesian) meant an hereditary incurable disease, which is a disgrace for the family.

Shortage of local paramedical and medical personnel

As in many other developing countries, one of the problems is how to reach the epileptic patient, with few physicians and nurses available. Much help was received with the inauguration of the new Indonesian health care system in 1974. In this system every district (with approximately 20 000 inhabitants on Java and 10 000 inhabitants outside Java) has at least one health centre, with one nurse and one doctor. These district health centres feed into regional hospitals (C hospitals) which are staffed by one surgeon, one internist, one gynaecologist and one pediatrician, and which are capable of dealing with the common medical and surgical problems. The regional hospitals in turn will feed into provincial hospitals (B hospitals), which are fully staffed and usually connected with a medical school. In these B hospitals there is usually a department of neurology, with an EEG. At the top of this health referral system are the two teaching hospitals in Jakarta and Surabaya (A hospitals), which can offer all the facilities of modern neurology. Since this system was established, the staff of the department of neurology has frequently visited and given post-graduate lectures and demonstrations for the doctors working in the regional hospitals and the district health centres. The rationale behind this scheme was that excellent neurological health care could only be given if the doctors staffing these hospitals were sufficiently and regularly upgraded on the advances and capabilities of modern epileptology.

The use of teachers in helping identify patients

In Indonesia, every child between 6 and 12 years is obliged to attend an elementary school. As there is at least one school in every district, which is usually used in two shifts (one in the morning and one in the afternoon), it was easy to ask the help of the teachers in identifying epileptic patients, as was done by Edoo (1978). As each school was visited at least once a month by the district physician, he could examine and treat if necessary the suspected epileptic patients. After four years experience it could be observed that elementary school teachers were a reliable and fruitful source of referral of epileptic children.

ETIOLOGICAL FACTORS

From clinical surveys done in rural areas and in big towns like Surabaya, it is evident that several factors play an important role in the pathogenesis and causation of epilepsy.

Birth injury

Especially in rural areas, birth injury to the brain was a leading cause of epilepsy. This was especially the case in areas in which a health centre had only recently been established and where deliveries formerly were done by nonmedically trained witch-women (*dukun*). With the establishment of district health centres, which offer better obstetrical and prenatal care, it is certain that this cause of seizures could be prevented. During discussions with local physicians it was stressed repeatedly, that, by simply offering better obstetrical and prenatal care and thereby preventing anoxia, epilepsy could be prevented in many children.

Meningoencephalitis

As in many other developing countries, both in rural and urban areas meningitis is frequently seen. During the acute phase, but more often as sequella, convulsions do appear. It was therefore repeatedly stressed to general physicians that they should be aware of meningitis and treat it as rapidly and vigorously as possible to prevent convulsions and hydrocephalus. An appeal was made to the paediatricians to do a lumbar puncture in children suspected of having meningitis. With these measures it was hoped to suppress the incidence of these postmeningial fits.

Post-traumatic fits

Year by year the number of traumatic brain injuries is rising and with it the number of post-traumatic convulsions. In Indonesia most of the casualties are caused by collisions and falls of motor cycle drivers, because they do not wear helmets (as in most other countries). It has therefore been stressed and emphasized to students and doctors alike that they should use helmets and give an example to the layman on how to protect the brain.

Alcohol is luckily not an important factor in Indonesia, because drinking alcohol is forbidden by the Islamic religion.

Febrile seizures (Chandra 1978)

As in many other developing countries, infectious diseases are very frequent and, because of this, febrile seizures are so common that many parents don't pay much attention to them. This fact combined with the large distances between the patient's home and the doctor's office or health centres, is the reason why prolonged convulsions are often not adequately treated (diazepam by intravenous injection). With these frequent prolonged convulsions the danger of complex partial seizures (psychomotor) later in life is significant and cannot be ignored. It has therefore been stressed to paediatricians and general practitioners alike that, if the parents are living far from a health centre or the doctor's office and the child has more than two febrile seizures, if he is younger or older than the usual age for febrile convulsions, or if the child has already a neurological defect, then he should be treated with prophylactic phenobarbitone because of the difficulty in suppressing rapidly these prolonged convulsions. These prolonged febrile fits are more frequent, because many parents in Indonesia lack medical knowledge and do not suppress quickly a rising body temperature with tepid water, but instead cover the child in a thick woollen blanket. Even in large towns, it is still a common sight to see a child with high fever coming into the doctor's office wrapped in a thick blanket.

CLINICAL MANAGEMENT

Clinical management of epileptic patients may be divided into three sections.

Diagnosis

Ideally every new patient with seizures should be seen and examined by a neurologist (Aird & Woodbury 1974, see also Ch. 5). This is difficult to achieve in developing countries because of the large number of patients and the lack of neurologists. The following scheme has been used with success in East Java. The diagnosis may be considered under three headings.

Is it epilepsy?

As the diagnosis of epilepsy is made mainly on clinical grounds, it should be possible to give the responsibility of managing this section to the general practitioner, who has followed a special course on epileptology. This course should be given before the general practitioner departs for the health centre. It should be stressed that taking an extensive history (from the patient, from family, friends, fellow students or workers) is a prerequisite of establishing a good diagnosis.

Periodic attacks of neurological symptoms without diminishing consciousness are usually not epilepsy. For instance transient ischaemic attacks, tetany and migraine can be differentiated by detailed questioning. Also the often encountered hyperventilation syndrome can be easily recognized.

If the attacks are accompanied by a lowering of consciousness then a differential diagnosis should be made with syncope, by observing the following points:

1. Did the patient collapse after a strong emotional stress or did it happen in a room filled with people to a patient who had not eaten sufficient breakfast?
2. How long was the duration of the attack? Syncope usually lasts some seconds, while the duration of an epileptic attack is between 5 to 15 minutes.
3. Did the attack begin with a cry? Grand mal attacks sometimes begin with a cry, syncope never.
4. Was there urinary incontinence? Convulsions often are accompanied by incontinence, syncope never.
5. Was there tongue biting? Epilepsy often shows tongue biting, syncope never.
6. How was the patient's face? During convulsions the patient's face is often flushed, in syncope the patient is pale.
7. Was the patient lying in bed when the attack began? Syncope, while the patient is lying, is rare. A grand mal attack can occur anywhere.
8. How was the patient after the convulsion? An epileptic patient is often confused and sleepy after a convulsion, a patient with a syncope is alert.

9. Carry out an EEG in cases of doubt. The record of a grand mal patient often shows spikes, while the record of a patient with syncope is normal.

Generalized seizures have to be differentiated from psychogenic fits. In this respect the following points are worth observing:

1. How long was the duration of the attack? Psychogenic seizures may last hours or even days, a grand mal attack usually lasts between 5 to 15 minutes, except in patients with status epilepticus.
2. Was there urinary incontinence? In grand mal epilepsy incontinence is rather common, in hysterical seizures it is never seen.
3. In generalized seizures injuries caused by tongue biting or falling are frequent, in psychogenic pseudoseizures they are never seen.
4. In grand mal attacks the movements follow a certain (constant) pattern, while in hysterical seizures the movements are bizarre and inconsistent.
5. An 'unconscious' patient because of an hysterical seizure can be aroused by pain, a grand mal patient will remain unconscious.
6. Generalized seizures may occur anywhere, psychogenic seizures often occur in circumstances where they may attract a large audience.
7. After the convulsion, the grand mal patient is confused and sleepy (post-ictal phase), the patient with pseudoseizures is fully alert.

In children the differential diagnosis of convulsions with breath-holding attacks may be difficult.

In breath-holding spells the child usually does not move his arms or legs as during convulsions, but cries loudly and then stops breathing in the expiration phase. Because of this an anoxaemia develops and the child becomes unconscious. The child then becomes flaccid, starts breathing regularly and falls asleep. The good observer will note that there are no real convulsions in breath-holding attacks.

Which type of epilepsy?

It is the duty of a neurologist to distinguish between the various types of epilepsy. Points worth observing are as follows.

Some neurologists working only in the big cities have the impression that absences (pure petit mal attacks) are rare in developing countries. Like Edoo (1978) the author has the experience that, if a persistent search is made for patients with absences, by surveying the schools (with the help of the teachers) and testing the suspected children with an EEG, it will show that the frequency of petit mal in developing countries is the same as in Europe or the United States.

Because of clouding of consciousness, patients with psychomotor epilepsy are often referred to psychiatrists. To help these patients it is recommended that regular courses are given to general practitioners and psychiatrists about the symptoms of temporal lobe epilepsy. It must be stressed in these courses that patients with lowered consciousness, who do seemingly purposeful movements, who smack their lips or chew repeatedly, should be referred to a neurologist, who by arranging an EEG can establish the right diagnosis. Often only a sleep record will reveal the temporal lobe abnormality.

Etiology

In Indonesia and in other South East Asian countries, focal seizures are often caused by arteriovenous malformations. Therefore, in any unexplained focal seizure, arteriography is often necessary to establish the right diagnosis.

Compared with Europe or the United States, meningoencephalitis is still one of the main causes of convulsions. In developing countries, fever and convulsions are always an indication for a lumbar puncture to exclude an inflammatory disease.

Section 1 should be the responsibility of the general practitioner in the local health centre. The few cases, in which the general practitioner cannot decide whether it is epilepsy or not, he should refer to the neurologist in the hospitals. Sections 2 and 3 should be in the hands of the neurologist, who has an EEG machine.

Treatment

In general the principles of treatment are similar

to that in other countries, except for some constraints.

The lack of physicians and paramedical personnel in developing countries makes effective treatment of prolonged convulsions often difficult. Intravenous injections with diazepam have to be administered by nurses or physicians. Until now, no other drug is known which is as effective as diazepam in stopping prolonged convulsions, but which can be injected intramuscularly. Because phenobarbitone cannot be given at the same time as diazepam (respiration difficulties) the general practitioners have been warned not to use phenobarbitone to stop prolonged convulsions or status epilepticus.

In most developing countries, the so-called front-line drugs like diazepam, phenytoin, carbamazepine and phenobarbitone are available. The newer drugs like clonazepam or sodium valproate are often not available or difficult to get.

Estimation of serum drug levels is often not possible. In Indonesia only the top-referral hospitals (A hospitals) have facilities for monitoring serum drug levels, but the B hospitals, where most of the epileptic patients are treated, cannot do serum level monitoring.

In most developing countries health insurance is still in an embryonic stage or non-existent. Because most of the epileptic patients are poor and antiepileptic therapy lasts several year, the doctors have to choose not only the most effective drug for the seizure type, but also have to consider the price of the drug the patient can afford to pay.

In Indonesia, like in many developing countries, liver diseases are frequent, therefore, every doctor treating epileptic patients has to realize the influence of the liver metabolism on the pharmacokinetics of antiepileptic drugs, before adjusting the dosage.

As most of the patients visiting an epileptic clinic are simple village people, extra effort and time is required to educate the patients regarding the long-term nature of antiepileptic therapy. For good results in the management of epilepsy, intelligent co-operation of the patient is required.

Treatment of status epilepticus

As in other developing countries, status epilepticus is often seen in Indonesia. In the author's experience status epilepticus often occurs because of:

1. Sudden discontinuance of antiepileptic therapy.
2. Meningoencephalitis
3. Subarachnoid or intracerebral bleeding
4. Acute electrolyte disturbances

As for other unconscious states, the first task of a doctor, when confronted with a patient in status epilepticus should be to maintain an open airway with sufficient respiratory ventilation. After that, a slow intravenous injection of diazepam (10 mg) should be given, which may be repeated after two hours if necessary. A combination of diazepam and phenobarbitone should be avoided to prevent respiratory difficulties. Immediately after control of the convulsions, phenytoin should be given to ensure better control, because diazepam is a short acting drug. After the convulsions have ceased, the patient should be admitted to hospital for a complete work-up.

Interictal antiepileptic treatment

The interictal treatment of patients with epilepsy will be discussed under three headings:

1. When to start antiepileptic treatment
2. The technique of treatment
3. When to stop treatment

When to start antiepileptic treatment. In developing countries the decision to start antiepileptic treatment should be taken by a neurologist because:

1. Antiepileptic treatment is a long term treatment, which means a heavy burden for the usually uninsured patient.
2. The epileptic patient needs regular supervision, which again means loss of time and more expense.
3. The treatment of the different types of epilepsy is not the same and therefore before starting the treatment the physician should first determine the electro-clinical type of epilepsy, from which the patient is suffering. This means an EEG is required and a neurologist to read the record.

In the department of neurology, Airlangga University, we have decided not to give antiepileptic drugs to a patient:

1. Who has had only one attack
2. Who has less than one seizure a year, provided the interictal EEG is normal

The technique of treatment. Once it has been decided to start treatment, the following rules should be used:

1. Always start with one drug. Because in developing countries serum levels of the antiepileptic drug cannot be estimated, the drug used is usually increased in dosage until the convulsions are controlled or until signs of intoxication develop. If more than one drug is used, observation of these signs will be more difficult. Monotherapy will also be of advantage if a drug allergy develops. The third reason why monotherapy is advised is that, if one uses more than one drug, one has to take into account the drug interactions.

2. *Always start with a low dose.* Many antiepileptic drugs will give side-effects at first. By starting with a low dose these side-effects will be fewer.

3. Increase the dosage of the drug slowly, and only change the dosage after there is a stabilization of the serum drug level. As the serum drug level only becomes stable after four times the half-life of the drug used, the half-life of each antiepileptic drug should be known. Phenobarbitone with a half-life of 96 hours, will only reach a stable serum level after 16 days.

4. Every neurologist is advised to use only the antiepileptic drugs with which he has had experience. Because in developing countries estimation of drug level is often not possible, one should increase the dosage slowly until the convulsions cease or until toxic complications develop. Therefore every physician working with antiepileptic drugs should know these complications and he should only work with the drugs with which he is familiar.

5. As most of the patients are people living in the villages, who are busy all day and do not pay enough attention to the regular intake of the antiepileptic drugs, one has to instruct the patient and family to put the daily dosage in a small box. This box should be filled each evening to diminish errors through forgetting.

6. In developing countries, control of patients' compliance cannot be done by measuring drug levels. Instead, the doctor has to advise patients to bring to the doctor's office all tablets which are left when they come for their monthly physical examination.

7. As most of the developing countries have a tropical climate, it is advisable not to prescribe antiepileptic drugs in the form of a suspension or syrup, as the concentration may change because of evaporation. It is much better to use capsules or tablets.

8. In grand mal patients, the first choice of an epileptic drug should be phenytoin. If it does not help it may be combined with carbamazepine. The same choice should be made in case of focal motor attacks. In case of absences the first choice should be ethosuximide. If it does not help one should search for clonazepam or sodium valproate, which are both difficult to get in developing countries. In minor motor attacks, one should try first sodium valproate and clonazepam as a second drug if sodium valproate does not decrease the attacks. In temporal lobe epilepsy the first drug used should be carbamazepine.

9. As there is a wide variation in body weight between people living in rural and urban areas, it is advisable to administer antiepileptic drugs on a mg/kg basis.

When to stop treatment. When the patient has been free of attacks for three years, one may decrease the dosage of the antiepileptic drug slowly and try to stop it after six months. In cases of grand mal attacks usually no recurrence of convulsions is seen, but in complex partial seizures one often has to continue giving drugs for a longer time.

Prognosis

The prognosis depends upon the following outlined below.

1. *The etiology* – in cases of infections (meningoencephalitis) the prognosis is often better than in cases of trauma, neoplasms or vascular disease

2. *The type of epilepsy* – myoclonic epilepsy is difficult to control
3. *The age of the patient* – attacks of secondary generalized epilepsy in early childhood are often resistent to therapy

PREVENTION

As in many other diseases, prevention is very important. In developing countries many factors can be corrected easily, if the patient pays enough attention. Several factors which may be improved are as follows.

Better obstetrical care

In many infants, convulsions are caused by cerebral bleedings, which develop during parturition. In breech presentation of the baby, it is often better to deliver the baby by the abdominal route than by the vaginal one. Vaginal delivery may cause more lacerations to the cerebral blood vessels. The aim of every doctor should not only be to deliver a living baby but a healthy baby.

Combat meningoencephalitis

Every physician working in a developing country should be aware that infections are still frequent. Especially in children, the doctor should diagnose and treat meningitis by doing a lumbar puncture in every suspected case. Only this aggressive approach will decrease the postencephalitic convulsions which are so common in developing countries.

Decrease the incidence of traumatic brain injuries

The incidence of traumatic brain injuries, with its consequent rise in post-traumatic convulsions, is increasing faster in developing countries than in the United States. In three years the incidence of traumatic brain injuries in the general hospital in Surabaya, which is the only hospital which receives emergency traffic accidents, has risen by 100%. Although it is not entirely the duty of the doctor to lower this extremely high figure, the authorities should be advised regarding the following points:

1. As most of the head injuries occur to motor bike riders, who do not use a helmet, everyone riding one should be strongly advised to use a helmet. Doctors and medical students should set an example
2. Decrease the speed limit
3. Make separate lanes for rapid moving cars and the slower traffic, consisting of bicycles, oxcarts etc
4. Persuade the general public, not to drive a motor vehicle, when they feel ill

Febrile convulsions

This factor has been explained in the section on etiology.

REHABILITATION

As a physician, one should be aware, that besides treating the patient with drugs, one should always try to restore the patient to society. This vocational rehabilitation is usually not present in developing countries, although it is needed more than in Europe or the United States. The large professional workshops, who do this rehabilitation so efficiently in Europe, usually are non-existent and the neurologist has to ask the help of volunteers to arrange small programmes. What one can do is usually to help in the placement of the patients.

School problems in epilepsy

Because of misinformation, children with epilepsy are often refused admittance in schools. To alter this, courses were given to the school teachers with the purpose of changing their attitude. In these courses explanation was given in simple terms regarding the nature of epilepsy. It was stressed that the epileptic child needed a normal school and not a special school, where overprotection easily developed.

Marriage problems in epileptic patients

More than in advanced countries, the belief is widely held in developing countries that epilepsy is a hereditary disease and that marriage with an epileptic patient should be avoided. We have tried to change this ignorance by:

1. Giving courses to district doctors, in the hope that they in turn explain to teachers and district chiefs the modern concepts of epilepsy
2. Distributing leaflets explaining in simple terms the fundamental aspects of epilepsy
3. Playing cassette-recorders in waiting rooms of hospitals with essential information regarding the nature of epilepsy

It is hoped that in this manner superstition and confusion regarding epilepsy and convulsions will decrease.

Employment problems in epileptic patients

In developing countries, more than in the United States and Europe it is very difficult for an epileptic patient to get work. First of all because jobs, even for normal people, are not abundant, but also because of wrong public attitudes based upon poor information. This has tried to be overcome by giving leaflets to big firms and important businessmen and stimulating hospitals and medical schools to set an example by using epileptic patients for jobs, whenever possible.

SUMMARY

This section has tried to highlight the importance of epilepsy in developing countries and the problems facing a neurologist when working with epileptic patients. A health referral scheme has been advocated which may be used in developing countries to treat epilepsy on a wide basis with the limited resources available. Much still needs to be done but, by hard work and the intelligent use and distribution of doctors, nurses and facilities, after some time the same results with antiepileptic treatment can be achieved as in more affluent countries.

REFERENCES

Aird R B, Woodbury D M 1974 The management of epilepsy. Thomas, Springfield p 239
Chandra B 1978 Management of febrile convulsions. In: Meinardi H, Rowan A J (eds) Advances in epileptology. Swets & Zeitlinger, Amsterdam, p 308
Edoo B B 1978 Absences in Ghanaian children – The problem of diagnosis in a developing country. In: Meinardi, H, Rowan A J (eds) Advances in epileptology. Swets & Zeitlinger, Amsterdam, p 420
Tower D B 1978 Epilepsy: a world problem. In: Meinardi, H Rowan A J (eds) Advances in epileptology. Swets & Zeitlinger, Amsterdam, p 2

PART TWO
EPILEPSY IN LATIN AMERICA
P. R. M. Bittencourt

LATIN AMERICA AND WORLD EPILEPTOLOGY

A review of some of the major neuroscience journals (Epilepsia, Neurology, Archives of Neurology, Annals of Neurology, Brain, Journal of Neurology, Neurosurgery and Psychiatry, Journal of Neurological Sciences and Acta Neurologica Scandinavica) revealed no more than ten epilepsy related papers by Latin American groups in the period 1979–1985. A search of the quoted references in the second edition of this textbook (Laidlaw & Richens 1982) produced four publications by Latin American groups, three of which were on epidemiology. Of between 300 and 500 abstracts presented at the 12th, 13th, 14th, 15th and 16th Epilepsy International Symposia, which took place at Florence (1979), Copenhagen (1980), Kyoto (1981), London (1982), Washington DC (1983) and Hamburg (1985), respectively 7, 5, 5, 6, 11 and 18 were by Latin American investigators. Practically all these publications, which achieved international status, came from the same groups in Mexico City, São Paulo, Curitiba, Montevideo, Buenos Aires and Santiago. No controlled trial of antiepileptic drugs has been reported from Latin America recently (Porter 1982, Richens 1982). Arquivos de Neuro-Psiquiatria, the major Brazilian neuroscience journal, published approximately 100 papers on epilepsy between 1943 and 1982. The majority were replications of studies carried out previously in the Northern Hemisphere or were clinical observations. It is clear how little importance epilepsy research originating in Latin America currently has in world epileptology.

There was until recently little information on any aspect of epilepsy in the South American continent. A prospective protocol to investigate various aspects of epilepsy was started in 1982 in Curitiba, Brazil, and closed in 1984 when some 600 patients had been assessed (The Curitiba Prospective Study on Epilepsy). Data collected included past seizure frequency by type according to the International League Against Epilepsy Classification (Commission 1981), history of birth injury, trauma, CNS infection, surgery or other events, family history, laboratory, radiological and EEG examinations, as well as past drug history. Also noted were seizure frequency and drug treatment after patients were included in the study. Similar data on children have recently been collected retrospectively by Sakamoto (1985) in Ribeirão Prêto, in the same geographical area as Curitiba. The present review will be based on these studies and on other Latin American reports published recently.

BASIC SCIENCE

At the moment scientists active in epilepsy related fields are based in Mexico City and São Paulo. The latter group has been set up recently and has devoted itself to work related to neurotransmitters and experimental models (Campos & Cavalheiro 1980). The difficulties involved in developing basic research in Latin America are illustrated in

a comparison of the number of papers by Latin American authors while working in Europe (Bortolotto et al 1985, Czuczwar et al 1985, Turski et al 1985a, b) to the number of papers published based on work carried out locally (Campos & Cavalheiro 1979, Campos et al 1980, Cavalheiro et al 1981). Mexican researchers have a long tradition in the fields of experimental epilepsy and neurotransmitters (Tapia et al 1979, Velasco et al 1979, Velasco et al 1980, Benitez et al 1982).

SOCIAL ASPECTS

The most common attitude towards epilepsy in Latin America is one of prejudice, creating a powerful stigma towards the term. Bigarella et al (1984), in a study of the prevalence of epilepsy in schools in Curitiba, found that the population did not know what epilepsy is. They initially interviewed teachers and their 1239 students in five special schools for the retarded and in two large schools for 'normal' children. As ignorance about the definition of epilepsy was the rule rather than exception, a questionnaire had to be developed with the objective of finding epileptic patients by all their possible denominations. Data were obtained on 226 retarded subjects of various ages and on 607 children aged 3 to 14 years, 402 of whom attend an upper class and 205 a lower class school. Various descriptions were used for possible epileptic subjects, such as 'dysrythmic', 'carriers of attacks', of 'petit-mal', of 'absences'. The results are summarized in Table 14.1. A great number of retarded subjects and of lower class schoolchildren received regular antiepileptic drugs.

Table 14.1 Prevalence of subjects denominated as epileptic, dysrythmic, other denominations suggestive of epilepsy (single seizures, febrile seizures, absences, petit-mal, attacks, etc) and of subjects on regular antiepileptic drugs (AED) in schools in Curitiba, Brazil. Data from Bigarella et al (1984)

	Special schools	Lower-class school	Upper-class School
Epileptic	20.0%	0.5%	0.0%
Dysrythmic	5.5%	2.5%	4.0%
Other	11.0%	5.0%	3.0%
On AED	37.0%	6.5%	2.5%
Population	226	205	402

The term 'epilepsy' was rarely, if at all, used for non-retarded subjects. They were considered carriers of a variety of pseudoneurological states such as 'cerebral dysrythmia'.

This state of affairs was partly the fault of physicians who either gave antiepileptic drugs to nonepileptic subjects or made a diagnosis of epilepsy without informing their patients or their parents. Furthermore, overtreatment with antiepileptic drugs was more common in lower than in upper-class students. The fact that only one out of 607 school children was regarded as 'epileptic' by their parents or teachers, although 24 were on regular antiepileptic medication, is indicative of the power of the stigma surrounding the term epilepsy with respect to patients, their relations and their physicians.

The origins of the term 'dysrythmia' are related to overemphasis on the EEG diagnosis of epilepsy (Caleffi 1984). Its continued use to the present day is related to the antiepilepsy stigma so prevalent in less developed countries, but also to its continued use in widely read texbooks (Walton 1985). The consequences of the 'dysrhythmia' tradition are many: a large number of patients with behavioural disorders, migraine, single seizures, transient ischaemic attacks or cardiovascular syndromes are diagnosed as 'dysrhythmic' and receive antiepileptic drugs, usually phenobarbitone (Bittencourt 1985). Table 14.1 shows that the most common reason for antiepileptic drug treatment in Curitiba, and the most likely throughout Latin America, is 'cerebral dysrhythmia'.

Ferreira et al (1984) found no difference between intelligence quotients of epileptic outpatients and controls, using a Brazilian version of the WAIS. After breaking down the groups, they found that employment, male sex and secondary education were related to significantly higher IQs than those of unemployed, female and uneducated subjects. The differences were statistically significant when the three variables were taken separately, showing that epilepsy is a lesser handicap in southern Brazil than lack of schooling or belonging to the female sex.

Factors related to employment of epileptic patients in Uruguay have been evaluated by de Pasquet et al (1976a, 1984). They found that 37% of epileptic patients were unemployed, as compared to 6.7% in the country as a whole and 9.6% in the same general hospital's population. A higher rate of unemployment was observed in 'mentally retarded' epileptic patients (76%) than in those of 'normal' intelligence (21%).

Rehabilitation of epileptic patients through the Brazilian national health scheme has been examined by Madallozzo et al (1984). Over ten years their centre evaluated 573 epileptic patients representative of the city of Curitiba who had left a variety of jobs, 395 of which entered the rehabilitation scheme. Re-employment occurred in 61% of these cases, through the efforts of a large multidisciplinary team. One year after successfuly leaving the rehabilitation scheme into employment, 54% of 215 patients were employed, 38% were lost to follow-up and 7% were unemployed.

EPIDEMIOLOGY

Usual demographic techniques may be inaccurate in determining epidemiological data with respect to epilepsy in developing countries, since neither the public nor physicians know what epilepsy is. Correct prevalence and incidence rates can thus be found only if trained epileptologists interview large samples of the population. These considerations possibly underlie the erratic figures published with respect to Latin America, such as prevalence rates above 19 per 1000 inhabitants in Colombia (Gomez et al 1978) or Chile (Chiofalo et al 1979) and 3.5 in Mexico (Olivares 1972). Zielinski (1982) concluded that most reliable studies indicated prevalence rates for epilepsy between 2.3 and 7.8 per 1000 inhabitants in areas as different from each other as Guam, Iceland, Rochester and Warsaw.

An idea of the methodological complexities of epidemiological studies is given by Chiofalo and colleagues in Chile, who found the prevalence rate for 9-year-old children in 1979 to be 31 per 1000 inhabitants (Chiofalo et al 1979) considering single seizures as epilepsy. When they repeated the study considering two seizures as diagnostic the rate decreased to 17 per 1000 (Chiofalo et al 1985).

Almeida Filho (1980) reviewed his own and other epidemiological studies on epilepsy, finding prevalence rates between 1 and 20 per 1000 inhabitants in various urban populations in Colombia, Chile, Peru, Argentina and Brazil. Santana (1978) and Almeida Filho (1980) studied respectively populations of 5 to 14 years of age and above 15 years in the same suburb of the city of Salvador in Brazil. Screening was carried out by trained medical students and cases of suspected mental disorders including epilepsy were interviewed by fully trained psychiatrists. The prevalence rates found were 1 and 8 per 1000 respectively, which, for a single population, contrasts with Zielinski's finding (1982) of between 4 and 10 per 1000 in over half of all epidemiological studies. A similar study including screening of 7603 inhabitants of a São Paulo suburb by medical students with subsequent interview of suspected epilepsy cases by a trained physician was carried out by Marino & Cukiert (1986). Again the prevalence rate of 11.9 per 1000 inhabitants was outside Zielinski's (1982) average range.

In summary, therefore, the South American studies indicate a prevalence rate of epilepsy in the general population to be twice as high as those in northern hemisphere countries.

ETIOLOGY

The frequencies of the various causes of epileptic seizures are relatively well worked out in northern hemisphere countries (Marsden & Reynolds 1982, Roger et al 1985). Data for the southern hemisphere are much more scanty and biased due to local sampling problems (Osuntokum 1977).

The major study in Latin America before the era of CT scanning was that of de Pasquet et al (1976a) who assessed 500 patients aged 14 years or more at a specialized clinic. Genetically related causes were found in 9% of the cases, perinatal in 8.5%, traumatic in 8%, vascular in 5%, infectious in 4% and miscellaneous in another 6.5%. The remaining 59% of the cases were labelled 'cryptogenetic'. It is interesting that only 5 cases of parasitosis were found even though the same group was able to collect 100 cases of operated cerebral hydatid cysts, 5 of which developed epilepsy (de Pasquet et al 1976b). It would thus appear that hydatid cysts lead to epilepsy more frequently after surgical resection, and then rarely.

Table 14.2 Frequency of etiology of epilepsy as found in the Curitiba Prospective Study of Epilepsy. 'Unclear' includes all cases in whom a definite cause could not be ascertained as well as 'familial' epilepsy. Cranial trauma includes at least definite loss of consciousness for more than 15 minutes with hospital admission. Perinatal includes fetal and new-born distress syndromes with clear asphyxia. Data adapted from Bittencourt et al (1983)

Aetiology	Number	Percentage
Unclear	100	68.0%
Perinatal	16	11.0%
Cranial Trauma	19	13.0%
Neurosurgery	2	1.5%
Cysticercosis	6	4.0%
Vascular	4	2.5%
TOTAL	147	100%

The Curitiba Prospective Study on Epilepsy. included all patients seen at a neurological outpatient clinic who were investigated according to a predetermined schedule. Table 14.2 shows data concerning 147 patients aged 13 years or more in whom the neurologist was satisfied as far as etiological investigation. They all had a detailed history, physical examination, skull X-rays, routine cerebrospinal fluid examination, blood tests and EEG. Whenever judged necessary, they were admitted for further investigation including CT scanning. The results cannot be taken as final because not all patients had a CT scan and because of the special nature of 'familial' epilepsy in areas such as Brazil. The fact that relatives have fits does not necessarily imply a genetic factor, since cysticercosis, malnutrition and perinatal asphyxia also strike families. As an example of 'familial' epilepsies in Brazil, Sakamoto (1985) found that 26% of 259 patients aged 1 month to 15 years had a positive history. Similarly, in Uruguay 17% of 500 patients aged 14 years or more had at least one epileptic close relative (de Pasquet et al 1976a).

Sakamoto (1985) evaluated retrospectively 455 patients aged under 15 years seen at a neurological outpatient clinic over a two-year period because of isolated or recurrent non-febrile seizures. They were investigated when judged necessary with routine blood and cerebrospinal fluid tests, EEG and skull X-rays. Table 14.3 shows the possible etiologies found. Although Sakamoto's data suffer from the major drawbacks of being retro-

Table 14.3 Possible etiology of epilepsy in 455 patients aged 1 month to 15 years (some had 2 possible etiologies) investigated in the pre-CT scan era (adapted from Sakamoto 1985). CNS infections includes pre- and postnatal events

Aetiology	Number	Percentage
Unclear	286	63%
CNS malformation	9	2%
Prematurity	8	2%
Toxaemia of pregnancy	5	1%
Perinatal anoxia	49	11%
CNS infection	22	5%
Cranial trauma	14	3%
Neurocysticercosis	60	13%
Miscellaneous	10	2%
TOTAL	463	102%

spective and collected previous to CT scan availability, the results are comparable with those of the Curitiba Prospective Study (Table 14.2) except for an even higher frequency of neurocysticercosis. This cannot be an artifact, as only 126 of Sakamoto's patients had cerebrospinal fluid studies and 344 had skull X-rays, while all subjects in the Curitiba Study had these tests and all diagnoses of vascular disease or neurocysticercosis were complemented by CT scanning.

A retrospective study on the etiology of epilepsy in patients aged 25 years or more was carried out in Uruguay by de Pasquet et al (1972) before CT scanning became available. Of 155 patients presenting primarily with seizures, 43 had clinical evidence of further CNS involvement such as pyramidal, frontal, visual, verbal or oculomotor disturbances. Eighteen were taken to surgery because of tumours (10), cranial trauma (4) or intracranial haemorrhage (4). Etiology remained obscure in 52% and was genetic in 7%. The most common cause of secondary epilepsy was vascular disease (13%) followed by cranial trauma (12%), tumours (11%), alcoholism (3%) and infectious diseases (2%).

It becomes clear from the Brazilian and Uruguayan studies that a large number of cases of epilepsy have etiologies which are potentially preventable. The high frequency of trauma, cysticercosis and perinatal disorders is the reason behind the belief of Latin American physicians that epilepsy is more common than in the Northern Hemisphere.

DIAGNOSIS OF SEIZURE TYPE

Clinical data

The relative frequency of seizure types in Rochester and Warsaw, and surveys of outpatient notes in Warsaw and Marseilles, have indicated that partial seizures outnumber generalized by approximately three to one (Zielinski 1982). Conflicting reports from Bogotá (Gomez et al 1978) and Santiago (Chiofalo et al 1985) claimed a 1 to 3 ratio. In Uruguay the rate was approximately 1:1 (de Pasquet et al 1976a). Two studies from Brazil substantiate the Warsaw, Rochester and Marseilles results. Table 14.4 shows data from the Curitiba Prospective Study (Bittencourt et al 1983) and from Ribeirão Prêto (Sakamoto 1985). The latter was based on retrospective review of notes, while the former used a standardized and prospective form for history taking. The results are probably comparable and representative of adult (Curitiba) and childhood (Ribeirão Prêto) populations in the south of Brazil.

Table 14.4 Frequency of seizure types according to the ILAE classification in the Curitiba (patients aged 13 to 63 years) and Ribeirão Prêto studies (patients aged 1 month to 15 years). Data respectively from Bittencourt et al (1983) and Sakamoto (1985); in the latter 5 patients (2%) had unclassified seizures

Seizure type	Curitiba No.	%	Ribeirão Prêto No.	%
Simple partial	3	0.8	11	4
Complex partical	45	12	73	28
Partial with generalization	155	41	27	10.5
Generalized	124	34.2	27	10.5
Mixed types	46	12	115	45
TOTAL	373	100	253	98

Speciali (1973, 1985) studied the clinical and electroencephalographic manifestations of the Lennox-Gastaut syndrome and described a variety of seizures hoping to define therapeutic and prognostic guidelines. The results, like those of Gastaut et al (1973), are difficult to interpret in the light of evidence that specific types of seizures may be a result of antiepileptic drug therapy in patients with the Lennox-Gastaut syndrome (Bittencourt & Richens 1981).

Table 14.5 Frequency of inconclusive (normal or irregular) and epileptiform records by seizure type in an adolescent and adult population of epileptic patients (same as Table 14.4, Curitiba group)

Seizures	Patients	EEGs	Inconclusive	Epileptifrom
Simple Partial	3	3	3 (100%)	0
Simple Partial + Generalization	80	96	63 (66%)	33(34%)
Complex Partial	45	56	35 (62%)	21 (38%)
Complex Partial + Generalization	75	92	58 (63%)	34 (37%)
Primary Generalized	101	134	83 (62%)	51 (38%)
Generalized (sleep)	23	23	18 (78%)	5 (22%)
Mixed types	46	61	26 (43%)	35 (57%)
TOTAL	373	465	286 (61.5%)	179(38.5%)

EEG data

The routine 8-channel EEG is the most widely used neurological investigational method in Latin America. Its role in diagnosis has been overemphasized due to the proliferation of laboratories unaccompanied by similar proliferation of experienced neurophysiologists (Bittencourt 1985). EEG is practically restricted to routine 8 or 16 channel recordings. Although video monitoring, telemetry and ambulatory EEG have consistently shown higher yields of abnormalities, there are few such laboratories in Latin America (Turner 1983).

The Curitiba Prospective Study showed EEG records to be 'epileptiform' in about 40% of epileptic adolescent and adult outpatients in a neurological clinic (Table 14.5). An 'epileptiform' record was one that showed focal or generalized spike or spike-wave discharges, focal spikes, sharp waves or pathological slowing. The other 60% of the records were 'normal' or 'irregular'. Sakamoto's study (1985), in patients under 15 years of age, found 37% of routine EEGs of 222 patients to be normal and 59% to show 'epileptiform' discharges; indicating that patients under 14 years of age have more 'epileptiform' abnormalities than found in the Curitiba group of adolescents and adults. These results show that, in a great number of cases, seizure description alone will indicate seizure type. Other authors have shown that after repeated recordings of patients with frequent seizures a significant number will remain undiagnosed as to the nature of the epileptic discharges (Ajmone-Marsan & Zivin 1970).

Data in Table 14.5 show a low yield of 'epileptiform' records in patients with nocturnal tonic-clonic seizures. The decision whether a nocturnal seizure is secondarily generalized or not is a common problem faced by physicians. The Curitiba Prospective Study looked into EEGs of patients whose seizures were thought to be primarily generalized on history taking and found that the majority of 'epileptiform' discharges were of focal nature (Table 14.6).

The electroclinical characteristics of the Lennox-Gastaut syndrome were evaluated by Speciali (1985), who concluded that K complexes and

Table 14.6 Frequency of specific EEG abnormalities in 45 patients with 'epileptiform' records and seizures which by history were primary generalized. They were taken from the group in Tables 14.4 and 14.5

EEG abnormality – Focal		Generalized	
Spikes	38%	Regular spike-wave	5%
Sharp waves	15%	Irregular	11%
Slowing	21%	Polyspikes	2%
Mixed focal and generalized abnormalities	8%		

sleep spindles indicated good prognosis. Multi-focal 'epileptogenic' activity, burst suppression, repetitive 8–10 Hz polyspikes and paroxysms of varying morphology suggested a bad outcome. These findings, already suggested by Gastaut et al (1973), were disputed by reports that burst suppression and repetitive spikes were drug-induced phenomena, albeit found only in patients with the Lennox-Gastaut syndrome (Bittencourt & Richens 1981).

Other investigational methods

Routine laboratory methods are available in Latin America. Determination of antiepileptic drug concentrations is possible in major cities but reliability is doubtful, because of the absence of international quality control. Computerized tomography has proliferated rapidly to become available in most Brazilian cities of more than 300 000 inhabitants. There are no positron emission tomography scanners in the area. Magnetic resonance imaging (MRI) is available in São Paulo.

DIAGNOSIS OF EPILEPTIC SYNDROMES

Recently a working, albeit controversial, classification of epileptic syndromes and epilepsies became available (Commission of the International League Against Epilepsy 1985). It is anticipated that this complex list of clinical entities will take a long time to become common knowledge among Latin American neurologists. One evidence of this difficulty is that a recent publication of the Asociacion Colombiana de Neurologia (Jimenez 1985) presented the 1981 Classification of Seizures of the International League Against Epilepsy as a classification of the epilepsies.

The greatest difficulty of the 1985 Classification is created by the sophistication necessary for the diagnosis of the subtypes of 'symptomatic localization related epilepsies'; presently a privilege of investigators using depth-electrodes. There are two groups performing routine epilepsy surgery in Latin America (Marino 1983, Martins 1984). Furthermore, there is an inherent weakness in applying the concept of 'syndrome' to seizure types ('frontal lobe, supplementary motor, cingulate epilepsies'). Nonetheless, word of the new classification is being spread throughout Latin America (Bittencourt 1986, Turner 1985) and it is hoped that the results of discussions and studies within the continent will be taken into account in its final format.

THERAPY

There are many peculiarities in the treatment of epilepsy in Latin America. One of them is the concept of prophylatic treatment of non-febrile seizures. In the study of Sakamoto (1985), 50% of 288 patients were started on drugs upon their first seizure. The criteria for this attitude are unclear, but the numbers reflect the widespread habit in the continent of considering a single non-febrile seizure as indicative of epilepsy.

A second peculiarity is that the single most commonly used treatment of seizures is phenobarbitone, a habit related to an oversimplification of epilepsy as an uniform clinical entity to which a single therapeutic manoeuvre may be applied. Contributing factors are simplicity of use, apparent lack of side-effects and early efficacy, as well as low cost. At any rate, the reality in Brazil and most likely throughout Latin America is that 'cerebral dysrhythmia' rather than epilepsy is the most frequent diagnosis (Bigarella et al 1984) and phenobarbitone alone (Bittencourt 1985) or in combination with phenytoin (de Pasquet et al 1976a) its obvious treatment.

An idea of the frequency and implications of widespread phenobarbitone prescribing is given by the 52 patients on barbiturates collected by the Curitiba Prospective Study over a period of two years (Gorz et al 1986). The problem faced by these patients was either previously unrecognized side-effects or refractoriness of seizures after a period of some years. When examined in detail, 71% of the patients had partial seizures with or without secondary generalization. A dramatic decrease in seizure frequency was observed when patients were switched to carbamazepine, phenytoin or sodium valproate (Gorz et al in press).

The magnitude of the phenobarbitone for 'cerebral dysrhythmia' habit in Brazil stimulated a campaign by the Brazilian branches of the International League Against Epilepsy and of the International Society of EEG and Neurophysiology (Bittencourt 1985, Caleffi 1984) aimed at educating the public as well as physicians about the two erroneous assumptions. This effort was made more difficult by the barrier of the economics of epilepsy, which includes the high cost of carbamazepine and sodium valproate as well as the unavailability and cost of reliable routine antiepileptic drug monitoring. The Curitiba Prospective Study tackled these peculiarities through the development of a safe schedule for therapeutic substitution in barbiturate-refractory epilepsy (Gorz et al in press) and by looking into the comparative efficacy of monotherapy without determination of serum levels (Bittencourt et al 1986). In the latter study clinical observation of side-effects without serum level monitoring was used to adjust dosage of phenobarbitone, phenytoin or carbamazepine in 80 previously untreated patients. After a follow up of 20 ± 9 (mean ± SD) months 77.5% were seizure-free. There was no difference in seizure control or frequency of side-effects in the three groups (Table 14.7).

An analysis of three studies carried out in developed countries which used routine antiepileptic drug monitoring (Shorvon et al 1978, Strandjord & Johannessen 1980, Turnbull et al 1982) showed that 80–90% of the patients were fully controlled on monotherapy with phenytoin,

sodium valproate or carbamazepine. The severity of epilepsy and length of follow-up are generally similar to that of the study of Bittencourt et al (1986), in which up to 85% of the patients were fully controlled (Table 14.7). The latter authors concluded that socioeconomic factors such as lack of available drugs were more likely to underlie the small difference in efficacy than lack of antiepileptic drug monitoring.

Such trials of comparative efficacy of antiepileptic drugs as those of Shorvon et al (1978) or Turnbull et al (1982) have not been reported from Latin America apart from the study of Bittencourt et al (1986). Uncontrolled open studies in mixed populations of untreated and already treated patients, with or without determination of serum antiepileptic drug concentrations, have claimed benefit with valproic acid (de Pasquet et al 1973), carbamazepine (Scaramelli & de Pasquet 1985) and phenytoin (Galdames et al 1980).

Epilepsy surgery has been available in Brazil for the past decade or so (Marino 1983). The complexities and cost of maintaining the multidisciplinary team needed for surgical procedures prevent the multiplication of such centres in Latin America (Martins 1984). Large epilepsy centres with inpatient facilities and multidisciplinary teams for rehabilitation do not exist. Similarly, outpatient care is provided by isolated units of the national health system, medical schools or by private hospitals in Brazil (Madallozzo et al 1984, Saraiva 1983, Bittencourt et al 1986). The very severe segment of the epileptic population in Brazil survives in large psychiatric hospitals and in outpatient institutions for the mentally handicapped.

Table 14.7 Demographic and prognostic factors, as well as length of follow-up, rate of full seizure control and of presence of side-effects in 80 patients on monotherapy with carbamazepine (CBZ), phenytoin (DPH) or phenobarbitone (PHB). Data from Bittencourt et al (1986)

	CBZ	PHB	DPH
Number	27	33	20
Age (years)	25 ± 10	26 ± 12	32 ± 15
Sex (male)	41%	58%	70%
Neuropsychiatric features	19%	12%	20%
Abnormal EEG	40%	25%	22%
Multiple seizure types	26%	6%	20%
Partial or secondarily generalized seizures	72%	31%	67%
Follow-up (months)	19 ± 10	22 ± 10	18 ± 8
Full seizure control	75%	85%	70%
Side-effects	7%	9%	10%

CONCLUSIONS

Medical care in Latin America mirrors its social and economic realities. Large urban conglomerates such as São Paulo, Mexico City and Buenos Aires offer medical standards comparable to those of major cities in North America, Europe or Japan. Distant communities in the Andes, Amazon or Tierra del Fuego regions are comparable to the poorest areas of the planet. There is little to be done apart from waiting for political changes which in their own time-scale will bring improvement to medical care.

Meanwhile, much may be done in the research fields related to epilepsy. Research has not followed the pace of modern clinical medicine in the continent. The present situation is one of isolation of the Latin American would-be scientist from his or her peers in the developed world, partly due to local deficiencies but also to the rarified atmosphere created in the scientific means of communication controlled by investigators in the developed world. Organizations such as Epilepsy International, International League Against Epilepsy and World Health Organization can take a leading role in decentralizing epileptological know-how, presently controlled by and feeding back into the developed world. As an example, the Commission on Classification on Epilepsies and Epileptic Syndromes of the International League Against Epilepsy (1985) stated that its proposal for an international classification 'would have to reflect' the 'pluralism of science' in order to be 'scientifically valid'. Nonetheless, the six members of this Commission are based solely in Japan, Western Europe and North America, as were all the specialists consulted by the Commission, a fact contrary to their own statement of the nature of a scientifically valid classification.

ACKNOWLEDGEMENT

Drs C E S Silvado, A M Gorz and D. de Paola participated in the Curitiba Prospective Study on Epilepsy. Funds were made available by private donations, by the National Society for Epilepsy (United Kingdom), Biogalênica Quimica e Farmacêutica Ltda. (São Paulo) and by Sanofi Pharma International (Paris). Drs. Francisco Rubio-Donnadieu (Mexico), Edith Gerstle de Pasquet (Uruguay), Marcos Turner (Argentina), Nelly Chiofalo (Chile), Arthur Cukiert, Esper Cavalheiro, Raul Marino Jr, A. C. Sakamoto and Ms Janice Meister (Brazil) contributed in locating the reviewed material. Some of the data reviewed were personal communications from these authors amplifying the abstracts of symposium presentations.

REFERENCES

Ajmone Marsan C, Zivin L S 1970 Factors related to the occurrence of typical paroxysmal abnormalities in the EEG records of epileptic patients. Epilepsia 11: 361–381

Almeida Filho N 1980 Epidemiologia social das epilepsias no Brasil. In: Sena P G (ed.) Novas achegas sôbre a epilepsia. Centro Editorial e Didático da Universidade Federal da Bahia, Salvador, pp 57–78

Benitez A S, Briones R, Guardiola H F 1982 Purkinje cell responses to a cerebral penicillin-induced epileptogenic focus in the cat. Epilepsia 23: 597–606

Bigarella M M, Dóro M P, Bittencourt P R M 1984 Epilepsia e escola. In: Bittencourt P R M (ed.) Epilepsia-1984: Palestras do II Simpósio Paranaense de Epilepsia, Publicações Capitulo Paranense da Liga Brasileira de Epilepsia, pp 89–97

Bittencourt P R M 1985 Disritmia cerebral, termo maldito. Journal da SBENC 9:4

Bittencourt P R M 1986 A nova classificação internacional das epilepsias. In: Bittencourt P R M (ed.) Epilepsia-1986, Palestras do III Simpósio Paranaense da Liga Brasileira de Epilepsia (in press)

Bittencourt P R M, Richens A 1981 Anticonvulsant-induced status epilepticus in Lennox-Gastaut syndrome. Epilepsia 22: 129–134

Bittencourt P R M, Silvado C E S, Gorz A M, de Paola D 1983 Frequência dos tipos de crise epiléptica e correlação com eletroencefalograma. Revista Neurologica Argentina 95:39

Bittencourt P R M, Gorz A M, Silvado C E S, Caropreso V 1986 Monotherapy without serum levels for epilepsy. Proceedings, Epilepsia Panamericana ' 86, p 100

Bortolotto Z A, Mello L E M, Turski L, Cavalheiro E A 1985 Effects of 2-chloroadenosine on amygdaloid and hippocampal kindled seizures. Archives Internationales de Pharmacodynamie et de Therapie 277: 313–320

Caleffi G H 1984 A posição do eletroencelografista. In: Bittencourt P R M (ed.) Epilepsia-1984: Palestras do II Simpósio Paranaense de Epilepsia, Publicações Capitulo Paranaense da Liga Brasileira de Epilepsia, pp 38–41

Campos C J R, Cavalheiro E A 1979 The paradoxical effect of lidocaine on an experimental model of epilepsy. Archives Internationales de Pharmacodynamie et de Thérapie 241: 01–08

Campos C J R, Cavalheiro E A 1980 Modificações do método 'kindling' para obtenção de status epilepticus experimental em ratos. Arquivos de Neuro-Psiquiatria 38: 81–88

Campos C J R, Cavalheiro E, Izquierdo I 1980 A study of the action of anticonvulsant drugs on an experimental model of epilepsy. Acta Physiologica Latinoamericana, 30: 239–243

Cavalheiro E A, Elisabetsky E, Campos C J R 1981 Effect of brain serotonin level on induced hippocampal paroxysmal activity in rats. Pharmacology Biochemistry and Behavior 15: 363–366

Chiofalo N, Schoenberg B, Kirschbaum A et al 1985 Neuroepidemiological study on epilepsy in Chile. Abstracts, 16th Epilepsy International Congress, Hamburg p 90

Chiofalo N, Kirschbaum A, Fuentes A, Cordero M L, Madsen J 1979 Prevalence of epilepsy in children of Melipilla, Chile. Epilepsia 20: 261–266

Commission on Classification and Terminology of the International League Against Epilepsy 1981 Proposal for revised clinical and electroencephalographic classification seizures. Epilepsia 22: 489–501

Commission on Classification and Terminology of the International League Against Epilepsy 1985 Proposal for classification of epilepsies and epileptic syndromes. Epilepsia 26: 268–278

Cowan C M, Cavalheiro E A 1980 Epilepsy and membrane Na$^+$K$^+$ ATPase: changes in activity using an experimental model of epilepsy. Acta Physiologica Latinoamericana 30: 253–258

Czuczwar S J, Cavalheiro E A, Turski L, Turski W A, Kleinrok Z 1985 Phosphonic analogues of excitatory amino acids raise the threshold for maximal electroconvulsions in mice. Neuroscience Research 3: 86–90

de Pasquet E G, Pietra M, Gaudin E S 1972 Etiologia de la epilepsia tardia. Acta Neurologica Latinoamericana 18: 256–275

de Pasquet E G, Gomensoro J B, Bustos L F, Tenzer S M 1973 Ensayo de un nuevo antiepileptico el dipropilancetato de magnesio. Acta Neurologica Latinoamericana 19: 119–128

de Pasquet E G, Pietra M, Bonnevaure S, Silva N P, Gomensoro J B, Tenza M 1976a Estudio epidemiológico de 500 epilépticos adultos procedentes de una población hospitalaria. Acta Neurologica Latinoamericana 22: 50–65

de Pasquet E G, Pietra M, Iñiquez R A 1976b Epileptic seizures as an early complication of neurosurgery. Acta Neurologica Latinoamericana 22: 144–151

de Pasquet E G, Avondet M, Castelli Y, Tenzer M 1984 Employment and employability among epileptic patients of Uruguay. In: Porter R J et al (ed.) Advances in epileptology. XVth Epilepsy International Symposium. Raven Press, New York, pp 615–618

Ferreira A A C P, Silvado C E S, Bittencourt P R M 1984 Epilepsia e inteligência. In: Bittencourt P R M (ed.) Epilepsia-1984 : Palestras do II Simpósio Paranaense de Epilepsia, Publicações Capitulo Paranaense da Liga Brasileira de Epilepsia pp 98–103

Galdames D G, Saavedra I N, Ortiz M A, Aguilera L I, Valenzuela A L, Concha G L, Droguett P A, Morales E R 1980 Plasma levels of diphenylhydantoin and the control of adult epileptic seizures: a Chilean experience. Epilepsia 21: 467–474

Gastaut H, Dravet C, Loubier D, Giove C, Vianif, Gastaut J A, Gastaut J L 1973 Evolution clinique et prognostic de Syndrome de Lennox-Gastaut. In: Lugaresi E, Pazzaglia R, Tassinari C A (eds) Evolution and prognosis of epilepsies. Gaggi Edituore, Bologna, pp 134–154

Gomez J G, Arciniegas E, Torres J 1978 Prevalence of epilepsy in Bogotá, Colombia. Neurology 28: 90–94

Gorz A M, Silvado C E S, Bittencourt P R M 1986 Barbiturate-refractory epilepsy: safe schedule for therapeutic substitution. Arquivos de Neuro-Psiquiatria 44: 225–231

Jimenez I R 1985 Classificación de la epilepsia. Acta Neurológica 1: 03–04

Laidlaw J, Richens A 1982 A textbook of epilepsy. Churchill Livingstone, Edinburgh

Madallozzo L E, Oliveira Z F, Santos J M B 1984 Epilepsia e trabalho. In: Bittencourt P R M (ed.) Epilepsia-1984:

Palestras do II Simpósio Paranaense de Epilepsia, Publicações Capitulo Paranaense da Liga Brasileira de Epilepsia, pp 105–111

Marino Jr R 1983 O tratamento cirúrgico das epilepsias. In: Marino Jr R (ed.) Epilepsias, Sarvier, São Paulo, pp 77–82

Marino Jr R Cukiert A 1986 Aspectos epidemiológicos da epilepsia em Sõ Paulo – um estudo da prevalência. Arquivos de Neuro-Psiquiatria 44: 243–252

Marsden C D, Reynolds E H 1982 Neurology: part one. In: Laidlaw J and Richens A (eds) A textbook of epilepsy. Churchill Livingstone, Edinburgh pp 90–131

Martins L F 1984 Dificuldades na instalação de um serviço de cirurgia de epilepsia. In: Bittencourt P R M (ed.) Epilepsia-1984: Palestras do II Simpósio Paranaense de Epilepsia, Publicações Capitulo Paranaense da Liga Brasileira de Epilepsia, pp 83–88

Olivares L 1972 Epilepsy in Mexico: a population study. The epidemiology of epilepsy: a workshop. In: Milton A and Hauser W A (eds) NINDS Monograph no. 14 DHEW, Washington DC, pp 53–58

Osuntokum B O 1977 Epilepsy in the African continent. In: Penry J K (ed.) Epilepsy: the eighth International Symposium, Raven Press, New York, pp 365–378

Porter R J 1982 Clinical efficacy and use of antiepileptic drugs. In: Woodbury D M, Penry F K, Pippinger C E (eds) Antiepileptic drugs. 2nd edn. Raven Press, New York pp 167–176

Richens A 1982 Clinical pharmacology and medical treatment. In: Laidlaw J, Richens A (eds) A textbook of epilepsy. Churchill Livingstone, Edinburgh, pp 292–348

Roger J, Dravet C, Bureau N, Dreifuss F E, Wolf P (eds) 1985 Epileptic syndromes in infancy, childhood and adolescence. John Libbey Eurotext, London, p 335

Santana V 1978 Estudo epidemiológico das doenças mentais em um bairro de Salvador – nordeste de Amaralina. Tese de Mestrado, Universidade Federal da Bahia, p 67

Sakamoto A C 1985 Estudo clinico e prognóstico das crises epilépticas que iniciam na infância numa população brasileira. Tese de doutorado, Universidade de Sõ Paulo, Ribeirõ Prêto, p 74

Saraiva M C S 1983 As implicações sociais em ser epiléptico. In: Marino Jr R (ed.) Epilepsias, Sarvier, Sõ Paulo, pp 77–82

Scaramelli A, de Pasquet E G 1985 Monoterapia com carbamazepina. Communication to the Sociedad de Neurologia y Neurocirurgia del Uruguay

Shorvon S D, Chadwick D, Galbraith A W, Reynolds E H 1978 one drug for epilepsy. British Medical Journal 1: 474–476

Speciali J G 1973 Contribuição ao estudo das manifestações epilépticas na sindrome de Lennox-Gastaut. Tese de mestrado. Universidade de São Paulo, Ribeirão Prêto, p 45

Speciali J G 1985 Achados eletroencefalográficos durante o sono na sindrome de Lennox-Gastaut. Tese de Livre Docência, Universidade de São Paulo, Ribeirão Prêto 1:82

Strandjord R E and Johannessen S I 1980 Single-drug therapy with carbamazepine in patients with epilepsy: serum levels and clinical effect. Epilepsia 21: 655–666

Tapia R, Colin R R D, Ruiz G M, Duran L, Levi G 1979 Neurophysiological and neurochemical studies on the action of the anticonvulsant y-Hydroxy, y-Ethyl, y-Phenyl-Butyramid. Epilepsia 20: 135–145

Turnbull D M, Rawlins M D, Wightman D, Chadwick D W 1982 A comparison of phenytoin and valproate in previously untreated adult epileptic patients. Journal of

Neurology, Neurosurgery, and Psychiatry 45: 55–59

Turner M 1983 Comparative analysis of 100 cases of suspected epileptic seizures studied with routine EEG and with prolonged ambulatory EEG (PAE). Abstracts, 15th Epilepsy International Symposium, Washington DC, 1983, p 141

Turner M 1985 Epilepsia Argentina. Editorial 2:18

Turski L, Ikonomidau C, Cavalheiro E H, Kleinrok Z, Czuczwar S J, Turski W A 1985a Effects of morphine and naloxone on pilocarpine – induced convulsions in rats. Neuropeptides 5: 315–318

Turski W A, Cavalheiro E A, Ikonomidou C, Mello L E A M, Bortolotto Z A, Turski 1985a Effects of aminophylline and 2-chloroadenosine on seizures produced by pilocarpine in rats: morphological and electroencephalographic correlates. Brain Research 361: 309–323

Turski L, Schwarz M, Cavalheiro E A, Turski W A,

Ikonomidou C, Sontag K H 1985b Nigral gabaergic modify the development of seizures produced by pilocarpine in rats: behavioural, electroencephalographic and neuroanatomical guidance. Journal of Cerebral Blood Flow and Metabolism 5: 363–364

Velasco F, Velasco M, Maldonado H, Romo R, Villanueva F E 1979 Specific and nonspecific multiple unit activities during the onset of pentylenotetrazol seizures. III. Animals with ablations of the cerebral cortex. Epilepsia 20: 635–642

Velasco A F, Olivares N, Rivas F, Velasco M, Velasco F 1980 Alumina cream-induced focal motor epilepsy in cats. Archives of Neurology 37: 287–290

Walton J 1985 Brain's diseases of the nervous system. 9th edn. Oxford Medical Publications, Oxford, p 701

Zielinski J J 1982 Epidemiology. In: Laidlaw J, Richens A (eds) A textbook of epilepsy. Churchill Livingstone, Edinburgh, pp 16–33

PART THREE
EPILEPSY IN DEVELOPING COUNTRIES
H. Meinardi

The problem of epilepsy in developing countries is also a challenge for countries that have attained greater sophistication in their health care. This is particularly justified since their progress has been made possible by affluence often derived from exploitation of the resources of colonies. With independence, these colonies did not inherit the instruments necessary to achieve a standard of living equal to that of their former rulers. Apart from this consideration, it is obvious that an appeal for assistance has to be complied with for purely humanitarian reasons.

This section is based on the experience of the author and does not pretend to give an overview of all existing policies and resources available.

THE WORK OF THE INTERNATIONAL BUREAU FOR EPILEPSY

There are two international organizations concerned with epilepsy, the International League Against Epilepsy (ILAE), founded in 1909, which primarily has scientific and health care objectives, and the International Bureau for Epilepsy (IBE)

founded in 1961, which primarily has social and welfare objectives.

The International Bureau was the first to receive requests for educational assistance from developing countries. It was decided to meet the requests for educational assistance by organizing a travelling educational team. Mr George Burden, at that time Secretary-General of the International Bureau, initiated and planned a series of workshops, first in Africa and subsequently in South-East Asia and Oceania. The travelling team consisted of a neurologist, a clinical neurophysiologist, a neuropsychiatrist, a paediatrician and a social worker, all actively engaged in the fight against epilepsy in their respective countries.

However, both before as well as after these travelling workshops there were heated debates over the investment for travel and leave of absence, and whether the cost was warranted in view of other dire needs in developing countries. In response to this criticism, it was argued that, not only is it inhumane to neglect a minority group of sufferers simply because all efforts and resources are usually used solely to combat major plagues, but also it is doubtful whether certain resources would become available if they were not earmarked for a specific purpose like the fight against epilepsy or the fight against leprosy and so on.

A second controversy concerned the wisdom of requesting people accustomed to working under sophisticated conditions in an affluent society to teach their way of handling a disease and its consequences to an audience that would not be able to afford the necessary diagnostic or therapeutic hardware. Nor could such an audience expect their patients to be able to cope with the therapeutic advice offered. Much of the success of such an undertaking depends on the quality of the dialogue between the invited experts and their audience. On the one hand, it is necessary to indicate the level of success that can be achieved given excellent conditions so that desirable goals can be established; on the other hand, through discussions and drawing on experiences from both sides, strategies can be developed which are appropriate to the circumstances in the developing country.

PROMOTING PRIMARY HEALTH CARE

After the world conference in Alma Ata in 1978, organized by the World Health Organization (WHO) and the United Nations Children's Fund (Unicef) most developing countries accepted the Primary Health Care declaration which partly replaced the Basic Health Services (BHS) strategy (Van Praag & Varkevisser 1986).

These services are characterized by a pyramidal structure with a Ministry of Health at the top advised by a medical faculty (and university hospital staff) and possibly a national medical association. From there, facilities of decreasing sophistication are spread over the country. In the villages, there are the health centres and dispensaries which, typically of the BHS, are run by paramedics. Often advised by Western policy makers, governments have created separate services for dealing with malaria, tuberculosis, leprosy, vaccination programmes, mother and child care and family planning; each with an independent budget and a separate staff.

This hierarchical organization did not seem to be effective in the more peripheral parts of the countries. Health workers trained in assisting to solve specific problems often get frustrated when they are confronted with other demands from the villagers they visit. The villagers may want to be provided first with help over health or social problems which are beyond the scope of the health workers and beyond their duty. On the other side of the coin, villagers often have little patience with visits from authorities which come to tell them how to immunize their children against future diseases while the acute problems of surviving, e.g. against gastrointestinal disorders or sheer famine cannot be solved.

Many papers have been written in the past two decades about epilepsy in developing countries. Quite a number of these have come from Nigeria. The International Bureau for Epilepsy even tried to set up an African Branch, the Epilepsy Bureau for Africa, in Lagos, Nigeria. This endeavour, however, failed. Perhaps this proves that a successful model of health care in one culture is not necessarily applicable in another. Many of the papers describing epilepsy in Africa stress the fact that follow-up is difficult and that the demand for non-traditional assistance, especially where young children are concerned, is probably rather low.

The WHO definition of Primary Health Care is 'essential health care, made universally accessible to individuals and families by means acceptable to them, through their full participation at a cost the community and the country can afford'.

A prerequisite for therapy of epilepsy 'by means acceptable to the people, through their full participation' is therefore an intensive enlightenment programme which will explain the true nature of epilepsy to the people and what they can expect of therapy. The feasibility of such an approach has recently been demonstrated in Sri Lanka.

THE SRI LANKAN PROJECT

On the occasion of its centenary, a Dutch charity, The Christian Society for the Care of People with Epilepsy (CSCPE), decided to provide funds for people with epilepsy in countries where, in essence, conditions still prevailed similar to those which existed in The Netherlands at the time the society was founded. According to the principle mentioned above, which was adopted by the CSCPE, primary health care for epilepsy is only feasible if knowledge about epilepsy is disseminated at grassroots level. In Sri Lanka, an excellent partner was found to put this principle into practice, namely, the Sarvodaya Shramadana movement.

This movement was started in 1958 by Dr A. T. Ariyaratne. Although the movement is non-sectarian, its principles are derived from Buddhism, the spiritual background of its leader. Dr Ariyaratne is convinced that the roots of society are in the rural community and that these roots should be healthy. A major tool to keep a community healthy and worthwhile for its members is mutual assistance. For effective co-operation, however, some degree of organizational capability should be available, and this is what the movement provides.

Sri Lanka is divided into 26 districts, each with a small staff supported through programme money provided by Developmental Aid Agencies and contributions from the villages. There are meetings with the people in the villages in which their needs are assessed. Next, the neighbourhood is mobilized to participate in a volunteer working party to achieve the objectives selected. On a more permanent basis, Sarvodaya believes in continuous education of the people and has selected the preschool class as a tool. Preschool classes can usually be maintained, even in the smallest village, since both parents often have to go out to work. The preschool teacher is in frequent communication with the young adults of the village, the parents of preschool children. She or he is therefore pre-eminently suited to disseminate ideas about hygiene, child raising and so on. Periodically, the preschool teachers convene for training programmes at an intermediate level in the district organization, the so-called Gramodaya centres. Special programmes promoted nationwide by Sarvodaya are an antimalaria programme and a programme for adapted agricultural technology. Thus there are trained senior healthworkers available at the district level.

After preliminary talks in 1981 and a fund-raising campaign in 1982, a contract was signed by Prof. A. J. van't Klooster on behalf the CSCPE and by Dr A. Ariyaratne for the Sarvodaya Shramadana Movement in June 1983. This formed a commitment to try and inform the villagers in one district about modern concepts of epilepsy and about the facilities available in Sri Lanka to treat the condition.

The Sarvodaya Programme: 'Epilepsy control through people's participation'

The Sarvodaya Shramadana movement decided to set up an experiment in the Kandy district to see if epilepsy can be better controlled by simple community health education and follow up. The Kandy district was chosen because of its size and the availability of a centrally located general hospital connected with the Medical Faculty of Peradeniya University. Prof. Nimal Senanayake of this faculty had an established interest in epilepsy and volunteered to co-operate closely with Sarvodaya.

Programme design

The first step was to prepare a handbook on epilepsy written in Sinhala and Tamil, suitable for use by the senior health workers, preschool teachers and the village people. This book was first prepared in the English language with the help of available WHO material, and was checked by Drs Senanayake and Meinardi. The style was kept as simple as possible and richly illustrated with simple drawings. In addition, a questionnaire was prepared to assess the degree of knowledge of the senior health workers and preschool teachers. Subsequently, an intensive three-day course was inaugurated.

The trainees participated in a regular Epilepsy Clinic at the General Hospital in Peradeniya. Guidelines were provided for the identification of the patient, the collection of data and the recognition of concomitant disease. At the end of the course, the knowledge acquired was formally evaluated and tested in a sociodrama in which the trainers working in pairs acted as patient and preschool teacher.

A preparatory course on the teaching of preschool teachers was included in the programme for senior health workers. They also assisted in the preparation of a survey form which the trained preschool teachers would use in their service area.

The preschool teachers incorporated into their sessions: first aid methodology; recognition of commonly used antiepileptic drugs; and general knowledge about the appropriate use and the possible side-effects of these drugs. Furthermore, special attention was given to the recognition of social problems connected with epilepsy.

During the sessions, two video films produced in the Peradeniya University were used, one showing different seizures, the other the interview techniques. When the first group of 22 preschool teachers had received their training, the survey form was tested in five villages by the trainees under the supervision of eight senior health-workers. A total of 19 senior health workers and 214 preschool teachers were trained, as well as 30 preschool instructors. These instructors operate at an intermediate level in the district, the so-called Gramodaya centres, of which the Kandy district has 12. They usually train and assist approximately 5 to 20 preschool teachers. They in turn report to a senior instructor operating at the district level. The neurologist only participated in the training of the health workers and senior instructors.

Results

At the start of the training, 30% of the trainees was not aware of epilepsy as an illness. They believed it to be an affliction due to supernatural forces. 68% had come across a patient suffering from epilepsy at one time or another but 32% had never seen a patient having a seizure. 90% believed that epilepsy cannot be cured. None of the trainees had ever seen the drugs used for the treatment of epilepsy.

In general, the study received a positive response from the villagers. In some places, people from outside would specially visit the village to offer information. In contrast certain persons of marriageable age only revealed their epilepsy after they had become sufficiently confident that the information about them was treated in strict confidence and when they saw the benefit of the programme.

It turned out to be important that plans had been made to direct patients to appropriate medical facilities. For this purpose 11 government hospitals corresponding with the 12 Gramodaya districts had been informed of the programme and had been asked for their support. Amongst many respondents there was resentment about previous surveys by university students on tuberculosis, filariasis, malaria etc as these were not associated with an immediate medical care programme.

Although only 54% of the population of the Sarvodaya villages in the Kandy district were subjected to the survey, i.e. 51 751 persons, 586 positive cases of epilepsy and 114 suspected cases were identified. Of these 114 suspected cases, 70 have now attended a hospital service and in 69 cases the diagnosis was confirmed. Of these 700 people with known or suspected epilepsy, 326 took Western medicine and 374 did not take any medicine at all.

Apparently, when prescribing medication for their seizures, the doctors in the congested government hospital did not have sufficient time to give a full explanation about the condition and to stress the need for regular and continuous use of medication. The recurrence of seizures due to the irregular intake of drugs (some only took their pills immediately after a seizure) caused dissatisfaction with the power of the Western medicines and after similar bad results with local remedies they believed that epilepsy must be the result of supernatural forces which cannot be influenced.

The seizure histories of the people identified are now being continuously recorded by the preschool teachers, where necessary assisted by the Gramodaya instructors.

SUMMARY AND CONCLUSIONS

The phase of identifying the size of the problem of epilepsy in developing countries should now be considered behind us. WHO has repeatedly emphasized the need to provide care for people with epilepsy. In 1968 Bernard and Kugler (Bernard & Kugler 1969) prepared an outline of the organization of care for patients with epilepsy in developing countries. The WHO technical report series no. 629 (1978) pays attention to epilepsy in developing countries, and the manual about community-based rehabilitation (WHO 1983) for developing countries published in 1983 includes a training package for a family member of a person who has fits. However, there is as yet no consistent worldwide programme for epilepsy control in the form of education of the people. There is also still great controversy about the use of phenobarbitone: i.e. whether, on account of economic reasons, the exclusive use of this drug should be advocated in developing countries, notwithstanding its well-known deficiencies, or whether efforts should be intensified to provide more appropriate medication at reasonable cost.

Cost-benefit analyses will be indispensable but are notoriously difficult to perform.

Voluntary organizations like epilepsy leagues of professionals concerned with epilepsy and epilepsy associations for people with epilepsy themselves and their relatives, are to play an important role in the development of epilepsy care in developing countries.

REFERENCES

Bernard P, Kugler J 1969 consultantship to WHO (personal communication)
Van Praag E, Varkevisser C 1986 Primary health care. Medisch Contact 2:41
WHO 1978 Technical report series no. 629, Geneva
WHO 1983 Training disabled people in the community. Manual RHB/83.1, Emar Helander, Padmani Mendis, Gunnel Nelson, Geneva

15

Some special problems of epilepsy

PART ONE
EPILEPSY AND MENTAL HANDICAP
J. Corbett

INTRODUCTION

Epilepsy is one of the most frequent additional major handicaps in people with mental retardation, coexistence of the two impairments tending to compound the disability rather than being merely additive. Even when the symptom is well controlled, the label of epilepsy often places the person with a mental handicap at an increased social disadvantage. It is therefore important that the handicapped person has access to the same modern services for the treatment of epilepsy as his or her fellows which will enable him or her to live as normal a life as possible.

No longer is epilepsy associated with the inevitability of mental deterioration. Although subtle impairments of cognitive function are seen in people receiving long-term treatment (see Ch. 11), marked and sustained deterioration, following a period of apparently normal development, is only seen in a minority. Most people with well-controlled seizures function within the normal range of intelligence.

PREVALENCE

The frequency of epilepsy in people with intellectual impairment provides a good indicator of the degree of underlying cerebral dysfunction and hence the organicity of the learning difficulties. The percentage of people having more than one seizure in the past year increases progressively with the degree of retardation. Estimates are most readily available for children of school age, where a number of studies has shown that epilepsy defined in this way occurs in between 0.4% and 0.7%, (Ross & Peckham 1983, Corbett & Pond 1986).

In children with mild mental retardation (IQ 50–76) a rate between 3% and 6% (depending on whether simple or complicated seizure patterns are seen) has been reported from the National Child Development Study (Peckham 1974).

In people with learning disability who were in contact with mental handicap services, most estimates were derived from institutional studies and these were influenced by the fact that severe epilepsy was one cause of long-term hospitalization.

Recently the pattern has changed, with a move towards community care, and there are now two epidemiological studies related to epilepsy and mental retardation which provide more accurate data (Corbett et al 1975, Richardson et al 1981). These are both based on case register studies, in Camberwell in South London and Aberdeen respectively, and include long-term follow-up data extending into early adult life. Although comprising somewhat different age and IQ-related population samples, the findings from these two studies are remarkably similar and provide a clearer picture of epilepsy and mental handicap than was previously available.

In Camberwell, for children under the age of 14 functioning in the severely retarded range (IQ <50), the percentage with seizures in the year prior to the initial study was nearly 20%, with a lifelong history of seizures in 30%. In children with the most severe brain damage, functioning in the profoundly handicapped range (IQ <20), almost 50% had had a seizure sometime during life.

When this cohort of 150 children was followed up for 14 years (until 14–28 years of age) the number still suffering from epilepsy (defined as at least one seizure in the year prior to study) was similar. Although the seizures had remitted in a number, they were replaced by a similar proportion who developed seizures for the first time in adolescence. (Corbett 1983).

These findings were confirmed in the Aberdeen study. The population, which comprised more mildly retarded people than in Camberwell, was followed up until a minimum of 22 years of age: 24% had a history of persistent seizures, which had occurred in 19% in the preschool years and 13% in each subsequent period of early-, late- and postschool years. Of the young people with *severe* mental retardation, that is with an IQ of less than 50, 44% had experienced one or more seizures by the age of 22 years compared with 19% of those with IQ's of 50 or more who were in contact with the mental retardation services. For those with some history of seizures there was no significant association between IQ and degree of seizure impairment, but 40% had experienced seizures for more than 10 years and only 21% for less than one year; attesting to the chronicity of epilepsy in people with a mental handicap.

ETIOLOGY

Epilepsy and mental retardation are outward manifestations of a common underlying brain dysfunction and the age at which they are first seen gives a guide to both underlying pathology and prognosis. Some of the main syndromes associated with epilepsy are listed in Table 15.1.

Convulsions with onset in the first year of life associated with gross evidence of pre- or perinatal brain damage have a poor prognosis for subsequent mental development and persistence

of seizures (Matsumoto et al 1983, Cavazzuti et al 1984). The same general principle applies with infantile spasms occurring between 3 and 18 months of age (Jeavons et al 1973, Lombroso 1983) and in the severe myoclonic epilepsies of early childhood, particularly the Lennox Gastaut Syndrome (onset 1 to 6 years) (O'Donohoe 1985). In each case, the progress tends to be worse if the epilepsy is symptomatic of some underlying brain pathology such as congenital malformation, perinatal brain damage, infection, biochemical disorder or progressive condition e.g. tuberous sclerosis.

The same poor prognosis may be anticipated in cases of infantile or febrile convulsions associated with status epilepticus and encephalopathy. In many of these situations it is difficult to distinguish between the effects of the underlying neuropathology on intellectual functioning and the damaging effect of subsequent seizures, particularly if these are frequent or prolonged.

The apparently beneficial effect of steroids in infantile spasms and other difficult-to-control epilepsies of early childhood (Corbett et al 1975, Snead et al 1983) suggests a specific link with biochemical changes occurring in the brain during seizures, and supports the idea that the seizures themselves may play a part in further damaging the brain. However, ACTH (adrenocorticotrophic hormone) tends to be of most benefit in 'idiopathic' infantile spasms which are likely to have a better prognosis.

PREVENTION

There is considerable scope for the prevention of mental retardation by early and energetic prophylaxis of prolonged infantile convulsions; the early diagnosis and treatment of bacterial meningitides; protection of the head from repeated injury in myoclonic astatic epilepsy in childhood; the early recognition and treatment of subconvulsive status (minor status epilepticus); and increased awareness of the iatrogenic dangers of prolonged antiepileptic medication to the developing brain. It is conceivable that if our present knowledge of the

Table 15.1 Epilepsy particularly associated with specific mental retardation syndromes

	Epilepsy	West's syndrome	Lennox-Gastaut syndrome	Epilepsy with onset in later childhood or adolescence
Perinatal brain injury	+		+	
Metabolic abnormalities				
Phenylketonuria	+	+	+	
Maple Syrup urine disease	+	+		
Hyperornithaemia	+	+		
Isovaleric acidaemia	+	+		
Non-ketotic hyperglycaemia	+	+		
Pyridoxine dependency	+	+		
Leucine-sensitive hypoglycaemia	+	+	+	
Tay-Sachs disease	+	+		
Lipoidosis GM 1 & GM 3	+		+	
Metachromatic leucodystrophy	+		+	+
Homocysteinuria			+	
Dysplastic conditions				
Tuberous sclerosis	+	+	+	+
Sturge-Weber syndrome	+	+	+	+
Megalencephaly	+		+	
Other cerebral malformations	+	+	+	
Aicardi syndrome	+	+		
Prenatal infections				
Cytomegalovirus	+	+		
Syphillis	+	+		
Toxoplasmosis	+	+		
Postnatal infections				
Purulent meningitis	+		+	+
Acute encephalitis	+		+	+
Subacute sclerosing panencephalitis	+		+	
Postimmunization encephalopathy	+	+		
Post-traumatic	+			+
Chromosomal abnormalities				
Down's syndrome		+		
Autistic syndromes	+	+		+
Others				
Retts syndrome	+			+

potential for prevention of childhood epilepsy was to be effectively applied in practice this would be one of the most important contributions to the medical prevention of mental retardation.

Conversely, it follows that strategies primarily directed to preventing underlying brain damage leading to mental retardation will have a significant impact on the overall prevalence of epilepsy. These will include general improve-ments in antenatal care and maternal screening to prevent genetic disorders; reduction in perinatal morbidity resulting from prematurity, anoxia, intracerebral haemorrhage, biochemical disorders such as hypoglycaemia and hypocalcaemia and infections. Postnatal prevention will comprise infantile screening and prevention of later onset encephalopathies resulting from dehydration, infection and head injury.

DIAGNOSIS AND TREATMENT

The general principles of diagnosis and treatment in people with a mental handicap are similar to those employed in people with epilepsy who are not otherwise disabled. However, a number of general and specific points do need to be borne in mind.

In the past, health and social services for those with a mental handicap were predominantly provided separately from the mainstream services. This has led to a labelling of people as 'the mentally handicapped' in a similar fashion to the labelling of people as 'epileptics' rather than as people first. A major consequence has been that people with a mental handicap and epilepsy have tended to be denied access to specialized services for the investigation and treatment of epilepsy. This has been compounded by the tendency to base specialized services for people with mental handicap in institutions which have also been their only home.

With an increasing trend towards community care, there is both an increasing recognition of the need to improve access of people with mental handicap to generic services but it has also meant that some people with epilepsy in the community who have not needed admission to institutions have had difficulty in obtaining services for epilepsy. This situation will only be resolved by improving the education of personnel working in the primary health care, social services and specialized hospital services about both epilepsy and mental retardation.

Greatest importance will be attached to the developmental history and description of the person's skills, behaviour and additional handicaps in interview with the parents or carer of the handicapped person. It must be remembered that there are likely, by definition, to be difficulties in obtaining a clear account from the disabled persons themselves of subjective experiences associated with seizures. The account obtained from an observer will be influenced by pre-existing neurological abnormality giving rise, for example, to other forms of movement disorder such as motor stereotypes or tics. Absence attacks or brief complex partial seizures are particularly difficult to detect in people whose attention and concentration may be impaired for other reasons. Ictal events with a basis in the temporal lobe or elsewhere in the limbic system may be profoundly disturbing to the handicapped person who is unable to give an account of the subjective experience. The introduction of ambulatory monitoring has produced evidence that, while the seizure itself may be quite brief, prolonged aggressive outbursts and other disturbed restless behaviour may be seen pre- or post-ictally.

Because of the difficulty in obtaining subjective accounts of the seizures and carrying out EEGs it was said, in the past, that temporal lobe epilepsy did not occur in people with mental handicap. It is clear that this is not the case: with careful observation and the help of EEG technicians with particular experience of mentally handicapped people, most can be trained to wear EEG leads without the need for sedation or anaesthesia. In occasional cases, where the person is very disturbed or frightened by the investigations, light anaesthesia while the leads are being applied with recording continuing into the recovery phase may be preferable to sedation with barbiturates or epileptogenic major tranquillisers, which may only increase the disturbed behaviour. Blood may also be taken at this time for screening of the more comon mental retardation syndromes and for antiepileptic drug levels.

TREATMENT

As with non-handicapped people, the mainstay of treatment of the seizure disorder is antiepileptic drug therapy, but it should be remembered that young handicapped people are particularly vulnerable to isolated seizures or even self-limiting episodes. For example, febrile convulsions may occur in early childhood in those with pre-existing brain damage, and isolated seizures in adolescence occur in up to 30% of severely handicapped people with symptoms of childhood autism. In each case a careful judgement needs to be made between the advantages of early treatment limiting the chance of recurrence, with reduction in parental or staff anxiety, and the disadvantages of committing a person who already has learning difficulties to lengthy treatment with drugs which may suppress brain activity and impair learning further.

It is always essential to consider alternative or additional strategies of management which will reduce the need to depend totally on pharmacological treatments. First and most essential is the reduction of anxiety in the child's caring network and a realization that the presence of a handicapped child in the family will have already been experienced as a partial bereavement. The occurrence of seizures, particularly of a generalized tonic-clonic variety, is likely to compound this anxiety. A parent may take a handicapped child in to their own bed for fear that they may not awake when seizures occur at night and this may lead to increased anxiety when the dependency needs cannot be met. This may engender fear in the child and contribute to an increase in seizure frequency; these anxieties have to be weighed against the fact that seizures are now the main cause of death in childhood in the severely and profoundly handicapped.

Such considerations will extend to the person's total network of dependent relationships and care staff and teachers may, understandably, be even more reluctant than parents to allow the handicapped person the dignity of risk to lead as normal a life as possible while maintaining sensible precautions.

Nowadays, swimming with staff trained in both life saving and the emergency treatment of seizures, respite care in homelike environments or with foster families who are familiar with the child's individual needs and whom parents can trust, and a range of other normative experiences should be available. These will not only enrich the quality of the disabled person's life, but by reducing anxiety help to minimize seizures.

The role of diet and behavioural strategies of management of seizures remain controversial and experimental. There is little doubt that in some brain-damaged people sensitivity to particular dietary components, such as food additives, gluten and stimulants, may provoke both episodic behaviour disturbance and precipitate seizures.

In some handicapped people with drug-resistant seizures a trial of ketogenic diet using medium triclyceride oil may also be considered (De Vivo 1983 and O'Donohoe 1985). It is also well established that even quite severely handicapped people can learn strategies to avoid seizure precipitants and abort attacks. It is, however, generally true that in our present state of knowledge these techniques can only very rarely be relied upon as the sole strategy of seizure management and may be more usefully viewed as an adjuvant to drug treatment, rather than an alternative.

COMPLICATIONS

A distinction must be made between the complications of epilepsy and the treatment of secondary handicaps associated with mental retardation and the underlying neurological damage. An understanding of the interaction between these influences calls for careful detective work and assessment of the situation in an individual patient.

It is well recognized that the side-effects of antiepileptic medication, such as slowing, inattention, apparent confusion, restlessness, dysarthria, ataxia and movement disorder, may be difficult to distinguish from the signs of underlying neurological disorder. (Reynolds & Travers 1974). It is likely that the damaged brain is more vulnerable to the side-effects of antiepileptic medication. Phenobarbitone can provoke hyperkinetic and irritable aggressive behaviour. Prolonged use of phenytoin may lead to a 'subacute encephalopathy' with few gross neurological signs and serum antiepileptic drug levels within the normal range (Corbett et al 1985). Diazepam derivatives may release disinhibited or aggressive behaviour and, with sustained use, tolerance develops, so that these compounds may become ineffective in the treatment of status epilepticus.

Adverse behavioural and cognitive side-effects occur in a minority of people receiving carbamazepine and sodium valproate and there are many interactions between these drugs which need to be borne in mind. There is a need for monitoring and constant re-evaluation using careful records to reduce the number of drugs to a minimum.

Finally, little is known about the side-effects of

long-term antiepileptic drug treatment. People tend to be labelled as 'epileptic' long after their seizures have remitted, and judicious and careful withdrawal should be considered after a seizure-free period of two to three years, avoiding vulnerable periods of brain development such as the adolescent growth spurt.

A small minority of people with epilepsy, receiving long-term medication, show either progressive cognitive deterioration or arrest in development. Recent research suggests that this is more likely to occur in people with pre-existing brain damage and particularly complicated and drug-resistant seizure patterns. As mentioned earlier, a number of factors may be incriminated. These tend to interact so that it may be difficult to tease them out in an individual patient. (Corbett et al unpublished). This may add to the burden of handicap but severe impairment is fortunately rare and it must constantly be restated that epilepsy is not inevitably linked with mental deterioration or abnormality of personality.

CONCLUSION

It can be seen that there is a close association between seizure disorders and mental retardation. This presents a particular challenge in terms of prevention and treatment and an increased awareness and sensitivity on the part of primary health care workers, paediatricians, psychiatrists and neurologists meeting the needs of disabled people. It also necessitates a continuing dialogue with community mental handicap teams who will be concerned with linking these services.

REFERENCES

Cavuzzuti G B, Ferrari P, Lalla M 1984 Follow-up study of 482 cases with convulsive disorders in the first year of life. Developmental Medicine & Child Neurology 26: 425–437

Corbett J A 1983 Epilepsy and mental retardation – a follow-up study. In: Parsonage M, Grant R H E, Craig A G et al (eds) Advances in epileptology. XIVth Epilepsy International Symposium. Raven Press, New York, pp 207–214

Corbett J A, Harris R, Robinson R 1975 Epilepsy. In: Wortis J (ed.) Mental retardation and developmental disabilities vol VII. Raven Press, New York, pp 79–111

Corbett J A, Trimble M R, Nicol T 1985 Behavioural and cognitive impairments in children with epilepsy; the long term effects of anticonvulsant therapy. Journal of American Academy of Child Psychiatry 24: 17–23

Corbett J A, Pond D A 1986 The management of epilepsy. In: Craft M, Bicknell J, Hollis S (eds) Mental Handicap. Baillière Tindall Cox, London

De Vivo D C 1983 How to use other drugs (steroids) and the ketogenic diet. In: Maselli P L, Pippenger C E, Penry J K (eds) Antiepileptic drug therapy in paediatrics. New York, Raven Press, pp 283–292

Jeavons P M, Bower B D, Dimitrakoudi M 1973 Long term prognosis of 150 cases of 'West's Syndrome'. Epilepsia 141: 153–164

Lombroso C T 1983 A prospective study of infantile spasms; clinical and therapeutic correlations. Epilepsia 24: 135–158

O'Donohoe N V 1985 Epilepsies of childhood. 2nd edn. Butterworths, London

Matsumoto A, Watanabe K, Sugiura M, Negoro, Takaesu E, Iwase K 1983 Long term prognosis of convulsive disorders in the first year of life: mental and physical development and seizure persistence. Epilepsia. 24: 321–329

Peckham C S 1974 National child development study (1958 cohort) personal communication.

Reynolds E H, Travers R D 1974 Serum anticonvulsant concentrations in epileptic patients with mental symptoms. A preliminary report. British Journal of Psychiatry 124: 440–445

Richardson S A, Koller H, Katz M, McLaren J 1981 A functional classification of seizures and its distribution in a mentally retarded population. American Journal of Mental Deficiency 85: 457–446

Ross E M, Peckham C S 1983 School children with epilepsy. In: Parsonage M, Grant R H E, Craig A G et al (eds) Advances in epileptology. XIVth Epilepsy International Symposium. Raven Press, New York, pp 215–220

Snead O C, Benton J N, Myers G J 1983 ACTH and prednisolone in childhood seizure disorder. Neurology 33: 966–97

PART TWO
SOME ASPECTS OF EPILEPSY IN WOMEN
P. G. Cleland
M. L. E. Espir

The management of epilepsy in women is dominated by the problems associated with pregnancy. However, there are other important issues such as the effects of fits and antiepileptic drugs on appearance, catamenial epilepsy, contraception, marriage and fertility. In this section we explore those aspects of epilepsy which are particularly relevant to women.

APPEARANCE

It is unfortunate that antiepileptic drugs may adversely affect appearance. The most common of these cosmetic side-effects are listed in Table 15.2.

Coarsened features with thickening of the lips and of the subcutaneous tissues of the face and scalp, broadening of the nose and hirsutism have been recognized for many years. These changes were graphically demonstrated by Falconer & Davidson (1973) in their study of two pairs of identical twins, one of each pair suffering from epilepsy. In their study of 222 institutionalized patients, Lefebvre et al (1972) found coarsened features in about 60%. The most affected group had a more severe seizure disorder and had higher antiepileptic drug levels. Phenytoin was the drug most commonly used, often in combination with phenobarbitone, primidone or ethosuximide. In some patients, cosmetic changes are the result of

Table 15.2 Effects of epilepsy and antiepileptic drugs on appearance

Manifestation	Antiepileptic drugs
Coarsened features	Phenytoin; phenobarbitone
Gum hyperplasia	Phenytoin
Hirsutism	Phenytoin
Chloasma	Phenytoin; phenobarbitone
Weight Gain	Sodium valproate
Alopecia	Sodium valproate; carbamazepine
Acne	?Phenytoin; ?phenobarbitone
Other skin rashes	Carbamazepine; and others

trauma from recurrent fits. However, phenytoin is thought to inhibit the metabolism of collagen by collagenase, thereby leading to coarsened features from the deposition of an insoluble scleroprotein (Houck et al 1972).

In her study of the residents of the Chalfont Centre for Epilepsy, Walshe (1972) found that the incidence of acne was 35%. Phenytoin was the usual offending drug, but acne did occur in some patients given phenobarbitone. However, a more recent study (Greenwood et al 1983) has suggested that acne and sebum excretion are no different in patients with epilepsy as compared with controls. Chloasma-like pigmentation of the face occurred in 2.7% of the men and 9.6% of the women in Walshe's series. In addition, nearly one-third of the women had facial hirsutism, usually on the chin and upper lip, which occasionally was associated with generalized hirsutism. Phenytoin was the principal offending drug.

Gum hyperplasia is a well-known side-effect of phenytoin treatment which is present to some extent in many patients taking this drug (see Part Three). There is no close relationship between phenytoin dose or duration of treatment. The mechanism may be a combination of excessive collagen deposition and recurrent gingivitis associated with phenytoin-induced reduction of salivary IgA (Aarli 1976). Special attention to oral hygiene and folate supplementation (5 mg per week) may help to prevent this problem in patients on long-term phenytoin therapy (Inoue & Harrison 1981).

Weight gain is a specific side effect of sodium valproate treatment which may occur when higher doses are used. In their study of 100 children taking this drug Egger & Brett (1981) found weight gain in 44 and this was excessive in three children. The mechanism is probably via increased appetite but the cause of this is not known. The most likely explanation is a direct effect of sodium valproate or its metabolite on the hypothalamus. This may cause a problem for weight-conscious women and one should be cautious about prescribing sodium valproate for women who are already overweight.

Thinning of the hair may occur with sodium valproate and occasionally with carbamazepine. Six children in Egger and Brett's series had transient hair loss and in three the hair subsequently became curly. In some patients a change to curliness may occur without preceding alopecia (Jeavons et al 1977) and the new hair may be paler or darker (Herranz et al 1981). The mechanism of hair loss is not known but it is usually mild and transient. Herranz et al speculated that as sodium valproate is structurally similar to mimosine, a toxic amino acid, it may cause alopecia by chelation of metals and inhibition of enzymes needed for hair growth and keratinization processes.

Drug rashes may be caused by any antiepileptic drug but occur most frequently with carbamazepine. This drug can cause many different types of skin rashes, including a photosensitive dermatitis and an SLE-like syndrome (Sillanpää 1981).

Thus, although phenytoin is the antiepileptic drug which has been most extensively studied, it is also the one which causes the most worrying cosmetic effects. It is kinder therefore to avoid prescribing phenytoin to women and particularly to adolescent girls.

CATAMENIAL EPILEPSY

Fit frequency is influenced by many factors but the relationship with the menstrual cycle has attracted particular interest. Cyclical variations in fit frequency were originally thought to be due to the influence of the moon; indeed, belief in the association of epilepsy with the moon was so widespread that a patient with epilepsy was considered to be suffering from 'the disease of the moon'. Similarly, the moon was considered responsible for other periodic disorders of the mind, hence giving rise to the term 'lunatic'. In 1853, the great French neurologist Romberg said 'The planetary influence of the moon (especially of the new and full moon) upon the course of epilepsy was known to the ancients, and although here and there doubts have been raised against this view, the accurate observations of others have established its correctness' (Lennox 1960). It was not until a century later that this view was finally disproved by Pastrňák (1967).

Speculation about the association between epilepsy and menstruation dates back thousands of years. Hippocrates stated that 'cessation of the menstrual flux is a cause of seizures', which led to the belief that 'a good menses would prevent epilepsy' (Temkin 1971). In the nineteenth century it was realized that fits sometimes occurred more frequently at the time of menstruation and this was felt to be an hysterical phenomenon. In 1857, Locock said 'there was also a form of hysterical epilepsy connected with the menstrual cycle, and as periodic as that function. This form of the disease was very difficult to treat. The attacks only occurred during the catamenial period, except under otherwise strong exciting causes'.

Menarche is a common time for epilepsy to begin and many women believe that there is a connection between menstruation and fit frequency. Strictly speaking, catamenial epilepsy should apply only to those patients who have seizures only during menstruation. However, as few patients fall into this category it is more useful to include patients with exacerbations of fits during a consistent phase of the menstrual cycle, not restricted to the time of menstrual flow.

There are considerable difficulties in trying to assess the incidence of catamenial epilepsy. The menstrual cycle is one of many influences determining fit frequency and some women show cyclical variations independent of menstruation (Bandler et al 1957). Moreover men and prepubescent girls may also have monthly exacerbations (Griffiths & Fox 1938). Gowers (1885), who was the first to investigate the problem, found that in 46 of 82 patients fits were more frequent around the time of menstruation, usually just before and during menstrual flow. Since then, the majority of studies, but not all (Almquist 1955), have supported the existence of catamenial epilepsy, but have given a widely varying incidence of between 10% and 75%. This variation is due to a number of factors including poor study design (too few women, too few cycles, reliance on a questionnaire); lack of consistent definition of catamenial epilepsy; and different ideas of what constitutes an exacerbation of fits (for a good review see Newmark & Penry 1980). However, one of the most comprehensive and convincing studies was carried out by Laidlaw (1956) on 50 women at St Faith's Hospital for epileptics at

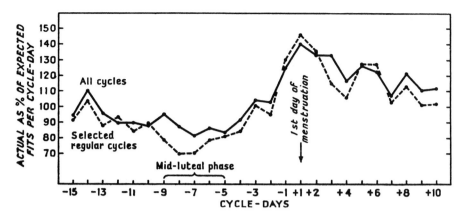

Fig. 15.1 The catamenial exacerbation of epilepsy. The distribution of fits according to day of the menstrual cycle. The distribution is similar for women with either regular or irregular periods (from Laidlaw 1956, reproduced with kind permission of the author and the editor)

Brentwood; these patients had 33 468 fits in 939 patient-years. He found an increased incidence of fits immediately before, during and after menstruation with a reduced incidence during the luteal phase (Fig. 15.1). The same pattern occurred irrespective of whether or not menstruation was regular. A more recent outpatient study by Rościszewska (1981) on 69 outpatients showed increased fit frequency in the seven days before menstruation, with the peak on the first menstrual day; thereafter there was a rapid decrease in fit frequency.

There is uncertainty about the cause of catamenial epilepsy and a number of different mechanisms have been proposed. It is clear that the type of fit, as well as the underlying cause of epilepsy, is not important (Schelp & Speciali 1983a, b). Some studies have suggested that women with more frequent fits tend to have catamenial epilepsy, but this is not always the case. Psychological factors were originally considered to be relevant, emphasizing the relationship felt to exist between female sexuality, menstruation, hysteria and fit frequency. However, there is little evidence to suggest that women with catamenial epilepsy have more emotional lability or suffer from a greater degree of premenstrual tension. Fluid retention occurs premenstrually and an excess of body water may provoke fits. However, women with catamenial epilepsy retain no more sodium and water than women with non-catamenial epilepsy and there is no correlation

between fit frequency and the degree of fluid retention (Ansell & Clarke 1956a).

Attention has recently been focused on the role of sex hormones in determining fit threshold during the menstrual cycle. In the rat, the hippocampus and amygdala show cyclical changes in excitability which correlate with stages of the oestrus cycle. Ovariectomized animals do not show this pattern, but oestradiol dipropionate restores it to some extent (Terasawa & Timiras 1968). In humans, there are minor changes in cerebral excitability during the menstrual cycle. The background rhythm of the EEG shows a slight increase in alpha rhythm during the luteal phase; in addition, patients with catamenial epilepsy may show increased seizure activity on the EEG at time of menstruation (Logothetis et al 1959).

There is good evidence that oestrogens lower and progesterone raises the fit threshold. For example, oestrogens can induce fits when applied to the cerebral cortex of rabbits and they also lower the electroshock threshold (Woolley & Timiras 1962); parenteral administration of oestrogens increases epileptiform activity in the EEG in humans. Progesterone, on the other hand, tends to decrease epileptiform activity on the EEG and it gives some protection against the development of audiogenic seizures (Werboff & Corcoran 1961).

The fluctuating levels of oestrogen and progesterone could provide an explanation for the varying fit threshold during the menstrual cycle (Fig. 15.2). Laidlaw (1956) speculated that the reduction in fit frequency during the luteal phase was due to the protective action of progesterone: as the level falls premenstrually, so the fit threshold falls. This view has received some recent support from Rościszewska et al (1986) who found a negative correlation between fit frequency and pregnanediol excretion. In their study, urinary excretion of oestrogens did not correlate with fit frequency, but Bäckström (1976), in a small number of patients, showed a positive correlation

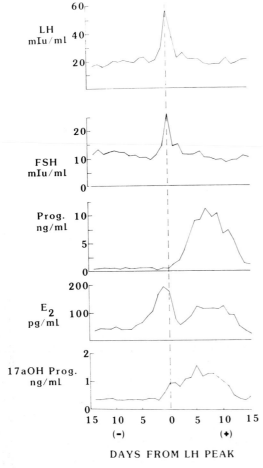

Fig. 15.2 Mean values of LH, FSH, progesterone, oestradiol (E2) and 17 Hydroxyprogesterone during the menstrual cycle. Day 0 is the midcycle LH peak, corresponding to ovulation. Progesterone levels rise after ovulation, then start to fall about 6 days before menstruation. Oestrogen levels peak at ovulation and again during the luteal phase, before falling just before menstruation (from Thorneycroft et al 1971, reproduced with kind permission of the editors)

between oestrogen: progesterone serum ratio and the frequency of generalized fits. There is therefore good evidence to show that oestrogen and progesterone play some part in determining fit frequency at various stages in the menstrual cycle. The epileptogenic effect of oestrogen might also explain the increased fit frequency at ovulation in some women, as well as the frequent onset of epilepsy at menarche and its occasional improvement at the menopause. However, this still leaves unexplained the high fit frequency on the first day of menstruation.

Another contributory factor might be variations in antiepileptic drug levels during the menstrual cycle. Phenytoin and phenobarbitone share a common metabolic pathway with many endogenous steroids; thus competition between sex hormones and antiepileptic drugs might result in higher antiepileptic drug levels during the luteal phase when oestrogen and progesterone levels are high. Towards menstruation, as the levels of sex hormones fall, more enzyme would be available for antiepileptic drug metabolism with a consequent decrease in serum level. Although Bäckström & Jorpes (1975) found no significant variations in antiepileptic drug levels, two recent studies (Shavit et al 1984, Rościszewska et al 1986) have suggested that phenytoin levels are lower at menstruation, particularly in patients with catamenial epilepsy. Further studies are needed to look at free phenytoin levels, as well as the levels of other antiepileptic drugs, in relation to sex hormone blood levels and fit frequency.

Treatment

Treatment for catamenial epilepsy dates back to the use of bromide, reported by Locock in 1857. In the early part of the twentieth century, oophorectomy was occasionally performed with uncertain results. Ansell & Clarke (1956b) reported favourably on the use of acetazolamide and, more recently, Goetting (1985) found it useful for treating catamenial exacerbations of action myoclonus. However, no trials of this drug have been carried out for the treatment of catamenial epilepsy. There are strong theoretical arguments for the use of progesterone and, indeed, there have been several case reports claiming its success

(Zimmerman et al 1973, Hall 1977). A recent preliminary study showed some benefit in women treated with oral medroxyprogesterone acetate, but the dose needed to be large enough to cause amenorrhoea (Mattson et al 1984). However, a double-blind, randomized and placebo-controlled study of high-dose and low-dose norithesterone in nine patients with catamenial epilepsy failed to show any advantage over placebo (Dana-Haeri & Richens 1983).

An alternative therapy is the 1,5-benzodiazepine clobazam at a dose of 20–30 mg daily. This should be given only for 7–10 days each month as tolerance develops (Feely et al 1982).

So what practical advice can be given to patients with catamenial epilepsy? First, the relationship of fits to the menses should be confirmed with a diary of events over at least six months. In many patients it is possible to improve the situation by establishing the best drug regimen. If there is a fall in antiepileptic drug level at the time of increased fits, that would justify increasing the dose over that period. Alternatively, clobazam or acetazolamide may be tried. The neurologist and gynaecologist should resist all pleas for a hysterectomy or oophorectomy which should be performed only on gynaecological grounds.

CONTRACEPTION

Epilepsy per se is not usually a contraindication to pregnancy; however, occasionally, there are reasons for advising against it in some women permanently, in others at least for a time (Table 15.3). Some women with epilepsy will themselves decide to have no children or to limit the number to one or two. Effective contraception is therefore

Table 15.3 Reasons why a woman with epilepsy might avoid pregnancy

Patient is unable to look after her baby because of:	physical handicap mental handicap severe, frequent fits liability to status epilepticus
High genetic risk Antiepileptic drugs:	toxic effects (large doses, polytherapy) concern about teratogenicity

an important matter and sterilization is sometimes justified.

Oral contraception

Many women are naturally concerned that oral contraceptives may increase fit frequency. In the majority of women there is no adverse effect (Espir et al 1969). Those with severe epilepsy seem to be most at risk and caution should be exercised in this group (Bickerstaff 1975). If, within a short time of starting oral contraception, epilepsy appears to have been provoked or aggravated, then alternative methods of contraception should be considered.

There are theoretical reasons why oral contraceptives might influence fit frequency, for sex hormones do alter seizure threshold in animals and humans (see section on catamenial epilepsy): oestrogens have epileptogenic properties whereas progesterone is a weak anticonvulsant. It might therefore be more appropriate to use progesterone-based contraceptives in women with severe epilepsy; however, these contraceptives are less reliable and tend to cause irregular bleeding.

It has become clear over the last ten years that antiepileptic drugs can reduce the efficacy of oral contraceptives (Coulam & Annegers 1979) and women should be warned of this possibility. The actual risk of an unplanned pregnancy is difficult to assess, but it is probably about the same as that with the modern copper intrauterine device, which has a Pearl Index (number of pregnancies per 100 women years) of 0.3–2.0. In women taking phenytoin, phenobarbitone, primidone or carbamazepine, 'pill failure' may result from increased metabolism of oestrogen due to hepatic enzyme induction by these drugs. Thus, levels of ethinyloestradiol fall in women treated with these drugs, and women on replacement oestrogen therapy may require a larger oestrogen dose if antiepileptic drugs are started (Notelovitz et al 1979). Sodium valproate is not a liver-enzyme inducer and there is no evidence that it interferes with oestrogen metabolism; it would appear therefore that sodium valproate is the safest drug in this context (Sonnen 1983).

One consequence of increased oestrogen metabolism is that breakthrough bleeding and spotting may occur if a low dose of oestrogen is used. This is a warning of inadequate contraception therefore additional contraceptive measures should be taken (Hempel & Klinger 1976) and the oestrogen dose should be increased. The initial dose should contain the equivalent of 50 μg ethinyloestradiol (Orme 1983); women may be reassured that, because of its increased metabolism, there is no increased risk of side-effects from the higher oestrogen dose. However, the other risk factors such as age, smoking, obesity and cardiovascular problems must not be ignored.

MARRIAGE AND FERTILITY

Little attention has been given to the effects of epilepsy and antiepileptic drugs on fertility. Women with epilepsy have fewer children than expected and there are a number of reasons for this.

Patients with epilepsy are less likely to marry, especially when epilepsy starts in the first decade. This is particularly true for men, but Dansky and her colleagues (1980) found that the marriage rate among women whose fits started in the first decade was 58% of expected, compared with 89% if fits started in the second decade. These marriage rates are higher than those reported in earlier studies reflecting better treatment of epilepsy and the changing attitude of society to the patient with epilepsy. Reasons for the reduced marriage rate include physical and mental handicaps in some women; in others, marriage opportunities may be restricted by lesser degrees of handicap or by overprotective parents. Another factor is reduced sexual drive, which may occur in both sexes (Taylor 1969).

The majority of women with epilepsy who marry do reproduce. In the series reported by Dansky et al (1980), 85.2% of married women with epilepsy reproduced during marriage; however, the actual number of liveborn children was less than expected, compared with the general population. This difference did not stem from an excess of spontaneous abortions or stillbirths, although women with epilepsy did have a greater number of therapeutic abortions and illegitimate

births. Interestingly, the more recently the woman with epilepsy had married, the closer was her fertility to the expected value.

There are likely to be medical and social factors responsible for the reduced number of liveborn children in women with epilepsy who marry. Such women may choose not to have children or to restrict the number; it is probable, however, that women with epilepsy do have reduced fertility, i.e. reduced ability to conceive and complete a pregnancy. It has been known for many years that women with epilepsy may have irregular menstrual periods and anovulatory cycles (Bäckström 1976). This may be due to the effect of fits on the neuroendocrine system: individual fits are known to cause a transient rise in prolactin levels (Trimble 1978) and patients with temporal lobe epilepsy have abnormal responses to intravenous luteinizing hormone releasing hormone (Herzog et al 1982). These changes are unlikely to be caused by medication for they may occur before antiepileptic treatment is started. Indeed, low doses of phenytoin have been used as an ovulation inducer (Gautray et al 1978).

PREGNANCY

Epilepsy is the most common neurological disorder requiring treatment in pregnancy and is not without hazards both for the mother and the baby. A woman with epilepsy who is planning a pregnancy is thus likely to be concerned about a range of matters involving her epilepsy and its possible effects on the fetus, pregnancy, delivery and care of the baby. These require special consideration, both before and during pregnancy, and preconception counselling should play a vital part in the prevention of, or preparation for, many of the potential problems (British Medical Journal 1981).

Genetic factors

Most parents with epilepsy worry about its possible transmission to any children they may have and request advice on its genetic aspects. These are covered in greater detail in Chapter 3 and in this section we shall merely give some practical advice.

Occasionally, epilepsy is the manifestation of an hereditary disease such as tuberous sclerosis, in which case the risk of transmission of the underlying disease must be assessed. In the majority of patients, this is not the case and the risks must be assessed on the basis of the type of epilepsy and the family history. It is important to remember that the EEG abnormality is more strongly inherited than its clinical manifestations and it is the latter on which parents require advice. In general, the children of women with epilepsy have a greater risk of developing epilepsy than do the children of affected males.

For partial epilepsy, if there is a well-defined cause such as head injury, then the risk is small. It is, however, greater than normal, implying that there are also hereditary factors in those who develop post-traumatic epilepsy (Gerken et al 1977). The inherited predisposition to temporal lobe epilepsy seems to stem largely from its relation to febrile convulsions and, if the parent acquired his or her epilepsy following recurrent febrile convulsions, then the risk to the child is probably greater.

There is, therefore, some increased risk of epilepsy in the offspring of a parent with epilepsy, but this is small and not sufficiently serious to inhibit those who want to have children. The only exception is when both parents suffer from epilepsy, in which case they should be made fully aware of the risks. Where epilepsy does occur within families it tends to be relatively mild and often responds to medication.

Effects of pregnancy on epilepsy

Women with epilepsy in pregnancy can be divided into two groups: those who already have epilepsy prior to conception and those who develop epilepsy during pregnancy.

First fit in pregnancy

Many women will have their first fit during the reproductive years and this may happen coincidentally in pregnancy. There is no convincing evidence that epilepsy is more likely to start in pregnancy. If the fit occurs without toxaemia or other detectable cause antiepileptic drug treatment can be withheld unless there is a second fit. Investigations should include routine blood tests and an EEG. Unless there are manifestations of raised intracranial pressure or focal signs, CT (computerized tomography) scanning can be deferred at least until after the pregnancy. If there are neurological signs, CT scanning will probably be required, depending on the stage of pregnancy and the likely cause (see Table 15.4). Occasionally, one or more fits without toxaemia or other detectable cause occur only during the pregnancy or the puerperium and the term 'gestational epilepsy' has been applied to this phenomenon (Dimsdale 1959, Knight & Rhind 1975). This is a diagnosis which can only be made in retrospect, for one cannot predict whether fits will recur outside pregnancy. Such patients may have a lowered fit threshold in pregnancy and may have a fit (or fits) in one or more pregnancies but not in all of them.

Table 15.4 Cause of seizure occurring for the first time in pregnancy

Primary generalized epilepsy	
Symptomatic epilepsy	Angioma
	Tumour
Complication of pregnancy	Eclampsia
	Cortical thrombophlebitis
	Cerebral venous thrombosis
Gestational epilepsy	

Fit frequency in pregnancy

There have been a number of prospective and retrospective studies to investigate the effect of pregnancy on fit frequency, and these have given similar results. Figure 15.3 shows the pooled results from seven studies published between 1975 and 1983.

In the most recent prospective study, Schmidt et al (1983) followed 136 pregnancies in 122 women. They found that pregnancy did not influence fit frequency in 68 pregnancies (50%); the number of fits increased in 37% and in two-thirds of these patients this was associated with non-compliance or sleep deprivation. Fit frequency

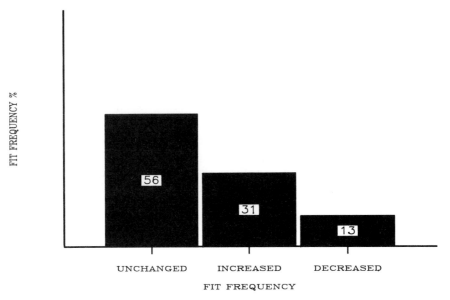

Fig. 15.3 Effect of pregnancy on fit frequency figures based on retrospective studies (Schmidt 1982, Knight & Rhind 1975, Svigos, 1984) and prospective studies (Bardy, 1982, Canger et al 1982, Schmidt et al 1982, 1983)

decreased in pregnancy in 13% and in a significant number of these patients this improvement was related to correction of inadequate therapy or of non-compliance before pregnancy and avoidance of sleep deprivation.

There are, unfortunately, no reliable clinical features which are helpful in predicting whether fits may increase in a particular patient; indeed, they may increase in one pregnancy but not in the next. Although early studies (Baptisti 1938, Knight & Rhind 1975) found that patients with more severe epilepsy (i.e. more than one fit per month before pregnancy) were likely to deteriorate, these were retrospective and drug levels were not available. Recent studies (Bardy 1982, Schmidt et al 1982) have shown that deterioration may not occur, even when epilepsy is severe. However, in over half the patients who do deteriorate, the increase occurs in the first trimester which is probably a reflection of poor compliance in early pregnancy (Schmidt et al 1983).

Pregnancy therefore appears to have only a minimal effect on the course of epilepsy, provided that good medical attention is given. Failure to recognize non-compliance and also that antiepileptic drug requirements increase in pregnancy (see section on pharmacokinetics) probably account for the increased fit frequency in many women.

Effect of epilepsy on pregnancy

Pregnancy tests

There is some evidence that patients on carbamazepine may have false negative pregnancy tests (Lindhout & Meinardi 1982). This does not apply to other antiepileptic drugs.

Pregnancy complications

Early studies on this problem suggested that women with epilepsy had an increased risk of complications during pregnancy and labour and that the babies were more frequently born prematurely and of low birth weight (Bjerkedal & Bahna 1973, Sabin & Oxorn 1956). However, these early studies were retrospective and no account was taken of the older age and lower socio-economic class of women with epilepsy – factors which are likely to contribute to the increased complication rate.

Two recent prospective studies (Battino et al 1982, Hiilesmaa et al 1985) have indicated that pregnancy complications are no greater in women with epilepsy. Hiilesmaa et al followed 139 women with epilepsy through 150 pregnancies and they were compared with 150 control pregnancies matched for age, parity, social class and fetal sex. Pregnancy complications (hypertension, breech presentation, premature live birth, diabetes) occurred with the same frequency in both groups. Inductions, vacuum or forceps extractions and caesarian sections were performed equally in the two groups and no difference was observed in the duration of labour or in the amount of bleeding at delivery. An Apgar score of less than seven was given to four live-born infants of mothers with epilepsy and to infants of seven matched controls. There were, however, five perinatal deaths in the epileptic group and two in the control group. Although this difference is not significant it is consistent with other studies which have shown a two-to three-fold increase in perinatal death in the offspring of mothers with epilepsy (Andermann et al 1982). Although birth weights were not mentioned in the study of Hiilesmaa et al (1985), there is some evidence that the offspring of mothers with epilepsy tend to be of lower birth weight (Yerby et al 1985). Further prospective studies are needed on these aspects.

Women with epilepsy therefore have an obstetric performance equal to that of other women. There is no need for more than the usual rate of caesarian section or forceps extraction for obstetric reasons, provided the mother has been under proper antenatal, neurological and obstetric care. Indications for caesarian section in women with epilepsy may include major seizures during labour; neurological or mental handicap that might reduce co-operation during the vaginal delivery; poor seizure control in late pregnancy, and previous severe seizures during physical or mental stress.

The effect of fits on pregnancy

There are potential risks of adverse effects on fetal development or abortion due to major fits in early pregnancy. Teramo et al (1979) showed that a major fit during labour can cause fetal asphyxia; however, Hiilesmaa et al (1985) found that none of the 170 generalized fits in 48 pregnancies was followed within 24 hours by any obstetric complications.

Management of fits in pregnancy

The same principles apply as for fits in non-pregnant patients; an adequate airway is vital to prevent not only maternal anoxia but also fetal asphyxia. Control of fits can usually be achieved with intravenous diazepam. The possibility of eclampsia should be considered, checking blood pressure and urine for protein.

Status epilepticus in pregnancy

Status epilepticus, although uncommon in pregnancy, carries serious risks for both mother and baby and intensive treatment is essential (Dalessio 1985). Termination of pregnancy may be required, but only as a last resort.

Malformations

A major concern for the mother is the risk of malformations in her child. There is general agreement that the incidence of congenital abnormalities in the children of mothers with epilepsy on treatment is two to three times greater than normal (Bjerkedal & Bahna 1973, Shapiro et al 1976, Monson et al 1973, Nakane et al 1980). The most common malformations are cleft lip and palate and congenital heart disease (usually atrial or ventricular septal defect). Other malformations include microcephaly, neural tube defects, skeletal abnormalities and intestinal atresia.

Various factors influence the malformation rate and are shown in Figure 15.4. As a general rule, older women with more severe epilepsy on large doses of multiple antiepileptic drugs, with a family history of malformations, are at greatest risk of producing a malformed child (Danksy et al 1982b, Lindhout et al 1982).

Antiepileptic drugs

Animal research has shown that all antiepileptic drugs are teratogenic and there is a correlation with antiepileptic drug levels: phenytoin, for

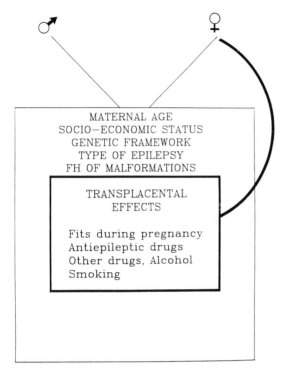

Fig. 15.4 Potential interaction of genetic, parental and transplacental factors in the production of malformations

the high risk of this syndrome, which causes developmental delay, craniofacial anomalies and congenital heart defects (Feldman et al 1977). The diones should therefore not be used in pregnancy and, in any case, they have been superseded by newer drugs.

Phenytoin This has been the most widely used antiepileptic drug in pregnancy and has long come under suspicion as having a teratogenic effect. However, there is little evidence that it causes major malformations in humans. Until recently, most patients were treated with several antiepileptic drugs, which makes it difficult to evaluate the effect of an individual drug. An important study from an analysis of data collected in the Collaborative Perinatal Project has suggested that the malformation rate is not influenced by phenytoin treatment in pregnancy (Shapiro et al 1976). The total malformation rate in 305 children born to mothers with epilepsy was 10.5%, as against 6.4% in children born to mothers without epilepsy. When the figures were analysed according to whether or not the mother received phenytoin in pregnancy, little difference was seen in the various groups: for example, the malformation rate in children exposed regularly, antenatally, to phenytoin was 11.8%, as opposed to 11.3% in unexposed children. A recent study, however, has suggested that a genetic defect of detoxification of arene oxide metabolites of phenytoin may increase the risk of the baby having major birth defects (Strickler et al 1985).

A more controversial issue is the 'fetal hydantoin syndrome'. This term was introduced by Hanson & Smith (1975) to describe the pattern of abnormalities observed in neonates whose mothers were exposed to phenytoin, usually in combination with phenobarbitone. The constellation of abnormalities they described are shown in Table 15.5. The most consistent abnormality is a variable degree of hypoplasia and irregular ossification of the distal phalanges, giving rise to short misshapen ends to the fingers and toes. The hypoplasia is more severe in the ulnar digits.

In a prospective study of 35 infants exposed prenatally to hydantoins (in 15 phenytoin was the sole antiepileptic drug) Hanson et al (1976) found that 11% had features of the 'fetal hydantoin syndrome'; an additional 31% displayed some

example, produces malformations in mice, depending on the strain of mouse and doses given. One of the malformations it causes in mice is cleft palate and this is the most common malformation seen in the offspring of humans with epilepsy. An interesting approach to this problem has been to culture rat embryos for 48 hours on sera from epileptic patients (Chatot et al 1984). Sera from subjects taking phenytoin, valproic acid and carbamazepine had comparable frequencies of cultured embryo abnormalities, whereas sera from subjects taking phenobarbitone produced abnormalities less frequently. It is therefore not surprising that there has been considerable interest and concern about the possible teratogenic effects of antiepileptic drugs.

Trimethadione A specific fetal disorder which is firmly established is the 'fetal trimethadione syndrome'. German et al (1970) reported a family in which four malformed babies were born to an epileptic mother taking this drug; she subsequently had two normal children following its discontinuation. Further studies have confirmed

Table 15.5 Fetal hydantoin syndrome

Intrauterine and postnatal growth retardation	Cranio-facial features	Hypoplasia of phalanges and nails
Microcephaly Mental retardation	Broad depressed nasal bridge Short upturned nose Long philtrum Hypertelorism Epicanthic folds Ptosis Malformed and low-set ears Wide mouth with prominent lips	Abnormal dermal ridge patterns Variations in palmar creases

features of this condition. A recent prospective study (Kelly et al 1984a) has also shown that 30% of children similarly exposed antenatally to phenytoin had minor craniofacial and digital changes. They did not, however, show any growth or mental retardation, and in the majority of cases the minor abnormalities disappeared in the first few years of life.

The fetal hydantoin and fetal alcohol syndromes have many features in common and combined syndromes have been described (Wilker & Nathenson 1982). This suggests that concurrent exposure in utero may have an additive effect in producing fetal malformations. Tumours (ganglioneuroblastoma, neuroblastoma, Wilm's tumour) have been found to coexist in the same individual exposed either to alcohol or phenytoin in utero (Ramilo & Harris 1979, Ehrenbard & Chaganti 1981). Twin studies (Phelan et al 1982, Loughnan et al 1973) have shown discordant expression of the fetal hydantoin syndrome in dizygotic and heteropaternal twins (twins having a different father) indicating that genetic predisposition has a role in fetal susceptibility. There are no reports of the fetal hydantoin syndrome in monozygotic twins.

Many features of the 'fetal hydantoin syndrome' are subjective and are open to observer bias: it is difficult, for example, to define a broad nose or low-set ears. The facial features do not appear specific to phenytoin treatment, for they have been described in the offspring of women taking other antiepileptic drugs including sodium valproate (Diliberti et al 1984); indeed, some of the features were described before the introduction of phenytoin (Paskind & Brown 1936). Digital abnormalities have also been described in patients not exposed antenatally to phenytoin and it is there-

fore unlikely that the fetal hydantoin syndrome is a specific entity caused exclusively by phenytoin.

Sodium valproate Sodium valproate is a relatively new drug and there were few data on the effects of exposure in utero until recently. It is known to be teratogenic at high doses in rats, mice and rabbits; in humans it crosses the placenta freely in late pregnancy to give higher values in the neonate than in the mother.

An early prospective study (Hiilesmaa et al 1980) of 12 infants exposed antenatally to sodium valproate showed that all were normal. However, around that time, sporadic case reports of neural tube defects began to appear. These prompted a retrospective survey of all cases of spina bifida entered into a regional birth defect registry in the Rhône–Alpes region of France: between August 1979 and August 1982 there were 72 infants with neural tube defects, 9 of whom were born to mothers taking sodium valproate; 4 had received other antiepileptic drugs and in 2 instances another case of neural tube defect was reported in the family (Bjerkedal et al 1982). On the basis of these figures it was calculated that the risk of a woman with epilepsy on sodium valproate giving birth to a child with a neural tube defect is about 1.2%; a comparable risk is faced by a woman who has already had a child with such a defect.

One must, however, be cautious about accepting these data uncritically; there is inevitable bias in any such retrospective study and further prospective studies are needed in patients on monotherapy with sodium valproate. Unfortunately, the manufacturers of sodium valproate have information on only 200 women who took this drug in pregnancy; in 89 women sodium valproate was the sole antiepileptic drug.

So what advice can be given to a woman contemplating pregnancy who is taking sodium valproate? If she has been seizure-free for two years or more gradual withdrawal of the drug may be justified. If her epilepsy is not controlled, then treatment with sodium valproate should be continued; at the present time there is not sufficient justification to switch drugs. At 18 weeks of pregnancy the mother should have an ultrasound examination and serum alpha-feto protein estimation. Amniocentesis should be considered, bearing in mind that this examination itself carries a fetal mortality of 1%. It is important that information on the outcome of all pregnancies in which the mother takes sodium valproate is given to the manufacturers. Where elective abortion is both safe and acceptable, women receiving valproate should be informed of the possible risk and offered counselling (WHO 1984, Committee on Safety of Medicines 1983).

Phenobarbitone There is little information about the teratogenicity of phenobarbitone; in the earlier studies most women were taking a combination of phenytoin and phenobarbitone. There is some experimental evidence to suggest that phenobarbitone might be less teratogenic than other antiepileptic drugs (Chatot et al 1984) and in humans Shapiro et al (1976) found that phenobarbitone caused no increase in malformation rate when taken for reasons other than epilepsy. Now that phenobarbitone is used less often in the treatment of epilepsy, it is unlikely we will ever find the answer.

Carbamazepine Carbamazepine has not been implicated in any major malformations but it may cause fetal head growth retardation. Hiilesmaa et al (1981) in their study of 133 women showed that carbamazepine alone or in combination with phenobarbitone caused such retardation; no definite correlation with intellectual development was shown. Kaneko et al (1983) found that antiepileptic drugs lowered both T4 and TSH levels in cord blood and postulated that this might explain the fetal head growth retardation.

Summary

There is a small teratogenic risk with all the antiepileptic drugs. The use of a single drug with an optimum serum level is likely to be less hazardous than a combination of drugs. Although carbamazepine cannot be cleared from teratogenic risks, at the moment it does seem to be the safest antiepileptic drug from this point of view.

In view of the possibility that the teratogenicity of antiepileptic drugs may be related to their effect on folate metabolism, even though this has not been proven, the routine provision of folate supplements to pregnant women who are taking antiepileptic drugs, preferably starting before conception, may be recommended.

Parental factors

There are a number of parental factors which might influence the incidence of congenital malformations. Many women with epilepsy have characteristics associated with an increased malformation rate (Monson et al 1973): they are often older, come from a lower socio-economic class, and they are more restricted in their choice of husband; hence their offspring may have a poor genetic background. However, even when these factors are taken into account, it is clear that parental epilepsy itself increases the malformation rate. There are two ways of investigating the problem: first, to look at the offspring of parents with epilepsy receiving no treatment; secondly, to analyse the prevalence of epilepsy among the parents of children with facial clefts, the most common malformation.

The malformation rate in the offspring of untreated women with epilepsy is higher than that in the general population (Nakane et al 1980); however, it is not generally as high as the risk from a treated pregnancy (Table 15.6). It is difficult to know whether this increase is due solely to the medication or to the more severe epilepsy suffered by those women requiring medication. Another interesting observation is that the malformation rate appears to be increased in the offspring of fathers with epilepsy: Shapiro et al (1976), for example, found the malformation rate among offspring of fathers with epilepsy was 8.3% as opposed to 10.5% for the offspring of mothers with epilepsy.

Friis (1979) has looked at the prevalence of epilepsy among parents of children with facial

Table 15.6 Malformation rates in live births of mothers with epilepsy related to whether or not antiepileptic drug treatment was given in pregnancy

Author	Drug-treated mothers will epilepsy		Untreated mothers with epilepsy	
	No. of Pregnancies	Malformation rate (%)	No. of pregnancies	Malformation rate (%)
Monson et al (1973)	205	5.3	101	2.9
Annegers et al (1974)	141	7.1	56	1.8
Nakane et al (1980)	3703	7.1	825	4.5
Dansky et al (1982)	114	15.9	50	6.5
Lindhout et al (1982)	170	9.9	14	7
Koch et al (1982)	89	10	20	10

clefts: he found 18 parents with epilepsy among 391 live-born children with facial clefts; this was three times the expected number. Of these 18, 7 were fathers and 11 were mothers and only two-thirds were on antiepileptic drug treatment. If there is an association between epilepsy and facial clefts, this could either be a direct effect of epilepsy or the presence of a common genetic link between epilepsy and facial clefts. This latter possibility gains some support from a study by Kelly et al (1984b): among 175 families with a proband with a facial cleft, there were 13 parents with epilepsy (11 mothers and 2 fathers) and only 6 of these received drug treatment in pregnancy. Of the 13 families in which a parent had epilepsy, 10 had other family members with epilepsy and 9 had other family members with facial cleft. In the remaining 162 families in which neither parent had epilepsy, 17% had a family history of epilepsy and 21% a family history of facial clefts. This finding, however, is in contrast with a study by Friis et al (1986) which suggests that the most important factor in determining facial clefts is the presence of maternal epilepsy, particularly if this is treated during pregnancy. Further studies are needed on this aspect.

Effect of fits

Another factor which might be important is the effect of fits on the developing fetus. There is conflicting evidence as to whether maternal convulsions during pregnancy are associated with malformations. Shapiro et al (1976), for example, found that the malformation rate was similar in children born to mothers with epilepsy who had

convulsions in pregnancy, compared with those who did not. However, in a report from a collaborative study in Japan of 516 live births of mothers with epilepsy (Nakane et al 1980) the malformation rate in the children of mothers not taking antiepileptic drugs was lowest (1.8%) when the mother had no fits during pregnancy, but was 5.3% in those whose mothers had had fits in the first trimester. The malformation rate in children of mothers who were taking antiepileptic drugs was 11.5% when the mothers had no fits during the first trimester, and 13.6% if they did (Table 15.7).

Table 15.7 Malformation rates in live births of mothers with epilepsy related to whether or not maternal fits occurred in pregnancy (from Nakane et al 1980)

Mothers with epilepsy	Malformation rates in live births	
	No fits during pregnancy	Fits during first trimester
Not on antiepileptic drug treatment	1.8%	5.3%
On antiepileptic drug treatment	11.5%	13.6%

These figures could be taken to support the view that antiepileptic drugs have a teratogenic effect and, in addition, suggest that maternal fits during the first trimester may also contribute in a small way to the malformation rate. Presumably, however, the women taking antiepileptic drugs, and particularly those whose fits are not controlled, have more severe forms of epilepsy which may themselves be associated with a higher malformation rate.

Pharmacokinetics of antiepileptic drugs in pregnancy

An important factor responsible for loss of seizure control in some pregnant women is a decline in serum antiepileptic drug level when the oral dose is kept constant. This seems to be true for all antiepileptic drugs but especially for phenytoin, which has been the drug most extensively studied. While there is considerable variation between patients and in the same patient, there is usually a 30–50% fall in serum phenytoin level. It is, however, more meaningful to measure phenytoin clearance (this is the ratio of dose and steady-state concentration) as the dose of phenytoin may be increased during pregnancy. Clearance rates for phenytoin increase in early pregnancy and tend to rise throughout pregnancy, reaching about twice the preconception values in the last few weeks of pregnancy (Bardy et al 1982); however, sometimes, they remain at about the same increased level during the whole of pregnancy (Dansky et al 1982a). Clearance may fall within a few days of delivery but usually it falls gradually over a two to three month period. Phenobarbitone, carbamazepine and sodium valproate levels also fall during pregnancy, but not usually to the same extent as phenytoin levels.

There are a number of possible reasons for the fall in antiepileptic drug levels in pregnancy (Fig. 15.5). Reduced compliance certainly occurs in some patients, often from fear of the teratogenic effects of antiepileptic drugs. Reduced phenytoin absorption has been reported in pregnancy (Ramsay et al 1978), but this is unlikely to be an important factor because the mean oral bioavailability of phenytoin is 90% of the intravenous bioavailability (Lander et al 1984). Increased blood

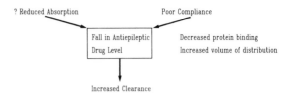

Fig. 15.5 Factors which may influence antiepileptic drug levels in pregnancy

volume and body weight with consequent increased volume of distribution of the drug might contribute to the lower levels in pregnancy; they would not, however, account for the fall in early pregnancy, or the considerable variation in the fall in serum level between different antiepileptic drugs.

The most likely explanation for the fall in antiepileptic drug levels in pregnancy is a combination of reduced protein binding and increased metabolic clearance (Table 15.8). Phenytoin and sodium valproate are highly protein bound and the pharmacologically active unbound or free drug constitutes only a small percentage of the total concentration. The fall in serum albumin level in pregnancy leads to a reduction in total antiepileptic drug level; however, the unbound drug level remains constant, leading to a rise in the unbound fraction (Perucca et al 1981, Chen et al 1982). Carbamazepine is 75% bound but its metabolite, 10,11-epoxide, is only 50% protein bound. Surprisingly, there is no decrease in protein binding of carbamazepine in pregnancy and therefore no increase in the unbound fraction.

In practical terms, the increased unbound fraction of phenobarbitone, phenytoin and sodium valproate in pregnancy means that estimations of the total levels will tend to underestimate the free levels: for phenytoin, a 25% fall in serum albumin

Table 15.8 Protein binding and clearance of antiepileptic drugs in pregnancy

Drug	% Protein bound non-pregnant	Protein binding in pregnancy	Total level in pregnancy	Unbound fraction in pregnancy	Clearance
Phenobarbitone	45%	−	−	+	+
Phenytoin	90%	−	−	+	+
Carbamazepine	75%	unchanged	−	unchanged	+
Sodium Valproate	90%	−	−	+	probably +

+ increase
− decrease

concentration results in an approximate 25% increase in unbound phenytoin fraction; for sodium valproate the changes are even greater. Ideally, free levels of phenytoin in either blood or saliva should be measured; if total drug levels are measured, then the serum albumin should also be estimated, so that an appropriate allowance can be made. Another consideration is that, after a single loading dose, the reduced binding capacity could result temporarily in higher free levels with enhanced therapeutic effect.

There is good evidence that metabolic clearance of antiepileptic drugs is increased in pregnancy: free phenytoin levels, for example, fall by about 30% (they do not fall as much as the total level). Total carbamazepine levels fall despite unaltered protein binding and the epoxide:carbamazepine ratio increases, suggesting enhanced metabolism (Dam et al 1979). It seems likely that the increased clearance is due to enhanced hepatic metabolism perhaps stimulated by high circulating progesterone levels (Davis et al 1973). It is possible that the feto-placental unit is also capable of some drug metabolism.

Antiepileptic drugs are transferred across the placenta: phenytoin concentrations are identical in cord and maternal serum at term (Mirkin 1971). The half-life of phenytoin in the newborn ranges from 55 to 69 hours, with elimination usually complete by the fifth day. The greatest concentration of phenytoin is in the liver. Phenobarbitone levels are also similar in the mother and newborn, and elimination occurs within two to seven days, depending on the length of time of exposure. Carbamazepine levels are also similar in the mother and newborn and the half life in the newborn ranges from 8–28 hours, which is similar to the adult half-life (Rane et al 1975). Sodium valproate levels are higher in the cord serum than in maternal serum and the mean elimination half-life is 47 ± 15 hours; this is about four times the value in adults (Nau et al 1981).

Management of epilepsy before and during pregnancy

The management of epilepsy during pregnancy is likely to be more satisfactory if potential problems have been considered beforehand. Time is required for preconception counselling, as much important advice and reassurance can be given at this stage. Many women are reluctant to voice their concerns and a gentle enquiry will often lead to a string of anxious questions.

Preconception counselling

The majority of women can be reassured that, with proper supervision, there is unlikely to be any problem with their fit control or pregnancy. An attempt should be made to assess the risks of a child developing epilepsy or having a malformation and this should be discussed with the prospective parents. Parents should be told that the majority of malformations are minor and are due in part to factors associated with parental epilepsy and not just to its treatment. Fear of the teratogenic risks of antiepileptic drugs often results from exaggeration of these risks and as a result some women stop treatment once they become pregnant. The need for compliance during pregnancy should be emphasized for those women in whom continuation of treatment is considered essential.

Patients on combinations of drugs and with serum drug levels higher than necessary may be at greater risk from teratogenicity. In women who need drug treatment, rationalization to the optimum should be achieved before conception, preferably using only one antiepileptic drug. If she has been seizure-free for two years, then gradual withdrawal of treatment could be considered. Ideally, one would try to avoid starting drug treatment during the important first three to four months of pregnancy when organogenesis is most active; when fits have been mild and infrequent it may be justifiable to withhold treatment at least over this period. However, potentially serious risks to both the fetus and mother from uncontrolled fits, and particularly from status epilepticus, must be considered and balanced against the teratogenic risks.

The possibility that folate and vitamin supplements given prior to conception and during pregnancy might prevent or reduce the incidence of fetal malformations is currently undergoing a multicentre trial (Smithells et al 1980). Pending the results of this trial, the authors advocate this supplementation for all women taking antiepileptic drugs if they are about to embark on pregnancy.

Managment of pregnancy

Maternity hospitals delivering 2000–3000 babies annually can expect 10–15 of the mothers to have epilepsy or a history of fits; this justifies special arrangements for their antenatal care along the lines of the highly successful clinics for diabetes (Espir & Hytten 1983). A rapid reliable drug monitoring service with report of the results (as with blood glucose) while the patient is still in the clinic is now possible and should be provided. Close collaboration between the general practitioner, neurologist, obstetrician and biochemist is important, and should greatly improve the prospects of women with epilepsy and their babies.

Once a woman with epilepsy is pregnant, in addition to her obstetric care, she should be seen every month, or more frequently if her epilepsy is severe, for assessment of her epilepsy and counselling; the blood levels of her antiepileptic drugs should be followed. The fall in antiepileptic drug blood level in pregnancy does not necessarily lead to a recurrence or increased frequency of fits and, in principle, the dose should not be increased just because the levels fall. However, in some patients, fit control before pregnancy will have been shown to be dependent on the blood level being above a certain level. In these patients, if the level falls during pregnancy, it would seem sensible to increase the dose to maintain the level, above that known to be critical, rather than to wait for fits to recur or increase in frequency (see case report below).

Morning sickness and more severe hyperemesis may interfere with antiepileptic drug treatment; this may be avoided by adjusting the time that the drug is given in order to ensure its absorption. Phenytoin may be given as effectively in a single dose at night.

General advice Iron and folic acid should be given throughout pregnancy. Care should be taken with diet to avoid excessive weight gain and women should avoid smoking, alcohol, aspirin (Stuart et al 1982), anti-emetics and other drugs.

Labour

Extra care is needed during labour, when pain, anxiety, lack of sleep and poor absorption of antiepileptic drugs may combine to cause fits. In women requiring drug treatment during pregnancy, it is essential to ensure that treatment is continued in the last stages of pregnancy and during labour.

Management of fits in labour

The initial management of the fit is the same, whatever the underlying cause. An intravenous bolus of diazepam 10–20 mg should be given: this may cause hypotonia and hypothermia in the neonate (Cree et al 1973) but these effects are not long lasting. If fits recur, then an infusion of intravenous diazepam or chlormethiazole should be given. In addition 1 g loading dose of phenytoin should be given intravenously, at a rate of 50 mg/min. Once the fits are under control, attention can be directed to their cause. The management of eclampsia (see below) consists of rigorous control both of blood pressure (this should be kept below 170/110 mmHg) and of fits. Patients should be nursed in a quiet room with minimal sensory input. Once the blood pressure is under control, most obstetricians will carry out a caesarian section. Whatever the cause of fits in labour, a careful assessment of the state of the fetus is needed. Fetal asphyxia may occur and changes in fetal heart rate are usually observed (Hiilesmaa et al 1985). Reduced maternal co-operation post-ictally may also make vaginal delivery difficult.

The puerperium

Careful follow-up postpartum is necessary as the factors leading to a fall in antiepileptic drug levels during pregnancy are reversed in the puerperium. If the patient has required higher doses of drugs during the pregnancy, these may have to be continued in the puerperium for two or three weeks; the blood levels should, however, be checked weekly to avoid drug toxicity. It may take six to ten weeks until the pre-pregnancy state is restored, and gradual reduction of the dose may be necessary to maintain an optimum blood level.

Breast feeding

The occurrence of fits in the puerperium is unrelated to the mode of baby feeding and it is therefore not necessary to discourage a mother from breast feeding. Antiepileptic drugs are excreted in breast milk but rarely cause any problems. Phenytion, carbamazepine and sodium valproate levels in breast milk are usually small; the levels of phenobarbitone are variable while those of ethosuximide tend to be high (Table 15.9). If the baby seems unduly drowsy, this may be drug related and a trial of artificial feeding should resolve this. If drowsiness persists, measurement of drug levels in maternal blood and breast milk and the baby's blood may provide the answer.

Table 15.9 Antiepileptic drugs in breast milk (modified from Kaneko et al 1979, with kind permission of the editors)

Drug	Milk/serum concentration (%)	No. of Patients
Phenytoin	18.1 ± 5.9	9
Phenobarbitone	45.9 ± 24.9	8
Primidone	80.9 ± 17.6	12
Carbamazepine	39.4 ± 19.3	3
Ethosuximide	78.8 ± 32.8	4
Sodium valproate (Nau et al 1981)	3	6

The main danger to the baby is if the mother has a fit and causes an injury to the baby for example while feeding. It is advisable therefore for someone else to be present at such times.

Eclampsia and peripartum convulsions

When a convulsion occurs in late pregnancy or during delivery the diagnosis of eclampsia must always be considered (for a good review see Donaldson 1978, Symonds 1986). Routine antenatal care has reduced the incidence of eclampsia; however, mothers with eclampsia may present as unbooked emergencies, having concealed their pregnancy.

The diagnosis of eclampsia is usually easy because of the progression of symptoms from mild pre-eclampsia to severe pre-eclampsia and then to the preconvulsive stage. However, the signs may be very slight and present for only a few days before the convulsion. There are recorded cases of normal blood pressure, absent oedema and no proteinuria occurring a few days before eclamptic convulsions; however, in most cases a careful history will elicit the typical symptoms of impending eclampsia – frontal headache, dimness of vision or flashes of light, and epigastric pain. These symptoms are usually present for 12 hours before the convulsion and they are associated with a rapid rise in blood pressure and proteinuria. The first convulsion occurs before labour in 25%, during labour in 50% and after delivery in 25%. It is very unusual for eclamptic convulsions to occur more than 24 hours after delivery and an alternative cause should then be considered. In some cases, only one convulsion occurs and the mother appears quite well when she regains consciousness. In other cases repeated convulsions occur – up to 200 have been reported.

Differential diagnosis

Epilepsy is the most likely source of confusion in the differential diagnosis; if there is any previous history of convulsions then epilepsy is most likely, although the two conditions may occur together. In epilepsy, there will be no preceding symptoms of the preconvulsive stage, little or no proteinuria and no sustained rise in blood pressure. Spontaneous subarachnoid haemorrhage, from an aneurysm or arteriovenous malformation may occur at any time in pregnancy or during delivery. The usual presentation is of sudden, severe headache and loss of consciousness. There may occasionally be a convulsion, but recurrent convulsions are uncommon. Patients have neck stiffness and some elevation of blood pressure; there is, however, no proteinuria.

Cerebral venous thrombosis and cortical thrombophlebitis usually occur from three days to four weeks after childbirth, often in the second or third postpartum weeks (Carroll et al 1966). It may, however, occur at any stage in pregnancy. The usual symptoms are headaches and focal fits followed by focal neurological signs and papilloedema. There is no significant proteinuria and the blood pressure is only mildly elevated.

Thrombotic thrombocytopenic purpura is a rare syndrome consisting of thrombocytopenic purpura,

Coomb's negative haemolytic anaemia with fragmented red cells, fever, renal dysfunction and various neurological manifestations. These consist of headache, seizures, altered level of consciousness and fluctuating focal neurological signs due to cerebral petechiae. The infant is usually macerated or stillborn and following delivery the condition of the mother deteriorates.

Water intoxication may cause seizures and the most likely cause of this is misuse of oxytocin. A low serum sodium confirms the diagnosis. Occasionally, convulsions may be caused by toxicity of local anaesthetics used for regional nerve blocks. Seizures are preceded by confusion, dysarthria and blurred vision (Foldes et al 1965). The reaction to lignocaine lasts about 20 minutes.

The newborn

Expert neonatal care should be available to deal with any problems during this period. Maternal and neonatal blood levels of the commonly used antiepileptic drugs (except sodium valproate which has a higher level in the neonate) are approximately equal at birth and, if possible, the umbilical cord blood level should be checked at birth.

Infants exposed to phenytoin or phenobarbitone derivatives in utero may develop bleeding disorders within the first 24 hours of life. This is due to depletion of vitamin K dependent clotting factors (Bleyer & Skinner 1976) and should be distinguished from the physiological deficiency which usually occurs between the second and fifth day after birth. The bleeding disorder may be serious and occasionally life threatening. It is likely that phenytoin reduces the clotting factors in an analogous way to warfarin, by competitive action with vitamin K. Women with epilepsy should be given phytomenadione 2 mg intravenously or intramuscularly before delivery. Vitamin K is well and rapidly absorbed when given orally and Deblay et al (1982) advocate giving mothers with epilepsy oral supplements of vitamin K, 20 mg daily for the last two weeks of pregnancy. In addition an injection of 1 mg should be given to the newborn immediately after birth. Clotting studies should be performed two hours later and, if they remain abnormal, or if there is any evidence of bleeding, further doses of phytomenadione should be given intravenously. Occasionally, it may be necessary to give fresh frozen plasma or an exchange transfusion with fresh frozen plasma.

Phenobarbitone withdrawal symptoms may occur in infants exposed in utero to phenobarbitone, even when the dose is as low as 90 mg daily (Desmond et al 1972). Symptoms occur within a few days of birth and consist of irritability, restlessness and vomiting. Seizures do not usually occur and the symptoms gradually resolve. Management consists of a regimen of frequent feeding, diminished input of environmental stimuli and mild sedation.

Care of the child

The doctor and health visitor should give some practical advice to the young mother with epilepsy; for example, she may be unwise to bath the baby in an adult or baby bath; it might be better to wash the baby on a mat in the cot with a bowl of water outside the cot. If fits are frequent and occur without warning then it would be hazardous to carry the baby. Extra help may be required during this time.

As the child becomes older, safety measures both in the house and garden need attention. The British Epilepsy Association produce a pamphlet 'Mother with Epilepsy' which gives useful advice.

Case report
A 29-year-old woman had a subarachnoid haemorrhage from a right frontal arterio-venous malformation in January 1973. She made a good recovery following operation for this and had no neurological deficit. She was treated with phenytoin 100 mg tds but this was tailed off after 8 weeks and stopped in April 1973. She remained well until April 1978 when she had two fits and was restarted on phenytoin 100 mg tds. In October 1979 she became pregnant and continued treatment with phenytoin 100 mg tds throughout pregnancy. She had no fits, the drug levels were not measured and she had a normal full-term delivery of a normal baby in August 1980. In September 1980, for reasons which are not clear, she was started on sodium valproate and the phenytoin was reduced initially to 200 mg daily and in October 1980 to 100 mg daily. She had two further fits in September and November 1980. Sodium valproate was stopped and she was restarted on phenytoin 100 mg tds. On 23 March 1981 she missed a dose of phenytoin and the following day she had a fit.

In April 1981 she became pregnant again and was referred to the National Hospital. She was taking phenytoin 100 mg tds and was advised to adjust this to 100 mg in the morning and 200 mg at night. The serum level on the 27

Serum phenytoin concentration μmol/l

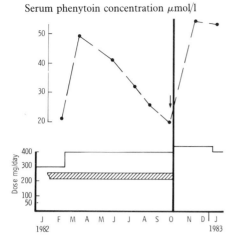

Fig. 15.6 Phenytoin levels in pregnancy and after delivery (see case report); the arrow indicates a fit.

May was 10 μmol/l (therapeutic range 40–80 μmol/l). She had a fit on 5 June (she had not missed any doses of phenytoin) and a few days later she had a spontaneous abortion. The dose of phenytoin was kept unchanged at 100 mg in

the morning and 200 mg at night and serum levels on 26 August and 25 November were 40 and 42 μmol/l.

In January 1982 she became pregnant again still taking phenytoin 100 mg in the morning and 200 mg at night. On 24 February, the serum level was 21 μmol/l and on 1 March the dose of phenytoin was increased to 200 mg in the morning and 200 mg at night. Serum levels during and after the pregnancy are shown in Figure 15.6. By 6 October the level had fallen to 20 μmol/l and on 11 October she had a fit. The dose of phenytoin was increased on 13 October by 100 mg on alternate days. The baby was born at term on 18 October with a normal delivery. The baby was normal and was breast-fed for five weeks without any problems.

The dose of phenytoin was reduced back to 200 mg bd in January 1983 and she has continued with this subsequently. The serum phenytoin level in March 1985 was 63 μmol/l and when last seen in February 1986 she was well and had had no further fits.

The fall in serum phenytoin level during pregnancy is striking in spite of increasing the dose of phenytoin from 300 to 400 mg daily. There was clearly a liability for her to have a fit when the serum levels of phenytoin were low. The rise in level postpartum is also shown, although this might have been partly due to the slight increase in the dose of phenytoin following the fit which she had shortly before her delivery.

REFERENCES

Aarli J A 1976 Phenytoin-induced depression of salivary IgA. Epilepsia 17: 283–391

Almquist R 1955 The rhythm of epileptic attacks and its relationhsip to the menstrual cycle. Acta Psychiatrica Scandinavica (suppl. 105) 30: 1–116

Andermann E, Dansky L, Kinch R A 1982 Complications of pregnancy, labour and delivery in epileptic women. In: Janz D, Bossi L, Dam M, Helge H, Richens A, Schmidt D (eds) Epilepsy, pregnancy and the child. Raven Press, New York, pp 61–74

Annegers J F, Elveback L R, Hauser W A, Kurland L T 1974 Do anticonvulsants have a teratogenic effect? Archives of Neurology 31: 364–373

Ansell B, Clarke E 1956a Epilepsy and menstruation. The role of water retention. Lancet 2: 1232–1235

Ansell B, Clarke E 1956b Acetazolamide in treatment of epilepsy. British Medical Journal 1: 650–654

Bäckström T 1976 Epileptic seizures in women related to plasma estrogen and progesterone during the menstrual cycle. Acta Neurologica Scandinavica 54: 321–347

Bäckström T, Jorpes P 1975 Serum phenytoin, phenobarbital, carbamazepine, albumin; and plasma estradiol, progestrone concentrations during the menstrual cycle in women with epilepsy. Acta Neurologica Scandinavica 59: 63–71

Bandler B, Kaufman I C, Dykens J W, Schleifer M, Shapiro L N 1957 Seizures and the menstrual cycle. American Journal of Psychiatry 113: 704–708

Baptisti A 1938 Epilepsy and pregnancy. A review of the literature and a study of 37 cases. American Journal of Obstetrics and Gynaecology 35: 818–824

Bardy A H 1982 Seizure frequency in epileptic women during pregnancy and the puerperium: results of the prospective Helsinki study. In: Janz D, Bossi L, Dam M, Helge H, Richens A, Schmidt D (eds) Epilepsy, pregnancy and the child. Raven Press, New York, pp 27–32

Bardy A H, Teramo K, Hiilesmaa V K 1982 Apparent plasma clearance of phenytoin, phenobarbitone, primidone and carbamazepine during pregnancy: results of the prospective Helsinki study. In: Janz D, Bossi L, Dam M, Helge H, Richens A, Schmidt D (eds) Epilepsy, pregnancy and the child. Raven Press, New York, pp 141–145

Battino D, Bossi L, Canger R et al 1982 Obstetric monitoring of pregnancy in 59 patients with epilepsy. In: Janz D, Bossi L, Dam M, Helge H, Richens A, Schmidt D (eds) Epilepsy, pregnancy and the child. Raven Press, New York, pp 99–101

Bickerstaff E R 1975 Neurological complications of oral contraceptives. Clarendon Press, Oxford, pp 87–90

Bjerkedal T, Bahna S L 1973 The course and outcome of pregnancy in women with epilepsy. Acta Obstetrica et Gynaecologica Scandinavica 52: 245–248

Bjerkedal T, Czeizel A, Goujard J et al 1982 Valproic acid and spina bifida. Lancet 2:1096

Bleyer W A, Skinner A L 1976 Fatal neonatal haemorrhage after maternal anticonvulsant therapy. Journal of the American Medical Association 235: 626–627

British Medical Journal 1981 Preconception clinics 283: 685

Canger R, Avanzini G, Battino D, Bossi L, Franceschetti S, Spina S 1982 Modifications of seizure frequency in pregnant patients with epilepsy: a prospective study. In: Janz D, Bossi L, Dam M, Helge H, Richens A, Schmidt D (eds) Epilepsy, pregnancy and the child. Raven Press, New York, pp 33–38

Carroll J D, Leak D, Lee H A 1966 Cerebral thrombophlebitis in pregnancy and the puerperium. Quarterly Journal of Medicine 35: 347–368

Chatot C L, Klein N W, Clapper M L et al 1984 Human serum teratogenicity studied by rat embryo culture: epilepsy, anticonvulsant drugs, and nutrition. Epilepsia 25(2): 205–216

Chen S, Perucca E, Lee J, Richens A 1982 Serum protein binding and free concentrations of phenytoin and phenobarbitone in pregnancy. British Journal of Clinical Pharmacology 13: 547–552

Committee on Safety of Medicines 1983 Sodium valproate (Epilim) and congenital abnormalities. Current Problems No 9

Coulam C B, Annegers J F 1979 Do anticonvulsants reduce the efficacy of oral contraceptives? Epilepsia 20: 519–526

Cree J E, Meyer J, Hailey D M 1973 Diazepam in labour: its metabolism and effect on the clinical condition and thermogenesis of the newborn. British Medical Journal 4: 251–255

Dalessio D J 1985 Seizure disorders and pregnancy. New England Journal of Medicine 312: 559–563

Dam M, Christiansen J, Munck O, Mygind, K I 1979 Antiepileptic drugs: metabolism in pregnancy. Clinical Pharmacokinetics 4: 53–62

Dana-Haeri J, Richens A 1983 Effect of norithesterone on seizures associated with menstruation. Epilepsia 24: 377–381

Dansky L V, Andermann E, Andermann F 1980 Marriage and fertility in epileptic patients. Epilepsia 21: 261–271

Dansky L, Andermann E, Sherwin A L, Andermann F 1982a Plasma levels of phenytoin during pregnancy and the puerperium. In: Janz D, Bossi L, Dam M, Helge H, Richens A, Schmidt D (eds) Epilepsy, pregnancy and the child. Raven Press, New York, pp 155–162

Dansky L, Andermann E, Andermann F, Sherwin A L, Kinch R A 1982b Maternal epilepsy and congenital malformations: correlation with maternal plasma anticonvulsant levels. In Janz D, Bossi L, Dam M, Helge H, Richens A, Schmidt D (eds) Epilepsy, pregnancy and the child. Raven Press, New York, pp 251–258

Davis M, Simmons C J, Dordoni B, Maxwell I D 1973 Induction of hepatic enzymes during normal human pregnancy. Journal of Obstetrics and Gynaecology 80: 690–694

Deblay M F, Vert P, Andre M, Marchal F 1982 Transplacental vitamin K prevents haemorrhagic disease of infant of epileptic mother. Lancet 1:1247

Desmond M M, Schwanecke R P, Wilson G S, Yasunaga S, Burgdorff I 1972 Maternal barbiturate utilisation and neonatal withdrawal symptomatology. Journal of Pediatrics 80(2): 190–197

Diliberti J H, Farndon P A, Dennis N R, Curry C J R 1984 The fetal valproate syndrome. American Journal of Medical Genetics 19: 473–481

Dimsdale H 1959 The epileptic in relation to pregnancy. British Medical Journal 28: 1147–1150

Donaldson J O 1978 Neurology of Pregnancy. W B Saunders, Philadelphia pp 211–250

Egger J, Brett E M 1981 Effect of sodium valproate in 100 children with special reference to weight. British Medical Journal 283: 577–581

Ehrenbard L T, Chaganti R S K 1981 Cancer in the fetal hydantion syndrome. Lancet 2:97

Espir M, Hytten F E 1983 Pregnancy with epilepsy – the need for combined care. British Journal of Obstetrics and Gynaecology 90: 1105–1106

Espir M, Walker M E, Lawson J P 1969 Epilepsy and oral contraception. British Medical Journal 1: 294–295

Falconer M A, Davidson S 1973 Coarse features in epilepsy as a consequence of anticonvulsant therapy. Lancet 2: 1112–1114

Feely M, Calvert R, Gibson J 1982 Clobazam in catamenial epilepsy. A model for evaluating anticonvulsants. Lancet 2: 71–73

Feldman G L, Weaver D D, Lovrien E W 1977 The fetal trimethadione syndrome. Report of an additional family and further delineation of this syndrome. American Journal of Diseases of Childhood 131: 1389–1392

Foldes F F, Davidson G M, Duncalf D, Kuwabara S 1965 The intravenous toxicity of local anaesthetic agents in man. Clinical Pharmacology and Therapeutics 6(3): 328–335

Friis M L 1979 Epilepsy among parents of children with facial clefts. Epilepsia 20: 69–76

Friis M L, Holm N V, Sindrup E H, Fogh-Anderson P, Hauge M 1986 Facial clefts in sibs and children of epileptic patients. Neurology 36: 346–350

Gautray J P, Jolivet A, Goldenberg F, Tajchner G, Eberhard A 1978 Clinical investigation of the menstrual cycle. II. Neuroendocrine investigation and therapy of the inadequate luteal phase. Fertility and sterility 29: 275–281

Gerken H, Kiefer R, Doose H, Völzke E 1977 Genetic factors in childhood epilepsy with focal sharp waves. I. Clinical data and familial morbidity for seizures. Neuropüdiatrie 8: 3–9

German J, Ehlers K H, Kowal A, DeGeorge F V, Engel M A, Passarge E 1970 Possible teratogenicity of the methadione and paramethadione. Lancet 2: 261–262

Goetting M G 1985 Catamenial exacerbation of action myoclonus: successful treatment with acetazolamide. Journal of Neurology, Neurosurgery and Psychiatry 40: 1304–1305

Gowers W R 1885 Epilepsy and other chronic convulsive disorders, their causes, symptoms and treatment. William Wood, New York, p 164

Greenwood R, Fenwick P B C, Cunliffe W J 1983 Acne and anticonvulsants. British Medical Journal 287: 1669–1670

Griffiths G M, Fox J T 1938 Rhythm in epilepsy. Lancet 2: 409–416

Hall S M 1977 Treatment of menstrual epilepsy with a progesterone-only oral contraceptive. Epilepsia 18: 235–236

Hanson J W, Smith D W 1975 The fetal hydantion syndrome. Journal of Pediatrics 87: 285–290

Hanson J W, Myrianthopoulos N C, Harvey M A S, Smith D W 1976 Risks to the offspring of women treated with hydantion anticonvulsants, with emphasis on the fetal hydantion syndrome. Journal of Pediatrics 89(4): 662–668

Herranz J L, Arteaga R, Armijo J A 1981 Change in hair colour induced by valproic acid. Developmental Medicine and Child Neurology 23: 386–387

Hempel E, Klinger W 1976 Drug stimulated biotransformation of hormonal steroid contraceptives: clinical implications. Drugs 12: 442–448

Herzog A G, Russell V, Vaitukaitis J L, Geschwind N 1982 Neuroendocrine dysfunction in temporal lobe epilepsy. Archives of Neurology 39: 133–135

Hiilesmaa V K, Bardy A H, Granström M-L, Teramo K A W 1980 Valproic acid during pregnancy. Lancet 1:883

Hiilesmaa V H, Bardy A, Teramo K 1985 Obstetric outcome in women with epilepsy. American Journal of Obstetrics and Gynaecology 152(5) 499–503

Hiilesmaa V K, Teramo K, Granstrom M L 1981 Fetal head growth retardation associated with maternal antiepileptic drugs. Lancet 2: 165–167

Houck J C, Cheng R F, Waters M D 1972 In: Woodbury D W, Penry J K, Schmidt D (eds) Antiepileptic drugs, Raven Press, New York, pp 267–274

Inoue F, Harrison J V 1981 Folic acid and phenytoin hyperplasia. Lancet 2:86

Jeavons P M, Clark J E, Harding G F A 1977 Valproate and curly hair. Lancet 1:359

Kaneko S, Hirano T, Fukushima, Sato T, Nomura Y, Shinagawa S, Ogawa Y 1983 Foetal head growth retardation due to antiepileptic drugs: with reference to GH, TSH, T4, T3 and reverse T3 concentrations. Folia Psychiatrica et Neurologica 37 (1): 25–32

Kaneko S, Sato T, Suzuki K 1979 The levels of anticonvulsants in breast milk. British Journal of Clinical Pharmacology 7: 624–626

Kelly T E, Edwards P, Rein M, Miller J Q, Dreifuss F E 1984a. Teratogenicity of anticonvulsant drugs. II: A prospective study. American Journal of Medical Genetics 19: 435–443

Kelly T E, Rein M, Edwards P 1984b Teratogenicity of anticonvulsant drugs. IV The association of clefting and epilepsy. American Journal of Medical Genetics 19: 451–458

Knight A H, Rhind E G 1975 A study of 153 pregnancies in 59 patients. Epilepsia 16: 99–110

Koch S, Hartmann A, Jäger-Roman E, Rating D, Helge H 1982 Major malformations in children of epileptic parents – due to epilepsy or its therapy? In Janz D, Bossi L, Dam M, Helge H, Richens A, Schmidt D (eds) Epilepsy, Pregnancy and the child. Raven Press, New York, pp 313–315

Laidlaw J 1956 Catamenial epilepsy. Lancet 271: 1235–1237

Lander C M, Smith M T, Chalk J B, de Wytt C, Symoniw P, Livingstone I, Eadie M J 1984 Bioavailability and pharmacokinetics of phenytoin during pregnancy. European Journal of Clinical Pharmacology 27: 105–110

Lefebvre E, Haining R G, Labbe R F 1972 Coarse facies, calvarial thickening and hyperphosphatasia associated with long-term anticonvulsant therapy. New England Journal of Medicine 286: 1301–1302

Lennox W G 1960 Epilepsy and related disorders vol. 2. Little, Brown, Boston, p 6646

Lindhout D, Meinardi H 1982 False-negative pregnancy test women taking carbamazepine. Lancet 2:505

Lindhout D, Meinardi H, Barth P G 1982. Hazards of fetal exposure to drug combinations. In: Janz D, Bossi L, Dam M, Helge H, Richens A, Schmidt D (eds) Epilepsy, pregnancy and the child. Raven Press, New York, pp 275–281

Locock C 1857 Discussion of Sieveking H Analysis of fifty two cases of epilepsy observed by the author. Lancet 1: 527–528

Logothetis J, Harner R, Morrell F, Torres F 1959 The role of estrogens in catamenial exacerbation of epilepsy. Neurology 9: 352–360

Loughnan P M, Gold H, Vance J C 1973 Phenytoin teratogenticity in man. Lancet 1: 70–72

Mattson R H, Cramer J A, Caldwell B V, Siconolfi B C 1984 Treatment of seizures with medroxyprogesterone acetate:

preliminary report. Neurology 34: 1255–1258

Mirkin B L 1971 Diphenylhydantion: placental transport, fetal localisation, neonatal metabolism and possible teratogenic effects. Journal of Pediatrics 78: 329–337

Monson R R, Rosenberg L, Hartz S C, Shapiro S, Heinonen O P, Slone D 1973 Diphenylhydantion and selected congenital malformations. New England Journal of Medicine 289: 1049–1052

Nakane Y, Okuma T, Takahashi R et al 1980 Multi-institutional study on the teratogenicity and fetal toxicity of antiepileptic drugs: a report of a collaborative study group in Japan. Epilepsia 21: 663–679

Nau H, Rating D, Koch I, Häuser I, Helge H 1981 Valproic acid and its metabolites: placental transfer, neonatal pharmàcokinetics, transfer via mothers milk and clinical status in neonates of epileptic mothers. Journal of Pharmacology and Experimental Therapeutics 219: 768–777

Newmark M E, Penry J K 1980 Catamenial epilepsy: a review. Epilepsia 21: 281–300

Notelovitz M, Tjapkes J, Ware M 1979 Interaction between estrogen and dilantin in a menopausal woman. New England Journal of Medicine 304: 788–789

Orme M 1983 Oral contraceptives and anticonvulsant drugs. British Journal of Clinical Practice. (symp. suppl. 2) 26–30

Paskind H A, Brown M 1936 Constitutional differences between deteriorated and non deteriorated patients with epilepsy. Archives of Neurology and Psychiatry 36: 1037–1044

Pastrňák M 1967 The influence of lunar and seasonal periodicity on epileptic seizures. Československá Neurologie 30: 268–276

Perucca E, Ruprah M, Richens A 1981 Decreased serum protein binding of diazepam and valproic acid in pregnant women. British Journal of Clinical Pharmacology 12:276

Phelan M C, Pellock J M, Nance W E 1982 Discordant expression of fetal hydantion syndrome in heteropaternal dizygotic twins. New England Journal of Medicine 307(2): 99–101

Ramilo J, Harris V J 1979 Neuroblastoma in a child with the hydantion and fetal alcohol syndrome. The radiographic features. British Journal of Radiology 52: 993–995

Ramsay R E, Strauss R G, Wilder J, James L 1978 Status epilepticus in pregnancy: effects of phenytoin malabsorption on seizure control. Neurology 28: 85–89

Rane A, Bertilsson L, Palmér L 1975 Disposition of placentally transferred carbamazepine (tegretol) in the newborn. European Journal of Clinical Pharmacology 8: 283–284

Rościszewska D 1981 Analysis of seizure dispersion during menstrual cycle in women with epilepsy. Monographs in Neural Sciences 5: 280–284

Rościszewska D, Buntner B, Guz I, Zawisza L 1986 Ovarian hormones, anticonvulsant drugs, and seizures during the menstrual cycle in women with epilepsy. Journal of Neurology, Neurosurgery and Psychiatry 49: 47–51

Sabin M, Oxorn H 1956 Epilepsy and pregnancy. Obstetrics and Gynecology 7(2): 175–179

Schelp A O, Speciali J G 1983a Estudo clinico da epilepsia catamenial. Tipos clinicos das crises epilepticas. Arquivos de Neuro-Psiquiatria 41 (2): 152–157

Schelp A O, Speciali J G 1983b Estudo clinica da epilepsia catamenial. Signficado da presença de lesao cerebral previa. Arquivos de Neuro-Psiquiatria 41 (2): 158–162

Schmidt D, Beck-Mannagetta G, Janz D, Koch S 1982 The effect of pregnancy on the course of epilepsy: a prospective study. In: Janz D, Bossi L, Dam M, Helge H, Richens A, Schmidt D (eds) Epilepsy, pregnancy and the child. Raven Press, New York, pp 39–49

Schmidt D 1982 The effect of pregnancy on the natural history of epilepsy: review of the literature. In: Janz D, Bossi L, Dam M, Helge H, Richens A, Schmidt D (eds) Epilepsy, pregnancy and the child. Raven Press, New York, pp 3–14

Schmidt D, Canger R, Avanzini G, Battino D, Cusi C 1983 Change in seizure frequency in pregnant epileptic women. Journal of Neurology, Neurosurgery and Psychiatry 46: 751–755

Shapiro S, Hartz S C, Siskind V et al 1976 Anticonvulsants and parental epilepsy in the development of birth defects. Lancet 1: 272–275

Shavit G, Lerman P, Korczyn A D, Kivity S, Bechar M, Gitter S 1984 Phenytoin pharmacokinetics in catamenial epilepsy. Neurology 34: 959–961

Sillanpää M 1981 Carbamazepine. Pharmacology and clinical uses. Acta Neurologica Scandinavica (suppl. 88) 64: 148–150

Smithells R W, Sheppard S, Schorah C J et al 1980 Possible prevention of neural-tube defects by periconceptional vitamin supplementation. Lancet 1: 339–340

Sonnen A E H 1983 Sodium valproate and the contraceptive pill. British Journal of Clinical Practice (symp. suppl. 27) 31–36

Strickler S M, Miller M A, Andermann E, Dansky L V, Seni M, Spielberg S P 1985 Genetic predisposition to phenytoin-induced birth defects. Lancet 2: 746–749

Stuart M J, Cross S J, Elrad H, Graeber J E 1982 Effects of acetylsalicylic-acid ingestion on maternal and neonatal and hemostasis. New England Journal of Medicine 307: 909–912

Svigos J M 1984 Epilepsy and pregnancy. Australia and New Zealand Journal of Obstetrics and Gynaecology 24: 182–185

Symonds E M 1986 Fits and hypertension in pregnancy. Hospital Update February: 103–108

Taylor D C 1969 Sexual behaviour and epilepsy. Archives of Neurology. 21: 510–516

Temkin O 1971 The falling sickness. 2nd edn. Johns Hopkins, Baltimore, p 32

Teramo K, Hiilesmaa V, Bardy A, Saarikoski S 1979 Foetal heart rate during a maternal grand mal epileptic seizure. Journal of Perinatal Medicine 7: 3–6

Terasawa E, Timiras P S 1968 Electrical activity during the oestrus cycle of the rat: cyclic changes in limbic structures. Endocrinology 83: 207–216

Thorneycroft I H, Mishell D R, Stone S C, Kharma K M, Nakamura R M 1971 The relation of serum 17-hydroxyprogesterone and estradiol -17B levels during the human menstrual cycle. American Journal of Obstetrics and Gynaecology 111: 947–951

Trimble M R 1978 Serum prolactin in epilepsy and hysteria. British Medical Journal 2:1682

Walshe M M 1972 Cutaneous drug effects in epilepsy. Transactions of St John's Hospital Dermatological Society 58: 269–281

Werboff J, Corcoran J B 1961 Effects of sex hormone manipulation on audiogenic seizures. American Journal of Physiology 201: 830–832

World Health Organization 1984 Valproate and pregnancy. WHO Drug Information Bulletin

Wilker R, Nathenson G 1982 Combined fetal alcohol and hydantion syndromes. Clinical Pediatrics 21 (6): 331–334

Woolley D E, Timiras P C 1962 Estrus and circadian periodicity and electroshock convulsions in rats. American Journal of Physiology 202: 379–382

Yerby M, Koepsell T, Daling J 1985 Pregnancy complications and outcomes in a cohort of women with epilepsy. Epilepsia 26(6) 631–635

Zimmerman A W, Holden K R, Reiter E O, Dekaban A S 1973 Medroxyprogesterone acetate in the treatment of seizures associated with menstruation. Journal of Pediatrics 89: 959–963

PART THREE
DENTAL PROBLEMS IN EPILEPSY
M. Addy

The dental care of both normal, healthy individuals and those with a variety of medical disorders, has in recent years been facilitated by a greater understanding of the etiology of the major dental diseases; namely, caries (tooth decay) and periodontal (gum) disease. Such knowledge has provided the possibility of preventing these prevalent conditions through public health measures, including water fluoridation and individual advice and instruction, notably on oral hygiene methods and the use of fluoride toothpastes. Furthermore, modern equipment and advances in dental materials have improved and extended the range of restorative dental treatment available for patients attending the dental surgery. Despite these factors, certain individuals provide particular problems to the dental profession and include those with epilepsy. These problems are not unique to epilepsy, but can be considered under the headings of

1. Routine dental care
2. Drug-induced oral changes
3. Traumatic injuries
4. Collapse in the dental surgery

ROUTINE DENTAL CARE

From a dental care point of view, it is important to consider individuals who suffer from epilepsy which is not associated with other physical or mental handicaps as essentially normal. Patients with epilepsy have invariably been well assessed medically before presenting for dental treatment (Hassel et al 1979). For this reason, there are no contraindications to performing operative dental procedures under local anaesthesia on an out-patient basis as for normal individuals. General anaesthesia also is not contraindicated for these patients, but a decision to use this should be made after discussion with the anaesthetist and also be based upon its requirement for the dental surgical procedure rather than the fact that the patient has epilepsy.

Ideally, the dental practitioner should be provided with the necessary information concerning the epileptic patient, either directly or through the consulting physician. Information concerning the type, frequency and severity of seizures, including the duration of episodes and known precipitating factors, are most useful to treatment planning and timing. Details of the drug regimen must be known by the dental practitioner, particularly as this may relate to drug interactions and, most importantly, the problems of gingival overgrowth associated with phenytoin.

Preventive advice and instruction is often more important for the epileptic patients than for normal individuals, particularly as it may relate to the prevention of occurrence or recurrence of gingival overgrowth. Gingival inflammation (chronic gingivitis) is caused by the accumulation of bacterial plaque at the gum margin (Löe et al 1965) and is highly prevalent in most populations by the early teens (Sheiham 1969). Progression of the inflammation to the supporting structures (chronic periodontitis) occurs in significant numbers of individuals and is a major cause of tooth loss in adults (Ramfjord et al 1968). Advice on effective toothbrushing should be established at an early age. For the person with epilepsy this may be more difficult to attain because of the greater attention paid to the neurological disorder than to personal hygiene or because of the reduction in mental and physical capabilities associated

with epilepsy or the prescribed medication (Reynolds 1975). Certainly, poor oral hygiene has been frequently reported in studies on the dental health of epileptic children and adolescents (Ass 1963, Lundstrom et al 1982, O'Neil & Figures 1982) and is an indication of the need for preventive care in this group.

Whilst there is little evidence to indicate that epileptic children are more prone to dental caries (Lundstrom et al 1982), despite in some cases drug-induced reduced saliva flow and salivary buffering capacity (Lundstrom et al 1982, Babcock & Nelson 1964), they are not any less susceptible than the normal population. Dental caries essentially results from the metabolism on the tooth surface of dietary refined carbohydrate, particularly sucrose, by bacterial plaque to produce acid (Hartles & Leach 1975). The most effective preventive approach to date has been directed towards decreasing the susceptibility of the tooth to such attack by the use of fluoride administration, either via the water supply or, as fluoride supplements, in particular toothpastes (Murray 1976). In the absence of water fluoridation, the use of such supplements should be encouraged at an early age, together with dietary advice concerning a reduction in the frequency of refined carbohydrate intake. Such information and advice should be given, where necessary, to parents or guardians of epileptic children. Additionally, sugar-free medicines should be prescribed, since prolonged therapy with sugar-containing syrups may itself become a regular source of sugar intake with well established detrimental effects to the dentition.

Restorative dental treatment for epileptic patients should be directed towards conserving an intact dentition. If possible, the provision of partial dentures should be avoided. This is not only because of the remote danger of inhalation of the whole or part of the prosthesis during a seizure, but also because of the extra burden such an appliance places on the maintenance of satisfactory oral hygiene (Bates & Addy 1978). Complex restorative treatment for such patients must be determined on the merits of each case, and factors relative to the epileptic condition, oral hygiene and drug-induced changes must all be taken into account when planning treatment for such patients. Orthodontic treatment for the adolescent or adult epileptic similarly has to be judged on the same grounds and is certainly not necessarily contraindicated. However, it is advisable that each case be assessed by a specialist or consultant orthodontist.

DRUG INDUCED ORAL CHANGES

Phenytoin gingival enlargement

Phenytoin, despite having many side-effects (Reynolds 1975), is widely used in the management of epilepsy because of well-established clinical benefits. Gingival enlargement or hyperplasia associated with phenytoin medication is arguably the most common dental problem of epilepsy and was first described in 1939 (Kimball 1939). Variable gingival enlargement occurs in approximately half the patients receiving phenytoin (Panuska et al 1961, Babcock 1965) but prevalence figures of 3% to 78% have been reported (Lennox 1940, Gardner et al 1962) and up to 93% for institutionalized groups (Kapur et al 1973). Gingival overgrowth commences within two to three months of the start of medication and usually stabilizes by 12 to 18 months (Livingston et al 1979). Complete or partial regression may follow cessation of phenytoin use (Lundstrom et al 1982). Although not finally proven, the balance of evidence suggests that phenytoin dosage and, more importantly, serum phenytoin levels do not correlate with either the incidence or severity of hyperplasia (Hassel et al 1984). Institutionalized groups are stated to be more commonly affected, as are individuals commencing therapy in childhood as opposed to in adulthood. Males have in some studies been found to be more commonly affected than females (Hassel et al 1984). However, the importance of co-variables in the aetiology of phenytoin hyperplasia, notably oral hygiene differences, do not permit absolute conclusions to be drawn as to the importance of environment, age or sex to the prevalence and severity of phenytoin gingival enlargement.

Drug-induced gingival hyperplasia typically affects the dentate areas and enlargement of the interdental papillae is the most characteristic feature. Rarely has phenytoin induced gingival enlargement been reported before tooth eruption (Church & Brandt 1983) or in edentulous areas of the mouth (Dreyer & Thomas 1978), and even in these cases the possibility of an alternative aetiology must be considered. In most cases of gingival enlargement, the patient's history and the clinical findings are sufficient to confirm the diagnosis. However, drug-induced gingival enlargement is not unique to phenytoin and recently has been noted with the immunosuppressant cyclosporin A (Adams & Davies 1984) and the angina prophylactic drug nifedipine (Lucas et al 1985). Histologically the gingival enlargement produced by cyclosporin A and nifedipine is similar to that associated with phenytoin. Pathogenesis of gingival enlargement produced by phenytoin is still not clearly established and appears to be dependent on the interaction of a number of variables. The major factors are considered to be the susceptibility of the individual and this may in part be genetically determined (Hassell & Gilbert 1983), the direct effect of phenytoin or one of its metabolites on connective tissue elements and the oral hygiene and related gingival inflammation present (Hassel 1981). Certainly, the relationship of poor oral hygiene and increased gingival hyperplasia has been consistently noted.

Ideally, the complete control of phenytoin gingival enlargement would require the use of alternative antiepileptic drugs. Effective drugs, including sodium valproate and carbamazepine, appear not to produce any oral changes even in the presence of poor oral hygiene (Lundstrum et al 1982, Eeg-Olofsson et al 1983). However, the choice of medication must be based upon effectiveness in controlling epilepsy rather than the oral side-effects. Despite this, when phenytoin is to be used there is evidence to indicate that improvements in oral hygiene can prevent or markedly reduce gingival enlargement (Ciancio et al 1972). Unfortunately, the findings were based on closely supervised oral hygiene by professionals, which may be impractical for most individuals. Moreover, it is known that initial improvements in home plaque control are not maintained (Sheiham 1970). Despite this, there would appear a need for close liaison between the physician and dental practitioner. Improvements in oral hygiene for epileptic patients who are to receive, or have commenced, phenytoin, should be made at an early stage particularly as gingival enlargement, if it is to occur, commences within two to three months of the start of therapy (Livingston et al 1979).

The use of chemical plaque control measures as an adjunct to toothbrushing should also be considered in the prevention of the occurrence of gingival hyperplasia. A 10 ml dose of 0.2% chlorhexidine gluconate mouthwash used twice daily is well established as the most effective antiplaque agent available (Addy 1986) with benefits reported in the prevention of phenytoin gingival overgrowth (O'Neil & Figures 1982). The antiseptic can be safely employed for extended periods and is free of systemic side-effects. Unfortunately, local side-effects, including taste disturbance and more importantly progressive brown discoloration of the teeth, may limit prolonged use in some individuals. Nevertheless, the brown discoloration, which is related to the dietary intake of chromogenic beverages such as tea (Addy & Moran 1985), can be removed by a professional polishing of the teeth at intervals.

In established phenytoin gingival enlargement the decision concerning possible lines of treatment are dependent upon associated aesthetic or functional problems. Furthermore, the likelihood of recurrence of the enlargement following surgical removal must be appreciated. First therefore, it is appropriate to discuss with the consulting physician the possibility of using alternative antiepileptic therapy for an individual patient but, again, the effectiveness of the present drug regime in controlling the epilepsy must take precedence. If alternative drug therapy is possible then a decision concerning surgical removal of the enlarged gingiva should be delayed for a period to determine whether some natural remission in the enlargement will occur. When alternative therapy is not possible and there are aesthetic and/or functional problems, the gingivectomy procedure can be used to remove excessive gingival tissue. In view of the likelihood of recurrence, it is sensible to limit the surgical removal of tissue only to those areas of the mouth which are creating the problem. Thus, typically where aesthetic difficulties are present, surgical removal of gingiva from the upper or lower anterior teeth is the usual

course of action. A decision concerning further surgical intervention can be made at a later date dependent upon the stability of the treated areas. Both before and after surgical intervention, oral hygiene practices by the patient must be improved and maintained. Here again, the use of a chlorhexidine gluconate mouthwash is a useful adjunct to plaque control (O'Neil & Figures 1982).

Dental abnormalities

Although phenytoin gingival hyperplasia is the most common oral problem associated with this drug, the changes appear only part of a more widespread connective tissue reaction (Reynolds 1975). Reduced skeletal growth and premature epiphyseal fusion has been noted in children receiving phenytoin; the condition appears to be a pseudohypoparathyroidism (Robinson et al 1983). Associated with this, dental changes, including smaller teeth, delayed shedding of the deciduous dentition and delayed eruption of permanent teeth, have been noted (Girgis et al 1980, Robinson et al 1983). Root resorption may also occur (Harris & Goldhaber 1974) and in part accounts for the smaller crown:root ratio seen in patients receiving phenytoin (Girgis et al 1980). Since these dental irregularities are largely developmental, as are the skeletal changes, their control is dependent upon the initial decision to use phenytoin in the management of each individual.

TRAUMATIC INJURIES

During epileptic seizures, traumatic injuries to the oral mucosae may occur as a result of collapse against a hard surface or biting of tissue, particularly the tongue. Such injuries are easily diagnosed; however, the possibility of foreign bodies within the tissues must be considered and may include tooth fragments. If in doubt, soft tissue radiographs should be obtained. Most intra-oral lacerations heal without problems, although occasionally they may require suturing. The use of a chlorhexidine gluconate mouth rinse may be useful to reduce bacterial contamination of the wounds and help maintain oral hygiene during a phase when toothbrushing may be difficult due to discomfort (Addy 1986). Similarly, damage to the teeth may occur as a result of either collapse or excessive biting forces during the period of seizure. Fractures of the crowns of teeth are readily diagnosed and require treatment in the appropriate manner. Root fractures, cracked cusps or split roots are not always so easily discovered and it is advisable, where there is the possibility of such damage, that the patient be referred to a dental practitioner for clinical and radiographic examination. Facial lacerations and fractures of the jaws and facial skeleton may also occur as a result of collapse and, here again, patients should be referred to the appropriate hospital department for diagnosis and management.

COLLAPSE IN THE DENTAL SURGERY

An epileptic seizure is one form of collapse in the dental surgery for which a dental practitioner and his or her staff should be prepared. Management of this problem is primarily directed towards preventing the patients injuring themselves and avoiding airway obstruction. At the first sign of a fit, all possible equipment or material must be immediately removed from the patient's mouth and the chair should be tilted to the low-line position. No attempt should be made to restrain the patient nor should a gag be placed between the patient's teeth. Equipment on the bracket trays or satellite units should be moved away from the dental chair. At most, the patient's movements should be guided by the dental surgeon or the assistant. Partially set impression material in trays must not be removed, but the tray fixed against the appropriate jaw and guided with movements of the patients. After a seizure, the patients should be allowed a period of rest and arrangements made for them to be escorted home once recovery is considered complete.

In cases of status epilepticus occurring in the dental surgery, management will depend on the experience of the dental surgeon and the facilities available. In most instances expert medical assistance should be summoned. A slow intravenous injection of diazepam may be given and an approximate total dose of 0.2 mg/kg is usually sufficient to control such cases although larger doses may be required.

REFERENCES

Adams D, Davies G 1984 Gingival hyperplasia associated with Cyclosporin A. British Dental Journal 157: 89–91

Addy M, Moran J 1985 Extrinsic tooth discolouration by metals and chlorhexidine. II. Clinical staining produced by chlorhexidine, iron and tea. British Dental Journal 159: 331–334

Addy M 1986 Chlorhexidine compared with other locally delivered antimicrobials – a short review. Journal of Clinical Periodontology 13: 957–964

Ass E 1963 Hyperplasia gingivae diphenylhydantoinea. A clinical, histological and biochemical study. Acta Odontologica Scandinavica 21 (suppl. 34)

Babcock J P, Nelson G H 1964 Gingival hyperplasia and Dilantin content of saliva: a pilot study. Journal of the American Dental Association 68: 195–198

Babcock J R 1965 Incidence of gingival hyperplasia associated with Dilantin therapy: Journal of the American Dental Association 71: 1447–1450

Bates J F, Addy M 1978 Partial dentures and plaque accumulation. Journal of Dentistry 6: 285–293

Church L F, Brandt S K 1983 Phenytoin-induced gingival overgrowth resulting in delayed eruption of the primary dentition. Journal of Periodontology 55: 19–21

Ciancio S G, Yaffe S J, Catz C C 1972 Gingival hyperplasia and diphenylhydantoin. Journal of Periodontology 43: 411–414

Dreyer W P, Thomas C J 1978 Diphenylhydantoinate-induced hyperplasia of the masticatory mucosa in an edentulous epileptic patient. Oral Surgery 45: 701–704

Eeg-Olofsson O, Lundstrom A, Hamp A S 1983 Oral state of children with epilepsy on treatment with sodium valproate. Scandinavian Journal of Dental Research 91: 219–223

Gardner A F, Gross S G, Wynne L E 1962 An investigation of gingival hyperplasia resulting from diphenylhydantoin sodium therapy in seventy-seven mentally retarded patients. Experimental Medicine and Surgery 20: 133–158

Girgis S S, Staple P H, Miller W A, Sedransk N, Thompson T 1980 Dental root abnormalities and gingival overgrowth in epileptic patients receiving anticonvulsant therapy. Journal of Periodontology 51: 474–482

Harris M, Goldhaber P 1974 Root abnormalities in epileptics and the inhibition of parathyroid hormone induced bone resorption in vitro. British Journal of Pharmacology 50: 405–408

Hartles R, Leach S A 1975 Effect of diet on dental caries. British Medical Bulletin 31: 137–141

Hassel T M, Dudley K H, Hirsch P F, Hutchens L H, Johnston M C, Moriarty J D 1979 Summary of an international symposium on phenytoin-induced teratology and gingival pathology. Journal of the American Dental Association 99: 652–655

Hassell T 1981 Epilepsy and the oral manifestations of phenytoin therapy. In: Myres H M (eds) Monographs in oral science vol 9. S Karger, Basel

Hassell T, Gilbert G H 1983 Phenytoin sensitivity of fibroblasts as the basis for susceptibility to gingival enlargement. American Journal of Pathology 112: 218–223

Hassell T, O'Donnell J, Pearlman J, Tesini D, Murphy T, Best T 1984 Phenytoin induced gingival overgrowth in institutionalised epileptics. Journal of Clinical Periodontology 11: 242–253

Kapur R N, Girgis S, Little T M, Masotti R E 1973 Diphenylhydantoin-induced gingival hyperplasia: its relation to dose and serum level. Developmental Medicine and Child Neurology 15: 483–487

Kimball O P 1939 The treatment of epilepsy with sodium diphenylhydantoinate. Journal of the American Dental Association 112: 1244–1245

Lennox W G 1940 The drug therapy of epilepsy. Journal of the American Medical Association 114: 1347–1351

Livingston S, Pruce S, Pauli L L, Livingston H L 1979 The medical treatment of epilepsy: Managing side effects of anti-epileptic drugs. Paediatric Annals 8: 261–265

Löe H, Theilade E, Jensen S B 1965 Experimental gingivitis in man. Journal of Periodontology 36: 177–187

Lucas R M, Howell L P, Wall B A 1985 Nifedipine-induced gingival hyperplasia. Journal of Periodontology 56: 211–215

Lundstrom A, Eeg-Ofofsson O, Hamp S E 1982 Effects of anti-epileptic drug treatment with carbamazepine or phenytoin on the oral state of children and adolescents. Journal of Clinical Periodontology 9: 482–488

Murray J J 1976 Fluorides in caries prevention. Dental practitioner handbook no 20. John Wright, Bristol, pp 60–80

O'Neil T C A, Figures K H 1982 The effects of chlorhexidine and mechanical methods of plaque control on the recurrence of gingival hyperplasia in young patients taking phenytoin. British Dental Journal 152: 130–133

Panuska H J, Gorlin R J, Bearman J E, Mitchell D F 1961 The effects of anticonvullsant drugs upon the gingiva – a series of analyses of 1048 patients. Journal of Periodontology 32: 15–19

Ramfjord S P, Emslie R O, Green J C, Held A J, Waerhaug J 1968 Epidemiological studies of periodontal diseases. American Journal of Public Health 58: 1713–1722

Reynolds E H 1975 Chronic anti-epileptic toxicity: a review. Epilepsia 16: 319–352

Robinson P B, Harris M, Harvey W 1983 Abnormal skeletal and dental growth in epileptic children. British Dental Journal 154: 9–13

Sheiham A 1969 The prevalence and severity of periodontal disease in Surrey school children. Dental Practice 19: 232–238

Sheiham A 1970 Dental cleanliness and chronic periodontal disease: studies on populations in Britain. British Dental Journal 129: 413–418

16

Social aspects of epilepsy

A. Craig
J. Oxley

INTRODUCTION

A philosophy of health care

The study of the epilepsies is already so diverse, and expanding so rapidly, that it cannot be easily encompassed by a single physician's competence, however skilled he or she may be. We believe it is only right, therefore, for epilepsy services to adopt a multiprofessional team approach. This means that equal emphasis must be given to clinical and social aspects of the epilepsies and their consequential impact on those around the person with epilepsy, in the family, at school, at work and in the wider community. Already health care workers other than doctors, for instance nurse practitioners, are beginning to function in some countries as the key workers for people with chronic conditions and disabilities (Stilwell 1986). For people with established, treated epilepsy, Bowman et al (1984) have argued that use of specialist nurses can reduce dependence on medical facilities while at the same time increasing opportunities for patient education, counselling and support; the needs for which often persist past the stabilization of seizures. Recent recommendations for community health services in the United Kingdom, especially the Cumberlege Report on Neighbourhood Nursing (DHSS 1986), reinforce the argument for many people with long-term conditions such as epilepsy to be helped by a circle of professionals much wider than doctors. We hope that they, as well as medical practitioners, will find the following discussion of the social aspects of epilepsy useful in approaching the comprehensive care of people with epilepsy.

Neurology, psychiatry and psychology; the sociology of health and illness; health economics and social anthropology; genetics and endocrinology; paediatrics and gerontology; aspects of the civil and criminal law; and considerable portions of social policy and administration – these are the aspects of the epilepsies in the modern world which demand teamwork for effective mastery (Hermann 1980). The individual doctor, nurse, social worker, psychologist, health educationist, teacher or other professional worker needs to be aware of the matrix of expertise available and be able to exploit it with enthusiasm if all those affected by the epilepsies are to gain optimum benefit (Beintema 1983, Betts 1983, Parsonage 1983).

The conventional approach to this objective is to seek more funding for professional staff and clinical facilities. This is increasingly untenable in world economic terms (O'Neill 1983). Even the wealthiest countries have found that they cannot sustain indefinitely heavily resourced, high technology, comprehensive epilepsy programmes, much less expand them uniformly. Even if less developed countries could afford it, this model for epilepsy services is not appropriate for the bulk of the world's population who live in countries far removed from even relative affluence. For them, progress will most probably come with the development of services within the domain of primary health care (WHO 1978). The training manual on epilepsy in the World Health Organization publication *Training Disabled People in the Community* (Helander et al 1983) is an example of the primary health care approach which does not depend on high-level investment in professional skills or technology.

An emphasis on primary health care for epilepsy

is also very relevant in the more developed nations. It can help reach sectors of the population whose needs in relation to epilepsy may be poorly served by secondary (hospital-based) epilepsy services, and thus contribute towards the achievement of general targets for improving the quality of life for disabled people (WHO 1985). In the United Kingdom there should be more emphasis on improving the expertise and enthusiasm for managing the epilepsies within general practice and primary health care teams, with appropriate involvement of consultants with a special interest in epilepsy and, where necessary, liaison and referral to special diagnostic and rehabilitation centres (DHSS 1986).

Expertise and enthusiasm are two parts of the professional's ideal approach to the epilepsies. The third key input is empathy; all the more attractive because it can be combined with the first two elements without additional resources. This is not a plea for sympathy. It is an exhortation to the professional worker first to seek understanding of the personal impact of epilepsy and then to use this as the foundation on which to establish a partnership in which treatment can be initiated, pursued and modified as necessary to cope with the inevitable vicissitudes of living with epilepsy (Scambler & Hopkins 1986, Buchanan 1982, Mostofsky 1978).

In 1891, the American physician and jurist Oliver Wendell Holmes wrote: 'If I wished to show a student the difficulties of getting at truth from medical experience, I would give him the history of epilepsy to read' (Holmes 1891). The study of epilepsy, or more accurately of the epilepsies, is undoubtedly a vehicle for imparting wider understanding. It can open 'a window on the mechanisms of the brain' (Lockard & Ward 1980). Paradoxically, and despite considerable advances in recent decades in diagnosis and management, Gowers' verdict (1901) that 'the ultimate course of epilepsy can never be foreseen' remains instructive. This holds true as much for the social course of epilepsy as it does for its physiological course.

Were he alive today, Dr Holmes would no doubt emphasize to his enquiring student several transcendent themes in the case histories of people with epilepsy: adjustment to an unpredictable and sometimes disabling disorder; coping with hurtful

social misconceptions and eroded self-esteem; and often having to struggle against the misplaced certainties expressed by some professional workers about 'epileptics'. Recently, in the course of compiling a video programme about attitudes to epilepsy, the author interviewed a cross-section of people with epilepsy. One feature that stood out from all these interviews was a self-identified sense of 'loss' because of having epilepsy. Some of the things these people with epilepsy felt they had lost were:

1. Driving licence
2. Job
3. Promotion at work
4. Friends
5. Marriage
6. Confidence
7. Self-esteem

The most obvious loss was the driving licence, or the right to hold one for at least two years. Not all had lost jobs, but many had, and others felt that having epilepsy had held them back at work in the career and promotions stakes. This all added up to a pervading sense of lowered self-esteem. The professional epilepsy worker must become skilled in the exercise of empathy in order to identify and take account of such recurring themes. He or she must also, of course, possess the expertise to offer appropriate guidance. It is cause for concern, therefore, that in a recent survey of more than 100 British neurologists, Hopkins & Harvey (1983) found widespread confusion and sometimes lamentable ignorance about laws relating to driving and epilepsy. This needs to be interpreted in the context of each neurologist in Britain being expected to cope with about 900 people with epilepsy (McLellan 1986b). Clearly, greater expertise is needed in this particular area. Loss of a driving licence often has an obvious and profound impact on a person with epilepsy's employability and social status. The professional helper will need empathy in order to appreciate and interpret the impact of this. How many readers of this chapter would cope well both practically and psychologically with the sudden loss of their driving licence, a development which is often poorly explained and for which no alternative assistance is readily available?

Attitudes of helpers and helped

Of course any professional epilepsy worker is from time to time likely to be placed in situations in which a particular person's problem seems largely of his or her own making. Reacting by 'victim blaming' is a danger, as it may prematurely rule out the possibility that the professional's interventions, however overtly knowledgeable and well-intentioned, may not be appropriate (Buchanan 1982). Lance (1977) has suggested that the attitudes of the doctor in particular may be reflected in the patient's self-perception and his or her understanding of the place of epilepsy in his or her life. This interpretation affords considerable scope for enhancing or depressing the quality of life as a significant consequence of medical attitudes.

Reviewing recent Australian experiences, Beran (1983) found that people with epilepsy generally had confidence in their doctors and looked to them for advice and support. However, the attitudes of general practitioners (GPs) in particular, the doctors most often in contact with people with epilepsy, were often negative in the degree of support offered in the social sphere, especially employment matters. He also found anxieties amongst GPs stemming from supposed high rates of work-related accidents and the likelihood of psychological instability in their patients with epilepsy. Such findings bear out the evidence submitted to the Commission for the Control of Epilepsy and its Consequences in the USA (1978) that professional expertise and attitudes cannot be assumed to be automatically a positive factor in the life of people with epilepsy. This may in part stem from the situation recently described by McLellan (1986b) that, 'Britain has no defined establishment of consultants in rehabilitation medicine who have neurological training and a neurological bias'. This deficit rebounds both on the GP and the person with epilepsy who may be making a considerable effort to maintain a management regime in the community.

Faced with problems of professional attitudes in particular, suggestions have been made (Appolone et al 1979, Shapiro 1983) that all health workers concerned with epilepsy should be encouraged to acquire and then actively taught the skills to examine and, if necessary, to correct their perceptions about epilepsy, in order to enable them to relate to the people with epilepsy in a more lucid and comfortable manner. Effective communication between doctor and patient is obviously central to an empathetic relationship. It is worrying, therefore, that a recent study (Maguire et al 1986) highlighted serious weaknesses in young hospital doctors' skills in communication and a reluctance to explore psychosocial aspects of patients' conditions.

While the essential search continues for new techniques to gain control of established epilepsy, and to prevent the onset of new cases, the parallel search for techniques to stimulate and sustain positive attitudes in people with epilepsy, the community and professional workers must receive even greater attention (West 1983). It is in this latter domain that the battle will ultimately be won or lost. The irony is that if no one with epilepsy had another fit from tomorrow but retained the diagnosis, it would still constitute for a considerable number a real impediment in their lives. One of the aims of this chapter is to help professional workers to shed distancing and self-protecting roles. We believe this is the best way to put expertise, enthusiasm and empathy to their optimum therapeutic use and to strive towards the goal stated by Porter (1984): 'the degree of social adaptation in work, school and recreation is the final criterion for health care delivery to the patient with epilepsy'.

EDUCATION

Introduction

This section is only partly concerned with the clinical details and prognoses of the epilepsies of childhood, and the neuropsychological correlates of various seizure types on learning or behaviour. Primarily, it seeks to identify the potential impact of these factors on the educational process and the relationships between schools, teachers, children and young people with epilepsy, their families and friends. It discusses the steps which might be taken to promote normal educational and personal development, insofar as this is possible in individual cases.

Sweeping statements about 'children with epilepsy', or worse about 'epileptic children', are less helpful than information about a particular child or young person with epilepsy and the factors which might be influential in his or her development. The potential for discrimination inherent in formulating policies for school activities such as swimming, gymnastics or school trips based on generalizations about 'children with epilepsy' should be self-evident, but a positive and informed approach is required if it is to be finally eradicated. The desire to comprehend the impact of what having epilepsy means for each child is made more difficult by two factors in particular: first, the lack of precision in estimating the prevalence of established epilepsy in young people of school age, which stems mainly from the varying criteria used by major epidemiological studies, even in developed countries; and secondly, the perils of trying to predict outcomes or calculate degrees of 'risk' in relation to specific activities (Hackney 1976, 1977, 1985, Radley 1985).

On the basis of epidemiological studies (see Ch. 2) it is probable that between six and eight children in every 1000 in the United Kingdom have the experience of epilepsy during their school years. We believe that, for practical purposes, when considering the impact of epilepsy on education, it is necessary to consider a prevalence rate somewhat higher than the 4 per 1000 for established, non-febrile recurrent seizures in children revealed by the National Childhood Development Study (NCDS) (Ross et al 1980). The reality of children's epilepsy is never as tidy as a well-controlled epidemiological study. The onset of epilepsy for the child, family and school environment is of no less portent, whether it subsequently persists for only a single year or throughout schooling. To focus exclusively on the prevalence figures for established cases would be to underestimate the impact of epilepsy during the childhood years. That being said, however, it is encouraging to note (Ross & Peckham 1983) that the substantial majority (67%) of the children with epilepsy in the NCDS cohort were attending ordinary schools at the age of 11, though for secondary education this number had reduced to 58% by the age of 15.

The law on special educational needs

In England and Wales, all steps taken to identify and meet special educational needs of children and young people of school age now relate in some way to the 1981 Education Act, described as 'an Act to make provision with respect to children with special educational needs'. Scotland has separate equivalent legislation, but this has not been extended to Northern Ireland. The 1981 Act became law on 30 October 1981, but did not come into force until 1 April 1983. It is often known as the 'Warnock legislation' because it incorporates several key concepts from the Report of the Committee of Enquiry into the Education of Handicapped Children and Young People chaired by Mary Warnock (Warnock Report 1978). With respect to epilepsy the Warnock Committee's report entitled Special Educational Needs argued (para 11.43) that:

> the great majority of children who have seizures experience them only for brief periods of time, or at very long intervals. Only those who have repeated seizures, or who need continuous anti-convulsants, can justifiably be described as children with epilepsy. Most such children are educated in ordinary schools, but not all are known to their teachers. This may be because society's attitudes to epilepsy makes some parents reluctant to pass on or let their doctors pass on to the school information which they think might be embarrassing to the children. In other cases the epilepsy may be so well controlled and so much a part of everyday life that parents and children consider it hardly worth mentioning. We consider that every effort should be made to inform staff in schools and colleges about the facts of epilepsy, how it may be controlled by drugs, what the side effects of these drugs may be and how to manage seizures should they occur, in order to create the right attitudes to chidren with epilepsy. Lack of full knowledge may cause a child's activity to be unduly restricted and if the school does not know about the existence of the condition the child may run unnecessary risks. This is an instance where mutual confidence and understanding between parents, doctors and teachers is particularly important.

We have quoted this section at length to illustrate the humane and commonsense approach to epilepsy taken by the Warnock Report. It is to be regretted, therefore, that the 1981 Education Act was, perhaps inevitably, somewhat reduced in vision. Warnock was fundamentally concerned with identifying special needs stemming from the interrelationship of a wide range of health and other factors. It sought to depart from the old medically conditioned and diagnostically related concept of 'special education' identifying a place (e.g. a 'special school') where a particular type of education was provided. This older view was embodied in the 1944 Education Act (Section 8(2)(c)) and the 1959 Handicapped Pupils and Special Schools Regulations which defined ten categories of disability (blind, partially sighted, deaf, partial hearing, delicate, educationally subnormal, epileptic, maladjusted, physically handicapped and those suffering from speech defects) which might indicate a need for a special education placement.

Warnock estimated that for various reasons as many as one in five of the total school population might have educational needs requiring special help in the ordinary school from time to time. This might encompass 'the whole range and variety of additional help, whether it is provided on a full or part-time basis, by which children may be helped to overcome educational difficulties, however they are caused' (Para 3.38). Further, Warnock recognized the importance of postschool provision in order to continue meeting special educational needs. A major weakness of the 1981 Educational Act, however, is that it does not apply to further education or to other postschool activities such as Adult Training Centres and Day Centres maintained by local authorities or other bodies. The 16–19 year old with epilepsy who might have special educational needs, will only be covered by the 1981 Act if he or she remains at school; and the 1944 Education Act makes specific provision for this if requested. While staying on past the age of 16 may have undoubted advantages in terms of increasing both cognitive and social skills, there is a strong disincentive to remaining at school for many families of disabled young people. This is often because current social security regulations prohibit pupils, handicapped or not, attending ordinary schools from claiming either Supplementary Benefit or Severe Disablement Allowance if they are over the age of 16. The DHSS regulations do permit such claims if young people are in further education or outside education altogether. This is a prime example of antagonism between education law and social security law which works to the disadvantage of young adults with special needs of an educational nature. They should be able to benefit from appropriate educational provision, whether or not they are still at school, in further education or in any other postschool learning environment without compromising their social security entitlements.

Although Warnock advocated a global approach (as did the authors of the USA's Education of All Handicapped Children Act of 1975, whose implementation can be followed for comparison purposes in Vaughan & Shearer 1986), the 1981 Education Act has many shortcomings. Nonetheless, it can and should be used fully; there are potential benefits in the legislation for children, parents, teachers and school authorities, provided that the law is understood and utilised. Paediatricians, general practitioners and community nurses in particular are ideally placed to provide necessary information, especially since Health Authorities have statutory duties under the Act.

The 1981 Education Act

The following discussion seeks to identify the key concepts in the law on special educational needs and to point the reader towards sources of expanded discussion (Cox 1985, Male & Thompson 1985). The key to the 1981 Act's application is the identification of 'special educational needs' (SEN), which is no longer taken as synonymous with the existence of physical or mental impairment. Section 1(1) of the Act defines a child as having SEN if 'he has a learning difficulty which calls for special educational provision to be made for him', The Act considers a child any person up to the age of 19 years who is registered at school. The Act defines 'learning difficulty' (Section 1(2)) as present if (subject to certain exceptions concerned with mother tongues and the language of the school):

1. he has a significantly greater difficulty in learning than the majority of children of his age; or
2. he has a disability which prevents him from making use of educational facilities of the kind generally provided in schools in the Local Education Authority; or
3. he is under 5 and may fall into either of the above categories when over that age.

Clearly, some children and young people with epilepsy may, and just as easily may not, have learning difficulties in comparison with their peers, and hence have special educational needs in particular cases. As the Warnock Report believed that as many as 20% of all children might have SEN at one time or another, there is every reason to explore the potential value of this legislation for the individual child with epilepsy, even if there is no obvious problem with schooling. The Act lays great stress on assessments for discovering the existence of special needs and the role of parents, at all stages, in initiating such assessments. The Spastics Society has recently published simple guidelines (Wolfendale et al 1986) to help parents ask the important questions concerning the educational development of younger and older children. Professionals in all disciplines dealing with school-age children should be familiar with these in order to assist parents wishing to initiate an assessment for their child with epilepsy. Where a Health Authority believes that a child has, or is likely to have, SEN by school age, they are obliged by law to bring this fact to the parent's attention and to facilitate the parent's discussion of the possible implications prior to referring the case to the local education authority. Further, if the Health Authority believes that a particular voluntary body, such as an epilepsy association, is likely to be able to assist the parent with information or advice, they have a statutory duty to inform the parent accordingly.

The majority of children with epilepsy do not have obvious handicaps. If they had, and if as a result special school placements were historically the norm for such children, then the implications of the 1981 Education Act would be much more straightforward. The wide variability of epilepsy and the likely changing nature over time of a particular child's needs mean that there are no short cuts in relation to this legislation; especially as about 80% of children and young people with epilepsy are already in mainstream schools. It should not be forgotten, however, that the philosophy of the Warnock Report was that special educational needs constituted a continuum and that the focus should always be on individual assessment and reassessment at key intervals during the school career.

The statutory instrument and various circulars issued in connection with the 1981 Education Act make it clear that only the 2% of children already placed in special schools are likely automatically to be given the legal protection of a statement of their special educational needs, which is prescriptive on the local education authority. Obviously, a proportion of these children, especially those with mental handicap, will also have epilepsy and will undoubtedly benefit from the careful scrutiny afforded by a statement. However, this leaves 18% of Warnock's estimated 20% of all children who might have special needs who will probably not receive a formal statement. Their special needs, if they are identified, will be met within the ordinary provision of mainstream schools. There is potentially a major problem here for many children with epilepsy (Craig 1985). Unless there is positive intervention – most probably by parents – to have an individual child assessed, he or she, if already attending an ordinary school, may legitimately be excluded from the legally enforceable provisions of a statement of SEN. It should not be forgotten that the Act is meant to extend to all children with SEN, not just those with a formal statement. It is most likely, therefore, that a child with epilepsy will not have a formal statement, unless the epilepsy is severe or concomitant with serious mental or physical handicap. The subtleties of educational problems related to epilepsy may be overlooked in an overly bureaucratic interpretation of this legislation. Therefore it is incumbent on parents, teachers, educational psychologists, school governors and health professionals to see that this does not happen by using the assessment provisions of the Act early and to the optimum degree.

A number of guides to the legislation and its implications are available for teachers and parents (National Union of Teachers 1984, Royal Association for Disability and Rehabilitation 1984). A survey conducted in late 1985 by the National Association of Schoolmasters/Union of Women Teachers (Guardian 25.11.85) showed that only 4985 children out of 4.5 million at school in 61 Local Education Authorities had been assessed under the 1981 Act and that formal 'statements' of SEN under the 1981 Act had been made on only 54% of children already attending special schools. Obviously, it will take time to assess all children thought likely to have SEN, but authorities must not use this and the need for additional resources as reasons for undue delay in fully implementing the Act. Parents, together with school governors, have power under this legislation to press forward its objectives. The Spastics Society's Centre for Studies on Integration in Education (CSIE) is monitoring the implementation of the 1981 Education Act and publishes reports on progress. These should be the starting place for anyone wishing to find out what a particular Local Education Authority has done under this legislation (CSIE 1986).

The 1981 Act also involves children below the usual school age. This can be as relevant to a young child with epilepsy as the provision for remaining at school until the age of 19 can be for a young adult with epilepsy. For children under 5 years of age, Section 6 of the Act gives education authorities the power to carry out assessments if it is thought that special educational needs will be present by school age. For children under the age of 2, this assessment is mandatory if requested by the parent. If SEN are likely to be present, then the provisions that authorities are required to make include support and advice to help parents help their own children, e.g. mother and toddler groups and other forms of opportunities provided by social services or voluntary bodies in an educational context. From the earliest time that epilepsy is diagnosed in a child, therefore, full use should be made of these provisions in the Act concerning children under school age. It is particularly important that parents be informed of these provisions so that the benefits of early assessment and intervention for the child with epilepsy can be realised.

The research background

In the UK, the National Child Development Study (NCDS), based on a cohort of children born in 1958 and reviewed at ages 7, 11 and 16 years provides the most comprehensive picture of the range and implications of epilepsy for school age children (Rose et al 1980). Broadly speaking, results obtained from this enquiry confirm the distribution of children with epilepsy into two

groups: those with epilepsy only, for whom it may or may not constitute a problem in school terms from time to time; and those whose epilepsy is complicated by other factors. The latter have traditionally tended to be segregated in special schools where their educational progress was often disappointing and their opportunities to experience the usual experiences of growing up in the everyday world were limited (Kurtz & Bennett 1981). Undoubtedly, for some children who are more handicapped by their epilepsy and other problems, special schools, especially residential special schools for children with epilepsy, will continue to be the most appropriate place for their special educational needs to be met. Where such facilities are retained, it is imperative that they should have close links with specialist medical facilities; involvement on a regular basis with parents; and a wider range of educational provision, e.g. links with further education colleges nearby. The pattern of special schooling is changing, and the trend in the UK, as in other developed nations, is for optimum integration of children with special educational needs into ordinary, 'mainstream' schools. In tackling the objective of integrated schooling, the experiences of other countries deserve close study (Vaughan & Shearer 1986).

A brief summary of the NCDS findings about epilepsy cannot do justice to the educational implications of factors such as the degree and location of structural brain abnormality; possible cognitive or behavioural effects of seizures and/or antiepileptic medication; the appropriateness of educational placements and pedagogical techniques; attendance records; family perceptions of epilepsy; degree (or lack) of stigma; level of self-esteem and so on, which may be encountered in particular children. The evidence is not complete and should not be used dogmatically to make generalizations. We still need to know much more about why some children with epilepsy have problems while others perform normally; and what specific measures might be taken to help particular individuals whose problems in respect of learning have been identified and assessed. However, in terms of commonly measured school attainments, Ross & West (1978) found that the children with epilepsy in the NCDS cohort at the age of 11 who were attending ordinary school performed non-academic tasks, e.g. copying designs, as well as children without epilepsy; though their scores on reading and mathematics tests were lower. School absence was also identified as a problem for this group of children with epilepsy, 13% having missed at least one month in their eleventh year compared to only 6% without epilepsy. At the age of 16, the group in ordinary schools remaining in the study were tested for reading and mathematical ability, scoring on average within 5% of the norms of their age groups (Ross et al 1980).

Teachers, in particular, need to be aware of research findings pointing to possible relationships between the epilepsies and factors affecting school performance. In a pioneering neuropsychiatric study of schoolchildren on the Isle of Wight, Rutter et al (1970) found specific reading deficits in children with uncomplicated epilepsy ranging up to three times that which might be expected. In this study, children with epilepsy were approximately 12 months behind in reading attainment for their age, and 18% of the epilepsy group were retarded in respect of reading by two years or more. Holdsworth & Whitmore (1974) studied children with epilepsy attending ordinary schools and, from the information provided by head-teachers, also concluded that poor progress was widespread, with only about one-third performing at or above the level their teachers believed appropriate for their age. Their study also revealed the equally worrying fact that almost 40% of teachers said they were previously unaware of the particular child's epilepsy.

Key work in Britain on educational implications of the epilepsies has been done by Stores and colleagues at the Park Hospital for Children in Oxford, which is the UK's National Centre for Children with Epilepsy. Stores & Hart (1976) pursued the relationship between reading skills and generalized and focal epilepsy in children attending ordinary schools and concluded that reading skills were significantly poorer in boys than in girls with epilepsy; though uniform liability to learning problems was discovered for children with epilepsy generally. The general implication for teachers would seem to be that individuals, whether or not they have epilepsy, who are behind in development of basic skills such

as reading will have a greater likelihood of being educationally disadvantaged in a school curriculum heavily biased in favour of communications skills based on reading and writing.

Reading skills, while no doubt a good general indicator of ability to perform well in school terms, are not the sole measure of performance. In a review of the literature Yule (1980) called additionally for measurements to be made of mathematical skills accompanied by more analysis of results by sex; together with attention to social factors and the wider clinical context. It is very much to be hoped that more comprehensive approaches will be adopted to the assessment of educational achievement for children with epilepsy, perhaps stimulated by the 1981 Education Act. The relevance and accessibility of research findings to those responsible in the classroom for the educational progress of the individual child must also improve. As yet, the only comprehensive source of guidance for the teacher who is not a specialist in this field is the National Society for Epilepsy's resources package 'Children and Young People with epilepsy' (Craig et al 1985).

Before summarizing possible relationships between organic epileptic activity and specific learning problems, it is salutary to note the results of a survey carried out by Stores (1982) on a series of 100 inpatients with established epilepsy referred mainly by paediatricians. Sixty-two were boys aged 4 to 16 with varying seizure patterns and a range of onset from neonatal to 13 years. Half the children were in the normal intelligence range, with both extremes represented. All social classes were represented, but with a preponderance from upper socio-economic groups. Although the usual reason for referral was stated as poor seizure control (only one child coming specifically because of family problems), on assessment an enormous range of other factors emerged: 95% had behaviour problems, over half being aggressive, and boys were over-represented in this group, over half were markedly distractable; and a third were said to be lethargic or socially isolated by their own choice (as distinct from the 20% said to be rejected by others). Other behaviour disorders found included; attention seeking; anxiety; low self-esteem; and extreme restlessness. Psychotic behaviour was rare, being found in only 5 children, though speech and language problems of a serious nature were diagnosed in 23 and severe clumsiness in 16. The researchers found that 'the most common difficulty within the family was serious inadequacy in the parents' ability to control or otherwise deal with their child's problems. Seventeen mothers had a history of serious psychiatric disorder'. Though by no means representative of all children and young people with epilepsy, this study underlines the need to look beyond the seizure disorder and its degree of control, since significant improvements in these, as this study revealed, may be possible if related behavioural, developmental and familial problems are identified and addressed in a multiprofessional manner.

In an important Dutch study of epilepsy and learning behaviour in children attending ordinary schools, Aldenkamp (1983) offered a useful corrective to overconcentration on strictly objective measures of school performance which neglect to assess the price some children with epilepsy may be paying in order to perform at or above the level of their peers. He found that 'those children with normal intelligence levels reported more school problems than were obtained by using objective measures'. As a result of asking the children with epilepsy in this sample whether they themselves experienced problems at school, it was concluded that 'a number of children do meet the requirements at school, but not without experiencing considerable difficulties and subjective discomfort'. Information for professionals about epilepsy and education has so far scarcely touched on these aspects, yet we believe they can be powerful factors affecting overall performance and preparation for adult life.

Organic causes of learning difficulties

There is growing evidence to suggest a number of relationships between specific organic epileptic disturbances and a range of learning problems (Stores 1981), However, this is not to say that learning problems always accompany specific disorders, or that, if they do, they necessarily have an organic cause. The suggested relationships are as follows.

1. Involvement of the hemisphere dominant for speech (usually the left) may result in impairment or delay in verbal skills, giving rise to poorer performance in a curriculum heavily based on language skills and reading.

2. Perceptual skills may be affected if the epileptic activity generally affects the non-dominant hemisphere.

3. Specific epileptic activity in the left temporal lobe, in both boys and girls, seems to be associated with a range of behaviour disturbances. Such children may be more anxious, inattentive, overactive or socially isolated; they may be more dependent on parents than other children. In very general terms, boys may be more vulnerable, for a combination of biological and cultural reasons, than girls in this respect.

4. More common than specific verbal or non-verbal deficits, are problems of attentiveness resulting from brief, generalized bursts of epileptic activity throughout the cerebral area. These are not always accompanied by observable features such as loss of consciousness or jerking, but they can markedly affect concentration or behaviour in the classroom. Long-term EEG monitoring techniques, which may be used in the ordinary school setting, can help detect such occurrences which may not be apparent to the casual observer or may be mistaken by a teacher for daydreaming or carelessness.

5. The underlying cause of the epilepsy itself, e.g. a structural brain abnormality or brain disease, may result in intellectual retardation. Perhaps some 40% of mentally handicapped children also have epilepsy, but it should also be remembered that in children with epilepsy only, or in association with a physical handicap such as cerebral palsy or spina bifida, the epilepsy itself is no predictor of intellectual capacity. In a recent American study, Ellenberg et al (1986) found that non-febrile seizures caused no significant deterioration in full-scale IQ scores except in children who had experienced neurologic abnormalities prior to the onset of epilepsy.

6. Finally, there may be adverse effects on school performance stemming from the consequences of antiepileptic drug (AED) therapy, aspects of which are discussed elsewhere in this volume. Sometimes these are not entirely avoidable, but often a reassessment combined with

measurement of drug levels can result in a rationalization of therapy and a decrease in the drowsiness, restlessness or inattentiveness which caused a problem in the classroom. The role of teachers is central to identifying aspects, such as complaints about having a poor memory or feeling unsteady, which may stem from inappropriate therapy. Where drug changes are not the answer, allowing more time on certain parts of lessons or allowing the child to work at his or her own pace may help. Special consideration needs to be given well in advance to coping with public examinations, and examining bodies will generally take epilepsy into consideration if the individual circumstances are discussed with them by the school early enough. It needs to be stressed that great care must to be exercised in attempting to reduce or withdraw AEDs at around the school-leaving age. The occurrence of a fit at this time could prejudice career plans and would undoubtedly negate the chances of a young person obtaining a driving licence, which to many is seen as a passport to normality and equality with peers.

Learning problems thought to be related to specific epileptic activity need the same remedial attention from teachers that the same problem originating from another source would require (Hackney 1985). It also should be emphasized that a range of other factors may be indicated in school-related problems, amongst which the following are most usually identified.

Some non-organic causes of learning problems

1. There may be a dysfunction in the family of the child with epilepsy. Often this is associated with an inability to come to terms with the diagnosis, and the parents' usually negative assessment of its implications, in a child who may otherwise appear normal. The unpredictability of epileptic attacks may also inhibit the family's ability to form healthy relationships with the child or with or between siblings (Hodgman et al 1979, Long & Moore 1979). Some parents and children may believe seizures will result in crippling injuries or even death (Ward & Bower 1978). The resulting fear may lead to parental overprotection with long-term consequences for normal social development (Ziegler 1981, Lechtenberg 1984).

2. The family's culture may contain beliefs or attitudes distorting the significance of epilepsy. In some African and Asian societies, epilepsy is still thought to be an inherited mental illness, deeply humiliating to the family, leading to attempts to conceal their 'shame' by keeping a child away from school and the usual range of activities outside the home. In the UK, considerably more work is needed on this aspect, so that teachers and social workers, as well as health care personnel, will be alert to such potential problems in some ethnic minority families.

3. The child or young person may have a poor self-image resulting either from lack of knowledge, rejection or frustration or a combination of such factors. Sometimes incontinence can accompany a fit, and if this occurs at school it is a cause of considerable embarrassment. Equally, having to take medication during school hours may lead to teasing about being a 'junkie' or having to 'have a fix'. Unjustified, as opposed to legitimate, restrictions on school activities can be just as damaging to the development of self-esteem as cosseting in a misguided attempt to avoid precipitation of seizures. Age-appropriate experiences are important for children and young people with epilepsy. These should include both successes and failures, if feelings of differentness and inferiority are to be combatted from an early stage. Epilepsy organizations generally provide a range of informative literature for parents and teachers discussing these vital points.

The role of professionals and parents

Caution should always be exercised in extrapolating from specific research findings. Samples are often based on highly selected populations, such as children attending a special centre for epilepsy or referred for other reasons. Most children with epilepsy remain under the care of general practitioner. When they do attend hospital, they may encounter a seemingly endless round of junior doctors. The result is that continuity of care, one of the essentials of rational management, may be sadly lacking. General guidance directed to all professionals concerned with children and young people is therefore probably more valuable in this section than detailed information about clinical aspects of paediatric epilepsy. The spirit with which we have made the following suggestions takes its cue from many quarters, but this (translated) statement by the French League Against Epilepsy (Ligue française contre l'épilepsie 1980) embodies a model approach to the whole family:

> Taking account of the essential elements of the dynamics of the family, and having an understanding of the repercussions of epilepsy – and of the person with epilepsy – on each of the family members, are the central elements in an ideal therapeutic programme. However, one must remember that the equilibrium of a family based on 'coping with the sick person' may be upset should that person's condition improve. These breaks in family stability, the inability of certain family members to adapt and cope when there is a change, favourable or not, in the condition, may suggest a productive course for family therapies. In all instances it is justifiable to make the parents the object of therapy, taking into account the pain caused to them and their wounded self-esteem. They deserve to be listened to in the same way as the child is listened to, since what they say is at least as important because their concept of the 'sickness' of their child is always present in what they have to say.

For all concerned, at whatever age, but especially during the school years, having epilepsy means much more than simply 'having fits'. That does not mean that parents or teachers should have to become highly expert in the epilepsies. Rather they should seek to utilize networks of information and help that may be available, so that understanding and plans appropriate to individual children and young people with epilepsy may be devised. The special educational needs legislation seeks to facilitate this. Teachers and parents are ideally placed, much more so than doctors, to observe children who might on investigation be found to have genuine epilepsy. Just as importantly, they can and should take a leading role in supporting and monitoring the educational progress and personal development of those children and young people whose epilepsy is already known. A good descriptive record is essential in making both an initial diagnosis with conviction, and the periodic reassessments which a potentially changeable condition in a maturing person requires. Although the label 'epilepsy' should never be applied lightly (and 'epileptic' only to the seizure itself, never the person), equally there is strong justification in some cases for seeking to remove it if the diagnosis is suspect. The question

'is it really epilepsy?' may need to be asked more than once during the school years and beyond, especially if the seizures remain uncontrolled. That is why a primary objective of the role teachers and parents can play should be to prevent the diagnosis from dominating the young person and distorting normal development, though of course account must be taken of any additional physical or mental impairment.

In its resources package for teachers, other educational staff and parents in the UK (Craig et al 1985), the National Society for Epilepsy states that the common psychological reactions to chronic conditions, such as anxiety and depression, are over-represented in the population with epilepsy. Anxiety may stem most often from worrying when the next fit might occur, especially if the diagnosis is concealed by the family or the reasons for the epilepsy are not understood (Scambler 1984). Anxiety may be accompanied by guilt feelings ('Why does this happen to me? What did we do wrong for this to happen to our child?' etc). Depression may result. Sometimes the phenomenon of 'learned helplessness' is also seen (De Villis et al 1980), where the person exhibits a fatalistic attitude to events which they have come to consider as unpredictable or unavoidable in their consequences. Specialized counselling directed at the whole family is indicated in such circumstances (Udall 1985, Booth 1985).

In addition to these problems, teachers and parents in particular may encounter other, and rarer, inappropriate psychological reactions to epilepsy which may have a fundamental bearing on schooling and family life. These include the following.

1. Expressions of anger as a 'safety valve' to relieve frustrations or anxiety, especially if seizures are not controlled. The approach to treatment should be flexible enough to take account of the legitimate need in some people to express the emotion of anger at having epilepsy, but care should be taken not to misinterpret it initially as violence or aggression, especially if it is part of a teenager's natural desire to demonstrate independence. But neither should this reaction be indulged by parents or school authorities.

2. Denial of the diagnosis of epilepsy as a negative means of coping. Sometimes denial may be associated with risk taking as a way of 'proving', perhaps to oneself or to peers, that the diagnosis is wrong. The need to demonstrate independence may also be a factor.

3. Fear of losing seizures. Ironically in a few instances this can lead to non-compliance if an established way of living is seen to be 'threatened' by the prospect of gaining control over the condition.

The presence of any handicap in a child may alter the normal dynamics in a family and lead to the child being overprotected or, much less frequently, rejected. Parental overprotection in particular is an understandable reaction, particularly if the seizures are accompanied by injury, but it is harmful in the long run in terms of normal development. Some parents may urge teachers to try and protect the child from stress if they believe this precipitates attacks. We believe that a more productive approach would be to teach all the family members the skills necessary to cope with stress, since it forms an inevitable part of everyday life.

Some schools may voice concern about the safety of the child or young person with epilepsy in workshops, laboratories or during sporting activities. Blanket restrictions are unacceptable. Risks, if there are any, to each child or to others in the vicinity should a seizure occur, must be assessed individually on the basis of accurate knowledge of that child's epilepsy. If attacks are completely controlled or only occur during sleep, we can see no justification for restrictions. Even if fits occur during the day, almost all activities, including swimming and climbing, can be undertaken, provided there is adequate supervision and due care and attention is exercised in order to comply with the policy of the Local Education Authority or school governing body. Most children with epilepsy can watch television and use computers with visual display units quite safely. It is sensible, however, to advise teachers to find out beforehand, through the school doctor or nurse if the parents are not forthcoming, if the child is known to be sensitive to flashing lights.

Careers advice and leaving school

The question of what to do when approaching the usual time for leaving school is addressed far too late in many instances, which undoubtedly has a bearing on the unacceptably high number of post-16 year olds with epilepsy who are unemployed and overly dependent on their families. In more favourable economic times, when job placements were far less difficult, even if not always easy, there was a danger that the job chosen would be below the young person's aptitudes or without prospects of further training or advancement. Given the likely continuing depression in the European youth employment market, therefore, there are some advantages in remaining registered at school after the age of 16, or else attending a college of further education in order to gain maturity and skills. The Education Act of 1944 (Section 8b) places a duty on Local Education Authorities to make school places available which are suitable for pupils up to the age of 19 years. This applies to pupils with disabilities as well.

Careers advice from a Careers Officer (or where epilepsy constitutes a real handicap, from a Specialist Careers Officer) or a teacher specializing in careers guidance should be sought early in the secondary school years. Nothing is more distressing than a young person whose career ambitions, for which they are otherwise admirably suitable, have been shattered by finding out much too late that epilepsy is a barrier to a particular occupation. The implications of epilepsy for certain types of employment are discussed later in this chapter, and it should not be forgotten that the various epilepsy organizations are also able to advise on careers matters (Aspinall 1985b).

The school leaver whose epilepsy is complicated by a mental handicap needs a particularly skilled approach from teachers, and from lecturers in further education colleges whose experience of this combination of disabilities may be very limited. Bicknell (1985) describes a model approach for the relationship of teachers to the adolescent student with a mental handicap and epilepsy which stresses the facilitation of self-development and the utilization of a range of services for mentally handicapped people which can be brought to bear within the general educational system catering for post-16 year olds. The expertise of the National Bureau for Handicapped Students can also be helpful in examining the whole range of post-school educational possibilities.

The management of epilepsy by doctors, school nurses, teachers and parents in the ordinary school setting will continue to be a primary focus for concern. Not only are the majority of children and young people with epilepsy already in 'mainstream' education, but recent legislation promoting educational integration lays specific duties on professionals working in the school setting. The role of the school health service is crucial in this regard (Ross et al 1983, Ross & Bommen 1983) working in close partnership with those responsible for the everyday management of children with epilepsy in schools (Kangesu et al 1984, Hall & Jolly 1984). We believe that the school nurse should be a key worker in this partnership. Indeed, her role in school health care generally has recently been singled out for development (Whitmore 1985, Nash et al 1985). Particular emphasis should be given to the school nurse's role in co-ordinating and monitoring services, and in initiating and supporting appropriate health education about epilepsy in the school in close liaison with teacher colleagues. This type of collaboration between professional services could be implemented with little or no expenditure increase.

Conclusion

The Report of the Working Group on Services for People with Epilepsy in England and Wales (DHSS 1986) underlined the need for the assessment of each child's epilepsy 'to be seen as a continuous process with regular reviews of the educational and other implications' (p. 36) which can only be achieved by better co-ordination between education, social services and health authorities. This report reiterates in policy terms the conclusions of the NCDS (Ross & Peckham 1983) that:

> if children with epilepsy are to make the most of their school years, it is vital that a comprehensive medical, social, and educational assessment is carried out, and that those with problems receive early and appropriate help. Many seem to develop an ability to cope and do well at school, and these children have the greatest tendency to stop having seizures. The difficulty is to determine whether this improvement is the result of cessation of seizures, or

whether the well-adjusted child has a greater ability to stop having seizures than one who has to face unmitigated social problems.

Although there is no single or simple answer to this conundrum, we believe it is nevertheless appropriate to include in this section the guidance contained in a ten-point plan for the future of children and young people with epilepsy, originally devised by epilepsy associations in North America, but relevant to children, parents and professional workers in all countries:

1. If a child has epilepsy, there are two possibilities for the future. He may grow out of it. He may not. Ideally, we should act as if he will, and make provision for the eventuality that he doesn't

2. Never make the epilepsy an excuse for lowering our expectations of his performance.

3. Make sure that life does not revolve around him and his epilepsy, and that we don't use it as an excuse – or as a scapegoat

4. Discuss epilepsy with him when necessary, and make sure he knows he has epilepsy and understands what it is and what it isn't. The older he is, the more factual information will be required

5. Don't talk about him as if he weren't there, or talk about his epilepsy in whispers or behind closed doors

6. Help him along the path between timidity and aggression, defeatism and overambition

7. Encourage any activity that improves his self-image. Concentrate on what he can do, rather than what he can't, and help him to increase the scope of his interests

8. From an age well in advance of leaving secondary school, guide him towards a choice of career or job that is realistic for him, but do it without stressing his limitations. The importance of inner reserves of self-esteem will become apparent if he is not able to find work either because of the epilepsy or the general economic situation facing young people seeking employment

9. There are 365 days in the year. If he has an average of one fit a week, that leaves 313 days in which, unless he is otherwise handicapped, he should be capable of living life to the full.

Encourage him to count the days that he's seizure-free, rather than those that may be spoilt by having an attack

10. Always remember that he may stop having fits, either because the treatment has become more accurate at controlling them or because they have ceased of their own accord, as sometimes happens. His acceptance then by the community will depend on his ability to form relationships, to take responsibility as a member of the community, and to live a productive and independent life, not on his past history of having epileptic attacks.

At a multiprofessional symposium on 'Epilepsy and Education – Changing Attitudes' held in London in May 1986, speakers were asked to identify an 'action point' which was practical and achieveable. The list which resulted is reproduced below. We believe it offers an important selection of goals for the multiprofessional approach to this subject which is the essence of real and lasting advances:

1. There should be routine communications between the parents, teachers and other professionals concerned with all children with epilepsy
2. There should be early identification of difficulties at school and also areas of success, so that remedial action can be taken about the former, and reinforcement can be offered to the latter
3. Good communications in respect of epilepsy and education are everybody's business, and not the preserve of professional workers
4. All children with epilepsy need and deserve a careful and comprehensive medical assessment
5. Full use should be made of services provided by the epilepsy associations
6. Full use should be made of the assessment and statementing provisions of the 1981 Education Act for children with epilepsy, to stimulate the sharing of knowledge about particular children
7. There should be greater knowledge about what specialized services are already available in respect of the educational implications of epilepsy
8. There should be counselling of the entire

family at the time of diagnosis of a child's epilepsy
9. There is as much a need to assess social behaviour as well as the medical aspects of the epileptic disorder
10. Urgent progress needs to be made on identifying a 'named person' in each school who could monitor the progress of children with epilepsy
11. There is a need for reassessment during the teenage years, and especially at the time of leaving school in order to plan continuing care.

EMPLOYMENT

Introduction

Finding and keeping work is becoming increasingly difficult for everyone, but in the competition for employment, people with disabilities have faired less well. There is good evidence, however, that once a disabled person has got a job, his ability to keep it is just as good as anyone else's (Kettle & Massie 1982, Manpower Services Commission 1984). However, in view of the present and persistent high level of unemployment and the decline in traditional manufacturing industries in the UK and most other developed nations, alternatives to traditional employment, especially in the service industries, as well as the constructive use of leisure time, may become more relevant for more people with epilepsy. Nevertheless, for most, paid employment, be it open or sheltered, is the desired objective; it confers both personal and social status as well as financial reward.

The research background

The research findings on epilepsy and employment recently reviewed by Floyd (1986) are not conclusive, but we believe one valuable general observaton from UK studies is that an individual with skills and talents and a strong sense of self-esteem is often much more employable, despite seizures, than someone else with few or even no seizures, but who has no skills and an eroded self-image (Scambler & Hopkins 1980, Tillotson & Stanley 1982, Floyd 1983).

A recent survey by Lisle & Waldron (1986) on employees with epilepsy in 48 Health Authorities in the National Health Service, showed a prevalence rate of known people with epilepsy in employment of 1.35/1000, much lower than the estimated prevalence of active epilepsy in adults. Undoubtedly, there were a number of undisclosed cases in this study, since it has been suggested (Scambler & Hopkins 1980) that only about one in ten people with epilepsy always disclose their condition to employers. Perhaps the explanation for the under-reporting stems from the anxiety described by Gloag (1985): 'people fear . . . that their job applications will not be considered on their merits if they admit a history of epilepsy and . . . their medical history will not be assessed by anyone knowledgeable'. From the standpoint of the role of an occupational health department, particularly within the National Health Service, Peake (1984) has described the steps which may be taken to assist the disabled worker in terms of policies and their practical application. A key element in this is the maintenance of confidentiality in respect of health information. This should be elicited from applicants on separate forms and should only be available to appropriately qualified occupational health staff. We support the view of Floyd & Espir (1986) that such forms should be scrutinized by those qualified to do so 'only after suitability for the post, on grounds other than health, has been established'.

Against this understandable anxiety must be set very positive findings about the performance of people with epilepsy in the workplace in comparison with workmates without epilepsy. These suggest that a person whose seizures are completely controlled and who has acquired skills appropriate for their age should not, other things being equal, be adversely affected in the job market (Dasgupta et al 1982, MacIntyre 1976). Specific exceptions to this are discussed below. A great deal also depends on the person with epilepsy knowing how to present epilepsy to an employer and having the knowledge and skills to correct misinformation. If attacks continue despite appropriate treatment, then the person with epilepsy may well be handicapped in seeking work. The degree of handicap may be composed of many factors: incidence and severity of seizures, adverse effects of drugs; pres-

ence of other disabilities; lack of skills; poor educational achievements; or low self-esteem. Often these factors interact. Simply knowing that someone has epilepsy, therefore, is not a very useful baseline from which to begin to assess an individual's employment prospects. Zielinski & Rader (1984) reviewed this complex field and concluded that factors such as availability of local employment opportunities, public transport and individual needs and qualities in the person with epilepsy were as important as seizure history in determining rehabilitation or improved employment status of an individual.

As in all questions connected with epilepsy, generalizations concerning employability and suitability for particular types of work must be avoided. Rather than 'is the person with epilepsy employable?', we believe a better approach would be 'is this individual employable in this post, and is the presence of epilepsy relevant?' Practical job-related questions such as, 'is it reasonable to stop people with epilepsy from using machinery if they are allowed to drive a car?' need to be asked (McLellan 1986a). Open-ended questions may predispose to stereotyped answers about 'epileptics'. Competition for certain types of jobs in certain areas is stiff and job seekers must have the qualities that make them attractive to an employer. These might be related to age, educational or technical qualifications, experience or good references from a previous employer. The job seeker's attitude and enthusiasm, coupled with the ability to 'sell oneself' at interview, are also vitally important. All job seekers, whether or not they have epilepsy, must be realistic about their employment prospects. If the person with epilepsy is suitable for a particular job in other respects, but is not successful, the temptation just to blame the epilepsy should be resisted. Undoubtedly however, having epilepsy will make getting many jobs more difficult, though a great deal depends on the nature and severity of the condition and whether the job seeker has any additional disabilities.

Disclosure of epilepsy

Dogmatism should be avoided on the question of what and when to tell an employer and fellow workers about epilepsy; though individuals should be aware that deliberate failure to disclose information in certain circumstances can be held to be legitimate grounds for dismissal should epilepsy subsequently be shown to be an impediment to the performance of a particular job. Many people with epilepsy are convinced that the declaration of the condition will deter employers. In general, however, we believe that more problems are likely to arise from not telling than from revealing epilepsy in the right way at the right time. The sociological evidence for this view has been discussed by Scambler (1984), who strongly suggests that non-disclosure and concealment, though often feasible in many social and employment settings, increases the person with epilepsy's fears of stigmatization and that this is potentially a greater source of personal anguish and unhappiness than actual discrimination because of epilepsy. Encouraging people with epilepsy, tacitly or otherwise, to believe that having epilepsy is automatically a 'passport to prejudice' may diminish both their degree of social adaptation and the chances for an open and productive relationship with their professional helpers (Scambler & Hopkins 1986).

At one extreme, the 1974 Health and Safety at Work Act, which puts obligations of information disclosure on employer and employee, could be cited as grounds for dismissal if an application form was inaccurately completed, whether or not there was intentional deception about the presence of epilepsy. It is unlikely that there would be successful recourse to an Industrial Tribunal in such a case. Of course, epilepsy should not be overemphasized either. No one wants to employ a person who has only epilepsy to offer and who describes all the 'problems' at work which this may entail. It is important, therefore, for the employee to understand his or her own epilepsy in the context of a particular employment, so that accurate personal information can be given. Once in the job, the occupational health service or the personnel department can help inform workmates about epilepsy in a positive way. We believe that if a person's seizures are completely controlled, it is a matter of individidual decision whether colleagues are told anything, though the employer's occupational health staff must be aware of the medical history. If attacks are likely to occur during working hours, those around need to know what to do. How they are told is a matter of using common sense and weighing up the circumstances of the individual's work situation.

Finding employment

Most people with epilepsy get jobs in the normal way without the need for any specialist help. It is advisable for job seekers with epilepsy to have their medical condition stabilized at the earliest opportunity. The young adult leaving school whose attacks are not controlled will be at a disadvantage compared to someone of the same age whose epilepsy was controlled much earlier. Where specialist employment help is required, early self-referral is probably the best course. Parents should request the help of a Specialist Careers Officer through the Careers Service of the local education authority if the epilepsy constitutes a significant problem. For those who have left school, the services of the Disablement Resettlement Officer (DRO), contacted through the nearest Jobcentre, can often be helpful, especially with placement on appropriate training schemes. The DRO should also be able to advise on the availability of sheltered work for those people who are severely disabled by epilepsy or associated conditions. For most people with epilepsy, however, the mainstream employment outlets such as Jobcentres, personal contacts, newspaper advertisements and employment agencies will probably produce the best results. Finally, doctors in particular should make use of the Employment Medical Advisory Service (EMAS) which is available to assist individuals as well as employers and occupational health personnel. EMAS will give free and confidential opinions about particular types of work where epilepsy is concerned.

Legislation

In addition to the barriers described below, there are several general requirements in law regarding the employment of disabled people. These are discussed further in the Code of Good Practice on the Employment of Disabled People (Manpower Services Commission 1984). Briefly, The Disabled

Persons (Employment) Acts of 1944 and 1958 established a voluntary register of disabled people (the so-called 'green card' system). The earlier legislation placed certain duties and obligations on employers with 20 or more employees relating to those registered under the Acts, in particular the duty to employ a quota of registered disabled people (currently 3%) of the total workforce. There are many ways to secure exemption from even these minimal requirements, however, and major employers such as Government Departments and the National Health Service are not bound by these laws.

The Companies (Directors' Report) (Employment of Disabled Persons) Regulations of 1980, which form part of the Companies Acts 1948–1983, require all companies covered by these Acts and employing on average 250 people to state in the annual report of their Board of Directors the company's policy applied during the previous financial year in respect of fair consideration for disabled people applying for jobs; for continuing the employment of employees who have become disabled; and for the training, career development and promotion of disabled employees. Useful though this requirement is in bringing the employment of disabled people to the attention of larger private sector employers, the regulations do not apply to public sector employers which are often the largest in any locality.

The Commission of the European Communities (1986) is promoting recommendations and a model code on vocational training and employment of those with disabilities. The UK's Code of Good Practice on the Employment of Disabled People (Manpower Services Commission 1984), though non-statutory, is nonetheless an excellent beginning towards the achievement of European goals in this field.

Barriers to employment

The reality of barriers to the employment of people with epilepsy must be admitted though, that having been said, there must be an effort to disentangle their complexity. We have proposed elsewhere a conceptual framework (Craig & Oxley 1986), Table 16.1, which differentiates between the intentional and unintentional, and indicates whether the barriers are either intrinsic to the people with epilepsy or extrinsic, i.e. in other people or due to external circumstances. We believe this approach helps to distinguish those barriers which are legitimate from those which are discriminatory and may be amenable to change. It also helps to direct educational or other persuasion campaigns more accurately. In this sense, it is an example of the application of the kind of problem analysis advocated in the section on health education about epilepsy later in this chapter.

We have set the commonly encountered problems within this framework and discuss some of the strategies which may be adopted to bring about change; a process which is itself not without problems from time to time. The list of potential barriers to people with epilepsy in employment is formidable and may give the impression that any individual with epilepsy is likely to encounter overwhelming obstacles. Clearly this is not the case. In attempting to evaluate any problem area it is vital to be specific and to consider a particular person in terms of a particular job. All assessments must conform to this individual model. Comments on some of the items listed in the framework will serve to illustrate this principle.

Table 16.1 Barriers to employment – a conceptual framework

OVERT/INTENTIONAL	COVERT/INTENTIONAL
Intrinsic	Intrinsic
Extrinsic	Extrinsic
OVERT/UNINTENTIONAL	COVERT/UNINTENTIONAL
Intrinsic	Intrinsic
Extrinsic	Extrinsic

Overt/intentional

Intrinsic:
none – this would negate the possibility of employment and the person with epilepsy would not be in the labour market.

Extrinsic:
1. Regulations backed by Act of Parliament, statutory instrument or a statutory body
2. Recruitment and selection policies barring those with epilepsy

3. Superannuation schemes barring people with a diagnosis of epilepsy
4. Scarcity of sheltered employment

Overt/unintentional

Intrinsic:

1. Low educational achievement of job seeker
2. Lack of appropriate work skills/experience
3. Previous periods of unemployment
4. Inadequate personal knowledge/inappropriate presentation of epilepsy to potential employer
5. Intractable fits and/or drug side effects affecting performance or acceptability in the workplace
6. Presence of handicaps additional to epilepsy, e.g. mental handicap, psychiatric problems, physical disability

Extrinsic:

1. Inadequate medical treatment of epilepsy prior to job search
2. Inappropriate professional guidance (medical and vocational)
3. Lack of access to counselling to identify and overcome any psychosocial problems
4. History of previous dismissal related to seizures
5. Disincentives to seeking employment, e.g. the 'poverty trap' of welfare benefits relative to low wages
6. Lack of public transport
7. Problems stemming from physical design of the workplace
8. Depressed local job market

Covert/intentional

Intrinsic:
None identified

Extrinsic:

1. Custom and practice not to engage people with epilepsy in certain occupations or workplaces/the effects of 'word of mouth' recruitment policies
2. Discrimination by staff responsible for recruitment and selection and/or management prejudice against disabled workers based on:
 i. inaccurate understanding of epilepsy
 ii. unjustified concerns about safety, insurance cover or trades union reactions
 iii. ignorance of productivity and attendance records of disabled employees generally
3. Use of 'quota' of 3% disabled employees as a maximum rather than a minimum
4. Unofficial 'quota' of employees with epilepsy operated by some organizations

Covert/unintentional

Intrinsic:

1. Unrealistic ambitions and expectations of employment
2. Personality problems/negative attitudes about self and others
3. Restricted mobility (physical and/or psychological in origin)

Extrinsic:

1. Employer ignorance of good practices in the employment of people with disabilities and of sources of help and guidance
2. Prevalence of 'myths about epileptics' held by some members of the public, and some professionals, such as:
 i. they have a high accident rate and are a danger to themselves and others
 ii. they put others in the workplace at risk if they have a fit at work
 iii. they have lower performance and productivity rates
 iv. they are often absent from work because of fits
 v. they have difficult personalities
 vi. they require higher employer insurance premiums

Intentional barriers

The UK has no central source of information about what restrictions might apply to a particular person with epilepsy in respect of types of employment. We have compiled a list of statutory prohibitions from many sources (Table 16.2), but this may be incomplete.

In addition to these 'statutory barriers', the common law is not infrequently used to avoid employing someone with epilepsy (Carter 1986). It would seem to be logical that for the UK, the

Table 16.2 Some occupations affected by statutory barriers

Occupation	Regulations	Effect
Aircraft pilot	Manual of Civil Aviation Medicine produced by International Civil Aviation Organisation	Applicants shall have no established medical history or clinical diagnosis of epilepsy
Ambulance driver	Follow PSV regulations (see below)	Barrier if fit occurred since age of 5 for drivers or crew. Clerical work available to those who develop epilepsy in employment
Armed services: Army	Army Act 1955; Manual of Military Law	Applicants are rejected on grounds of epilepsy and likely to be discharged if they develop epilepsy during employment. If they have had no fits since childhood, each case is considered individually
Navy		Medical regulations state any attacks at any age would debar from entry
RAF	Recruiting regulations in Air Force Act 1955 as amended in Army and Air Force Act 1961 and the Armed Forces Acts of 1966, 1971 and 1976	Proven epilepsy with a few exceptions is bar to recruitment. People developing epilepsy during service are given a medical employment standard which limits their employment
Coastguard	Civil Service Medical Advisory Service policy based on individual merit	Coastguards come into a category which requires special physical qualifications, therefore medical examination is arranged in all cases to determine fitness to undertake the full range of duties
Diver	Health & Safety at Work Act 1974. Diving Operations at Work Regs. 1981 (SI 1981/399)	Any history of fits (apart from febrile convulsions) will preclude granting a Certificate of Medical Fitness to Dive which must be renewed every 12 months
Fire brigade	Fire Service Act 1947: Fire Services Appointments (and Promotion) Regs. 1965	A history of epilepsy renders a man unsuitable for operational fire duties
HSV & PSV & Taxi driver	Statutory Instrument 1309 HGV (Drivers' Licences) Regs. 1977. Amendment 429, 1982 – consolidated in 1984, 1925 Reg. 4 Section 22 Public Passenger Vehicle Act 1981 PSV 1985, Statutory Instrument 214 Reg. 5a	Absolute barrier if fit occurred after attaining age of 5. Immediate loss of licence to existing licence holder
Merchant Seaman	DoT Merchant Shipping (Med. Exam) Regs. 1983 Statutory Instrument 1983 No. 808, Merchant Shipping Notice M1144	Absolute barrier on applicants with history of fits since age 5. Serving seamen who develop epilepsy may be employed after 2 years free of seizures on a ship carrying a Medical Officer and provided they are not involved in the safety of ship or passengers.
Nurse & Midwife	Nurses, Midwives & Health Visitors Act 1979 SI 1983/873 – midwives only	Epilepsy is not mentioned specifically. Nurses: each training authority sets own standards. Midwives: prospective trainees must provide evidence that they are not knowingly suffering from any disabilities which might preclude them from carrying out the duties of a midwife.
Police	Statutory qualifications contained in Police Regulations 1979. Regulation 14(1) (C) relates to general health criteria for entry – not specific to epilepsy.	Applicants currently having fits not recruited. Those with past history dealt with on individual basis. Also applies to traffic wardens, drivers, etc.

Continued

Table 16.2 (*Cont'd*)

Occupation	Regulations	Effects
Prison Service	No Statutory Instrument regarding health standards for prison service.	Recent history of epilepsy debars an applicant on grounds of security for posts at Prison Officer Grade. Applicants to other grades of prison service are considered individually.
Teacher in state school	Education (Teachers) Regulations, 1982.	Applicants must be 3 years free of seizures. Teachers in post may be barred from teaching PE, Craft, Science and Home Economics.
Train driver	No statutory requirements for medical fitness	Absolute barrier if fit ever occurred (London Regional Transport) or if fit occurred since age 5 (British Rail). Also applies to LRT guards and track operatives.

Health and Safety Executive should be the agency first to collate and provide existing information about statutory barriers to employment; secondly, to examine their validity from time to time in the light of current practices; and thirdly, to issue guidance in general terms about the suitability for employment of those with epilepsy. Leaving this to legislative pronouncements and the inevitable variations of different regulatory or employing authorities only perpetuates confusion, to the disadvantage of the job seeker with epilepsy.

The matter of intentional and declared barriers must include reference to superannuation schemes and the provision of sheltered employment. The Occupational Pensions Board (OPB 1977) concluded that the principle 'fit for the job, fit for the pension scheme' should apply to all disabled workers. However, some employers still justify refusing employment on the spurious grounds that the person with epilepsy is ineligible for the company's occupational pension scheme. Recent Government proposals for legislative changes in the social security system may be disadvantageous to people with epilepsy in terms of their access to pension cover. As seems likely, much more emphasis in the future will be placed on individual employees taking responsibility for making their own pension arrangements rather than relying on the present state earnings-related scheme. Private sector pension plans, therefore, will need clear guidance and incentives on the subject of epilepsy if discrimination is not to result. We believe that specific safeguards will be needed for people with disabilities in employment, and for job seekers with disabilities, in terms of their rights of access to private pension schemes on equal terms with other employees.

The provision of sheltered employment is determined by government social and economic policies expressed through the allocation of funds for disabled persons' employment services. In 1984/85, the Manpower Services Commission's total allocation for services for this group was £118.1 m, of which £78.9 m (66.8%) was spent on sheltered employment schemes. The number of severely disabled people in sheltered employment rose by 600 to 15 600 during that year, largely due to an increased number employed under the Sheltered Placement Scheme. However, over 6000 severely disabled people remain on the unemployed register, indicating a continuing inadequacy of sheltered employment. From a European standpoint, the Commission of the European Communities has agreed (1986) that sheltered workshops should not be established except at designated assessment centres. Preference should instead be given to promoting the availability of sheltered employment, whether particular posts or groups of workers, within normal enterprises, in an effort to reduce segregation of disabled workers. These policies illustrate the scope for expansion in the sheltered employment field in areas of activity which are both personally stimulating and commercially viable. Greater government commitment, followed by higher levels of investment, is needed to realize them.

Some intentional barriers, of course, are not declared. Such practices are deplorable and help to perpetuate myths about epilepsy and employment. If there are sound practical reasons why a person with epilepsy should not be employed in a particular job, these should be clearly stated and justified.

Unintentional barriers

The majority of unintentional barriers to employment stem either from wrong information or from inappropriate perceptions and expectations. Both people with epilepsy and their professional helpers may be implicated. Recent Australian work (Beran & Read 1980) suggests that people with epilepsy perceive the attitudes of others in a widely varying way, but that the community in general is frequently seen as unaccepting and employers, as a segment of the community, are perceived as hostile, fearful or indifferent. Undoubtedly this is only true in limited circumstances, but as a generally held belief among the sample of people with epilepsy studied it is very worrying. This study also found that a high percentage of those interviewed believed that job opportunities generally were very restricted for people with epilepsy. Starting out in the job market with such perceptions invites the creation of self-fulfilling prophecies when employment is not obtained. It also illustrates one of the critical areas in which appropriate counselling at an early stage could markedly improve opportunities for employment. Without such interventions, and in a deteriorating job market, the prospects for those with such negative views must be grim.

A recent study of people with epilepsy in nine Northern Ireland general practices (Dowds 1983) asked about their experiences of counselling and perceptions of work. Of a group of 182 adults assessed as able to comment on their own condition and its effects on their lives, some 35% claimed to have had no counselling or social support from any source, even their own family. Moreover, secrecy about epilepsy at work and in social settings was widespread. Nevertheless, 76% of those available for employment had jobs, although there was a commonly reported feeling amongst them that having epilepsy meant reduced opportunities for promotion and pay. Half of those in this study who were unemployed were young people under the age of 30 without educational qualifications. Of course, these figures

must be interpreted in the light of unusually high unemployment in that part of the UK, but the study is nevertheless a good illustration of the complex interconnections of unintentional factors which can constitute powerful barriers to employment.

The importance of inappropriate psychosocial adjustment in some people with epilepsy, of which difficulties in employment are often only a symbol, cannot be overemphasized when discussing employment and the subtle prerequisite of employability. The use of psychological measures to gain a better understanding of the adjustment levels of individuals with epilepsy is gaining momentum (see Ch. 11). Much more use could and should be made of these approaches in order to identify factors such as poor emotional adjustment to epilepsy, which may not be immediately obvious, before it is concluded that some people with epilepsy are simply 'failures' in the employment stakes (Cofield & Austin 1984).

Inappropriate professional advice on employment is an equally potent impediment. Some trades unions state that they follow the guidance of the International Labour Office's (ILO) Encyclopaedia of Occupational Health and Safety concerning epilepsy (ILO 1983). This states that: 'work entailing exposure to heat, noise, radiation or glare, etc., work requiring rapid reactions or distribution of attention to several matters at the same time (e.g. despatch, control desk work, conveyer work) or work necessitating permanent contact with a large number of people should not be entrusted to epileptics'. This virtual blanket exclusion constitutes a powerful barrier to employment that should be amenable to modification to reflect current best practices.

In the UK, both the Confederation of British Industry (CBI) and the Trade Union Congress (TUC) have policies on employing disabled people which are wholly positive (TUC 1983, CBI 1983). An enquiry made by the authors to all trades unions affiliated to the TUC showed that of the 30% of unions responding, only a few could produce information on specific problems which their members with epilepsy had encountered. A number of unions remarked, however, on a general inadvisability of people with epilepsy working with or near machinery, without making any reference to the type of epilepsy they had in mind or the type of machinery they felt constituted a hazard. This is cause for concern on two grounds. It shows that epilepsy is still often perceived in employment contexts as a single, usually convulsive, and unchanging entity. The view of working near machinery ignores the fact that all machinery must be adequately guarded in order to comply with safety regulations for the protection of all workers. This in normal circumstances, and providing due care and attention has been taken in deciding on the type and location of the work to be undertaken, should be adequate to prevent injury should a seizure happen in the vicinity. Special adaptations, if required, often can be made with grants obtainable from the Manpower Services Commission via the Disablement Resettlement Service.

The campaign for employability

It has often been suggested that disabled people need the protection of statute law against discrimination in employment, similar to legislation which exists in the areas of racial and sexual equality. Precedents for such legislation exist in other countries, and a majority (61%) of the British public sampled in a Gallup poll commissioned by the Disablement Income Group in 1983 favoured it. The last major discussion of this matter in Parliament in the UK was in late 1983, when a Private Member's Bill to amend the 1970 Chronically Sick and Disabled Person's Act to prohibit discrimination against disabled people was defeated on a second reading (Hansard col 1092, 19 Nov 1983). As one of its proponents argued in debate, 'some discrimination is intentional but much of it – probably most of it – is unintentional and is caused by ignorance, but it is still hurtful and degrading to the disabled'. Two examples of specific discrimination against people with epilepsy at work were highlighted: one was a merchant seaman who had only experienced one fit, and the other was a man who fell asleep during his lunch break on a hot day and unintentionally revealed his epilepsy by having a sleep seizure. Both were dismissed (Hansard col 1093, 19 Nov 1983). Opponents claimed that 'if all employers were to take up the quota of 3% registered

disabled workers, there would not be enough disabled people to fill it', thus highlighting the relative failure of what little positive discrimination employment legislation exists (Ibid col 1095). In a questioning political climate, Ministers claimed agnosticism, especially as one opponent put it, the Bill would 'create a new crime of discriminating against disabled people and this would especially affect small business people, who are the key figures in providing employment' (Ibid col 1111). This sentiment is obnoxious, implying that disabled people are merely 'passengers' who can only be carried by large employers.

Although it is unlikely that a legislative remedy will be provided, in this country at least, for many of the extrinsic barriers to employment, the campaign to improve employment chances for people with disabilities is very active. The Spastics Society has recently reviewed the problems in this sphere and suggested a new basis for broad-based efforts, though still calling attention to the persistence of a wider pattern of discrimination in employment (Spastics Society 1985, 1986). Several organisations including the Royal Association for Disability and Rehabilitation (RADAR), the CBI, the TUC and the Royal College of Nursing (RCN) have published positive guidance on the recruitment or employment of disabled people in which the sections on epilepsy reflect current best practices (Kettle & Massie 1982, CBI 1983, TUC 1985, RCN 1985). RADAR's EMPLOYABILITY '85 campaign stressed that 'very few employers deliberately discriminate against disabled people, but sometimes recruitment policies discourage disabled people from applying'. This emphasis, away from 'employer and public bashing' and towards identifying specific aspects of recruitment and retention policies amenable to change, is a positive step and one for which the MSC's Code of Good Practice on the Employment of Disabled People (Manpower Services Commission 1984) is an excellent foundation. The experience of the National Society for Epilepsy is that both employers and professionals concerned with employment are not yet well enough aware of the Code and thus how it can act as a support rather than as a restraint for them. Nor is sufficient use made of the wide range of services and incentives administered by the MSC which can assist the job seeker and employee with epilepsy. For example, the MSC's Job Introduction Scheme, which seeks to overcome initial employer reservations by providing financial assistance in the early weeks of engagement of a disabled worker, can be an excellent tool for getting people with epilepsy into work. Failure to make maximum use of such an existing scheme must constitute one of the most regrettable, but most easily remedied, barriers to employment.

THE LAW

This section concerns the following aspects of epilepsy and the law: the criminal law; the law controlling antiepileptic drugs (AEDs); legal aspects of certain social security matters; and the law on driving. Information on epilepsy and legal aspects of employment, other than driving, and on epilepsy and education are found in a preceding section. Unless otherwise stated, the discussion refers exclusively to the United Kingdom.

The criminal law

Gunn (1981) has reviewed the medicolegal and sociomedical problems most usually encountered in relation to epilepsy. He concluded that although 'no neat general conclusions can be drawn . . . epilepsy does show very nicely that legal and social issues have a considerable impact upon clinical practice'. Most people with epilepsy are completely law abiding. Those few who commit crimes do so for the same reasons that motivate other people. However, a very few people with epilepsy have the misfortune to do something in a confused state after a fit which may be misunderstood as a criminal act. These events are rare and usually trivial, such as picking up an object in a shop (which may lead to prosecution for 'shoplifting') or undressing in a public place. Normally, if it is known that the person has had an epileptic attack, no action will result. Difficulties can and do occasionally arise, however, if the person is not known in the locality or is unaccompanied or, very unusually, if an aggressive act occurs resulting in physical injury. Actions committed during a seizure are automatisms and

it is generally agreed that persons in such a confused state have no control over what they do. Important social aspects relating to the criminal law and epilepsy which are outside the scope of this chapter are discussed by Gunn (1977), Oliver (1981) and Channon (1982).

This clinically difficult situation was made more complicated by a ruling in the House of Lords in February 1984 (Regina v. Sullivan) which abolished the legal distinction between this view of automatisms due to an epileptic attack and insanity. If, therefore, a person pleads 'not guilty' to a charge on the grounds that the action took place during an epileptic automatism, the law treats the plea as one of 'not guilty by reason of insanity'. If this plea is successful, the court may have no choice but to order the person to be detained compulsorily in a psychiatric hospital. This judgment does not apply to Scotland, but there the end result of such a plea is the same (Her Majesty's Advocate v. James Cunningham 1963). The current situation was summed up by a leading barrister (Swift 1985) at a recent symposium on epilepsy and the law:

> in the eyes of the law, there can be no exception to the McNaughten Rules where the definition of insanity is concerned. This means that if an epileptic commits an act but does not realise it, or if he commits an act not knowing the quality and nature of that act, or if he commits an act knowing the quality and nature of that act, but does not know he is doing wrong, then for the purposes of the criminal law he is to be regarded as temporarily insane.

The situation following the Sullivan Case is clearly unsatisfactory and grossly discriminatory against the, admittedly small, number of people with epilepsy likely to be affected by it (Brahams 1983a). While efforts are being made to bring about a change in the law to reflect clinical understanding of what happens during an epileptic attack, it is strongly recommended that expert legal advice be sought by or for anyone charged with an offence committed during an epileptic automatism. Especially worrying is the possibility described by Aspinall (1985c) of improving social attitudes towards people with epilepsy being set back because this judgment equated epilepsy with 'a disease of the mind'. However, there are also potential disadvantages in the prospect of a change in the law which would allow a plea of 'not guilty by reason of an epileptic automatism', since this could easily be abused both by those with and by those without epilepsy and involve clinicians in even greater amounts of time trying to establish the presence or absence of epilepsy for the courts. A multiprofessional conference held at the Royal College of Physicians in London in 1984, recommended changes in the laws of England and Scotland (Fenwick & Fenwick 1985). Its summary of recommendations (Lancet 30 June 1984, 1481) is given below.

1. The distinction between insane and non-insane automatism should be removed. Although it was appreciated that this might cause difficulty in states of self-induced drug and alcohol intoxication, it was felt that it was not beyond the resource of the legislature to take this into account
2. An alternative special verdict of 'not guilty by reason of automatism' should be made available as an alternative to the special verdict of 'not guilty by reason of insanity' in cases where it was clearly inappropriate to suggest that the defendant was insane
3. Should a plea of 'not guilty by reason of automatism' succeed, the judge's powers should be varied so that he could have wide discretion ranging from making no order at all, to detention in a secure hospital at the Home Secretary's discretion

Proposals of this type have been made in the UK from time to time since the publication of the Report of the Committee on Mentally Abnormal Offenders (The Butler Report) in 1975. In the light of the judgment in the Sullivan Case, the need for reform of the law through Parliament is even more urgent, a view which has recently been endorsed by the Faculty of Community Medicine (Golding 1985).

Control of antiepileptic drugs

All drugs used in the UK for the control of epilepsy are classed as Prescription Only Medicines (POMs) and are thus obtainable only through a registered medical practitioner. Additionally, the Misuse of Drugs Act (1971), in an attempt to restrict the availability of barbiturates which may be abused, now controls phenobarbitone (Luminal), methylphenobarbitone (Prominal) and compounds containing phenobarbitone. However, because phenobarbitone is not a drug of abuse, and because of its special use in the treatment of epilepsy, it is exempted from some of the provisions of this Act.

In practice, therefore, it is not necessary for doctors to handwrite prescriptions, though preprinted prescriptions and ones written by a receptionist are acceptable only if they are signed (not stamped) by the doctor. Additionally, it is necessary for the prescription to be hand-dated and for the amount of the drug to be dispensed to be stated in letters and figures. Pharmacists are, however, able to dispense phenobarbitone without a prescription in an emergency. In certain circumstances, the police may wish to be satisfied that a person in possession of phenobarbitone is legally entitled to it. The National Society for Epilepsy (NSE) has, therefore recommended that everyone who takes phenobarbitone for the treatment of epilepsy has a statement to that effect signed by their doctor. The NSE and other epilepsy associations provide epilepsy identification cards, on to which full details of a person's seizure pattern and treatment can be entered.

In 1985, the Government restricted the number of drugs in certain pharmaceutical categories which may be prescribed under the National Health Service. The benzodiazepines were included in this 'limited list', but the majority of those used to treat epilepsy are still permitted. However, one benzodiazepine, clobazam (Frisium) can now only be prescribed under the NHS to treat epilepsy, and prescriptions for it must be identified with the code 'S3b'. The matter of the 'limited list' is still under discussion between the professions and the Health Departments.

People taking medication regularly for the control of epilepsy are exempt from prescription charges for all drugs, not just those for epilepsy, dispensed under the NHS. They should complete Form P. 11 which should be available from the local Family Practitioner Committee (FPC) in England and Wales or Health Board in Scotland, social security offices, or dispensing chemists and give it to their doctor after completion.

Epilepsy and social security

If epilepsy results from an injury sustained, for example, at work or in a road traffic accident, then compensation can be sought in the usual way through the civil courts, if third party negligence can be proved. If it results from a criminal act, e.g. head injury during an assault, then compensation may be obtainable from the Criminal Injuries Compensation Board. Information on these and other aspects of the complex of social security legislation may be found in Matthewman & Lambert (1985).

In the rare cases where epilepsy has occurred as a result of vaccination and has caused severe disablement, a claim for payment under the Vaccine Damage Payments Scheme may be made. Application should be made to the Vaccine Damage Payments Unit, DHSS, North Fylde Central Office, Norcross, Blackpool, within a period of six years of a child's second birthday, or the date of the vaccination.

If the disability due to epilepsy is severe, then Attendance Allowance (DHSS Leaflet NI. 205) may be claimed. If attacks occur frequently at night the higher rate 24-hour allowance may apply. However, this allowance is less likely to be granted if the person is capable of looking after him or herself between attacks. The Severe Disablement Allowance (DHSS Leaflet NI. 252) may apply if a person is incapable of work and is at least 80% disabled. Unpredictable, frequent or severe seizures may be grounds for claiming this benefit. If a severely disabled person in receipt of Attendance Allowance requires constant care from another person, then it may be possible for the carer to claim an Invalid Care Allowance (DHSS Leaflet NI. 212). On the other hand, Mobility Allowance (DHSS Leaflet NI. 211) is not normally awarded to people with epilepsy, however frequent the attacks, unless there is also a physical impairment which renders the person unable or virtually unable to walk.

Under the Chronically Sick and Disabled Persons Act (1970), extended to Scotland in 1972 and Northern Ireland in 1978, local authorities are required to maintain a register of disabled people in their locality and provide as required 'assistance . . . in arranging for the carrying out of any works of adaption in his home or . . . any additional facilities to secure his greater safety, comfort or convenience'. Some people with epilepsy with very severe attacks or additional incapacities are able to obtain assistance under this legislation, for example, to install a telephone to maintain contact with relatives or the doctor. Other aids and adaptations may be available by virtue of this legislation, but the degree of implementation of the legislation is highly variable from area to area. The local authority must first acknowledge that a need exists, and that can be the most difficult part of the process. The epilepsy organizations, and major voluntary agencies such as MIND (The National Association for Mental Health) and MENCAP (The Royal Society for Mentally Handicapped Children and Adults) have specialized advice departments which can offer guidance in relation to social security legislation and, where appropriate, take up individual cases with the local authority.

The Disabled Persons (Services, Consultation and Representation) Act which became law in July 1986 may prove a useful tool to 'bring representation into rehabilitation', as one of its parliamentary supporters termed it. This statute, which also applies to Scotland, aims to give disabled people and their representatives a considerably expanded voice in arrangements which may be made for them in the community in terms of assessments and services. Although it has yet to be tested in practice, it may also go a long way towards closing the gap in the 1981 Education Act between school and community or further education described earlier in this chapter. It may also serve to clarify the intent of the 1970 Chronically Sick and Disabled Persons Act by putting beyond doubt that local authorities have a duty to consider the need of the disabled for services if so requested by the disabled person, or his or her representative carer (Hansard 4 July 1986, cols 1306 ff). The major voluntary organizations for disabled people will undoubtedly be issuing guidance concerning this important new legislation in the near future. It will be highly relevant to people disabled by epilepsy or who have additional problems.

The whole field of welfare rights is now very specialized, and the Government has proposed sweeping changes in the social security system during the next several years. Given their other concerns, it is unlikely that doctors, nurses or most other health workers can claim particular expertise in this sphere, especially when epilepsy might just be one strand in a combination of problems to do with employment, accommodation and health matters. The Child Poverty Action Group produces guides through this maze, e.g. the annual National Welfare Benefits Handbook and the Rights Guide to Non-Means-tested Social Security Benefits, and the Disability Alliance publishes annually the invaluable Disability Rights Handbook which covers benefits and services for disabled people. We recommend these publications as the best places for professionals or people with epilepsy to start when faced with a social welfare problem possibly related to epilepsy. Given the known links between poor health and economic and social disadvantage, this dimension of comprehensive care cannot be overlooked.

Driving

It should be stressed at the outset that laws regulating the holding of driving licences by people with epilepsy vary from country to country, and even within countries, e.g. amongst the American and Australian states. This section is not concerned with the vital questions of clinical judgement which must underlie the initial assignment of a diagnosis of epilepsy and its inevitable statutory consequences for an individual's fitness to drive (Espir 1983a). Rather, it describes the relevant law in the UK and usual pattern of its application.

In the UK, nearly half the population, i.e. some 24 million people, hold a driving licence. Of these it has been estimated there are about 130 000 adults with epilepsy who are potential drivers. A study of 1605 police- reported accidents involving collapse at the wheel but minimal injury was reported by Taylor (1982). Epilepsy, or suspected epileptic attack, was the most common cause of collapse at the wheel leading to an accident (38% involved a witnessed generalized seizure; 23% were 'blackouts' of which probably half were due to epilepsy). It is very worrying that of those collapsing due to a witnessed generalized seizure,

70% had not declared their epilepsy and 12% were experiencing a first attack.

Ordinary driving

On 21 April 1982 the Motor Vehicles (Driving Licences) (Amendment) (No 3) Regulations 1982 came into operation. These Regulations introduced new conditions (Statutory Instrument No. 423, 1982) for granting licences to persons with epilepsy. For ordinary vehicle licences, the relevant law now reads:

> Epilepsy is prescribed for the purposes of section 87(3)(b) of the Act of 1972 [the Road Traffic Act as amended in 1974] and an applicant for a licence suffering from epilepsy shall satisfy the conditions that –
> (a) he shall have been free from any epileptic attack during the period of 2 years immediately preceding the date when the licence is to have effect; or
> (b) in the case of an applicant who has had such attacks whilst asleep during that period, he should have had such attacks only whilst asleep during a period of at least 3 years immediately preceding the date when the licence is to have effect; and
> (c) the driving of a vehicle by him in pursuance of the licence is not likely to be a source of danger to the public.

Previously, a three-year rule had applied both when awake or asleep, with or without treatment. When a person with epilepsy wishes to drive for the first time, the normal application form must be completed in full. When received by the Driver and Vehicle Licensing Centre (DVLC) in Swansea, a further form will be sent to the applicant requesting details about the epilepsy, and information will also be requested from the applicant's doctor. Provided that the applicant fulfils all the usual and epilepsy related criteria, a licence will be issued but this may be for a reduced period in the first instance. If someone already holding a driving licence is diagnosed as having epilepsy, that person must notify DVLC and stop driving until further directed by DVLC. A licence will not be reissued until the person fulfils the above requirements. Reapplication may be made to the DVLC after the appropriate period, at which time further medical information will be requested.

A licence will be withdrawn from a person known to have epilepsy if any seizures occur during wakefulness. From the point of view of the Driving Regulations, which are the law as enacted by Parliament and enforced by the DVLC, auras and epileptic myoclonic jerks are counted as an epileptic attack. Despite the Regulations, a number of people who continue to have attacks while awake, also continue to drive. Many excuses are advanced – 'I've never had a seizure whilst driving', 'I always know when I'm going to have an attack', 'I get such a long warning that I can stop the car' etc. None of these carry any weight in law and may lead to prosecution if the person has been told that he or she is driving illegally while medically unfit and that his or her circumstances should be reported to DVLC. Physicians must avoid misleading patients into thinking that the regulations do not apply to them or that they can be waived in the light of individual circumstances (O'Brien 1986).

The onus of responsibility to inform DVLC rests with the licence holder, or licence applicant, and not with the doctor. Anyone who continues to drive once the diagnosis of epilepsy has been made does so illegally until the requirements are fulfilled. Car insurance, including third-party cover, is invalid if a person drives illegally. The matter of confidentiality is frequently raised in regard to information about fitness to drive. Doctors and nurses should always observe the rules of confidentiality established by their professional or statutory body, except in the exceptional circumstance in which every effort to obtain the person with epilepsy's consent to disclose information voluntarily has failed, and in which disclosure is judged to be in the best interests of the person with epilepsy or the public. The doctor may then disclose confidential information directly to a Medical Adviser at the DVLC.

This being said, however, doctors and other professionals must be able to exercise a sense of empathy and react sensitively to the considerable socio-economic implications of losing a driving licence. The advice offered by a doctor following a first seizure – and before a diagnosis of epilepsy is made – is crucial. In terms of practical advice, we would endorse the conclusion of Espir (1983b) that:

> in these cases, if there is no evidence of any other cause, then it may be considered that there is no disability for the ordinary licence holder or applicant to declare to the DVLC. However, driving should be stopped pending

specialist advice, and it is suggested that the doctor writes personally to the Medical Adviser at the DVLC seeking the opinion of the Honorary Medical Advisory Panel, without disclosing the patient's name unless consent is given.

In such cases, it is usual for a licence to be suspended for 12 months only. A second medical opinion about the diagnosis can always be sought by the person with epilepsy via his or her general practitioner and the DVLC's decision not to grant, or to withdraw, a licence may be contested by lodging an appeal at a Magistrate's Court within 30 days of the decision having been notified. If an employee is unable to continue in a job because he or she can no longer drive, the employer should make every effort to re-deploy that person within the same firm. The Manpower Services Commission's Code of Good Practice on the Employment of Disabled People (1984) discusses this further, though it does not have the force of law. Much can be achieved by expert counselling at such critical junctures.

Vocational and professional driving

Stringent special provisions apply to vocational and professional drivers who are required to hold a Heavy Goods Vehicle (HGV) or Public Service Vehicle (PSV) licence. Although covered by different legislation, the same rules are applied to taxi drivers. The regulations regarding HGV (exceeding 7.5 metric tonnes laden weight) and PSV (nine or more seats for hire or reward) licences were amended in 1982 (Road Traffic Act. The Heavy Goods Vehicles (Drivers' Licences) (Amendment) Regulations 1982). An individual is now barred from holding a vocational licence if he or she:

1. has suffered an epileptic attack since attaining the age of 5 years; and
2. has any medical condition likely to cause the driving by him or her of a HGV or PSV to be a source of danger to the public.

Thus a single epileptic seizure occurring since the age of 5 will debar a person from holding an HGV, PSV or taxi driver's licence. A single seizure occurring in a person already holding such a vocational licence will result in its immediate and permanent withdrawal. The situation regarding professional driving is less clear-cut. Many people with epilepsy hold ordinary licences quite legally and some may be required to drive vehicles, not covered by the HGV or PSV regulations, as part of their employment duties. Such activity is only covered by the statutory regulations pertaining to ordinary driving licences. However, since its inception in 1956 the Honorary Medical Advisory Panel on Epilepsy has reasoned that a person who has experienced an attack of epilepsy in early adulthood should not drive professionally. Occupations likely to be affected by this recommendation include ambulance drivers, mini-bus and mini-cab drivers and commercial delivery vehicle drivers.

The whole area of epilepsy and driving is one in which doctors in particular will be expected to give guidance, often on less than clear clinical evidence. An excellent review of the subject is Godwin-Austen & Espir (1982). All physicians should also be familiar with the latest version of Medical Aspects of Fitness to Drive (Raffle 1986).

LEISURE

Health professionals are often called on to give opinions about the risk of a particular person with epilepsy engaging in a leisure activity. Although this is a common request, no systematic study has been made of such areas of ordinary daily activity. Individual assessment of both the person concerned and the proposed activity is highly desirable, but not always practical. We have, therefore, formulated general guidance which can at least be a starting point to aid the individual concerned, the teacher or other responsible person organizing the activity.

Using leisure in a constructive way is important, especially as paid employment is becoming harder to find and time that might formerly have been filled by working needs to be taken up by other activities. If work is not possible for a person with epilepsy, or is not appropriate because of age or other circumstances, then a positive use of leisure time helps to prevent an erosion of physical health and self-esteem. Children with epilepsy at school should be included in the full range of ordinary team sports and other recreational activities,

unless the disorder is severe or other impairments prevent this. Some local regulations may still be over-restrictive in this area and based on outmoded assumptions. Simply knowing that a child or adult has epilepsy says nothing about suitability for sports and other activities.

The age of onset of epilepsy is a strong factor in the perception the person with epilepsy may take of 'alternative' activities. For example, an adult used to using a car, but who can no longer drive because of epilepsy, may already have well-developed leisure interests which can be pursued and developed further with minimal inconvenience. Indeed, it may be an impetus to beginning some new activity for which there was not time before and possibly in the company of new people. There is a potential for making positive changes in life patterns at a time when much that is valued appears threatened. An adult is also less dependent on others, who may tend to be over-restrictive because of their own anxieties about epilepsy. It is crucial, however, and regardless of age of onset, to avoid blaming everything on the epilepsy. Ordinary living involves both successes and failures, and it is 'ordinary living', after all, that should be the objective.

Before any activity is undertaken, the individual with epilepsy should ask 'is this realistic given my particular circumstances?' The list of activities below are those about which questions are most often asked. We believe that if the activity is suitable on health and safety grounds, then attitudes (both of others and the person with epilepsy) may be the deciding factor. Undoubtedly, the more the person with epilepsy can be seen to have something positive to offer and the confidence to back this up, the easier social integration will be. Most problems where epilepsy and leisure activities are concerned stem from misinformation coupled with general anxiety about taking risks. An informed person may need to ensure that these are corrected beforehand, especially if the question of the 'risk' of an individual having a seizure during the activity (which might range from virtually nil to highly probable) is confused with estimating the 'danger' which might result to the individual and others should the seizure happen.

One-off accidents can happen to anyone, whether epilepsy is present or not. If a seizure occurs during an activity, this is not an automatic signal that something tragic will follow and that future participation must be barred. Over-reaction to an attack is understandable on some occasions, but it can lead to over-restriction and its psychological consequences. Anxiety is normal where epileptic attacks may happen, but sensible provision for dealing with one should it occur can go a long way towards making most activities safe. Individual assessment and an informed decision about participation are always needed.

Swimming

In properly managed swimming pools there is little or no extra risk. Some local authority pool managements, and some schools, insist that people with epilepsy wear a coloured swimming cap. We feel this is more stigmatizing than helpful, though it is only right to inform the responsible authority at the swimming bath or for a teacher to keep a special check on a child with epilepsy in the water. The 'buddy system' is extensively used in some countries, and places responsibility for safety in the water on pairs of children. We believe this is well suited to epilepsy where a fit might occur. The general subject is discussed in the Sports Council's free publication 'Swimming and Epilepsy'. Swimming alone in the sea, rivers or lakes or in very cold water is not recommended. We firmly believe that every person with epilepsy should have the benefit of learning to swim and enjoying themselves in the water with others.

Water sports

The range is very wide and guidance varies with the particular sport. Subaqua diving is not advised for the person prone to epileptic seizures. Guidance is available in the excellent review by Croucher (1981)

Cycling

Where attacks are controlled there should be no increased risk. If seizures still occur, busy roads are best avoided and a companion would be advisable. Young children all want to ride bicycles, and a blanket restriction will probably result in covert riding in unsupervised settings, resulting in a greater danger than properly managed cycling.

Horse riding

Normal hard riding hats should be worn by all riders. The organization Riding for the Disabled maintains local groups and facilities where the person with epilepsy wishing to ride can be catered for, especially if he or she is additionally handicapped.

Boxing

All activities in which injury to the head is likely to occur are not advisable for people with epilepsy. Field sports involving possible head contact need individual assessment.

Climbing

Climbing frames and trees cannot be avoided, even if forbidden by well-meaning parents or schools. Most informed opinion now favours the benefits of these normal childhood activities. For organized climbing see the review by Croucher (1981).

Yoga

The physical and psychological aspects of yoga may be highly beneficial. The controlled deep breathing associated with the more common forms of yoga should not present any problems to the majority of people. Any of the national yoga associations can provide further guidance.

Discos

These are a normal part of growing up and should not be needlessly avoided by the young person with epilepsy who seeks a full social life. Some people may find flashing or flickering lights unpleasant, but generally it is only bright white 'strobe' lights operating at more than five flashes per second that may, in some individuals with photosensitive epilepsy, induce a seizure. Most local authorities have policies governing use of such lighting. It should be remembered that the majority of those with epilepsy are not photosensitive; if a fit should occur in a disco, it may well be spontaneous or due to another cause.

Television and videogames

A few people who are photosensitive may have a seizure while watching television or staring directly at the flashing screen of a videogame. If a particular game causes problems, then a different game should be chosen without the same stimulus on its screen. A television set used as a monitor for a computer or a videogame at home may present the same hazard. If normal television viewing is the problem, it should be watched in a well-lit room, more than eight feet away from the set. The susceptible person should avoid approaching the set to make adjustments, or should cover one eye (thus reducing the photic stimulation by half) while doing so (Jeavons 1985). Seizures due to television flicker are more common in Europe than in North America because of the differing electricity supply cycles, and consequently the slower flash rates on European screens.

Social drinking

Some people with epilepsy choose not to drink alcohol at all. But for most it seems that the occasional drink should cause no problems. It is well known, though, for over-indulgence in alcohol to cause seizures as a withdrawal symptom. Drinking bouts should be avoided, especially as they are usually associated with irregular sleeping patterns.

Travel

Difficulties may be encountered in some countries in obtaining exactly the same antiepileptic drugs used in one's own country, and of course the proprietary names of most AEDs differ from country to country. Drugs supplied in the UK by the National Health Service can usually be prescribed for no longer than one month's absence abroad. We strongly recommend that all people with epilepsy should carry accurate written information about their epilepsy and any drugs being taken. The various epilepsy associations can supply cards and forms for this purpose which can be signed by the doctor. The UK has reciprocal health arrangements with a number of countries, including all EEC countries. However, in order to obtain treatment and have the costs reimbursed at home, Form E 111 must be completed before travelling. It is obtainable from any DHSS office. The relevant publication is Leaflet SA. 30 which discusses reciprocal health arrangements. Adequate travel insurance for everyone is essential. The epilepsy associations can advise on companies which do not discriminate. If lack of sleep leads to attacks, then long-distance journeys overnight are not advisable. Flying does not cause fits, though disrupted sleeping and eating patterns may make them more likely in some people. Cabin staff should always be told in advance if a person's seizures are poorly controlled. Abrupt changes in tablet-taking regimes should be avoided and alternatives necessitated by new time zones should be phased in gradually after arrival.

Special holiday schemes

There are special holiday schemes for people who are either physically or mentally handicapped. Some people with epilepsy may sometimes need these special services. The Royal Association for Disability and Rehabilitation (RADAR) maintains lists of holidays for people with physical disabilities. The organization Physically Handicapped and Able-Bodied (PHAB) runs over 250 'PHAB Clubs' in the UK as well as residential holidays to bring handicapped and able-bodied people together on equal terms. The Royal Society for Mentally Handicapped Children and Adults (MENCAP) supports the Gateway Clubs scheme which include holidays for this special group amongst a wide range of other activities.

HEALTH EDUCATION

The practice of health education presents the epilepsy worker with considerable opportunities for co-ordinating expertise, enthusiasm and empathy. It also presents considerable challenges. There are snares for the unwary in health education's undoubted attractiveness. The thought of being able to facilitate people with epilepsy to acquire more information and thereby (it is often implicitly assumed) exercise greater self-care in the management of their condition is tempting to the professsional, who is perhaps more used to encountering social problems and non-compliance. However, in order to avoid one's initial enthusiasm for health education turning into cynicism after a first attempt that may fall short of achieving its objectives, it is advisable at the outset to consider some principles and practices before deciding on the appropriateness of various strategies.

The steps in identifying the components of a specific programme of health education in epilepsy have been discussed by Craig (1982). A prerequisite for planning is an awareness of the dynamics of health in both the natural and the social dimensions (Fig. 16.1).

Health is not static and human behaviour is a key factor linking its natural and social dimensions. Of course, behaviour itself is a composite force, the product of many influences (environmental, economic, ideological etc) acting upon and in addition to personal lifestyle. It is necessary to make this obvious statement in order to remind ourselves how easy it is to forget behaviour's complex antecedents when people don't do as we, or they, might otherwise have hoped or expected. For example, in the management of epilepsy, nothing is more common than for an outcome dependent on patient behaviour, such as compliance with prescribed drug therapy, not to be achieved. Since the desired outcome has by definition been identified as medically desirable, non-compliance can all too easily be identified with 'failure' by the patient and even with the assignment of blame for this predicament. Later in this section we discuss the assumptions underlying this view which may prejudice the success of a health education programme.

Impairment, disability and handicap

The World Health Organization (WHO) has promulgated widely adopted concepts of impairment, disability and handicap which help to explain the interrelationships between the dimensions of health (WHO 1980). Returning to Figure

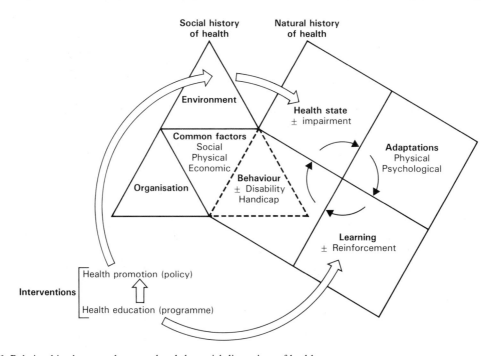

Fig. 16.1 Relationships between the natural and the social dimensions of health

16.1, we can say that from the standpoint of epilepsy, in the natural history of health, the given health state is one of neurological impairment. The impairment, i.e. the loss or dysfunction at organ or system level, expresses itself in the individual's tendency to experience recurrent paroxysmal cerebral disturbances. In response to this, most individuals will seek to make adaptations in the physical and/or psychological aspects of their lives, whether or not medical treatment is available, offered or followed. The learning process through which such adaptations become established will be reinforced positively or negatively by repetition, experimentation and change. Some new pattern of behaviour will eventually become dominant. The context in which this is expressed may reveal a dislocation of function at the level of the whole person. This whole-person problem constitutes a disability, i.e. a state of literally not being able to do something physical or mental that would otherwise be achieveable if the impairment were not present. The spectrum of disability is very wide, especially in the epilepsies, and susceptible to improvement or deterioration for many reasons.

The reactions of others in society (both in the formal, bureaucratic sense and the informal, personal sense) to the person with epilepsy may produce a state of relative disadvantage. This is termed 'handicap', i.e. a state which is the product of the interaction in a social setting between impairment and disability. A person's adaptive behaviour in response to a handicap may be the achievement of a new steady state in which, other things being equal, no further compensations are felt to be needed. In many instances, however, adjusting to handicap because of epilepsy means that something approaching a new equilibrium in one's life is achieved only by paying a high, if involuntary, price. The quality of life may be eroded; opportunities for personal development may be lost; reserves of confidence and self-esteem may dwindle. Health education in epilepsy should be proactive in recognizing and seeking to prevent this handicapping process wherever possible. Doing this effectively in the social dimension of health requires knowledge of the forces which might be brought to bear there, together with a clear set of objectives. We believe

that in many cases these objectives need not be medically defined, and neither should professionals always be in control of the process leading to their achievement.

Medical care is only one, and not always the most important, factor operating in the social dimension of the health of the person with epilepsy. No one exists in splendid isolation with only their doctor for company. As shown in Figure 16.1, the social, physical and economic aspects of the environment, the organization of its institutions and, of course, personal lifestyle, are all potential determinants of health behaviour in the social sphere. To illustrate this consider a single man in his early thirties whose attacks began about five years previously following a motor-cycle accident. The advent of epilepsy would most probably not have had a significant effect on his socialization into adult life or his acquisition of work skills. Though not completely controlled, his average of one complex partial attack and the occasional generalized seizure every few months does not stop him from performing well in the employment sphere. However, uncontrolled epilepsy does prevent him from retaining a driving licence. Depending largely on where he lives and what sort of work he does, and the social life he wants to have, he might or might not consider that his epilepsy constitutes a disability. If he lives in a city with good public transport and numerous leisure possibilities, and if he has a job that is adequately paid, then he might consider that not being able to drive is a fairly minor inconvenience. The same young man, however, would be severely handicapped as a result of epilepsy barring him from driving if he lived in a rural area where social isolation was compounded by lack of mobility, which in turn prejudiced his chances of finding and holding down employment in the surrounding area.

The dividing line between disability and handicap is not always clear cut. This is often the case where epilepsy is the major factor in the equation. To continue with the above example, the young man unable to drive and socially isolated in a rural area would certainly be handicapped in terms of job opportunities if no effort were made by statutory or voluntary agencies to identify his needs and seek to meet them by, for example, providing transport to work on a regular basis or organizing a placement in some type of work scheme which would enable him to earn an adequate income. The alternative would probably be reliance on inadequate social security benefits, itself felt to be stigmatizing by many disabled people. Of course, should his seizure control improve to the extent that he obtained a driving licence, then, other things being equal, the handicap stemming from epilepsy should largely disappear with the return of mobility and wider social contacts, possibly linked to relationships formed at work.

Handicap, then, need not be static. Its dynamic and relative nature has been described by the Inner London Education Authority (1985):

> disabilities and difficulties become more or less handicapping depending on the expectations of others and on social contexts. Handicaps thus arise from the mismatch between the intellectual, physical, emotional and social behaviour and aspirations of the individual and the expectations, appropriate or otherwise, of the community and society at large. Individuals with disabilities or significant difficulties may be handicapped by their own attitude to them and by the attitudes of others. Of equal significance, the degree to which the individual is handicapped is determined by the educational, social, physical and emotional situations which he or she encounters. Handicapping effects will vary from situation to situation and may change over time. (Educational Opportunities for All? para 1.1.25)

Deterioration as well as improvement is possible in response to the complex of factors operating in the social dimension of health. To conclude our example, the boredom and frustration of an unemployed and socially isolated young man might be associated with a worsening in his seizure control. As a result of more frequent, possibly more disabling, attacks he might become depressed about his state of health, thus reinforcing already lowered chances of mixing socially or finding work. Of course generalizing from a particular, and fictional, example is not valid. However, in times of general economic recession which severely affects parts of the country and types of traditional employment, individuals with a disability may be more likely to experience handicap stemming from reduced or withdrawn services, rejection or restrictions whose equity society may be less inclined to question than when opportunities are more widespread.

Problem analysis

Tackling complex problems such as outlined above calls for a systematic analysis of the interrelationship between factors in both the social and natural histories of the particular person's epilepsy. This is even more true if one intends to devise a programme which will be on offer to groups of people with epilepsy. We have modified a well-known approach to programme development in health education (Fig. 16.2) (Green et al 1980). This is usually known as the 'PRECEDE model'. PRECEDE is an acronym for Predisposing, Reinforcing, and Enabling Causes in Educational Diagnosis and Evaluation, and describes the steps in problem analysis which should literally precede attempts at implementation. This is particularly important given the vulnerability of health education programmes to failure if undertaken without a thorough understanding of the wider context of the presenting problem.

The attractiveness of the PRECEDE model is that it allows the planner to start with the 'here and now' social problem, probably identified by the person with epilepsy or someone close to him, such as no job, feelings of discrimination, low achievement, social security needs, lack of mobility, overprotection, general fears about epilepsy etc. The planner may then work through several antecedent stages to try and identify what lies behind that problem. With reference to Figure 16.2, the planner might ask such questions as: What are the problem's health components? What are its behavioural components? What factors in the individual's knowledge or attitudes towards epilepsy, in his general value system, his perceptions of himself and others, and the social norms of his environment might predispose to the appearance of this problem? What form of access to the intended client will be possible? What resources might be used and how? What referral network might be indicated? How will the programme, once begun, be reinforced? What will be the effect of the attitudes and behaviour of other people, lay and professional, to the success of the health education programme? Are health professionals primarily needed to achieve the programme's objective(s)? Attempting systemati-

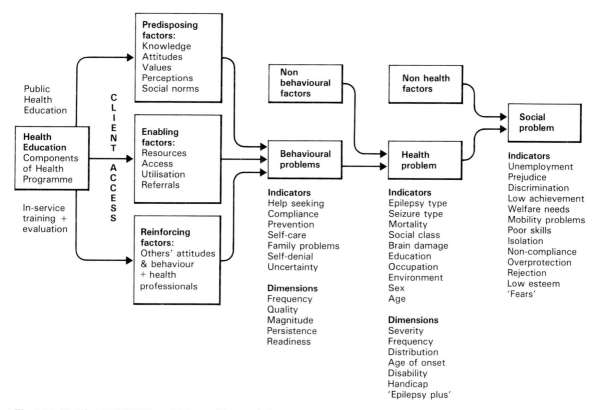

Fig. 16.2 Modified PRECEDE model for problem analysis

cally to answer questions such as these with the benefit of the PRECEDE model can, we believe, make it easier to identify the components which should go into the health education programme itself. Otherwise, the temptation might be to use whatever resources are already available, mainly for reasons of convenience rather than because they were particularly suited to the achievement of the desired outcomes in terms of changes in knowledge, skills, attitudes or behaviour of a particular individual or group receiving the programme.

For an example of the relevance of this approach, it is helpful to note that recent British social research suggests that some adults with epilepsy may, in effect, self-deny themselves employment opportunities because of reduced self-perceptions and their pessimistic expectations about the likely reactions of others in work situations. One study (Scambler & Hopkins 1980) concluded that this self-denial of opportunities might rank as high in creating life problems for this sample as overt stigmatization by others and

legitimate exclusion from some activities because of severity or frequency of attacks.

Taking 'self-denial of employment opportunities' as the presenting social problem for a particular individual, the PRECEDE model approach might suggest that factors lying behind this handicapping attitude included such things as a history of frequent partial epileptic attacks which tended to be misunderstood by lay observers as psychological disturbances. The person experiencing them might have a poor educational achievement record, which itself is often linked with a low social status and a history of dependency on social security. All of these factors may contribute to eroded self-esteem. Further probing might reveal predisposing factors in the individual's knowledge and beliefs about epilepsy. If these are negative or fatalistic, then it is not surprising that employment chances will be seen as relatively unattainable and employers and workmates as inherently prejudiced towards those with epilepsy. There might be a pattern of erratic communications between this individual and a succession of doctors, resulting in frequent changes in drug treatment and a poor grasp on the person with epilepsy's part of his or her role in helping to prevent the recurrence of seizures, for instance by keeping more regular hours or cutting down on alcohol consumption or taking medication as prescribed.

A detailed description of a programme of health education in epilepsy planned along these lines is beyond the scope of this chapter. However, it is encouraging to see the growing influence of systematic approaches to programme design in the efforts of leading epilepsy organizations whose projects were displayed at the Public Education Seminar as part of the 1985 XVIth Epilepsy International Symposium (Aspinall 1985a).

Types of health education

Analysis, however important, is only the first stage, and often a fairly mechanical one, in the construction of an appropriate health education programme. Arangio (1978) has suggested that the professional epilepsy worker in attempting to offer help and support should also strive to acknowledge the need of the person with epilepsy to be seen as:

1. A person
2. A person who has seizures
3. A person who may be viewed in various ways as different, because of his or her disorder
4. A person born into a cultural milieu that possesses some information about epilepsy that is already qualitatively and quantitatively defined
5. An offspring, or perhaps a sibling, or even a parent who is part of a family which may or may not have experience of epilepsy, but who have for themselves and for the person with epilepsy a set of needs, wishes, goals, aspirations and desires now complicated by the impact of epilepsy
6. A consumer of professionally delivered health and allied services
7. A consumer of institutional services such as schooling

Craig (1983) has discussed the contrast between professional and consumer objectives and needs, and suggested a typology for epilepsy health education. This illustrates the potential disparity of perspectives on epilepsy, and underscores the advantages of seeking a partnership in treatment, especially from the standpoint of encouraging compliance with rational antiepileptic therapy. Just as polypharmacy continues too often to masquerade as good treatment, so too a plethora of 'paper pills' exhorting and directing people with epilepsy to be 'good patients' often passes uncritically for effective health education. It needs to be said frequently that health education is not simply an adjunct to medical procedures. In the view of the World Health Organization (1969):

> the focus in health education is on people and action. In general its aims are to persuade people to adopt and sustain healthy life practices, to use judiciously and wisely the health services available to them, and to take their own decisions both individually and collectively, to improve their health status and environment

With this objective in mind, we believe that what health education in epilepsy should seek to do is to help the individual to attain an optimum level of functioning rather than to strive exclusively towards some absolute state of physical and mental wellbeing. In this approach, the active participation, if possible, of the person with seizures, and of the family and those closely around him or her, is strongly associated with success (Shope 1980, Schulman & Swain 1980). Three main approaches to health education in epilepsy are identified in the following typology (Craig 1983).

Type One Health Education

Objective	maximum patient compliance with treatment
Mode of operation	giving selected information to achieve compliance
Locus of control	external; doctor in control
Programme	giving 'facts' and implications of diagnosis
Resources	doctor talking plus printed information
Evaluation	informal/anecdotal
Modification	marginal success may produce 'victim' blaming and devalue health education

Type Two Health Education

Objective	preventive problem solving for 'good patients'

Mode of operation	selected fact giving to achieve remediation
Locus of control	external; multiprofessional 'experts' in control
Programme	recognizing and reporting problems (patient's role) and problem solving (professional role)
Method	persuasion/counselling to adopt attitudes of a 'good patient' and accept professional guidance and objectives
Resources	multi-media patient education; one-to-one and group work in hospital and community settings
Evaluation	patient attitude and behaviour changes measured against professionally-set objectives
Modification	changes in materials and techniques to increase success in terms of treatment objectives

Type Three Health Education

Objective	optimum functioning and treatment partnership with professional helpers
Mode of operation	provides conceptual framework for thinking, feeling and doing by the person in relation to everyday environment
Locus of control	internal; shared with 'experts' who may not be health professionals, including others with epilepsy
Programme	uses alternatives to 'medical model' of epilepsy; stresses wellness rather than illness
Method	person-centred learning strategies and agenda setting with appropriate professional input
Resources	'self-help groups', health education games and simulations, assertiveness training
Evaluation	parallel patient and professional measurements of success against individually set objectives
Modification	away from 'illness management' towards 'health maintenance' and optimum functioning despite disability

Type One is probably the most common on offer in all countries. It reflects the traditionally pre-eminent role of the medical profession in controlling access to health information. It relies on authority models and the doctor–patient relationship to transmit preselected information with, more often than not, compliance with medical instructions as the objective. Within a medical model of epilepsy and its management, compliance equals 'good patient behaviour' (Burkitt 1983, Black 1979). This is not to criticize the sincerity behind such an 'information giving' approach, but simply to state that it is not likely to achieve the global results usually hoped for it, except in the highly competent and motivated. It is naive to rely on an educational style alone, in the hope that inculcating more facts about epilepsy and its implications will somehow automatically lead to 'correct' behaviour. This is especially true when information is only presented verbally. This type of health education usually takes little or no account of the individual's readiness to learn and the circumstances in which learning might take place, the quality and quantity of existing health knowledge and factors from the physical and social dimensions of health which may strongly influence behaviour (Becker & Rosenstock 1984). It is particularly weak at recognizing such barriers when they lie behind non-compliance, especially when failure to follow a doctor's instructions might stem from the person with epilepsy's perception of the limits of the medical role (West 1976, Haynes et al 1979).

Type Two also provides information previously selected by a professional helper, but its objective is remedial and preventive rather than simply control through compliance. Its leading figure is usually, though not necessarily, a doctor. Everyone knows that otherwise 'good patients' often encounter problems with their treatment or other aspects of life, and usually seek professional help in devising solutions once the problem has been recognized and reported. Central to this, of course, is a constructive doctor–patient relationship. For this type of health education to succeed, the doctor 'should never forget that his *medical explanation* will always be *interpreted* by his hearers in their own particular way' (Ligue française contre l'épilepsie 1980). Even with this level of sophistication, the desired outcome, however, is still defined largely in medical objective terms, which it is assumed that 'good patients' implicitly share.

Both of the foregoing types of health education share a weakness which can affect even carefully constructed programmes. This stems from the relatively small attention, sometimes none, paid to factors influencing patient behaviour outside the medical model of epilepsy. People with epilepsy are not 'empty buckets' waiting to be filled with information chosen for them by professionals (Mittan 1982). Though considerable variations are possible, especially with Type Two, something more is needed that will bridge what is often a perceptual gap between the professional's objectives and expectations of treatment and the individual's rather more personal and concrete goals. This alternative approach can be found in Type Three health education about epilepsy. It is not primarily concerned with 'fact giving' or even with solving the problems of otherwise compliant patients, though these things are often by-products of its techniques. Rather, it is primarily concerned with facilitating wider understanding by the person with epilepsy, according to an agenda he or she sets him or herself with appropriate professional guidance. This is taken together with the development of coping skills to increase self-esteem and help the individual to act in a more 'self-empowered' manner in respect of aspects of life (and they are the majority) beyond the strictly medical.

Central to Type Three health education is some degree of 'power sharing' in devising and directing the therapeutic programme. Marinker (1981) amongst others has argued that the growth of information technology alone may mean that the 'distribution of power and control between patient and doctor will . . . be radically shifted towards a new equilibrium. The patient will be capable of making choices which are more informed than we now believe either possible or prudent'. It should be stressed, however, that Type Three health education as we conceive it is based not on competition but on partnership with the professional helper. It seems likely that those with epilepsy who feel they have more control over their own lives, and their treatment, as opposed to having feelings of relative powerlessness (De Villis et al 1980), may be more motivated to follow medical directions (de la Sota et al 1982). The reasons for this seem to be not because they have been ordered to do so, but because they have played a part in formulating a plan both they and their doctors and other helpers are all following (Wallston et al 1976). It also appears possible to teach individuals to improve their sense of being in control of their own bodies (having a stronger 'internal locus of control') in ways which also improve self-esteem (Lefcourt 1976). This is especially important in epilepsy, because the factor of self-esteem has been identified (Ekermo 1975) as aiding some people to 'withstand the attitudes of persons in their surroundings . . . and also interpret the reactions of others more positively than those with lower degrees of self-esteem'.

With the increasing use and sophistication of psychosocial measurement instruments in epilepsy (Dodrill et al 1983), undoubtedly the importance of health education strategies aimed at increasing self-esteem and assertiveness in individuals with epilepsy will be highlighted (Tan 1983, Cofield & Austin 1984). We believe that, in the longer term, approaches inspired by Type Three health education stand the best chance of engendering the awareness, attitudes and skills necessary to motivate and sustain the majority of people with epilepsy to acquire the sort of factual information which the Type One approach seeks to impart at the outset, often with only marginal success.

CONCLUSION: THE NEED FOR A COMPREHENSIVE APPROACH

Considerable progress could be made towards the goal of optimum social adaptation for people with epilepsy on the basis of existing knowledge and expertize, if more attention were devoted to organizing and delivering services in a comprehensive and multiprofessional way. The failings in the British National Health Service to meet the needs of the disabled population have recently been highlighted by the Royal College of Physicians (1986). Ironically, many young people with disabilities have fewer contacts with specialist health and social support services just as they are entering adulthood and could possibly benefit considerably from a complete reassessment of their need for medical, educational and social services (Thomas et al 1985). But progressive policies and better integrated services, and even more so the resources which no one doubts are needed, would in themselves be inadequate if divorced from an awareness of the factors shaping the community's understanding of epilepsy. Research suggests that social attitudes towards people with epilepsy are strongly conditioned by overexposure to the highly visible extremes of the epilepsy spectrum, i.e. where seizures are uncontrolled or where the people with epilepsy have a physical or mental handicap noticeable to others (Hansson & Duffield 1976, West 1979). Not surprisingly, this can lead to the popular notion that epilepsy is a catastrophe that only happens to 'other people'. Of course, nothing could be further from the truth, but the 'evidence' of everyday experience is very persistent. As epilepsy organizations are learning (Scherer 1983), merely asserting that people with epilepsy are the same as everyone else, is often ineffective because it contradicts powerful lay knowledge (Schneider & Conrad 1980, 1983).

Helping people without epilepsy to get things into perspective requires, above all, that people with epilepsy are enabled to make their collective presence felt in the everyday world; their role is indispensable in a comprehensive approach. Here again teamwork is required. Some countries have made considerable strides in focusing professional skills and the initiatives of voluntary organizations for people with epilepsy, their families and friends (Shorvon 1983). People who only a few years ago would not have dared to put their careers or reputations at risk by admitting their epilepsy are now proudly stating that they, too, are 'a person with epilepsy'. The self-help movement in epilepsy is the context in which such developments most often occur. It is at its strongest as an impetus for change (though still evolving even in developed countries) when professionals and the consumers of epilepsy services begin to unite for common objectives (Hartman et al 1983). There should be more such alliances worldwide, and it is highly relevant to consider why the self-help movement should be more advanced in some countries than in others.

Today it is undoubtedly becoming easier for an ever increasing number of people with epilepsy to get their seizures under control. But, of course, having epilepsy is more than 'just having fits'. There is not likely to be any 'magic tablet' treatment to counteract the subtle intertwining of psychological, sociocultural and economic aspects of this most variable of conditions. To meet these challenges what will always be needed is the appropriate marshalling of essentially human skills – empathy, skilled and knowledgeable communication and sensitive counselling and support (Baron 1981). From the standpoint of enabling individuals to achieve the fullest lives possible in spite of epilepsy, these skills can have as much, and sometimes more, impact than high-technology interventions, and at a fraction of the cost. If, by using this approach, epilepsy can be demystified on a personal level, then the atavistic misconceptions which still surround it on a social level will be more amenable to change. If the experiences of people with epilepsy can be shown to be part of the universal range of human experiences, then they will cease to be regarded as products of medical misfortune. If this chapter has kindled a wish to know more about these wider aspects of epilepsy, then it will have made a small contribution to the preconditions for a change in attitudes which will benefit everyone.

APPENDIX 16.1: SOME USEFUL ADDRESSES

Not all, or probably even most, people with epilepsy will need the services provided by the agencies listed below. However, because the epilepsies are broad and variable in their effects, it is essential that health professionals, especially doctors, have a basic knowledge of the range and expertize of such agencies for specialist advice and possible referral purposes. The list is selective and drawn from our own professional experiences.

Association of Carers
Medway Homes
Balfour Road
Rochester, Kent ME4 6QU
Tel. (0634) 813981
Offers advice, support and opportunities for self-help to carers of disabled and/or elderly people and represents their needs to statutory services and other agencies.

Association of Disabled Professionals
The Stables
73 Pound Road
Banstead, Surrey SM7 2HU
Tel. (07373) 52366
A pressure group which aims to ensure that the abilities of severely disabled people are fully used by securing improved opportunities for them as full members of society.

Association of Parents of Vaccine Damaged Children
2 Church Street
Shipston-on-Stour, Warwickshire CV36 4AP
Tel. (0608) 61595
A campaigning body concerned with obtaining compensation and appropriate services for children and families injured by the complications of immunisation.

Association for Spina Bifida and Hydrocephalus
22 Upper Woburn Place
London WC1H OEP
Tel. (01) 388 1382
Pursues both welfare and research connected with these conditions and offers social work, advice, education and training, education and employment services as well as other aspects of support and care.

British Epilepsy Association
Anstey House
40 Hanover Square
Leeds LS3 1BE
Tel. (0532) 439393
Offers educational and social work services across the range of needs related to epilepsy as well as maintaining a nationwide (England, Wales and Northern Ireland) network of self-help 'Action Groups'. Regional offices in Birmingham, Cardiff, Belfast, Leeds, Reading and London.

Centre on Environment for the Handicapped
126 Albert Street
London NW1 7NF
Tel. (01) 482 2247
Works to make architects and other professionals concerned with design and the environment more aware of special needs of disabled people. Offers a consultancy and information service on access issues.

Centre for Studies on Integration in Education (CSIE)
c/o The Spastics Society
12 Park Crescent
London W1N 4EQ
Tel. (01) 636 5020
Promotes good practice in integration in education for all children with special educational needs, collects information on implementation of the 1981 Education Act and disseminates up to date advice.

Child Poverty Action Group
1 Bath Street
London EC1 V9PY
Tel. (01) 253 3406
Research and publication of facts relating to causes of family poverty in relation to the social security benefits system. Offers an information service to professionals, including advice on appeals procedures.

Children's Legal Centre
20 Compton Terrace
London N1 2UN
Tel. (01) 359 6251
Offers free advice and information service by letter or telephone concerning legal rights and interests of children and young people; monitors and makes representations on matters of law and policy affecting these groups.

Disability Alliance Educational and Research Association
25 Denmark Street
London WC2 8NJ
Tel. (01) 240 0806
Runs a welfare rights advice service and produces publications on social security for people with disabilities and their advisers.

Disabled Living Foundation
380–384 Harrow Road
London W9 2HV
Tel. (01) 289 6111
Provides an information service on all a pects of living with disabilities, with an emphasis on practical help with daily tasks including special aids and equipment.

Epilepsy Association of Scotland
48 Govan Road
Glasgow G51 1JL
Tel. (041) 427 4911
Besides Strathclyde, EAS also has offices in the Central, Grampian, Lothian and Tayside Regions offering a comprehensive education and social work service for lay people and professionals.

Health and Safety Executive
Local offices of the HSE (see telephone directory under 'Health and Safety Executive') will provide contacts for the Employment Medical Advisory Service, which is able to advise on any questions about aspects of health and safety concerning a particular disabled person and the need for any special provision.

Irish Epilepsy Association
249 Crumlin Road, Dublin
Tel. Dublin 516500/516371
The national voluntary association for epilepsy in the Republic of Ireland, offering a comprehensive social work, education and training and advisory service to lay people and professionals.

Manpower Services Commission (Disabled Persons Services)
MSC Head Office
Moorfoot, Sheffield S1 4PQ
Tel (0742) 753275
General information on full range of services for disabled persons; also contactable via local Jobcentre (Disablement Resettlement Officer).

Medicalert Foundation
9 Hanover Street
London W1R 9HF
For a small fee this foundation provides a useful service to those liable to require emergency attention because of epilepsy. The person wears either a bracelet or a necklet on which epilepsy is identified, together with a personal serial number and emergency telephone number. Any authorized person may thus contact Medicalert by phone, reversing the charges, from anywhere in the world and obtain information, provided by the person's doctor, from a central file.

MIND (The National Association for Mental Health)
22 Harley Street
London W1N 2ED
Tel. (01) 637 0741
Offers educational, advocacy and advisory services on all aspects of mental health issues.

National Bureau for Handicapped Students
336 Brixton Road
London SW9 7AA
Tel. (01) 733 77977
Provides an information and advice service on all aspects of education and handicap.

National Federation of Gateway Clubs
117 Golden Lane
London EC1Y 0TJ
Tel (01) 253 9433
Co-ordinates and develops the work of Gateway Clubs, a national network of clubs providing widely varying activities including sports, music, drama, arts and crafts, visits and holidays for mentally handicapped people.

National Head Injuries Association (HEADWAY)
17–21 Clumber Avenue
Sherwood Rise
Nottingham NG5 1AG
Tel. (0602) 622382

National Society for Epilepsy
Chalfont Centre for Epilepsy
Chalfont St Peter, Buckinghamshire SL9 0RJ
Tel. (02407) 3991
Maintains the Chalfont Centre for Epilepsy offering, in the Main Centre, long and intermediate term care for approximately 400 people who are maintained by their local authorities and, in the Special Centre, a 45-bedded assessment unit funded by the National Health Service on a supra-regional basis for 3–6 month assessment of epilepsy and its attendant problems. The NSE also provides a health education and information service to professionals and publishes a wide range of educational packages, videos and leaflets.

Opportunities for the Disabled
1 Bank Buildings
Princes Street
London EC2R 8EV
Tel. (01) 762 4963

An organization funded by employers whose senior staff are on secondment from industry and commerce. It offers help with recruitment, rehabilitation and career development of disabled employees. Offices also in Birmingham, Leicester and Manchester.

PHAB (Physically Handicapped and Able-Bodied)
Tavistock House North (2nd floor)
Tavistock Square
London WC1H 9HX
Tel. (01) 388 1963

Provides and promotes opportunities for the physically handicapped and the able-bodied to come together on equal terms in a range of activities centred in some 450 'PHAB' Clubs and holiday schemes throughout the country.

Riding for the Disabled Association
Avenue 'R'
National Agricultural Centre
Kenilworth, Warwickshire CV8 2LY
Tel. (0203) 56107

Through a nationwide membership group scheme, provides opportunities for disabled adults and children to ride and thus benefit their general health and sense of well-being.

Royal Association for Disability and Rehabilitation (RADAR)
25 Mortimer Street
London W1N 8AB
Tel. (01) 637 5400

Co-ordinates some 400 local member associations and acts as a pressure group on central and local government. Has an active legal and parliamentary committee. RADAR is concerned with all aspects of disability, but particularly with access, education, employment, holidays, housing, mobility and welfare. Extensive range of publications which are useful to professionals and clients alike.

Royal Society for Mentally Handicapped Children and Adults
(MENCAP)
Mencap National Centre
123 Golden Lane
London EC1Y 0RT
Tel. (01) 253 9433

Offers support for mentally handicapped people and their families through a network of 450 local societies and regional offices, as well as financing research and providing specialist information and advisory services to lay people and professional workers.

Spastics Society
12 Park Crescent
London W1N 4EQ
Tel. (01) 636 5020

Maintains a network of local groups and supports schools, education centres, industrial units etc for people with cerebral palsy. Also runs a family services and assessment centre and a comprehensive network of social services.

SPOD (Association to Aid the Sexual and Personal Relationships of the Disabled)
286 Camden Road
London N7 0BJ
Tel. (01) 607 8851/2

Provides information and advice on problems in sex and personal relationships which disability can cause. Publishes leaflets and gives individual advice on request or through a network of counsellors. Provides an information and training service for professional workers.

REFERENCES

Aldenkamp A P 1983 Epilepsy and learning behaviour. In: Parsonage M, Grant R H E, Craig A G, Ward A A (eds) Advances in epileptology: the XIVth Epilepsy International Symposium. Raven Press, New York, pp 221–228

Appolone C, Romeis J, Gibson P, McLean W, Howard G 1979 An epilepsy workshop for professionals. Epilepsia 20: 129–132

Arangio A J 1978 An assessment model: a systemic examination of the psychosocial needs of patients with epilepsy. Patient Counselling and Health Education 1(2): 75–80

Aspinall A (ed) 1985a An International approach to educational campaigns about epilepsy. Public Education Seminar Organizing Committee, Hamburg, unpublished

Aspinall A 1985b Careers advice, further education and employment prospects for ordinary school leavers with epilepsy. In: Craig A G, Oxley J, Dowds C (eds) Children and young People with epilepsy: an educational package for teachers. National Society for Epilepsy, Chalfont St Peter, pp. 1–2

Aspinall A 1985c The change in the law and its effect on the community. In: Fenwick P, Fenwick E (eds) Epilepsy and the law. Royal Society of Medicine (symposium series No 81), London, pp 29–34

Baron J 1981 The development of counselling and education service for people with epilepsy. Counselling 38: 26–29

Becker M H, Rosenstock I M 1984 Compliance with medical advice. In: Steptoe A, Matthews A (eds) Health care and human behaviour. Academic Press, London, pp 153–178

Beintema D J 1983 Comments from nonmedical professionals. In: Parsonage M, Grant R H E, Craig A G, Ward A A (eds) Advances in epileptology: the XIVth Epilepsy International Symposium. Raven Press, New York, pp 31–34

Beran R G 1983 Attitude of doctors toward patients with epilepsy. In: Parsonage M, Grant R H E, Craig A G, Ward A A (eds) Advances in epileptology: the XIVth Epilepsy International Symposium. Raven Press, New York, pp 9–16

Beran R G, Read T 1980 Patient perspectives of epilepsy. Clinical and Experimental Neurology 17: 59–69

Betts T A 1983 What the patient needs to know. In: Parsonage M, Grant R H E, Craig A G, Ward A A (eds) Advances in epileptology: the XIVth Epilepsy International Symposium. Raven Press, New York, pp 17–23

Bicknell D J 1983 A community-based service for mentally-handicapped adults with epilepsy. British Journal of Clinical Practice (Symp. suppl. no 27): 131–134

Bicknell D J 1985 The teacher and the adolescent student with mental handicap and epilepsy. In: Craig A G, Oxley J, Dowds C (eds) Children and young people with epilepsy: An educational package for teachers. National Society for Epilepsy, Chalfont St Peter, pp 3–7

Black D 1979 The paradox of medical care. Journal of the Royal College of Physicians 13: 57–65

Booth P 1985 Parental attitudes towards a child with epilepsy. In: Craig A G, Oxley J, Dowds C (eds) Children and young people with epilepsy: an educational package for teachers. National Society for Epilepsy, Chalfont St Peter, pp 8–11

Bowman T, Leppik I, Loewenson R, Pepin S, Beniak T 1984 Nurse clinician availability decreases use of medical facilities by persons with epilepsy. Paper presented at XVth Epilepsy International Symposium, Washington DC, unpublished

Brahams D 1983a Epilepsy and legal insanity – R v. Sullivan. Practitioner 227: 421–423

Brahams B 1983b Epilepsy and insanity at common law. Lancet 5 February: 309

Buchanan N 1982 Treatment of epilepsy: whose right is it anyway? British Medical Journal 1:173

Burkitt A 1983 Health education. In: Clark J, Henderson J (eds) Community health. Churchill Livingstone, Edinburgh, pp 29–39

Carter T 1986 Health and safety at work: implications of current legislation. In: Edwards F, Espir M, Oxley J (eds) Epilepsy and employment: a medical symposium on current problems and best practices. Royal Society of Medicine (symposium series no 86), London, pp 9–17

Centre for Studies on Integration in Education (CSIE) 1986 Caught in the act – a survey and handbook. Spastics Society, London

Channon S 1982 The resettlement of epileptic offenders. In: Gunn J, Farrington D P (eds) Abnormal offenders, delinquency and the criminal justice system. John Wiley, London, pp 339–373

Cofield R, Austin J K 1984 Psychosocial adjustment of adults with epilepsy. Patient Counselling and Health Education 6(3): 125–130

Commission for the Control of Epilepsy and its Consequences 1978 4 vols. US Department of Health, Education and Welfare Pub. No. (NIH) 78–276, Washington DC

Commission of the European Communities 1986 Memorandum of the commission to the council concerning the employment of disabled people in the European Community (COM (86) 9 final) Brussels

Confederation of British Industry 1983 Employing disabled people. CBI, London

Cox B 1985 The law of special educational needs. Croom Helm, London

Craig A G 1982 Increasing the effectiveness of epilepsy health education. British Journal of Clinical Practice (symposium supplement no. 18): 121–129

Craig A G 1983 Health education and epilepsy. In: Rose F C (ed) Research progress in epilepsy (Progress in neurology series). Pitman, London, pp 564–571

Craig A G 1985 Epilepsy and the 1981 education act: some implications for teachers, parents and children. In: Craig A G, Oxley J, Dowds C (eds) Children and young people with epilepsy: an educational package for teachers. National Society for Epilepsy, Chalfont St Peter, pp 12–15

Craig A G, Oxley J 1986 Statutory and non-statutory barriers to the employment of people with epilepsy. In: Edwards F, Espir E, Oxley J, Epilepsy and employment: a Medical symposium on current problems and best practices. Royal Society of Medicine (symposium series no 86), London, pp 21–31

Craig A G, Oxley J, Dowds C eds 1985 Children and young people with epilepsy: an educational package for teachers. National Society for Epilepsy, Chalfont St. Peter.

Croucher N 1981 Outdoor pursuits for disabled people Woodhead-Faulkner, London

de la Sota A, Herfindahl L, Lee J, Clark M, Treiman D M 1982 'Circles of Decisions': a new epilepsy patient education programme. In: Akimoto H, Kazamatsuri H, Seino M, Ward A A (eds) Advances in epileptology: the XIIIth Epilepsy International Symposium. Raven Press, New York, pp 471–473

Dasgupta A K, Saunders M, Dick D J 1982 Epilepsy in the British Steel Corporation: an evaluation of sickness, accident and work records. British Journal of Industrial Medicine 39: 145–148

Department of Health and Social Security 1986 Report of the Working Group on Services for People with Epilepsy. HMSO, London

Department of Health and Social Security 1986 neighbourhood nursing – a focus for care (the Cumberlege report). HMSO, London

De Villis R F, De Villis M, Wallston S, Wallston K A 1980 Epilepsy and learned helplessness. Basic and Applied Social Psychology 1(3): 241–253

Dodrill C B 1983 Psychosocial characteristics of epileptic patients. Research Publications of the Association for

Research in Nervous and Mental Disease 61: 341–353

Dowds N, McCluggage J R, Nelson J 1983 A survey of the socio-medical aspects of epilepsy in a general practice population in Northern Ireland. Department of General Practice, Queen's University/British Epilepsy Association, Belfast

Ellenberg J H, Hirtz D G, Nelson K B (1986) Do seizures in children cause intellectual deterioration? New England Journal of Medicine 314: 1085–1088

Ekermo E 1975 What it means to have epilepsy: emotional experience and social reality. In: Janz D (ed.) Epileptology: proceedings of the seventh internationl symposium on epilepsy (West Berlin). Thieme, Stuttgart, pp 91–96

Espir M L E 1983a Fitness to drive: additional guidance on epilepsy. Health Trends 15: 46–47

Espir M L E 1983b The present regulations and their application. In: Godwin-Austen R B, Espir M L E (eds) Driving and epilepsy – and other causes of impaired consciousness. Royal Society of Medicine (symposium series no 60), London, pp 29–33

Fenwick P, Fenwick E (eds) 1985 Epilepsy and the law – a medical symposium on the current law. Royal Society of Medicine (symposium series no 81), London

Fitzpatrick P, Hinton J, Newman S, Scambler G, Thomson J 1984 The experience of illness. Tavistock, London

Floyd M 1983 Draft Report on an exploratory study on epilepsy and employment. Tavistock Institute of Human Relations, London (unpublished)

Floyd M 1986 A review of published literature on epilepsy and employment. In: Edwards F, Espir M, Oxley J (eds) Epilepsy and employment: a medical symposium on current problems and best practices. Royal Society of Medicine (symposium series no 86), London, pp 3–7

Floyd M, Espir M L E 1986 Assessment of medical fitness for employment: the case for a code of practice. Lancet 26 July: 207–209

Gloag D 1985 Epilepsy and employment. British Medical Journal 291: 2–3

Godwin-Austen R B, Espir M L E 1983 Driving and epilepsy – and other causes of impaired consciousness. Royal Society of Medicine (symposium series no 60), London, pp 29–33

Golding A M B 1985 The law relating to epilepsy and allied disorders. Community Medicine 7: 278–281

Gowers W 1901 Epilepsy and other chronic convulsive diseases. 2nd edn. Churchill, London, p 302

Green L W, Kreuter M W, Deeds S G, Partridge K B 1980 Health education planning: a diagnostic approach. Mayfield, Palo Alto

Gunn J 1977 Epileptics in prison. Academic Press, London

Gunn J 1981 Medico-legal aspects of epilepsy. In: Reynolds E H, Trimble M R (eds) Epilepsy and psychiatry. Churchill Livingstone, Edinburgh, pp 165–174

Hackney A 1976 Epilepsy and the ordinary school. Special Education-Forward Trends 3(1): 12–15

Hackney A 1977 Emotional problems of children with epilepsy. Education in the North 14: 55–58

Hackney A 1985 Awareness of epilepsy in schools: why teachers need it and how it can be developed. In: Craig A G, Oxley J, Dowds C (eds) Children and young people with epilepsy: an educational package for teachers. National Society for Epilepsy, Chalfont St Peter, pp 16–19

Hall M B, Jolly H 1984 The child with a handicap. Blackwell, Oxford

Hansson R O, Duffield B J 1976 Physical attractiveness and the attribution of epilepsy. Journal of Social Psychology 99: 233–240

Hartman E, Arntson P, Droge D, Norton R 1983 Initial results from a questionnaire for people who have experienced seizure activity. Epilepsy in the Urban Environment Project/Center for Urban Affairs and Policy Research, Northwestern University, Evanston, Ill

Harvey P, Hopkins A 1983 Neurologists, epilepsy and driving. In: Godwin-Austen R B, Espir M L E (eds) Driving and epilepsy – and other causes of impaired Consciousness. Royal Society of Medicine (symposium series no 60), London, pp 9–15

Haynes R B, Taylor D W, Sackett D L 1979 Compliance in health care. Johns Hopkins, Baltimore, Md

Helander E, Mendis P, Nelson G 1983 Training disabled people in the community: a manual on community-based rehabilitation for developing countries. WHO, Geneva

Hermann B P (ed) 1980 A multidisciplinary handbook of epilepsy. Thomas, Springfield, p 111

Hodgman C H, McAnarney E , Myers G J et al 1979 Emotional complications of adolescent grand mal epilepsy. Journal of Pediatrics 95(2): 309–312

Holdsworth L, Whitmore K 1974 A study of children with epilepsy attending ordinary schools 1. their seizure patterns, progress and behaviour in school; 2. information and attitudes held by their teachers. Developmental Medicine and Child Neurology 16(6): 746–758, 759–765

Holmes O W 1891 Medical essays. Houghton, Mifflin, Boston, p 192

Inner London Education Authority (1985) Educational opportunities for all? The report of the committee reviewing provision to meet special educational needs. ILEA, London

International Labour Office 1983 Encyclopaedia of Occupational Health and Safety (Parmeggiani L ed.). 3rd edn. ILO, Geneva, pp 1769–1770

Jeavons P M 1985 The management of photosensitivity in school-aged children and young adults. In: Craig A G, Oxley J, Dowds C (eds) Children and young people with epilepsy: an educational package for teachers. National Society for Epilepsy, Chalfont St Peter, pp 20–23

Kangesu E, McGowan M E L, Eheh J 1984 Management of epilepsy in schools. Archives of Disease in Childhood 59(1): 45–47

Kettle M, Massie B (eds) 1982 An employer's guide to disabilities. RADAR, London

Kurtz Z, Bennett A E 1981 Services for young people with epilepsy. DHSS, London (unpublished)

Lance J W 1977 Empathy with epilepsy. Medical Journal of Australia 25: 907–908

Lechtenberg R 1984 Epilepsy and the family. Harvard University Press, Cambridge

Lefcourt H M 1976 Locus of control. Laurence Erlbaum, Princeton

Ligue Française contre L'epilepsie 1980 Epilepsies et epileptiques, Paris

Lisle J, Waldron H A 1986 Employees with epilepsy in the National Health Service. British Medical Journal 292: 305–306

Lockard J S, Ward A A (eds) 1980 Epilepsy: a window to brain mechanisms. Raven Press, New York

Long C G, Moore J R 1979 Parental expectations for their epileptic children. Journal of Child Psychology and Psychiatry 20: 299–312

MacIntyre I 1976 Epilepsy and employment. Community Health 7: 195–204

McLellan D L 1986a British Medical Journal 7 June 1986 292:1530

McLellan D L 1986b Medical needs of young physically handicapped people. Lancet 21 June 1986:1446

Maguire P, Fairbairn S, Fletcher C 1986 Consultation skills of young doctors. British Medical Journal 292: 1573–1578

Male J, Thompson C 1985 The educational implications of disability. RADAR, London

Manpower Services Commission 1984 Code of good practice on the employment of disabled people. MSC, London

Marinker M 1981 '2010' Journal of the Royal College of General Practitioners 31(230): 540–546

Matthewman J, Lambert N 1985 Social security and state benefits. Tolley, London

Mittan R J, Wasterlain C G, Locke G E 1982 Fear of seizures. In: Akimoto H, Kazamatsuri H, Seino M, Ward A A eds. Advances in epileptology: the XIIIth Epilepsy International Symposium. Raven Press, New York, pp 459–461

Mostofsky D I 1978 Epilepsy: action for improving socialization and family support, and reducing stigma and negative attitudes. In: Perlman L G (ed.) The role of vocational rehabilitation in the 1980s serving those with invisible handicaps such as cancer, cardiac illness and epilepsy. National Rehabilitation Association, Washington DC, pp 46–61

National Union of Teachers 1984 Meeting special educational needs in ordinary schools: NUT, London

Nash W, Thurston M, Baly M 1985 Health at school – caring for the whole child. Heinemann, London

O'Brien S 1986 The controversy surrounding epilepsy and driving: a review. Public Health 100: 21–27

Occupational Pensions Board 1977 Occupational pension scheme cover for disabled people (Cmnd 6849). HMSO, London

Oliver M J 1981 Epilepsy, crime and delinquency: a sociological account. Sociology 14(4): 417–440

O'Neill P 1983 Health crisis 2000. WHO/Heinemann, London

Parsonage M 1983 Education of medical undergraduates and postgraduates about epilepsy. In: Parsonage M, Grant R H E, Craig A G, Ward A A (eds) Advances in epileptology: the XIVth Epilepsy International Symposium. Raven Press, New York, pp 1–8

Peake G 1984 Assisting the disabled worker. Nursing 32 (2nd series): 939–941

Porter R J 1984 Epilepsy – 100 elementary principles. Saunders, Great Yarmouth

Radley R 1985 The management of epilepsy in the classroom and during school related activities. In: Craig A G, Oxley J, Dowds C (eds) Children and young People with epilepsy: an educational package for teachers. National Society for Epilepsy, Chalfont St Peter, pp 23–25

Raffle A (ed.) 1986 Medical aspects of fitness to drive. 4th edn. Medical Commission on Accident Prevention, London

Ross E M, West P B 1978 Achievements and problems of British eleven year olds with epilepsy. In: Meinhardi H, Rowan A J (eds) Advances in epileptology 1977. Swets and Zeitlinger, Amsterdam, pp 34–37

Ross E M, Peckham C S, West P B, Butler N R 1980 Epilepsy in childhood: findings from the National Child Development Study. British Medical Journal 280: 207–210

Ross E M, Kurtz Z, Peckham C S 1983 Children with epilepsy: implications for the school health service. Public Health 97(2): 75–81

Ross E M, Peckham C S 1983 School children with epilepsy. In: Parsonage M, Grant R H E, Craig A G, Ward A A (eds) Advances in epileptology: the XIVth Epilepsy International Symposium. Raven Press, New York, pp 215–220

Ross E M, Bommen M 1983 An epilepsy clinic for children: analysis of a year's work. British Journal of Clinical Practice (symposium suppl. no 27): 131–134

Royal Association for Disability and Rehabilitation 1984 Guide to the education act 1981. RADAR, London

Royal College of Nursing 1985 Health screening of entrants for nurse training: report of the working party of the RCN society of occupational health nursing. RCN, London

Royal College of Physicians 1986 Physical disability in 1986 and beyond. RCP, London

Rutter M, Graham P, Yule W 1970 A neuropsychiatric study in childhood. Spastics International Medical Publications/Heinemann, London

Scambler G, Hopkins A 1980 Social class, epileptic activity and disadvantage at work. Journal of Epidemiology and Community Health 34(2): 129–133

Scambler G, Hopkins A 1986 Being epileptic: coming to terms with stigma. Sociology of Health and Illness 8(1): 26–46

Scambler G 1984 Perceiving and coping with stigmatizing illness, 203–226. In: Fitzpatrick P, Hinton J, Newman S, Scambler G, Thomson J (eds) The experience of illness, Tavistock, London

Scherer A 1983 Epilepsy and public attitudes: strategies for change. In: Parsonage M, Grant R H E, Craig A G, Ward A A (eds) Advances in epileptology: the XIVth Epilepsy International Symposium. Raven Press, London, pp 63–70

Schneider J W, Conrad P 1980 In the closet with illness: epilepsy, stigma potential and information control. Social Problems 28: 32–44

Schneider J W, Conrad P 1983 Having epilepsy: the experience and control of illness. Temple University Press, Philadelphia

Schulman B A, Swain M A 1980 Active patient orientation. Patient Counselling and Health Education 2(1): 32–37

Shapiro H L 1983 Training of nonmedical professionals through clinical treatment, monitoring, and evaluation of people with epilepsy. In: Parsonage M, Grant R H E, Craig A G, Ward A A (eds) Advances in epileptology: the XIVth Epilepsy International Symposium, Raven Press, New York, pp 35–40

Shope J T 1980 Intervention to improve compliance with pediatric anticonvulsant drug therapy. Patient Counselling and Health Education 2(3): 135–141

Shorvon S D 1983 Specialized services for the non-institutionalized patient with epilepsy: developments in the US and the UK. Health Trends 15: 40–45

Spastics Society 1985 Discrimination and disabled people. Spastics Society, London

Spastics Society 1986 An equal chance for disabled people? Spastics Society, London

Stilwell B 1986 Nurses as co-practitioners: threat or promise? The Practitioner 230: 501–503

Stores G, Hart J 1976 Reading skills of children with generalized or focal epilepsy attending ordinary school. Developmental Medicine and Child Neurology 18: 705–716

Stores G 1981 Learning and emotional problems in children with epilepsy. In: Reynolds E H, Trimble M R (eds)

Epilepsy and psychiatry. Churchill-Livingstone, Edinburgh, pp 33–48

Stores G 1982 Psychosocial preventive measures and rehabilitation of children with epilepsy. In: Akimoto H, Seino M, Kazamatsuri H, Ward A A (eds) Advances in epileptology: the XIIIth Epilepsy International Symposium. Raven Press, New York, pp 437–439

Swift L 1985 The present law. In: Fenwick P, Fenwick E (eds) Epilepsy and the law. Royal Society of Medicine (symposium series no 81), London, pp 9–13

Tan S-Y 1983 Psychological functioning of epileptic patients referred for psychological intervention. In: Parsonage M, Grant R H E, Craig A G, Ward A A (eds). Advances in epileptology: the XIVth Epilepsy International Symposium. Raven Press, New York, pp 79–87

Taylor J 1982 Epilepsy and other causes of collapse at the wheel. In: Godwin-Austen R B, Espir M L E (eds) Driving and epilepsy – and other causes of impaired consciousness. Royal Society of Medicine (symposium series No 60), London, pp 5–7

Thomas A, Bax M, Coombes K, Goldson E, Smyth D, Whitmore K 1985 The health and social needs of physically handicapped young adults: are they being met by the statutory services? Developmental Medicine and Child Neurology (suppl. 50) 27(4)

Tillotson A, Stanley P J 1982 Epilepsy in the community school of social studies. Leeds Polytechnic (unpublished)

Trades Union Congress 1985 TUC guide on the employment of disabled people. TUC, London

Udall R 1985 Family adjustment and the role of counselling. In: Craig A G, Oxley J, Dowds C (eds) Children and young people with epilepsy: an educational package for teachers. National Society for Epilepsy, Chalfont St Peter, pp 31–33

Vaughan M, Shearer A 1986 Mainstreaming in Massachusetts. Centre for Studies in Integration/Spastics Society, London

Wallston B S, Wallston K A, Kaplan G D, Maides S A 1976 Development and validation of the health locus of control (HLC) scale. Journal of Consulting and Clinical Psychology 44(4): 580–585

Ward F, Bower B D 1978 A study of certain social aspects of epilepsy in childhood (suppl. 39 to Developmental Medicine and Child Neurology vol 20). Spastics

International Medical Publications/Heinemann, London

Warnock Report – Special Educational Needs 1978 The Report of the Committee of Enquiry into the Education of Handicapped Children and Young People. HMSO, London

West P B 1976 The physician and the management of childhood epilepsy. In: Wadsworth M, Robinson D (eds) Studies in everyday medical life. Martin Robertson, London, pp 13–31

West P B 1979 An investigation into the social construction and consequences of the label epilepsy. Sociological Review 27(4): 719–741

West P B 1983 Acknowledging epilepsy: improving professional management of stigma and its consequences. In: Parsonage M, Grant R H E, Craig A G, Ward A A (eds) Advances in epileptology: the XIVth Epilepsy International Symposium. Raven Press, New York, pp 41–50

Whitmore K 1985 Health services in schools – a new look. Spastics International Medical Publications, London

Wolfendale S et al 1986 Advice on your child. Spastics Society RADAR, London

World Health Organization 1969 Planning and evaluation of health education services (technical report series no 409). WHO, Geneva.

World Health Organization 1978 Alma-Ata 1978: Primary health care. (Health for all series no 1). WHO, Geneva

World Health Organization 1980 International Classification of impairments, disabilities and handicaps. WHO, UNICEF, Geneva

World Health Organization 1985 Targets for health for all: targets in support of the European regional strategy of health for all. WHO, Copenhagen

Yule W 1980 Educational achievement, epilepsy and behaviour. Workshop on the psychological assessment of persons with epilepsy. Swets and Zeitlinger, Amsterdam, pp 162–168

Ziegler R G 1981 Impairments of control and competence in epileptic children and their families. Epilepsia 22: 339–346

Zielinski J J, Rader B 1984 Employability of people with epilepsy: difficulties of assessment. In: Porter R J, Mattson R H, Ward A A, Dam M (eds) Advances in epileptology: the XVth Epilepsy International Symposium. Raven Press, New York, pp 577–581

17

Medical services

S. D. Shorvon

INTRODUCTION

The planning and provision of services for epilepsy in any community depend broadly on the following considerations.

1. The epidemiological characteristics of the epileptic population
2. The range of needs of the epileptic patients
3. The adequacy and range of the general medical, neurological and paediatric services, with which the epilepsy services must interrelate
4. The funding and the level of care which the community is able and willing to provide for the epileptic patient.

Circumstances vary in different countries, in all these aspects, and generalizations applicable to all communities are therefore possible only in the very broadest terms. The needs of epileptic patients, for instance, depend on the level of support received from family and others; and on the patient's perception of his or her rights and requirements. The adequacy of the medical services in any country must also be related to the general standard of living and the social network in the community. The funding of health care provision is largely a political matter, and one which of course will have a profound effect on the level of services ultimately provided. This chapter will concentrate mainly on the provision of services in the United Kingdom and then briefly draw comparisons with the concerns and structure of services in two other countries, with markedly constrasting priorities, the United States and Kenya, based on experience in all three countries. This review is very much a personal one and is not intended to provide comprehensive coverage.

Only the adult services and those provided within the medical context will be considered in any detail.

EPIDEMIOLOGICAL ASPECTS

A discussion of services for any condition can only be usefully conducted with an understanding of the epidemiological characteristics of the condition. This is complicated in regard to epilepsy as the severity, etiology, prognosis and extent of associated handicap may vary enormously. Thus, simple vital statistics should be interpreted with care, and detailed information about the characteristics of epilepsy in a population is as important as the prevalence or incidence. Furthermore, although epilepsy is perhaps the most common serious neurological disorder, exact incidence and prevalence figures have varied considerably in different studies because of differences in inclusion criteria, diagnostic criteria and case ascertainment methods; evaluation is therefore difficult (Sander & Shorvon 1987). If for instance, febrile seizures, neonatal seizures, single seizures or seizures in acute illnesses are included, the figures may be elevated by several fold. Similarly, if active seizures only are counted in prevalence studies, a figure several times lower than the lifetime prevalence will be found. Many studies have been retrospective and based on hospital records, and the selection bias introduced in such investigations may result in a distorted view of the clinical characteristics of the condition (as for instance severe and partial epilepsies may be over-represented in hospital clinics) and a significant underestimate of the true number of cases in any community. Some patients are unaware that they have seizures; and in one survey in metropolitan London, for instance, less than 20% of patients presenting with seizures expected the diagnosis (Hopkins & Scambler 1977). In a community survey in Warsaw, one-third of cases identified had never been treated, and one-quarter had not consulted a doctor (Zielinski 1974). It is clear, therefore, that any interpretation of epidemiological figures requires a detailed understanding of the study methodology.

In most studies, the overall incidence of epilepsy (excluding febrile seizures and single seizures, and sometimes neonatal seizures and seizures in acute illnesses) has been found to lie between 20 and 80 cases per 100 000 persons. About 1% of all neonates are said to have seizures, and about 5% of all children, by the age of 5 years, have febrile convulsions. The prevalence of epilepsy in a community has been usually found to lie between 3 to 10 cases per 1000 persons, depending on the methods of investigation (Sander & Shorvon 1987). In most patients developing epilepsy, the condition remits, and the lifetime prevalence (the number of patients who have ever had the condition) is estimated at between 2% and 5% (excluding febrile convulsions) – considerably higher than the actual prevalence found where only active cases are included (see Table 17.1). Incidence rates are highly age specific, and well over half of patients developing seizures do so before the age of 15, and thus while they are in the age range covered by paediatric services.

The characteristics of epilepsy in a general population have been poorly studied, and large-scale investigations are currently under way. The US Commission for the Control of Epilepsy and its Consequences (1978) attempted to quantify such aspects as the requirement for medical services, the frequency and type of seizures, and the presence of associated handicap, and these and other estimates are shown in Table 17.2. Although these should be taken as an approximate guide only, they do indicate the scale of the health care needed. As not all patients with epilepsy carry the same economic load, the commission divided the cases into five groups, as shown in Table 17.3; and this classification is useful for the planning of services. Thus, of the estimated 10 persons per 1000 with epilepsy, 6 will require little medical attention (groups 4 and 5 - comprising mainly those with seizures in remission, those with mild seizures or undiagnosed cases); 3 will require regular medical care, which is usually provided by both community and hospital services (group 3); and 1 will require institutional care or its equivalent (groups 1 and 2). An aetiology is found for the epilepsy in about one-third of cases only; the sex incidence is roughly equivalent, and the condition is slightly more common in the lower socio-economic classes.

Table 17.1 Prevalence findings from a survey of epilepsy amongst 6000 persons in a single general practice in Tonbridge, Kent, UK (derived from Goodridge & Shorvon 1983)

Seizures	Per 1000 persons
Lifetime prevalence*	20.3
Recurrent seizures**	17.0
Active epilepsy† and/or on treatment	10.5
Active epilepsy†	5.3

* Defined and the number of persons in the population who have ever had a non-febrile seizure.
** Lifetime prevalence of recurrent seizures
† Defined as those who had a seizure within the previous 24 months

Table 17.3 Classification of patients with epilepsy for analysis of service requirements (from Commission for the Control of Epilepsy and its Consequences 1978)

Group	Prevalence rate
Group 1 Institutionalized patients (including those in nursing homes, institutions for the mentally retarded, state mental homes etc)	0.04%
Group 2 The residential equivalent (patients in the community requiring or waiting for institutional care)	0.03%
Group 3 Patients in the community requiring regular medical attention for their epilepsy	0.33%
Group 4 Patients in the community requiring only occasional medical care for their epilepsy	0.26%
Group 5 The unidentified patient in the community whose epilepsy is unreported	0.34%

Table 17.2 The characteristics of epilepsy and medical manpower in a typical British region of 1 000 000 persons

	Generalized	Partial
Prevalence and incidence of seizure disorders		
New cases of epilepsy each year (incidence 50/100 000)		500
New cases of febrile seizures (incidence 50/100 000)		500
New cases of single seizures (incidence 20/100 000)		200
Cases of active epilepsy (prevalence 5/1000)		5 000
Cases who have ever had a seizure (lifetime prevalence 20/1000)		20 000
Requirement for medical care (for grouping, see text)		
Group 1: Cases in institutions (0.4/1000)		400
Group 2: Residential equivalent (0.3/1000)		300
Group 3: Cases requiring ongoing medical attention (3.3/1000)		3 300
Group 4: Cases requiring occasional medical attention (2.6/1000)		2 600
Characteristics of the epilepsy (for the 3600 persons in the community under active medical care, groups 2 and 3)		
Seizure type and etiology:		
generalized seizures only		2 000
partial seizures only		700
mixed partial and generalised seizures		700
others		200
Seizure frequency (seizures/year):	Generalized	Partial
one or less a year	450	50
between one a month and one a year	1650	400
more than one a month	600	950
Associated neurological or psychiatric disorders:		
epilepsy only		900
intellectual disability also		1 600
behavioural disability also		1 800
neurological disability also		350
Medical manpower provision (approximate mean figures)		
General practitioners		465
Consultant psychiatrists (mental illness)		22
Consultant general physicians		21
Consultant paediatricians		11
Specialists in community medicine		6
Consultant psychiatrists (mental handicap)		3
Consultant neurologists		3
Consultant neurosurgeons		2
Consultant clinical neurophysiologists		1

(Approximate estimates only, derived from a variety of sources, see text).

Extrapolating these figures to a UK population, there would be about 500 000 persons with epilepsy, including 20 000 in institutions (group 1). Of those in the community, 180 000 would need on-going (usually community and hospital based) medical treatment (groups 2 and 3) and a further 130 000 would require occasional medical treatment (usually provided by the community services). Figures of severity and additional handicap are a very rough approximation only, and have been based on small often selected samples; community-based studies are currently in progress. From currently available information, it can been estimated that about 37 000 patients in the UK will have more than one major attack

a month and 55 000 more than one minor attack a month. Similarly, about 175 000 reported cases and an equal number of unreported cases have epilepsy as the only problem, and 150 000 have additional intellectual or behavioural handicap. Figures, computed for a representative region of one million inhabitants, are shown in Table 17.4.

The US Commission also attempted to estimate the cost of epilepsy, and their figures are shown in Table 17.4. These again can be considered very rough estimates only and are based on 1975 values. Unemployment is calculated on the basis of an average salary for a non-handicapped person with the same demographic characteristics, and is calculated for the number in excess of the national

Table 17.4 The estimated overall cost of epilepsy in the US in 1975 (from The Commission for the Control of Epilepsy and its Consequences 1978)

Cost areas	Cost in US dollars
Unemployment (groups 2,3)	516 000 000
Unemployment (group 1)	317 000 000
Underemployment (group 3)	517 000 000
Excess mortality (groups 1,2,3)	435 000 000
Treatment (groups 2,3)	333 000 000
Institutionalization (group 1)	908 000 000
Residential care (group 2)	370 000 000
Drugs (groups 1,2,3,4)	110 000 000
Vocational rehabilitation and special education (groups 1,2,3)	77 000 000
Research	38 000 000
Total	3 621 000 000

See Table 17.3 for description of groups

unemployment rate (8.5% at that time). The costs of underemployment were based on the assumption that the average person in the community earned 20% less than his or her unaffected colleague. Excess mortality rates are based on the costs of lost production. Treatment costs include all professional care (excluding drugs which are calculated separately). Institutional and rehabilitation costs are based on the excess costs of epilepsy over and above the cost of institutionalization and rehabilitation for other reasons (e.g. mental or physical handicap). In 1975, therefore, the annual cost to the community was estimated to be over 3000 million dollars. Other authorities arrived at higher figures, such as the 4.37 billion dollars calculated by the Epilepsy Foundation of America. Although these figures are approximate estimates only, and can not be accurately extrapolated to the UK, it is clear that the condition carries with it an enormous economic liability. No similar figures are available for the UK, but only with such data can rational decisions about the allocation of resources be made.

Traditionally, and properly, epilepsy lies within the province of neurology, and recently in the US, there has been considerable debate about the numbers of neurologists needed to provide an adequate service. The structure of health care in the US, of course, is very different from that in the UK, as are the numbers of neurologists and their role in the provision of care. Nevertheless, a comparison is illuminating. There are about

450 000 active medical practitioners in the US, about 1 per 600 persons in the population (and this compares with 68 000 in the UK, or about 1 per 800 persons). About 1.5% of these practitioners are neurologists compared with 0.2% in the UK. Furthermore, the future (1990) national need for neurologists has been recently considered by a number of authorities (all groups with vested interests) and their estimates have diverged widely: the Joint Commission on Neurology of the American Neurological Association/American Academy of Neurology calculated a need for 14 000 neurologists for direct patient needs (or 17.27 million neurologist hours per year); the Graduate Medical Education National Advisory Panel 62 000, the Delphi panel 11 200, and Kurtze et al 12 600 neurologists (Kurtze et al 1986). These are rates of between 3.44 and 6.76 neurologists per 100 000 population, compared with the current UK figure of about 0.27. Kurtze et al (1986) analysed these needs by neurological condition, and concluded that a neurologist (including one assumes paediatric neurologists) will need annually 340 hours for outpatient consultations for patients with epilepsy for every 100 000 population; 74 hours for single seizures; and 52 hours for febrile seizures (out of a total of 2100 hours per annum per neurologist). The epilepsy figures, for example, are based on the assumption that the annual incidence of epilepsy is 50 per 100 000; that the condition lasts for a mean of 13 years, that between 75% and 99% of new cases and 50% of old cases will be seen by a neurologist; and that 50 minutes should be spent on a first consultation, 120 minutes per new case for the next 12 months and 40 minutes per old case per year. Similar figures are not available for the UK and comparisons are not easily made. In the UK, primary care facilities are much better developed than in the US, and much of the consultation time spent by neurologists would in the UK be spent by general practitioners. The neurologist in the UK takes much more of a consulting role and is seldom involved in the 'total care' of patients or in routine follow-up to the extent of his or her American colleague. Furthermore, in the UK, children with epilepsy are usually dealt with by paediatricians and not paediatric neurologists. Nevertheless, these figures

give an approximate idea of the American neurologist's perception of the time needed to care for patients with seizure disorders.

EPILEPSY SERVICES IN THE UNITED KINGDOM.

The principle of specialization

In the UK, there has been, since the 1939–45 war, a series of government-sponsored reports concerned with the provision of services for epilepsy. These include *Welfare of handicapped persons: the special needs of epileptics and spastics* (Ministry of Health, 1953), *Medical care of epileptics. (The Cohen report)* (Central Health Services Council 1956), *People with epilepsy. (The Reid Report)* (Central Health Services Council 1969), *The development of services for epilepsy in the 1970's* (Morgan & Bennett unpublished), *Services for young people with epilepsy* (Kurtz & Bennett unpublished), *Report of the working group on services for people with epilepsy* (DHSS 1986). These reports are a chronicle of English social history and mirror the conceptual evolution of health planning in the post-war years. The most ambitious was the Reid report of 1969, which was a high watermark of British Welfare State philosophy. The most recent DHSS Working Group report is a substantial retrenchment; reflecting the current retreat from the view that the State should provide for all medical needs. Many good recommendations have been made in these various documents but, sadly, many have been ignored or shelved, due to lack of funding or political will; the failure to act on the substance of these reports deserves further examination (Shorvon 1983).

Since 1948, and the inception of the National Health Service, medical care of patients with epilepsy has been carried out largely by the general NHS facilities, and the private and voluntary agencies have played a relatively minor role. An issue crucial to the development of services within this system is that of *specialization*. This must be clearly appreciated, for the need to accept the principle of specialization is implicit in many of the recommendations made by the Reid committee and the later reports.

In the UK, epilepsy is treated in hospitals usually by the neurological and paediatric services and the general disinclination to accede to this principle has perhaps more than any other factor, inhibited the development of specific epilepsy services (Shorvon 1983). Furthermore, in the current political climate, new initiative is unwelcome and any radical restructuring of the service provision is most unlikely to occur. A particular example of this has been the fate of the suggestion (made in 1969 by the Reid committee amongst others) that specialized epilepsy clinics be set up on a regional or district level (see below). At present, a few such clinics exist but their development has been piecemeal and largely due to the enthusiasm of a local consultant, without any central administrative support (Espir et al 1987). It has been the decision to maintain epilepsy services within the general neurological provision which has impeded such developments. Ironically, the Reid report proved very influential elsewhere, and the development in the 1970s of epilepsy services in the US for instance were due more to this report than were developments in the UK. Having said this, however, the general medical services in the UK are well developed, and much has been achieved. The advances in the care of all patients with chronic disease have been paralleled in the undeniable improvement in the care of those with epilepsy.

Framework of care for epilepsy in the UK

General practice

A great strength of medical care provision in the UK is the structure of general practice. All persons in the community are registered with and have free access to a general practitioner (GP), who acts as that patient's personal physician and who has a legally binding responsibility for his primary medical care. The GP may refer a patient to a specialist of his or her choice, and a report of the consultation will be retained in the general practice notes which should therefore contain the patient's lifetime medical records. A single physician, therefore, has overall charge of a patient's medical care over long periods, and this opportunity for continuity of care is a major advantage for the patient with epilepsy.

Table 17.5 The role of the general practitioner in epilepsy

Initial referral to specialist for
  diagnosis
  classification
  investigation
  treatment recommendations

Medical surveillance:
  Monitor effectiveness of antiepileptic drugs
  Monitor side effects of antiepileptic drugs
  Prescription of antiepileptic drugs
  Monitor compliance
  Monitor neurological developments
  Emergency treatment

Re-referral to specialist:
  seizures return after a remission
  unacceptable seizure frequency
  medical complications of epilepsy or treatment
  neurological deterioration
  treatment review or treatment withdrawal
  specific developments eg. pregnancy, surgery
  counselling

Counselling and long-term support:
Co-ordination of primary health care services

The role of the GP in epilepsy is summarized in Table 17.5. The GP is the first doctor a patient with newly developed epilepsy will normally see, and the GP is therefore likely to be the first doctor to suspect the diagnosis of epilepsy. An average practitioner with 2000 patients may expect to see two new cases of non-febrile epileptic seizures a year, and may have ten patients with active epilepsy and 30 with a history of epilepsy on his list. Usually the new patient will be referred for a specialist opinion for confirmation of the diagnosis, and for advice regarding treatment. For the patient with established epilepsy, the GP will be responsible for the continued medical supervision of the patient, sometimes in concert with the hospital clinic (in practice, the hospitals are involved in the care of less than one-half of patients with active epilepsy), and will be normally the source for prescription of the patient's medication. The GP is in the best position to obtain a witnessed account of the seizures and, to monitor seizure frequency, compliance, the effectiveness and side-effects of the medication and other medical developments. In cases where care is shared with the hospital services, a co-operation card has been suggested (as used in diabetic clinics); but as yet no such a scheme has been tried. The GP should be well versed in the emergency treatment of seizures, including febrile convulsions, and should probably carry rectal diazepam with his or her emergency equipment.

The GP is also the person best placed to counsel a patient concerning medical and non-medical aspects of epilepsy (Table 17.6), whether this entails a detailed discussion of the implications of the seizure disorder or simply a sympathetic ear. He or she should also take a lead in the co-ordination of the efforts of other community-based services (see below). An audit of care has been recommended to GPs to cover various aspects of epilepsy, and has been tried in a number of practices (Table 17.7). Patients who are seizure-free (on or off medication) or who are stabilized may be quite satisfactorily supervised by the general practitioner, but facilities for re-referral should be available for all patients for advice.

Table 17.6 Counselling checklist in epilepsy

Medical	*Social*
Basic facts about nature of epilepsy and seizures	Education
Seizures – practical management of a seizure	Employment
– emergency action	Leisure and sport
– precipitating factors	Marriage and domestic life
EEG and other investigations	Driving
Prognosis	
Inheritance	
Treatment – objectives	
– limitations	
– toxicity	
Other aspects – contraception and pregnancy	
– intercurrent illness	
– surgery	

Other community based medical, paramedical, nursing and social work facilities

Other community-based health care facilities which may be of value to patients with epilepsy include the school medical service; the occupational health service; and the community nursing and psychological services. For those with additional mental handicap, the district mental handicap team can be a valuable asset. Again, in the absence of a well-defined specialized epilepsy service, the efforts of these groups are often unco-ordinated and overlapping, which is wasteful of resources and expertise. The GP has an important role in co-ordinating the activities of these other primary care agencies.

The community social work agencies have an important part to play in assisting those significantly handicapped by their epilepsy (largely groups 2 and 3 of the US Commission report). They can provide guidance and counselling; help in housing, employment and financial aspects; and support in times of personal crisis. Individual

Table 17.7 The audit of care in general practice

1. The following questions could be entered initially on to an audit card.
   Date of first seizure and pattern of subsequent epilepsy
   Description of epileptic seizures
   Classification of seizures
   Aetiology
   Seizure precipitation and timing
   Previous episodes of status
   Other neurological features
   Other psychological features
   Drug treatment (drug/dose/regimen): current/past
   Side-effects of treatment: current/past
   Hospital attendance (dates/hospital/consultant): current/past
   Investigation: EEG
                 CT
                 Serum antiepileptic levels
                 Other (e.g. Fbc, folate, calcium, LFTs)
   Counselling checklist; (see Table 17.6)

2. The following aspects entered onto the card during on-going review (depending on the clinical situation, but usually every 6–12 months).
   Seizure occurrence
   Treatment (drug, dose, regimen)
   Side effects
   Serum levels (if required)
   Other investigations
   Compliance
   Hospital attendance
   New developments

patients have individual needs, and the professional social worker's training, with its emphasis on individual case work, is well suited to assistance in these areas. The extent to which social workers are able to provide succour to handicapped patients has been underestimated in the past, and their important role should be fully recognized.

The DHSS Working Group (1986) felt, as did the Reid committee, that a patient with epilepsy 'should not be dealt with on the basis of the medical diagnosis, but on the basis of the extent to which they are, or are not, handicapped in their daily lives'. For this reason, they should not be treated as a separate client group, but rather within the general framework of facilities for the handicapped. In this sense, the need for specialization advocated for the medical care of patients is not mirrored in the nursing, psychology or social work services. This is inappropriate and is a reflection of the different models of disability taken by different disciplines. In practice, no such specialization occurs, and according to one survey for instance (Morgan & Bennett 1980), only one of the 118 directorates of social work in England and Wales have special policies for the care of those with epilepsy. They concluded that 'whilst there might be a general philosophical framework which departments work within, there is certainly no coherent policy, no generally operated code of practice'. Whether there should be some sort of coherent policy is debatable, but the principle of treating a person as an individual rather than a case is correct. Nevertheless, identified individual social workers should be encouraged to take a special interest and gain special experience in epilepsy; and, within districts, the client load should be great enough to make this feasible. In 1984, 70% of main-grade social workers were professionally qualified, compared with 40% in 1976, so there is a high level of expertise available. It is of vital importance to co-ordinate social work and medical efforts, and again this role falls most appropriately to the general practitioner.

Voluntary agencies

Voluntary agencies have been active in the field of epilepsy for over a century, and there are now

Table 17.8 The role of the voluntary agencies

Individual patient care – counselling and support:
    Individual volunteers
    Professional workers
    Promotion and organization of self-help groups
    Organization of local activities

Educational activities – public and professional:
    Written and audiovisual material
    Organization of meetings and seminars
    Professional education officers

The provision of residential accommodation and day centres:
    Institutional accommodation
    Community housing
    Day centre support

Research:
    Research funding
    Research projects

a number of independent organizations (see appendix). Table 17.8 lists the traditional roles of the voluntary sector, but in the current climate of central and local government financial restraint, charitable funding of much of what previously was regarded as a statutory responsibility is increasingly necessary. An important feature of the work of the voluntary agencies is that they approach the problems of epilepsy with a non-medical perspective, and this is a useful counterbalance to the medical domination of service provision. On an individual level, volunteer workers and self-help groups can support and sustain epileptic patients in a way which the professional medical and paramedical personnel often overlook. On a broader level, the voluntary agencies should provide public and professional education and training. Another primary function of several of the voluntary organizations is the provision and administration of a range of residential accommodation and day-care facilities. Finally, the voluntary sector supports research into epilepsy.

The activities of the voluntary sector in the field of epilepsy in the UK have been of variable success. Whilst the residential functions have been well run, the educational, public relations and research roles have been deficient, when compared with both the voluntary epilepsy agencies abroad and the charities involved in other medical fields in the UK. A considerable opportunity has been wasted here.

Hospital-based facilities.

Initial referral, assessment and follow up The role of the hospital medical services is summarized in Table 17.9. The Reid report (1969) recommended that all patients who develop seizures should be referred for a specialist opinion, and this recommendation is now widely accepted. In a survey of general practice in 1960, Pond et al (1960) estimated that approximately 70% of newly diagnosed patients were referred for specialist opinion; and in a more recent survey of practice in Southern England, over 90% of patients were referred (Goodridge & Shorvon 1983). Initial referral is important to confirm the diagnosis of epilepsy; to classify the seizures and establish an aetiology; and to make initial treatment recommendations. Counselling is also important at this stage (Table 17.6) and assessment should be made of associated handicaps. Many patients will not require more than a straightforward medical

Table 17.9 The role of the hospital medical service

New patients:
    Confirm diagnosis of epileptic seizures
    Classify seizures
    Establish etiology
    Assess associated handicaps
    Institute necessary investigations
    Institute initial treatment
    Monitor treatment in initial stages (efficacy and toxicity)
    Make long-term treatment recommendations
    Follow-up of selected patients

Patients with epilepsy in remission (group 4*):
    Review the need for treatment

Patients with chronic active epilepsy (groups 1,2,3,4*):
    Review diagnosis and etiology
    Institute further investigations as necessary
    Review treatment and decide on antiepileptic drug changes
    Make long term antiepileptic drug treatment
    recommendations
    Consider surgical treatment
    Follow-up of selected patients

All patients:
    Provide facilities for emergency treatment
    Refer to other specialists as required
    Provide re-referral facilities to general practitioners
    Counsel patients as required
    Co-ordinate input from other medical and non-medical
    services

* See Table 17.3 for description of groups
Some of these fucntions could be carried out most effectively in a specialized epilepsy clinic

evaluation and, once treatment is stabilized, their follow-up can be best continued by the GP. For other patients, inpatient assessment, continual outpatient follow-up or further referral are necessary.

Electroencephalographic (EEG) facilities (see Ch. 8) A variety of EEG techniques now exist for the diagnosis and evaluation of epilepsy. The great majority of new cases require a routine 16-channel EEG recording, for purposes of diagnosis and classification. Routine EEG is available in all regions in the country, sited sometimes, for historical reasons, in psychiatric rather than general hospitals, and the EEGs are usually reported by consultant neurophysiologists.

In a small number of cases, differential diagnosis may be difficult and more specialized EEG may be necessary, including prolonged recording using ambulatory EEG or video EEG telemetry (Table 17.10). EEG telemetry is also used for quantification of seizure activity, for sleep studies and for ITU uses. In the few hospitals in the country with telemetry facilities, these are situated within special units, often funded or part funded from research grants. Facilities should also exist for sleep recordings, and for sphenoidal EEG recordings, again on a supraregional basis. Specialized EEG (including telemetry, sphenoidal and invasive EEG) recording is also needed where

Table 17.10 Use of EEG telemetry in epilepsy

1. To record seizures:
   Differential diagnosis of epileptic seizures (e.g. from psychogenic seizures or syncope or cardiac dysrhythmia)
   Localize seizure onset, for classification purposes. This is important for treatment purposes, and in particular as part of presurgical investigation (sometimes with intracerebral or sphenoidal electrode placement)
   Identify precipitating factors

2. To minimize EEG temporal sampling error:
   Identify interictal abnormalities, not seen on routine EEG recordings, for diagnosis and classification (e.g. the recording of natural light sleep for the detection of interictal spikes in partial epilepsy).
   Quantify epileptic activity
   Identify diurnal patterns of seizure activity

3. Other applications:
   Sleep studies in epilepsy
   ITU monitoring of acute epilepsy
   Teaching and research

epilepsy surgery is carried out, and this should also be provided on a supraregional basis.

Serum antiepileptic drug level monitoring Facilities for monitoring antiepileptic drug levels are also required to provide a useful epilepsy service, and these are now available in most districts. With all techniques of measurement (e.g. gas liquid chromatography), quality control is an important issue and may be deficient in a laboratory where levels are only occasionally measured. A voluntary nationwide scheme for monitoring quality control exists, administered from the epilepsy unit at the University Hospital of Wales in Cardiff; and national laboratories have been urged to participate. A quick service, in which results are available in the clinic within a few minutes of venupuncture, greatly improve efficiency, cutting down patient visits and correspondence, and this should be provided where possible. Again, this is only likely to prove feasible in the context of a dedicated epilepsy clinic. Antiepileptic drugs requiring routine serum level monitoring are phenytoin, carbamazepine, ethosuximide, and phenobarbitone (and phenobarbitone derived from primidone).

Other diagnostic facilities The other investigational requirements for epilepsy are shared with other medical and, in particular, neurological departments. These are largely biochemical and radiological and are required for the investigation of etiology. Many patients will require a CT (computerized tomography) scan, usually on a non-urgent basis; and for a few patients angiography or other neuroradiological investigations may be needed. These facilities are widely available in all regions, as part of the neurological or paediatric service. Specialized laboratory facilities for the investigation of rare biochemical defects for instance are also required, and are available on a supraregional basis. Neuropsychological evaluation is helpful in complex cases, and is an absolute requirement in the assessment of surgical cases, and again this service is available on a regional basis.

The dedicated epilepsy clinic and the epilepsy unit The concept of specialized care for at least some epileptic patients has been supported in each of the government sponsored reports. The Cohen committee (Central Health Services Council 1956) suggested that this should be organized on a regional basis, but the Reid committee (Central Health Services Council 1969) recommended a far more ambitious scheme, with the introduction of dedicated epilepsy clinics on a regional or district level staffed by a 'multidisciplinary team', the recommendation to set up epilepsy clinics was also endorsed by the report of the recent DHSS working group (1986). Following the publication of the Reid report, Regional Hospital Boards and Area Health Authorities were asked to comment on the advisibility of specialized epilepsy clinics. Morgan & Bennet (1980) examined the replies received and exposed a clear divergence of opinion. Of the 54 Area Health Authorities who replied, 31 were against the concept, usually because they were judged to offer no advantages over existing arrangements. The concept of the multidisciplinary team seems to have attracted particular criticism, and some respondents felt that the resources would not be able to support such a scheme; that the dedicated clinic might stigmatize patients; or simply that the problems of epilepsy were not distinct enough to require special provision. A selection of quotations from individuals at Area level was compiled by Morgan & Bennett (1980) and these give a flavour of the responses received (Table 17.11)

Thus, the Reid report did not fire professional opinion with enthusiasm; indeed, its publication produced an almost total silence in the British medical press. As a result, little action was taken to develop special clinics and no concerted expansion occurred in specialized services. It is not clear how much of the indifference was due to the hostility induced by the concept of the multidisciplinary team or to the mistaken view that the Reid committee felt that *all* patients should be treated in these clinics. What is certain, however, is that an important opportunity for the development of services for epilepsy was lost. The Reid report was a comprehensive and detailed review which did not deserve this professional indifference. The recent report of the DHSS Working Group (1986) also supported the establishment of dedicated epilepsy clinics, although sensibly without the full panoply of a 'multi-disciplinary team' and for selected patients only; it is to be

Table 17.11 Quotations from the replies from Area Health Authorities in response to enquiries about the need for dedicated epilepsy clinics (from Morgan & Bennett 1980)

It is my particular view that the phrase 'multi-disciplinary team' introduces an unnecessary and at times even unhealthy atmosphere in the conduct of an essentially practical clinic. Clearly in our hospital, we have the support of all the available services; clinical, radiological, medical and social, but there is no place for the inclusion of all representatives of these many departments in the day-to-day running of the clinic

Consultant neurologist

It is not necessary nor desirable to have a designated clinic since there still tends to be a stigma attached to the word epileptic

Consultant physician

I think most of us in community medicine in the area would feel that there is little justification for regarding epilepsy as giving rise to unique problems, and requiring special provision outside the general ambit of neurology

Area medical officer

It is important to realise that epilepsy is not the sole prerogative of the neurologist

Paediatrician

It would not be a pleasant clinic to run; I doubt if it would help in the long-term management of these unfortunate patients

Consultant physician

hoped that this report will receive a more favourable response.

Parallels have been drawn between the services provided for epilepsy and those provided for diabetes. There is general agreement that the institution of dedicated diabetic clinics has greatly improved the standard of care of diabetic patients and, indeed, so successful have such clinics been that they are now established widely throughout the country. Similar success has been achieved for instance with the introduction of antenatal clinics and asthma clinics. Diabetic clinics have been organized in a fashion very similar to that envisaged by Reid for epilepsy clinics. As noted elsewhere (Goodridge & Shorvon 1983):

Diabetes and epilepsy share many characteristics: both are very common conditions in which are intermingled a number of medical, surgical and psychosocial aspects, both require long term potentially toxic medication that may be monitored biochemically; both vary considerably in severity; and both are prone to serious complications. These parallels have been recognised in other countries, and epilepsy clinics are now widespread in North America and Europe for instance.

The structure and functions of a dedicated epilepsy clinic are outlined in Table 17.12, although these will depend to some extent on existing local arrangements. In most settings, the clinic will be set up within an existing neurological department and there must be close ties between the neurology and the epilepsy service. The clinic will usually be run by a consultant neurologist and a consultant paediatrician where a joint clinic is possible. The clinic need not be multidisciplinary in the sense envisaged by Reid, and other staff should include junior medical staff, nursing or administrative staff. On the medical side, it is important to ensure as much continuity of care as is feasible and a clinical assistant (perhaps a local GP) or a neurophysiologist might usefully have sessions in the clinic on a long-term basis. In order to ensure that appropriate services are available for individual patients, the clinic should develop links with agencies (e.g. social work departments, Disablement Rehabilitation Officer, local education authorities, voluntary organizations etc) and one clinic member, perhaps on the nursing or administrative side, should be designated for these co-ordinating tasks. Close links should be set up with the psychiatric services, the hospital social workers, the hospital psychologists, the obstetric and family planning services, and the mental handicap services. While the clinic itself need not have a multidisciplinary structure, communication with these other professionals is important and, if possible, a particular social worker, psychologist and psychiatrist should be identified as having particular responsibility for the epilepsy clinic referrals.

The main function of the clinic is the follow-up of patients with severe or complicated epilepsy, who form a minority of cases with epilepsy

Table 17.12 The dedicated epilepsy clinic

Advantages over existing arrangements:
 Concentration of resources and thus their more efficient utilization and expansion

Situation:
 Hospital outpatient setting, with access to a small number of hospital beds, often in an existing neurological unit, and in close association with the medical, psychiatric and paediatric services

Functions:
 Follow-up and management of severe or complicated epilepsy (groups 1,2,3*)
 Initial medical assessment and diagnosis of epilepsy (the extent to which this is necessary depends on local arrangements)
 Co-ordination of medical and non-medical services

Staffing:
 Consultant neurologist and/or paediatrician with overall responsibility for the clinic
 Junior medical staff (or general practitioners or clinical assistants)
 Nursing staff
 Administrative staff, including a clinic co-ordinator
 Other staff available to the clinic as required should include a psychiatrist, social worker, psychologist, and other specialists depending on local arrangements

Referrals:
 From general practitioners or hospital doctors

Facilities:
 Access to EEG and serum level monitoring, preferably with a same-day on-site service
 Access to other hospital medical and neurological services

Education/counselling; there should be available:
 Educational material
 Counselling facilities
 The voluntary agencies may be involved in this aspect of the clinic work, depending on local arrangements

Teaching:
 The clinic should be a focus for in-service medical and para-medical teaching

Research:
 The opportunity for clinical research should be actively exploited

* See Table 17.3 for description of groups

attending hospital. To what extent the clinic should provide initial assessment and diagnosis will depend on local arrangements and the manner in which the clinic meshes into the neurological and paediatric facilities.

The main advantage of the dedicated clinic is that it can concentrate resources and in so doing improve and extend the use made of these resources. On-site EEG and serum level measurement, for instance, should be available, if possible with a same-day service; much as the diabetic clinic doctor has the blood-sugar measurement to hand. Leaflets, literature and other information services should also be provided for patient education; and voluntary organizations should be invited to contribute to the clinic in this area. Organized in this way, the epilepsy clinic should become a focus for teaching and in-service training of medical and paramedical staff, and also a natural focus for research activities. Here the parallels with diabetic clinics are strong.

Where the organization of epilepsy services has been highly developed, epilepsy units have been established, often in a university setting. The unit in the University Hospital of Wales, run by Professor Alan Richens, is an example of such a unit which provides a broad-based epilepsy service. The unit runs five epilepsy clinics each week and has designated inpatient facilities with on-site same-day serum level monitoring and EEG. The British Epilepsy Association provides voluntary staff, and a co-ordinator, social worker and nursing and technical staff are also present in the clinic. Research is a major activity of the unit, concerned largely with antiepileptic drug development, and this provides a substantial contribution to the funding of the unit. Education of patients and staff is considered a major part of the work of the unit, and strong links have been formed with the British Epilepsy Association and other voluntary organizations. The unit is highly successful, referrals are drawn from a wide area, and over half of the patients seen are out of the hospital district. The emphasis is on comprehensive care, and the standards achieved are very high.

Neurosurgical facilities for epilespy Neurosurgery has an important part to play in the care of a small number of patients with epilepsy. The hospital neurosurgical and neuroradiological services in the UK provide a good service for routine diagnostic and therapeutic purposes; for instance, in the treatment of cerebral tumour, hydrocephalus, cerebral trauma, cerebrovascular disease and so on; and such units are provided on a national basis. Specialized stereotactic or resective surgery for epilepsy itself though is not widely available, and regular epilepsy surgery takes place probably in only three or four centres in the country. An important reason for this is the lack of the special medical and, in particular, EEG facilities. These include EEG telemetry, with sphenoidal EEG or intracerebral recording in some cases; skilled neuropsychological assessment, including the facilities for carotid amytal testing; and a high standard of modern neuroradiological investigation. The investigation of a patient for surgery is labour intensive and time consuming and requires the close co-operation of specialists in different disciplines and co-ordination of their efforts. Such a service provision is really only practical in a specialized epilepsy service. As such services are not widely available in the UK, surgery is often delayed or deferred.

Information concerning the hospital services available for epilepsy on a national basis in the UK is remarkably scarce and, without a full appreciation of the spread of facilities, rational planning is difficult. A pilot survey of services for adults in one UK region (North East Thames Region) has been carried out and the findings reported by Espir et al (1986). In this region, there is a fair spread of neurological provision, with consultant neurologist sessions in 14 of the 15 districts, 9 consultant neurophysiologists with sessions in the region, and access to 5 neurosurgical units; EEG is available in 10 hospitals, and antiepileptic drug serum level measurements in 14. Specialized EEG is also available, including ambulatory EEG in 4 units and video EEG telemetry in one. 4 dedicated epilepsy clinics are being held, each organized at the initiative of the consultant in charge. Junior staff support is provided in only one clinic and in none are clinical assistants employed; on-site EEG is available in three clinics, and some of these clinics are situated in the EEG department itself. Same-day antiepileptic drug measurements are not available and no clinic had formal links with voluntary agencies or a service co-ordinator. These clinics are therefore less well supported than those envisaged in the DHSS Working Group (1986) report, and the hospital has provided minimal extra resources for their running. Epilepsy surgery is carried out in a neighbouring region, and referral to this unit, to a specialized medical epilepsy unit and to a Special Centre for Epilepsy is regularly made. How the services in this region compare with others in the country is unknown. The North East Thames Region has a relatively high concentration of neurological services, and four undergraduate and postgraduate teaching hospitals are situated in the region. In spite of this, it is interesting to note that the four epilepsy clinics are all in situated in non-teaching districts.

Special assessment centres for epilepsy

In the Reid report (Central Health Services Council 1969), another far-reaching recommendation was made, 'that special centres should be provided for those people with epilepsy whose management presents particular problems' (largely group 3 patients, see Table 17.3). These patients were those 'whose fits have not been effectively controlled', and also those who 'require medical supervision under everyday living conditions'. The centres should be for those whose primary disability is epilepsy, and patients 'with mental disorder or severe physical handicap should receive care within the general arrangements for these groups rather than at the special centres for epilepsy'. The Reid committee suggested that these centres should have two components: the first a hospital neurological and neurosurgical unit, to provide all the medical facilities necessary for diagnosis, assessment and treatment; and the second a residential unit in which patients could be admitted, after full assessment by the associated hospital unit. It was also recommended that these units should form 'focal points for research and teaching about epilepsy'. The report suggested that as an initial step, six such units should be established in England and Wales on a supraregional basis. This suggestion was accepted provisionally by the DHSS, and three centres were created: at The Chalfont Centre for Epilepsy

in Buckinghamshire; Bootham Park Hospital in York; and the Park Hospital for Children in Oxford (see Appendix). As suggested by the committee each of these designated centres was set up within already existing facilities.

The Special Assessment Unit at the Chalfont Centre for Epilepsy may be taken as an example. It has 45 beds, there are about 160 admissions each year, and the average patient's stay in the centre is several months. The unit is located in the Chalfont Centre for Epilepsy, which provides residential care, in an asylum setting administered by a charity, the National Society for Epilepsy. Medical sessions are provided by a consultant neurologist (a linked post with the Institute of Neurology and National Hospital), Senior House Officer (on rotation with the National Hospital), a research funded registrar (linked with the Institute of Neurology), and a consultant psychiatrist (linked with the National Hospital). The unit is funded from an allocation from the National Hospital, whose medical facilities are freely available, and the beds are administered jointly by the National Hospital and the National Society for Epilepsy. There is a full complement of nursing and auxillary nursing staff and a part-time social worker. Outpatients clinics are held at the Centre and the National Hospital. Other facilities are shared with the residential centre and include: routine EEG and EEG ambulatory monitoring; on-site serum antiepileptic drug monitoring; the services of a clinical psychologist and speech therapist; and rehabilitation facilities such as a therapeutic workshop.

As the unit has evolved, it has four main roles. Outlined below. It provides

1. A comprehensive medical assessment: this aspect of work has become more prominent than envisaged in the Reid report, perhaps because of the failure of the hospital service to provide epilepsy clinics on a nationwide basis. The assessment includes a detailed review of the medical history, EEG and other investigations, and treatment history. Further investigation routinely includes EEG, serum antiepileptic drug level monitoring and psychometric evaluation, and other investigations as needed. A comprehensive assessment should be also made by the social work, nursing and rehabilitation staff. On the

basis of this assessment, during admission the diagnosis may be re-examined, treatment adjusted, further investigations carried out, and recommendations made for future medical management after discharge.

2. A realistic appraisal of the patient's overall abilities, in the educational, vocational and psychosocial fields: this assessment may take several months of inpatient observation, and during this time short-term remedial programmes may be carried out. For a young person with severe epilepsy, the opportunity to live independently away from family and to make new social relationships is often as useful as formal training.

3. Recommendations for long-term assistance: these include recommendations regarding work, day time occupation, psychosocial help and, where necessary, long term residential arrangements. Close liason with local medical and social services is essential, and if the patient is a young adult, work with the families is important.

4. Postgraduate teaching, professional training and research: these are activities which have increased in recent years, and both research and educational departments have been set up in the Centre. The research department is linked to the University Department of Clinical Neurology at the Institute of Neurology, through the joint appointment of the Senior Lecturer/Consultant Neurologist. Such links were envisaged by the Reid report and a considerable expansion of research activities has been possible. The educational department has been funded by the National Society for Epilepsy, and has expanded its activities into the production of visual and written material and the organization of courses and seminars.

The evolution of the special centres has therefore been largely along the lines conceived by the Reid Committee. A review of the special centres was commissioned by the DHSS (Morgan & Bennett 1980), and the findings were considered by the recent DHSS Working Group (1986). The Working Group fully endorsed the value of the Assessment Centres. They considered their particular advantages to be that assessment and treatment can be undertaken on an intensive basis; the assessment period can be prolonged according

to individual needs; and that a range of disciplines with special expertise in epilepsy can be brought together. The Working Group recommended 100 adult places and the opening of two more centres (a downgrading of the estimates made by the Reid committee in the expansionist atmosphere of 1969), and that the Supraregional Services Advisory Group should be asked to consider the designation of Special Assessment Centres as supraregional, and hence eligible for direct funding by the DHSS.

In the future, the relative lack of special provision for epilepsy in general hospitals will require that the special centres carry out a more medically orientated function than originally envisaged; as is the case in epilepsy centres in Holland for instance. This is a development which should be welcomed and it has several advantages: a higher quality of medical and paramedical staff will be attracted than might be the case if the centre was wholly devoted to rehabilitation, and this will help maintain a higher level of service. The Special Assessment Centres should not take on long-term rehabilitation, as this is best carried out in residential epilepsy units (see below) and other units on a regional, rather than supraregional, basis. The rehabilitation needs of handicapped persons with epilepsy will, in the great majority of cases, be met within the facilities provided for other handicaps, and funded accordingly. The role of the Special Assessment Centres in this regard is very much to provide recommendations for future care, based on the detailed assessment, rather than the provision of extensive rehabilitation.

The need for Special Assessment Centres for children was also endorsed by the Working Group, run along the lines of the adult centres described above, but with specialist teaching staff in attendance to provide for the educational needs. In general the aim of the units should be to enable the children to return home for continuing care and wherever possible education in an ordinary school. To this end close ties with local health, education and social services are vital, and the group recommended that a new Special Assessment Centre for children should be established in addition to the present centre at the Park Hospital Oxford.

Residential facilities

Residential schools The great majority of children with epilepsy are educated in normal schools and recent legislation has emphasized that handicapped children should, wherever possible, be schooled with their healthy peers. Nevertheless, a small number of children with epilepsy do require residential schooling, and there are five schools for epileptic children in the UK, all of which are residential (see Appendix). The DHSS Working Group (1986) noted that the children referred are increasingly more intellectually retarded, reflecting the improved care for epilepsy in the community and the increasing efforts to provide community care and normal schooling for the handicapped. Indeed, epileptic seizures are now seldom the main reason for boarding-school provision. Traditionally, the schools fulfil not only an educational role, but also provide a medical and social assessment, and an environment in which even children with severe and frequent seizures can develop their full potential. The roles of the special epilepsy schools are also expanding in response to changing needs, and short term educational and social assessment are now offered in some as an advisory service, in addition to residential care. The Working Group welcomed this development, and also urged that the schools keep close ties with the local medical and social facilities, and with the special medical services for epilepsy.

Residential care for adults Epilepsy colonies were first established in the nineteenth century in the UK, as part of the philanthropic movement of the times. The colonies were run by benevolent organizations to provide shelter and care and also, no doubt, to remove troublesome problems from the public gaze. They were certainly in advance of their time, and provided accommodation and care for handicapped persons long before general welfare services took on this task. In the post-war years, of course, the situation has radically changed. The 1948 National Assistance Act placed the responsibility to provide residential accommodation for those who were in need of care (part III accommodation) on local authorities and since that time, the state has recognized a statutory obligation to provide for those with epilepsy who are unable to live independently (groups 1 and 2,

see Table 17.3.). The local authorities were empowered to sponsor places in existing colonies, and this was a common pattern of referral; although of course many epileptic patients were and are also cared for in other institutions, not specifically earmarked for epilepsy.

In 1969, the Reid Committee noted that eight epilepsy homes or colonies were in existence, with 2250 beds; three were run by local authorities and five by voluntary organizations, funded largely by sponsorship for individual patients by the local authorities; five were housed in buildings constructed between 1888 and 1905 and two more in hospitals established by the Metropolitan Asylums Board between 1910 and 1920; most provided dormitory accommodation, little in the way of rehabilitation and were situated in rural areas. The Reid Committee felt that in many ways this pattern of care was increasingly inappropriate. The committee predicted that, as medical and social facilities improved, and as the prevailing social philosophy was to move away from residential care in distant institutions towards supervision in small local units, the need for residential care in colonies would fall dramatically. This prediction has proved partly correct, although the rate at which this has happened was overestimated. In 1969, there were about 400 admissions to colonies from 175 local authorities, and the committee felt it would take 20 or more years before the need for part III accommodation in colonies would disappear altogether. In 1984, five centres in England (the term 'colony' has fallen from favour) remain; four of which are administered by voluntary organizations, with a total of about 1100 residents (see Appendix). The DHSS Working Group (1986) endorsed the modern philosophy of promoting care in the community and avoiding residential placement in large institutions where possible, and it does seem likely that referrals will continue to fall.

The reason that the residential centres continue to exist at all is because of the failure of local authorities to keep pace with the demand for the local facilities for the handicapped (a statutory obligation), and because of the excellent standards set by the modern centres. The Working Group did feel that there would remain a place for residential epilepsy centres on a smaller scale; first to provide a more extended programme of assessment and rehabilitation than is possible in the Special Assessment Centre (and this can be best offered when the two facilities are on the same site); and, secondly, for a small number of severe cases for whom there is no satisfactory alternative and for whom care in the community is not feasible, whatever the level of social service support.

The main emphasis therefore, as in all establishments caring for the mentally ill, has shifted from passive custodial care to a more active role, in which rehabilitation and training are important aspects of the work. Whether the residential centres will manage this transition is unclear. Certainly, it will be possible only with extra funding and this will need to be provided from central sources. It is clear, nevertheless, that the local authorities will have to increase greatly the level of provision of supervised housing in the community before some patients will be actually better off in the community than in the well-run epilepsy centres.

The DHSS Working Group recognized that the following groups of patients will require a range of local residential facilities if placement in residential epilepsy centres is to be avoided.

1. Children who require residential care, but not special residential education, might be placed in ordinary children's home, with foster families or in homes for handicapped children
2. Young people might be offered transitional placement in a hostel or with a family
3. Adults might be placed in local authority, voluntary or private homes for handicapped people, sheltered housing, hostels or homes, or provided with local day care centres
4. The elderly may be accommodated in homes for elderly people

The residential epilepsy centres currently supply these needs, in addition to the residential care of those whose seizure disorder is so severe that placement in any other setting is unrealistic.

Private health services

There has been a great expansion of private health care facilities in the UK over the past few years,

and this has been encouraged by government policy and financial assistance. In general terms, the private health insurance agencies, however, will not provide cover for epilepsy for any known epileptic patient and, as epilepsy usually starts in childhood or adolescence, this automatically excludes many people. Furthermore, even if a person develops the condition after taking up insurance, the insurance will not usually cover the costs of follow-up. Nor will the insurance companies support prolonged inpatient assessment or residential care. The NHS therefore provides medical care for the vast majority of cases and will continue to do so. As in many areas of medicine in the UK, the private sector is currently concerned mainly with the financially attractive provision of one-off acute medical care, which has little to do with the main burden of epilepsy work. It has contributed very little to overall medical surveillance in national terms.

EPILEPSY SERVICES IN OTHER COUNTRIES

It is of course invidious and misleading to contrast the services provided in different countries, as many factors bear on these and a simple comparison hides as much as it reveals. Nevertheless, certain observations may be made about the structure of individual services and the broad sweep of facilities, and the author has chosen to discuss briefly aspects of the epilepsy services in two countries, the United States and Kenya.

The United States

Medical care in the United States is generally geared towards a high-tech, high-cost approach, and this is certainly demonstrated in the services for epilepsy. First, it is worth noting that the principle of subspecialization has been fully accepted and, within the broad sweep of neurology, there exists the well-defined discipline of epileptology and a number of physicians deal only with epileptic patients. There are epilepsy units in many locations and specialized epilepsy clinics in all major neurological centres. In most of the larger epilepsy units, there are facilities for video EEG telemetry and beds earmarked for epilepsy work. Parallel with this elaboration of telemetry systems, there has been a considerable expansion of interest in epilepsy surgery, which is now carried out on a regular basis in 10–20 neurosurgical units specializing in epilepsy work. Intracerebral EEG recording is now also routinely carried out in several centres, as a presurgical investigation. The impetus for these developments has been the existence of epileptology as a subspecialty in its own right, as well as the greater resources available, and the lucrative nature of work in this area.

Two particular developments in US services can be specifically noted. The first is the establishment of officially designated 'Intensive Monitoring Units'; by 1980 for instance 29 such units were in existence and a marked expansion was under way. The units form a hospital-based epilepsy service, staffed by neurologists, psychiatrists and paramedical staff, working in close association with the hospital neurological and neurosurgical services. Each unit runs a video EEG telemetry system and has access to the full range of neurological services. The units are organized autonomously, run epilepsy clinics, have inpatient facilities. and form the core of the specialized epilepsy services in the US. A second development has been the more ambitious 'Comprehensive Epilepsy Programs'. These programs were established in 1975 and a total of ten are either planned or in existence. Their thrust is to provide a comprehensive service for epilepsy, with a multidisciplinary approach. The program at the University of Virginia may be cited as an example (Dreifuss 1980). It is centred around a 15-bed inpatient intensive monitoring unit, with facilities which include two video EEG monitoring systems; and there are close administrative links with the neurological facilities of the University Department of Neurology. In addition to the medical personnel, unit staff include specially trained nurses, a social worker, psychologist, education officer, vocational rehabilitation counsellor, occupational therapist and EEG technician. The comprehensive program conducts outpatient clinics both in the University hospital and in outreach clinics in neighbouring rural communities, and is active in epilepsy education and training. The other comprehensive programs differ in their detailed arrangements, but share the same broad conception. The advantages of defining programmes such as these is that resources and efforts may be concentrated towards well-defined objectives, and that service, teaching and research activities may be intermingled to their mutual benefit.

A comparison between these facilities and those in the UK is not easy. Undeniable advantages of the UK arrangements are the system of primary care and the principle of free medical care. Nevertheless, the willingness to accept the principles of specialization; the establishment of officially designated and well-defined programmes and facilities; and the greater material resources in the US, have permitted a much more ambitious epilepsy service to develop. Until resources can be specifically earmarked for epilepsy in the same way in the UK and other countries, and until the anonymous and non-specialist structure of service provision in the the UK is changed, patient care will advance only slowly. Finally, it is worth noting the much more aggressive role played by the voluntary organizations in promoting health care in the US. The Epilepsy Foundation of America runs national advertising campaigns, regularly lobbies central government, and is active in teaching and research at a level which the British voluntary agencies do not emulate. The public awareness of epilepsy is higher, a greater proportion of government resources are devoted to epilepsy, and there can be little doubt that this is in part due to the efforts of the voluntary groups.

Kenya

The epilepsy services in Kenya are an interesting contrast to those in the UK or the US, reflecting different concerns and priorities. Resources are of course fewer, as are qualified personnel. The country has one physician for every 8000 persons and medical specialization is not a high priority. Indeed, there is only one accredited neurologist in the country (but several neurosurgeons) and epilepsy is treated by general practitioners, general physicians and psychiatrists. The great majority of specialist resources are concentrated in Nairobi and about 75% of all doctors practice from Nairobi. Primary care is carried out from health centres, which in towns are administered by the municipalities and are staffed by paramedical personnel. Treatment is limited, and pheno-barbitone, but no other antiepileptic drugs, may be officially prescribed from these centres by apppointed paramedical staff. Patients may be referred from these primary care facilities to district hospitals, then regional hospitals and, finally, to the Central Government Hospital in Nairobi. The district hospitals are very basic, and a typical 300-bed unit will be staffed by only two doctors. EEG is available only in Nairobi and there are no cranial CT facilities in the country. Epilepsy is not a government health care priority and there are, indeed, more pressing problems. What specialized medical provision there is has been developed as the result of individual effort. There is for instance an epilepsy clinic in the provincial town of Nakuru, set up by a psychiatrist (one of the only six working outside Nairobi), who has a particular interest in the condition. A major force in epilepsy work is the Kenyan Epilepsy Association, a lay organization which is extremely active in the education and welfare fields. The Association also runs its own epilepsy clinics in four locations (two of which are in Nairobi), staffed by volunteers, including two doctors, a psychologist and social workers; 750 patients a month may be seen in these clinics.

A major concern in Kenya, and indeed in many third world countries, is the supply of antiepileptic drugs. The government hospitals are supplied from central sources, and the supply is notoriously unreliable. This is due, on the governments own admission, to 'poor planning, unsuitable procurement policies, shortage of foreign exchange, and pilferage' (Anon 1986). It is therefore common for a hospital, even a large hospital, pharmacy to run out of antiepileptic drugs or for a supply of, say, phenobarbitone suddenly to be replaced with phenytoin; which may of course result in a catastrophic withdrawal reaction. The problem of drug supply is often misrepresented, and yet is a crucial and fundamental consideration in everyday practice. Drugs may also be supplied by private physicians who have access to a wider selection, and the situation has of course encouraged unregulated dispensing on a large scale.

The whole question of government drug policies world wide has been the subject of recent debate. The World Health Organization (WHO) has recently made efforts 'to penetrate into government national drug policies' in order to direct these towards rational drug prescribing, and to take up a leadership role, without becoming a 'supranational manipulator of Governments' (Anon 1985); but, needless to say, this is a fine distinction and there has been a heated debate about these new initiatives. A series of guidelines for rational drug use (an *Essential Drug List*), has been produced to act as a formulary for appropriate prescribing. In *The Use of Essential Drugs*. (World Health Organization 1985), diazepam, ethosuximide, phenobarbitone and phenytoin are included in the main list, and carbamazepine and valproate in the complementary drug list ('for use when drugs in the main list are known to be ineffective or inappropriate for a given individual'). Whether or not this list is appropriate is surely a matter of concern. Phenobarbitone is the most comonly used and the cheapest antiepileptic drug but it has a number of disadvantages: it is a drug of abuse; sudden withdrawal may be extremely hazardous; it may interact with alcohol; overdose is dangerous; and it may produce serious mental depression in adults and hyperactivity in children. The Kenyan government has responded to the problems of drug supply by supplying rural health care facilities with an 'essential drugs kit', based on the essential drug list, comprising 40 essential drugs, of which phenobarbitone is the only oral antiepileptic drug. This scheme was devised to combat the problems of drug shortage and has been applauded by the WHO, and yet it has proved only partly successful. It has had little influence on the day-to-day treatment of epilepsy, and underlines the difficulties introduced by a restrictive and rigid drug policy.

APPENDIX 17.1
Special Assessment Centres, special schools, and agencies and professional agencies in the UK

Special assessment centres for epilepsy

Bootham Park Hospital
Bootham
York Y03 7BY

Chalfont Centre for Epilepsy
Chalfont St Peter
Bucks SL9 ORJ

Park Hospital for Children
Oxford OX3 7LQ

Other units offering specialized in-patient assessment

David Lewis Centre
Alderley Edge
Cheshire SK9 7UD

Maudsley Hospital
Epilepsy Unit
Denmark Hill
London SE5 8AZ

Special schools for children with epilepsy

David Lewis Centre
Alderley Edge
Cheshire SK9 7UD

Lingfield Hospital School
St Piers Lane
Lingfield
Surrey RH7 6PN

St Elizabeth's School
Much Hadham
Herts SG10 6EW

Residential centres for epilepsy

Chalfont Centre for Epilepsy
Chalfont St Peter
Bucks SL9 ORJ

David Lewis Centre
Alderley Edge
Cheshire SK9 7UD

Meath Home for Women and Girls with Epilepsy
Westbrook Rd
Godalming
Surrey GU7 2QJ

The Maghull Homes
Deyes Lane
Maghull
Merseyside L31 6DJ

Quarrier's Home
Bridge of Weir
Renfrewshire OA11 3SA

St Elizabeth's Home
Much Hadham
Herts SG10 6EW

National voluntary organisations

British Epilepsy Association
Anstey House
40 Hanover Square
Leeds LS3 1BE

Epilepsy Association of Scotland
48 Govan Rd
Glasgow GS1 1JR

Epilepsy Wales
142 Whitchurch Road
Cardiff CF4 3NA

Irish Epilepsy Association
249 Crumlin Rd
Dublin W12

National Society for Epilepsy
Chalfont Centre for Epilepsy
Chalfont St Peter
Bucks SL9 ORJ

International League Against Epilepsy

Dr D. C. Chadwick
Honorary Secretary
ILAE British Branch
Walton Hospital
Liverpool

REFERENCES

Anon 1985 WHO meeting on rational drug strategy. Lancet ii: 1350–1351

Anon 1986 New drug supplies management system for rural health facilities in Kenya (presentation of Kenya's drug kit to the WHO conference of Experts on the Rational Use of Drugs, Nairobi 1985). Medicus 13–18

Central Health Services Council 1956 Report on the Sub-committee on the Medical Care of Epileptics (Chairman: H Cohen). HMSO, London

Central Health Services Council 1969 People with epilepsy: report of the joint sub-committee of the Standing Medical Advisory Committee and the Advisory Committee of the Health and Welfare of Handicapped persons (Chairman J A Read). HMSO, London

Commission for the Control of Epilepsy and its Consequences 1978 Plan for nationwide action on epilepsy vols 1–4. DHJEW publication no. (NIH) 78–279, US Department of Health Education and Welfare, Bethesda Md.

DHSS Working Group 1986 A report of the working group on Services for People with Epilepsy. A report to the Department of Health and Social Security, Department of Education and Science and the Welsh Office. HMSO, London

Dreifuss F 1980 Development of a comprehensive epilepsy program. In: Robb P (ed) Epilepsy updated: causes and treatment. Year book medical publishers, Chicago

Espir M L E, McCarthy M, Shorvon S D 1987 A survey of specialised hospital services for adults with epilepsy in the North East Thames Region. Neuroepidemiology (in press)

Goodridge D M G, Shorvon S D 1983 Epileptic seizures in a population of 6000. 1: Demography, diagnosis and role of the hospital services. 2: treatment and prognosis. British Medical Journal 287: 641–647

Hopkins A, Scambler G 1977 How doctors deal with epilepsy. Lancet i: 183–186

Kurtze J F, Bennett D R, Berg B O et al 1986 On national needs for neurologists in the United States. Neurology 36: 383–388

Ministry of Health 1953 Welfare of handicapped persons: The special needs of epileptics and spastics. HMSO, London

Morgan J D, Bennett A E 1980 Specialised services for people with epilepsy (the Bennett report). (unpublished)

Pond D A, Bidwell B H, Stein L 1960 A survey of epilepsy in fourteen general practices. 1. Demographic and medical data. Psychiatrica Neurologia Neurochirugia 63: 217–236

Sander J W A S, Shorvon S D 1987 Incidence and prevalence studies in epilepsy and their methodological problems: a review. Journal of Neurology, Neurosurgery and Psychiatry 50: 829–839

Shorvon S D 1983 Specialised services for the non-institutionalised patient with epilepsy; developments in the US and UK. Health Trends 15: 40–45

World Health Organization 1985 The use of essential drugs. Second report of the WHO expert committee. World Health Organization technical report series 722. World Health Organization, Geneva

Zielinski J J 1974 Epileptics not on treatment. Epilepsia 15: 203–210

18

People with epilepsy

J. Laidlaw
M. V. Laidlaw

INTRODUCTION

In this chapter, we try to make the patient the subject, the Person with Epilepsy: how does *HE* react; what does *HE* need; how does *HE* feel about his seizures? Although People with Epilepsy should seldom be considered as being ill, for the sake of simplicity we will refer usually to the Person with Epilepsy as the patient or sometimes as *HE*. We will hope to bring to life *HIS* problems by reproducing five stories about People with Epilepsy. (Laidlaw & Laidlaw 1984.)

WHAT DOES *HE* EXPECT FROM HIS DOCTOR?

HE needs to understand and be understood

When he or his family are presented with the diagnosis of epilepsy it should never be thought of as a disaster, although it may seem to be a tragedy. Similar feelings may be aroused by the diagnosis of cancer or of impending death, but in these cases it is seldom necessary for the doctor to spell out his diagnosis until the patient has a very good idea of it himself. In the case of epilepsy, the patient would not want his doctor to wrap up his diagnosis in meaningless and confusing euphemisms. Rather it is the doctor's responsibility over a period to help his patient to overcome his irrational fears and understand the condition with which he will have to live, possibly for the rest of his life. Epilepsy, like diabetes, requires the greatest possible co-operation of the patient and/or his family. Nevertheless, although diabetes is probably the more dangerous disease,

it is epilepsy that is feared the more. The doctor must appreciate not only that this fear exists but understand why it exists, so that he may help to exorcise it.

When a patient and his family are faced for the first time with the diagnosis of epilepsy, there is almost invariably this feeling of shock, of inevitable disaster. This is probably the worst possible time to try to discuss the implications: both the patient and his family are likely to be so overwrought that they are unable to absorb anything which is said to them. Long afterwards, the doctor, who may have spent some time trying to help, may hear that he has been accused, altogether unjustifiably, of never having explained anything. It is much more sensible for the doctor to send the patient away with a few soothing words and to make an appointment to see him again in a week or two, telling him in the meantime to think out any questions which he would like to discuss.

Nowadays, in developed countries, most patients will be referred to a neurological (or neuropsychiatric) hospital department to confirm the diagnosis and in some cases to exclude a remediable lesion. Any competent second-year registrar can cope with 90% of the work involved in excluding gliomas or picking up rare cases of tuberous sclerosis. However, it is the consultant who bears the total responsibility not only for establishing the diagnosis and advising on treatment, but also for overall management. The patient has the right to expect him – with his experience and authority – to be available to answer questions and to help him with his problems.

One of *HIS* fears

Although it is seldom voiced spontaneously, there are many patients who have the considerable covert anxiety that having epilepsy means that they are, or will become, in some way mad or peculiar. The doctor should be prepared to bring this fear out into the open; appreciate how it arose; and explain to the patient that it is without foundation. If he does not, it may well grow, nurtured by gossip and anecdote, and become a belief so firmly held that it is difficult or impossible to eradicate later.

A major fit is a dramatic event. All too often it is taken as the common factor of that wide variety of conditions causing fits; termed 'epilepsy', it carries with it associations with all these conditions. Severe mental deficiency often associated with corresponding physical stigmata is commonly complicated by major convulsions, i.e. epilepsy. May not the patient presented with the diagnosis of epilepsy, conjure up, not altogether irrationally if it is has not been explained to him, a picture of a convulsing brain-damaged person with severe mental handicap, in a way that the symptom of a hacking cough, diagnosed as tracheitis, does not evoke fears of the putrefying lung of phthisis or bronchial carcinoma? It is fairly easy for the doctor to explain to his patient that fits are (probably) due to a combination of a congenital brain sensitivity (or liability to fits), and acquired brain damage; which in only the extreme case results in significant mental handicap.

The word 'seizure' describes an epileptic attack much more aptly than 'fit'. In nearly every case, the patient is quite unable to prevent or control his ictus. Literally, he seems to have been seized by something not only outside his control but which he cannot see or begin to understand. It is all too easy for him to believe that this something is supernatural or, if he is more sophisticated, that it is something apart from his physical self; something in his mental self – his mind. It is not difficult to understand the basic idea of an EEG recording and patients may often be reassured by seeing a seizure on the EEG.

Further explanations

Although some may be nervous or embarrassed, most patients find examination by the doctor reassuring. However, special investigations such as the EEG or (computerized tomography) CT scan with complex and formidable equipment can be very frightening. The doctor needs to do more than dismiss them as harmless and painless. An equally important problem is that the patient is often confused as to why such tests are being carried out. The neurologist will be quite clear that the EEG may be of some help in arriving at the diagnosis of epilepsy or in determining the type; whereas CT scan is only called for if he feels that a potentially remediable lesion needs to be excluded. This is in no way obvious to the patient unless it is explained to him. Particularly at the time of diagnosis, a patient's epilepsy is of paramount importance to him and, between his outpatient appointments, he and his family are likely to have absorbed a great deal of quasi-information from the library, from friends or from acquaintances who knew someone who had fits and had this that or the other done. If the doctor explains fully to his patient why certain tests are necessary, whereas others are not, he will not only relieve his anxieties but retain his confidence.

MAY *HE* FACE PREJUDICE?

Popular prejudice has become part of the dialect used in talking about epilepsy. Not an adjuvant, all too often it is adduced as the main cause of a patient's problems or of his failures. To mention it in a textbook is not superfluous; to consider it carefully is essential.

Prejudice is an emotive word. It raises spectres of apartheid and ghettoes. Almost invariably linked with ignorance, it is inflated to imply brutish stupidity or even overt brutality. However, the prejudice is always described as popular. But surely the general public is also described as remarkable for its common sense, tolerance and kindness and, in particular, for its anxiety to help the disabled? The white stick of the blind man evokes almost embarrassing sympathy and desire to help. If, then, epilepsy evokes in the same general public stupid, intolerant and unkind prejudice, this atypical response needs examination. Either it does not exist or, if it does, there must be some reason for its existence. We would suggest that popular prejudice is not nearly as widespread as it is supposed to be and that, when it does exist, it is not irrational but based on genuine fear.

No longer would anyone maintain that the person with epilepsy was a dangerous fiend, a creature possessed of the devil, but there are ways in which a fit may be fearsome and awesome to the onlooker. The first witness of a friend or a colleague seized by a major convulsion needs comment. We all expect life to be consequential: an action to provoke a reaction. The intense drama of a major fit is the more frightening because it is quite inconsequential. It comes out of the blue; only exceptionally is there any apparent proximate cause. This proposition is to some extent substantiated by the differing reactions to so-called symptomatic and idiopathic epilepsy. An artisan engineer, who fractures his skull in a motor car accident, later develops epilepsy and returns to his firm as a storeman will arouse less unease when he has an occasional fit than an unknown young man with 'idiopathic' epilepsy who is found a job in the same firm by his welfare officer. The effect of complex partial seizures on the observer will be considered in the last section of this chapter.

We would suggest that prejudice is a good deal less widespread than many patients fear and that it is easier to prevent it developing than to remove it once it has become established. The patient should be warned not, himself, to prejudge, not to anticipate non-existent difficulty and adopt a scratchy abrasive mien to those around him. His associates may not be put off by his epilepsy but may be by his own attitude to it and to them. Those around him will reflect the patient's own attitude to his fits and the patient will reflect the attitude of his doctor. It is sensible to advise him to talk quite openly about the seizures (although not, of course, to the point of obsession since they are of less interest to others than to himself) to give some explanation of when they may occur, describe what form they usually take and what help he may need. If he does so, he is more than likely to meet kindness, understanding and help which he did not expect, rather than the prejudice

which he feared. If he is fortunate enough to be in work, he must be warned in the strongest possible terms against using his epilepsy as a crutch, as an excuse for avoiding difficult jobs or for getting special concessions. If others help him out, he must be more than prepared to give them a hand in other ways.

DOES *HE* FEEL OVERPROTECTED?

It is a simple biological instinct of parents to protect their young. A young person who is disabled requires more protection, and a disability such as epilepsy may call for special precautions. In our experience most parents try hard to approach the hazards of fits in a sensible way and to control their fears. It does not require much imagination to put oneself in the position of someone responsible for a person subject to frequent seizures. It is only reasonable to assert that there is overprotection when the protection is more than is needed, is exercised stupidly, or in some way harms the patient.

Doctors can do a great deal to guide parents. The general practitioner will be the one to give detailed advice since he should be in closer touch with the family circumstances and personalities. However, the specialist consultant has an important role in guiding the family doctor and offering him the support of his authority. It may be very difficult for even the most sensible parent to know just where to draw the line, and it is really not adequate for the doctor, whether general practitioner or specialist, to dismiss the subject with: 'Treat Johnnie like the other children but, of course, take reasonable care.' It is essential that he should take the time to discuss the whole position with the family, including the patient if he is old enough and intelligent enough to understand. He must define necessary limitations specifically and explain why they are necessary. If he does this, he will be able to accept the responsibility for any improbable misfortunes. If he does not, and if something goes wrong, the family will have to bear an intolerable burden of guilt. The doctor in his surgery or in the outpatient clinic is able to make his assessment and give his specific advice in an objective way which is not possible for the family who are involved so personally and subjectively.

The effect of environment upon fits is well known. There is no situation more epileptogenic than the family whose whole life revolves around the unfortunate patient: the fits which he may have and the disasters which may occur; and, consequently, the fits which he does have and the disasters which are only too likely to occur. How many patients whose fits are well controlled in hospital or in a Centre for Epilepsy, spend their weekend leave having serial seizures? For that matter, how many patients in status asthmaticus recover on admission to hospital without specific treatment? If families are overprotective, it is because they are worried and anxious, and it is their uncertainties that may exacerbate the patient's seizures.

The doctor can do a great deal to advise parents how to approach the protection of a young person with seizures. As children grow older they need less looking after as they become more independent. It is an easy mistake for parents, because a child needs looking after on account of his fits, to treat him as being much younger than his years, since considering him as a younger child is the only way they understand of exercising the degree of supervision he needs. Inevitably this approach arouses great resentment; not because his activities are being restricted, but because his dignity has been offended by being treated as a younger child. Not only should the parents talk things over with the child as an equal but, whenever possible, he should be included in discussions with the doctor. This applies more particularly to adolescents, who are especially sensitive. The patient should help to work out plans for his own protection. Handled in the proper way, this should not be too difficult because he is often frightened himself by his attacks and their consequences. Risks must be taken and they should be explained to the young person. However, we would advise that very great care should be taken concerning fire. Broken bones usually mend and lacerations heal, but many patients with severe epilepsy suffer mutilating burns, which, particularly if they affect the face, cause permanent disfigurement that will have profound psychosocial effects on his relationships with other people throughout his life. In assessing

risks it is important to remember that seizures are more likely to occur when patients are relaxed and it may well be more dangerous to browse over a book in front of the fire with the room full of people than it is to cross a busy road on one's own.

Important as it is for parents to understand the problem of their child with epilepsy, it is equally important for the child to appreciate parental anxiety.

Personal situation

16-year-old Sue just could not understand it, and she was becoming irritated and just a little worried. Her mother had always been there when she got back from school, at least until today she had. Now it was nearly six o'clock. Her father was away on business. Her older brother, unemployed, was lolling in an armchair, quite unconcerned. Her older sister had settled down to her homework. She should be doing the same because she had important exams coming up soon, but she could not settle. Where was her mother?

Sue had epilepsy with rare major fits, usually at night, and occasional partial attacks in the daytime. They were a bit of a nuisance and sometimes she grumbled about them but most of the time she pretended that she did not have attacks. She was growing up and determined that everyone should know it. Yes, she really was an adult, not a child who had to be looked after because she had fits. Just now she felt very much like a child, she wanted her mother and she was getting very worried indeed. She was always there when she got back from school.

At half past seven the front door bell rang. For the past hour and a half she had been fidgeting about, staring at her school books, getting up, wandering about, sitting down again and having another go at starting. All the time it was getting clearer, something terrible had happened to her mother. She knew exactly what would happen. They would not telephone. A policeman would call to break the news personally. He would ring the front door bell. Within seconds Sue had opened the front door to Penny, her brother's latest girlfriend.

Sue had been home from school for three and a half hours when her mother opened the front door and walked in. The release of Sue's pent up anxieties overflowed into a furious verbal assault on her mother. It was some time later when the family sat down quietly to talk it all over. For months Mrs M. had asked Sue to let her know when she would be home, what she was planning to do, or where she was going, and to telephone if there was any sudden change in plan. It was only polite, and Mrs M. could not help worrying about Sue's attacks. But Sue was not having any therefore she saw it as a threat to her independence, an attempt to baby her. She was not mature enough or secure enough to realize that to keep in touch as her mother had asked would have been the behaviour of an independent adult.

Comment

The occasion which we have just described had, of course, been set up by Mrs M. and her two other children. It was the occasion when Sue grew up.

HOW SHOULD *HE* COPE WITH STRESS?

It is accepted that most patients are less likely to have fits when they are alert, and that a moderate degree of anxiety may be a useful alerting stimulus. It has been our experience that, when a patient is faced with a single stress with which he is competent to deal, he does not fit. Patients seldom have seizures when they come for a consultation and it is rare for children to have fits during examinations. An exception being that myoclonic jerks often seem to be particularly sensitive to simple stress. In other cases, it seems probable that epilepsy is exacerbated by an excessive stress, whether physical or psychological, with which the patient cannot cope. This applies particularly to prolonged stresses and when the patient feels encompassed by an environment which he finds intolerable: when there is a long-term build up of multiple pressures of adverse circumstance. It is as if, when there is no single superable difficulty, he withdraws altogether and opts out of trying. Out of touch with his environment, unoccupied, unmotivated, he retires into a vegetative hopelessness, devoid of stimuli and at risk of having a greatly increased number of fits.

If these propositions are accepted, it follows that the patient should if possible avoid excessive physical or mental stresses with which he is unlikely to be able to deal. Equally, it is important that he should learn to deal with stress, since it is impossible to live effectively in the ordinary environment, filled with problems and difficulties, without being subject to greater or lesser stresses. The problem of learning to deal with stress is not so likely to arise with someone who develops epilepsy in later life; it is particularly important for the child who develops epilepsy early. It is within the security of a good family that he will have the chance, which he may never have again, of learning not to avoid or be protected from, but rather to face up to difficult situations, so that in later life even minor stresses do not prove too much for him; do not provoke fits. The following story dramatizes a situation which, unfortunately, is not rare.

Personal situation

Bill was 11 years old when he had his first fit. As they watched him convulsing on the dining-room floor, his parents were convinced that he was dying. In the agonizingly long interval between the last jerking movement and the first deep breath back to normality, they were certain that he was dead. Bill was to have a number of attacks and, whether or not they were aware of it, those fears were always there in the back of their minds.

Their family doctor confirmed the diagnosis. There was no need for reference to hospital. He spent a long time telling the parents all about epilepsy. If he was not very reassuring at least he was very kind. As they left his surgery his final words were: 'Take great care not to upset the lad, you don't want to bring on one of his attacks.' They accepted his advice without question.

Bill was not worried by his fits. He had never witnessed one and only knew that he had had one because he had a slight headache and felt a bit achey. On the contrary, being an intelligent boy, it was not long before he realized that there were distinct advantages in having epilepsy. No longer was he forced to do any of his household chores; the flimsiest excuse let him off. He had always had frequent rows with his younger brother and sister, who irritated him. Now he could indulge his irritations: it was they who got punished. Even at school life was much easier. There was no comeback when his homework was not handed in on time. Careless and untidy work was accepted without comment.

Apparently immune from sanctions, Bill became increasingly irresponsible. He found he could manipulate people and situations, he found his new·power rather fun. He did not realize that he was become increasingly unpopular. Other children came to play, but not with him. His parents felt that the strain of 'living with epilepsy' was beginning to tell on them. Perhaps, this was what epilepsy was all about. The doctor had introduced the diagnosis in a subdued, almost sepulchral voice.

The parents talked it over many times. The father began to have his doubts: were they tackling Bill in the right way? The mother was not so sure. The father felt that Bill should be treated a bit more like the other children. The mother repeated the doctor's final warning. One evening Bill was reminded to clean his shoes ready for school the next day. He was told to do them at once because friends were coming to supper. Bill made it quite clear that he didn't want to clean his shoes, now or ever. The father insisted. The mother was in the kitchen preparing the supper. Bill made no move to clean his shoes. The father insisted again. Bill had his fit. Did the mother say: 'I told you so?' We do not know. The father stormed out of the house, frustrated. Bill recovered quickly from his fit. He had plenty of time to clean his shoes, but he didn't. Next morning his shoes were clean and ready for him to go to school. The father had cleaned them at midnight after the guests had left.

Six years later Bill – referred to by some behind his back as 'That Bloody Willie' – was having more and more seizures in a special unit for delinquent adolescents with epilepsy. The parents were both on tranquillizers and quite uncertain how to steer their normal younger children through the perils of early adolescence. Was epilepsy, after all, a diagnosis of doom and disaster?

Comment

Did the kindly family doctor say, 'I told you so', or should we say to the kindly family doctor, 'We could have told you so?'

HE NEEDS APPROVAL OF ACHIEVEMENT

Success, a sense of achievement, is one of the strongest stimuli to further effort: a very basic need for a gregarious animal such as man. If we are honest with ourselves, how many of us are not only encouraged by, but dependent upon, attitudes of approval: applause, private congratulations, spontaneous comment – 'You explained that very well' or 'You do look nice today'.

The average person with epilepsy may have considerable ability but very often his performance is impaired in some measure by the lesion responsible for his fits, by the occurrence of subclinical electrocerebral disturbances, or by the antiepileptic drugs which he is taking. A patient once described this as, 'Feeling like a powerful motor car with the brakes half on'. He appreciated that he was not stupid, he knew what he wanted to do, but he was frustrated by his inability to achieve his purpose. Within the environments of school, family, social life or at work, these people may never really succeed, never achieve what they expect of themselves or feel that others expect of them. The great majority are not beset by prejudice or intolerance, they meet sympathy, understanding and support, albeit too often flavoured with patronage. May it not be that what they need even more is the opportunity to achieve even limited success, to merit genuine praise. Without these things, they lack a very real stimulus and are at risk of slipping into disinterested apathy. This problem is often the greater for the children of intelligent and sophisticated families. True, they are more likely to receive enlightened understanding and well-structured support; but is the understanding really enlightened and are they getting the kind of support they need? It is so much more difficult for them to compete with their more talented brothers and sisters; to play a positive role in the life of the family: when there is conversation, they are talked at; they have the sense of being second-class citizens. Perhaps no-one would suggest that they are failures, but they do not feel that they are successes.

It is important that *HE* should not feel that he is being treated as a fool. If his features are coarsened and his responses slowed down by antiepileptic drugs, he is probably a good deal more intelligent than he looks. Behind a mask, perhaps of indifference, perhaps of truculence, he may well be hypersensitive and he is very likely deeply to resent being patronized. He should have the opportunity to discuss the factors which may limit his opportunities – the nature and frequency of his seizures and the effects of his treatment. Having done so, he should be able to identify and be encouraged to develop those abilities which he has, rather than feel that emphasis is being placed on what he cannot do. If he feels hemmed in by prohibitions, he is liable to opt out and fall back on the cushion of welfare benefits. If he can see opportunities and possibilities of success, however small, if he can be encouraged to realize that it is worth trying, then his desire to prove himself, to achieve together with his need for approval and appreciation may well confound the gloomy estimates of the experts.

Unless a patient is permanently handicapped by a significant degree of brain damage, for by far the greater part of his life he is capable and in control of his destiny; but for a tiny percentage of his life, he is seized by ictal and peri-ictal events or by subclinical electrocerebral disturbance, when he is almost entirely incapable and there is nothing that he can do about it. Although it may not always be possible to validate by formal testing, it would seem probable that, if toxic doses of antiepileptic drugs can impair performance seriously, even therapeutic doses cannot be wholly without some effect. Cerebral lesions causing epilepsy are seldom global. The normal parts of the brain may find it difficult to appreciate the limitations imposed by those parts which are damaged. For all these reasons, the person with epilepsy is in a position different from the person who is globally mentally handicapped. He may at once be at risk of failing to achieve his ambitions and at the same time aware of and frustrated by his failure.

HE IS SWALLOWING THE PILLS

Nowadays much care is taken to adjust the dose of antiepileptic drugs with serum levels, to avoid polypharmacy, to watch for side-effects and to adjure the patient to absolute compliance. This would seem straightforward enough and it might sometimes be thought that there was little need to involve the patient so long as he took the pills prescribed. However, the patient needs to be involved actively in two ways.

He needs to know

If he is to be taking antiepileptic drugs for many years, it is only sensible to spend a few minutes with the doctor finding out how they work. For example:

1. Although he may become dependent on them, he need not fear addiction. To some, *drugs* raise the spectre of heroin or cocaine addicts.
2. Compliance is important, but most antiepileptic drugs are eliminated relatively slowly. To forget the midday dose and take it with the evening one is unlikely to be pharmacologically (although if not explained it may be psychologically) disastrous.
3. Although these drugs control fits, increasing the recommended dose will not necessarily control fits better, and quite often will make them worse.

How does he feel?

1. Antiepileptic drugs are potent. While the toxic and side-effects are well known, what may be appreciated less is the way the patient who is taking them feels in himself. Slight alterations in dose or quite small changes in regimen may alter significantly those inner feelings in a way he finds it difficult to describe but which may disturb and alarm him.
2. Different drugs seem to suit different patients, although they may have the same kind of seizures. The patient should have the opportunity of discussing with his doctor what drug or even, dare we say it, what dose is best for him. It is not rare to find that an intelligent, conscientious patient, who is non-compliant, *knows better*.

HOW IS *HE* AFFECTED BY HIS SEIZURES

To assess the effect of a tonic-clonic convulsion on the patient, or on a friend with him, does not require much imagination and needs little elaboration: a cataclysmic event of which the patient is unaware, although he may live in fear of the occurrence and suffer from its consequences, whether of headache and sore muscles or lacerations and even fractures. *HE* who lives with continuing major fits has courage. Such a seizure in a public place cannot but be an embarrassment to his friend. But it is a happening which is clearly a major crisis, which is understandable as such; an event which calls for action from sympathetic if horrified onlookers. The companion is likely to be occupied ensuring that these actions are not inappropriate: that cups of hot sweet tea console the crowd and do not choke the unconscious patient.

Understanding the complex partial seizure

With adequate treatment major fits should be rare events. Various forms of complex partial seizures are much more difficult to control and are common. After the initial impact of the grotesque and obviously abnormal, it is easier to accept the generalized convulsion than the subtle, often barely perceptible, deviations from the usual, which may imbue the lesser attack with an eerie unreality: is he going mad or am I? To awake one morning to find one's garden trampled down by the neighbour's cows would cause shock and horror. To look out to see that some of yesterday's yellow daffodils were blue, would evoke an awesome fear, not of the daffodils, but of one's own sanity.

Not only may complex partial seizures be fearsome to the onlooker but often they remain undiagnosed and are misinterpreted as aberrant and unacceptable behaviour.

Personal situations

Mrs W. lived with her sister Mrs Y. in a respectable suburb of a large city. They had much in common, including their widowhood. Mrs W. suffered from epilepsy, but only occasionally did this disturb the settled regularity of their lives.

However, at first their happily adjusted relationship nearly foundered on the rocks of Mrs W's epilepsy. Mrs Y. could not understand why her usually easy-natured sister unpredictably should be so frankly unkind, even rude. Perhaps their decision to live together had been a disaster. However, money was tight and Mrs Y. could not move out until she had time to make new plans. The delay was fortunate, since she came to realize that her sister's uncharacteristic and hurtful behaviour was related to her fits.

Mrs Y. began to watch her sister more closely. When other people were present she seemed to fade out of the conversation. She became inaccessible, her face paled then her lips seemed to be blue and she started making chewing movements. Soon her normal colour returned but she would start to fumble clumsily with her clothes or anything else to hand. If she had been knitting, she would get into a terrible mess. These episodes would last only two or three minutes, but for at least 20 minutes she would be different: she would be irritable and abrasive. Back to her usual self, she would have no memory of what had happened.

Comment

Mrs W. had been having complex partial seizures with alteration of consciousness. She was in no way responsible for her behaviour. It must have been difficult for Mrs Y. to understand what had been happening, but once she did appreciate the bizarre nature of her fits, the two widows lived happily ever after. The odd 20 minutes, now and again, could be ignored as just one of those things.

Psychic clothes

It may be said that we all wear psychic clothes. These clothes make it possible for us to present ourselves, not as we are, but as we would like to be: kind, intelligent, a good fellow, beautiful, fearless or sophisticated. Most of us are continuously in touch with our environment, affected by it, trying to relate to it, to manipulate or rather to control it. Our psychic clothes are an essential part of our relationships with our environment: putting them on should not be criticized and dismissed as an empty charade. What we imagine ourselves, or would like, to be, is almost invariably better than what we are. It is no better or no worse to adjust the psychic dress than it is to glance in the mirror before going off to work or to shave on the morning of one's execution. As time goes on, we come to fit these clothes better and we are the better for them.

Almost inevitably, a seizure involves a loss or significant alteration of consciousness, a break in the continuity of contact with and, therefore, control of environment: the inescapable removal of psychic clothes. The prospect of the slow involuntary undressing which may occur during a complex partial seizure is one with which it is difficult to live.

Personal situation

The von Z.s lived in North London, perhaps just a little too far North, but not so far North that the 'von' would not be appreciated. Now both in late middle age, some ten years before they had moved imperceptibly into their modest cottage with its delightful garden. They were known to everyone and they had many good acquaintances: that is everyone knew Mrs von Z. at the Bridge Club and the Horticultural Society. Mr von Z. remained aloof. Invariably polite and courteous, he would go on regular shopping expeditions and, of course, to the library where he ordered books not usually in demand. Everyone realized that they did not have much money, but their cottage was full of treasures from the past. To the locals, they were still People of Importance. No one knew that Mr von Z. suffered from complex partial seizures; few would have known what they were. Anyway, now he was getting older, he was having few attacks. Soon he should be able to get back his driving licence and he would forget about the whole thing.

Mrs von Z. had finished the washing up. It was a lovely day and she went out into the garden. Mr von Z had gone off to the library. She stopped the motor mower to empty the grass box, and then she heard the telephone. Miss B., the librarian, was distraught and it was difficult to make out what she was saying: 'Mr von Z. has gone mad. He tried to rape me.'

By the time she reached the library the worst of the panic was over. Her husband was sitting hunched up, alone, pale and very shaken. Miss B. was also sitting alone looking pale and very shaken. At the far end of the room the local doctor was trying to explain things to the local policeman against opposition from a group of local experts. It did not take Mrs von Z. long to find out what had happened. When he handed in his books, Mr von Z. had been his usual charming self. He had smiled at the young librarian and patted her arm. She was a favourite of his. Some minutes later she was startled to feel an arm round her waist. Mr von Z. was at her side of the counter trying to kiss her. He looked flushed, his eyes were glazed and his trousers were undone. In the event she had had little difficulty in avoiding the advances. Mr von Z. had appeared to lose interest and had wandered off aimlessly to sit in a corner. Miss B. was now shamefaced that she had panicked and rushed to the telephone. The doctor had told her about the attack which Mr von Z. had had and how he would not have known what he was doing for a few minutes afterwards. It was not long before a general attitude of shamefacedness spread through the neighbourhood. Everyone tried hard to be kind and was more than understanding which was the last thing that Mr von Z. wanted. He wanted his psychic clothes back again.

Comment

Mr and Mrs von Z. moved and settled in a small village near Cambridge, as Mr and Mrs Z.

The lost half hour

Although *HE* may be able to react purposefully, or semipurposefully, during a complex partial seizure, afterwards he is unlikely to be able to remember what happened during the attack. He may be very deeply concerned about what he may have done when he had lost control of his environment. Apart from reassuring him that the distorted appreciation of sensory input, which may have been experienced during his state of altered consciousness, is not a portent of impending insanity, it is useful to encourage him to discuss his attacks with people who have witnessed them. To surround his seizures with a well-meaning conspiracy of silence often arouses deep-seated fears that his behaviour must in fact have been unspeakable. At other times the lost half hour may result in some harmless embarrassment.

Personal situation

Mr R. was a 35-year-old civil servant. For 10 years he had been married. His wife worked as a ward sister at the Infirmary. They lived in Edinburgh in a third-floor flat of a high-class, if 90-year-old, tenement within easy walking distance of their work. Mrs R. was in charge of the flat and of Mr R. as well as her ward. Mr R. did not resent this. He suffered from complex partial seizures which might last up to 10 minutes and be followed by several minutes of confusion. However, he knew when they were coming on and he was able to retire to a quiet place where his inappropriate behaviour did not embarrass his colleagues. Nevertheless, he never knew quite when they would hit him and appreciated the support to his insecurity that he got at work and from his wife.

Two years ago they decided that they had saved up enough to be able to afford to start a family, although they would have to do without Mrs R.'s salary. Timothy was three months old and a bonny baby. His feeding demands had been creating tensions which all too often became frank rows. Mr R. took to spending the early evenings with his friends in the pub and, as Mrs R. insisted all too frequently, this did not do his fits any good. Mr R. was more at home with his wife's undivided attention than with her criticism. Mrs R. was lonely, isolated, and getting more and more fed up with washing, sheets and baby clothes. The one thing in the world which she wanted was a washing machine. The R.s were very fond of each other and one evening, after a particularly long and fruitless argument, they stopped quite suddenly and laughed. It was all too silly, they must start again. Mr R. promised faithfully to come straight home. They would save for the washing machine.

Mr R. kept to his resolution, Timothy became less demanding and they had enough saved for the washing machine. All went well, that is to say until a Friday afternoon when Timothy was nearly five months old. The telephone rang. It was the office: 'Is Mr R. all right? We have not seen him since lunchtime'. Mrs R. became more and more worried. By the time her husband returned at 7 p.m. she was so frantic that she said all sorts of things which she should not have said. When it was clear that, although not drunk, he had been drinking, she said a lot more. Mr R. denied vehemently that he had been drinking. It is not on record what happened after that, but on Saturday morning they took a walk with Timothy and bought a washing machine.

On Monday morning two men struggled up three flights of stairs, rang the bell and, totally exhausted, delivered a washing machine. Mrs R. resuscitated them with tea and her delight. She then washed. In early afternoon she was feeding Timothy, happily, when the door bell rang. Two more men, who were totally exhausted, delivered a washing machine.

Comment

During the Friday lunch break Mr R had had quite a severe complex partial seizure and during his confused period he had left the office and gone for a walk to clear his head. On recovering full consciousness, he had acted quite normally: he fulfilled their decision to buy a washing machine; perhaps, he celebrated with a pint of beer. He had, of course, no memory of what had happened and was quite honest when he said that he had not been drinking. The memory of the pint had not registered any more than that of buying the washing machine.

It is not recorded how the second washing machine got down three flights of stairs.

★　★　★　★　★　★　★　★

Sadly many People with Epilepsy still face formidable medical and social problems. This new edition will prove a success if it enables the experts to go some way to solve them.

REFERENCE

Laidlaw M V, Laidlaw J 1984 People with epilepsy. Churchill Livingstone, Edinburgh

Index